EXPERIMENTAL DESIGNS

NONTRADITIONAL RESEARCH DESIGNS

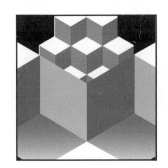

The Practice of
NURSING
RESEARCH

The Practice of
NURSING
RESEARCH

Conduct, Critique, & Utilization

4th Edition

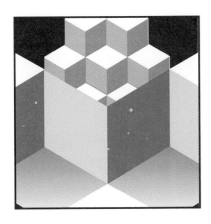

Nancy Burns, Ph.D., R.N., FAAN
Jenkins Garrett Professor
School of Nursing
University of Texas at Arlington
Arlington, Texas

Susan K. Grove, Ph.D., R.N., C.S., A.N.P., G.N.P.
Professor of Nursing
Assistant Dean, Graduate Nursing Program
School of Nursing
University of Texas at Arlington
Arlington, Texas

W.B. SAUNDERS COMPANY
An Imprint of Elsevier Science
Philadelphia • London • New York • St. Louis • Sydney • Toronto

W.B. SAUNDERS COMPANY
An Imprint of Elsevier Science

The Curtis Center
Independence Square West
Philadelphia, Pennsylvania 19106

Library of Congress Cataloging-in-Publication Data

Burns, Nancy, Ph.D.
The practice of nursing research: conduct, critique, & utilization / Nancy Burns, Susan K. Grove—4th ed.

p. cm.

Includes bibliographical references and index.

ISBN 0–7216–9177–3

1. Nursing—Research—Methodology. I. Grove, Susan K. II. Title.
    [DNLM: 1. Nursing Research. WY 20.5 B967p 2001]

RT81.5.B86 2001
610.73′072—dc21   00-047072

Vice President, Nursing Editorial Director: Sally Schrefer
Executive Editor: Barbara Nelson Cullen
Developmental Editor: Victoria Legnini
Supervising Copy Editor: Jodi von Hagen
Production Manager: Frank Polizzano
Illustration Specialist: Walt Verbitski
Book Designer: Jonel Sofian
Illustrator: Lisa Weischedel

THE PRACTICE OF NURSING RESEARCH:
CONDUCT, CRITIQUE, & UTILIZATION   ISBN 0–7216–9177–3

Last digit is the print number: 9   8   7   6   5   4   3   2

To our readers, nationally and internationally, who are the future of nursing research.

PREFACE

Research is a major force in the nursing profession and is used to change practice, education, and health policy. Our aim in developing the fourth edition of *The Practice of Nursing Research* is to increase the excitement about research and to facilitate the quest for knowledge through research. The depth and breadth of content presented in this edition reflect the increase in research activities and the growth in research knowledge since the last edition. Nursing research is introduced at the baccalaureate level and becomes an integral part of graduate education and clinical practice. An increasing number of nurses are involved in research activities such as critiquing research, utilizing research findings in practice, and conducting sophisticated quantitative and qualitative studies.

Content New to the Fourth Edition

The fourth edition of our text provides comprehensive coverage of nursing research and is focused on the learning needs and styles of today's nursing student. The exciting new areas of the fourth edition include a comprehensive chapter that addresses designing interventions for nursing studies. Intervention research has become a major focus in the profession, and this chapter facilitates the examination of the effectiveness of treatments on patient outcomes. The literature review chapter now emphasizes electronic searching of literature and the use of the Internet to generate current information for relevant practice problems. The ethics chapter includes an expanded discussion of scientific misconduct and current regulations guiding research that are available on the Internet. The statistical content was significantly reorganized into five versus four chapters, with titles and information that will facilitate student reading and understanding of statistical techniques. The chapters are now entitled

Introduction to Statistical Analysis (Chapter 18), *Using Statistics to Describe* (Chapter 19), *Using Statistics to Examine Relationships* (Chapter 20), *Using Statistics to Predict* (Chapter 21), and *Using Statistics to Examine Causality* (Chapter 22). The chapter on qualitative research methods was reorganized and revised to reflect methodologies currently being used by nurse researchers, such as storytelling and narrative analysis. The nursing research literature now stresses the importance of evidence-based practice, best practices, and standardized guidelines for practice. Thus, the old utilization chapter was revised to include these new concepts and a model to facilitate evidence-based practice in a chapter now entitled *Utilization of Research to Promote Evidence-Based Practice*. The fourth edition is organized to facilitate ease in reading, understanding, and implementing the research process. The major strengths of this text include:

- A clear, concise writing style that is consistent among the chapters to facilitate student learning
- A nursing perspective and framework that links research to the rest of nursing
- Comprehensive coverage of both quantitative and qualitative research techniques
- Electronic references and websites that direct the student to an extensive array of information that is important for conducting studies and using research findings in practice
- Rich and frequent illustration of major points and concepts from the most current nursing research literature
- Exciting coverage of research utilization, best practices, and evidence-based practice—topics of vital and growing importance in a health care arena focused on quality and cost-effectiveness of patient care

Many examples from current published studies are used to illustrate points under discussion clearly and to demonstrate the direct connection between research and clinical practice. The book continues to be based on a strong conceptual framework that links nursing research with practice, theory, knowledge, and philosophy.

Our text provides a comprehensive introduction to nursing research for graduate and practicing nurses. At the master's and doctoral level, the text provides not only substantive content related to research but also practical applications based on the authors' experiences in conducting various types of nursing research, familiarity with the research literature, and experience in teaching nursing research at various educational levels.

The fourth edition of our text is organized into four units, containing 29 chapters. Unit I introduces the reader to the world of nursing research. The content and presentation of this unit have been designed to assist the reader in overcoming the barriers frequently experienced in understanding the language used in nursing research. The unit also includes a classification system for types of quantitative and qualitative research and introduces the reader to these types of research.

Unit II provides an in-depth presentation of the research process for both quantitative and qualitative research. As with previous editions, this text provides extensive coverage of the many types of quantitative and qualitative research. Unit II includes a new chapter entitled *Intervention Research* (Chapter 13) to facilitate the conduct of studies to generate evidence-based practice.

Unit III addresses the implications of research for the discipline and profession of nursing. Content is provided to direct the student in critiquing both quantitative and qualitative research. Specific steps are provided to direct nurses in using research findings to improve practice. Nursing and medical practice guidelines are also addressed as essential aspects of implementing evidence-based advanced nursing practice roles as nurse practitioner, clinical nurse specialist, nurse anesthetist, and midwife.

Unit IV addresses seeking support for research. Readers are given direction for developing quantitative and qualitative research proposals and seeking funding for their research.

An *Instructor's Manual* for the fourth edition is now on a CD-ROM, rather than in printed form. The transparencies for the third edition of the *Instructor's Manual* have been developed into a "LectureView," or PowerPoint presentations with the extensive addition of new slides. The CD and the use of PowerPoint also make it possible to include a variety of visuals on the slides. The LectureView slides are also viewable for those who do not use PowerPoint. The Manual includes test items, syllabi, and classroom activities that are provided in both rich text format and ASCII, making it easy for the faculty member to access and print them through most word processing software.

The changes in the fourth edition of this text reflect the advances in nursing research and also incorporate comments from outside reviewers, colleagues, and students. Our desire to promote the continuing development of the profession of nursing was the incentive for investing the time and energy required to develop this new edition.

Nancy Burns, Ph.D., R.N., FAAN
Susan K. Grove, Ph.D., R.N., C.S., A.N.P., G.N.P.

ACKNOWLEDGMENTS

Writing the fourth edition of this textbook has allowed us the opportunity to examine and revise the content of the previous edition based on input from the literature and a number of scholarly colleagues. A textbook such as this requires synthesizing of the ideas of many. We have attempted to extract from the nursing literature the essence of nursing knowledge related to the conduct of nursing research. Thus, we would like to thank those nursing scholars who shared their knowledge with the rest of us in nursing, and who made this knowledge accessible for inclusion in this textbook.

The ideas from the literature were synthesized and discussed with our colleagues to determine their contribution to the fourth edition. Thus, we would like to express our appreciation to Dean Elizabeth Poster, Associate Dean Carolyn Cason, and faculty of the School of Nursing at The University of Texas at Arlington for their support during the long and sometimes arduous experiences that are inevitable in developing a book of this magnitude. We would like to extend a special thanks to Helen Hough for her scholarly input regarding the literature review chapter. We would also like to thank the following nurse researchers who provided critiques during various stages of the development of the intervention chapter: Dr. Mary Duffy, Dr. Dorothy J. Stuppy, Dr. Karin Kirchhoff, and Dr. Cheryl Stetler. We would also like to express gratitude to our students for the questions they raised regarding the content of this text.

We would also like to recognize the excellent reviews of the colleagues who helped us make important revisions in this text; a list of their names appears on p. 11.

A special thanks is extended to the people at the W.B. Saunders Company, who have been extremely helpful to us in producing an attractive, appealing text. The people most instrumental in the development and production of this book include Thomas Eoyang, former Editorial Manager, Nursing Division, and Victoria Legnini, Developmental Editor.

On a personal note, development of this text would not have been possible without the constant support and stimulating discussion with our husbands Jerry Burns and Jack R. Suggs. We appreciate their positive attitude and endurance during the times of intense work.

Nancy Burns, Ph.D., R.N., FAAN
Susan K. Grove, Ph.D., R.N., C.S., A.N.P., G.N.P.

REVIEWER LIST

Patricia L. Ackerman, Ph.D., R.N.
California State University
Sacramento, California

**Judith W. Alexander, Ph.D., R.N.,
M.B.A., CNAA**
University of South Carolina
Columbia, South Carolina

Carole Ann Bach, Ph.D., R.N., CRRN
Vanderbilt University School of Nursing
Nashville VA Medical Center
Nashville, Tennessee

Ann Harley, Ed.D., M.S.N., R.N.
Division of Nursing
Carson-Newman College
Jefferson City, Tennessee

Donna K. Hathaway, Ph.D., R.N., FAAN
University of Tennessee, Memphis
Memphis, Tennessee

Sharon L. Jacques, Ph.D., R.N.
Western Carolina University
Cullowhee, North Carolina

Kathleen A. Sullivan, Ph.D., R.N.
La Roche College
Pittsburgh, Pennsylvania

CONTENTS

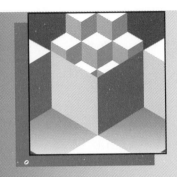

INTRODUCTION TO
NURSING RESEARCH

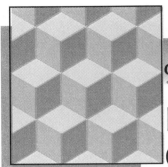

CHAPTER 1

DISCOVERY OF THE WORLD OF NURSING RESEARCH

Welcome to the world of nursing research. You might think it is strange to consider research a "world," but research is truly a new way of experiencing reality. Entering a new world requires learning a unique language, incorporating new rules, and using new experiences to learn how to interact effectively within that world. As you become a part of this new world, your perceptions and methods of reasoning will be modified and expanded. To many nurses, research is a relatively new world, and we believe this textbook can facilitate entry into it.

The purpose of this chapter is to explain broadly the world to be explored. A definition of nursing research is provided, and the significance of research to nursing is addressed. The chapter concludes with the presentation of a framework that connects nursing research with the rest of nursing. This framework introduces concepts and relationships that are further developed throughout the text.

DEFINITION OF NURSING RESEARCH

The root meaning of the word research is "search again" or "examine carefully." More specifically, *research* is diligent, systematic inquiry or investigation to validate and refine existing knowledge and generate new knowledge. The concepts *systematic* and *diligent* are critical to the meaning of research because they imply planning, organization, and persistence. Systematic, diligent inquiry is

necessary for researchers to address the following questions:

- What needs to be known?
- What research methods are needed to validate, refine, and generate this knowledge?
- What meaning can be extracted from the studies in a discipline to build a sound knowledge base?

Many disciplines conduct research, so a question often raised is "What distinguishes nursing research from research in other disciplines?" In some ways, there is no difference, because the knowledge and skills required for research do not vary from one discipline to another. However, looking at a different dimensions of research in a discipline reveals that there are distinctions. The research in nursing must address the questions relevant to nurses and must develop a unique body of knowledge for practice. Nursing involves providing holistic care to promote health in patients and families. Therefore, nursing studies focus on the understanding of human needs and the use of therapeutic interventions to promote health, prevent illness, and treat illness. The holistic perspective influences the development and implementation of nursing studies and the interpretation of the findings (Stevenson, 1988).

There are differing views about the realm of nursing knowledge. One view is that nursing research should focus on knowledge that is directly useful in clinical practice. Another view is that nursing research includes studies of nursing education, nursing administration, health services, and the

3

characteristics of nurses and nursing roles as well as clinical situations. Those who support this second view argue that findings from such studies indirectly influence nursing practice and thus add to nursing's body of knowledge. Educational research is necessary to provide an efficient, effective educational background for nurses. Studies of nursing administration, health services, and nursing roles are necessary to promote quality in the health care system.

The ultimate goal of nursing is to provide evidence-based care that promotes quality outcomes for patients, families, health care providers, and the health care system (Omery & Williams, 1999). *Evidence-based practice* involves the use of collective research findings in (1) promoting the understanding of patients' and families' experiences with health and illness, (2) implementing effective nursing interventions to promote patient health, and (3) providing quality, cost-effective care within the health care system. For example, research related to a chronic health problem could be critiqued and synthesized to develop practice guidelines that might be implemented by nurse practitioners, thus providing quality, cost-effective care to patients experiencing that chronic problem (Brown, 1999). Therefore, nursing research is needed to generate knowledge that will directly and indirectly influence nursing practice. In this text, *nursing research* is defined as a scientific process that validates and refines existing knowledge and generates new knowledge that directly and indirectly influences nursing practice.

SIGNIFICANCE OF NURSING RESEARCH

Nursing research is essential for the development of scientific knowledge that enables nurses to provide evidence-based health care (Brown, 1999; Omery & Williams, 1999). Broadly, nursing is accountable to society for providing quality, cost-effective care and for seeking ways to improve that care. More specifically, nurses are accountable to their patients to promote a maximum level of health. A solid research base will provide evidence of the nursing actions that are effective in promoting positive patient outcomes (Hegyvary, 1991). Developing

an evidence-based practice will require conducting studies with varied methodologies to describe, explain, predict, and control phenomena essential to nursing.

Description

Description involves identifying and understanding the nature of nursing phenomena and, sometimes, the relationships among them (Chinn & Kramer, 1998). Through research, nurses are able to (1) describe what exists in nursing practice, (2) discover new information, (3) promote understanding of situations, and (4) classify information for use in the discipline.

For example, Jacobs (2000) conducted a study to describe the informational needs of surgical patients after discharge. The findings from this study could be used to develop discharge instruction guidelines for surgical patients. The study found that discharge instructions must include content on activity levels, pain management, and prevention of complications (Jacobs, 2000). Research focused on description is essential groundwork for studies that will provide explanation, prediction, and control of nursing phenomena.

Explanation

Explanation clarifies the relationships among phenomena and identifies the reasons why certain events occur. For example, Pronk and associates (1999) studied the relationships between modifiable health risks (physical inactivity, obesity, and smoking) and health care charges and found that adverse health risks translate into significantly higher health care charges. Thus, managed health care plans and payers seeking to reduce health care charges need to identify and implement interventions that will effectively modify adverse health risks. This study illustrates how explanatory research is useful in identifying relationships among variables and in linking nursing interventions with patient outcomes. Identifying relationships among nursing phenomena provides a basis for conducting research for prediction and control.

Prediction

Through *prediction,* one can estimate the probability of a specific outcome in a given situation (Chinn & Kramer, 1998). However, predicting an outcome does not necessarily enable one to modify or control the outcome. With predictive knowledge, nurses could anticipate the effects that nursing interventions would have on patients and families. For example, Defloor (2000) conducted a study to determine the effect of position and mattress type on skin pressure of persons lying in bed. The researcher found that the 30-degree semi-Fowler position and polyethylene-urethane mattress produced a significant reduction in skin pressure. Further research is needed to determine whether controlling position and type of mattress will decrease the incidence of pressure ulcers in patients at bed rest. Predictive studies isolate independent variables that require additional research to ensure that their manipulation results in successful outcomes, as measured by designated dependent variables (Omery et al., 1995).

Control

If one can predict the outcome of a situation, the next step is to control or manipulate the situation to produce the desired outcome. Dickoff and colleagues (1968) described *control* as the ability to write a prescription to produce the desired results. Nurses could prescribe specific interventions to assist patients and families in achieving their health goals.

Parker and colleagues (1999) conducted a study that implemented a prescribed intervention to prevent further abuse of pregnant women. They found that significantly less violence was reported by women in the intervention group than by women in the comparison group. Thus, implementing this intervention manipulated or controlled the situation to produce the positive outcome of reduced abuse (Omery et al., 1995).

A limited number of studies have developed knowledge that is useful for prediction and control in nursing practice. However, the extensive clinical studies conducted in the last two decades have greatly expanded the scientific knowledge needed for description, explanation, prediction, and control of phenomena within nursing.

FRAMEWORK LINKING NURSING RESEARCH TO THE WORLD OF NURSING

In the exploration of nursing research, a framework is helpful to establish connections between research and the various elements of nursing. A framework linking nursing research to the world of nursing is presented in the following pages and is used as an organizing model for this textbook. In the framework model (see Figure 1–1), nursing research is not an entity disconnected from the rest of nursing but rather is influenced by and influences all other nursing elements. The concepts in this model are pictured on a continuum from concrete to abstract. The discussion of this model introduces this continuum and progresses from the concrete concept of the empirical world to the most abstract concept of nursing philosophy.

Concrete–Abstract Continuum

Figure 1–1 presents the components of nursing on a concrete–abstract continuum. This continuum demonstrates that nursing thought flows both from

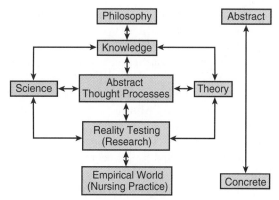

FIGURE 1–1 ■ Framework linking nursing research to the world of nursing.

concrete to abstract thinking and from abstract to concrete thinking.

Concrete thinking is oriented toward and limited by tangible things or by events that are observed and experienced in reality. The focus of concrete thinking is immediate events that are limited by time and space. In the past, nursing was seen as a "doing" profession rather than as a "thinking" profession. The nurse was expected to do the work, not to ask why. Therefore, nurses tended to be concrete, "practical" thinkers. This type of thinking and behavior was valued and rewarded. Problem solving was considered important only if the effect was immediate. The rudiments of these values are still present to some extent in nursing education and practice.

Abstract thinking is oriented toward the development of an idea without application to, or association with, a particular instance. Abstract thinkers tend to look for meaning, patterns, relationships, and philosophical implications. This type of thinking is independent of time and space. In the past, nurses who were able to think in abstract ways were often considered dreamers. Their behaviors were regarded as impractical, and their skills in problem solving and decision making were discouraged. Currently, abstract thinking is fostered in graduate nursing education and is an essential skill for developing theory and research. Abstract thinking is also evolving as a valuable skill for responding to problem situations in clinical practice. For example, the nurse practitioner must explore *why* patients are experiencing symptoms, examine the patients' perceptions of their symptoms, and determine patterns among these symptoms before he or she can accurately diagnose and manage the patients' health care problems.

Nursing research requires skills in both concrete and abstract thinking. Abstract thought is required to identify researchable problems, design studies, and interpret findings. Concrete thought is necessary in both planning and implementing the detailed steps of data collection and analysis. This back-and-forth flow between abstract and concrete thought may be one reason why nursing research seems foreign and complex.

Empirical World

The *empirical world* is experienced through our senses and is the concrete portion of our existence. It is what is often called *reality,* and "doing" kinds of activities are part of this world. There is a sense of certainty about the empirical or real world; it seems understandable, predictable, controllable. This world also appears to have more substance to it than do ideas, and it feels safe and secure. Concrete thinking is focused on the empirical world; words associated with this thinking include "practical," "down-to-earth," "solid," and "factual." Concrete thinkers want facts. Whatever they know must be immediately applicable to the current situation.

The practice of nursing takes place in the empirical world, as demonstrated in Figure 1–1. Some components of the research process also take place in the empirical world. For example, research ideas, which are developed into research problems, are primarily derived from the empirical world. Data collection involves actually measuring some aspect of the empirical world (measurement of reality). In a study, a blood pressure cuff, a weight scale, or an interview and observation might be used to measure reality. The findings generated through research are used in clinical practice, which is within the empirical world.

Reality Testing

People tend to *validate* or test the reality of their existence through their senses. In everyday activities, they constantly check out the messages received from their senses. For example, they might ask, "Am I really seeing what I think I am seeing?" Sometimes their senses can play tricks on them. This is why instruments have been developed to record sensory experiences more accurately. For example, does the patient just feel hot or actually have a fever? Thermometers were developed to test this sensory perception accurately.

Research is a way of validating reality. This measurement of reality is performed in terms of the researcher's perception. For example, the researcher might ask, "Do patients consume more oxygen when they use a bedside commode than when they use a bedpan?" Our senses would tell us that getting up to use a bedside commode would use more oxygen, but nurse researchers have found that this assumption is not accurate (Winslow et al., 1984). Thus, nursing research is a way of testing reality— a way of understanding what really goes on in the empirical world.

Abstract Thought Processes

Abstract thought processes influence every element of the nursing world. In a sense, they link all the elements together. Without skills in abstract thought, a person is trapped in a flat existence in the empirical world, an existence in which that world can be experienced but not understood (Abbott, 1952). Through abstract thinking, theories (which explain the nursing world) can be tested and included in the body of scientific knowledge. Abstract thinking also allows scientific findings to be developed into theories. Abstract thought enables both science and theories to be blended into a cohesive body of knowledge, guided by a philosophical framework, and applied in clinical practice.

Abstract thinking is actually more useful in clinical practice than one might think. For example, an abstract thinker is often the one who will recognize patterns in the incidence of infection in patients receiving a specific treatment and who will contemplate ideas about the relationships between the infection and other elements of the patient's care.

Three major abstract thought processes—introspection, intuition, and reasoning—are important in nursing (Silva, 1977). These thought processes are used in practicing nursing, developing and evaluating theory, critiquing and using scientific findings, planning and implementing research, and building a body of knowledge.

INTROSPECTION

Introspection is the process of turning your attention inward toward your own thoughts. It occurs at two levels. At the more superficial level, you are aware of the thoughts you are experiencing. You

have a greater awareness of the flow and interplay of feelings and ideas that occur in constantly changing patterns. These thoughts or ideas can rapidly fade from view and disappear if they are not quickly written down. When you allow introspection to occur in more depth, you examine your thoughts more critically and in detail. Patterns or links between thoughts and ideas emerge, and you may recognize fallacies or weaknesses in your thinking. You may question what brought you to this point in your thinking and find yourself really enjoying the experience.

Imagine the following clinical situation in which you have just left John Brown's home. John has a colostomy and has been receiving home health care for several weeks. Although John is caring for his colostomy, he is still reluctant to leave home for any length of time. You experience feelings of irritation and frustration with this situation. You begin to review your nursing actions and to recall other patients who have reacted in similar ways. What were the patterns of their behavior?

You have an idea—perhaps the patient's behavior is linked to the level of family support. You feel unsure about your ability to help the patient and family deal with this situation effectively. You recall other nurses describing similar reactions in their patients, and you wonder how many patients with colostomies have this problem. Your thoughts jump to reviewing the charts of other patients with colostomies and reading relevant ideas discussed in the literature. Some research has been conducted on this topic recently, and you could critique the findings for use in practice. If the findings are inadequate, perhaps other nurses would be interested in studying this situation with you.

INTUITION

Intuition is an insight or understanding of a situation or event as a whole that usually cannot be logically explained (Rew & Barrow, 1987). Because intuition is a type of knowing that seems to come unbidden, it may also be described as a "gut feeling" or a "hunch." Because intuition cannot be explained with ease scientifically, many people are uncomfortable with it. Some even say that it does not exist. Sometimes, therefore, the feeling or sense is suppressed, ignored, or dismissed as silly. However, intuition is not the lack of knowing; it is rather a result of deep knowledge — tacit knowing or personal knowledge (Benner, 1984; Polanyi, 1962, 1966). The knowledge is incorporated so deeply within that it is difficult to bring it consciously to the surface and express it in a logical manner (Beveridge, 1950; Kaplan, 1964).

Intuition is generally considered unscientific and unacceptable for use in research. In some instances, that consideration is valid. For example, a hunch that there is a significant difference between one set of scores and another set of scores is not particularly useful as an analytical technique. However, even though intuition is often unexplainable, it has some important scientific uses. Researchers do not always need to be able to explain something in order to use it. A burst of intuition may identify a problem for study, indicate important variables to measure, or link two ideas together in interpreting the findings. The trick is to recognize the feeling, value it, and hang on to the idea long enough to consider it.

Imagine the following situation. You have been working in an outpatient cardiac rehabilitation unit for the past 3 years. You and two other nurses working on the unit have been meeting with the clinical nurse specialist to plan a study to determine the factors important in promoting positive patient outcomes in the rehabilitation program. The group has met several times with a nursing professor at the university, who is collaborating with the group to develop the study. At present, the group is concerned with identifying the factors that need to be measured and how to measure them.

You have had a busy morning. Mr. Green, a patient, stops by to chat on his way out of the clinic. He chats and you listen, but not attentively. You then become more acutely aware of what he is saying. While listening, you begin to have a feeling about one variable that should be studied. You cannot really explain the origin of this feeling. You cannot identify any specific thing that Mr. Green said that triggered the idea, but somehow, the flow of his words stimulated a burst of intuition. The

variable you have in mind has not been studied previously. You feel both excited and uncertain. What will the other nurses think? If it has not been studied, is it really significant? Somehow, you feel that it is important to consider.

REASONING

Reasoning is the processing and organizing of ideas in order to reach conclusions. Through reasoning, people are able to make sense of both their thoughts and their experiences. This type of thinking is often evident in the verbal presentation of a logical argument in which each part is linked together to reach a logical conclusion. Patterns of reasoning are used to develop theories and to plan and implement research. Barnum (1998) identified four patterns of reasoning as being essential to nursing: (1) problematic, (2) operational, (3) dialectic, and (4) logistic. An individual uses all four types of reasoning, but frequently one type of reasoning is more dominant than the others. Reasoning is also classified by the discipline of logic into inductive and deductive modes (Chinn & Kramer, 1998; Omery et al., 1995).

Problematic Reasoning

Problematic reasoning involves (1) identifying a problem and the factors influencing it, (2) selecting solutions to the problem, and (3) resolving the problem. For example, nurses use problematic reasoning in the nursing process to identify nursing diagnoses and to implement nursing interventions to resolve these problems. Problematic reasoning is also evident in the identification of a research problem and the successful development of a methodology to examine it.

Operational Reasoning

Operational reasoning involves the identification of and discrimination among many alternatives and viewpoints. The focus is on the process (debating alternatives) rather than on resolution (Barnum, 1998). Nurses use operational reasoning in developing realistic, measurable goals with patients and families. Nurse practitioners use operational reasoning in debating which pharmacological and nonpharmacological treatments to use in treating patient illnesses. In research, operationalizing a treatment for implementation and debating which measurement methods or data analysis techniques to use in a study both require operational thought (Omery et al., 1995).

Dialectic Reasoning

Dialectic reasoning involves looking at situations in a holistic way. A dialectic thinker believes that the whole is greater than the sum of the parts and that the whole organizes the parts (Barnum, 1998). For example, a nurse using dialectic reasoning would view a patient as a person with strengths and weaknesses who is experiencing an illness, and not just as the "gallbladder in room 219." Dialectic reasoning also involves examining factors that are opposites and making sense of them by merging them into a single unit or idea that is greater than either alone. For example, analyzing studies with conflicting findings and summarizing these findings to determine the current knowledge base for a research problem require dialectic reasoning.

Logistic Reasoning

Logic is a science that involves valid ways of relating ideas to promote understanding. The aim of logic is to determine truth or to explain and predict phenomena. The science of logic deals with thought processes, such as concrete and abstract thinking, and methods of reasoning, such as logistic, inductive, and deductive.

Logistic reasoning is used to break the whole into parts that can be carefully examined, as can the relationships among the parts. In some ways, logistic reasoning is the opposite of dialectic reasoning. A logistic reasoner assumes that the whole is the sum of the parts and that the parts organize the whole. For example, a patient states that she is cold, and the nurse logically examines the following parts of the situation and their relationships: (1) room temperature, (2) patient's temperature, (3) patient's clothing, and (4) patient's activity. The room temperature is 65°F, the patient's temperature is 98.6°F, and the patient is wearing lightweight pajamas and drinking ice water. The nurse concludes that the patient is cold because of external environmental factors (room temperature, lightweight pajamas, and drinking ice water). Logistic reasoning is used frequently in research to develop a study design, plan and implement data collection, and conduct statistical analyses.

Inductive and Deductive Reasoning. The science of logic also includes inductive and deductive reasoning. People use these modes of reasoning constantly, although the choice of types of reasoning may not always be conscious (Kaplan, 1964). *Inductive reasoning* moves from the specific to the general, whereby particular instances are observed and then combined into a larger whole or general statement (Bandman & Bandman, 1995; Chinn & Kramer, 1998). An example of inductive reasoning follows:

> A headache is an altered level of health that is stressful.
> A fractured bone is an altered level of health that is stressful.
> A terminal illness is an altered level of health that is stressful.
> Therefore, all altered levels of health are stressful.

In this example, inductive reasoning is used to move from the specific instances of altered levels of health that are stressful to the general belief that all altered levels of health are stressful. The testing of many different altered levels of health through research to determine whether they are stressful is necessary to confirm the general statement that all types of altered health are stressful.

Deductive reasoning moves from the general to the specific or from a general premise to a particular situation or conclusion (Chinn & Kramer, 1998). A *premise* or *hypothesis* is a statement of the proposed relationship between two or more variables. An example of deductive reasoning follows:

Premises

All human beings experience loss.
All adolescents are human beings.

Conclusion

All adolescents experience loss.

In this example, deductive reasoning is used to move from the two general premises about human beings experiencing loss and adolescents being human beings to the specific conclusion, "All adolescents experience loss."

However, the conclusions generated from deductive reasoning are valid only if they are based on valid premises. Consider the following example:

Premises

All health professionals are caring.
All nurses are health professionals.

Conclusion

All nurses are caring.

The premise that all health professionals are caring is not valid or an accurate reflection of reality. Research is a means to test and confirm or refute a premise so that valid premises can be used as a basis for reasoning in nursing practice.

Science

Science is a coherent body of knowledge composed of research findings and tested theories for a specific discipline. Science is both a product (end point) and a process (mechanism to reach an end point) (Silva & Rothbart, 1984). An example from the discipline of physics is Newton's law of gravity, which was developed through extensive research. The knowledge of gravity (product) is a part of the science of physics that evolved through formulating and testing theoretical ideas (process). The ultimate goal of science is to be able to explain the empirical world and thus to have greater control over it. To accomplish this goal, scientists must discover new knowledge, expand existing knowledge, and reaffirm previously held knowledge in a discipline (Andreoli & Thompson, 1977; Greene, 1979; Toulmin, 1960).

The science of a field determines the accepted process for obtaining knowledge within that field. Research is an accepted process for obtaining scientific knowledge in nursing. Some sciences rigidly limit the types of research that can be used to obtain knowledge. The acceptable method for developing a science is the traditional research process, or *quantitative research*. According to this process, the information gained from one study is not sufficient for its inclusion in the body of science. A study must be repeated (replicated) several times and must yield similar results each time before that information can be considered a *fact* (Toulmin, 1960).

Consider the research on the relationship between smoking and lung damage and cancer. Numerous studies of animals and humans have been conducted, and the findings all indicate a relationship between smoking and lung damage. Everyone who smokes experiences lung damage, although not everyone who smokes has lung cancer. However, enough research has been conducted so that it is now considered a fact that smoking causes lung damage and is a major factor in the development of lung cancer.

Facts from studies are systematically related to one another in a way that seems to best explain the empirical world. Abstract thought processes are used to make these linkages. The linkages are called *laws, principles,* or *axioms,* depending on the certainty of the facts and relationships within the linkage. Laws are used to express the most certain relationships. The certainty depends on the amount of research conducted to test it and, to some extent, on skills in abstract thought processes. The truths or explanations of the empirical world reflected by these laws, principles, and axioms are never absolutely certain and may be disproved by further research.

Nursing science has been developed through the use of predominantly quantitative research methods. However, since 1980, a strong qualitative research tradition has evolved in nursing. *Qualitative research* is based on a philosophical orientation toward reality that is different from that of quantitative research (Kikuchi & Simmons, 1994). Within the qualitative research tradition, many of the long-held tenets about science and ways of obtaining knowledge are questioned. The philosophical orientation of qualitative research is holistic, and the purpose of this research is to examine the whole rather than the parts. Qualitative researchers are more interested in understanding complex phenomena than in determining cause-and-effect relationships among specific variables. Both quantitative research and qualitative research have proved valuable in the development of nursing knowledge (Clarke, 1995; Dzurec & Abraham, 1993; Omery et al., 1995). For this reason, this textbook provides a background for conducting different types of both quantitative research and qualitative research.

Nursing is in the beginning stages of developing a science, because a limited number of original studies and replications have been conducted (Bednar, 1993). Major studies with findings significant to nursing practice must be replicated. If researchers find similar study results through replication, they believe they are accurately describing the empirical world. The cluster of findings from replicated research then becomes a part of science (Beck, 1994).

Theory

A *theory* is a way of explaining some segment of the empirical world and can be used to describe, explain, predict, or control that segment (Dubin, 1978). A theory consists of a set of concepts that are defined and interrelated to present a view of a phenomenon. For example, Selye developed a theory about stress; Freud, a theory of human personality; and Maslow, a theory about human needs.

A theory is developed from a combination of personal experiences, research findings, and abstract thought processes. Findings from research may be used as a starting point, with the theory emerging as the theorist organizes the findings to best explain the empirical world. Alternatively, the theorist may use abstract thought processes, personal knowledge, and intuition to develop a theory of a phenomenon. However these theories are developed, it is essential that there be a variety of them to give nurses new insights into patient care and to stimulate the development of innovative interventions (Levine, 1995).

Research is conducted either to develop or to test theory. However, many nurse researchers do not recognize or value the linking of theory and research. Thus, many nursing studies are not based on theory, and their findings are not linked to theory (Moody et al., 1988). To be useful, information acquired through nursing research must be linked to nursing theories. Isolated facts gleaned from a study are not useful alone; they must be linked within nursing's knowledge base to form theories.

The theories explain the meaning of research findings and require further testing to enhance their usefulness in nursing practice. Of course, not all nursing theory is originally developed from research findings. Sometimes, a theory originates as an idea, and then research is conducted to test its accuracy. Either way, research has a role in furthering the development of nursing theories (Chinn & Kramer, 1998; Fawcett & Downs, 1986; Meleis, 1990).

Knowledge

Knowledge is a complex, multifaceted concept. For example, you may say that you "know" your friend John, "know" that the earth rotates around the sun, "know" how to give an injection, and "know" pharmacology. These are examples of knowing—being familiar with a person, comprehending facts, acquiring a psychomotor skill, and mastering a subject. There are differences in types of knowing, yet there are also similarities. Knowing presupposes order or imposes order on thoughts and ideas (Engelhardt, 1980). People have a desire to know what to expect (Russell, 1948). There is a need for certainty in the world, and individuals seek it by trying to decrease uncertainty through knowledge (Ayer, 1966). Think of the questions you ask a person who has presented some bit of knowledge: "Is it true?" "Are you sure?" "How do you know?" Thus, knowledge is acquired in a variety of ways and is expected to be an accurate reflection of reality.

WAYS OF ACQUIRING NURSING KNOWLEDGE

An additional expectation of knowledge is that it be acquired through acceptable and accurate means (White, 1982). Nursing has historically acquired knowledge through (1) traditions, (2) authority, (3) borrowing, (4) trial and error, (5) personal experience, (6) role-modeling and mentorship, (7) intuition, (8) reasoning, and (9) research. Intuition, reasoning, and research were discussed earlier in this chapter; the other ways of acquiring knowledge are briefly described in this section.

Traditions

Traditions consist of "truths" or beliefs that are based on customs and past trends. Nursing traditions from the past have been transferred to the present by written and verbal communication and role-modeling and continue to influence the present practice of nursing. For example, many of the policy and procedure manuals in hospitals and other health care facilities contain traditional ideas. In addition, nursing interventions are commonly transmitted verbally from one nurse to another over the years. Traditions can positively influence nursing practice, because they were developed from effective past experiences. For example, the idea of providing a patient with a clean, safe, well-ventilated environment originated with Florence Nightingale.

However, traditions can also narrow and limit the knowledge sought for nursing practice. For example, nursing units are frequently organized and run according to set rules or traditions. Tradition has established the time and pattern for giving baths, evaluating vital signs, giving medications, and selecting needle length for giving injections. The nurses on patient care units quickly inform new staff members about the accepted or traditional behaviors for the unit.

Traditions are difficult to change because they have existed for long periods and are frequently supported by people with power and authority. Many traditions have not been evaluated or tested for accuracy or efficiency. However, even those traditions that have not been supported through research tend to persist. For example, many cardiac patients are required to take basin baths throughout their hospitalization despite the findings from nursing research, which has shown "that the physiologic costs of the three types of baths (basin, tub, and shower) are similar; differences in responses to bathing seem more a function of subject variability than bath types; and many cardiac patients can take a tub bath or shower earlier in their hospitalization" (Winslow et al., 1985, p. 164). Nursing's body of knowledge needs to have an empirical rather than a traditional base. Through the use of evidence-based interventions, nurses can exert a powerful, positive effect on the health care system and patient outcomes.

Authority

An *authority* is a person with expertise and power who is able to influence opinion and behavior. A person is given authority because it is thought that she or he knows more in a given area than others do. Knowledge acquired from authority is illustrated when one person credits another person as the source of information. Nurses who publish articles and books or develop theories are frequently considered authorities. Students usually view their instructors as authorities, and clinical nursing experts are considered authorities within their clinical settings. However, persons viewed as authorities in one field are not authorities in other fields. An expert is an authority only when addressing his or her area of expertise. To be considered a source of knowledge, authorities in nursing must have both expertise and power. The use of only power and control does not make someone an authority.

Many customs or traditional ways of knowing are maintained by authorities, but the knowledge obtained from these authorities can be inaccurate. Like tradition, the knowledge acquired from authorities frequently has not been validated, and although it may be useful, it must be verified through research.

Borrowing

Some nursing leaders have described part of nursing's knowledge as information borrowed from disciplines such as medicine, psychology, physiology, and education (Andreoli & Thompson, 1977; McMurrey, 1982). *Borrowing* in nursing involves the appropriation and use of knowledge from other fields or disciplines to guide nursing practice.

Nursing has borrowed knowledge in two ways. For years, some nurses have taken information from other disciplines and applied it directly to nursing practice. This information was not integrated within the unique focus of nursing. For example, some nurses have used the medical model to guide their nursing practice, thus focusing on the diagnosis and treatment of disease. This type of borrowing continues today as nurses use advances in technology to become highly specialized and focused on the detection and treatment of disease, to the exclusion of health promotion and illness prevention.

Another way of borrowing, which is more useful in nursing, is the integration of information from other disciplines within the focus of nursing. Because disciplines share knowledge, it is sometimes difficult to know where the boundaries exist between nursing's knowledge base and that of other disciplines. There is a blurring of boundaries as the knowledge bases of disciplines evolve (McMurrey, 1982). For example, information about self-esteem as a characteristic of the human personality is associated with psychology, but this knowledge of self-esteem also directs the nurse in assessing the psychological needs of patients and families. However, borrowed knowledge has not been adequate for answering many questions generated in nursing practice.

Trial and Error

Trial and error is an approach with unknown outcomes that is used in a situation of uncertainty, when other sources of knowledge are unavailable. Because each patient responds uniquely to a situation, there is uncertainty in nursing practice. Because of this uncertainty, nurses must use trial and error in providing care. However, with trial and error, there is frequently no formal documentation of effective and ineffective nursing actions. When this strategy is used, knowledge is gained from experience but often is not shared with others. The trial-and-error way of acquiring knowledge can also be time-consuming, because multiple interventions might be implemented before one is found to be effective. There is also a risk of implementing nursing actions that are detrimental to a patient's health.

Personal Experience

Personal experience involves gaining knowledge by being personally involved in an event, situation, or circumstance. In nursing, personal experience enables one to gain skills and expertise by providing care to patients and families in clinical settings.

Learning occurs during personal experience and enables the nurse to cluster ideas into a meaningful whole. For example, students may be told how to give an injection in a classroom setting, but they do not "know" how to give an injection until they observe other nurses giving injections to patients and actually give several injections themselves.

The amount of personal experience affects the complexity of a nurse's knowledge base. Benner (1984) described five levels of experience in the development of clinical knowledge and expertise: (1) novice, (2) advanced beginner, (3) competent, (4) proficient, and (5) expert. *Novice* nurses have no personal experience in the work that they are to perform, but they have preconceived notions and expectations about clinical practice that are challenged, refined, confirmed, or contradicted by personal experience in a clinical setting. The *advanced beginner* has just enough experience to recognize and intervene in recurrent situations. For example, the advanced beginner nurse is able to recognize and intervene to meet patients' needs for pain management.

Competent nurses frequently have been on the job for 2 or 3 years, and their personal experiences enable them to generate and achieve long-range goals and plans. Through experience, the competent nurse is able to use personal knowledge to take conscious, deliberate actions that are efficient and organized. From a more complex knowledge base, the *proficient* nurse views the patient as a whole and as a member of a family and community. The proficient nurse recognizes that each patient and family respond differently to illness and health. The *expert* nurse has an extensive background of experience and is able to identify accurately and intervene skillfully in a situation.

Personal experience increases an expert nurse's ability to grasp a situation intuitively with accuracy and speed. The dynamics of expert nursing practice need to be clarified through research. In addition, the methods that facilitate meaningful personal experiences need to be identified for use in nursing education.

Role-Modeling and Mentorship

Role-modeling is learning by imitating the behaviors of an exemplar. An exemplar or role model is regarded as knowing the appropriate and rewarded roles for a profession, and these roles reflect the attitudes and include the standards and norms of behavior for that profession (Bidwell & Brasler, 1989). In nursing, role-modeling enables the novice nurse to learn through interaction with, or following examples set by, highly competent nurses. Examples of role models are "admired teachers, practitioners, researchers, or illustrious individuals who inspire students through their examples" (Werley & Newcomb, 1983, p. 206).

An intense form of role-modeling is *mentorship.* In a mentorship, the expert nurse or *mentor* serves as a teacher, sponsor, guide, exemplar, and counselor for the novice nurse (*mentee*) (Vance, 1982). Both the mentor and the mentee invest time and active involvement, which results in a close, personal mentor-mentee relationship. This relationship promotes a mutual exchange of ideas and aspirations relative to the mentee's career plans. The mentee assumes the values, attitudes, and behaviors of the mentor while gaining intuitive knowledge and personal experience.

Body of Knowledge for Nursing

To summarize, in nursing, a body of knowledge must be acquired (learned), incorporated, and assimilated by each member of the profession and collectively by the profession as a whole. This body of knowledge guides the thinking and behavior of the profession and individual practitioners and provides direction for further development and interpretation of science and theory in the discipline. Nursing's development of a body of knowledge will give nurses the confidence that they know what they are doing. This knowledge base is necessary for the recognition of nursing as a science by health professionals, consumers, and society.

Philosophy

Philosophy provides a broad, global explanation of the world. It is the most abstract and most all-encompassing concept in the model (see Figure 1–1). Philosophy gives unity and meaning to nursing's world and provides a framework within which thinking, knowing, and doing occur (Kikuchi &

Simmons, 1994). Nursing's philosophical position influences its knowledge. How nurses use science and theories to explain the empirical world depends on their philosophy. Ideas about truth and reality as well as beliefs, values, and attitudes are part of philosophy. Philosophy asks questions such as, "Is there an absolute truth, or is truth relative?" "Is there one reality, or is reality different for each individual?" "What are my purposes in life?"

Everyone's world is modified by her or his philosophy as a pair of eyeglasses would modify vision. Perceptions are influenced first by philosophy and then by knowledge. For example, if what you see is not within your ideas of truth or reality, if it does not fit your belief system, you may not see it. Your mind may reject it altogether or may modify it to fit your philosophy (Scheffler, 1967).

Philosophical positions commonly held by the nursing profession include the view of human beings as holistic, rational, and responsible. Nurses believe that people desire health and health is considered to be better than illness. Quality of life is as important as quantity of life. Good nursing care facilitates improved patterns of health and quality of life. In nursing, truth is seen as relative and reality tends to vary with perception (Kikuchi et al., 1996; Silva, 1977). For example, because nurses believe that reality varies with perception and that truth is relative, they would not try to impose their views of truth and reality on patients. Rather, they would accept patients' views of the world and help them seek health from within those world views.

Nursing's philosophical positions have a strong influence on the research conducted (Kikuchi & Simmons, 1994; Omery et al., 1995). These philosophical positions support the use of both quantitative research and qualitative research in the development of a scientific knowledge base for nursing. The research problems selected for study, the methodologies implemented in research, and the interpretations of research findings are influenced by nursing's philosophy.

In conclusion, the most abstract concept, philosophy, links in a direct and meaningful way with the most concrete concept, the empirical world. Our philosophy directs how we view and interact with others in the world around us. Figure 1–1 demonstrates that research is not off to the side, disconnected from the rest of nursing. In order to utilize nursing's body of knowledge in practice, one must incorporate all the elements of the nursing world. If one element is missing, the rest of the elements lose meaning. One cannot be only concrete, only abstract, only theoretical, or only scientific. One cannot attend only to clinical practice and disregard the rest of the nursing world—not if one is a nurse in the whole sense of the word.

■ SUMMARY

The purpose of this chapter is to introduce the reader to the world of research. *Research* is defined as diligent, systematic inquiry to validate and refine existing knowledge and generate new knowledge. Defining nursing research requires examining differing views about what is relevant knowledge for nursing. One view is that nursing research should be limited to only those studies that generate knowledge that is directly useful in clinical practice. Another view is that nursing research includes studies of nursing education, nursing administration, health services, and the characteristics of nurses and nursing roles as well as clinical situations. Those who support this second view argue that findings from such studies indirectly influence nursing practice. In this textbook, *nursing research* is defined as a scientific process that validates and refines existing knowledge and generates new knowledge that directly and indirectly influences nursing practice.

Nursing research is essential for the development of scientific knowledge that enables nurses to provide evidence-based health care to patients and their families. This knowledge base is derived from the focus or unique perspective of the discipline and provides an organizing framework for nursing practice. The knowledge generated through research is essential for description, explanation, prediction, and control of nursing phenomena.

This chapter presents a framework that links nursing research to the world of nursing and provides an organizing model for this textbook. The concepts in this framework range from concrete to abstract and include concrete and abstract thinking, empirical world (nursing practice), reality testing (research), abstract thought processes, science, theory, knowledge, and philosophy.

Nursing thought flows along a continuum of concrete thinking and abstract thinking. *Concrete thinking* is oriented toward tangible things or events. *Abstract thinking* is oriented toward the development of an idea without application to, or association with, a particular instance. The *empirical world* is the concrete portion of human existence experienced through the senses and is validated through reality testing. Research is a form of reality testing that requires skills in both concrete thinking and abstract thinking. Abstract thought processes influence every element of the nursing world. Three major abstract thought processes—introspection, intuition, and reasoning—are important in nursing. These thought processes are used in practicing nursing, developing and evaluating theory, critiquing and using scientific findings, planning and implementing research, and building a body of knowledge.

Science and theory are two different but interdependent concepts that are linked by abstract thought processes. *Science* is a coherent body of knowledge composed of research findings and tested theories for a specific discipline. It is both a process (scientific methods) and a product (body of knowledge). Nursing science is slowly developing with the utilization of a variety of both quantitative and qualitative research methods. *Theory* is a way of explaining some segment of the empirical world. Theories are developed and tested through research, and when they are adequately tested, they become part of science.

Science and theory contribute to the development of a body of knowledge in a discipline. In nursing, a body of knowledge must be acquired (learned), incorporated, and assimilated by each member of the profession and collectively by the profession as a whole. Nursing has historically acquired knowledge through traditions, authority, borrowing, trial and error, personal experience, role-modeling and mentorship, intuition, reasoning, and research. There is a growing need for nursing knowledge to be validated, refined, and expanded through research.

The most abstract element of the framework is philosophy. Philosophy gives unity and meaning to the world of nursing and provides a structure within which thinking, knowing, and doing occur. Nursing's philosophical positions, such as the holistic perspective and the importance of quality of life, have a strong influence on the research conducted and the knowledge developed in the discipline. The framework demonstrates that nursing research is not an entity disconnected from the rest of nursing but, rather, is influenced by and influences all other aspects of nursing.

• •

REFERENCES

Abbott, E. A. (1952). *Flatland.* New York: Dover Publications.

Andreoli, K. G., & Thompson, C. E. (1977). The nature of science in nursing. *Image—Journal of Nursing Scholarship, 9*(2), 32–37.

Ayer, A. J. (1966). *The problem of knowledge.* Baltimore: Penguin.

Bandman, E. L., & Bandman, B. (1995). *Critical thinking in nursing* (2nd ed.). Norwalk, CT: Appleton & Lange.

Barnum, B. S. (1998). *Nursing theory: Analysis, application, evaluation* (5th ed.). Philadelphia: Lippincott–Williams & Wilkins.

Beck, C. T. (1994). Replication strategies for nursing research. *Image—Journal of Nursing Scholarship, 26*(3), 191–194.

Bednar, B. (1993). Developing clinical practice guidelines: An interview with Ada Jacox. *ANNA Journal, 20*(2), 121–126.

Benner, P. (1984). *From novice to expert: Excellence and power in clinical nursing practice.* Menlo Park, CA: Addison-Wesley.

Beveridge, W. I. B. (1950). *The art of scientific investigation.* New York: Vintage Books.

Bidwell, A. S., & Brasler, M. L. (1989). Role modeling versus mentoring in nursing education. *Image—Journal of Nursing Scholarship, 21*(1), 23–25.

Brown, S. J. (1999). *Knowledge for healthcare practice: A guide to using research evidence.* Philadelphia: W. B. Saunders.

Chinn, P. L., & Kramer, M. K. (1998). *Theory and nursing: A systematic approach* (5th ed.). St. Louis: Mosby–Year Book.

Clarke, L. (1995). Nursing research: Science, visions, and telling stories. *Journal of Advanced Nursing, 21*(3), 584–593.

Defloor, T. (2000). The effect of position and mattress on interface pressure. *Applied Nursing Research, 13*(1), 2–11.

Dickoff, J., James, P., & Wiedenbach, E. (1968). Theory in a practice discipline: Practice oriented theory (Part I). *Nursing Research, 17*(5), 415–435.

Dubin, R. (1978). *Theory building* (Rev. ed.). New York: Free Press.

Dzurec, L. C., & Abraham, I. L. (1993). The nature of inquiry: Linking quantitative and qualitative research. *Advances in Nursing Science, 16*(1), 73–79.

Engelhardt, H. T., Jr. (1980). Knowing and valuing: Looking for common roots. In H. T. Engelhardt & D. Callahan (Eds.), *Knowing and valuing: The search for common roots* (Vol. 4, pp. 1–17). New York: Hastings Center.

Fawcett, J., & Downs, F. S. (1986). *The relationship of theory and research.* Norwalk, CT: Appleton-Century-Crofts.

Greene, J. A. (1979). Science, nursing and nursing science: A conceptual analysis. *Advances in Nursing Science, 2*(1), 57–64.

Hegyvary, S. T. (1991). Issues in outcomes research. *Journal of Nursing Quality Assurance, 5*(2), 1–6.

Jacobs, V. (2000). Informational needs of surgical patients following discharge. *Applied Nursing Research, 13*(1), 12–18.

Kaplan, A. (1964). *The conduct of inquiry.* New York: Harper & Row.

Kikuchi, J. F., & Simmons, H. (1994). *Developing a philosophy of nursing.* Thousand Oaks, CA: Sage Publications.

Kikuchi, J. F., Simmons, H., & Romyn, D. (1996). *Truth in nursing inquiry.* Thousand Oaks, CA: Sage Publications.

Levine, M. E. (1995). The rhetoric of nursing theory. *Image—Journal of Nursing Scholarship, 27*(1), 11–14.

McMurrey, P. H. (1982). Toward a unique knowledge base in nursing. *Image—Journal of Nursing Scholarship, 14*(1), 12–15.

Meleis, A. I. (1990). *Theoretical nursing: Development and progress* (2nd ed.). Philadelphia: Lippincott–Williams & Wilkins.

Moody, L. E., Wilson, M. E., Smyth, K., Schwartz, R., Tittle, M., & Van Cott, M. L. (1988). Analysis of a decade of nursing practice research: 1977–1986. *Nursing Research, 37*(6), 374–379.

Omery, A., & Williams, R. P. (1999). An appraisal of research utilization across the United States. *Journal of Nursing Administration, 29*(12), 50–56.

Omery, A., Kasper, C. E., & Page, G. G. (1995). *In search of nursing science.* Thousand Oaks, CA: Sage Publications.

Parker, B., McFarlane, J., Soeken, K., Silva, C., & Reel, S. (1999). Testing an intervention to prevent further abuse to pregnant women. *Research in Nursing & Health, 22*(1), 59–66.

Polanyi, M. (1962). *Personal knowledge.* Chicago: University of Chicago Press.

Polanyi, M. (1966). *The tacit dimension.* New York: Doubleday.

Pronk, N. P., Goodman, M. J., O'Connor, P. J., & Martinson, B. C. (1999). Relationship between modifiable health risks and short-term healthcare charges. *JAMA, 282*(23), 2235–2239.

Rew, L., & Barrow, E. M. (1987). Intuition: A neglected hallmark of nursing knowledge. *Advances in Nursing Science, 10*(1), 49–62.

Russell, B. (1948). *Human knowledge, its scope and limits.* Brooklyn: Simon & Schuster.

Scheffler, I. (1967). *Science and subjectivity.* Indianapolis, IN: Bobbs-Merrill.

Silva, M. C. (1977). Philosophy, science, theory: Interrelationships and implications for nursing research. *Image—Journal of Nursing Scholarship, 9*(3), 59–63.

Silva, M. C., & Rothbart, D. (1984). An analysis of changing trends in philosophies of science on nursing theory development and testing. *Advances in Nursing Science, 6*(2), 1–13.

Stevenson, J. S. (1988). Nursing knowledge development: Into era II. *Journal of Professional Nursing, 4*(3), 152–162.

Toulmin, S. (1960). *The philosophy of science.* New York: Harper & Row.

Vance, C. (1982). The mentor connection. *Journal of Nursing Administration, 12*(4), 7–13.

Werley, H. H., & Newcomb, B. J. (1983). The research mentor: A missing element in nursing? In N. L. Chaska (Ed.), *The nursing profession: A time to speak* (pp. 202–215). New York: McGraw-Hill.

White, A. R. (1982). *The nature of knowledge.* Totowa, NJ: Rowman and Littlefield.

Winslow, E. H., Lane, L. D., & Gaffney, F. A. (1984). Oxygen consumption and cardiovascular response in patients and normal adults during in-bed and out-of-bed toileting. *Journal of Cardiac Rehabilitation, 4*(8), 348–354.

Winslow, E. H., Lane, L. D., & Gaffney, F. A. (1985). Oxygen uptake and cardiovascular responses in control adults and acute myocardial infarction patients during bathing. *Nursing Research, 34*(3), 164–169.

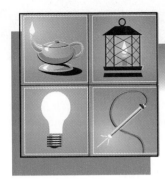

CHAPTER 2

THE EVOLUTION OF RESEARCH IN NURSING

Initially, research evolved slowly in nursing from the investigations of Florence Nightingale in the nineteenth century to the studies of nursing education in the 1930s and 1940s and the research of nurses and nursing roles in the 1950s and 1960s. However, in the late 1970s and 1980s, numerous studies were conducted that focused on improving nursing practice. This emphasis continued in the 1990s with the conduct of research to promote improved patient outcomes. The goal in the new millennium is the development of an evidence-based practice (EBP) for nursing, with nurses using the current, best research findings in their delivery of health care.

Over the years, a variety of scientific methodologies have been implemented to develop nursing knowledge. Initially, empirical nursing knowledge was generated through quantitative research. In the late 1970s, a group of nurses began conducting qualitative research to generate a holistic understanding of nursing phenomena. Since 1980, nurses have conducted both quantitative and qualitative research to build a sound knowledge base for nursing practice. In the 1990s, outcomes research emerged as an important methodology for generating knowledge about the end-results of patient care. Outcomes research is conducted to examine both short-term and long-term results of health care, such as patient health status, quality of care, and cost-effectiveness of care. Another emerging methodological trend for the new millennium is the conduct of intervention research, which examines the effectiveness of nursing actions in promoting healthy outcomes for patients and families.

In this chapter, the historical events relevant to nursing research are identified; the problem-solving process and nursing process are discussed as a basis for the research process; and the types of quantitative and qualitative research methods important to the generation of nursing knowledge are introduced. The chapter concludes with a discussion of two new methodologies, outcomes research and intervention research, that are being conducted to generate essential knowledge for the implementation of evidence-based nursing care.

HISTORICAL DEVELOPMENT OF RESEARCH IN NURSING

Some people think that research is relatively new to nursing, but Florence Nightingale initiated nursing research more than 140 years ago (Nightingale, 1859). Following Nightingale's work (1850–1910), research received minimal attention until the mid-1900s. From the 1960s, the recognition that nursing research is of value gradually increased, but few nurses had the educational background to conduct studies until the 1970s. However, in the 1980s and 1990s, research became a major force in developing a scientific knowledge base for nursing practice. Table 2–1 identifies some of the key historical events that have influenced the development of nursing research. These events are discussed in the following section.

TABLE 2–1
HISTORICAL EVENTS INFLUENCING NURSING RESEARCH

Year	Historical Event
1850	Nightingale, first nurse researcher
1900	*American Journal of Nursing* first published
1923	Teacher's College at Columbia University offers the first educational doctoral program for nurses
1929	First Master of Nursing degree is offered at Yale University
1932	The Association of Collegiate Schools of Nursing is organized
1950	American Nurses' Association (ANA) study of nursing functions and activities
1952	*Nursing Research* first published
1953	Institute of Research and Service in Nursing Education established
1955	American Nurses Foundation established to fund nursing research
1963	*International Journal of Nursing Studies* first published
1965	ANA sponsored first nursing research conferences
1967	*Image* (Sigma Theta Tau publication) first published
1970	ANA Commission on Nursing Research established
1972	ANA Council of Nurse Researchers established
1973	First Nursing Diagnosis Conference held
1978	*Research in Nursing & Health* first published *Advances in Nursing Science* first published
1979	*Western Journal of Nursing Research* first published
1982–83	*Conduct and Utilization of Research in Nursing (CURN) Project* (published)
1983	*Annual Review of Nursing Research* first published
1985	National Center for Nursing Research (NCNR) established within the National Institutes of Health
1987	*Scholarly Inquiry for Nursing Practice* first published
1988	*Applied Nursing Research* first published *Nursing Science Quarterly* first published
1989	Agency for Health Care Policy and Research (AHCPR) established Clinical practice guidelines first published by the AHCPR
1992	*Healthy People 2000* published by U.S. Department of Health and Human Services
1993	NCNR renamed the National Institute of Nursing Research (NINR)
1994	*Qualitative Nursing Research* first published
1999	AHCPR renamed Agency for Healthcare Research and Quality (AHRQ)
1999	American Association of Colleges of Nursing position statement on nursing research
2000	NINR identified mission and funding priorities for 2000–2004 (*http://www.nih/gov/ninr*)
2000	AHRQ identified mission and funding priorities (*http://www.ahrq.gov*)

Florence Nightingale

Nightingale has been described as a reformer, reactionary, and researcher who has influenced health care in general and nursing specifically. Nightingale's book, *Notes on Nursing* (1859), described her initial research activities, which focused on the importance of a healthy environment in promoting the patient's physical and mental well-being. She identified the need to gather data on the environment, such as ventilation, cleanliness, temperature, purity of water, and diet, to determine their influence on the patient's health (Herbert, 1981).

Nightingale is most noted for her data collection and statistical analyses during the Crimean War. She gathered data on soldier morbidity and mortality and the factors influencing them and presented her results in tables and pie diagrams, a sophisticated type of data presentation for this period (Palmer, 1977). Nightingale's research enabled her to instigate attitudinal, organizational, and social changes. She changed the attitudes of the military and society toward the care of the sick. The military began to view the sick as having the right to adequate food, suitable quarters, and appropriate medical treatment. These interventions drastically reduced mortality from 43% to 2% in the Crimean War (Cook, 1913). She improved the organization of army administration, hospital management, and hospital construction. Because of Nightingale's influence, society began to accept responsibility for testing public water, improving sanitation, preventing starvation, and decreasing morbidity and mortality (Palmer, 1977).

Early 1900s

From 1900 to 1950, research activities in nursing were limited, but a few studies advanced nursing education. These studies included the Nutting Report, 1912; Goldmark Report, 1923; and Burgess Report, 1926 (Abdellah, 1972; Johnson, 1977). On the basis of recommendations of the Goldmark Report, more schools of nursing were established in university settings. The baccalaureate degree in nursing provided a basis for graduate nursing education, with the first Master of Nursing degree offered by Yale University in 1929. Teachers College at Columbia University offered the first doctoral program for nurses in 1923 and granted a degree in education (Ed.D.) to prepare teachers for the profession. The Association of Collegiate Schools of Nursing, organized in 1932, promoted the conduct of research to improve education and practice. This organization also sponsored the publication of the first research journal in nursing, *Nursing Research*, in 1952 (Fitzpatrick, 1978).

A research trend that started in the 1940s and continued in the 1950s focused on the organization and delivery of nursing services. Studies were conducted on the numbers and kinds of nursing personnel, staffing patterns, patient classification systems, patient and personnel satisfaction, and unit arrangement. Types of care such as comprehensive care, home care, and progressive patient care were evaluated. These evaluations of care laid the foundation for the development of self-study manuals, which are similar to the quality assurance manuals of today (Gortner & Nahm, 1977).

Nursing Research in the 1950s and 1960s

In 1950, the American Nurses' Association (ANA) initiated a 5-year study on nursing functions and activities. The findings of this study were reported in *Twenty Thousand Nurses Tell Their Story*. As a result of this study, ANA developed statements on functions, standards, and qualifications for professional nurses in 1959. Also during this time, clinical research began expanding as specialty groups, such as community health, psychiatric, medical-surgical, pediatrics, and obstetrics, developed standards of care. The research conducted by ANA and the specialty groups provided the basis for the nursing practice standards that currently guide professional nursing practice (Gortner & Nahm, 1977).

Educational studies were conducted in the 1950s and 1960s to determine the most effective educational preparation for the registered nurse. Montag developed and evaluated the 2-year nursing preparation (associate degree) in the junior colleges. Student characteristics, such as admission and retention patterns and the elements that promoted success in

nursing education, were studied (Downs & Fleming, 1979).

In 1953, an Institute for Research and Service in Nursing Education was established at Teacher's College, Columbia University, which provided research learning experiences for doctoral students (Werley, 1977). The American Nurse's Foundation, chartered in 1955, was responsible for receiving and administering research funds, conducting research programs, consulting with nursing students, and engaging in research. In 1956, a Committee on Research and Studies was established to guide ANA research (See, 1977).

A Department of Nursing Research was established in the Walter Reed Army Institute of Research in 1957. This was the first nursing unit in a research institution that emphasized conducting clinical nursing research (Werley, 1977). Also in 1957, the Southern Regional Educational Board (SREB), the Western Interstate Commission on Higher Education (WICHE), and the New England Board of Higher Education (NEBHE) were developed. These organizations are actively involved in promoting research and disseminating the findings. ANA sponsored the first of a series of research conferences in 1965, and the conference sponsors required that the studies presented be relevant to nursing and be conducted by a nurse researcher (See, 1977). These ANA conferences continue to be an important means of disseminating research findings today.

In the 1960s, a growing number of clinical studies focused on quality care and the development of criteria to measure patient outcomes. Intensive care units were being developed, which promoted the investigation of nursing interventions, staffing patterns, and cost-effectiveness of care (Gortner & Nahm, 1977).

Nursing Research in the 1970s

In the 1970s, the nursing process became the focus of many studies, with the investigations of assessment techniques and guidelines, goal-setting methods, and specific nursing interventions. In 1973, the first Nursing Diagnosis Conference was held; these conferences continue to be held every 2 years. Studies are being conducted to identify appropriate diagnoses for nursing and to generate an effective diagnostic process (Carlson-Catalano & Lunney, 1995).

The educational studies of the 1970s were concerned with the evaluation of teaching methods and student learning experiences. A number of studies were conducted to differentiate the practices of nurses with baccalaureate and associate degrees. These studies, which primarily measured abilities to perform technical skills, were ineffective in differentiating between the two levels of education.

In the service setting, primary patient care was the trend of the 1970s; studies were conducted in relation to its implementation and outcomes. The number of nurse practitioners (NPs) and clinical nurse specialists (CNSs) with master's degrees increased rapidly during the 1970s. Limited research has been conducted on the CNS role; however, the NP and nurse midwifery roles have been researched extensively to determine their positive impact on productivity, quality, and cost of health care (Brown & Grimes, 1995). In addition, those clinicians with master's degrees were provided the background to conduct research and to use research findings in practice.

In the late 1960s and 1970s, nursing scholars began developing models, conceptual frameworks, and theories to guide nursing practice. These nursing theorists' works provided direction for future nursing research. In 1978, a new journal, *Advances in Nursing Science,* began publishing the works of nursing theorists and the research related to their theories.

The number of doctoral programs in nursing and the number of nurses prepared at the doctoral level greatly expanded in the 1970s (Jacox, 1980). Nurses with doctoral degrees increased the conduct and complexity of nursing research; however, many of these nurses did not become actively involved in research. In 1970, the ANA Commission on Nursing Research was established; in turn, this commission established the Council of Nurse Researchers in 1972 to advance research activities, provide an exchange of ideas, and recognize excellence in research. The commission also prepared position papers on subjects' rights in research and on federal guidelines concerning research and human subjects,

and sponsored research programs nationally and internationally (See, 1977).

Federal funds for nursing research increased significantly, with a total of just over $39 million awarded for research in nursing from 1955 to 1976. Even though federal funding for nursing studies rose, the funding was not comparable to the $493 million in federal research funds received by those doing medical research in 1974 alone (de Tornyay, 1977).

The dissemination of research findings was a major issue in the 1970s. Sigma Theta Tau, the International Honor Society for Nursing, sponsored national and international research conferences, and the chapters of this organization sponsored many local conferences to promote the dissemination of research findings. *Image,* a journal initially published in 1967 by Sigma Theta Tau, contains many nursing studies and articles about research methodology. A major goal of Sigma Theta Tau is to advance scholarship in nursing by promoting the conduct, communication, and utilization of research in nursing. The communication of research findings was also facilitated by the addition of two new research journals in the 1970s, *Research in Nursing & Health* in 1978, and *Western Journal of Nursing Research* in 1979.

Nursing Research in the 1980s and 1990s

The conduct of clinical nursing research was the focus of the 1980s and 1990s. A variety of clinical journals (*Cancer Nursing*; *Cardiovascular Nursing*; *Dimensions of Critical Care Nursing*; *Heart & Lung*; *Journal of Obstetric, Gynecologic, and Neonate Nursing*; *Journal of Neurosurgical Nursing*; *Pediatric Nursing*; and *Rehabilitation Nursing*) published an increasing number of studies. One new research journal was published in 1987, *Scholarly Inquiry for Nursing Practice*, and two in 1988, *Applied Nursing Research* and *Nursing Science Quarterly*. Even though the body of empirical knowledge generated through clinical research grew rapidly in the 1980s, little of this knowledge was used in practice.

During 1982 and 1983, the materials from a federally funded project, Conduct and Utilization of Research in Nursing (CURN), were published to facilitate the use of research to improve nursing practice (Horsley et al., 1983). In 1983, the first volume of the *Annual Review of Nursing Research* was published (Werley & Fitzpatrick, 1983). This annual publication contains experts' reviews of research in selected areas of nursing practice, nursing care delivery, nursing education, and the profession of nursing. It continues to be published each year, promoting the use of research findings in practices and identifying directions for future research.

Many nurses obtained master's and doctoral degrees during the 1980s and 1990s, and postdoctoral education was encouraged for nurse researchers. The ANA Cabinet on Nursing Research identified the research participation for various levels of educational preparation. As indicated in Figure 2–1, nurses at all levels of education have a role in research (ANA, 1989). Educational preparation encourages:

- The nurse with an associate degree to assist with problem identification and data collection.
- The nurse with a baccalaureate degree to use research findings in practice.
- The nurse with a master's degree to collaborate in research projects.

- The nurse with a doctoral degree to conduct independent, funded research projects.

The researcher's role expands with advanced education, so that the nurse with a postdoctoral preparation has the background to develop and coordinate funded research programs (ANA, 1989). These research expectations for each level of nursing education were supported by the American Association of Colleges of Nursing (AACN)'s 1999 position statement on nursing research (AACN, 1999).

Another priority of the 1980s and 1990s was to obtain greater funding for nursing research. Most of the federal funds in the 1980s were designated for studies involving the diagnosis and cure of diseases. Therefore, nursing received a very small percentage of the federal research and development (R&D) funds (approximately 2–3%) compared with medicine (approximately 90%), even though nursing personnel greatly outnumber medical personnel (Larson, 1984). However, ANA achieved a major political victory for nursing research with the creation of the National Center for Nursing Research (NCNR) in 1985. This center was created after years of work and two presidential vetoes (Bauknecht, 1986). The purpose of NCNR was to sup-

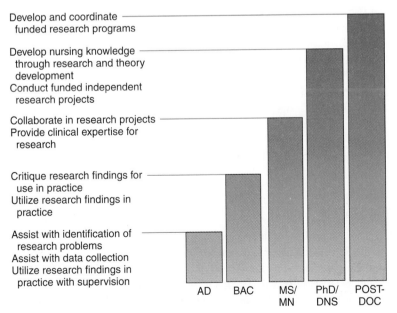

FIGURE 2–1 ■ Research participation at various levels of education preparation. (Adapted from Maxine E. Loomis, Ph.D., R.N., C.S., F.A.A.N., unpublished work, 1989, by American Nurses Association [1989]. *Education for participation in nursing research*. Kansas City, MO: American Nurses Association.)

port the conduct of basic and clinical nursing research and the dissemination of findings. The NCNR, established under the National Institutes of Health (NIH), provided visibility for nursing research at the federal level. In 1993, during the tenure of its first director, Ada Sue Hinshaw, Ph.D., R.N., the NCNR became the National Institute of Nursing Research (NINR). This change in title enhanced the recognition of nursing as a research discipline and expanded the funding for nursing research.

Outcomes research emerged as an important methodology for documenting the effectiveness of health care services in the 1980s and 1990s. This effectiveness research evolved from the quality assessment and quality assurance functions that originated with the professional standards review organizations (the PSROs) in 1972. Outcomes research was promoted during the 1980s by William Roper, director of the Health Care Finance Administration (HCFA), for the purpose of determining quality and cost-effectiveness of patient care.

In 1989, the Agency for Health Care Policy and Research (AHCPR) was established to facilitate the conduct of outcomes research (Rettig, 1991). AHCPR also had an active role in communicating research findings to health care practitioners and was responsible for publishing the first clinical practice guidelines in 1989. Several of these guidelines, including the latest research findings with directives for practice, were published in the 1990s. The Healthcare Research and Quality Act of 1999 reauthorized the AHCPR, changing its name to the Agency for Healthcare Research and Quality (AHRQ). This significant change positioned the AHRQ as a scientific partner with the public and private sectors to improve the quality and safety of patient care (*http://www.ahcpr.gov/*).

Nursing Research in the 21st Century

The vision for nursing in the twenty-first century is the development of a scientific knowledge base that enables nurses to implement an evidence-based practice (EBP) (Brown, 1999; Omery & Williams, 1999). This vision is consistent with the mission of NINR, which is to "support clinical and basic research to establish a scientific basis for the care of individuals across the lifespan—from management of patients during illness and recovery to the reduction of risks for disease and disability, the promotion of healthy lifestyles, promoting quality of life in those with chronic illness, and care for the individuals at the end of life" (*http://www.nih.gov/ninr/*). NINR is seeking expanded funding for nursing research and is encouraging the use of a variety of methodologies (quantitative, qualitative, outcomes research, and intervention research) to generate essential knowledge for nursing practice.

The AHRQ has been designated the lead agency supporting research designed to improve the quality of health care, reduce its cost, improve patient safety, decrease medical errors, and broaden access to essential services. AHRQ sponsors and conducts research that provides evidence-based information on health care outcomes, quality, cost, use, and access. This research information is needed to promote effective health care decision making by patients, clinicians, health system executives, and policymakers. More nurse researchers need to collaborate with practitioners of other disciplines in seeking funding from AHRQ to have an impact on the future of health care services.

The focus of health care research and funding is expanding from the treatment of illness to include health promotion and illness prevention interventions. *Healthy People 2000,* a government document published by the U.S. Department of Health and Human Services, has increased the visibility of and identified priorities for health promotion research. In the twenty-first century, nurses can have a major role in the development of interventions to promote health and prevent illness in individuals, families, and communities.

To ensure an effective research enterprise in nursing, the discipline must:

1. Create a research culture.
2. Provide quality educational (baccalaureate, master's, doctoral, and postdoctoral) programs to prepare a work force of nurse scientists.
3. Develop a sound research infrastructure.
4. Obtain sufficient funding for essential research. (AACN, 1999)

The remaining sections of this chapter were developed to promote an understanding of the research process and the scientific methodologies that are important to the future development of nursing knowledge.

BACKGROUND FOR THE RESEARCH PROCESS

Research is a process similar in some ways to other processes. Therefore, the background acquired early in nursing education in problem solving and the nursing process is also useful in research. A process consists of a purpose, a series of actions, and a goal. The purpose gives direction to the process, and the series of actions are organized into steps to achieve the identified goal. A process is continuous and can be revised and reimplemented to reach an end point or goal.

The steps of the problem-solving process, nursing process, and research process are presented in Table 2–2. Relating the research process to problem-solving and nursing processes can help the beginning researcher use familiar ways of thinking to facilitate the incorporation of new knowledge and skills.

Comparison of the Problem-Solving Process and the Nursing Process

The *problem-solving process* is the (1) systematic identification of a problem, (2) determination of goals related to the problem, (3) identification of

possible approaches to achieve those goals, (4) implementation of selected approaches, and (5) evaluation of goal achievement. Problem solving is frequently used in daily activities and in nursing practice. For example, a nurse uses problem solving when selecting clothing, deciding where to live, turning a patient with a fractured hip, and treating a patient for hypertension.

The *nursing process* is a subset of the problem-solving process. The steps of the nursing process are (1) assessment, (2) diagnosis, (3) plan, (4) implementation, (5) evaluation, and (6) modification. Assessment involves the collection and interpretation of data for the development of nursing diagnoses. These diagnoses guide the remaining steps of the nursing process, just as the step of defining the problem directs the remaining steps of the problem-solving process. The planning step in the nursing process is the same as that in the problem-solving process. Both processes involve implementation, or putting the plan into action, and evaluation, or determination of the effectiveness of the process. The problem-solving process and the nursing process are cyclical. If the process is not effective, all steps are reviewed and revised (modified), and the process is reimplemented.

Comparison of the Nursing Process and the Research Process

Having experience with the nursing process facilitates an understanding of the research process.

TABLE 2–2
COMPARISON OF THE PROBLEM-SOLVING PROCESS, NURSING PROCESS, AND RESEARCH PROCESS

Problem-Solving Process	Nursing Process	Research Process

Data collection	Assessment
	  Data collection
	  Data interpretation
		Knowledge of the world of nursing
		  Clinical experience
		  Literature review

Problem definition	Nursing diagnosis	Problem and purpose identification

Plan
  Goal setting
  Identifying solutions
	Plan
	  Goal setting
	  Planned interventions
		Methodology
		  Design
		  Sample
		  Methods of measurement

Implementation	Implementation	Data collection and analysis
Evaluation and revision of process	Evaluation and modification	Outcomes and dissemination of findings

Both processes involve abstract, critical thinking and complex reasoning that enable one to identify new information, discover relationships, and make predictions about phenomena. In these two processes, information is gathered, observations are made, problems are identified, plans are developed (methodology), and actions are taken (data collection and analysis) (Blumer, 1969; Whitney, 1986). Both processes are reviewed for effectiveness and efficiency—the nursing process is evaluated, and outcomes are determined in the research process (see Table 2–2). These processes are also iterative and spiraling, which means that implementing them expands and refines the user's knowledge. With this growth in knowledge, the user is able to implement increasingly complex nursing processes and studies.

The research and nursing processes also have definite differences in focus, purpose, and outcomes. The research process requires a broad understanding of nursing, use of a unique language, and rigorous application of a variety of scientific methods (Burns, 1989). The nursing process has a narrow focus, and its purpose is to organize and direct care for a particular patient and family. The purpose of research is to refine and generate knowledge that is shared with numerous nurses through presentations and publications.

The outcome of the nursing process is improved health for the patient and family. However, with the research process, the outcomes are focused on improved consumer health, delivery of quality care by health care providers, and implementation of a high-quality, cost-effective health care system. The knowledge developed through research has the potential to be used by practicing nurses to provide evidence-based care to numerous patients and families in a variety of health care systems. Knowledge development in nursing requires the conduct of many types of research methodologies.

NURSING RESEARCH METHODOLOGIES

Scientific method incorporates all procedures that scientists have used, currently use, or may use in the future to pursue knowledge (Kaplan, 1964). This definition eliminates the concept of "the" scientific method, or the belief that there is only one way to conduct research. This broad definition of scientific method includes quantitative and qualitative research and two relatively new methodologies used to generate knowledge for clinical practice: outcomes research and intervention research (Munhall, 1989; Rettig, 1991; Sidani & Braden, 1998; Silva, 1977; Tinkle & Beaton, 1983).

Introduction to Quantitative and Qualitative Research

Since 1930, many researchers have narrowly defined *scientific method* to comprise only quantitative research. This research method is based in the philosophy of logical empiricism or positivism (Norbeck, 1987; Scheffler, 1967). Therefore, scientific knowledge is generated through an application of logical principles and reasoning, whereby the researcher adopts a distant and noninteractive posture with the research subject to prevent bias (Newman, 1992; Silva & Rothbart, 1984).

Quantitative research is a formal, objective, systematic process in which numerical data are used to obtain information about the world. This research method is used to describe variables, examine relationships among variables, and determine cause-and-effect interactions between variables. Currently, the predominantly used method of scientific investigation in nursing is quantitative research. Some researchers believe that quantitative research provides a sounder knowledge base to guide nursing practice than qualitative research (Norbeck, 1987).

Qualitative research is a systematic, interactive, subjective approach used to describe life experiences and give them meaning (Leininger, 1985; Munhall & Boyd, 1999). Qualitative research is not a new idea in the social and behavioral sciences (Baumrind, 1980; Glaser & Strauss, 1967). However, nurses' interest in qualitative research is more recent, having begun in the late 1970s. This type of research is conducted to describe and promote understanding of human experiences such as pain, caring, and comfort. Because human emotions are difficult to quantify (assign a numerical value), qualitative research seems to be a more effective method than quantitative research for investigating these emotional responses. In addition, qualitative research focuses on discovery and understanding of the whole, an approach that is consistent with the holistic philosophy of nursing (Munhall & Boyd, 1999).

Comparison of Quantitative and Qualitative Research

Quantitative research and qualitative research complement each other because they generate different kinds of knowledge that are useful in nursing practice. The problem area to be studied determines the type of research to conduct, and the researcher's knowledge of both types of research promotes accurate selection of the methodology for the problem identified. Quantitative and qualitative research methodologies have some similarities, because both require researcher expertise, involve rigor in implementation, and result in the generation of scientific knowledge for nursing practice. Some of the differences between the two methodologies are presented in Table 2–3.

PHILOSOPHICAL ORIGIN OF QUANTITATIVE AND QUALITATIVE RESEARCH

Quantitative research is thought to produce a "hard" science that involves rigor, objectivity, and control. The quantitative approach to scientific inquiry emerged from a branch of philosophy called *logical positivism,* which operates on strict rules of logic, truth, laws, axioms, and predictions. Quantitative researchers hold the position that truth is absolute and that there is a single reality that one could define by careful measurement. To find truth, one must be completely objective, meaning that values, feelings, and personal perceptions cannot enter into the measurement of reality. Quantitative researchers believe that all human behavior is objective, purposeful, and measurable. The researcher needs only to find or develop the "right" instrument or tool to measure the behavior.

Today, however, many nurse researchers base their quantitative studies on more of a post-positivism philosophy (Clark, 1998). This philosophy evolved from positivism but focuses on the discovery of reality that is characterized by patterns and trends that can be used to describe, explain, and predict phenomena. With post-positivism philosophy, "truth can be discovered only imperfectly and in a probabilistic sense, in contrast to the positivist ideal of establishing cause-and-effect explanations of immutable facts" (Ford-Gilboe et al., 1995, p. 16). The post-positivism approach also rejects the idea of complete objectivity of the researcher toward what is to be discovered but continues to emphasize the need to control environmental influences (Newman, 1992).

Qualitative research is an interpretive methodological approach that is thought to produce more of

	TABLE 2–3	
	QUANTITATIVE AND QUALITATIVE RESEARCH CHARACTERISTICS	
Characteristic	**Quantitative Research**	**Qualitative Research**
Philosophical origin	Logical positivism	Naturalistic, interpretive, humanistic
Focus	Concise, objective, reductionistic	Broad, subjective, holistic
Reasoning	Logistic, deductive	Dialectic, inductive
Basis of knowing	Cause-and-effect relationships	Meaning, discovery, understanding
Theoretical focus	Tests theory	Develops theory
Researcher involvement	Control	Shared interpretation
Methods of measurement	Structured interviews, questionnaires, observations, scales, or physiological instruments	Unstructured interviews and observations
Data	Numbers	Words
Analysis	Statistical analysis	Individual interpretation
Findings	Generalization, accept or reject theoretical propositions	Uniqueness, dynamic, understanding of phenomena, and new theory

a "soft" science than quantitative research. Qualitative research evolved from the behavioral and social sciences as a method of understanding the unique, dynamic, holistic nature of human beings. The philosophical base of qualitative research is interpretive, humanistic, and naturalistic and is concerned with the understanding of the meaning of social interactions by those involved. Qualitative researchers believe that truth is both complex and dynamic and can be found only by studying persons as they interact with and within their sociohistorical settings (Munhall & Boyd, 1999).

FOCUS OF QUANTITATIVE AND QUALITATIVE RESEARCH

The focus or perspective for quantitative research is usually concise and reductionistic. Reductionism involves breaking the whole into parts so that the parts can be examined. Quantitative researchers remain detached from the study and try not to influence it with their values (objectivity). Researcher involvement in the study is thought to bias or sway the study toward the perceptions and values of the researcher, and biasing a study is considered poor scientific technique.

The focus of qualitative research is usually broad, and the intent of the research is to give meaning to the whole (holistic). The qualitative researcher has an active part in the study, and the findings from the study are influenced by the researcher's values and perceptions. Thus, this research approach is subjective, but the approach assumes that subjectivity is essential for the understanding of human experiences.

UNIQUENESS OF CONDUCTING QUANTITATIVE AND QUALITATIVE RESEARCH

Quantitative research is conducted to describe and examine relationships, and determine causality among variables. Thus, this method is useful in testing a theory by testing the validity of the relationships that compose the theory. Quantitative research incorporates logistic, deductive reasoning as the researcher examines particulars to make generalizations about the universe.

Qualitative research is conducted to generate knowledge concerned with meaning and discovery. Inductive and dialectic reasoning are predominant in these studies. For example, the qualitative researcher studies the whole person's response to pain; this is accomplished by examining premises about human pain and by determining the meaning that pain has for a particular person. Because qualitative research is concerned with meaning and understanding, the findings from these studies can be used to identify the relationships among the variables, and these relational statements are used in theory development.

Quantitative research requires control (see Table 2–3). The investigator uses control to identify and limit the problem to be researched and attempts to limit the effects of extraneous or outside variables that are not being studied. For example, one might study the effects of nutritional education on serum lipid levels (total serum cholesterol, low-density lipoprotein [LDL], and high-density lipoprotein [HDL]). The researcher would control the educational program by manipulating the type of education provided, the teaching methods, the length of the program, the setting for the program, and the instructor. Other extraneous variables, such as subject age, history of cardiovascular disease, and exercise level, would be controlled because they might affect the serum lipid levels. The intent of this control is to provide a more precise examination of the effects of nutritional education on serum lipid levels.

Quantitative research also requires the use of (1) structured interview, questionnaires, or observations; (2) scales; or (3) physiological instruments that generate numerical data. Statistical analyses are conducted to reduce and organize data, determine significant relationships, and identify differences among groups. Control, instruments, and statistical analyses are used to render the research findings an accurate reflection of reality, so the study findings can be generalized.

Generalization involves the application of trends or general tendencies (which are identified by studying a sample) to the population from which the research sample was drawn. For example, a controlled, quasi-experimental study has indicated that nutrition education was effective in lowering the total serum cholesterol and LDL levels and raising the HDL level in a selected sample of adult males. Therefore, the researcher generalizes that nutrition education is an effective treatment for positively changing the serum lipid values of "similar" adult males. Researchers must be cautious in making generalizations, because a sound generalization requires the support of many studies.

Qualitative researchers use unstructured observations and interviews to gather data. The data include the shared interpretations of the researcher and the subjects, and no attempts are made to control the interaction. For example, the researcher and subjects might share their experiences of powerlessness in the health care system. The data are subjective and incorporate the perceptions and beliefs of the researcher and the subjects (Munhall & Boyd, 1999).

Qualitative data take the form of words and are analyzed in terms of individual responses or descriptive summaries, or both. The researcher identifies categories for sorting and organizing the data (Miles & Huberman, 1994; Munhall & Boyd, 1999). The intent of the analysis is to organize the data into a meaningful, individualized interpretation, framework, or theory that describes the phenomenon studied. The findings from a qualitative study are unique to that study, and it is not the intent of the researcher to generalize the findings to a larger population. However, understanding the meaning of a phenomenon in a particular situation is useful for understanding similar phenomena in similar situations.

Use of Triangulation to Combine Quantitative and Qualitative Research Methodologies

Beginning in the mid-1980s, some nurse researchers discussed the use of triangulation to study the complex, dynamic human health phenomena relevant to nursing science (Duffy, 1987; Mitchell, 1986; Morse, 1991). The idea of triangulation is not new to social scientists and was first used by Campbell and Fiske in 1959 (Denzin, 1989). *Trian-*

gulation is the use of multiple methods, usually quantitative and qualitative research, in the study of the same research problem (Denzin, 1989). "When a single research method is inadequate, triangulation is used to ensure that the most comprehensive approach is taken to solve a research problem" (Morse, 1991, p. 120). The problem investigated is usually complex, like the human ability to cope with chronic illness, and requires in-depth study from a variety of perspectives to capture the reality.

Triangulation is a complex method that usually requires a research team of quantitative and qualitative researchers to maintain the integrity of both methodologies. The philosophical basis and assumptions for both quantitative and qualitative research must be maintained when these methodologies are combined, if the findings are to be meaningful (Dootson, 1995; Kimchi et al., 1991). The design of triangulation research is discussed in Chapter 10.

Types of Quantitative and Qualitative Research

Research methods can be classified in many different ways. The classification system for this textbook, presented in Table 2–4, includes both quantitative and qualitative research methodologies. The quantitative research methods are classified into four categories: (1) descriptive, (2) correlational, (3)

TABLE 2–4
CLASSIFICATION SYSTEM FOR NURSING RESEARCH METHODOLOGIES

Types of quantitative research:
    Descriptive research
    Correlational research
    Quasi-experimental research
    Experimental research
Types of qualitative research:
    Phenomenological research
    Grounded theory research
    Ethnographic research
    Historical research
    Philosophical inquiry:
        Foundational inquiry
        Philosophical analyses
        Ethical analyses
    Critical social theory methodology

quasi-experimental, and (4) experimental. These types of research are used to validate theories and knowledge; they are discussed briefly in this section and described in more detail in Chapter 3.

The qualitative research methods included in this textbook are (1) phenomenological research, (2) grounded theory research, (3) ethnographic research, (4) historical research, (5) philosophical inquiry, and (6) critical social theory. These approaches, all methodologies for discovering knowledge, are introduced in this section and described in depth in Chapters 4 and 23. Unit II of this textbook focuses on understanding the research process and includes discussions of both quantitative and qualitative research.

QUANTITATIVE RESEARCH METHODS

Descriptive Research

Descriptive research provides an accurate portrayal or account of characteristics of a particular individual, situation, or group (Selltiz et al., 1976). Descriptive studies are a way of (1) discovering new meaning, (2) describing what exists, (3) determining the frequency with which something occurs, and (4) categorizing information. Descriptive studies are usually conducted when little is known about a phenomenon.

In descriptive research, investigators often use interviews, unstructured observation, structured observations (observations guided by a checklist), and questionnaires to describe the phenomenon studied. Descriptive studies provide the knowledge base and potential hypotheses to direct the conduct of correlational, quasi-experimental, and experimental studies.

Correlational Research

Correlational research involves the systematic investigation of relationships between or among two or more variables that have been identified in theories or observed in practice, or both. If the relationships exist, the researcher determines the type (positive or negative) and the degree or strength of the relationships. The primary intent of correlational studies is to explain the nature of relationships, not to determine cause and effect. However, correlational studies are the means for generating hypothe-

ses to guide quasi-experimental and experimental studies that do focus on examining cause-and-effect interactions.

Quasi-Experimental Research

The purposes of *quasi-experimental research* are (1) to explain relationships, (2) to clarify why certain events happened, or (3) to examine causal relationships, or (4) a combination of these (Cook & Campbell, 1979). These studies are a basis for testing the effectiveness of nursing interventions that can then be implemented to control the outcomes in nursing practice.

Quasi-experimental studies are less powerful than experimental studies because they involve a lower level of control in at least one of three areas: (1) manipulation of the treatment variable, (2) manipulation of the setting, and (3) selection of subjects. When studying human behavior, especially in clinical areas, researchers are commonly unable to manipulate or control certain variables. Also, subjects are not randomly selected but are selected on the basis of convenience. Thus, nurse researchers conduct more quasi-experimental than experimental studies.

Experimental Research

Experimental research is an objective, systematic, controlled investigation for the purpose of predicting and controlling phenomena. The purpose of this type of research is to examine causality (Kerlinger, 1986). Experimental research is considered the most powerful quantitative method because of the rigorous control of variables. Experimental studies have three main characteristics: (1) a controlled manipulation of at least one treatment variable (independent variable), (2) administration of the treatment to some of the subjects in the study (experimental group) and not to others (control group), and (3) random selection of subjects or random assignment of subjects to groups, or both. Experimental studies usually have very controlled settings in laboratories or research units in clinical agencies.

QUALITATIVE RESEARCH METHODS

Phenomenological Research

Phenomenological research is a humanistic study of phenomena that is conducted in a variety of ways according to the philosophy of the researcher. The aim of phenomenology is the description of an experience as it is lived by the study participants and interpreted by the researcher. Thus, the researcher's experiences, reflections, and interpretations during the study constitute the data (Munhall & Boyd, 1999). The outcomes are based on the researcher's interpretations and perceptions of reality. Thus, phenomenologists agree that there is no single reality; each person has his or her own reality. Reality is considered subjective, and the experience is unique to the individual. Phenomenological research is an effective methodology to discover the meaning of a complex experience as it is lived by a person, such as the lived experience of health or dealing with chronic illness (Omery, 1983).

Grounded Theory Research

Grounded theory research is an inductive research method initially described by Glaser and Strauss (1967). This research approach is useful in discovering what problems exist in a social scene and the process persons use to handle them. Grounded theory methodology emphasizes observation and the development of practice-based intuitive relationships among variables.

Throughout the study, the researcher formulates, tests, and redevelops propositions until a theory evolves. The theory developed is "grounded," or has its roots in, the data from which it was derived (Simms, 1981). Grounded theory research can also be used to evaluate a patient situation, health care program, or health care delivery system. This qualitative approach to evaluation can take into account the people and their experiences in the situation as well as the situation (Hutchinson, 1999).

Ethnographic Research

Ethnographic research was developed by the discipline of anthropology for investigating cultures through an in-depth study of the members of the culture. This type of research attempts to tell the story of people's daily lives while describing the culture they are part of. The ethnographic research process is the systematic collection, description, and analysis of data to develop a theory of cultural behavior. The researcher (ethnographer) actually lives in or becomes a part of the cultural setting to gather the data. Through the use of ethnographic research, different cultures are described, compared, and contrasted to add to the understanding of the impact of culture on human behavior and health (Germain, 1999; Leininger, 1985).

Historical Research

Historical research is a narrative description or analysis of events that occurred in the remote or recent past. Data are obtained from records, artifacts, or verbal reports. Through historical research, nursing has a way of understanding itself and interpreting the discipline and its contributions to others. The mistakes of the past can be examined to facilitate an understanding of and an effective response to present situations affecting nurses and nursing practice. In addition, historical research has the potential to provide a foundation for and to direct the future movements of the profession (Fitzpatrick, 1999). A limited amount of historical research has been conducted in nursing, with the majority of the studies focusing on past and current nursing leaders (Newton, 1965).

Philosophical Inquiry

Philosophical inquiry involves using intellectual analyses to (1) clarify meanings, (2) make values manifest, (3) identify ethics, and (4) study the nature of knowledge (Ellis, 1983). The philosophical researcher considers an idea or issue from all perspectives by extensively exploring the literature, examining conceptual meaning, raising questions, proposing answers, and suggesting the implications of those answers. The research is guided by philosophical questions that have been posed.

There are three categories of philosophical inquiry covered in this textbook: foundational inquiry, philosophical analyses, and ethical inquiry. *Foundational inquiries* involve the analyses of the structure of a science and the process of thinking about and valuing certain phenomena held in common by members of a scientific discipline. The purposes of *philosophical analyses* are to examine meaning and develop theories of meaning through concept analysis or linguistic analysis (Rodgers, 1989). *Ethical inquiry,* another type of philosophical inquiry, involves intellectual analysis of problems of ethics related to obligation, rights, duty, right and wrong, conscience, justice, choice, intention, and responsibility. Ethical inquiry is a means of striving for rational ends when other people are involved.

Critical Social Theory

Critical social theory provides the basis for research that focuses on understanding how people communicate and how they develop symbolic meanings in a society. Many of the meanings occur in a world where certain facts of the society are taken for granted, rather than being discussed or disputed. The established political, social, and cultural orders are perceived as closed to change and are not questioned.

The researcher attempts to "uncover the distortions and constraints that impede free, equal, and uncoerced participation in society" (Stevens, 1989, p. 58). Through research, power imbalances are exposed, and people are empowered to make changes (Newman, 1992). Empowerment involves (1) recognizing the contradictions in a situation, (2) reflecting on the reality of the situation, (3) moving to a state of action, and (4) making changes in the situation to correct the contradictions or imbalances. Critical social theory provides a philosophical basis for multiple research methods to generate knowledge that might promote empowerment and political change (Ford-Gilbe et al., 1995). Thus, critical social scientists might use both quantitative and qualitative research or a combination of the two, triangulation, because the knowledge generated can be the most persuasive to policymakers and the public.

Critical nursing science provides a framework from which one may examine how social, political, economic, gender, and cultural factors interact to influence health or illness experiences (Ford-Gilbe et al., 1995). Nurses need to be aware of constraints and power imbalances in society that affect areas such as access to care, care of the chronically ill, and pain management of the terminally ill. The patients' and families' health needs and the health care system developed to meet these needs are continuously influenced by the social system that surrounds them.

Outcomes Research

The spiraling cost of health care has generated many questions about the quality and effectiveness of health care services and the patient outcomes related to these services. Consumers want to know what services they are buying and whether these services will improve their health. Health care policymakers want to know whether the care is cost-effective and high quality. These concerns have promoted the development of outcomes research. An outcome is the end-result of care or a measure of the change in health status of the patient (Higgins et al., 1992; Jones, 1993; Rettig, 1991).

In the past, outcome measures have been negative, such as mortality, morbidity (iatrogenic complications), length of stay, infection rate, unscheduled readmission, unscheduled second surgery, and unnecessary hospital procedures. These outcomes are only short term and intermediate results of care and are focused primarily on hospital services (Johnson, 1993; Jones, 1993). In the future, outcomes research must include determination of short-term and long-term end-results of care as well as examination of negative and positive results of care throughout a variety of settings, such as hospitals, rehabilitation centers, clinics, and homes. Some of the positive patient outcomes are better quality of life, improved health status, increased functional status, improved mobility, patient satisfaction, and return to work or normal activities (Chinn & Kramer, 1999).

Jones identified four areas that require examination through outcomes research:

- Clinical patient response to medical and nursing interventions
- Functional maintenance or improvement of physical functioning
- Financial outcomes achieved with most efficient use of resources
- Perceptual patient's satisfaction with outcomes, care received, and providers (Jones, 1993, p. 146)

Nurses need to take an active role in the conduct of outcomes research and to participate in the multidisciplinary teams that are examining the outcomes of health care services. The conduct of quality outcomes research can influence (1) patient health status, (2) the delivery of practitioners' services, (3) the use of limited resources, (4) the development of public policy, and (5) purchaser demand (Davies et al., 1994). Key ideas related to outcomes research are addressed throughout the text, and Chapter 12 contains a detailed discussion of this methodology.

Intervention Research

An important methodology for refining and generating nursing knowledge in the 21st century will be intervention research. *Intervention research* involves the investigation of the effectiveness of a nursing intervention in achieving the desired outcome or outcomes in a natural setting. "Interventions are defined as treatments, therapies, procedures, or actions implemented by health professionals to and with clients, in a particular situation, to move the clients' condition toward desired health outcomes that are beneficial to the clients" (Sidani & Braden, 1998, p. 8). An intervention can be a specific treatment implemented to manage a well-defined patient problem or a program. A program intervention, such as a cardiac rehabilitation program, consists of multiple nursing actions that are implemented as a package to improve the health conditions of those participating in the program.

Intervention research is to be theory driven, which means that the theory determines (1) the nature of the intervention, (2) the health professionals to deliver the intervention, (3) the setting where the intervention is to be provided, (4) the type of patient to receive the intervention, and (5) the selection and measurement of the outcome variables. This type of research provides a methodology for determining how, when, and for whom an intervention works. Such knowledge is essential for generalizing the findings about the intervention, improving or refining the intervention, and using the intervention in practice.

The goal of intervention research is to generate sound scientific knowledge for nursing actions that can be used by nurses to provide evidence-based nursing care. The details of intervention research are discussed in Chapter 13.

■ SUMMARY

The focus of this chapter is the evolution of research in nursing. Reviewing the history of research in nursing enables one to better understand the cur-

rent status and project the future of nursing research. Historical events also provide a basis for the methods of scientific inquiry that are used in developing the empirical or research knowledge base for the discipline. Some people think that research is relatively new to nursing, but Florence Nightingale initiated nursing research more than 140 years ago. Nightingale's research enabled her to instigate attitudinal, organizational, and social changes. However, after her work, little research was conducted in nursing until the 1950s.

During the 1950s and 1960s, research became a higher priority, with the support of nursing leaders, development of graduate programs in nursing, and growing numbers of nurses with doctorates and masters' degrees. The number of research conferences held at the local and national levels increased, and the first research journal, *Nursing Research,* was published. The studies conducted during these two decades focused on topics such as nursing education, standards for nursing practice, nurses' characteristics, staffing patterns, and quality of care.

Research activities advanced extensively during the 1970s and 1980s. The major focus was on the conduct of clinical research to improve nursing practice. Several new research journals were initiated, numerous research conferences were held, and the educational level and research background of nurses were drastically improved. The National Center for Nursing Research (NCNR) was created in 1985 after years of work and two presidential vetoes. The purpose of NCNR was to support the conduct of basic and clinical nursing research and the dissemination of findings. Under the direction of Dr. Hinshaw, the NCNR became the National Institute of Nursing Research (NINR) in 1993. This change in title increased the recognition of nursing as a research discipline and expanded the funding for nursing research.

Outcomes research emerged as an important methodology for documenting the effectiveness of health care service in the 1980s and 1990s. In 1989, the Agency for Health Care Policy and Research (AHCPR) was established to facilitate the conduct of outcomes research (Rettig, 1991). AHCPR also had an active role in communicating research findings to health care practitioners and was responsible for publishing the first clinical practice guidelines in

1989. The AHCPR became the Agency for Healthcare Research and Quality (AHRQ) in 1999 and was designated as a scientific partner with the public and private sector to improve the quality and safety of patient care.

The vision for nursing in the 21st century is the development of a scientific knowledge base that enables nurses to implement an evidence-based practice (EBP). NINR is seeking expanded funding for nursing research and is encouraging a variety of methodologies (quantitative, qualitative, outcomes research, and intervention research) to be used to generate essential knowledge for nursing practice. To ensure an effective research enterprise in nursing, the discipline must: (1) create a research culture, (2) provide quality educational programs (baccalaureate, masters, doctoral, and postdoctoral) to prepare a work force of nurse scientists, (3) develop a sound research infrastructure, and (4) obtain sufficient funding for essential research (AACN, 1999).

Research is a process and is similar in some ways to other processes. Therefore, the background acquired early in nursing education in problem solving and the nursing process is also useful in research. A comparison of the problem-solving process, nursing process, and research process shows the similarities and differences in these processes and provides a basis for understanding the research process.

Scientific method comprises all procedures that scientists have used, currently use, or may use in the future to pursue knowledge. Nursing research incorporates both quantitative and qualitative research and two new methodologies: outcomes research and intervention research. Quantitative research is an objective, systematic process of using numerical data to obtain information about the world. This research method is used to describe, examine relationships, and determine cause-and-effect interactions. Qualitative research is a systematic, subjective approach used to describe life experiences and give them meaning. Knowledge generated from qualitative research provides meaning and understanding of (1) the specific, not the general, (2) values, and (3) life experiences.

Quantitative research and qualitative research complement each other, because they generate different kinds of knowledge that are useful in nursing practice. A comparison of quantitative and qualitative research methods is presented to clarify the similarities and differences of these two methods. Some researchers advocate combining quantitative and qualitative research methods in studying certain nursing problems. Combining research methods, called *triangulation,* is used to ensure that the most comprehensive approach is taken to solve a research problem. If the findings from triangulation research are to be meaningful, the philosophical basis and assumptions for both quantitative research and qualitative research must be maintained when these methodologies are combined.

Research methods can be classified in many different ways. In this textbook, three methodologies are identified: quantitative research, qualitative research, and outcomes research. Quantitative research is classified into four types: descriptive, correlational, quasi-experimental, and experimental. Six types of qualitative research are included in this text: phenomenological research, grounded theory research, ethnographic research, historical research, philosophic inquiry, and critical social theory.

The spiraling cost of health care has generated many questions about the quality and effectiveness of health care services and the patient outcomes related to these services. These concerns have promoted the development of outcomes research. Outcomes are the end-results of care or a measure of the change in health status of the patient. The conduct of quality outcomes research can influence (1) patient health status, (2) the delivery of practitioners' services, (3) the use of limited resources, (4) the development of public policy, and (5) purchaser demand.

Another important methodology for refining and generating nursing knowledge in the 21st century is intervention research. Intervention research involves the investigation of the effectiveness of a nursing intervention in achieving the desired outcomes in a natural setting. Intervention research provides a methodology for determining how, when, and for whom an intervention works. The goal of intervention research is to generate sound scientific knowledge for nursing actions that can be used by nurses to provide evidence-based nursing care.

REFERENCES

Abdellah, F. G. (1972). Evolution of nursing as a profession. *International Nursing Review, 19*(3), 219–235.

American Association of Colleges of Nursing. (1999). Position statement on nursing research. *Journal of Professional Nursing, 15*(4), 253–257.

American Nurses Association. (1950). Twenty thousand nurses tell their story. Kansas City, MO: Author.

American Nurses Association. (1989). *Education for participation in nursing research.* Kansas City, MO: Author.

Bauknecht, V. L. (1986). Congress overrides veto, nursing gets center for research. *American Nurse, 18*(1), 24.

Baumrind, D. (1980). New directions in socialization research. *American Psychologist, 35*(7), 639–652.

Blumer, H. (1969). *Symbolic interactionism: Perspective and method.* Englewood Cliffs, NJ: Prentice-Hall, Inc.

Brown, S. A., & Grimes, D. E. (1995). A meta-analysis of nurse practitioners and nurse midwives in primary care. *Nursing Research, 44*(5), 332–339.

Brown, S. J. (1999). *Knowledge for healthcare practice: A guide to using research evidence.* Philadelphia: W. B. Saunders.

Burns, N. (1989). The research process and the nursing process: Distinctly different. *Nursing Science Quarterly, 2*(4), 157–158.

Carlson-Catalano, J., & Lunney, M. (1995). Quantitative methods for clinical validation of nursing diagnoses. *Clinical Nurse Specialist, 9*(6), 306–311.

Chinn, P. L., & Kramer, M. K. (1999). *Theory and nursing: A systematic approach* (5th ed.). St. Louis: Mosby.

Clark, A. M. (1998). The qualitative-quantitative debate: Moving from positivism and confrontation to post-positivism and reconciliation. *Journal of Advanced Nursing, 27*(6), 1242–1249.

Cook, Sir E. (1913). *The life of Florence Nightingale* (Vol. 1). London: Macmillan.

Cook, T. D., & Campbell, D. T. (1979). *Quasi-experimentation: Design and analysis issues for field settings.* Chicago: Rand McNally.

Davies, A. R., Doyle, M. A. T., Lansky, D., Rutt, W., Stevic, M. O., & Doyle, J. B. (1994). Outcomes assessment in clinical settings: A consensus statement on principles and best practices in project management. *The Joint Commission Journal of Quality Improvement, 20*(1), 6–16.

Denzin, N. K. (1989). *The research act* (3rd ed.). New York: McGraw-Hill.

de Tornyay, R. (1977). Nursing research—the road ahead. *Nursing Research, 26*(6), 404–407.

Dootson, S. (1995). An in-depth study of triangulation. *Journal of Advanced Nursing, 22*(1), 183–187.

Downs, F. S., & Fleming, W. J. (1979). *Issues in nursing research.* New York: Appleton-Century-Crofts.

Duffy, M. E. (1987). Methodological triangulation: A vehicle for merging quantitative and qualitative research methods. *Image—Journal of Nursing Scholarship, 19*(3), 130–133.

Ellis, R. (1983). Philosophic inquiry. In H. H. Werley & J. J. Fitzpatrick (Eds.), *Annual review of nursing research* (Vol. 1, pp. 211–228). New York: Springer.

Fitzpatrick, M. L. (1978). *Historical studies in nursing.* New York: Teachers College Press.

Fitzpatrick, M. L. (1999). Historical research: The method. In P. L. Munhall & C. O. Boyd (Eds.), *Nursing research: A qualitative perspective* (pp. 359–371). New York: National League for Nursing.

Ford-Gilboe, M., Campbell, J., & Berman, H. (1995). Stories and numbers: Coexistence without compromise. *Advances in Nursing Science, 18*(1), 14–26.

Germain, C. P. (1999). Ethnography: The method. In P. L. Munhall & C. O. Boyd (Eds.), *Nursing research: A qualitative perspective* (pp. 237–268). New York: National League for Nursing.

Glaser, B. G., & Strauss, A. L. (1967). *The discovery of grounded theory: Strategies for qualitative research.* Chicago: Aldine.

Gortner, S. R., & Nahm, H. (1977). An overview of nursing research in the United States. *Nursing Research, 26*(1), 10–33.

Herbert, R. G. (1981). *Florence Nightingale: Saint, reformer or rebel?* Malabar, FL: Robert E. Krieger.

Higgins, M., McCaughan, D., Griffiths, M., & Carr-Hill, R. (1992). Assessing the outcomes of nursing care. *Journal of Advanced Nursing, 17*(5), 561–568.

Horsley, J. A., Crane, J., Crabtree, M. K., & Wood, D. J. (1983). *Using research to improve nursing practice: A guide; CURN Project.* New York: Grune & Stratton.

Hutchinson, S. A. (1999). Grounded theory: The method. In P. L. Munhall & C. O. Boyd (Eds.), *Nursing research: A qualitative perspective* (pp. 180–212). New York: National League for Nursing.

Jacox, A. (1980). Strategies to promote nursing research. *Nursing Research, 29*(4), 213–218.

Johnson, J. E. (1993). Outcomes research and health care reform: Opportunities for nurses. *Nursing Connections, 6*(4), 1–3.

Johnson, W. L. (1977). Research programs of the National League for Nursing. *Nursing Research, 26*(3), 172–176.

Jones, K. R. (1993). Outcomes analysis: Methods and issues. *Nursing Economics, 11*(3), 145–152.

Kaplan, A. (1964). *The conduct of inquiry: Methodology for behavioral science.* New York: Chandler.

Kerlinger, F. N. (1986). *Foundations of behavioral research* (3rd ed.). New York: Holt, Rinehart, & Winston.

Kimchi, J., Polivka, B., & Stevenson, J. S. (1991). Triangulation: Operational definitions. *Nursing Research, 40*(6), 364–366.

Larson, E. (1984). Health policy and NIH: Implications for nursing research. *Nursing Research, 33*(6), 352–356.

Leininger, M. M. (1985). *Qualitative research methods in nursing.* Orlando, FL: Grune & Stratton.

Miles, M. B., & Huberman, A. M. (1994). *Qualitative data analysis: A sourcebook of new methods* (2nd ed.). Beverly Hills, CA: Sage Publications.

Mitchell, E. S. (1986). Multiple triangulation: A methodology for nursing science. *Advances in Nursing Science, 8*(3), 18–26.

Morse, J. M. (1991). Approaches to qualitative-quantitative methodological triangulation. *Nursing Research, 40*(1), 120–123.

Munhall, P. L. (1989). Philosophical ponderings on qualitative research methods in nursing. *Nursing Science Quarterly, 2*(1), 20–28.

Munhall, P. L., & Boyd, C. O. (1999). *Nursing research: A qualitative perspective* (2nd ed.). Norwalk, CT: Appleton-Century-Crofts.

Newman, M. A. (1992). Prevailing paradigms in nursing. *Nursing Outlook, 40*(1), 10–13, 32.

Newton, M. E. (1965). The case for historical research. *Nursing Research, 14*(1), 20–26.

Nightingale, F. (1859). *Notes on nursing: What it is, and what it is not.* Philadelphia: J. B. Lippincott.

Norbeck, J. S. (1987). In defense of empiricism. *Image—Journal of Nursing Scholarship, 19*(1), 28–30.

Omery, A. (1983). Phenomenology: A method for nursing research. *Advances in Nursing Science, 5*(2), 49–63.

Omery, A., & Williams, R. P. (1999). An appraisal of research utilization across the United States. *Journal of Nursing Administration, 29*(12), 50–56.

Palmer, I. S. (1977). Florence Nightingale: Reformer, reactionary, researcher. *Nursing Research, 26*(2), 84–89.

Rettig, R. (1991). History, development, and importance to nursing of outcomes research. *Journal of Nursing Quality Assurance, 5*(2), 13–17.

Rodgers, B. L. (1989). Concepts, analysis and the development of nursing knowledge: The evolutionary cycle. *Journal of Advanced Nursing, 14*(4), 330–335.

Scheffler, I. (1967). *Science and subjectivity.* Indianapolis, IN: Bobbs-Merrill.

See, E. M. (1977). The ANA and research in nursing. *Nursing Research, 26*(3), 165–171.

Selltiz, C., Wrightsman, L. S., & Cook, S. W. (1976). *Research methods in social relations* (3rd ed.). New York: Holt, Rinehart, & Winston.

Sidani, S., & Braden, C. P. (1998). *Evaluating nursing interventions: A theory-driven approach.* Thousand Oaks, CA: Sage Publications.

Silva, M. C. (1977). Philosophy, science, theory: Interrelationships and implications for nursing research. *Image—Journal of Nursing Scholarship, 9*(3), 59–63.

Silva, M. C., & Rothbart, D. (1984). An analysis of changing trends in philosophies of science on nursing theory development and testing. *Advances in Nursing Science, 6*(2), 1–13.

Simms, L. M. (1981). The grounded theory approach in nursing research. *Nursing Research, 30*(6), 356–359.

Stevens, P. E. (1989). A critical social reconceptualization of environment in nursing: Implications for methodology. *Advances in Nursing Science, 11*(4), 56–68.

Tinkle, M. B., & Beaton, J. L. (1983). Toward a new view of science: Implications for nursing research. *Advances in Nursing Science, 5*(2), 27–36.

U.S. Department of Health and Human Services. (1992). Healthy people 2000. Washington, D.C.: Author.

Werley, H. H. (1977). Nursing research in perspective. *International Nursing Review, 24*(3), 75–83.

Werley, H. H., & Fitzpatrick, J. J. (Eds.) (1983). *Annual review of nursing research* (Vol. 1). New York: Springer.

Whitney, F. W. (1986). Turning clinical problems into research. *Heart & Lung, 15*(1), 57–59.

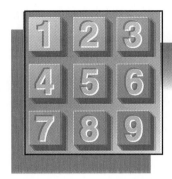

CHAPTER 3

INTRODUCTION TO QUANTITATIVE RESEARCH

What do you think of when you hear the word *research?* Frequently, the word *experiment* comes to mind. One might equate experiments with randomizing subjects into groups, collecting data, and conducting statistical analyses. Many people believe that an experiment is conducted to "prove" something, such as that one pain medicine is more effective than another. These common notions are associated with the classic experimental design originated by Sir Ronald Fisher (1935). Fisher is noted for adding structure to the steps of the research process with ideas such as the null hypothesis, research design, and statistical analysis.

Fisher's experimentation provided the groundwork for what is now known as experimental research. Throughout the years, a number of other quantitative approaches have been developed. Campbell and Stanley (1963) developed quasi-experimental approaches. Karl Pearson developed statistical approaches for examining relationships among variables, which increased the conduct of correlational research. The fields of sociology, education, and psychology are noted for their development and expansion of strategies for conducting descriptive research. The steps of the research process used in these different types of quantitative studies are the same, but the philosophy and strategies for implementing these steps vary with the approach.

A broad range of quantitative research approaches is needed to develop nursing's body of knowledge and provide evidence-based nursing care. Thus, quantitative research is a major focus throughout this textbook. This chapter provides an overview of quantitative research by (1) discussing concepts relevant to quantitative research, (2) identifying the steps of the quantitative research process, and (3) providing examples of different types of quantitative studies.

CONCEPTS RELEVANT TO QUANTITATIVE RESEARCH

Some concepts relevant to quantitative research are basic and applied research, rigor, and control. These concepts are defined and major points are reinforced with examples from quantitative studies.

Basic Research

Basic, or pure, *research* is a scientific investigation that involves the pursuit of "knowledge for knowledge's sake," or for the pleasure of learning and finding truth (Nagel, 1961). The purpose of basic research is to generate and refine theory and build constructs; thus, frequently the findings are not directly useful in practice. However, because the findings are abstract (theoretical in nature), they can be generalized to various settings (Wysocki, 1983).

Basic research is also conducted to examine the underlying mechanisms of actions of an intervention (Wallenstein, 1987). For example, what mediates the onset of cachexia-anorexia syndrome with tumor growth? Are the anorexigenic effects of interleukin-1 mediated in part by prostaglandins (PGs)? If so, would inhibitors of PG synthesis improve food intake and body weight in tumor-bearing rats? McCarthy (1999, p. 380) conducted basic research "to determine if administration of ibuprofen (ibu) or indomethacin (indo), which inhibit PG synthesis, would affect the food intake and body weight of tumor-bearing rats." The researcher found that ibu and indo failed to improve food intake in tumor-bearing rats. Thus, PG synthesis does not seem to play a major role in the onset of weight loss and anorexia in rats. However, a 20% reduction in the mass of the rats' tumors was noted with the administration of ibu. Thus, McCarthy (1999) recommended the conduct of additional basic research to determine the effects of PG inhibitors, such as ibu and indo, on the kinetics of tumor growth. This finding is consistent with other studies that identified 35%, 40%, and 50% reductions in rat tumor size with the use of PG inhibitors.

Basic research usually precedes or provides the basis for applied research. Thus, this example of basic research provides a basis for the conduct of applied studies to examine the effects of selected PG inhibitors on tumor growth in patients with cancer and the use of PG inhibitors in the prevention of cancer in humans.

Applied Research

Applied, or practical, *research* is a scientific investigation conducted to generate knowledge that will directly influence or improve clinical practice. The purpose of applied research is to solve problems, to make decisions, or to predict or control outcomes in real-life practice situations (Abdellah & Levine, 1994). Because applied research focuses on specific problems, the findings are less generalizable than those from basic research. Applied research is also used to test theory and validate its usefulness in clinical practice. Often, the new knowledge discovered through basic research is examined for usefulness in practice by applied research, making these approaches complementary (Bond & Heitkemper, 1987; Wallenstein, 1987).

Johnson and colleagues (2000) conducted an applied study to determine the effectiveness of a program to prevent smoking relapse on the outcomes of continuous smoking abstinence, daily smoking, and smoking cessation self-efficacy in postpartum women. The sample consisted of 254 women who had quit smoking during pregnancy, and they were randomly assigned to a treatment or control group. The treatment group received face-to-face, in-hospital counseling sessions at the births of their babies, followed by telephone counseling after discharge. At 6 months, the rate of continuous smoking abstinence was significantly higher in the treatment group (38%) than in the control group (27%). "Significantly more control (48%) than treatment (34%) group participants reported smoking daily. . . . The smoking cessation self-efficacy did not vary significantly between the two groups" (Johnson et al., 2000, p. 44). The implications for practice include the importance of providing a program to prevent smoking relapse in new mothers. Continuous smoking abstinence of postpartum women has major health implications for both mothers and children.

Many nurse researchers have chosen to conduct applied studies to produce findings that directly affect clinical practice. Commonly conducted applied studies focus on developing and testing the effectiveness of nursing interventions in the treatment of patient and family health problems. In addition, most federal funding has been granted for applied research. However, additional basic research is needed to expand the understanding of several physiological and pathophysiological variables, such as oxygenation, perfusion, fluid and electrolyte imbalance, acid-base status, eating patterns, and sleep disturbance (Bond & Heitkemper, 1987). Because the future of any profession rests on its research base, both basic research and applied research are needed to develop nursing knowledge.

Rigor in Quantitative Research

Rigor is the striving for excellence in research and involves discipline, scrupulous adherence to detail, and strict accuracy. A rigorous quantitative researcher constantly strives for more precise measurement methods, representative samples, and tightly controlled study designs. Characteristics valued in these researchers include (1) critical examination of reasoning and (2) attention to precision.

Logistic reasoning and deductive reasoning are essential to the development of quantitative research. The research process consists of specific steps that are developed with meticulous detail and logically linked together. These steps are critically examined and reexamined for errors and weaknesses in areas such as design, treatment implementation, measurement, sampling, statistical analysis, and generalization. Reducing these errors and weaknesses is essential to ensure that the research findings are an accurate reflection of reality.

Another aspect of rigor is precision, which encompasses accuracy, detail, and order. Precision is evident in the concise statement of the research purpose, detailed development of the study design, and the formulation of explicit treatment protocols. The most explicit use of precision, however, is evident in the measurement of the study variables. Measurement involves objectively experiencing the real world through the senses: sight, hearing, touch, taste, and smell. The researcher continually searches for new and more precise ways to measure elements and events of the world.

Control in Quantitative Research

Control involves the imposing of "rules" by the researcher to decrease the possibility of error and thus increase the probability that the study's findings are an accurate reflection of reality. The rules used to achieve control are referred to as *design.* Through control, the researcher can reduce the influence or confounding effect of extraneous variables on the research variables. For example, if a study focused on the effect of relaxation therapy on the perception of incisional pain, the extraneous variables, such as type of surgical incision and the timing, amount, and type of pain medicine administered after surgery, would have to be controlled to prevent their influencing the patient's perception of pain.

Controlling extraneous variables enables the researcher to identify relationships among the study variables accurately and examine the effects of one variable on another. Extraneous variables can be controlled by randomly selecting a certain type of subject, such as individuals who have never been hospitalized before or those with a certain medical diagnosis. The selection of subjects is controlled with sample criteria and sampling method. The setting can also be changed to control extraneous variables such as temperature, noise, and interactions with other people. The data collection process can be sequenced to control extraneous variables such as fatigue and discomfort.

Quantitative research requires varying degrees of control, ranging from uncontrolled to highly controlled, depending on the type of study (see Table 3–1). Descriptive studies are usually conducted without researcher control, because subjects are examined as they exist in their natural setting, such as home, work, or school. Experimental studies are highly controlled and often conducted on animals in laboratory settings to determine the underlying mechanisms for and effectiveness of a treatment. Some common areas in which control might be enhanced in quantitative research are (1) selection of subjects (sampling), (2) selection of the research setting, (3) development and implementation of a treatment, and (4) subjects' knowledge of the study.

SAMPLING

Sampling is a process of selecting subjects who are representative of the population being studied. In quantitative research, both random and nonrandom sampling methods are used to obtain study samples. Random sampling methods usually provide a sample that is representative of a population, be-

TABLE 3–1
CONTROL IN QUANTITATIVE RESEARCH

Type of Research	Researcher Control	Research Setting
Descriptive	Uncontrolled	Natural or partially controlled
Correlational	Uncontrolled or partially controlled	Natural or partially controlled
Quasi-experimental	Partially controlled or highly controlled	Partially controlled
Experimental	Highly controlled	Highly controlled, laboratory

cause each member of the population has a probability greater than zero of being selected for a study. Thus, random or probability sampling methods require greater researcher control and rigor than nonrandom or nonprobability sampling methods.

The research problem and purpose, the study design, and the number and type of subjects needed all affect the selection of a sampling method. Many studies in nursing have patients of different types as subjects in their study. Often, a nonprobability sampling method is used to obtain study subjects (frequently patients) to ensure the largest sample size that it is economically possible to obtain in a reasonable period. The concepts of sampling theory, such as population, representative sample, and sampling methods, are presented in Chapter 14.

RESEARCH SETTINGS

There are three common settings for conducting research: natural, partially controlled, and highly controlled (see Table 3–1). *Natural settings,* or field settings, are uncontrolled, real-life situations (Abdellah & Levine, 1994). Conducting a study in a natural setting means that the researcher does not manipulate or change the environment for the study. For example, the previously described study by Johnson and colleagues (2000) to test a program to prevent smoking relapse in postpartum women was conducted in the natural settings of hospital and home. The initial collection of baseline data and the implementation of the intervention of counseling were performed in the women's rooms in the hospital. A follow-up intervention of counseling was performed by telephone calls to the women's homes, and a final interview for data collection also was conducted in the home setting. These are considered natural settings, because there was no manipulation of the setting during the conduct of the study.

A *partially controlled setting* is an environment that is manipulated or modified in some way by the researcher. An increasing number of nursing studies are being conducted in partially controlled settings. Younger and associates (1995, p. 294) studied the "relationships among participation in outpatient rehabilitation, health locus of control, and mastery of stress with coronary artery disease." This was a two-phase study; Phase I took place in the hospital and Phase II in the rehabilitation center. Within the hospital, the researchers controlled the assessment of patient and family needs, provided appropriate teaching, and enrolled the patients in the rehabilitation program. However, the researchers did not control other aspects of the hospital environment, such as family support and different types of nursing care on the hospital units, which might have influenced the research variables, patients' decisions to participate in rehabilitation, health locus of control, and mastery of stress. In Phase II of the study, the participants were enrolled in a rehabilitation program that involved attending a 60-minute session 3 days a week in a rehabilitation center. The content and activities of these sessions were controlled, but no attempt was made to control the interactions of the participants as they exercised together, which could have influenced the research variables.

Highly controlled settings are artificially constructed environments that are developed for the sole purpose of conducting research. Laboratories, research or experimental centers, and test units are highly controlled settings for conducting research. This type of setting reduces the influence of extraneous and environmental variables, enabling the researcher to examine the effect of the independent variable on the dependent variable accurately. Only a limited number of nursing studies are conducted in highly controlled settings; most are conducted in natural settings.

The previously described study by McCarthy (1999), to determine whether inhibitors of prostaglandin synthesis would improve food intake or body weight in tumor-bearing rats, was conducted in a laboratory setting and used animals. McCarthy (1999) implemented precise control of (1) the selection of animals, (2) maintenance of their environment and nutrition, (3) implementation of the treatment, and (4) measurement of the dependent variables, as shown by the following description.

. . . .

"Male Buffalo rats (Harlan Sprague-Dawley, Houston, TX) weighing between 125 and 150 grams (at 6 weeks old) were maintained on 12-hour light-dark cycle, with lights off from 6 PM to 6 AM. They were housed individually with ad libitum access to food and water. The animals were fed a pulverized rat chow, and food intake was determined by weighing the dishes each morning. . . . A 1-mm tumor fragment was implanted between the scapulae with a trocar needle. . . . The area between the scapulae was palpated daily for growth of the implemented tumor fragment. Once it was palpable, the tumor was measured in mm at its longest axis and perpendicular to the axis using calipers. . . . The rats were weighed each morning and the tumor weight was subtracted to determine body weight. Animals were euthanized by intraperitoneal injection of an overdose (100 mg/kg) of pentobarbital." (McCarthy, 1999, p. 381) ▪

DEVELOPMENT AND IMPLEMENTATION OF STUDY INTERVENTIONS

Quasi-experimental and experimental studies are conducted to examine the effect of an independent variable or intervention on a dependent variable or outcome. More intervention studies are being conducted in nursing to establish an evidence-based practice. Controlling the development and implementation of a study intervention increases the validity of the study design and the credibility of the findings. A study intervention needs to be (1) clearly and precisely developed, (2) consistently implemented with protocol, and (3) examined for effectiveness through quality measurement of the dependent variables (Egan et al., 1992; Sidani & Braden, 1998). The development and implementation of intervention research is the focus of Chapter 13. Johnson and colleagues (2000) provided the following detailed description of the intervention in their study on preventing smoking relapse in postpartum women.

· ·

"A postpartum counseling intervention was designed to prevent or interrupt the relapse process by teaching skills to deal with high-risk situations and cognitive restructuring techniques to deal with lapses. The intervention was based on the following principles derived from Marlatt's Relapse model (Marlatt, 1985). . . .

"Nurses were hired and trained to provide the

one-to-one counseling intervention. The in-hospital component consisted of sharing information and beginning skill building. The nurse began by learning about the woman's smoking experiences and the context of the smoking cessation effort. . . . The skill-building component focused on teaching the woman to recognize high-risk situations in which she may be tempted to smoke, and to problem solve about how to manage those situations. . . . The counseling was augmented with materials developed for the study and tailored to the particular circumstances of postpartum women. . . .

"Eight subsequent at-home telephone counseling sessions were provided by the nurse who initially enrolled the participant. These sessions focused on efforts to maintain smoking cessation, review of high-risk situations and their management, possible lapses, guidance in problem solving, and support and encouragement. The telephone sessions were held weekly during the first month postpartum and biweekly during the second and third months." (Johnson et al., 2000, p. 47) ▪

SUBJECTS' KNOWLEDGE OF A STUDY

Subjects' knowledge of a study could influence their behavior and possibly alter the outcome. This creates a threat to the validity or accuracy of the study design.

An example of this type of threat to design validity is the *Hawthorne effect*, which was identified during the classic experiments at the Hawthorne plant of the Western Electric Company during the late 1920s and early 1930s. The employees at this plant exhibited a particular psychological response when they became research subjects: They changed their behavior simply because they were subjects in a study, not because of the research treatment. In these studies, the researcher manipulated the working conditions (altered the lighting, decreased work hours, changed payment, and increased rest periods) to examine the effects on worker productivity (Homans, 1965). The subjects in both the treatment group (whose work conditions were changed) and the control group (whose work conditions were not changed) increased their productivity. Even those subjects in a group for whom lighting was decreased showed an increase in productivity. The subjects seemed to change their behaviors (increase their productivity) just because they were part of a study.

There are several ways to strengthen a study design by decreasing the threats to design validity. They are addressed in Chapter 10.

STEPS OF THE QUANTITATIVE RESEARCH PROCESS

The quantitative research process involves conceptualizing a research project, planning and implementing that project, and communicating the findings. Figure 3–1 identifies the steps of the quantitative research process and shows the logical flow of this process as one step progressively builds on the last one. This research process is also flexi-

ble and fluid, with a flow back and forth among the steps as the researcher strives to clarify the steps and strengthen the proposed study. This flow back and forth among the steps is indicated in the figure by the two-way arrows connecting the steps of the process. Figure 3–1 also contains a feedback arrow, which indicates that the research process is cyclical, for each study provides a basis for generating further research in the development of a sound knowledge base for practice.

The steps of the quantitative research process are briefly introduced in this chapter and then presented in detail in Unit II, The Research Process (Chapters 5–22, 24, and 25). The descriptive correlational study conducted by Hulme and Grove (1994), on the symptoms of female survivors of child sexual abuse, is used as an example during this discussion and introduction of the steps of the research process; quotations from and descriptions of this study appear throughout the text.

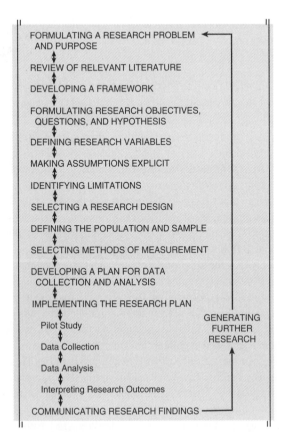

FIGURE 3–1 ■ Steps of the quantitative research process.

Formulating a Research Problem and Purpose

A *research problem* is an area of concern in which there is a gap in the knowledge base needed for nursing practice. The problem identifies an area of concern for a particular population and often indicates the concepts to be studied. The major sources for nursing research problems include nursing practice, researcher and peer interactions, literature review, theory, and research priorities. Using deductive reasoning, the researcher generates a research problem from a research topic or a broad problem area of personal interest that is relevant to nursing.

The *research purpose* is generated from the problem and identifies the specific goal or aim of the study. The goal of a study might be to identify, describe, explain, or predict a solution to a situation. The purpose often indicates the type of study to be conducted (descriptive, correlational, quasi-experimental, or experimental) and includes the variables, population, and setting for the study.

As the research problem and purpose improve in clarity and conciseness, the researcher is able to determine the feasibility of conducting the study.

Chapter 5 provides a background for formulating a research problem and purpose. Hulme and Grove (1994) identified the following problem and purpose for their study of female survivors of child sexual abuse.

• •

Problem

"The actual prevalence of child sexual abuse is unknown but is thought to be high. Bagley and King (1990) were able to generalize from compiled research that at least 20% of all women in the samples surveyed had been victims of serious sexual abuse involving unwanted or coerced sexual contact up to the age of 17 years. Evidence indicates that the prevalence is greater for women born after 1960 than before (Bagley, 1990).

"The impact of child sexual abuse on the lives of the girl victims and the women they become has only lately received the attention it deserves. . . . The knowledge generated from research and theory has slowly forced the recognition of the long-term effects of child sexual abuse on both the survivors and society as a whole. . . . Recently, Brown and Garrison (1990) developed the Adult Survivors of Incest (ASI) Questionnaire to identify the patterns of symptoms and the factors contributing to the severity of these symptoms in survivors of childhood sexual abuse. This tool requires additional testing to determine its usefulness in identifying symptoms and contributing factors of adult survivors of incest and other types of child sexual abuse." (Hulme & Grove, 1994, pp. 519–520)

Purpose

"Thus, the purpose of this study was twofold: (a) to describe the patterns of physical and psychosocial symptoms in female sexual abuse survivors using the ASI Questionnaire, and (b) to examine relationships among the symptoms and identified contributing factors." (Hulme & Grove, 1994, p. 520) ▪

The research purpose clearly indicates that the focus of this study is both descriptive and correlational.

Review of Relevant Literature

A *review of relevant literature* is conducted to generate a picture of what is known about a particular situation and the knowledge gaps that exist in it. *Relevant literature* refers to those sources that are pertinent or highly important in providing the in-depth knowledge needed to study a selected problem. This background enables the researcher to build on the works of others. The concepts and interrelationships of the concepts in the problem guide the researcher's selection of relevant theories and studies for review. Theories are reviewed to clarify the definitions of concepts and to develop and refine the study framework.

Reviewing relevant studies enables the researcher to clarify (1) which problems have been investigated, (2) which require further investigation or replication, and (3) which have not been investigated. In addition, the literature review directs the researcher in designing the study and interpreting the outcomes. The process for reviewing relevant literature is described in Chapter 6. Hulme and Grove's (1994) review of the literature covered relevant theories and studies related to child sexual abuse and its contributing factors and long-term effects, as shown in the following extracts.

• •

"Theorists indicated that . . . the act of child sexual abuse can be explained as an abuse of power by a trusted parent figure, usually male, on a dependent child, violating the child's body, mind, and spirit. The family, which normally functions to nurture and protect the child from harm, is viewed as not fulfilling this function, leaving the child to feel further betrayed and powerless. Acceptance of the immediate psychological trauma of child sexual abuse has given impetus for acknowledging the long-term effects.

"Studies of both nonclinical and clinical populations have lent support to these theoretical developments. When compared with control groups consisting of women who had not been sexually abused as children, survivors of child sexual abuse consistently have higher incidence of depression and lower self-esteem. Other psychosocial long-term effects encountered include suicidal plans, anxiety, distorted body image, decreased sexual satisfaction, poor general social adjustment, lower positive affect, negative personality characteristics, and feeling different from significant others. . . . The physical long-term effects suggested by research include gastrointestinal problems such as ulcers, spastic colitis, irritable bowel syndrome, and chronic abdominal pain; gynecological disorders; chronic headache; obesity; and increased lifetime surgeries." (Hulme & Grove, 1994, p. 521)

"Studies of contributing factors that may affect the traumatic impact of child sexual abuse are less in number and less conclusive than those that identify long-term effects. However, poor family functioning, increased age difference between the victim and perpetrator, threat or use of force or violence, multiple abusers, parent or primary caretaker as perpetrator, prolonged or intrusive abuse, and strong emotional bond to the perpetrator with betrayal of trust may all contribute to the increased severity of the long-term effects." (Hulme & Grove, 1994, pp. 521–522) ■

Developing a Framework

A *framework* is the abstract, logical structure of meaning that guides the development of the study and enables the researcher to link the findings to nursing's body of knowledge. In quantitative research, the framework is a testable midrange theory that has been developed in nursing or in another discipline, such as psychology, physiology, or sociology. The framework may also be developed inductively from clinical observations.

The terms related to frameworks are concept, relational statement, theory, and framework map. A *concept* is a term to which abstract meaning is attached. A *relational statement* declares that a relationship of some kind exists between two or more concepts. A *theory* consists of an integrated set of defined concepts and relational statements that presents a view of a phenomenon and can be used to describe, explain, predict, or control the phenomenon. The statements of the theory, not the theory itself, are tested through research.

A study framework can be expressed as a map or a diagram of the relationships that provide the basis for a study or can be presented in narrative format. The steps for developing a framework are described in Chapter 7. The framework for Hulme and Grove's (1994) study, described in the following quotation, is based on Browne and Finkelhor's (1986) theory of traumagenic dynamics in the impact of child sexual abuse.

· ·

Framework

"As shown in [Figure 3–2], child sexual abuse is at the center of the adult survivor's existence. Arising from the abuse are four trauma-causing dynamics: traumatic sexualization, betrayal, powerlessness, and stigmatization. These traumagenic dynamics lead to behavioral manifestations and collectively indicate a history of child sexual abuse. The behavioral manifestations were operationalized as physical and psychosocial symptoms for the purposes of this study. Piercing the adult survivor are the contributing factors, which are characteristics of the child sexual abuse or other factors occurring later in the survivor's life, that affect the severity of behavioral manifestations (Follette, Alexander, & Follette, 1991). The contributing factors examined in this study were age when the abuse began, duration of the abuse, and other victimizations. Other victimizations included past or present physical and emotional abuse, rape, control by others, and prostitution." (Hulme & Grove, 1994, pp. 522–523) ■

Formulating Research Objectives, Questions, and Hypotheses

Research objectives, questions, and hypotheses are formulated to bridge the gap between the more abstractly stated research problem and purpose and the study design and plan for data collection and analysis. Objectives, questions, and hypotheses are more narrow in focus than the purpose and often (1) specify only one or two research variables, (2) identify the relationship between the variables, and (3) indicate the population to be studied.

Some quantitative studies do not include objectives, questions, or hypotheses; the development of such a study is directed by the research purpose. Many descriptive studies include only a research purpose, and other descriptive studies include a pur-

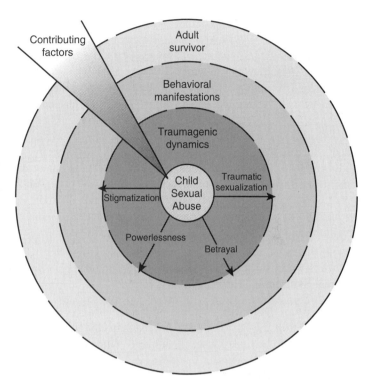

FIGURE 3–2 ■ Long-term effects of child sexual abuse. (From Symptoms of female survivors of sexual abuse. *Issues in Mental Health Nursing, 15*[5], 123. Hulme, P. A., & Grove, S. K. [1994]. Taylor & Francis, Inc., Washington, DC: reproduced with permission. All rights reserved.)

pose and objectives or questions. Some correlational studies include a purpose and specific questions or hypotheses. Quasi-experimental and experimental studies often use hypotheses to direct the development and implementation of the studies and the interpretation of findings. The development of research objectives, questions, and hypotheses is discussed in Chapter 8. Hulme and Grove (1994) developed the following research questions to direct their study.

• •

Research Questions

"1. What patterns of physical and psychosocial symptoms are present in women 18 to 40 years of age who have experienced child sexual abuse?

2. Are there relationships among the number of physical and psychosocial symptoms, the age when the abuse began, the duration of abuse, and number of other victimizations?" (Hulme & Grove, 1994, p. 523) ■

The focus of question 1 is description and that of question 2 is correlation, or examination of relationships.

Defining Research Variables

The research purpose and the objectives, questions, or hypotheses identify the variables to be examined in a study. Research *variables* are concepts of various levels of abstraction that are measured, manipulated, or controlled in a study. The more concrete concepts, such as temperature, weight, and blood pressure, are referred to as "variables" in a study. The more abstract concepts, such as creativity, empathy, and social support, are sometimes referred to as "research concepts."

The variables or concepts in a study are operationalized through the identification of conceptual and operational definitions. A *conceptual definition* provides a variable or concept with theoretical meaning (Fawcett & Downs, 1986) and either is derived from a theorist's definition of the concept or is developed through concept analysis. An *operational definition* is developed so that the variable can be measured or manipulated in a study. The knowledge gained from studying the variable will increase understanding of the theoretical concept that the variable represents.

A more extensive discussion of variables is provided in Chapter 8. Hulme and Grove (1994) provided conceptual and operational definitions of the study variables identified in their purpose and research questions: physical and psychosocial symptoms, age that abuse began, duration of abuse, and victimizations. Only the definitions for physical symptoms and victimizations are presented as examples here.

• •

Physical Symptoms

Conceptual Definition. "Behavioral manifestations that result directly from the traumagenic dynamics of child sexual abuse." (Hulme & Grove, 1994, p. 522)

Operational Definition. The ASI Questionnaire was used to measure physical symptoms.

Victimizations

Conceptual Definition. Adult survivor who has experienced multiple forms of abuse, including "past and present physical and emotional abuse, rape, control by others, and prostitution." (Hulme & Grove, 1994, p. 523)

Operational Definition. The ASI Questionnaire was used to measure victimizations. ■

Making Assumptions Explicit

Assumptions are statements that are taken for granted or are considered true, even though they have not been scientifically tested (Silva, 1981). Assumptions are often embedded (unrecognized) in thinking and behavior, and uncovering them requires introspection. Sources of assumptions include universally accepted truths (e.g., all humans are rational beings), theories, previous research, and nursing practice (Myers, 1982).

In studies, assumptions are embedded in the phil-osophical base of the framework, study design, and interpretation of findings. Theories and instruments are developed on the basis of assumptions that may or may not be recognized by the researcher. These assumptions influence the development and implementation of the research process. The recognition of assumptions by the researcher is a strength, not a weakness. Assumptions influence the logic of the study, and their recognition leads to more rigorous study development.

Williams (1980) reviewed published nursing studies and other health care literature to identify 13 commonly embedded assumptions:

1. People want to assume control of their own health problems.
2. Stress should be avoided.
3. People are aware of the experiences that most affect their life choices.
4. Health is a priority for most people.
5. People in underserved areas feel underserved.
6. Most measurable attitudes are held strongly enough to direct behavior.
7. Health professionals view health care in a different manner than do lay persons.
8. Human biological and chemical factors show less variation than do cultural and social factors.
9. The nursing process is the best way of conceptualizing nursing practice.
10. Statistically significant differences relate to the variable or variables under consideration.
11. People operate on the basis of cognitive information.
12. Increased knowledge about an event lowers anxiety about the event.
13. Receipt of health care at home is preferable to receipt of care in an institution. (Williams, 1980, p. 48)

Hulme and Grove (1994) did not identify assumptions for their study but the following assumptions seem to provide a basis for it: (1) the child victim bears no responsibility for the sexual contact, (2) a relatively large portion of the survivors remember and are willing to report their past child sexual abuse, and (3) behavioral manifestations are not indicative of optimal health and functioning.

Identifying Limitations

Limitations are restrictions in a study that may decrease the generalizability of the findings. The two types of limitations are theoretical and methodological.

Theoretical limitations restrict the abstract generalization of the findings and are reflected in the study framework and the conceptual and operational definitions. Theoretical limitations include the following:

1. A concept might not be clearly defined in the theory used to develop the study framework.
2. The relationships among some concepts might not be identified or are unclear in the theorist's work.
3. A study variable might not be clearly linked to a concept in the framework.
4. An objective, question, or hypothesis might not be clearly linked to the study framework.

Methodological limitations can limit the credibility of the findings and restrict the population to which the findings can be generalized. Methodological limitations result from factors such as unrepresentative samples, weak designs, single setting, limited control over treatment (intervention) implementation, instruments with limited reliability and validity, limited control over data collection, and improper use of statistical analyses. Limitations regarding design (see Chapter 10), sampling (see Chapter 14), measurement (see Chapter 15), and data collection (see Chapter 17) are discussed later in this text. Hulme and Grove (1994) identified the following methodological limitation.

. . . .

Methodological Limitation

"This study has limited generalizability due to the relatively small nonprobability sample. . . . Additional replications drawing from various social classes and age groups are needed to improve the generalizability of Brown and Garrison's (1990) findings and establish reliability and validity of their tool." (Hulme & Grove, 1994, pp. 528–529) ■

Selecting a Research Design

A research *design* is a blueprint for the conduct of a study that maximizes control over factors that could interfere with the study's desired outcome. The type of design directs the selection of a population, sampling procedure, methods of measurement, and a plan for data collection and analysis. The choice of research design depends on the researcher's expertise, the problem and purpose for the study, and the desire to generalize the findings (Brophy, 1981).

Designs have been developed to meet unique research needs as they emerge; thus, a variety of descriptive, correlational, quasi-experimental, and experimental designs have been generated over time. In descriptive and correlational studies, no treatment is administered, so the focus of the study design is improving the precision of measurement. Quasi-experimental and experimental study designs usually involve treatment and control groups and focus on achieving high levels of control as well as precision in measurement. The purpose of a design and the threats to design validity are covered in Chapter 10. Models and descriptions of several types of descriptive, correlational, quasi-experimental, and experimental designs are presented in Chapter 11.

In the study by Hulme and Grove (1994), a descriptive correlational design was used to direct the conduct of the study. A diagram of the design, presented in Figure 3–3, indicates the variables described and the relationships examined. The findings generated from correlational research provide a basis for generating hypotheses for testing in future research.

Defining the Population and Sample

The *population* is all the elements (individuals, objects, or substances) that meet certain criteria for inclusion in a given universe (Kaplan, 1964; Kerlinger & Lee, 1999). A study might be conducted to describe patients' responses to nurse practitioners as their primary care providers. The population could be defined in different ways: It could include all patients being seen for the first time in (1) a single

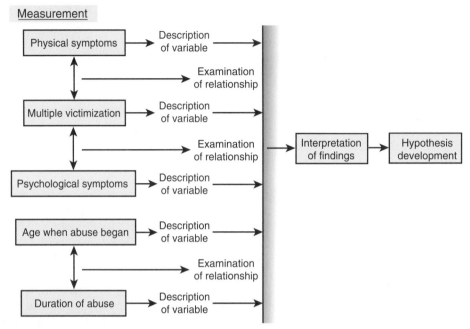

FIGURE 3–3 ■ Proposed descriptive correlational design for Hulme and Grove (1994) study of symptoms of female survivors of child sexual abuse.

clinic, (2) all clinics in a specific network in one city, or (3) all clinics in that network nationwide. The definition of the population depends on the sample criteria and the similarity of subjects in these various settings. The researcher must determine which population is accessible and can be best represented by the study sample.

A *sample* is a subset of the population that is selected for a particular study, and the members of a sample are the subjects. Sampling defines the process for selecting a group of people, events, behaviors, or other elements with which to conduct a study. A variety of probability and nonprobability sampling methods is used in nursing studies. In *probability sampling*, every member of the population has a probability greater than zero of being selected for the sample. With *nonprobability sampling*, not every member of the population has an opportunity for selection in the sample. Sampling theory and sampling methods are presented in Chapter 14. The following quotation identifies the sampling method, setting, sample size, population,

sample criteria, and sample characteristics for the study conducted by Hulme and Grove (1994).

. . . .

Sample

"The convenience sample [sampling method] was obtained by advertising for subjects at three state universities in the southwest [setting]. Despite the sensitive nature of the study, 22 [sample size] usable interviews were obtained. The sample included women between the ages of 18 and 39 years ($\overline{X}$ = 28 years, SD = 6.5 years) who were identified as survivors of child sexual abuse [population] [sample criteria]. The majority of these women were white (91%) and students (82%). A little more than half (54%) were single, seven (32%) were divorced, and three (14%) were married. Most (64%) had no children. A small percentage (14%) were on some form of public assistance and only 14% had been arrested. Although 27% of the subjects had stepfamily members, the parents of 14 subjects (64%) were still married. Half the fathers were working class or self-employed; the rest were professionals. Mothers were either working class or self-employed (50%), homemakers (27%), or professionals (11%). Most subjects (95%) had siblings, and 36% knew or suspected their siblings also had been abused [sample characteristics]." (Hulme & Grove, 1994, pp. 523–524) ■

Selecting Methods of Measurement

Measurement is the process of assigning "numbers to objects (or events or situations) in accord with some rule" (Kaplan, 1964, p. 177). A component of measurement is *instrumentation*, which is the application of specific rules to the development of a measurement device or instrument. An instrument is selected to examine a specific variable in a study. Data generated with an instrument are at the nominal, ordinal, interval, or ratio level of measurement. The level of measurement, with nominal being the lowest form of measurement and ratio being the highest, determines the type of statistical analyses that can be performed on the data.

Selection of an instrument requires extensive examination of its reliability and validity. *Reliability* is concerned with how consistently the measurement technique measures a concept. The *validity* of an instrument is the extent to which the instrument actually reflects the abstract concept being examined. Chapter 15 introduces the concepts of measurement and explains the different types of reliability and validity for instruments. Chapter 16 provides a background for selecting measurement methods for a study. Hulme and Grove (1994) provided the following description of the ASI Questionnaire that was used to measure their study variables.

. . . .
Measurement Methods

"The ASI Questionnaire contains 10 sections: demographics; family origin; educational history, occupational history and public assistance; legal history; characteristics of the child sexual abuse (duration, perpetrator, pregnancy, type, and threats); past and present other victimizations; past and present physical symptoms; past and present psychosocial symptoms; and relationship with own children. Each section is followed by a response set that includes space for 'other.' Content validity was established by Brown and Garrison (1990) using an in-depth review of 132 clinical records. . . . For this descriptive correlational study. . . content validity of the tool was examined by asking an open-ended question: Is there additional information you would like to share?" (Hulme & Grove, 1994, p. 524) ■

Developing a Plan for Data Collection and Analysis

Data collection is the precise, systematic gathering of information relevant to the research purpose or the specific objectives, questions, or hypotheses of a study. The data collected in quantitative studies are usually numerical. Planning data collection enables the researcher to anticipate problems that are likely to occur and to explore possible solutions. Usually, detailed procedures for implementing a treatment and collecting data are developed, with a schedule that identifies the initiation and termination of the process (see Chapter 17).

Planning data analysis is the final step before the study is implemented. The analysis plan is based on (1) the research objectives, questions, or hypotheses, (2) the data collected, (3) research design, (4) researcher expertise, and (5) availability of computer resources. A variety of statistical analysis techniques is available to describe the sample, examine relationships, or determine significant differences. Most researchers consult a statistician for assistance in developing an analysis plan.

Implementing the Research Plan

Implementing the research plan involves treatment or intervention implementation, data collection, data analysis, interpretation of research findings, and, sometimes, a pilot study.

PILOT STUDY

A *pilot study* is commonly defined as a smaller version of a proposed study conducted to refine the methodology (Van Ort, 1981). It is developed much like the proposed study, using similar subjects, the same setting, the same treatment, and the same data collection and analysis techniques. However, a pilot study could be conducted to develop and refine a variety of the steps in the research process (Prescott & Soeken, 1989). For example, a pilot study could be conducted to develop and refine a research treatment, a data collection tool, or the data collection process. Thus, a pilot study could be used to develop a research plan rather than to test an already developed plan.

Some of the reasons for conducting pilot studies are as follows (Prescott & Soeken, 1989; Van Ort, 1981):

■ To determine whether the proposed study is feasible (e.g., are the subjects available, does the researcher have the time and money to do the study?)
■ To develop or refine a research treatment
■ To develop a protocol for the implementation of a treatment
■ To identify problems with the design
■ To determine whether the sample is representative of the population or whether the sampling technique is effective
■ To examine the reliability and validity of the research instruments
■ To develop or refine data collection instruments
■ To refine the data collection and analysis plan
■ To give the researcher experience with the subjects, setting, methodology, and methods of measurement
■ To try out data analysis techniques

Prescott and Soeken (1989) reviewed 212 studies published in three research journals (*Nursing Research, Research in Nursing & Health,* and *Western Journal of Nursing Research*) during 1985 through 1987. Only 18 (8.8%) of these studies included a pilot study. In 13 of the 18 studies, a pilot study was conducted to assess instrument reliability. In the other 5 studies, the pilot studies were smaller versions of the published studies that were conducted to test the research plans.

Pilot studies can be used to improve the quality of research conducted, and their findings need to be shared through presentations and publications. Wilkie and associates (1995, p. 8) conducted a "pilot study to develop and test a method of COACH-

ING 18 patients with lung cancer to inform clinicians about their pain." COACHING is one method of improving clinicians' assessments of pain by encouraging patients to communicate their pain in ways that clinicians recognize. "Pilot study findings demonstrated feasibility of implementing the COACHING protocol and suggest a trend for COACHING to possibly be an effective method of reducing discrepancies between patients' self-reports and nurses' assessments of sensory pain" (Wilkie et al., 1995, p. 13). Thus, the focus of this pilot study was to test the completeness of the protocol for implementing the COACHING intervention and to determine the effectiveness of this intervention in increasing the recognition of cancer patients' pain.

DATA COLLECTION

In quantitative research, data collection involves the generation of numerical data to address the research objectives, questions, or hypotheses. In order to collect data, the researcher must obtain consent or permission from the setting or agency where the study is to be conducted and from potential subjects. Frequently, the subjects are asked to sign a consent form, which describes the study, promises the subjects confidentiality, and indicates that the subjects can stop participation at any time (see Chapter 9).

During data collection, the study variables are measured through the use of a variety of techniques, such as observation, interview, questionnaires, and scales. In a growing number of studies, nurses are measuring physiological variables with high-technology equipment. The data are collected and recorded systematically for each subject and are organized in a way to facilitate computer entry. Hulme and Grove (1994) identified the following procedure for data collection.

• •

"Although the tool can be self-reporting, it was administered by personal interview to allow for elaboration of 'other' responses. The interviews lasted about one hour and were conducted in a private room provided by The University of Texas at Arlington. Each interview started with a discussion of the study benefits and risks and included signing a consent form. Risks included possible painful memories and embarrassment during the interview as well as emotional and physical discomfort after the interview. Sources of public and private counseling were provided to assist subjects with any difficulties experienced related to the study." (Hulme & Grove, 1994, pp. 524–525) ■

DATA ANALYSIS

Data analysis is conducted to reduce, organize, and give meaning to the data. The analysis of data from quantitative research involves the use of (1) descriptive and exploratory procedures (see Chapter 19) to describe study variables and the sample and (2) statistical techniques to test proposed relationships (see Chapter 20), make predictions (see Chapter 21), and examine causality (see Chapter 22). Most analyses are performed by computer, so Chapter 18 provides a background for using computers in research.

The choice of analysis techniques implemented is determined primarily by the research objectives, questions, or hypotheses; the research design; and the level of measurement achieved by the research instruments. Hulme and Grove (1994) chose frequencies, percents, means, standard deviations, and Pearson correlations to answer their research questions.

. . . .

Results

"The first research question focused on description of the patterns of physical and psychosocial symptoms. Six physical symptoms occurred in 50% or more of the subjects: insomnia, sexual dysfunction, overeating, drug abuse, severe headache, and two or more major surgeries. . . . Eleven psychosocial symptoms occurred in 75% or more of the subjects: depression, guilt, low self-esteem, inability to trust others, mood swings, suicidal thoughts, difficulty in relationships, confusion, flashbacks of the abuse, extreme anger, and memory lapse. . . . Self-injurious behavior was reported by eight subjects (33%)." (Hulme & Grove, 1994, pp. 527–528)

"The second research question focused on the relationships among the number of physical and psychosocial symptoms and three contributing factors (age abuse began, duration of abuse, and other victimizations). There were five significant correla-

tions among study variables: physical symptoms with other victimizations ($r = .59$, $p = .002$), physical symptoms with psychosocial symptoms ($r = .56$, $p = .003$), age abuse began with duration of abuse ($r = .50$, $p = .009$), psychosocial symptoms with other victimizations ($r = .40$, $p = .033$), and duration of abuse with psychosocial symptoms ($r = .40$, p = .034)." (Hulme & Grove, 1994, p. 528) ■

INTERPRETING RESEARCH OUTCOMES

The results obtained from data analysis require interpretation to be meaningful. *Interpretation of research outcomes* involves (1) examining the results from data analysis, (2) forming conclusions, (3) considering the implications for nursing, (4) exploring the significance of the findings, (5) generalizing the findings, and (6) suggesting further studies. The results obtained from data analyses are of five types:

■ Significant as predicted by the researcher
■ Nonsignificant
■ Significant but not predicted by the researcher
■ Mixed
■ Unexpected

The study results are then translated and interpreted to become *findings*, and *conclusions* are formed from the synthesis of findings. The conclusions provide a basis for identifying nursing implications, generalizing findings, and suggesting further studies (see Chapter 24). In the excerpts that follow, Hulme and Grove (1994) provide a discussion of their findings, with implications for nursing and suggestions for further study.

. . . .

Discussion

"While this study may have limited generalizability due to the relatively small nonprobability sample, the findings do support previous research. . . . In addition, the findings support Browne and Finkelhor's (1986) framework that a wide range of behavioral manifestations (physical and psychosocial symptoms) comprise the long-term effects of child sexual abuse." (Hulme & Grove, 1994, p. 528)

"Brown and Garrison's (1990) ASI Questionnaire was effective in identifying patterns of physical and psychosocial symptoms in women with a history of child sexual abuse. . . . As data on the behavioral manifestations (physical and psychosocial symptoms) and the effect of each of the contributing factors accumulate, hypotheses need to be formulated to further test Browne and Finkelhor's (1986) framework explaining the long-term effects of child sexual abuse. . . . With additional research, the ASI Questionnaire might be adapted for use in clinical situations. This questionnaire might facilitate identification and delivery of appropriate treatment to female survivors of child sexual abuse in clinical settings." (Hulme & Grove, 1994, pp. 529–530) ▪

Communicating Research Findings

Research is not considered complete until the findings have been communicated. *Communicating research findings* involves the development and dissemination of a research report to appropriate audiences, including nurses, health professionals, health care consumers, and policymakers. The research report is disseminated through presentations and publication. The details for developing a research report and presenting and publishing the report are in Chapter 25.

TYPES OF QUANTITATIVE RESEARCH

Four types of quantitative research are described in this text: (1) descriptive, (2) correlational, (3) quasi-experimental, and (4) experimental. The type of research planned is influenced by the level of existing knowledge for the research problem. When little knowledge is available, descriptive studies are often conducted. As the knowledge level increases, correlational, quasi-experimental, and experimental studies are implemented. In this section, the purpose of each quantitative research approach is identified, and examples of the steps of the research process from published studies are presented.

Descriptive Research

The purpose of descriptive research is the exploration and description of phenomena in real-life situations. This approach is used to generate new knowledge about concepts or topics about which limited or no research has been conducted. Through descriptive research, concepts are described and relationships are identified that provide a basis for further quantitative research and theory testing. The study by Hulme and Grove (1994) on the symptoms of female survivors of child sexual abuse, which was used earlier in the chapter to illustrate the basic discussion of the steps of the quantitative research process, is a combined descriptive correlational study. The descriptive aspects of this study can be clearly identified in its purpose, research questions, design, data analysis, and findings.

Correlational Research

Correlational research is conducted to examine linear relationships between two or more variables and to determine the type (positive or negative) and degree (strength) of the relationship. The strength of a relationship varies from −1 (perfect negative correlation) to +1 (perfect positive correlation), with 0 indicating no relationship. The positive relationship indicates that the variables vary together, that is, the two variables either increase or decrease together. The negative or inverse relationship indicates that the variables vary in opposite directions; thus, as one variable increases, the other decreases. The descriptive correlational study conducted by Hulme and Grove (1994), presented earlier in this chapter, is an example of the steps of the quantitative research process for correlational research.

Quasi-Experimental Research

The purpose of quasi-experimental research is to examine cause-and-effect relationships among selected independent and dependent variables. Quasi-experimental studies in nursing are conducted to determine the effects of nursing interventions or treatments (independent variables) on patient outcomes (dependent variables) (Cook & Campbell, 1979). Hastings-Tolsma and colleagues (1993, p. 171) conducted a quasi-experimental study of the "effect of warm and cold applications on the resolution of IV infiltrations." The steps for this study are described here and illustrated with extracts from the study.

STEPS OF THE RESEARCH PROCESS IN A QUASI-EXPERIMENTAL STUDY

1: Research Problem

"It has been estimated that as many as 80% of hospitalized patients receive intravenous (IV) therapy each day (Millam, 1988). IV infiltration, or extravasation, occurs in as many as 23% of all IV infusion failures (MacCara, 1983) and is second only to phlebitis as a cause of IV morbidity (Lewis & Hecker, 1991). The resulting tissue injury depends on the clinical condition of the patient, the nature of the infusate, and the volume infiltrated, and may range from little apparent injury to serious damage. In addition, considerable patient suffering, prolonged hospitalization, and significant costs may be incurred. Despite the frequency and potential severity of injury, little is known about how to treat IV infiltration effectively once it is identified." (Hastings-Tolsma et al., 1993, p. 171)

2: Research Purpose

"The purpose of this research was to determine the effect of warm versus cold applications on the pain intensity and the speed of resolution of the extravasation of a variety of commonly used intravenous solutions." (Hastings-Tolsma et al., 1993, p. 172)

3: Review of Literature

The literature review for this study included relevant, current sources ranging in publication date from 1976 to 1991; the article describing the study was received by the journal in April 1992 and ac-

cepted for publication in January 1993. The signs and symptoms of IV infiltration were identified, and the tissue damage that occurs with an IV infiltration was described. The effects of the pH and osmolarity of different types of IV solutions on IV infiltration were also discussed. The literature review concluded with a description of the effects of a variety of treatments, including warm and cold applications, on the resolution of IV infiltrations. Hastings-Tolsma and colleagues (1993, p. 172) concluded that "examination of warm and cold application with less toxic infiltrates has not been studied carefully under controlled conditions."

4: Framework

Hastings-Tolsma and colleagues (1993) did not identify a framework for their study. They did identify relevant concepts (IV therapy, nature of infusate, vessel damage, extravasation, tissue damage, treatment, and resolution) and discuss the relationships among them in their review of literature.

A possible map for their study framework is presented in Figure 3–4. The map indicates that the more IV therapy patients receive, the more likely they are to experience vessel damage that leads to extravasation or IV infiltration. The nature of the IV infusate (IV solution) also affects the severity of the vessel damage and extravasation. The extravasation then leads to tissue damage, and the greater the extravasation, the greater the tissue damage. The treatment with warm and cold applications has an unknown effect on the extravasation and tissue damage. If the extravasation and tissue damage are decreased by either the cold or the warm treat-

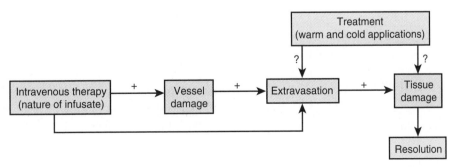

FIGURE 3–4 ▪ Proposed framework map in Hastings-Tolsma and colleagues' (1993) study of the effect of warm and cold applications on the resolution of intravenous infiltrations.

ment, then the patient experiences resolution of the extravasation.

5: Research Questions

"(a) What are the differences in tissue response as measured by pain, erythema and induration, and interstitial fluid volume between warm versus cold applications to infiltrated IV sites? (b) What is the effect of warm versus cold applications in the resolution of infiltrated solutions of varying osmolarity when pH is held constant?" (Hastings-Tolsma et al., 1993, pp. 172–173)

6: Variables

The independent variables were temperature applications (warm and cold) and osmolarity of the IV solution. The dependent variables were pain, erythema, induration, and interstitial fluid volume.

Independent Variable—Temperature Applications

Conceptual Definition. Topical warm and cold applications to the sites of extravasation to promote the reabsorption of infusate and resolution of the infiltration.

Operational Definition. Warm (43°C) or cold (0°C) topical applications using a thermostat-controlled pad to the sites of IV infiltration.

Independent Variable—Osmolarity of the IV Solution

Conceptual Definition. The osmolar concentration expressed as osmoles per liter of solution.

Operational Definition. IV solutions of ½ saline (154 mOsm), normal saline (308 mOsm), or 3% saline (1027 mOsm).

Dependent Variable—Pain

Conceptual Definition. Sensation of discomfort caused by tissue damage and the inflammatory response.

Operational Definition. Pain was measured with the Analogue Chromatic Continuous Scale (ACCS), which is a self-reported, unidimensional visual analogue scale for quantifying pain intensity.

Dependent Variable—Erythema

Conceptual Definition. Redness at the IV infiltration site due to inflammatory response.

Operational Definition. Indelible ink pen was used to mark the borders of erythema. Then a centimeter ruler was used to measure the widest perpendicular widths, and the two widths were multiplied to estimate the surface area of erythema.

Dependent Variable—Induration

Conceptual Definition. The swelling at the site of the IV infiltration created by the IV solution, tissue damage, and inflammatory response.

Operational Definition. Indelible ink pen was used to mark the borders of induration. Then a centimeter ruler was used to measure the widest perpendicular widths, and the two widths were multiplied to estimate surface area of induration.

Dependent Variable—Interstitial Fluid Volume

Conceptual Definition. The amount of fluid that leaks outside the damaged blood vessel into the surrounding tissues.

Operational Definition. Magnetic resonance imaging (MRI) was used to quantify the amount of infiltrate remaining at the IV site.

7: Design

The design most closely resembles an interrupted time series design (see Chapter 11), with each subject receiving both treatments of warm and cold applications.

8: Sample

"The sample was composed of 18 healthy adult volunteers. All participants were nonpregnant and taking no medications. . . . Of the 18 participants studied, 78% were female (n = 14) and 22% were male (n = 4), and they ranged in age from 20 to 45 years with a mean age of 35 years (SD = 7). All subjects were Caucasian. The research was approved by the Health Science Center Institutional Review Board for the Protection of Human Subjects. After the study was explained to interested individuals, written informed consent was obtained from volunteers. All individuals were offered financial compensation for their participation." (Hastings-Tolsma et al., 1993, p. 173)

9: Procedures

"All measurements were taken in the Health Science Center's Department of Radiology NMR Laboratory. After obtaining written informed consent, participants were taken to the MR imaging suite where infiltrations and subsequent measurements were made. . . . Total data collection time was approximately 3½ hours. One of three solutions was infiltrated into the cephalic vein of the forearm: ½ saline (154 mOsm), normal saline (308 mOsm), or 3% saline (1027 mOsm). These solutions were selected because of the varying osmolarity range, as well as relatively common clinical use. Solutions were infiltrated sequentially so that each participant was given a different solution in the order of recruitment into the study. Randomization was used to determine right or left arm, as well as which application, warm or cold, would be used." (Hastings-Tolsma et al., 1993, p. 174)

10: Results

"Warm and cold treatments to the infiltrated IV sites using three solutions revealed significant differences in tissue response as measured by the interstitial fluid volume. . . . For all three solutions, the volume remaining was always less with warm than with cold application, $F_{(1,15)} = 46.69$, $p < .001$.

"There was no difference in pain with warm or cold applications. . . . Surface area measurement failed to demonstrate the presence of erythema with any of the solutions. . . . Surface induration reflected a significant decrease over time, $F_{(2,16)} = 14.38$, $p = .001$, although accurate measurement of the infiltrate was nearly impossible after the first or second imaging period as the borders were so poorly defined. . . . There was no significant effect of warmth or cold on surface area." (Hastings-Tolsma et al., 1993, p. 175)

11: Discussion

This step of a research paper consists of the study conclusions, recommendations for further research, and the implications of the findings for nursing practice.

"These findings demonstrate that the application of warmth to sites of IV infiltration produces faster resolution of the extravasation than does cold, as monitored over one hour. . . . It is interesting to note that cold appeared to have a more immediate dramatic effect on the increase in interstitial edema than warmth when applied to the hyperosmolar infiltrate. Presumably this is due to osmosis of fluid from the plasma and surrounding tissues into the area of infiltration. . . . Other factors that might influence accurate assessment and treatment of infiltrations need to be examined. These should include the use of larger amounts of extravasate and other more varied and caustic solutions, as well as other treatments such as elevation, differing IV site placement, differing gauge needles, and the study of patients of varying ages and clinical conditions." (Hastings-Tolsma et al., 1993, p. 176)

"The nurse generally has responsibility for IV therapy and criteria for accurate assessment and appropriate intervention clearly are needed. Findings from this research support the use of warm application to sites of infiltration of noncaustic solutions of varying osmolarity, but raise questions about the adequacy of currently used indicators of IV infiltrations. Continued scientific scrutiny should contribute to the development of standards useful in the assessment and treatment of IV extravasation." (Hastings-Tolsma et al., 1993, p. 177) ■

Experimental Research

The purpose of experimental research is to examine cause-and-effect relationships between independent and dependent variables under highly controlled conditions. The planning and implementation of experimental studies are highly controlled by the researcher, and often these studies are conducted in a laboratory setting on animals or objects. Few nursing studies are "purely" experimental. McCarthy and associates (1997, p. 131) conducted an experimental study of "the effect of protein density of food on food intake and nutritional status of tumor-bearing rats."

Steps of the Research Process in an Experimental Study

1: Research Problem

"Anorexia and weight loss are significant concerns to cancer patients and their loved ones. . . .

The progressive decline in food intake and body weight are powerful negative prognostic indicators of survival in cancer patients. . . . The loss of lean body mass is a major aspect of the nutritional decline of cancer patients. The literature presents a uniform emphasis on increasing dietary protein intake with the expectation of preserving lean body mass of cancer patients. . . . However, it has been shown that healthy animals will reduce their food intake when protein density of their food is increased. . . . It is not known if this response to increased protein density of food will occur in hypophagic tumor-bearing rats.

"It also should be noted that tumor growth is associated with depressed serum levels of insulin associated with depressed serum levels of insulin-like growth factor 1 (IGF-1). . . . It is not known if serum levels of insulin or IGF-1 will improve in hypophagic tumor-bearing rats fed a diet of increased protein density." (McCarthy et al., 1997, pp. 130–132)

2: Research Purpose

The purpose of this laboratory study "was to determine (a) if increasing the protein density of food would affect food and total protein intake of tumor-bearing rats and (b) if increased protein intake would alter serum levels of insulin and IGF-1, two hormones requisite to protein synthesis and tissue anabolism." (McCarthy et al., 1997, p. 132)

3: Review of Literature

The literature review included mainly studies focused on the causes of tumor-induced anorexia and weight loss in cancer patients, the impact of high-calorie and high-density protein diets on healthy animals, and the link of tumor growth to serum levels of insulin and IGF-1.

4: Framework

This study has an implied framework that is a combination of physiology and pathology theories about nutrient utilization, tumor development, body response to tumor development, anorexia, nutritional treatment of anorexia, and body response to nutritional supplement.

5: Variables

The independent variable was a high-density protein diet. The dependent variables were serum insulin, serum IGF-1, food intake, protein intake, and body weight.

Independent Variable—High-Density Protein Diet

Conceptual Definition. Nutritional supplement to promote increased intake, nutrient utilization, and weight stabilization with cancerous conditions.

Operational Definition. The high-density protein diet was an isocaloric diet containing 40% casein protein (TD#93331, Harlan Tecklad, Madison, WI). A table in the article listed the specific ingredients of this diet.

Dependent Variable—Serum Insulin and IGF-1

Conceptual Definition. Serum indicators (serum insulin and IGF-1) are sensitive markers for nutritional status and play an important role in protein metabolism and tissue anabolism.

Operational Definitions. "Analysis of serum insulin was done using a radioimmunoassay (RIA) . . . . Serum IGF-1 was determined by RIA after the IGF binding proteins were removed by high-performance chromatography under acid conditions." (McCarthy et al., 1997, p. 133)

Dependent Variable—Food Intake and Protein Intake

Conceptual Definition. Nutrients consumed by healthy and tumor-bearing animals. ■

Operational Definitions. Food intake was operationalized as the number of grams of food eaten by both the healthy and tumor-bearing rats. Protein intake was operationalized as the number of milligrams of protein consumed by the healthy and tumor-bearing rats.

Dependent Variable—Body Weight

Conceptual Definition. Body mass of healthy and tumor-bearing rats.

Operational Definitions. Body weight in grams

of healthy and tumor-bearing rats at days 0, 15, 18, 24, and 27 of the experiment.

5: Design

This study has an experimental design that consisted of four groups of subjects (15 healthy rats in the control group on a regular diet, 15 healthy rats in a group on 40% protein diet, 15 tumor-bearing rats on a regular diet, and 15 tumor-bearing rats on 40% protein diet) with repeated measurements of three of the five dependent variables.

"The experimental period lasted for 27 days. For the first 15 days, all animals were maintained on a semipurified rodent diet containing 20% casein protein. . . . After day 15 of tumor growth, one half of the tumor-bearing [rats] and one half of the healthy controls were switched to an isocaloric diet containing 40% casein protein. The dependent variables of serum insulin and serum IGF-1 were measured on day 27 and the other dependent variables of food intake, protein intake, and body weight were measured at day 0, 15, 18, 24, and 27." (McCarthy et al., 1997, p. 133)

6: Sample and Setting

"A total of 60 randomly selected male Buffalo rats, weighing between 100 and 120 grams were housed individually and maintained on a 12-hour light-dark cycle commencing at 6:00 a.m. Food and water were freely available. The animals were conditioned to the housing for 5 days before the start of the experiment and were treated at all times in a manner consistent with Department of Health, Education, and Welfare Guidelines for the Care and Use of Laboratory Animals. . . . The animals were matched according to weight and a total of 30 were randomly selected for tumor implant, leaving 30 healthy animals as controls." (McCarthy et al., 1997, pp. 132–133)

7: Data Collection

"The food was placed in conical dishes inside a metal cup to catch any spillage. The dishes were weighed each morning on a portable electric digital scale which was zeroed before each weighing . . . . The rats were weighed daily and at the end of the experiment the tumors were excised and weighed. . . . On day 27 of tumor growth, animals were lightly anesthetized with ether fumes and exsanguinated by cardiac puncture between 8 and 10 a. m. to control for any circadian variations in plasma hormone levels. The blood was allowed to coagulate and serum samples for 48 animals were frozen at −20 C (12 specimens were inadvertently destroyed)." (McCarthy et al., 1997, p. 133)

8: Results

The extensive study results were presented in five figures and the narrative of the article.

"There was a significant main effect of tumor growth, $F_{(1,56)} = 26.6$, $p < .001$, diet, $F_{(1, 56)} = 4.1$, $p = .05$, and days, $F_{(4,224)} = 29.6$, $p < .001$, on the grams of food eaten by the rats. . . . Due to the effect of tumor growth on food intake, the tumor-bearing animals were consuming less protein than healthy controls by day 15, $F_{(1,59)} = 16$, $p < .001$. On day 18, 3 days after the diet switch, protein intake was significantly different by tumor, $F_{(1,59)} = 377$, $p < .001$, and by diet, $F_{(1,59)} = 176$, $p < .001$ . . . body weight of tumor-bearing rats was significantly less than controls over the course of the experiment, $F_{(1,56)} = 20.5$, $p < .001$ . . . there was a significant effect of tumor growth on mean serum insulin, $F_{(1,4)} = 4.7$, $p = .03$, but no effect of diet. . . . Similarly, serum IGF-1 was significantly lower in tumor-bearing rats than healthy controls, $F_{(1,47)} = 25.7$, $p < .001$, and was not affected by diet." (McCarthy et al., 1997, pp. 133–136)

9: Discussion: Findings and Suggestions for Further Research

"Increasing the protein density of food from the standard 20% formulation to 40% resulted in a decline in total grams of food intake, and an increase in total grams protein intake of both control and tumor-bearing rats. The increased protein intake of tumor-bearing animals fed the 40% protein diet did not affect the nutrient status of these animals as indicated by body weight, or serum levels of total protein, insulin, or IGF-1, nor did it affect tumor size in the tumor-bearing animals. . . . These data suggest that the lower serum levels of IGF-1 and insulin in hypophagic tumor-bearing animals are not the direct results of their reduced food, or in this case, protein intake. . . . Increasing the protein density of food resulted in a decrease in food intake in both healthy control and tumor-bearing animals." (McCarthy et al., 1997, p. 136)

"The regulation of food intake in humans is more complex than in animals which are maintained on standardized diets and feeding schedules. There is a need for studies to determine the effects of high calorie or high protein nutrition supplements on the total caloric and protein intake and, specifically, meal taking, of cancer patients. There is some evidence that use of nutritional supplements by patients with head and neck cancers results in a significant decline in food-derived calories and protein, though the caloric and protein density of the supplements produces a net increase in total calorie and protein intake. . . . However, there is little evidence that increased nutritional intake affects morbidity and mortality in weight-losing cancer patients. . . . Clearly, there is a need for further study of the metabolic impact of nutritional interventions, as well as the impact of calorie and/ or protein dense nutritional supplements on meal taking and food appetite of cancer patients." (McCarthy et al., 1997, p. 137) ▪

▪ SUMMARY

Quantitative research is the traditional research approach in nursing. Nurses use a broad range of quantitative approaches, including descriptive, correlational, quasi-experimental, and experimental, to develop nursing knowledge. Some of the concepts relevant to quantitative research are (1) basic and applied research, (2) rigor, and (3) control. *Basic,* or pure, *research* is a scientific investigation that involves the pursuit of "knowledge for knowledge's sake" or for the pleasure of learning and finding truth. *Applied,* or practical, *research* is a scientific investigation conducted to generate knowledge that will directly influence or improve clinical practice. Many of the studies conducted in nursing are applied because researchers have chosen to focus on clinical problems, such as developing and testing the effectiveness of nursing interventions. Because the future of any profession rests on its research base, both basic research and applied research are needed to develop nursing knowledge.

Conducting quantitative research involves *rigor,* which is the striving for excellence in research. Rigor involves discipline, scrupulous adherence to detail, and strict accuracy. A rigorous quantitative researcher constantly strives for more precise measurement tools, a representative sample, and tightly controlled study designs. *Control* involves the imposing of "rules" by the researcher to decrease the possibility of error and thus increase the probability that the study's findings are an accurate reflection of reality. Some of the mechanisms for enhancing control within quantitative research are (1) subject selection (sampling), (2) research setting selection, (3) development and implementation of study interventions, and (4) subject's knowledge of the study. *Sampling* is a process of selecting subjects who are representative of the population being studied. The three settings for conducting research are natural, partially controlled, and highly controlled. Controlling the development and implementation of a study intervention improves the validity of the study design and the credibility of its findings. Subjects' knowledge of a study could influence their behavior and possibly alter the study outcome, thus creating a threat to the validity and accuracy of the study design.

The quantitative research process involves conceptualizing a research project, planning and implementing that project, and communicating the findings. The steps of this research process are briefly introduced in this chapter and presented in detail in Unit II, The Research Process. The steps of the quantitative research process are as follows:

1. **Formulating a research problem and purpose.** The research *problem* is an area of concern in which there is a gap in the knowledge base needed for nursing practice. A problem stimulates interest and prompts investigation. The research *purpose* is generated from the problem and identifies the specific goal or aim of the study.
2. **Review of relevant literature:** The literature review is conducted to build a picture of what is known about a particular situation and identify the knowledge gaps in the situation.

3. **Developing a framework:** The *framework* is the abstract, logical structure of meaning that guides the development of the study and enables the researcher to link the findings to nursing's body of knowledge.

4. **Formulating research objectives, questions, and hypotheses:** Research objectives, questions, and hypotheses are formulated to bridge the gap between the more abstractly stated research problem and purpose and the study design and plan for data collection and analysis.

5. **Defining research variables:** *Variables* are concepts of various levels of abstraction that are measured, manipulated, or controlled in a study. Variables are operationalized by identifying conceptual and operational definitions.

6. **Making assumptions explicit:** *Assumptions* are statements that are taken for granted or are considered true even though they have not been scientifically tested. Assumptions influence the logic of the study, and their recognition leads to more rigorous study development.

7. **Identifying limitations:** *Limitations* are restrictions in a study that may decrease the generalizability of the findings. The two types of limitations are theoretical and methodological.

8. **Selecting a research design:** A *research design* is a blueprint for the conduct of a study that maximizes control over factors that could interfere with the study's desired outcome. The type of design directs the selection of a population, sampling procedure, methods of measurement, and a plan for data collection and analysis.

9. **Defining the population and sample:** The *population* is all elements that meet certain criteria for inclusion in a given universe. A *sample* is a subset of the population that is selected for a particular study and the members of a sample are the subjects. *Sampling* defines the process for selecting a group of subjects with which to conduct a study.

10. **Selecting methods of measurement:** *Measurement* is the process of assigning numbers to objects, events, or situations in accordance with some rule. An instrument or scale is selected to measure each variable in a study.

11. **Developing a plan for data collection and analysis:** *Data collection* is the precise, systematic gathering of information relevant to the research purpose or the specific objectives, questions, or hypotheses of a study. The data collected in quantitative studies are usually numerical. Planning of data analysis involves the selection of appropriate statistical techniques to analyze the study data.

12. **Implementing the research plan:** The *research plan* involves treatment implementation, data collection, data analysis, and interpretation of research outcomes. In some studies, implementation of the research plan includes a pilot study. Some reasons for conducting a pilot study are refining a research treatment, refining a data collection sheet, examining an instrument's reliability or validity, and identifying problems in the design. Data collection involves the generation of numerical data to answer the research objectives, questions, or hypotheses. *Data analysis* is conducted to reduce, organize, and give meaning to the data. *Interpretation of research outcomes* involves examining the results from data analysis, forming conclusions, considering the implications for nursing, exploring the significance of the findings, generalizing the findings, and suggesting further studies.

13. **Communicating findings:** Research is communicated by developing and disseminating a research report to appropriate audiences, including nurses, other health professionals, health care consumers, and policymakers. The research report is disseminated through presentations and publication.

Four types of quantitative research are introduced in this chapter: descriptive, correlational, quasi-experimental, and experimental. The purpose of each quantitative approach is identified. Examples from a published study are then used to illustrate the steps of the research process for the type of research being conducted.

. . . .

REFERENCES

Abdellah, F. G., & Levine, E. (1994). *Preparing nursing research for the 21st century: Evolution, methodologies, and challenges.* New York: Springer.

Bagley, C. (1990). Development of a measure of unwanted sexual contact in childhood, for use in community health surveys. *Psychology Reports, 66*(2), 401–402.

Bagley, C., & King, K. K. (1990). *Child sexual abuse: The search for healing.* New York: Travistock/Routledge.

Bond, E. F., & Heitkemper, M. M. (1987). Importance of basic physiologic research in nursing science. *Heart & Lung, 16*(4), 347–349.

Brophy, E. B. (1981). Research design: General introduction. In S. D. Krampitz & N. Pavlovich (Eds.), *Readings for nursing research* (pp. 40–48). St. Louis: C. V. Mosby.

Brown, B. E., & Garrison, C. J. (1990). Patterns of symptomatology of adult women incest survivors. *Western Journal of Nursing Research, 12*(5), 587–600.

Browne, A., & Finkelhor, D. (1986). Initial and long-term effects: A review of the research. In D. Finkelhor (Ed.), *A source book on child sexual abuse* (pp. 143–179). Beverly Hills, CA: Sage.

Campbell, D. T., & Stanley, J. C. (1963). *Experimental and quasi-experimental designs for research.* Chicago: Rand McNally.

Cook, T. D., & Campbell, D. T. (1979). *Quasi-experimentation: Design and analysis issues for field settings.* Chicago: Rand McNally.

Egan, E. C., Snyder, M., & Burns, K. R. (1992). Intervention studies in nursing: Is the effect due to the independent variable? *Nursing Outlook, 40*(4), 187–190.

Fawcett, J., & Downs, F. S. (1986). *The relationship of theory and research.* Norwalk, CT: Appleton-Century-Crofts.

Fisher, Sir R. A. (1935). *The designs of experiments.* New York: Hafner.

Follette, N. M., Alexander, P. C., & Follette, W. C. (1991). Individual predictors of outcome in group treatment for incest survivors. *Journal of Consulting and Clinical Psychology, 59*(1), 150–155.

Hastings-Tolsma, M. T., Yucha, C. B., Tompkins, J., Robson, L., & Szeverenyi, N. (1993). Effect of warm and cold applications on the resolution of IV infiltrations. *Research in Nursing and Health, 16*(3), 171–178.

Homans, G. (1965). Group factors in worker productivity. In H. Proshansky & B. Seidenberg (Eds.), *Basic studies in social psychology* (pp. 592–604). New York: Holt, Rinehart & Winston.

Hulme, P. A., & Grove, S. K. (1994). Symptoms of female survivors of child sexual abuse. *Issues in Mental Health Nursing, 15*(5), 519–532.

Johnson, J. L., Ratner, P. A., Bottorff, J. L., Hall, W., & Dahinten, S. (2000). Preventing smoking relapse in postpartum women. *Nursing Research, 49*(1), 44–52.

Kaplan, A. (1964). *The conduct of inquiry: Methodology for behavioral science.* New York: Chandler.

Kerlinger, F. N., & Lee, H. B. (1999). *Foundations of behavioral research.* New York: Harcourt Brace.

Lewis, G. B. H., & Hecker, J. F. (1991). Radiological examination of failure of intravenous infusions. *British Journal of Surgery, 78*(4), 500–501.

MacCara, M. E. (1983). Extravasation: A hazard of intravenous therapy. *Drug Intelligence and Clinical Pharmacy, 17*(10), 713–717.

Marlatt, G. A. (1985). Relapse prevention: Theoretical rationale and overview of the model. In G. A. Marlatt & J. R. Gordon (Eds.), *Relapse prevention: Maintenance strategies in the treatment of addictive behaviors* (pp. 3–70). New York: Guilford Press.

McCarthy, D. O. (1999). Inhibitors of prostaglandin synthesis do not improve food intake or body weight of tumor-bearing rats. *Research in Nursing & Health, 22*(5), 380–387.

McCarthy, D. O., Lo, C., Nguyen, H., & Ney, D. M. (1997). The effect of protein density of food on food intake and nutritional status of tumor-bearing rats. *Research in Nursing & Health, 20*(2), 131–138.

Millam, D. A. (1988). Managing complications of IV therapy. *Nursing 88, 18*(3), 34–42.

Myers, S. T. (1982). The search for assumptions. *Western Journal of Nursing Research, 4*(1), 91–98.

Nagel, E. (1961). *The structure of science: Problems in the logic of scientific explanation.* New York: Harcourt, Brace & World.

Prescott, P. A., & Soeken, K. L. (1989). Methodology corner: The potential uses of pilot work. *Nursing Research, 38*(1), 60–62.

Sidani, S., & Braden, C. J. (1998). *Evaluating nursing interventions: A theory-driven approach.* Thousand Oaks, CA: Sage.

Silva, M. C. (1981). Selection of a theoretical framework. In S. D. Krampitz & N. Pavlovich (Eds.), *Readings for nursing research* (pp. 17–28). St. Louis: C. V. Mosby.

Van Ort, S. (1981). Research design: Pilot study. In S. D. Krampitz & N. Pavlovich (Eds.), *Readings for nursing research* (pp. 49–53). St. Louis: C. V. Mosby.

Wallenstein, S. L. (1987). Research perspectives: A response. *Journal of Pain and Symptom Management, 2*(2), 103–106.

Wilkie, D. J., Williams, A. R., Grevstad, P., & Mekwa, J. (1995). COACHING persons with lung cancer to report sensory pain: Literature review and pilot study findings. *Cancer Nursing, 18*(1), 7–15.

Williams, M. A. (1980). Assumptions in research [Editorial]. *Research in Nursing & Health, 3*(2), 47–48.

Wysocki, A. B. (1983). Basic versus applied research: Intrinsic and extrinsic considerations. *Western Journal of Nursing Research, 5*(3), 217–224.

Younger, J., Marsh, K. J., & Grap, M. J. (1995). The relationship of health locus of control and cardiac rehabilitation to mastery of illness-related stress. *Journal of Advanced Nursing, 22*(2), 294–299.

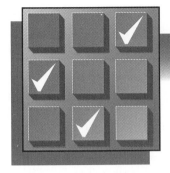

CHAPTER 4

INTRODUCTION TO QUALITATIVE RESEARCH

Qualitative research is a systematic, subjective approach used to describe life experiences and give them meaning (Leininger, 1985; Munhall, 1989; Silva & Rothbart, 1984). Qualitative research is not a new idea in the social or behavioral science (Baumrind, 1980; Glaser & Strauss, 1967; Kaplan, 1964; Scheffler, 1967). However, nursing's interest in qualitative research is relatively recent, having begun in the late 1970s.

Qualitative research is a way to gain insights through discovering meanings. However, these insights are obtained not through establishing causality but through improving our comprehension of the whole. Within a holistic framework, qualitative research is a means of exploring the depth, richness, and complexity inherent in phenomena. The insights from this process can guide nursing practice and aid in the important process of theory development for building nursing knowledge (Schwartz-Barcott & Kim, 1986).

Comprehension of qualitative research methodologies is necessary to critique the studies in publications and use the findings in practice. The terminology used in qualitative research and the methods of reasoning are different from those of quantitative research and are reflections of the philosophical orientations. The specific philosophical orientations differ with each qualitative approach and direct the methodology. Although each qualitative approach is unique, there are many commonalities. To facilitate comprehension of these methodologies, this chapter explores the logic underlying the qualitative approach, using gestalt change as a model. A general overview of the following qualita-

tive approaches is presented: phenomenological research, grounded theory research, ethnographic research, historical research, philosophical inquiry, and critical social theory.

THE LOGIC OF QUALITATIVE RESEARCH

The qualitative approaches are based on a world view that is holistic and has the following beliefs:

1. There is not a single reality.
2. Reality, based on perceptions, is different for each person and changes over time.
3. What we know has meaning only within a given situation or context.

The reasoning process used in qualitative research involves perceptually putting pieces together to make wholes. From this process, meaning is produced. However, because perception varies with the individual, many different meanings are possible (Munhall & Oiler, 1986). One can understand this reasoning process by exploring the formation of gestalts.

GESTALTS

The concept of gestalt is closely related to holism and proposes that knowledge about a particular phenomenon is organized into a cluster of linked ideas, a *gestalt*. A theory is a form of gestalt. If we are trying to understand something new and are offered a theory that explains it, our reaction may be "Now that makes sense" or "Oh, I see." The concept has "come together" for us.

One disadvantage of this process is that once we understand a phenomenon through the interpretation of a particular theory, it is difficult for us to "see" the phenomenon outside the meaning given it by that particular theory. Therefore, in addition to giving meaning, a theory can limit meaning. "Seeing" the phenomenon from the perspective of one point of view may limit our ability to see it from another point of view. For example, because Selye's theory of stress is so familiar to us as nurses, it would be difficult to examine the phenomenon of stress without using Selye's perception.

The purpose of qualitative research is to form new gestalts and, sometimes, to generate new theories. To accomplish this purpose, the researcher has to "get outside" any existing theories or gestalts that explain the phenomenon of interest. The researcher's mind must be open to new gestalts that emerge through abstract thinking processes while he or she is conducting the research.

Experiencing Gestalt Change

One qualitative researcher, Ihde (1977), has explained the process of (1) forming a gestalt, (2) "getting outside" that gestalt, and (3) developing a new gestalt in such a way that you can experience the process. According to the qualitative point of view, experiencing the process is the best way to understand it.

Ihde's extensive research has been conducted in the area of vision. He has studied how our eyes and brain perceive an image—for example, how our eyes sometimes see one line as shorter or longer than another when the lines are actually equal in length. Ihde has associated the vision of the eye with the way we "see" mentally. Consider the concrete thinking behind sayings such as "seeing makes it real," "seeing is believing," and "I saw it with my own eyes." It is easy to generalize from seeing to the other senses (hearing, touching, smelling, tasting), or empirical ways of knowing, and from there to perception. In fact, we often use phrases such as "I see" or "I hear" to mean "I understand."

Ihde (1977) proposes that we have an initial way of perceiving (or seeing) a phenomenon that is naive and inflexible but that we think is the one and only way of seeing that is real. "Seeing" occurs, however, within a specific context of beliefs, which Ihde calls a natural or *sedimented view*. In other words, we see things from the perspective of a specific frame of reference, world view, or theory. This is our reality, which gives us a sense of certainty, security, and control. Ihde uses line drawings to demonstrate this sedimented view. Examine the following line drawing:

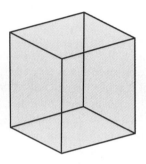

Most people who passively view this figure see a cube. If you continue to gaze at it, however, you will find that the cube reverses itself. The figure actually seems to move. It "jumps" and then becomes fixed again in your view. With practice, you can see first one view and then the other, and then reverse the cube again.

Ihde (1977) developed five alternative ways to view the following drawing and suggested that there are more. He refers to the smaller cube on the right as the "guide picture."

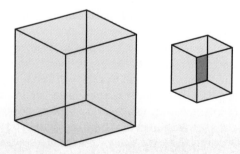

Suppose, now, that the cube drawing is not a cube at all, but is an insect in a hexagonal opening. . . . Suppose I tell you that the cube is not a cube at all, but is a very oddly cut gem. The central facet (the shaded area of the guide picture) is nearest you, and all the other facets are sloping downwards and away from it. . . . Now, suppose I tell you that the gem is also reversible. Suppose you are now inside the gem, looking upwards, so that the central facet (the shaded area of the guide picture) is the one farthest away from you, and the oddly cut side facets are sloping down towards you. (Idhe, 1977, pp. 96–98)

Ihde proposes that in order to see an alternative view of the drawing, you must first deconstruct your original sedimented view. You must then reconstruct another view. This activity involves the use of intuition. He regards this process as jumping from one gestalt to another.

Try examining the line drawing shown here. What is your sedimented view? Can you reconstruct another gestalt or view?

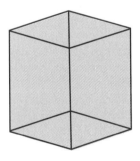

Ihde (1977) found that one of the important strategies in switching from one view of a drawing to another was to change one's focus. Try focusing on a different point of the drawing or looking at it as two-dimensional rather than as three-dimensional. If you concentrate and gaze for a long enough time, you can experience the change in gestalt. Ihde cautions that a new reconstruction tends to be considered odd at first and unnatural but attains stability and naturalness after a while.

Once you have accomplished this "jump," you are no longer naive; you cannot go back to the idea that the phenomenon you have observed can be seen in only one way. You have become more open

and receptive to experiencing the phenomenon; you can explore deeper layers of the phenomenon. Viewing these deeper layers requires a second-order deconstruction and an additional increase in openness. Ihde (1977) refers to this increase as *ascendance to the open context*. It allows you to see more depth and complexity within the phenomenon you examine; you have enlarged your capacity for insight. Ihde suggests that ascendance to the open context gives you multistability and greater control than the sedimented view.

Changing Gestalts in Nursing

Nursing has a strong traditional base. With this tradition comes a sedimented view of phenomena such as patients, illness situations, health, and nursing care and its effects. We are introduced to these sedimented views very early in our nursing experiences. Now in this era of nursing research we are beginning to question many of these long-held ideas, and the insights gained are changing nursing practice.

For example, for many years, nurses perceived the patient as being passive, dependent, and unable to take responsibility for his or her care. Now patients are more often perceived as participating in their care and being responsible for their health. Ascendance to the open context requires more than just switching from one sedimented view to another. The nurse functioning within an open context would be able to view the patient from a variety of perspectives, regarding him or her as passive and dependent in some ways, participating with health care givers in other ways, and directing his or her care in yet other ways.

Qualitative research provides a process through which we can examine a phenomenon outside the sedimented view. The earliest and perhaps most dramatic demonstration of the influence that qualitative research can have on nursing practice was the 4-year study conducted by Glaser and Strauss (1965, 1968, 1971), who are credited with developing a qualitative approach referred to as *grounded theory* for health-related topics. This study was reported in three books, entitled *Awareness of Dying*,

Time for Dying, and *Status Passage,* which described the social environment of dying patients in hospitals. At that time, the gestalt commonly held was that people could not cope with knowing that they were dying and must be protected from that knowledge. The environment of care was designed to keep from a dying patient the knowledge that he or she was dying.

Glaser and Strauss examined the meanings that social environment had to the patient. The study changed our gestalt. We now saw that instead of protecting the patient, traditional care of the dying was creating loneliness and isolation. We began to "see" the patient in a new light, and our care began to change. Kubler-Ross (1969), perhaps influenced by the work of Glaser and Strauss, then began her studies of the dying, using an approach similar to that of phenomenology. From this new orientation of caring for the dying, hospice care began to develop, and now, 30 years later, the environment of care for the dying is different.

PHILOSOPHY AND QUALITATIVE RESEARCH

In qualitative research, frameworks are not used in the same sense as they are in quantitative studies, because the goal is not theory testing. Nonetheless, each type of qualitative research is guided by a particular philosophical stance thought to be a paradigm. The philosophy directs the questions that are asked, the observations that are made, and how the data are interpreted (Munhall, 1989). These philosophical bases and their methodologies, developed outside nursing, will likely undergo evolutionary changes within nursing. The works of Parse (1981), Leininger (1985), Chenitz and Swanson (1984), and Artinian (1988), discussed later in the chapter, are illustrations of these changes.

RIGOR IN QUALITATIVE RESEARCH

Scientific rigor is valued because it is associated with the worth of research outcomes, and studies are critiqued as a means of judging rigor. Qualitative research methods have been criticized for lack of rigor. However, these criticisms have occurred because of attempts to judge the rigor of qualitative studies using rules developed to judge quantitative studies. Rigor needs to be defined differently for qualitative research because the desired outcome is different (Burns, 1989; Dzurec, 1989; Morse, 1989; Sandelowski, 1986).

In quantitative research, rigor is reflected in narrowness, conciseness, and objectivity and leads to rigid adherence to research designs and precise statistical analyses. In qualitative research, rigor is associated with openness, scrupulous adherence to a philosophical perspective, thoroughness in collecting data, and consideration of all the data in the subjective theory development phase. Evaluation of the rigor of a qualitative study is based, in part, on the logic of the emerging theory and the clarity with which it sheds light on the studied phenomenon.

In order to be rigorous in conducting qualitative research, the researcher must ascend to an open context and be willing to continue to let go of sedimented views (*deconstructing*). Maintaining openness requires discipline. The researcher will be examining many dimensions of the area being studied and forming new ideas (*reconstructing*) while continuing to recognize that the present reconstruction is only one of many possible ways of organizing data. Lack of rigor in qualitative research is due to problems such as (1) inconsistency in adhering to the philosophy of the approach being used, (2) failure to "get away from" older ideas, (3) poorly developed methods, (4) inadequate time spent collecting data, (5) poor observations, (6) failure to give careful consideration to all the data obtained, and (7) inadequacy of theoretical development from the data. Critique of qualitative studies is discussed in more detail in Chapter 26.

APPROACHES TO QUALITATIVE RESEARCH

Six approaches to qualitative research being used in nursing are presented here: phenomenological research, grounded theory research, ethnographic research, historical research, philosophical inquiry, and critical social theory. In some ways, these approaches are very different. Ethnography and historical research are broad and are the accepted methodologies for a discipline. Critical social theory is narrow in focus and controversial in its philosophical perspective. The world view of phenomenology is also controversial. However, in each method, the purpose is to examine meaning. The unit of analysis is words rather than numerical values.

Although the data are gathered through the use of an open context, this fact does not mean that the interpretation is value-free. Each approach is based on a philosophical orientation that influences the interpretation of the data. Thus, it is critical to understand the philosophy on which the method is based. In selecting a qualitative method, the researcher should consider the following:

- What is the most appropriate methodology and why?
- Which method of data collection will produce the richest set of data?
- How should the data be analyzed?
- What checks should be undertaken to maximize the accuracy of the findings? (Cutcliffe, 1997, p. 969)

Each approach is discussed in relation to the philosophical orientation, nursing knowledge, and a brief overview of research methodology. Data collection strategies and the process of qualitative data analysis are described in more detail in Chapter 23.

Phenomenological Research

Phenomenology is both a philosophy and a research method. The purpose of phenomenological research is to describe experiences as they are lived—in phenomenological terms, to capture the "lived experience" of study participants. The philosophers from whom phenomenology emerged include Husserl, Kierkegaard, Heidegger, Marcel, Sartre, and Merleau-Ponty (Boyd, 1993a; Munhall, 1989). The philosophical positions taken by phenomenological researchers are very different from those common in nursing's culture and research traditions and thus are difficult to understand. In fact, Holmes (1996) questions the fit between phenomenological philosophy and nursing philosophy. Discussions of this philosophical stance, which have

been appearing more frequently in the nursing literature, are introducing a broader audience to these ideas (Anderson, 1989; Beck, 1994; Boyd, 1993b; Hallett, 1995; Leonard, 1989; Munhall, 1989; Salsberry, Smith, & Boyd, 1989; Walters, 1995).

PHILOSOPHICAL ORIENTATION

Phenomenologists view the person as integral with the environment. The world is shaped by the self and also shapes the self. At this point, however, phenomenologists diverge in their beliefs. Heideggerian phenomenologists believe that the person is a self within a body. Thus, the person is referred to as *embodied.* "Our bodies provide the possibility for the concrete actions of self in the world" (Leonard, 1989, p. 48). The person has a world, which is "the meaningful set of relationships, practices, and language that we have by virtue of being born into a culture" (Leonard, 1989, p. 43). The person is *situated* as a consequence of being shaped by his or her world and thus is constrained in the ability to establish meanings through language, culture, history, purposes, and values. Therefore, the person has only *situated* freedom, not total freedom. A person's world is so pervasive that generally, he or she does not notice it, unless some disruption occurs. Not only is the world of each person different, but each person's concerns are qualitatively different. The body, the world, and the concerns, unique to each person, are the *context* within which that person can be understood. Husserlian phenomenologists believe that although self and world are mutually shaping, it is possible to bracket oneself from one's beliefs, to see the world firsthand in a naive way.

Heideggerians believe that the person experiences *being* within the framework of time. This is referred to as *being-in-time.* The past and the future influence the now and, thus, are part of being-in-time (Leonard, 1989). All phenomenologists agree that there is not a single reality; each individual has his or her own reality. Reality is considered subjective; thus, an experience is considered unique to the individual. This is true even for the researcher's experiences in collecting data for a study and analyzing the data. "Truth is an interpretation of some phenomenon; the more shared that interpretation is, the more factual it seems to be, yet it remains temporal and cultural" (Munhall, 1989). The researcher needs to invest considerable time exploring the various philosophical stances within phenomenology to select one compatible with his or her perspective.

Taylor (1995) provides an excellent description of her search for a compatible phenomenological perspective, discussing the methods of Langveld (1978), Heidegger (1962), Husserl (1960, 1964, 1970, 1980) and Gadamer (1975). According to Taylor (1995), "the search for the nature of a phenomenon begins with the people, in their place and time, and it leads to an explication of the aspects of a phenomenon. The nature of a phenomenon is a reflection of the nature of people as human beings, who find themselves within the context of a healthcare institution, who are living and making sense of their experiences. The language used by the people in the research not only illuminates the nature of the phenomenon of interest, but it also shows some of their own There-Being as human beings."

METHODOLOGY

The broad question that phenomenologists ask is, "What is the meaning of one's lived experience?" Being a person is self-interpreting; therefore, the only reliable source of information to answer this question is the person. Understanding human behavior or experience requires that the person interpret the action or experience for the researcher, and then the researcher must interpret the explanation provided by the person.

Developing Research Questions

The first step in conducting a phenomenological study is to identify the phenomenon to be explored. Next, the researcher develops a research question. Two factors need to be considered in developing the research question: "(1) What are the necessary and sufficient constituents of this feeling or experience? (2) What does the existence of this feeling or experience indicate concerning the nature of the human being?" (Omery, 1983, p. 55)

Sampling

After developing the research question, the researcher identifies sources of the phenomenon being studied and, from these sources, seeks individuals who are willing to describe their experiences with the phenomenon in question. These individuals must understand and be willing to express inner feelings and describe the physiological experiences that occur with the feelings.

Data Collection and Analysis

Data are collected through a variety of means: observation, interactive interviews, videotape, and written descriptions by subjects. Analysis begins when the first data are collected and then guides decisions related to further data collection. The meanings attached to the data are expressed within the phenomenological philosophy. The outcome of analysis is a theoretical statement responding to the research question. The statement is validated by examples of the data—often, direct quotes from the subjects.

NURSING KNOWLEDGE AND PHENOMENOLOGY

Phenomenology is the philosophical base for three nursing theories: Parse's (1981) theory of man-living-health, Paterson and Zderad's (1976) theory of humanistic nursing, and Watson's (1985) theory of caring. By virtue of the assumptions of her theory, Parse (1981, 1990) states that the only acceptable method of testing her theory is through qualitative research. She also holds that any qualitative method—phenomenological, ethnographic, exploratory, or case method—can be used because all of these methods are consistent with phenomenological theory (Parse, 1990). Parse (1987, 1995) has also developed a man-living-health research methodology, which "includes the processes of dialogical engagement (researcher-person dialogues), extraction-synthesis (transforming the data across levels of abstraction to the level of science), and heuristic interpretation (specifying the findings in the light of the man-living-health theory and integrating them into the language of the theory)" (Parse, 1990, p. 140).

A number of the published phenomenological nursing studies are based on the man-living-health theory. Parse (1990) regards these studies as clarifying or substantiating her theory. The following abstract is from a study using Parse's method.

· ·

"Parse's research method was used to investigate the meaning of serenity for survivors of a life-threatening illness or traumatic event. Ten survivors of cancer told their stories of the meaning of serenity as they had lived it in their lives. Descriptions were aided by photographs chosen by each participant to represent the meaning of serenity for them. The structure of serenity was generated through the extraction-synthesis process. Four main concepts—steering-yielding with the flow, savoring remembered visions of engaging surroundings, abiding with aloneness-togetherness, and attesting to a loving presence—emerged and led to a theoretical structure of serenity from the human becoming perspective. Findings confirm serenity as a multidimensional process." (Kruse, 1999, p. 143) ■

Grounded Theory Research

Grounded theory is an inductive research technique developed for health-related topics by Glaser and Strauss (1967). It emerged from the discipline of sociology. The term *grounded* means that the theory developed from the research is based on or has its roots in the data from which it was derived. Artinian (1998, p. 5) indicates that "grounded theory provides a way to transcend experience—to move it from a description of what is happening to understanding the process by which it happens."

PHILOSOPHICAL ORIENTATION

Grounded theory is based on symbolic interaction theory, which holds many views in common with phenomenology. George Herbert Mead (1934), a social psychologist, was a leader in the development of symbolic interaction theory. Symbolic interaction theory explores how people define reality and how their beliefs are related to their actions. Reality is created by people through attaching meanings to

situations. Meaning is expressed in terms of symbols, such as words, religious objects, and clothing. These symbolic meanings are the basis for actions and interactions.

Unfortunately, symbolic meanings are different for each individual. We cannot completely know the symbolic meanings of another individual. In social life, meanings are shared by groups. These shared meanings are communicated to new members through socialization processes. Group life is based on consensus and shared meanings. Interaction may lead to redefinition and new meanings, and can result in the redefinition of self. Because of its theoretical importance, the interaction is the focus of observation in grounded theory research (Chenitz & Swanson, 1986).

Grounded theory has been used most frequently to study areas in which little previous research has been conducted and to gain a new viewpoint in familiar areas of research. Because of the basic quality of theory generated through this methodology, however, further theory testing is not usually needed to enhance usefulness.

METHODOLOGY

The steps of grounded theory research occur simultaneously. The researcher observes, collects data, organizes data, and forms theory from the data at the same time. An important methodological technique in grounded theory research is the constant comparative process, in which every piece of data is compared with every other piece. The methodological techniques used in grounded theory research are explained in depth in two books, *Theoretical Sensitivity*, by Glazer (1978), and *From Practice to Grounded Theory: Qualitative Research in Nursing*, by Chenitz and Swanson (1986).

Data Collection and Analysis Techniques

Data may be collected by interview, observation, records, or a combination of these techniques. Data collection usually results in large amounts of handwritten notes or typed interview transcripts that contain multiple pieces of data to be sorted and analyzed. This process is initiated by coding and categorizing of the data.

Outcomes

The outcome is a theory explaining the phenomenon under study. The research report presents the theory supported by examples from the data. The literature review and numerical results are not used in the report. The report tends to be narrative discussions of the study process and findings.

NURSING KNOWLEDGE AND GROUNDED THEORY

Artinian (1988) has identified four qualitative modes of nursing inquiry within grounded theory, each used for different purposes: descriptive mode, discovery mode, emergent fit mode, and intervention mode.

The *descriptive mode* provides rich detail and must precede all other modes. This mode, ideal for the beginning researcher, answers questions such as What is going on? How are activities organized? What roles are evident? What are the steps in a process? What does a patient do in a particular setting?

The *discovery mode* leads to the identification of patterns in life experiences of individuals and relates the patterns to one another. Through this mode, a theory of social process, referred to as *substantive theory*, is developed that explains a particular social world.

The *emergent fit mode* is used to extend or refine substantive theory after it has been developed. This mode enables the researcher to focus on a selected portion of the theory, to build on previous work, or to establish a research program around a particular social process.

The *intervention mode* is used to test the relationships in the substantive theory. The fundamental question for this mode is How can I make something happen in such a way as to bring about new and desired states of affairs? This mode demands deep involvement on the part of the researcher or practitioner.

The following abstract is taken from a grounded theory study.

∙∙∙

"A naturalistic field study of low-income women (N = 17) in an intensive outpatient addiction recovery program addressed the question: What is the nature of addiction recovery for pregnant and parenting women in an addiction treatment program? Grounded theory methodology was used to determine the nature of the interpersonal and social processes that define addiction recovery for women in this study. Over 2 years, audiotaped semi-structured interviews, document reviews of medical records, treatment progress and group therapy notes, and participant observation notes were collected and analyzed. The constant comparison method of analysis involved an ongoing process of theoretical sampling, memoing, and open and then axial coding to identify, group, link, and reduce the categories produced. A developmental model of addiction recovery in pregnant and parenting women emerged that consisted of the dimensions of becoming drug and alcohol free, a partner in a relationship, a person, and a parent. These four dimensions parallel and transform each other, yielding different outcomes but similar patterns over time. This model of addiction recovery provides a beginning framework for understanding the transactional nature of addiction recovery for low-income women who are adapting to a drug and alcohol-free lifestyle and the task and role of parenting a newborn." (Nardi, 1998, p. 81) ■

As can be seen from the study described, grounded theory research examines a much broader scope of dimensions than is usually possible with quantitative research. The findings can be intuitively verified by the experiences of the reader. The clear, cohesive description of the phenomenon can allow greater understanding and, thus, more control of nursing practice.

Ethnographic Research

Ethnographic research provides a mechanism for studying our own culture and that of others. The word *ethnographic* means "portrait of a people." Although ethnography originated as the research methodology for the discipline of anthropology, it is now a part of the cultural research conducted by a number of other disciplines, including social psychology, sociology, political science, education, and nursing, and is also used in feminist research. Although all ethnography focuses on culture, not all cultural research is, or needs to be, ethnography. Ethnography describes and analyzes aspects of the ways of life of particular cultures, subcultures, or subculture groups. Ethnographic studies result in theories of culture. Ethnography has been associated with studies of primitive, foreign, or remote cultures. Such studies enabled the researcher to acquire new perspectives beyond his or her own ethnocentric perspective. Today, the emphasis has shifted to obtaining cultural knowledge within one's own society (Germain, 1993). Within nursing, one of the major contributions of ethnography may be to promote culturally specific care (Baillie, 1995).

PHILOSOPHICAL ORIENTATION

Anthropology, which began about the same time as the nursing discipline did, in the mid-19th century, seeks to understand people: their ways of living, ways of believing, and ways of adapting to changing environmental circumstances. The philosophical basis for anthropology has not been spelled out clearly, is in evolution, and needs considerable refinement (Sanday, 1983). *Culture*, the most central concept, is defined by Leininger (1970, pp. 48–49), a nurse anthropologist, as "a way of life belonging to a designated group of people . . . a blueprint for living which guides a particular group's thoughts, actions, and sentiments . . . all the accumulated ways a group of people solve problems, which are reflected in the people's language, dress, food, and a number of accumulated traditions and customs." The purpose of anthropological research is to describe a culture through examining these various cultural characteristics.

Anthropologists study the origin of people, their past ways of living, and their ways of surviving through time. These insights increase our ability to predict the future directions of cultures and the forces that guide their destiny or may provide opportunities to influence the direction of cultural development (Leininger, 1970). Many cultural aspects of our own society need to be understood in order to address issues related to health.

[C]ultures and subcultures in American society may be found in rural and urban ethnic and racial enclaves; non-

ethnic groups such as those located in prisons and bars; complex organizations; factories; the social institutions such as nursing homes, hospitals, or shelters for the homeless or the abused; community-based groups of various types such as street gangs, motorcycle gangs, and teenage groups such as jocks and skinheads; religious communities; and disciplines such as nursing and medicine. Thus, for example, nursing is a professional culture, a hospital is a sociocultural institution, and a unit of a hospital can be viewed as a subculture. (Germain, 1993, p. 238)

A number of dimensions of culture are of interest within anthropology. *Material culture* consists of all man-made objects associated with a given group. *Ethnoscientific* ethnography focuses on the ideas, beliefs, and knowledge that a group holds that are expressed in language, and may address aspects such as symbolic referents, the network of social relations, and the beliefs reflected in social and political institutions. Cultures also have ideals that the people hold as desirable, even though they do not always live up to these standards. A relatively new approach, referred to as *cognitive anthropology*, holds the view that culture is an adaptive system that is in the minds of people and is expressed in the language or semantic system of the group. Studies from this perspective examine observable patterns of behavior, customs, and ways of life. Anthropologists seek to discover the many parts of a whole culture and how these parts are interrelated, so that a picture of the wholeness of the culture evolves. Ethnographic research is used in nursing not just to increase ethnic cultural awareness but also to enhance the provision of quality health care for all cultures (Germain, 1993; Laugharne, 1995; Leininger, 1970).

METHODOLOGY

There are two basic research approaches in anthropology, emic and etic. The *emic approach* to research involves studying behaviors from within the culture. The *etic approach* involves studying behaviors from outside the culture and examining similarities and differences among cultures. The steps of ethnographic research are as follows: (1) identifying the culture to be studied, (2) identifying the significant variables within the culture, (3) literature review, (4) gaining entrance, (5) cultural immersion, (6) acquiring informants, (7) gathering data (elicitation procedures), (8) analysis of data, (9) description of the culture, and (10) theory development.

Literature Review

The purpose of a literature review in ethnographic research is to provide background for the study. The researcher is seeking a broad general understanding of the variables to be considered in a specific culture or subculture.

Data Collection and Analysis

Data collection involves primarily observation and interview. The researcher may become a participant/observer in the culture, so that he or she "becomes a part of the subculture being studied by physical association with the people in their setting during a period of fieldwork. . . . The researcher learns from informants the meanings they attach to their activities, events, behaviors, knowledge, rituals, and other aspects of their life-style" (Germain, 1993, p. 238).

Analysis involves identifying the meanings attributed to objects and events by members of the culture. These meanings are often validated by members of the culture before the results are finalized.

NURSING KNOWLEDGE AND ETHNOGRAPHY

A group of nurse scientists, lead by Madeleine Leininger, have developed a strategy of ethnonursing research, which emerged from Leininger's theory of transcultural nursing (Leininger, 1985, 1990, 1991, 1997). *Ethnonursing research* "focuses mainly on observing and documenting interactions with people of how these daily life conditions and patterns are influencing human care, health, and nursing care practices" (Leininger, 1985, p. 238). Munet-Vilero (1988) identifies three problems related to the use of ethnographic methodology by nurses. First, nurse researchers may not be sufficiently familiar with the cultural mores of the people being studied or their language. Second, studies sometimes use measures that are assumed, inaccurately,

to be equivalent among cultures. Third, interpretation of findings may be inadequate because of the limited knowledge of the culture being studied. These concerns should be carefully considered by nurse researchers who are planning ethnographic studies.

The following abstract is taken from an ethnographic study.

● ●

"Vigilance, or the close, protective involvement of families caring for hospitalized relatives, was explored in this study using holistic ethnography. Leininger's theory of cultural care diversity and universality provided direction for the researcher to generate substantive data about the meanings, patterns, and day-to-day experience of vigilance. Five categories of meaning were derived from the data: commitment to care, emotional upheaval, dynamic nexus, transition, and resilience. The research findings expand understanding of vigilance as a caring expression, suggest direction for nursing practice, and contribute to Leininger's theory of cultural care diversity and universality and the development of nursing science." (Carr, 1998, p. 74) ▪

Studies such as this provide insights that can be used in many clinical situations. Reading this type of study can lead the nurse to ask different questions about patients and their behavior.

Historical Research

Historiography examines events of the past. Many historians believe that the greatest value of historical knowledge is a greater self-understanding. Historical nursing research also increases nurses' understanding of their profession.

PHILOSOPHICAL ORIENTATION

History is a very old science that dates back to the beginnings of humankind. The primary questions of history are, Where have we come from? Who are we? Where are we going? Although the questions do not change, the answers do.

The most ancient form of history is the myth. The myth explains origins and gives justification to the order of existence. In the myth, past, present, and future are not distinguishable. Myths, which are a form of storytelling, provide an image of and legitimize the existing order.

History moved beyond the myth to the chronicling of events such as great deeds, victories, and stories about peoples and citizens. These descriptions blurred the distinction between the real and the ideal. Historians then moved to comparing histories, selecting histories on the basis of values, and identifying patterns of regularity and change.

More recently, there has been a move to interpretive history, an effort to make sense out of it, to search for meaning. Interpretation may be accomplished by concept development, by explaining causality through theory development, and by generalizing to other events and other times. Miller (1967, p. xxxi) suggests, "History is an estimate of the past from the standpoint of the present." Looking at history from the present, historians may see their role as that of patriots, as judges and censors of morals, or as detached observers. The values contained in each of these roles are reflected in the nature of the historical interpretation.

Philosophers found that understanding humankind as a historical phenomenon held out the promise of understanding the essence of humankind. To this extent, the development of a historical method was of interest to philosophy (Pflug, 1971). The initial philosophy of history and an associated research methodology were developed by Voltaire (Sakmann, 1971). His strategy was to look at general lines of development rather than to offer an indiscriminate presentation of details, the common practice of historians of his period. Using this strategy, Voltaire moved history from chronicling to critical analysis. He recognized that in history there can be no certainty, but he searched for criteria by which historical truth could be ascertained.

One of the assumptions of historical philosophy is that "there is nothing new under the sun." Because of this assumption, the historian can search throughout history for generalizations. For example, the question can be asked "What causes wars?" The historian could search throughout history for commonalities and develop a theoretical explanation of the causes of wars. The questions asked, the factors that the historian selects to look for throughout history, and the nature of the explanation are all based on a world view (Heller, 1982).

Another assumption of historical philosophy is that one can learn from the past. The philosophy of history is a search for wisdom, with the historian examining what has been, what is, and what ought to be. Historical philosophers have attempted to identify a developmental scheme for history, to explain all events and structures as elements of the same social process. Heller (1982) identifies three developmental schemes found in philosophies of history, as follows:

1. History reflects progression—the development from "lower" to "higher" stages.
2. History has a tendency to regress—development is from "higher" stages to "lower" stages; movement is toward a decrease in freedom and the self-destruction of our species.
3. History shows a repetition of developmental sequences in which patterns of progression and regression can be seen.

Fitzpatrick (1993, p. 361) suggests that "there is usually a tendency to justify historical research in professional fields like nursing from the standpoint of its helping to inform future decisions and to avoid repeating past mistakes. Such arguments have only slight merit because they serve a reductionist belief that historical facts can be distilled with a formula. History, although its goal is the establishment of fact that leads us to truth, cannot be reduced to statistical proof."

NURSING KNOWLEDGE AND HISTORIOGRAPHY

Christy (1978, p. 9) asks, "How can we in nursing today possibly plan where we are going when we don't know where we have been nor how we got here?" One criterion of a profession is that there is a knowledge of the history of the profession that is transmitted to those entering the profession. Until recently, historical nursing research has not been a valued activity, and few nurse researchers had the skills or desire to conduct it. Therefore, our knowledge of our past is sketchy. However, there is now a growing interest in the field of historical nursing research. Sarnecky (1990) suggests that the greater interest in historiography is related to the move from a total focus on logical positivism to a broader perspective that is fully supportive of the type of knowledge provided by historical research.

METHODOLOGY

The methodology of historical research consists of the following steps: (1) formulating an idea, (2) developing research questions, (3) developing an inventory of sources, (4) clarifying the validity and reliability of data, (5) developing a research outline, and (6) conducting data collection and analysis.

Formulating an Idea

The first step in historical research is selecting a topic. Some appropriate topics for historical research in nursing are "Origins, epochs, events treated as units; movements, trends, patterns over stated periods; history of specific agencies or institutions; broad studies of the development of needs for specialized types of nursing; biographies and portrayals of the nurse in literature, art, or drama" (Newton, 1965, p. 20).

As with many types of research, the initial ideas for historical research tend to be broad. Initial ideas must be clearly stated and narrowed to a topic that is precisely defined so that the time required to search for related materials is realistic. In addition to narrowing the topic, it is often important to limit the historical period to be studied. Limiting the period requires a knowledge of the broader social, political, and economic factors that would have an impact on the topic under study.

The researcher may spend much time extensively reading related literature before making a final decision about the precise topic. For example, Waring (1978) conducted her doctoral dissertation using historical research to examine the idea of the nurse experiencing a "calling" to practice nursing. In the following abstract from that dissertation, she describes the extensive process of developing a precise topic.

• •

"Originally my idea was to pursue concepts in the area of Puritan social thought and to relate concepts such as altruism and self-sacrifice to nurs-

ing. Two years after the formulation of this first idea, I finally realized that the topic was too broad. Reaching that point was slow and arduous but quite essential to the development of my thinking and the prospectus that developed as an outcome.

When I first began the process, it seemed that I might have to abandon the topic 'calling.' Now, since the clarification and tightening up of my title and the clarification of my study thesis, I open volumes fearing that I will find yet another reference, once overlooked. It is only recently that I have become convinced that there was a needle in the haystack and that I had indeed found it." (Waring, 1978, pp. 18–19) ■

In historical research, there frequently is no problem statement. Rather than being defined in a problem statement, the research topic is usually expressed in the title of the study. For example, the title of Waring's dissertation was *American Nursing and the Concept of the Calling*.

Developing Research Questions

After the topic has been clearly defined, the researcher identifies the questions to be examined during the research process. These questions tend to be more general and analytical than those found in quantitative studies. In the following excerpt, Evans, then a doctoral student, describes the research questions she developed for her historical study.

• •

"I propose to study the nursing student. Who was this living person inside the uniform? Where did she come from? What were her experiences as a nursing student? I use the word 'experience' in terms of the dictionary definition of 'living through.' What did she live through? What happened to her and how did she respond, or react, as the case may be? What was her educational program like? We have a pretty good notion of what nurse educators and others thought about the educational program, but what about it from the students' point of view?

What were the functions of rituals and rites of passage such as bed check, morning inspection, and capping?

What kind of person did the nursing student

tend to become in order to successfully negotiate studenthood? What are the implications of this in terms of her own personal and professional development and the development of the profession at large?" (Evans, 1978, p. 16) ■

Developing an Inventory of Sources

The next step is to determine whether sources of data for the study exist and are available. Many of the materials needed for historical research are contained within private archives in libraries or are privately owned. One must obtain written permission to gain access to library archives. Private materials are often difficult to ferret out, and when they are discovered, access to them may be a problem. However, Sorensen (1988) believes that the primary problem is the lack of experience of nurse researchers with the use of archival data. Sorensen (1988) and Fairman (1987) have identified the major sources of archival data for historical nursing studies (see Table 4–1). Lusk (1997) also provides an

---

TABLE 4–1
SOURCES OF ARCHIVAL DATA FOR HISTORICAL NURSING STUDIES

The American Journal of Nursing Company
Bellevue Hospital
Boston University, Mugar Memorial Library
Columbia University
Hampton University
Johns Hopkins University
Massachusetts General Hospital, The Palmer–Davis Library
The Museum of Nursing History, Inc.
National Archives
National League for Nursing, National Library of Medicine
New York Hospital—Cornell Medical Center
New York Public Library, Manuscript Division
New York State Nurses' Association Library
Rockefeller Archive Center
Schlesinger Library at Radcliffe College
Simmons College
Sophia Smith Women's History Archive at Smith College in Massachusetts
Stanford University, Lane Medical Library
State University of New York at Buffalo
University of California at San Francisco
University of Illinois
University of Pennsylvania
University of Texas at Austin
University of Wisconsin—Milwaukee
Yale University

---

extensive discussion of sources for historical researchers. Lusk suggests that the pleasure of the pursuit for sources should not be underrated. The assistance of a librarian in selecting appropriate indexes is recommended.

Historical materials in nursing, such as letters, memos, handwritten materials, and mementos of significant leaders in nursing, are being discarded because no one recognizes their value. The same is true of materials related to the history of institutions and agencies within which nursing has been involved. Christy (1978, p. 9) observes, "It seems obvious that interest in the preservation of historical materials will only be stimulated if there is a concomitant interest in the value of historical research."

Sometimes, when such material is found, it is in such poor condition that much of the data are unclear or completely lost. Christy describes one of her experiences in searching for historical data in the following excerpt.

. . . .

"M. Adelaide Nutting and Isabel M. Stewart are two of the greatest leaders we have ever had, and their friends, acquaintances, and former students were persons of tremendous importance to developments in nursing and nursing education throughout the world. Since both of these women were historians, they saved letters, clippings, manuscripts—primary source materials of inestimable value. Their friends were from many walks of life: physicians, lawyers, social workers, philanthropists—supporters and nonsupporters of nursing and nursing interests. Miss Nutting and Miss Stewart crammed these documents into boxes, files, and whatever other receptacles were available and—unfortunately—some of these materials are this very day in those same old boxes.

"When I began my research into the Archives in 1966, the files were broken, rusty, and dilapidated. Many of the folders were so old and ill-tended that they fell apart in my hands, the ancient paper crumbled into dust before my eyes. My research was exhilaratingly stimulating, and appallingly depressing at the same time; stimulating due to the gold mine of data available, and depressing as I realized the lack of care provided for such priceless materials. In addition, there was little or no organization, and one had to go through each document, in each drawer, in each file, piece by piece. . . . The boxes and cartons were worse, for materials bearing absolutely no relationship to each other were simply piled, willy-nilly, one atop the other. Is it any wonder that it took me eighteen months of solid work to get through them?" (Christy, 1978, pp. 8–9) ▪

Currently, most historical nursing research has focused on nursing leaders. However, Noel (1988, p. 107) suggests that "women in general are woefully underrepresented in the biographical form." She comments that worthy nurses are those controversial figures who have influenced broad segments of their cultures, although any life well told can help the reader understand and value the individual and his or her contributions. She suggests two prerequisites for selecting a subject, 'the biographers' interest, affinity, or fatal fascination for the subject (living or dead) . . . and the existence and availability of data" (Noel, 1988, p. 107).

Life histories can provide insight into the lives of significant nursing figures. Gathering data for life histories involves collecting stories and interpretations told by the individual being studied. This method allows the individuals to present their views of their lives in their own words. Life histories have been viewed with skepticism because findings are difficult to verify, results are vague, and generalization is very limited. In-depth and repeated interviews longitudinally overcome some of these drawbacks, but selective memory of the subject can be problematic. Triangulation of data collection methods and verification with other sources reduce this limitation (Admi, 1995).

Rosenberg (1987) has identified eight areas that are important to examine from a nursing history perspective: (1) history from below—the life of ordinary men and women in nursing, (2) gender and the professions, (3) knowledge and authority, (4) the role of technology, (5) the new institutional history, (6) the hospital as problematic, (7) the nurse as worker, and (8) history as meaning.

There seems to have been no examination of historical patterns of nursing practice. Because so much of nursing knowledge has been transmitted verbally or by role-modeling, we as nurses may lose much of the understanding of our roots unless studies are initiated to record them. We have no clear picture of how nursing practice has changed over the years (e.g., When, how, and for what reasons have nursing care patterns changed for individuals experiencing diabetes, cardiovascular disease, surgery, or stroke?). Changes in nursing procedures, such as bed baths, enemas, and the feeding of patients, could be examined. Procedure manuals, policy books, and nurses' notes in patient charts are useful sources for examining changes in nursing practice.

Some possible research questions are as follows:

1. Which nursing practice changes were due to medical actions, and which were nursing innovations?
2. What factors in nursing influence changes in nursing practice?
3. What are the time patterns for changes in practice?
4. Have the time patterns for changes in practice remained fairly consistent, or have they changed over the history of nursing?
5. What has been the influence of levels of education (LVN, ADN, Diploma, BSN) on nursing practice?
6. What has been the influence of advanced nursing roles (Clinical Nurse Specialist, Nurse Practitioner, Administrator) on nursing practice?
7. How has the quality of nursing care changed over the decade? Century?

This type of information might provide greater insight into future directions for nursing practice, research, and theory development. However, if quality historical research is to be conducted, those of us in the process of making history must accept responsibility for preserving the sources.

Philosophical Inquiry

Philosophy is not generally thought of as a discipline within which one conducts research, because philosophy is not a science. Philosophy does, however, have strong links with science. Most importantly, philosophy guides the methods within any given science; it is the foundation of science. Furthermore, philosophy is used to develop theories about science and to debate issues related to science. The purpose of philosophical inquiry is to perform research using intellectual analyses to clarify meanings, make values manifest, identify ethics, and study the nature of knowledge (Ellis, 1983).

PHILOSOPHICAL ORIENTATION

The philosophical researcher considers an idea or issue from all perspectives through an extensive exploration of the literature, examining conceptual meaning, raising questions, proposing answers, and suggesting the implications of those answers. The research is guided by philosophical questions that have been posed. As with other qualitative approaches, data collection in philosophical inquiry occurs simultaneously with analysis and focuses on words. However, because philosophy attends to ideas, meaning, and abstractions, the content the researcher seeks may be implied rather than clearly stated in the literature. It may be necessary for the researcher to come to some conclusions about what the author meant in a specific text. Ideas, questions, answers, and consequences are often explored or debated or both with colleagues during the analysis phase. The process is cyclical, with answers generating further questions, leading to further analysis. Therefore, the thoughtful posing of questions is considered more important than the answers.

To avoid bias in their analysis, philosophers cultivate detachment from any particular type of knowledge or method. Published reports of philosophical inquiries do not describe the methodology used but focus on discussing the conclusions of the analyses. There are three categories of philosophical inquiry: foundational inquiry, philosophical analyses, and ethical analyses.

FOUNDATIONAL INQUIRY

The *foundations* of a science are its philosophical bases, concepts, and theories. A new science tends to borrow elements from the foundations of other sciences, although sometimes they are a poor fit. Even those developed within the science may have problems, such as logical inconsistencies. *Foundational inquiries* examine the foundations for a science. The studies include analyses of the structure of a science, and of the process of thinking about and valuing certain phenomena held in common by the science. They are important to perform prior to developing theories or programs of research. The debates related to qualitative and quantitative research methods and triangulation of methods emerge from foundational inquiries.

Nursing Knowledge and Foundational Inquiry

Philosophical analyses are expected to be carried out by scientists within a particular field, such as nursing, rather than by philosophers as such. What is recommended is that the nurse scientist desiring to perform a philosophical study seek consultation with a philosopher. An example of a foundational analysis is presented in Chapter 23.

Purposes

The purposes for a foundational study include the following:

1. Compare different philosophical bases, different theories, and different definitions of concepts.
2. Seek common meanings in radically different theories.
3. Critically examine operational definitions of concepts.
4. Explore the relationship between the concept and the science being examined.
5. Define the boundaries of a specific science by showing what phenomena belong to the field and what do not (boundary delineation).
6. Assist in the development of programs of research capable of shaping the empirical content of the field.
7. Draw attention to differences in ways of exploring, explaining, proving, and valuing.
8. Explain the rationale or thoughtful consequences of choosing various ways to investigate phenomena.
9. Analyze the reasoning that underlies the science.
10. Describe productive reasoning activities from which the science may develop methods for conducting foundational inquiries as well as conceiving, planning, executing, and monitoring its programs of research.

Questions

Because philosophical questions are critical to the process of philosophical inquiry, the formation of questions of concern to the discipline is important. Ellis (1983, pp. 212, 224) identified the following questions that need to be addressed in nursing from the perspective of philosophical inquiry: "What does it mean to be human? What is the meaning of dignity? What does it mean to be compassionate, humane, and caring? What is nursing? . . . What views of humans are appropriate, for what purpose, and for what questions?"

PHILOSOPHICAL ANALYSIS

The primary purpose of *philosophical analysis* is to examine meaning and to develop theories of meaning. This is usually accomplished through concept analysis or linguistic analysis (Rodgers, 1989). In some cases, attempts are made to reconcile apparently different concepts. These analyses clarify the language of a science and use multiple concepts and their relationships to organize the phenomena of a science. Clarification of the process of theory development and the criteria for critiquing theories emerges from philosophical inquiry and is referred to as *metatheory*.

Critiques of these analyses are conducted to determine completeness, meaning, and an explanation of scientific significance. These analyses provide descriptions of the meaning of a word as it is used in theoretical models and in research programs using those models. Linguistic analysis requires an examination of the occasions, intentions, and practical consequences of using certain words relevant to the science. This examination includes (1) their function when applied to various research problems in different sciences, (2) their operational definitions, (3) the kinds of research methods they dictate, (4) their relationship with the theoretical goals and values of the science in which they function, and (5) most important, their possible relationship to the idea of nursing science (Manchester, 1986).

Nursing Knowledge and Philosophical Analysis

Ellis (1983) suggests that many of the "nursing theories" are actually philosophies of nursing even though they were not developed through the use of philosophical analysis. These philosophies of nursing were developed to express the essence of nursing and the desired goals of nursing. They are statements of the way nursing ought to be. Concept analyses are strengthening our nursing theories and providing conceptual definitions for our research. An example of a concept analysis using the methods of philosophical analysis is presented in Chapter 23.

ETHICAL INQUIRY

Ethics is the branch of philosophy that deals with morality. This discipline contains a set of propositions for the intellectual analysis of morality. The problems of ethics relate to obligation, rights, duty, right and wrong, conscience, justice, choice, intention, and responsibility. Ethics is a means of striving for rational ends when others are involved. The desirable rational ends are justice, generosity, trust, faithfulness, love, and friendship. These ends reflect respect for the other person. An ethical dilemma occurs when one must choose between conflicting values. In some cases, both choices are good, and in other cases, neither choice is good but one must choose even so (Steele & Harmon, 1983).

Methodology

In *ethical inquiry*, the researcher identifies principles to guide conduct on the basis of ethical theories. The research methodology is similar to other philosophical inquiries. The literature related to the problem is thoroughly examined. With the use of a selected ethical theory, an analysis is performed. The actions prescribed by the analysis may vary with the ethical theory used. The ideas are submitted to colleagues for critique and debate. Their conclusions reflect judgments of value, which are prescriptive in nature. They are associated with rights and duties rather than preferences.

Nursing Knowledge and Ethics

Curtin (1979), a nurse ethicist, claims that the goals of nursing are not scientific; they are moral and seek good. To her, nursing is not a science; it is an art. Scientific knowledge is used as a tool in the artful practice of nursing (Curtin, 1990). As such, ethical inquiry is a research method required to clarify the means and ends of nursing practice. Much of the ethical analyses in the nursing literature addresses the following three issues: (1) combining the roles of nurse and scientist, (2) protection of human subjects, and (3) peer and institutional review (Gortner, 1985). An example of a study using ethical inquiry is presented in Chapter 23.

Critical Social Theory

Another philosophy with a unique qualitative research methodology is critical social theory. Feminist research, which is receiving growing interest in nursing, uses critical social theory methods and could be considered a subset of critical social theory (Chinn & Wheeler, 1985; MacPherson, 1983). Allen (1985, p. 62) believes that critical social theory is important to nursing because nurses need to "be as conscious as possible about the constraints operating on both nurse and client." She also suggests that the way nurses define health, promote health, and define themselves as nurses is governed by factors explored within this philosophy (Allen, 1986).

The perspective of critical social theory has led to the development of a new approach to research called *participatory research*, in which representatives from the group are studied as members of the research team. This approach to research is described in Chapters 10 and 13. The intent of the research method is to give control of some aspects of the study, such as what is studied, how it is studied, and who is informed of the findings, to the participants. The study is designed to "empower" the participant group to take control of their life situations.

PHILOSOPHICAL ORIENTATION

Critical social theory contains the views of a number of philosophers, with its beginnings in Frankfurt, Germany, at the Institute for Social Research. In the 1920s and 1930s, critical social theory was influenced by the writings of Karl Marx. These philosophers, who contend that social phenomena must be examined within a historical context, believe that most societies function on the basis of closed systems of thought, which lead to patterns of domination and prevent personal growth of individuals within the society. In the late 1960s, a second generation of German philosophers, the most prominent being Habermas (1971), revised critical social theory, leading to a resurgence of interest in these ideas (Thompson, 1987).

From a critical perspective, knowledge is not something that stands alone or is produced in a vacuum by a sort of "pure" intellectual process. Instead, all knowledge is value laden and shaped by historic, social, political, gender, and economic conditions. Ideology—the taken-for-granted assumptions and values that usually remain hidden and unquestioned—creates a social structure that serves to oppress particular groups by limiting the options available to them. A fundamental assumption among critical researchers is that knowledge ought not be generated for its own sake but should be used as a form of social or cultural criticism. Critical scholars hold that oppressive structures can be changed by exposing hidden power imbalances and by assisting individuals, groups, or communities to empower themselves to take action. . . . A critical "agenda" then focuses on creating knowledge that has the potential to produce change through personal or group empowerment, alterations in social systems, or a combination of these. Implicit in this view is a valuing of people as the experts in their own lives, who have an important stake in how issues are resolved. Critical scholars . . . do not wish to control and predict, or to understand and describe, the world; they wish to change it. Hence, the type of knowledge sought must be capable of meeting this challenge (Berman et al., 1998, p. 2).

To accomplish this goal the researcher needs to construct a picture of society that exposes the prevailing system of domination, expresses the contradictions embedded in the domination, assesses society's potential for emancipatory change, and criticizes the system in order to promote that change (Stevens, 1989).

According to Berman and colleagues (1998), a critical social theory study has the following aims:

1. The study addresses an issue that is of concern to a group that is disadvantaged, oppressed, or marginalized in some way.
2. The research process or results have the potential to benefit the group, immediately or longer term.
3. The researcher's assumptions, motivations, biases, and values are made explicit and their influence on the research process is examined.

4. Prior scholarship is critiqued in an attempt to elucidate the ways in which biases, especially those related to gender, race, and class, have distorted existing knowledge.

5. Interactions between the researcher and participants convey respect for the expertise of the participants (Berman et al., 1998, p. 3).

An example of a study using critical social theory methods is presented in Chapter 23.

FRIERE'S THEORY OF CULTURAL ACTION

Friere (1972), a Brazilian educator, used critical social theory methodology to develop a theory of cultural action through his experiences in attacking illiteracy in his country. Friere's theory is beginning to attract the interest of nurse researchers. Friere sees the world not as a static and closed order but as a problem to be worked on and solved. He is convinced that every human being, no matter how "ignorant" or submerged in the "culture of silence," is capable of looking critically at the world in a dialogical encounter with others. "Provided with the proper tools for such an encounter, he can gradually perceive his personal and social reality as well as the contradictions in it, become conscious of his own perception of that reality, and deal critically with it" (Shaull, 1972, p. 12).

"Dialogue cannot exist, however, in the absence of a profound love for the world and for men" (Friere, 1972, p. 77). Redefining the world is an act of creation and is not possible if it is not infused with love.

Love is an act of courage, not of fear, love is commitment to other men. . . . If I do not love the world—if I do not love life—if I do not love men—I cannot enter into dialogue. On the other hand, dialogue cannot exist without humility. . . . How can I dialogue if I always project ignorance onto others and never perceive my own? How can I dialogue if I regard myself as a case apart from other men? . . . Dialogue further requires an intense faith in man, faith in his power to make and remake, to create and re-create, faith in his vocation to be more fully human. (Friere, 1972, pp. 78–79)

Shaull (1972) points out that a peasant can facilitate this process for his or her neighbor more effectively than a teacher brought in from outside.

In his book *Pedagogy of the Oppressed,* Friere (1972) describes the behavior of both the oppressed group and the oppressors. He describes an act of oppression as any act that prevents a person from being more fully human. He believes that both the oppressed and the oppressor must be liberated. If not, the liberated oppressed will simply become oppressors, because both oppressors and oppressed fear freedom, autonomy, and responsibility. However, a person cannot be liberated by others, but must liberate himself or herself. Friere sees the fight against oppression as an act of love.

Friere (1972) points out that education can be a tool of conformity to present social situations or an instrument of liberation. He advocates working with groups, which leads to cultural synthesis, rather than trying to manipulate groups, which leads to cultural invasion. In a true educational experience, both teacher and student learn, and all grow as a consequence. This type of education is the practice of freedom. Friere's ideas are currently being applied to nursing situations.

FEMINIST RESEARCH

Feminist research is considered by some to emerge from critical social theory. According to Rafael (1997), "Feminism is based on the premise that gender is a central construct in a society that privileges men and marginalizes women. . . . Feminist perspectives seek to equalize the power relations between men and women. . . . Critical social feminism emphasizes the social action required to bring about changes in social structures that are oppressive to women, whereas poststructural . . . feminism seeks to expose patriarchal power relations in societal institutions, particularly those that generate knowledge."

Feminist researchers use a broad range of research methodologies, both qualitative and quantitative. Although some feminists see themselves as speaking for all women, others, such as Baber and Allen (1992, p. 19) claim that "there is no woman's voice, no woman's story, but rather a multitude of voices that sometimes speak together but often must speak separately." Glass and Davis (1998) hold that "there is not one [philosophical] explanation for women's or nurses' oppression. Therefore, while general strategies aimed at transforming oppressive states may be appropriate in some contexts, consideration should always be given to individualized and context-specific experiences and subsequent strategies."

Sigsworth (1995), basing ideas on those of Harding (1987), suggests the following methodological conditions for feminist research:

1. Feminist research should be based on women's experiences, and the validity of women's perceptions as the "truth" for them should be recognized.
2. Artificial dichotomies and sharp boundaries are suspect in research involving women and other human beings. They should be carefully scrutinized as reflecting a logical positivist approach to research.
3. The context and relationship of phenomena, such as history and concurrent events, should always be considered in designing, conducting, and interpreting research.
4. Researchers should recognize that the questions asked are at least as important as the answers obtained.
5. Researchers should address questions that women want answered (i.e., the research should be for women).
6. The researcher's point of view (i.e., biases, background, and ethnic and social class) should be treated as part of the data. This involves ensuring that the researcher is on a plane with the person being researched. (Sigsworth, 1995, p. 897)

NURSING KNOWLEDGE AND CRITICAL SOCIAL THEORY

Cody (1998) expresses the following concern about the use of critical social theory in nursing research and practice:

Critical theorists seek to inspire their readers to action, either instrumental or communicative, toward social change in the direction of freedom and justice. In recent years nurse scholars have explicated critical theory in relation to the practice of nursing, the role of the nurse in society, the fact that most nurses are women, and the relation between nurses and those who are oppressed . . . . For those espousing the use of critical theory in nursing, action on the part of the nurse should promote emancipation from oppressive sociocultural systems. . . .

I would like to invite nurses who have considered using critical theories to guide their practice to consider an alternative. Critical theory evolved from sociology, and the phenomena of concern to critical theorists are, in the main, sociological phenomena—the dynamics of social systems, the rules that underpin stability and change in societies, and so on. Most scholars would concede that the goal of nursing and the goal of critical theory are different. The first plank of the American Nurses' Association *Code for Nurses* (1985) states in essence that the nurse provides care to any client without regard to individual or health-related characteristics that may offend the nurse. How does one, then, ethically, turn a critical eye on the reasoning, discourse, and practices of one's client? Much of the literature on critical theory that has appeared in nursing journals could be said to reflect the sociology of healthcare systems. Little or no literature on critical theory in nursing has linked critical theory to the theoretical discourse on self-care, interpersonal relations in nursing, goal attainment in nursing, the person as an adaptive biopsychosocial system, the conservation principles, humanistic nursology, cultural care, human-environment field patterning, human becoming, health as expanding consciousness, transpersonal caring, or nursing as caring. (Cody, 1998, pp. 44–45)

■ SUMMARY

Although the writings of qualitative researchers began to appear occasionally in nursing journals in the 1970s, it was not until the middle to late 1980s that these works were published with any regularity. This approach's concepts and methods of reasoning are very different from those of quantitative research. Some major concepts important to qualitative research are gestalt, sedimented view, and open context. A *gestalt* is a way of viewing the world that is closely related to holism. This view proposes that knowledge about a particular phenomenon is organized into a cluster of linked ideas. It is this clustering and interrelatedness that provides meaning. A gestalt is in some ways like a theory. A *sedimented view* is seeing things within a specific gestalt, frame of reference, or world view. This gives a sense of reality, certainty, and, seemingly, control. A sedimented view is a naive and inflexible way of perceiving a phenomenon. The opposite of a sedimented view is an *open context*. An open context requires deconstruction of the sedimented view, which allows you to see the depth and complexity within the phenomenon being examined. Ihde's (1977) work is cited as a way of helping the reader experience the jump from a sedimented view to an open context.

The conduct of qualitative research requires the rigorous implementation of qualitative research techniques, such as openness, scrupulous adherence to a philosophical perspective, thoroughness in collecting data, and inclusion of all the data in the theory development phase.

Six approaches to qualitative research are described in this chapter: phenomenological research, grounded theory research, ethnographic research, historical research, philosophical inquiry, and critical social theory. The goal of *phenomenological research* is to describe experiences as they are lived. *Grounded theory* is an approach for discovering what problems exist in a social scene and how the persons involved handle them. The research process involves formulation, testing, and redevelopment of propositions until a theory is developed. *Ethnographic research* is the investigation of cultures through an in-depth study of the members of the culture. The ethnographic research process consists of the systematic collection, description, and analysis of data to develop a theory of cultural behavior. *Historical research* is a narrative description or analysis of events that occurred in the remote or recent past. The data of past events are obtained from records, artifacts, or verbal reports. *Philosophical inquiry* consists of three types: foundational studies, philosophical analysis, and ethical analysis. *Foundational inquiry* provides analyses of the structures of a science, such as concepts and theories, and the process of thinking about and valuing certain phenomena held in common by the science. *Philosophical analyses* are used to examine conceptual meaning and develop theories of meaning. *Ethical inquiry* is intellectual analyses of morality. *Critical social theory* involves analysis of systems of thought that lead to patterns of domination and prevent personal growth of individuals within a society.

• •

REFERENCES

Admi, H. (1995). The life history: A viable approach to nursing research. *Nursing Research, 44*(3), 186–188.

Allen, D. G. (1985). Nursing research and social control: Alternative models of science that emphasize understanding and emancipation. *Image: The Journal of Nursing Scholarship, 17*(2), 58–64.

Allen, D. G. (1986). Using philosophical and historical methodologies to understand the concept of health. In P. L. Chinn (Ed.), *Nursing research methodology: Issues and implementation* (pp. 157–168). Rockville, MD: Aspen.

American Nurses Association. (1985). *Code for nurses with interpretive statements.* (ANA Publication) 1985 Jul; (G-56):1–17.

Anderson, J. M. (1989). The phenomenological perspective. In J. M. Morse (Ed.), *Qualitative nursing research: A contemporary dialogue* (pp. 15–26). Rockville, MD: Aspen.

Artinian, B. M. (1988). Qualitative modes of inquiry. *Western Journal of Nursing Research, 10*(2), 138–149.

Artinian, B. M. (1998). Grounded theory research: Its value for nursing. *Nursing Science Quarterly, 11*(1), 5–6.

Baber, K. M., & Allen, K. R. (1992). *Women and families: Feminist reconstructions.* New York: Guilford Press.

Baillie, L. (1995). Ethnography and nursing research: A critical appraisal. *Nurse Researcher, 3*(2), 5–21.

Baumrind, D. (1980). New directions in socialization research. *American Psychologist, 35*(7), 639–652.

Beck, C. T. (1994). Phenomenology: Its use in nursing research. *International Journal of Nursing Studies, 31*(6), 499–510.

Berman, H., Ford-Gilboe, M., & Campbell, J. C. (1998). Combining stories and numbers: A methodologic approach for a critical nursing science. *Advances in Nursing Science, 21*(1), 1–15.

Boyd, C. O. (1993a). Philosophical foundations of qualitative research. In P. Munhall and C. O. Boyd (Eds.), *Nursing research: A qualitative perspective* (2nd ed., pp. 66–93). New York: National League for Nursing Press.

Boyd, C. O. (1993b). Phenomenology: The method. In P. Munhall and C. O. Boyd (Eds.), *Nursing research: A qualitative perspective,* (2nd ed., pp. 99–132). New York: National League for Nursing Press.

Burns, N. (1989). Standards for qualitative research. *Nursing Science Quarterly, 2*(1), 44–52.

Carr, J. M. (1998). Vigilance as a caring expression and Leininger's theory of cultural care diversity and universality. *Nursing Science Quarterly,* 11(2), 74–78.

Chenitz, W. C., & Swanson, J. M. (1984). Surfacing nursing process: A method for generating nursing theory from practice. *Journal of Advanced Nursing, 9*(7), 205–215.

Chenitz, W. C., & Swanson, J. M. (1986). *From practice to grounded theory: Qualitative research in nursing.* Menlo Park, CA: Addison-Wesley.

Chinn, P. L., & Wheeler, C. E. (1985). Feminism and nursing. *Nursing Outlook, 33*(2), 74–77.

Christy, T. E. (1978). The hope of history. In M. L. Fitzpatrick (Ed.), *Historical studies in nursing* (pp. 3–11). New York: Teachers College.

Cody, W. K. (1998). Critical theory and nursing science: Freedom in theory and practice. *Nursing Science Quarterly, 11*(2), 44–46.

Curtin, L. L. (1979). The nurse as advocate: A philosophical foundation for nursing. *Advances in Nursing Science, 1*(3), 1–10.

Curtin, L. L. (1990). Integrating practice with philosophy, theory and methods of inquiry. *Proceedings: Symposium on knowledge development: I. Establishing the linkages between philosophy, theory, methods of inquiry and practice*, September 6–9, 1990. University of Rhode Island College of Nursing.

Cutcliffe, J. (1997). Qualitative research in nursing: A quest for quality. *British Journal of Nursing, 6*(17), 969.

Dzurec, L. C. (1989). The necessity and evolution of multiple paradigms for nursing research. *Advances in Nursing Science, 11*(4), 69–77.

Ellis, R. (1983). Philosophic inquiry. In H. H. Werley & J. J. Fitzpatrick (Eds.), *Annual review of nursing research* (Vol. I, pp. 211–228). New York: Springer.

Evans, J. C. (1978). Formulating an idea. In M. L. Fitzpatrick (Ed.), *Historical studies in nursing* (pp. 15–17). New York: Teachers College.

Fairman, J. A. (1987). Sources and references for research in nursing history. *Nursing Research, 36*(1), 56–59.

Fitzpatrick, M. L. (1993). Historical research: The method. In P. Munhall & C. O. Boyd (Eds.), *Nursing research: A qualitative perspective* (2nd ed., pp. 359–371). New York: National League for Nursing Press.

Friere, P. (1972). *Pedagogy of the oppressed* (M. B. Ramos, Trans.). New York: Herder and Herder.

Gadamer, H-G. (1975). *Truth and method.* Braden, G., & Cumming, J. (Trans). New York, NY: Seabury.

Germain, C. P. (1993). Ethnography: The method. In P. Munhall & C. O. Boyd (Eds.), *Nursing research: A qualitative perspective* (2nd ed., pp. 237–268). New York: National League for Nursing Press.

Glaser, B. G. (1978). *Theoretical sensitivity.* Mill Valley, CA: Sociology Press.

Glaser, B. G., & Strauss, A. (1965). *Awareness of dying.* Chicago: Aldine.

Glaser, B. G., & Strauss, A. (1967). *The discovery of grounded theory: Strategies for qualitative research.* Chicago: Aldine.

Glaser, B. G., & Strauss, A. (1968). *Time for dying.* Chicago: Aldine.

Glaser, B. G., & Strauss, A. (1971). *Status passage.* London: Routledge & Kegan Paul.

Glass, N., & Davis, K. (1998). An emancipatory impulse: A feminist postmodern integrated turning point in nursing research. *Advances in Nursing Science*, 21(1), 43–52.

Gortner, S. R. (1985). Ethical inquiry. In H. H. Werley & J. J. Fitzpatrick (Eds.), *Annual review of nursing research* (Vol. 3, pp. 193–214). New York: Springer.

Habermas, J. (1971). *Knowledge and human interests* (J. J. Shapiro, Trans.). Boston: Beacon.

Hallett, C. (1995). Understanding the phenomenological approach to research. *Nurse Researcher, 3*(2), 55–65.

Harding, S. (1987). *Feminism and methodology.* Bloomington, Indiana: Open University Press.

Heidegger, M. (1962). *Being and time* (J. Macquarrie & E. Robinson, Trans.). New York, New York: Harper & Row.

Heller, A. (1982). *A theory of history.* London: Routledge & Kegan Paul.

Holmes, C. A. (1996). The politics of phenomenological concepts in nursing. *Journal of Advanced Nursing, 24*(3), 579–587.

Husserl, E. (1960). *Cartesian meditations: An introduction to phenomenology.* (D. Carins, Trans.). The Hague: Martinus Nijhoff.

Husserl, E. (1964). *The idea of phenomenology.* (W. P. Alston & G. Nakhnikian, Trans.). The Hague: Martinus Nijhoff.

Husserl, E. (1970). *The crisis of the European sciences and transcendental phenomenology.* Evanston, IL: Northwestern University Press.

Husserl, E. (1980). *Phenomenology and the foundations of the sciences.* (T. E. Klein, & W. E. Pohl, Trans). The Hague: Martinus Nijhoff.

Ihde, D. (1977). *Experimental phenomenology: An introduction.* New York: Putnam.

Kaplan, A. (1964). *The conduct of inquiry: Methodology for behavioral science.* New York: Chandler.

Kruse, B. G. (1999). The lived experience of serenity: Using Parse's research method. *Nursing Science Quarterly, 12*(2), 143–150.

Kubler-Ross, E. (1969). *On death and dying.* New York: Macmillan.

Langveld, M. J. (1978). The stillness of the secret place. *Phenomenology and Pedagogy, 1*(1), 181–189.

Laugharne, C. (1995). Ethnography: research method or philosophy? *Nurse Researcher, 3*(2), 54–54.

Leininger, M. M. (1970). *Nursing and anthropology: Two worlds to blend.* New York: Wiley.

Leininger, M. M. (1985). *Qualitative research methods in nursing.* Orlando, FL: Grune & Stratton.

Leininger, M. M. (1990). Ethnomethods: The philosophic and epistemic basis to explicate transcultural nursing knowledge. *Journal of Transcultural Nursing, 1*(2), 40–51.

Leininger, M. M. (1991). *Ethnonursing: A research method with enablers to study the theory of culture care* (pp. 73–117). (NLN Publication #15–2402). New York: National League for Nursing.

Leininger, M. M. (1997). Transcultural nursing research to transform nursing education and practice: 40 years. *Image—the Journal of Nursing Scholarship, 29*(4), 341–347.

Leonard, V. W. (1989). A Heideggerian phenomenologic perspective on the concept of the person. *Advances in Nursing Science, 11*(4), 40–55.

Lusk, B. (1997). Historical methodology for nursing research. *Image—The Journal of Nursing Scholarship, 29*(4), 355–359.

MacPherson, K. I. (1983). Feminist methods: A new paradigm for nursing research. *Advances in Nursing Science, 5*(2), 17–25.

Manchester, P. (1986). Analytic philosophy and foundational inquiry: The method. In P. L. Munhall & C. J. Oiler (Eds.), *Nursing research: A qualitative perspective* (pp. 229–249). Norwalk, CT: Appleton-Century-Crofts.

Mead, G. H. (1934). *Mind, self and society.* Chicago: University of Chicago Press.

Miller, P. S. (1967) Introduction. In M. A. Fitzsimons, A. G. Pundt, & C. E. Nowell (Eds.), *The development of historiography* (pp. xxv–xxxii). Port Washington, NY: Kennikat.

Morse, J. M. (1989). Qualitative nursing research: A free-for-all? In J. M. Morse (Ed.), *Qualitative nursing research: A contemporary dialogue* (pp. 14–22). Rockville, MD: Aspen.

Munet-Vilaro, F. (1988). The challenge of cross-cultural nursing research. *Western Journal of Nursing Research, 10*(1), 112–116.

Munhall, P. L. (1989). Philosophical ponderings on qualitative research methods in nursing. *Nursing Science Quarterly, 2*(1), 20–28.

Munhall, P. L., & Oiler, C. J. (1986). *Nursing research: A qualitative perspective.* Norwalk, CT: Appleton-Century-Crofts.

Nardi, D. (1998). Addiction recovery for low-income pregnant and parenting women: A process of becoming. *Archives of Psychiatric Nursing, 12*(2), 81–89.

Newton, M. E. (1965). The case for historical research. *Nursing Research, 14*(1), 20–26.

Noel, N. L. (1988). Historiography: Biography of "Women Worthies" in nursing history. *Western Journal of Nursing Research, 10*(1), 106–108.

Omery, A. (1983). Phenomenology: A method for nursing research. *Advances in Nursing Science, 5*(2), 49–63.

Parse, R. R. (1981). *Man-living-health: A theory of nursing.* New York: Wiley.

Parse, R. R. (1987). *Nursing science: Major paradigms, theories, and critiques.* Philadelphia: W. B. Saunders.

Parse, R. R. (1990). Health: A personal commitment. *Nursing Science Quarterly, 3*(3), 136–140.

Parse, R. R. (Ed.) (1995). *Illuminations: The human becoming theory in practice and research.* New York: National League for Nursing.

Paterson, J. G., & Zderad, L. T. (1976). *Humanistic nursing.* New York: Wiley.

Pflug, G. (1971). The development of historical method in the eighteenth century. In G. Pflug, P. Sakmann, & R. Unger (Eds.), *History and theory: Studies in the philosophy of history* (pp. 1–23). Middletown, CT: Wesleyan University Press.

Rafael, A. R. F. (1997). Advocacy oral history: A research methodology for social activism in nursing. *Advances in Nursing Science, 2*(20), 32–44.

Rodgers, B. L. (1989). Concepts, analysis and the development of nursing knowledge: The evolutionary cycle. *Journal of Advanced Nursing, 14*(4), 330–335.

Rosenberg, C. (1987). Clio and caring: An agenda for American historians and nursing. *Nursing Research, 36*(1), 67–68.

Sakmann, P. (1971). The problems of historical method and of philosophy of history in Voltaire [1906]. In G. Pflug, P. Sakmann, & R. Unger (Eds.), *History and theory: Studies in the philosophy of history* (pp. 24–59). Middletown, CT: Wesleyan University Press.

Salsberry, P. J., Smith, M. C., & Boyd, C. O. (1989). Dialogue on a research issue: Phenomenological research in nursing— Commentary and responses. *Nursing Science Quarterly, 2*(1), 9–19.

Sanday, P. (1983). The ethnographic paradigm(s). In J. Van Maanen (Ed.), *Qualitative methodology* (pp. 19–36). Beverly Hills, CA: Sage. (Original work published 1979, in *Administrative Science Quarterly, 24,* 527–538.)

Sandelowski, M. (1986). The problem of rigor in qualitative research. *Advances in Nursing Science, 8*(3), 27–37.

Sarnecky, M. T. (1990). Historiography: A legitimate research methodology for nursing. *Advances in Nursing Science, 12*(4), 1–10.

Scheffler, I. (1967). *Science and subjectivity.* Indianapolis: Bobbs-Merrill.

Schwartz-Barcott, D., & Kim, H. S. (1986). A hybrid model for concept development. In P. L. Chinn (Ed.), *Nursing research methodology: Issues and implementation* (pp. 91–101). Rockville, MD: Aspen.

Shaull, R. (1972). Foreword. In P. Friere, *Pedagogy of the oppressed* (pp. 9–15). New York: Herder and Herder.

Sigsworth, J. (1995). Feminist research: Its relevance to nursing. *Journal of Advanced Nursing, 22*(5), 896–899.

Silva, M. C., & Rothbart, D. (1984). An analysis of changing trends in philosophies of science on nursing theory development and testing. *Advances in Nursing Science, 6*(2), 1–13.

Sorensen, E. S. (1988). Historiography: Archives as sources of treasure in historical research. *Western Journal of Nursing Research, 10*(5), 666–670.

Steele, S. M., & Harmon, V. M. (1983). *Values clarification in nursing* (2nd ed.). New York: Appleton-Century-Crofts.

Stevens, P. E. (1989). A critical social reconceptualization of environment in nursing: Implications for methodology. *Advances in Nursing Science, 11*(4), 56–68.

Taylor, B. (1995). Interpreting phenomenology for nursing research. *Nurse Researcher, 3*(2), 66–79.

Thompson, J. L. (1987). Critical scholarship: The critique of domination in nursing. *Advances in Nursing Science, 10*(1), 27–38.

Walters, A. J. (1995). The phenomenological movement: Implications for nursing research. *Journal of Advanced Nursing, 22*(4), 791–799.

Waring, L. M. (1978). Developing the research prospectus. In M. L. Fitzpatrick (Ed.), *Historical studies in nursing* (pp. 18–20). New York: Teachers College.

Watson, J. (1985). *Nursing: Human science and human care: A theory of nursing.* Norwalk, CT: Appleton-Century-Crofts.

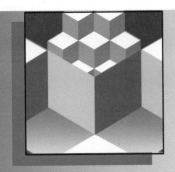

II

THE RESEARCH PROCESS

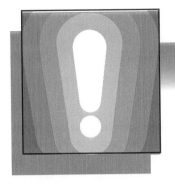

CHAPTER 5

RESEARCH PROBLEM AND PURPOSE

We are constantly asking questions to gain a better understanding of ourselves and the world around us. This human ability to wonder and ask creative questions about behaviors and situations in the world provides a basis for identifying research topics and problems. Identifying a problem is the initial step, and one of the most significant, in conducting both quantitative and qualitative research. The research purpose evolves from the problem and provides direction for the subsequent steps of the research process.

Research topics are concepts or broad problem areas that indicate the foci of essential research knowledge needed to provide evidence-based nursing practice. Research topics contain numerous potential research problems, and each problem provides the basis for developing several research purposes. Thus, the identification of a relevant research topic and a challenging, significant problem can facilitate the development of numerous study purposes to direct a lifetime of research. However, the abundance of research topics and potential problems frequently are not apparent to individuals struggling to identify their first research problems.

This chapter differentiates a research problem from a purpose, identifies sources for research problems, and provides a background for formulating a problem and purpose for study. The criteria for determining the feasibility of a proposed study problem and purpose are described. The chapter concludes with examples of research topics, problems, and purposes from current quantitative and qualitative studies.

WHAT IS A RESEARCH PROBLEM AND PURPOSE?

A *research problem* is an area of concern in which there is a gap in the knowledge base needed for nursing practice. Research is conducted to generate essential knowledge to address the practice concern, with the ultimate goal of providing evidence- or research-based nursing care. A research problem can be identified by asking questions such as: What is wrong or is of concern in this situation? What is known and not known about this situation? What information is needed to improve this situation? Will a particular intervention work in a clinical situation? Who is best to implement the intervention? Would another intervention be more effective? What changes need to be made to improve this intervention?

Through questioning and a review of the literature, a research problem emerges that includes a specific area of concern and the knowledge gap that surrounds this concern. The knowledge gap, or what is not known about this clinical problem, determines the complexity and number of studies needed to generate essential knowledge for nursing practice (Martin, 1994; Wright, 1999). Foster-Fitzpatrick and colleagues (1999) studied the effects of crossed legs on blood pressure measurement and identified the following research problem.

"Blood pressure monitoring is one of the most commonly used techniques in the diagnosis and treatment of various health care problems. Accurate measurement of blood pressure is especially crucial in the assessment of hypertension. Consequently, all efforts should be made to eliminate errors in measuring blood pressure.

"Numerous factors influence an individual's blood pressure measurement including medications, arm and body position, noise, extreme temperatures, constrictive clothing, faulty equipment, white-coat effect, attitude of the person taking the measurement, anxiety, improper cuff length or width, and talking. . . . Although not an acceptable practice, a single blood pressure measurement often is the basis for clinical decisions such as adjustment of a person's antihypertensive drug dosage. Thus, it is crucial to eliminate all possible sources of error in measuring a person's blood pressure." (Hill & Grim, 1991)

"Some guidelines for accurately measuring blood pressure specify that the patient should keep feet flat on the floor. However, research is lacking on the effect of crossing the leg at the knee during blood pressure measurement." (Foster-Fitzpatrick et al., 1999, pp. 105–106) ■

In this example, the first two paragraphs identify the area of concern for a particular population and provide background and significance for this concern. The concern is accurate blood pressure measurement and the population is individuals having their blood pressure measured. This is a significant problem because blood pressure measurement is used in the diagnosis and treatment of several health care problems, and there are numerous factors that influence accurate measurement. The last paragraph indicates limited research causing a knowledge gap for this clinical problem. In this example, the research problem includes concepts such as accurate measurement of blood pressure, factors influencing blood pressure measurement, and nursing intervention to promote accurate blood pressure measurement. The concept of interventions is abstract, and a variety of nursing actions could be implemented to determine their effects on blood pressure measurement. Thus, each problem provides the basis for generating a variety of research purposes. The knowledge gap regarding the effects of crossed legs on blood pressure measurement pro-

vides clear direction for the formulation of the purpose.

The *research purpose* is a concise, clear statement of the specific goal or aim of the study. The goal of a study might be to identify, describe, explain, or predict a solution to a clinical problem (Beckingham, 1974). The purpose usually indicates the type of study to be conducted and often includes the variables, population, and setting for the study. Every study should have an explicit or implicit purpose statement. Foster-Fitzpatrick and colleagues (1999) explicitly stated that the purpose of their study was . . .

• •

"to determine if blood pressure measurement is affected by the leg crossed at the knee as compared with feet flat on the floor." (Foster-Fitzpatrick et al., 1999, p. 106) ■

The goal of this study was to compare the effects of two positions (legs crossed at knees and feet flat on the floor) on blood pressure measurement. This quasi-experimental study was conducted to determine the effects of two independent variables or treatments (legs crossed at knees and feet flat) on the dependent variable or outcome of blood pressure measurement. The results indicated that systolic and diastolic blood pressure readings were significantly increased ($p < .0001$) with the crossed leg position. Thus, patients should be instructed to place their feet flat on the floor when their blood pressure is measured to eliminate a source of error (Foster-Fitzpatrick et al., 1999).

SOURCES OF RESEARCH PROBLEMS

Research problems are developed from many sources. However, one must be curious, astute, and imaginative to use these sources effectively. Moody and associates (1989) studied the source of research ideas and found that 87% came from clinical practice, 57% from the literature, 46% from interactions with colleagues, 28% from interactions with students, and 9% from funding priorities. These findings indicated that researchers often use more than one source to identify a research problem. The sources for research problems included in this text are (1) nursing practice, (2) researcher and peer interactions, (3) literature review, (4) theory, and (5) research priorities identified by funding agencies and specialty groups.

Nursing Practice

The practice of nursing must be based on knowledge generated through research. Thus, clinical practice is an extremely important source for research problems (Diers, 1979). Problems can evolve from clinical observations, such as watching the behavior of a patient and family in crisis and wondering what interventions a nurse might use to improve their coping skills. A review of patient records, treatment plans, and procedure manuals might reveal concerns or raise questions about practice that could be the basis for research problems. For example, what procedures should be followed in providing mouth care to cancer patients? What nursing intervention will facilitate communication with a patient who has had a stroke? What is the impact of home visits on the level of function, readjustment to the home environment, and rehospitalization pattern? What is the most effective treatment or treatments for acute and chronic pain? What is the best pharmacological agent or agents for treating hypertension in an elderly, African American, diabetic patient—β-blocker, angiotensin-converting enzyme inhibitor, angiotensin II receptor blocker, calcium channel blocker, α_1 antagonists, or diuretic, or a combination of these drugs? These significant clinical questions could direct research to generate essential evidence for use in practice.

Extensive patient data, such as diagnoses, treatments, and outcomes, are now computerized. Analyzing this information might generate research problems that are significant to a clinic, community, or nation. For example, why has the incidence of cancer increased in your patient population over the last 5 years? What pharmacological and nonpharmacological treatments have been most effective in treating common acute illnesses such as otitis media, sinusitis, and bronchitis in your practice or nationwide? What are the outcomes (patient health status and costs) for treating Type II diabetes in your practice?

Some students and nurses keep logs or journals of their practice that contain research ideas (Artinian & Anderson, 1980). They might record their experiences and thoughts and the observations of others. Analysis of these logs often reveals patterns and trends in a setting and facilitates the identification of patient care concerns. Some concerns might include the following: Do the priority needs perceived by the patient direct the care received? Why do patients frequently fail to follow the treatment plan provided by their nurse practitioner or physician? What is the involvement of family members in patient care and what impact does this care delivery have on the family unit?

Questions about the effectiveness of and the desire to improve certain interventions and health care programs have facilitated the development of intervention effectiveness research (Sidani & Braden, 1998). Studies have focused on specific interventions directed at alleviating well-defined clinical problems, such as the effects of a crossed leg position on blood pressure measurement (Foster-Fitzpatrick et al., 1999) and the effects of dynamic exercise on subcutaneous oxygen tension and temperature to promote wound healing (Whitney et al., 1995). The research might also focus on a program that includes a combination of interventions that address various aspects of patient health and are focused on improving overall health outcomes (Sidani & Braden, 1998). For example, a comprehensive care program for pregnant women was studied by Lowry and Beikirch (1998) to determine the impact of this program on pregnancy outcomes.

Health care is constantly changing in response to consumer needs and trends in society. Examples of current research focused on consumer needs include (1) examining nursing care for preterm infants (Brandon et al., 1999), (2) improving outcomes of residents in nursing homes (Anderson et al., 1999); and (3) implementing health promotion and illness prevention interventions (Morin et al., 1999). Research examining health care and societal trends includes studies of the impact of the nurse practitioner role on health outcomes (Brown & Grimes, 1995; Mundinger et al., 2000), the relationship of modifiable health risks (inactivity, obesity, and smoking) to health costs (Pronk et al., 1999), and health needs of different cultures (Waters, 1999).

Researcher and Peer Interactions

Interactions with researchers and peers are valuable sources for generating research problems. Experienced researchers serve as mentors and share their knowledge with novice researchers in the identification of research topics and the formulation of problems. Nursing educators assist students in selecting research problems for theses and dissertations. When possible, students conduct studies in the same area of research as the faculty. The faculty can share its expertise regarding its research program, and the combined work of the faculty and students can build a knowledge base for a specific area of practice. This type of relationship could also be developed between an expert researcher and a nurse clinician. Building a sound research knowledge base for nursing practice requires collaboration between nurse researchers and clinicians as well as collaboration with researchers from other health-related disciplines.

Beveridge (1950) identified several reasons for discussing research ideas with others. Ideas are clarified and new ideas are generated when two or more people pool their thoughts. Interactions with others enable researchers to uncover errors in reasoning or information. These interactions are also a source of support in discouraging or difficult times. In addition, another person can provide a refreshing or unique viewpoint, which prevents conditioned thinking or following an established habit of thought. A workplace that encourages interaction can stimulate nurses to identify research problems. Nursing conferences and professional organization meetings also provide excellent opportunities for nurses to discuss their ideas and brainstorm to identify potential research problems.

Communication among researchers and clinicians around the world has greatly expanded with access to the Internet for sharing information and ideas about areas of interest and proposing potential problems for research. For example, the Washington Area Nursing Research Resources (WANRR) website was developed in the fall of 1997 to encourage sharing of expertise and information among regional nurse researchers (Ailinger & Neal, 1999). This website (*http://www.gmu.edu/departments/nursing/wanrr/research.html*) and others exist to assist you in interacting with expert researchers in formulating a quality study. Interactions with others are essential to broaden the perspective and knowledge base of researchers and to provide support in identifying significant research problems and purposes.

Literature Review

Reviewing research journals—such as *Advances in Nursing Science, Applied Nursing Research, Clinical Nursing Research, Image—Journal of Nursing Scholarship, Journal of Advanced Nursing, Nursing Research, Research in Nursing & Health, Scholarly Inquiry for Nursing Practice: An International Journal,* and *Western Journal of Nursing Research*—and theses and dissertations will acquaint novice researchers with studies conducted in an area of interest. The nursing specialty journals, such as *Archives of Psychiatric Nursing, Cancer Nursing, Dimensions of Critical Care, Heart & Lung,* and *Journal of Pediatric Nursing: Nursing Care of Children & Families,* also place a high priority on publishing research findings. Reviewing research articles enables you to identify an area of interest and determine what is known and what is not known in this area. The gaps in the knowledge base provide direction for future research. The process of reviewing the literature is the focus of Chapter 6.

At the completion of a research project, an investigator often makes recommendations for further study. These recommendations provide opportunities for others to build on a researcher's work and strengthen the knowledge in a selected area. Foster-Fitzpatrick and colleagues (1999, p. 107) examined the effects of crossed leg position on blood pressure measurement and "recommended that their study be replicated on a larger sample that includes female hypertensives because the sample of all-male hypertensive veterans limits the generalization of this study." These researchers encouraged validation of their findings through replication and expansion of the findings by studying a different population.

REPLICATION OF STUDIES

Reviewing the literature is a way to identify a study to replicate. *Replication* involves reproducing or repeating a study to determine whether similar findings will be obtained (Taunton, 1989). Replication is essential for knowledge development because it (1) establishes the credibility of the findings, (2) extends the generalizability of the findings over a range of instances and contexts, (3) reduces the number of Type I and Type II errors, (4) provides support for theory development, and (5) decreases the acceptance of erroneous results (Beck, 1994). Some researchers replicate studies because they agree with the findings and wonder if the findings will hold up in different settings with different subjects over time. Others replicate studies because they want to challenge the findings or interpretations of prior investigators.

Four different types of replication are important in generating sound scientific knowledge for nursing: (1) exact, (2) approximate, (3) concurrent, and (4) systematic extension (Beck, 1994; Haller & Reynolds, 1986). An *exact,* or identical, *replication* involves duplicating the initial researcher's study to confirm the original findings. All conditions of the original study must be maintained; thus, "there must be the same observer, the same subjects, the same procedure, the same measures, the same locale, and the same time" (Haller & Reynolds, 1986, p. 250). Exact replications might be thought of as ideal to confirm original study findings but are frequently not attainable. In addition, one would not want to replicate the errors in an original study, such as small sample size, weak design, or poor quality measurement methods.

An *approximate,* or operational, *replication* involves repeating the original study under similar conditions, following the methods as closely as possible (Beck, 1994). The intent is to determine whether the findings from the original study hold up despite minor changes in the research conditions. If the findings generated through replication are consistent with the findings of the original study, these data are more credible and have a greater probability of being an accurate reflection of the real world. If the replication fails to support the original findings, the designs and methods of both studies should be examined for limitations and weaknesses, and further research needs to be conducted. Conflicting findings might also generate additional theoretical insights and provide new directions for research.

King and Tarsitano (1982) did an approximate replication of Lindeman and Van Aernam's (1971) landmark study of the effects of structured and unstructured preoperative teaching on patient outcomes. In the original study, Lindeman and Van Aernam developed the following research questions:

1. What are the effects of a structured and an unstructured preoperative teaching program upon the adult surgical patient's ability to deep breathe and cough 24 hours postoperatively?
2. What are the effects of a structured and an unstructured preoperative teaching program upon the adult surgical patient's length of hospital stay?
3. What are the effects of a structured and an unstructured preoperative teaching program upon the adult surgical patient's postoperative need for analgesia? (Lindeman & Van Aernam, 1971, p. 321)

King and Tarsitano's (1982) research questions were:

1. What are the results of a structured and unstructured preoperative teaching program on the adult surgical patient's postoperative recovery as measured by pulmonary function tests?
2. What are the results of a structured and unstructured preoperative teaching program on the adult surgical patient's length of hospital stay? (King & Tarsitano, 1971, p. 324)

King and Tarsitano elected to narrow the scope of the study to exclude the phenomenon of pain, as recommended by the original investigators. They also modified the measurement of respiratory function by including pulmonary function tests. They also controlled factors that were not controlled in the original study.

• •

"The sample was restricted to patients of three surgeons with similar techniques and to patients having lower or upper abdominal surgery. The structured preoperative teaching was conducted primarily by the principal investigator and associate and a checklist was used to indicate that the patients could perform the deep breathing, coughing and exercises." (King & Tarsitano, 1971, p. 324) ■

Findings from both studies indicated that structured preoperative instruction significantly improved the ability of patients to cough and breathe deeply postoperatively, which increases the credibility of this finding. However, King and Tarsitano found that structured preoperative instruction did not significantly decrease the length of hospital stay, which is contradictory to the findings of Lindeman and Van Aernam. Additional research is needed to clarify the conflicting findings.

A *concurrent,* or internal, *replication* involves the collection of data for the original study and its simultaneous replication to provide a check of the reliability of the original study (Beck, 1994; Brink & Wood, 1979). The confirmation, through replication of the original study findings, is part of the original study's design. For example, a research team might collect data simultaneously at two different hospitals and compare and contrast the findings. Consistency in the findings increases the credibility and ability to generalize the findings. Some expert researchers obtain funding to conduct multiple concurrent replications, in which a number of individuals are involved in the conduct of a single study but with different samples in different settings. As each study is completed, the findings are compiled in a report indicating the series of replications that were conducted to generate these findings (Brink & Wood, 1979).

A *systematic extension,* or constructive, *replication* is done under distinctly new conditions. The researchers conducting the replication do not follow the design or methods of the original researchers; rather, the second investigative team identifies a similar problem but formulates new methods to verify the first researchers' findings (Haller & Reynolds, 1986). The aim of this type of replication is to extend the findings of the original study and test the limits of the generalizability of such findings.

Beck (1994) conducted a computerized and manual review of the nursing literature from 1983 through 1992 and found only 49 replication studies. Possibly, the number of replication studies is limited because replication is viewed by some as less scholarly or less important than original research. However, the lack of replication studies severely limits the use of research findings in practice and the development of a scientific knowledge base for practice (Beck, 1994; Martin, 1995; Reynolds & Haller, 1986; Taunton, 1989). Thus, replicating a study should be respected as a legitimate scholarly activity for expert as well as novice researchers.

Replication provides an excellent learning opportunity for the novice researcher to conduct a significant study, validate findings from a previous study, and generate new information from different populations and settings. Students studying for their Master's degree could be encouraged to replicate studies for their theses, possibly to replicate faculty studies. When developing and publishing a replication study, you need to indicate that your study was a replication and designate the type of replication and how it was accomplished. You also need to identify the strengths and weaknesses of the original study and provide a rationale for the modifications made in the replication.

Landmark studies are significant research projects that generate knowledge that influences a discipline and sometimes society. These studies are frequently replicated or are the basis for the generation of additional studies. For example, Williams (1972) studied factors that contribute to skin breakdown, and these findings provided the basis for numerous studies on the prevention and treatment of pressure ulcers. Many of these studies are summarized in the document *Pressure Ulcers in Adults: Prediction and Prevention* published by the Agency for Health Care Policy and Research (Panel for the Prediction and Prevention of Pressure Ulcers in Adults, 1992).

Theory

Theories are an important source for generating research problems because they set forth ideas about events and situations in the real world that require testing (Chinn & Kramer, 1998). In examining a theory, one notes that it includes a number of propositions and that each proposition is a statement of the relationship of two or more concepts. A research problem and purpose could be formulated to explore or describe a concept or to test a proposition from a theory.

Some researchers combine ideas from different theories to develop maps or models for testing through research. The map serves as the framework for the study and includes key concepts and relationships from the theories that the researcher wants to study. Phillips and Wilbur (1995) developed the breast cancer screening model (see Figure 5–1) to examine the breast cancer screening practices of African American women. Their model was based on the health belief model (Becker, 1974), Ajzen and Fishbein's (1980) theory of reasoned action, and Cox's (1982) interaction model of client health behavior and provided a framework for their study. The purpose of the study was "to identify and com-

pare the adherence to breast cancer screening guidelines (monthly breast self-examination [BSE], age-related mammography, and yearly professional breast exam [PBE] among African American women of different employment status" (Phillips & Wilbur, 1995, p. 261). The following questions addressed in this study show a clear relationship to the framework model:

1. To what extent do demographic characteristics (age, education, marital status), social influence (healthcare provider recommendation), previous healthcare experiences (personal risk factors, previous instruction in breast cancer screening) and environmental resources (income, insurance) influence adherence to breast can-

Element of Client Singularity

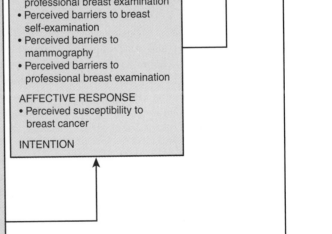

FIGURE 5–1 ■ Phillips' (1993) breast cancer screening model, adapted with permission from Cox (1982): Interaction model of client health behavior: Theoretical prescription for nursing. *Advances in Nursing Science* 5(1), 41–56. Copyright © 1982 Aspen Publishers, Inc. (Phillips, J. M., & Wilbur, J. [1995]. Adherence to breast cancer screening guidelines among African-American women of differing employment status. *Cancer Nursing, 18*[4], 260.)

cer screening guidelines (monthly BSE, age-related mammography, and yearly PBE)?

2. Do motivation (intrinsic motivation, BSE, self-efficacy), cognitive appraisal (knowledge of breast cancer, breast cancer screening, and benefits and barriers related to breast cancer screening), affective response (perceived susceptibility to breast cancer), and intention vary by employment status and age group?

3. How do motivation, cognitive appraisal, and intention influence adherence to breast cancer screening guidelines?

4. Which variables (demographic characteristics, social influence, previous healthcare experiences, environmental resources, motivation, cognitive appraisal, and affective response) are most predictive of the adherence to breast cancer screening guidelines? (Phillips & Wilbur, 1995, p. 261).

The findings from a study either lend support to or do not support the relationships identified in the model. Phillips and Wilbur (1995, p. 268) found that "the Breast Cancer Screening Model was useful in explaining 74% of the variance in monthly BSE, 15% of the variance in age-related mammography, and 42% of the variance in yearly PBE." Thus, the relationships in this model were supported by this study. With additional research, this model could be useful in practice for predicting patient behaviors, especially monthly BSE and yearly PBE. Further research is needed to determine the factors that will predict the behavior of obtaining a mammography. Once the factors for predicting the performance of BSE, obtaining a mammography, and receiving a PBE are determined, interventions can be developed based on these factors to improve women's behaviors related to breast cancer screening (BSE, mammography, and PBE). As a graduate student, you could use this model as a framework and test some of the relationships in your clinical setting.

Research Priorities

Since 1975, expert researchers, specialty groups, and funding agencies have identified nursing research priorities. The identification of research priorities for clinical practice was originally studied by Lindeman (1975, p. 434), who identified priorities such as "nursing interventions related to stress, care of the aged, pain, and patient education." Develop-

ing evidence-based nursing interventions in these areas continues to be a priority today.

Many professional organizations have websites and have used these sites to communicate their research priorities for 2000. For example, the American Association of Critical Care Nurses (AACN) determined initial research priorities for this specialty in the early 1980s (Lewandowski & Kositsky, 1983) and revised these priorities in 1993 (Lindquist et al., 1993) and 1999. The most current AACN research priorities are identified on their website (*http://www.aacn.org*) as (1) effective and appropriate use of technology to achieve optimal patient assessment, management, or outcomes, or a combination of these factors; (2) creating a healing, humane environment; (3) processes and systems that foster the optimal contribution of critical care nurses; (4) effective approaches to symptom management; and (5) prevention and management of complications. If your specialty is critical care, this website might assist you in identifying a priority problem and purpose for study.

The American Organization of Nurse Executives (AONE) has established research priorities for 2000 for nurses in executive practice (Beyers, 1997). The three areas for research and education identified were (1) work force, (2) patient care advocacy, and (3) technology. The work force topic includes research focused on diversity, composition, professional growth, accountability, and recruitment and retention. Patient care advocacy includes research to address areas such as relationships in the community, among health professionals, and in health care settings; efficient use of resources, new management methods, and techniques; and improvement in health care processes and outcomes across the continuum. In the area of technology, investigations need to focus on examining the outcomes of technological adaptations, systems improvement and infrastructure changes to accommodate new technology, and leadership in managing technological change. AONE provides a discussion of their research priorities for 2000 on their website (*http:// www.aone.org/practiceresearch/research_priorities. htm*).

As more health care is provided in the home, Albrecht (1992) recognized the importance of developing a list of the research priorities for home health nursing. These priorities were generated by surveying 50 experts in the field of home health care, and the top 10 research priorities identified were (1) outcomes of care, (2) cost of home care, (3) policy analysis and reimbursement, (4) client classification systems, (5) uniform data set, (6) predictors of care and managed care, (7) coordination of care and managed care, (8) productivity, (9) documentation, and (10) use of health care services.

A significant funding agency for nursing research is the National Institute of Nursing Research (NINR). A major initiative of NINR is the development of a national nursing research agenda that will involve identifying nursing research priorities, outlining a plan for implementing priority studies, and obtaining resources to support these priority projects. NINR has a budget of $70,053 for 2000, and 73% of the budget will be used for extramural research project grants. NINR has developed four goals to direct the institute's activities over the next 5 years (2000–2004). Goal 1 is to identify and support research opportunities that will achieve scientific distinction and produce significant contributions to health. The priority areas selected include end-of-life and palliative care research, chronic illness experiences, quality of life and quality of care, health promotion and disease prevention research, symptom management of illness and treatment, "telehealth" interventions and monitoring, and cultural and ethnic considerations in health and illness. Goal 2 is to identify and support future areas of opportunity to advance research of high-quality, cost-effective care and to contribute to the scientific base for nursing practice. The priorities related to this goal include research in chronic illness and long-term care, health promotion and risk behaviors, cardiopulmonary health and critical care, neurofunction and sensory conditions, immune responses and oncology, and reproductive and infant health. Goal 3 is to communicate and disseminate research findings resulting from NINR-funded research, and Goal 4 is to enhance the development of nurse researchers through training and career development opportunities. Details about the NINR mission, goals, and areas of funding are available on their website at *http://www.nih.gov/ninr.*

Another federal agency that is funding health care research is the Agency for Healthcare Research and Quality (AHRQ), formerly the Agency for Health Care Policy and Research (AHCPR). The purpose of AHRQ is to enhance the quality, appropriateness, and effectiveness of health care services, and access to such services, through the establishment of a broad base of scientific research and the promotion of improvements in clinical practice and in the organization, financing, and delivery of health care services. Some of the current funding priorities are research on the effectiveness of children's mental health and substance abuse; cancer prevention, screening, and care; care at the end of life; and primary care practice. For a complete list of funding opportunities and grant announcements, see the AHCPR website at *http://www.ahcpr.gov.*

Nursing research priorities are also being identified in Europe, Africa, and Asia. Some European countries (United Kingdom, Denmark, and Finland) have been conducting nursing research for more than 30 years, but most of the countries have been involved in such research for less than a decade. The European countries identified the following research topics as priorities: (1) promoting health and well-being across the life span, (2) symptom management, (3) care of the elderly, (4) cost-effectiveness evaluation, (4) restructuring health care systems, (5) self-care and self management of health and illness, and (6) developing knowledge for practice (Tierney, 1998). The two major priorities for nursing research in Africa are HIV/AIDS and health behaviors. In Asia, limited nursing research is being conducted, with the priorities focused on health service research, including human resources and health outcomes (Henry & Chang, 1998).

The World Health Organization (WHO) is encouraging the identification of priorities for a common nursing research agenda among countries. A quality health care delivery system and improved patient and family health have become global goals. By 2020, the world's population is expected to increase by 94%, with the elderly population increasing by almost 240%. Seven of every 10 deaths are expected to be caused by noncommunicable diseases, such as chronic conditions (heart disease, cancer, and depression) and injuries (unintentional and intentional). The six top priority areas for a common research agenda identified by WHO are (1) evaluation of the effects of health care reform; (2) comparative analysis of supply and demand of the health work force of different countries; (3) evaluation of health care organizations, work conditions, technology, and supervision on the motivation and productivity of nursing personnel; (4) analyses of the feasibility, effectiveness, and quality of education and practice of nurses; (5) comparative analysis of the effectiveness of education and quality of services provided by nurses; and (6) action research on delivery modes and necessary context for quality nursing care to vulnerable populations (Hirschfeld, 1998).

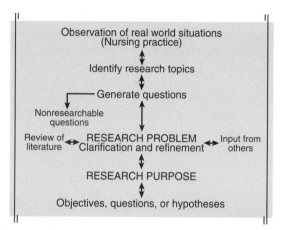

FIGURE 5–2 ■ Formulating a research problem and purpose.

FORMULATING A RESEARCH PROBLEM AND PURPOSE

Potential nursing research problems often emerge from observation of real-world situations, such as those in nursing practice. A *situation* is a significant combination of circumstances that occur at a given time. Inexperienced researchers tend to want to study the entire situation, but it is far too complex for a single study. Multiple problems exist in a single situation, and each can be developed into a study. A researcher's perception of what problems exist in a situation depends on that individual's clinical expertise, theoretical base, intuition, interests, and goals. Some researchers spend years developing different problem statements and new studies from the same clinical situation.

The exact thought processes used to extract problems from a situation have not been clearly identified because of the abstractness and complexity of the reasoning involved. However, the following steps are often implemented by researchers in formulating their study problems: the researcher examines the real-world situation, identifies research topics, generates questions, and ultimately clarifies and refines a research problem. From the problem, a specific goal or research purpose is developed for study. The flow of these steps is presented in Figure 5–2 and described in the following sections.

Research Topics

A nursing situation often includes a variety of research topics or concepts that identify broad problem areas requiring investigation. Some of the patient- and family-related topics frequently investigated by nurses include stress, pain, coping patterns, the teaching and learning process, self-care deficits, health promotion, rehabilitation, prevention of illness, disease management, and social support. Other relevant research topics focus on the health care system and providers, such as cost-effective care; advanced nursing practice role (nurse practitioner, clinical nurse specialist, midwife, and nurse anesthetist); managed care; and redesign of the health care system. Outcomes research is focused on topics of health status, quality of life, cost-effectiveness, and quality of care that require examination in research. A specific outcome study might focus on a particular condition such as terminal cancer and examine outcomes such as nutrition, hygiene, skin integrity, and pain control with a variety of treatments (Davies et al., 1994).

Generating Questions

Encountering situations in nursing stimulates the constant flow of questions. The questions fit into three categories: (1) questions answered by existing knowledge, (2) questions answered with problem solving, and (3) research-generating questions. The first two types of questions are nonresearchable and do not facilitate the formulation of research problems that will generate knowledge for practice. Some of the questions raised have a satisfactory answer within the nursing profession's existing body of knowledge, and these answers are available in the literature or from experts in nursing or other disciplines. For example, questions nurses have about performing some basic nursing skills, such as a protocol for taking a temperature or giving injections, are answered in the research literature and provided in procedure manuals. However, problems that focus on investigating new techniques to improve existing skills, patient responses to techniques, or ways to educate patients and families to perform techniques could add to nursing's knowledge base.

Some of the questions raised can be answered using problem solving or evaluation projects. Chapter 2 includes a comparison of the problem-solving process and the research process and indicates when and why to use each process. Many evaluation projects are conducted with minimal application of the rigor and control that are required in conducting research. These projects do not fit the criteria of research, and the findings are relevant for a particular situation. For example, quality assurance is an evaluation of patient care implemented by a specific health care agency; the results of this evaluation project are usually relevant only to the agency conducting the review.

The type of question that can initiate the research process is one that requires further knowledge to answer. Some of the questions that come to mind about situations include the following. Is there a need to describe concepts, to know how they are related, or to be able to predict or control some event within the situation? What is known and what is not known about the concepts? What are the most urgent factors to know? Research experts have found that asking the right question is frequently more valuable than finding the solution to a problem. The solution identified in a single study might not withstand the test of time or might be useful in only a few situations. However, one well-formulated question can lead to the generation of numerous research problems, a lifetime of research activities, and possibly significant contributions to a discipline's body of knowledge.

Clarifying and Refining a Research Problem

Fantasy and creativity are part of formulating a research problem, so imagine prospective studies related to the situation. Imagine the difficulties likely to occur with each study, but avoid being too critical of potential research problems at this time. Which studies seem the most workable? Which ones appeal intuitively? Which problem is the most significant to nursing? Which study is of personal interest? Which problem has the greatest potential to provide a foundation for further research in the field? (Campbell et al., 1982; Kahn, 1994; Wright, 1999)

The problems investigated need to have professional significance and potential or actual significance for society. A research problem is significant when it has the potential to generate or refine knowledge or influence nursing practice, or both (Wright, 1999). Moody and colleagues (1989) surveyed nurse researchers and identified the following criteria for significant research problems: They should be (1) focused on real-world concerns (57%), (2) methodologically sound (57%), (3) knowledge building (51%), (4) theory building (40%), and (5) focused on current or timely concerns (31%). The problems that are considered significant vary with time and the needs of society. The priorities identified earlier indicate some of the current, significant nursing research topics and problems.

Personal interest in a problem influences the quality of the problem formulated and the study conducted. A problem of personal interest is one that an individual has pondered for a long time or one that is especially important in the individual's nursing practice or personal life. For example, a researcher who has had a mastectomy may be particularly interested in studying the emotional impact of a mastectomy or strategies for caring for mastectomy patients. This personal interest in the topic can become the driving force needed to conduct a quality study (Beveridge, 1950).

Answering these questions regarding significance and personal interest often assists one in narrowing the number of problems. Without narrowing potential problems to only one idea, try some of the ideas out on colleagues. Let them play the devil's advocate and explore the strengths and weaknesses of each idea. Then begin some preliminary reading in the area of interest. Examine literature related to the situation, the variables within the situation, measurement of the variables, previous studies related to the situation, and supportive theories (Flemming, 1999). The literature review often enables one to refine the problem and clearly identify the gap in the knowledge base. Once the problem is identified, it must be framed or grounded in past research, practice, and theory. Thus, the refined problem has documented significance to nursing practice, is based on past research and theory, and provides direction for the development of the research purpose.

Research Purpose

The purpose is generated from the problem, identifies the goal or goals of the study, and directs the development of the study. In the research process, the purpose is usually stated after the problem, since the problem identifies the gap in knowledge in a selected area and the purpose clarifies the knowledge to be generated by a study. The research purpose needs to be stated objectively or in a way that does not reflect particular biases or values of the researcher. Investigators who do not recognize their values might include their biases in the research. This can lead them to generate the answers they want or believe to be true and might add inaccurate information to a discipline's body of knowledge (Kaplan, 1964). Based on the research purpose, specific research objectives, questions, or hypotheses are developed to direct the study (see Chapter 8).

The purpose of an outcomes research project is usually complex and requires a team of multidisciplinary health care providers to accomplish it. The

research team members are cautious in the identification of a purpose that will make a significant contribution to the health care system and yet be feasible. Some possible purposes for outcomes research projects include the following:

- Comparing one treatment with another for effectiveness in the routine treatment of a particular condition
- Describing in measurable terms the typical course of a chronic disease
- Using variations in outcomes to identify opportunities for improving clinical process
- Developing decision support programs for use with individual patients when choosing among alternative treatment options (Davies et al., 1994, p. 11)

EXAMPLE OF PROBLEM AND PURPOSE DEVELOPMENT

You might have observed the women receiving treatment at a psychiatric facility and noted that many were withdrawn and depressed and seemed to be unable to discuss certain events in their lives. Their progress in therapy was usually slow, and they seemed to have similar physical and psychological symptoms. Often, after a rapport was developed with a therapist, they would reveal that they were victims of incest as a child. This situation could lead you to identify research topics and generate searching questions. Research topics of interest include sexual abuse, childhood incest, physical and psychological symptoms of incest, history of incest, assessment of emotional problems, and therapeutic interventions. Possible questions include, What are the physical and psychological symptoms demonstrated by someone who has experienced childhood incest? How would one assess the occurrence, frequency, and impact of rape or incest on a woman? What influences do age and duration of abuse have on the woman's current behavior? How frequently is childhood sexual abuse a problem in the mentally disturbed adult female? How does a health care provider assess and diagnosis emotional problems of adult survivors of child sexual abuse? What type of treatment is effective in an individual who has experienced child abuse? Questions such as these might have been raised by Brown and Garrison (1990) as they developed the following problem, purpose, and questions for their investigation.

Research Problem

· ·

"There is evidence that one in four girls and one in seven boys are sexually abused in some way prior to their 18th birthday ... The long-term consequences of child sexual abuse make it one of the most severe offenses against a child's dignity and sense of well-being . . . Unreported, untreated child sexual abuse results in long-term dysfunctional behavior requiring therapy (Browne & Finkelhor, 1986). Gold (1986) suggested that histories of incest are not often obtained by a systematic interviewing protocol or by specifically trained interviewers. Thus, the need for a systematic assessment tool to identify childhood incest in this high-risk population is imperative." (Brown & Garrison, 1990, pp. 587–588) ■

Child sexual abuse is a significant health care topic because it occurs frequently and has a long-lasting impact on the victim's physical and emotional health. The problem statement that "a systematic assessment tool is needed to identify childhood incest in this high-risk population" is supported by past research, practice, and theory.

Research Purpose

· ·

"The purpose of this study was to (a) identify physical and psychosocial patterns of symptomatology in adult women incest survivors, and (b) design a systematic assessment instrument to identify incest early in nonreporting adult women survivors." (Brown & Garrison, 1990, p. 588) ■

This purpose clearly develops from the problem and identifies the goals of the study, which are to ascertain patterns of symptoms and design an assessment instrument. The variables studied are physical and psychosocial symptoms and an assessment instrument in a population of adult women incest survivors.

Research Questions

1. What patterns of physical symptoms are present in adult women incest survivors?
2. What patterns of psychosocial symptoms are present in adult women incest survivors?
3. Is there a correlation between the frequency of multiple victimization and the number of reported physical and psychosocial symptoms?
4. Is there a correlation between the age when the sexual abuse began and its duration? (Brown & Garrison, 1990, p. 588)

These research questions clearly develop from the first part of the purpose "to identify physical and psychosocial patterns of symptomatology." However, there is no link of the research questions to the second part of the purpose that focused on designing an assessment instrument. This is a break in the logical flow of this study and could lead to problems in the development of the remaining steps of the research process.

FEASIBILITY OF A STUDY

As the research problem and purpose increase in clarity and conciseness, the researcher has greater direction in determining the feasibility of a study. The *feasibility of a study* is determined by examining the time and money commitment; the researcher's expertise; availability of subjects, facility, and equipment; cooperation of others; and the study's ethical considerations (Flemming, 1999; Rogers, 1987).

TIME COMMITMENT

Conducting research frequently takes more time than is anticipated, which makes it difficult for any researcher, especially a novice, to estimate the time that will be involved. In estimating the time commitment, the researcher examines the purpose of the study; the more complex the purpose, the greater the time commitment. An approximation of the time needed to complete a study can be determined by assessing the following factors: (1) type and number of subjects needed, (2) number and complexity of the variables to be studied, (3) methods for measuring the variables (are instruments available to measure the variables or must they be developed?), (4) methods for collecting data, and (5) the data analysis process. A time commitment that is often overlooked is writing the research report for presentation and publication. The researcher must approximate the time needed to complete each step of the research process and determine whether the study is feasible.

Most researchers propose a designated period or set a specific deadline for their project. For example, an agency might set a 2-year deadline for studying the turnover rate of staff. The researcher needs to determine whether the identified purpose can be accomplished by the designated deadline; if not, the purpose could be narrowed or the deadline extended. Researchers are often cautious about extending deadlines because a project could continue for many years. The individual interested in conducting qualitative research frequently must make an extensive time commitment of years. Time is as important as money, and the cost of a study can be greatly affected by the time required to conduct it.

MONEY COMMITMENT

The problem and purpose selected are influenced by the amount of money available to the researcher. Potential sources for funding should be considered at the time the problem and purpose are identified. The cost of a research project can range from a few dollars for a student's small study to hundreds of thousands of dollars for complex projects. In estimating the cost of a research project, the following questions need to be considered:

1. **Literature:** What will the review of the literature—including computer searches, copying articles, and purchasing books—cost?
2. **Subjects:** Will the subjects have to be paid for their participation in the study?
3. **Equipment:** What will the equipment cost for the study? Can the equipment be borrowed, rented, bought, or obtained through donation? Is the equipment available, or will it have to be built? What type of maintenance will be required for the equipment during the study? What will the measurement instruments cost?

4. **Personnel:** Will assistants or consultants, or both, be hired to collect, computerize, and analyze the data and assist with the data interpretation? Will clerical help be needed to type and distribute the report and prepare a manuscript for publication?
5. **Computer time:** Will computer time be required to analyze the data? If so, what will be the cost?
6. **Transportation:** What will be the transportation costs for conducting the study and presenting the findings?
7. **Supplies:** Will any supplies—such as envelopes, postage, pens, paper, or photocopies—be needed? Will a beeper be needed to contact the researcher about potential subjects? Will long distance phone calls or overnight mailing be needed?

RESEARCHER EXPERTISE

A research problem and purpose must be selected based on the ability of the investigator. Initially, one might work with another researcher (mentor) to learn the process and then investigate a familiar problem that fits one's knowledge base or experience. Selecting a difficult, complex problem and purpose can only frustrate and confuse the novice researcher. However, all researchers need to identify problems and purposes that are challenging and collaborate with other researchers as necessary to build their research background.

AVAILABILITY OF SUBJECTS

In selecting a research purpose, one must consider the type and number of subjects needed. Finding a sample might be difficult if the study involves investigating a unique or rare population, such as quadriplegic individuals who live alone. The more specific the population, the more difficult it is to find. The money and time available to the researcher will affect the subjects selected. With limited time and money, the researcher might want to investigate subjects who are accessible and do not require payment for participation. Even if a researcher identifies a population with a large number of potential subjects, those individuals may be unwilling to participate in the study because of the topic selected for study. For example, nurses could be asked to share their experiences with alcohol and drug use, but many might fear that sharing this information would jeopardize their jobs and licenses. Researchers need to be prepared to pursue the attainment of subjects at whatever depth is necessary. Having a representative sample of reasonable size is critical to the generation of quality research findings (Kahn, 1994).

AVAILABILITY OF FACILITIES AND EQUIPMENT

Researchers need to determine whether their studies will require special facilities to implement. Will a special room be needed for an educational program, interview, or observations? If the study is conducted at a hospital, clinic, or school of nursing, will the agency provide the facilities that are needed? Setting up a highly specialized laboratory for the conduct of a study would be expensive and probably require external funding. Most nursing studies are done in natural settings like a hospital room or unit, a clinic, or a patient's home.

Nursing studies frequently require a limited amount of equipment, such as a tape recorder or video recorder for interviews or a physiological instrument such as a scale or thermometer. Equipment can often be borrowed from the facility at which the study is conducted, or it can be rented. Some companies are willing to donate equipment if the study focuses on determining the effectiveness of the equipment and the findings are shared with the company. If specialized facilities or equipment are required for a study, the researcher needs to be aware of the options available before actively pursuing the study.

COOPERATION OF OTHERS

A study might appear feasible but, without the cooperation of others, it is not. Some studies are conducted in laboratory settings and require the minimal cooperation of others. However, most nursing studies involve human subjects and are conducted in hospitals, clinics, schools, offices, or homes. Having the cooperation of people in the research setting, the subjects, and the assistants involved in data collection is essential. People are frequently willing to cooperate with a study if they view the problem and purpose as significant or if they are personally interested. For example, nurses would probably be interested in cooperating in a study that examined the cost-effectiveness of nursing care in that institution. Gaining the cooperation of others in a research project is discussed in Chapter 17.

ETHICAL CONSIDERATIONS

The purpose selected for investigation must be ethical, which means that the subjects' rights and the rights of others in the setting are protected. If the purpose appears to infringe on the rights of the subjects, it should be reexamined and may have to be revised or abandoned. There are usually some risks in every study, but the value of the knowledge generated should outweigh the risks. Ethics in research is the focus of Chapter 9.

QUANTITATIVE, QUALITATIVE, AND OUTCOMES RESEARCH TOPICS, PROBLEMS, AND PURPOSES

Quantitative and qualitative research approaches enable nurses to investigate a variety of research problems and purposes. Examples of research topics, problems, and purposes for some of the different types of quantitative studies are presented in Table 5–1. The research purpose usually reflects the type of study that is to be conducted. The purposes of descriptive research are to describe concepts, describe and identify relationships among variables, or compare and contrast groups on selected variables. The comparative descriptive study by Mundinger and associates (2000) described and compared the outcomes of patients treated by nurse practitioners and physicians and found the outcomes to be comparable. The purpose of correlational research is to examine the type (positive or negative) and strength of relationships among variables. In

TABLE 5–1
Quantitative Research: Topics, Problems, and Purposes

TYPE OF RESEARCH	RESEARCH TOPIC	RESEARCH PROBLEM AND PURPOSE
Descriptive Research	Primary care outcomes, health care providers (nurse practitioners, physicians)	Problem: "Studies have suggested that the quality of primary care delivered by nurse practitioners is equal to that of physicians. However, these studies did not measure nurse practitioner practices that had the same degree of independence as the comparison physician practices, nor did previous studies provide direct comparison of outcomes for patients with nurse practitioner or physician providers." (Mundinger et al., 2000, p. 59) Purpose: The purpose of this study was "to compare outcomes for patients randomly assigned to nurse practitioners or physicians for primary care follow-up and ongoing care after an emergency department or urgent care visit." (Mundinger et al., 2000, p. 59)
Correlational Research	Modifiable health risks (physical inactivity, obesity, and smoking), health care charges	Problem: "If physical inactivity, obesity, and smoking status prove to contribute significantly to increased health care charges within a short period of time, health plans and payers may wish to invest in strategies to modify these risk factors. However, few data are available to guide such resource allocation decisions." (Pronk et al., 1999, p. 2235) Purpose: The purpose of this study was to examine the relationship of modifiable health risks (physical inactivity, obesity, and smoking) to subsequent health care charges after controlling for age, race, sex, and chronic conditions." (Pronk et al., 1999, 2235)
Quasi-experimental Research	Perception, control, coping patterns, stress management, cognitive therapy, rheumatoid arthritis	Problem: "Rheumatoid arthritis (RA) is a chronic, unpredictable, systemic connective tissue disorder that manifests itself primarily in the joints. Approximately 1% of the U.S. population has RA, including people of all races, with three times as many women affected as men. (Shlotzhauer & McGuire, 1993) The treatment of RA is not curative, but palliative. It is an expensive and often debilitating disease, both in financial and psychosocial costs." (Sinclair et al., 1998, p. 315) Purpose: "The purpose of this quasi-experimental study was to test the effectiveness of a cognitive-behavioral intervention program designed to affect perceptions of control and coping patterns in women with RA." (Sinclair et al., 1998, p. 315)
Experimental Research	Sleep deprivation, wound healing	Problem: "Sleep is thought to be essential for recovery from injury, and lost or disturbed sleep is believed to hinder postinjury wound healing (tissue repair) . . . The consequences of lost sleep are of particular concern to nurses and other clinicians who provide or guide care for patients after acute surgical or accidental injury and are in a position to facilitate or educate patients about sleep. Questions regarding the possible effects of sleep loss on tissue repair and mechanisms by which sleep loss might negatively affect wound healing have been raised (Lee & Stotts, 1990), but no investigators have systematically evaluated the impact of sleep loss on tissue repair at cellular and subcellular levels." (Landis & Whitney, 1997, p. 259) Purpose: "The purpose of this study was to determine the effects of 72 hours of sleep loss on cellular markers of the proliferative and early collagen biosynthesis phases of wound healing. (Landis & Whitney, 1997, p. 261)

their correlations study, Pronk and colleagues (1999) found that modifiable health risks (physical inactivity, obesity, and smoking) were significantly related to health care charges. Nonsmokers with a body mass index (BMI) of 25 kg/m^2, who participated in physical activity 3 days per week, had mean annual health care charges that were approximately 49% lower than physically inactive smokers with a BMI of 27.5 kg/m^2 (Pronk et al., 1999). Quasi-experimental and experimental studies are conducted to examine causal relationships or to determine the effect of a treatment on designated outcomes. If little is known about a topic, the researcher usually starts with a descriptive study and progresses to the other types of studies.

The problems formulated for qualitative research identify an area of concern that requires investigation. The purpose of a qualitative study indicates the focus of the study and whether it is a subjective concept, an event, a phenomenon, or a facet of a culture or society. Examples of research topics, problems, and purposes from some different types of qualitative studies are presented in Table 5–2. Phenomenological research seeks an understanding of human experience from an individual researcher's perspective, such as the experience of living with the diagnosis of borderline personality disorder (Nehls, 1999). Nehls (1999) identified three themes important to these patients: (1) living with a label, (2) living with self-destructive behavior perceived as manipulation, and (3) living with limited access to care. This knowledge can facilitate increased understanding and management of patients with borderline personality disorder. Some of the types of research problems investigated with phenomenological research include "(1) the interpretation of the single, unique event; (2) the interpretation of a single, unique individual; and (3) the interpretation of a general or repetitive psychological process (e.g., anger, learning, etc.)" (Knaack, 1984, p. 111).

In grounded theory research, the problem identifies the area of concern and the purpose indicates the focus of the theory to be developed from the research. In ethnographic research, the problem and purpose identify the culture and the specific attributes of the culture that are to be examined and

described. The problem and purpose in historical research focus on a specific individual, a characteristic of society, an event, or a situation in the past and identify the period in the past that will be examined. The problem and purpose in philosophical inquiry identify the focus of the analysis, whether it is to clarify meaning, make values manifest, identify ethics, or examine the nature of knowledge. Of the three types of philosophical inquiry (foundational inquiry, philosophical analyses, and ethical analyses), only an example of philosophical analysis is provided with an analysis of the concept "rights" (Reckling, 1994). The problem and purpose in critical social theory identify a society and indicate the particular aspects of the society that will be examined to determine their influence on an event, situation, or system in that society.

Outcomes research is conducted to examine the end-results of care. Table 5–3 includes the topics, problem, and purpose from an outcomes study. Rudy and colleagues (1995) conducted a study to determine the outcomes for patients with chronic critical illness in the special care unit versus in the intensive care unit.

■ SUMMARY

A research problem is an area of concern in which there is a gap in the knowledge base needed for nursing practice. Thus, the problem identifies an area of concern for a particular population and indicates the concepts to be studied. The major sources for nursing research problems include nursing practice, researcher and peer interactions, literature review, theory, and research priorities identified by individuals, specialty groups, and funding agencies. Through the literature review, one might identify studies that require replication. Replication involves reproducing or repeating a study to determine whether similar findings will be obtained. Replication is essential to the development of a knowledge base and provides an excellent learning experience for novice researchers. Four types of replication are identified: exact, approximate, concurrent, and systematic.

The research purpose is a concise, clear state-

TABLE 5–2
QUALITATIVE RESEARCH: TOPICS, PROBLEMS, AND PURPOSES

TYPE OF RESEARCH	RESEARCH TOPIC	RESEARCH PROBLEM AND PURPOSE
Phenomenological Research	Borderline personality disorder, lived experience, phenomenon	Problem: "It is estimated that borderline personality disorder represents 15–25% of all reported psychiatric illness . . . For some individuals, borderline personality disorder is a disabling and life-threatening illness . . . Nearly 10% of patients with borderline personality disorder will kill themselves . . . What remains absent, however, from the voluminous literature on borderline personality disorder is the voice of patients. It has become increasingly clear that studying the lived experience of identified populations is of value." (Nehls, 1999, p. 285)
		Purpose: "The purpose of this interpretive phenomenological study was to generate knowledge about the experience of living with the diagnosis of borderline personality disorder." (Nehls, 1999, p. 285)
Grounded Theory Research	Mechanical ventilation, weaning process, patient's experience	Problem: "Mechanical ventilation and weaning present significant challenges for clinicians. A substantial minority of patients who receive mechanical ventilation support have considerable weaning difficulties and account for a disproportionate amount of health care costs . . . Predictors of weaning success have been studied extensively, primarily from physiologic and technologic perspectives. Less attention has been paid to patients' subjective experience of mechanical ventilation and weaning, even though psychologic factors have been proposed as important determinants of outcomes in some patients, particularly for those requiring prolonged ventilator support." (Logan & Jenny, 1997, p. 140)
		Purpose: "The purpose of this study was to examine patients' subjective experiences of mechanical ventilation and weaning to validate and extend previous work. The study also contributes another perspective to an evolving theory of ventilator weaning." (Logan & Jenny, 1997, p. 141)
Ethnography Research	Inner-city ghettos, survival, elders, drug activity	Problem: "In underserved, inner-city ghettos known for drug-related violence and crime, active participation in community life is dangerous and even life-threatening. This is especially true for elders burdened with the infirmities of aging and lacking the means to provide for alternatives to social isolation. Few researchers have ventured into inner-city communities known for troublesome and dangerous public spaces . . . Therefore, little is known about the social lives of people in these communities, in particular, vulnerable older people who are frequently victims of illegal drug activity." (Kauffman, 1995, p. 231)
		Purpose: "This urban ethnography was conducted over a period of 3 years in a predominantly African American inner-city ghetto. The main question to be answered was: How do elders survive in the midst of 'drug warfare' in an inner-city community known for its dangerous streets and public spaces?" (Kauffman, 1995, p. 231)
Historical Research	Spirituality, beliefs, morals, religion	Problem: "Rigid morals characterize the nineteenth century in the minds of most twentieth-century people . . . While Nightingale's moral beliefs are well documented, less is known about why she held them. Moral and spiritual are not necessarily the same . . . To simply define Florence Nightingale's beliefs, however, does not describe her spirituality—the force that motivated her life." (Widerquist, 1992, p. 49)

	TABLE 5–2	
QUALITATIVE RESEARCH: TOPICS, PROBLEMS, AND PURPOSES *Continued*		
TYPE OF RESEARCH	**RESEARCH TOPIC**	**RESEARCH PROBLEM AND PURPOSE**
Philosophical Analysis Research	Rights, human rights, patient rights, health care	Purpose: "An examination of Nightingale's life—what influenced her beliefs, how she arrived at them, and what she did about them—offers a deeper understanding of her spirituality and a greater awareness of the spiritual issues surrounding nursing." (Widerquist, 1992, p. 49) Problem: "Nurses encounter the word right(s) in many aspects of their personal and professional lives. Patients' rights documents are displayed in healthcare institutions . . . Yet the idea of rights often is not understood clearly. For instance, controversy exists regarding whether access to healthcare is a human right. Furthermore, individual rights are not always honored. Sometimes rights are in conflict, as when one individual's right to confidentiality conflicts with another's right to information." (Reckling, 1994, p. 309) Purpose: "Philosophers have analyzed the ontology and epistemology of rights: Do rights exist? If so, what constitutes them? How do we recognize one when we see it? Where do rights originate? What does having a right imply?." (Reckling, 1994, p. 311)
Critical Social Theory Research	Oppressed group behaviors	Problem: "The study of the behavior of others sometimes reflects our own behaviors." Purpose: "A study was carried out in the Federal Republic of Germany (FRG) to analyze the social, economic, and political factors affecting the nursing education system . . . Theoretical constructs from the work of critical social theorist Jurgen Habermas and adult educator Paulo Freire were used to achieve a deeper understanding of the interrelations between the cultural context and the nursing education system as well as to provide direction for conceptualizing ways to transcend oppressive circumstances." (Hedin, 1986, p. 53)

ment of the specific goal or aim of the study. The goal of a study might be to identify, describe, explain, or predict a solution to a situation. The purpose indicates the type of study to be conducted and often includes the variables, population, and setting for the study. Several purposes can be generated from each research problem.

The exact thought processes used to formulate a research problem and purpose have not been clearly identified because of the abstractness and complexity of the reasoning involved. The researcher examines the real-world situation, identifies research topics, generates questions, and ultimately clarifies and refines a research problem. From the problem, a specific goal or research purpose is developed for the study. The problem selected for investigation must have professional significance and be of personal interest to the researcher.

The purpose is generated from the problem and clearly focuses the development of the study. Based on the research purpose, specific research objectives, questions, or hypotheses are developed to direct the study. As the research problem and purpose become more clear and concise, the researcher has greater direction in determining the feasibility of a study. The feasibility is determined by examining the time and money commitments; researchers' expertise; availability of subjects, facility, and equipment; cooperation of others; and the study's ethical considerations.

Quantitative, qualitative, and outcomes research studies enable nurses to investigate a variety of re-

TABLE 5–3
OUTCOMES RESEARCH: TOPICS, PROBLEMS, AND PURPOSE

TYPE OF RESEARCH	RESEARCH TOPIC	RESEARCH PROBLEM AND PURPOSE
Outcomes Research	Patient outcomes, special care unit, intensive care unit, chronically critically ill	Problem: "The original purpose of intensive care units (ICUs) was to locate groups of patients together who had similar needs for specialized monitoring and care so that highly trained health care personnel would be available to meet these specialized needs. As the success of ICUs has grown and expanded, the assumption that a typical ICU patient will require only a short length of stay in the unit during the most acute phase of an illness has given way to the recognition that stays of more than one month are not uncommon . . . These long-stay ICU patients represent a challenge to the current system, not only because of costs, but also because of concern for patient outcomes . . . While ample evidence confirms that this subpopulation of ICU patients represents a drain on hospital resources, few studies have attempted to evaluate the effects of a care delivery system outside the ICU setting on patient outcomes, costs, and nurse outcomes.' (Rudy et al., 1995, p. 324) Purpose: "The purpose of this study was to compare the effects of a low-technology environment of care and a nurse case management care delivery system (specific care unit, SCU) with the traditional high-technology environment (ICU) and primary nursing care delivery system on the patient outcomes of length of stay, mortality, readmission, complications, satisfaction, and cost." (Rudy et al., 1995, p. 324)

search problems and purposes. In quantitative research, the problem identifies an area of concern, and the purpose reflects the type of study (descriptive, correlational, quasi-experimental, or experimental) to be conducted. The problems formulated for qualitative research also identify an area of concern. The purpose of a qualitative study indicates the focus of the investigation—whether it is a subjective concept, an event, a phenomenon, or a facet of a culture or society. The purpose of outcomes research is to examine the end-results of patient care.

• •

REFERENCES

Ailinger, R. L., & Neal, L. J. (1999). Developing a regional nursing research website. *Image—Journal of Nursing Scholarship, 31*(3), 249–250.

Ajzen, I., & Fishbein, M. (1980). *Understanding attitudes and predicting social behavior.* Englewood Cliffs, NJ: Prentice-Hall.

Albrecht, M. (1992). Research priorities for home health nursing. *Nursing & Health Care, 13*(10), 538–541.

Anderson, R. A., Su, H., Hsieh, P., Allred, C. A., Owensby, S., & Joiner-Rogers, G. (1999). Case mix adjustment in nursing

systems research: The case of resident outcomes in nursing homes. *Research in Nursing & Health, 22*(4), 271–283.

Artinian, B. M., & Anderson, N. (1980). Guidelines for the identification of researchable problems. *Journal of Nursing Education, 19*(4), 54–58.

Beck, C. T. (1994). Replication strategies for nursing research. *Image—Journal of Nursing Scholarship, 26*(3), 191–194.

Becker, M. H. (1974). *The health belief model and personal health behaviors.* Thorofare, NJ: Charles B. Slack.

Beckingham, A. C. (1974). Identifying problems for nursing research. *International Nursing Review, 21*(2), 49–52.

Beveridge, W. I. B. (1950). *The art of scientific investigation.* New York: Vintage.

Beyers, M. (1997). The American Organization of Nurse Executives (AONE) research column: Research priorities of the American Organization of Nurse Executives. *Applied Nursing Research, 10*(1), 52–53.

Brandon, D. H., Holditch-Davis, D., & Beylea, M. (1999). Nursing care and the development of sleeping and waking behaviors in preterm infants. *Research in Nursing & Health, 22*(3), 217–229.

Brink, P. J., & Wood, M. J. (1979). Multiple concurrent replication. *Western Journal of Nursing Research, 1*(1), 117–118.

Brown, B. E., & Garrison, C. J. (1990). Patterns of symptomatology of adult women incest survivors. *Western Journal of Nursing Research, 12*(5), 587–600.

Brown, S. A., & Grimes, D. E. (1995). A meta-analysis of nurse practitioners and nurse midwives in primary care. *Nursing Research, 44*(5), 332–339.

Browne, A., & Finkelhor, D. (1986). Impact of child sexual

abuse: A review of the research. *Psychological Bulletin, 99*(1), 66–77.

Campbell, J. P., Daft, R. L., & Hulin, C. L. (1982). *What to study: Generating and developing research questions.* Beverly Hills, CA: Sage.

Chinn, P. L., & Kramer, M. K. (1998). *Theory and nursing: Integrated knowledge development.* St. Louis: Mosby.

Cox, C. (1982). An interaction model of client health behavior: Theoretical prescription for nursing. *Advances in Nursing Science, 5*(1), 41–56.

Davies, A. R., Doyle, M. A. T., Lansky, D., Rutt, W., Stevic, M. O., & Doyle, J. B. (1994). Outcomes assessment in clinical settings: A consensus statement on principles and best practices in project management. *The Joint Commission Journal on Quality Improvement, 20*(1), 6–16.

Diers, D. (1979). *Research in nursing practice.* Philadelphia: Lippincott.

Flemming, K. (1999). Searchable questions. *Nursing Times Learning Curve, 3*(2), 6–7.

Foster-Fitzpatrick, L., Ortiz, A., Sibilano, H., Marcantonio, R., & Braun, L. T. (1999). The effects of crossed leg on blood pressure measurement. *Nursing Research, 48*(2), 105–108.

Gold, E. (1986). Long-term effects of sexual victimization in childhood: An attributional approach. *Journal of Consulting and Clinical Psychology, 54*(4), 471–475.

Haller, K. B., & Reynolds, M. A. (1986). Using research in practice: A case for replication in nursing: Part II. *Western Journal of Nursing Research, 8*(2), 249–252.

Hedin, B. A. (1986). A case study of oppressed group behavior in nurses. *Image—Journal of Nursing Scholarship, 18*(2), 53–57.

Henry, B. M., & Chang, W. Y. (1998). Nursing research priorities in Africa, Asia, and Europe. *Image—Journal of Nursing Scholarship, 30*(2), 115–116.

Hill, M. N., & Grim, C. M. (1991). How to take a precise blood pressure. *American Journal of Nursing, 91*(2), 38–42.

Hirschfeld, M. J. (1998). WHO priorities for a common nursing research agenda. *International Nursing Review, 45*(1), 13–14.

Kahn, C. R. (1994). Picking a research problem: The critical decision. *The New England Journal of Medicine, 330*(21), 1530–1533.

Kaplan, B. A. (1964). *The conduct of inquiry: Methodology for behavioral science.* New York: Harper & Row.

Kauffman, K. S. (1995). Center as haven: Findings of an urban ethnography. *Nursing Research, 44*(4), 231–236.

King, I., & Tarsitano, B. (1982). The effect of structured and unstructured preoperative teaching: A replication. *Nursing Research, 31*(6), 324–329.

Knaack, P. (1984). Phenomenological research. *Western Journal of Nursing Research, 6*(1), 107–114.

Landis, C. A., & Whitney, J. D. (1997). Effects of 72 hours sleep deprivation on wound healing in the rat. *Research in Nursing & Health, 20*(3), 259–267.

Lee, K. A., & Stotts, N. A. (1990). Support of the growth hormone-somatomedin system to facilitate healing. *Heart & Lung, 19*(2), 157–164.

Lewandowski, A., & Kositsky, A. M. (1983). Research priorities for critical care nursing: A study by the American Association of Critical Care Nurses. *Heart & Lung, 12*(1), 35–44.

Lindeman, C. A. (1975). Delphi survey of priorities in clinical nursing research. *Nursing Research, 24*(6), 434–441.

Lindeman, C. A., & Van Aernam, B. (1971). Nursing intervention with the presurgical patient: The effects of structured and unstructured preoperative teaching. *Nursing Research, 20*(4), 319–332.

Lindquist, R., Banasik, J., Barnsteiner, J., Beecroft, P. C., Prevost, S., Riegel, B., Sechrist, K., Strzelecki, C., & Titler, M. (1993). Determining AACN's research priorities for the 90s. *American Journal of Critical Care, 2*(2), 110–117.

Logan, J., & Jenny, J. (1997). Qualitative analysis of patients' work during mechanical ventilation and weaning. *Heart & Lung, 26*(2), 140–147.

Lowry, L. W., & Beikirch, P. (1998). Effect of comprehensive care on pregnancy outcomes. *Applied Nursing Research, 11*(2), 55–61.

Martin, P. A. (1994). The utility of the research problem statement. *Applied Nursing Research, 7*(1), 47–49.

Martin, P. A. (1995). More replication studies needed. *Applied Nursing Research, 8*(2), 102–103.

Moody, L., Vera, H., Blanks, C., & Visscher, M. (1989). Developing questions of substance for nursing science. *Western Journal of Nursing Research, 11*(4), 393–404.

Morin, K., Gennaro, S., & Fehder, W. (1999). Nutrition and exercise in overweight and obese postpartum women. *Applied Nursing Research, 12*(1), 13–21.

Mundinger, M. O., Kane, R. L., Lenz, E. R., Totten, A. M., Tsai, W., Cleary, P. D., Friedewald, W. T., Siu, A. L., & Shelanski, M. L. (2000). Primary care outcomes in patients treated by nurse practitioners or physicians: A randomized trial. *Journal of the American Medical Association, 283*(1), 59–68.

Nehls, N. (1999). Borderline personality disorder: The voice of patients. *Research in Nursing & Health, 22*(4), 285–293.

Panel for the Prediction and Prevention of Pressure Ulcers in Adults. (1992, May). *Pressure ulcers in adults: Prediction and preventions. Clinical practice guideline.* AHCPR Pub. No. 92–0047. Rockville, MD: Agency for Health Care Policy and Research, Public Health Service, U.S. Department of Health and Human Services.

Phillips, J. M., & Wilbur, J. (1995). Adherence to breast cancer screening guidelines among African-American women of differing employment status. *Cancer Nursing, 18*(4), 258–269.

Pronk, N. P., Goodman, M. J., O'Connor, P. J., & Martinson, B. C. (1999). Relationship between modifiable health risks and short-term health care charges. *Journal of the American Medical Association, 282*(23), 2235–2239.

Reckling, J. B. (1994). Conceptual analysis of rights using a philosophic inquiry approach. *Image: Journal of Nursing Scholarship, 26*(4), 309–314.

Reynolds, M. A., & Haller, K. B. (1986). Using research in practice: A case for replication in nursing: Part I. *Western Journal of Nursing Research, 8*(1), 113–116.

Rogers, B. (1987). Research corner: Is the research project feasible? *AAOHN Journal, 35*(7), 327–328.

Rudy, E. B., Daly, B. J., Douglas, S., Montenegro, H. D., Song, R., & Dyer, M. A. (1995). Patient outcomes for the chronically critically ill: Special care unit versus intensive care unit. *Nursing Research, 44*(6), 324–330.

Sidani, S., & Braden, C. P. (1998). *Evaluating nursing interventions: A theory-driven approach.* Thousand Oaks, CA: Sage.

Sinclair, V. G., Wallston, K. A., Dwyer, K. A., Blackburn, D. S., & Fuchs, H. (1998). Effects of a cognitive-behavioral intervention for women with rheumatoid arthritis. *Research in Nursing & Health, 21*(4), 315–326.

Taunton, R. L. (1989). Replication: Key to research application. *Dimensions of Critical Care Nursing, 8*(3), 156–158.

Tierney, A. J. (1998). Nursing research in Europe. *International Nursing Review, 45*(1), 15–18.

Waters, C. M. (1999). Professional nursing support for culturally diverse family members of critically ill adults. *Research in Nursing & Health, 22*(2), 107–117.

Whitney, J. D., Stotts, N. A., & Goodson, W. H. (1995). Effects of dynamic exercise on subcutaneous oxygen tension and temperature. *Research in Nursing & Health, 18*(2), 97–104.

Williams, A. (1972). A study of factors contributing to skin breakdown. *Nursing Research, 21*(3), 238–243.

Widerquist, J. G. (1992). The spirituality of Florence Nightingale. *Nursing Research, 41*(1), 49–55.

Wright, D. J. (1999). Developing an effective research question. *Professional Nurse, 14*(11), 786–789.

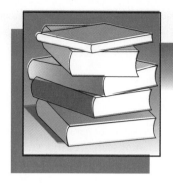

CHAPTER **6**

REVIEW OF RELEVANT LITERATURE

Reviewing the existing literature related to your study is a critical step in the research process. It is essential that a researcher's work be built upon the works of others (Kaplan, 1964). As Becker (1986, p. 140) puts it, "Science and humanistic scholarship are, in fact as well as in theory, cumulative enterprises. None of us invent it all from scratch when we sit down to write. We depend on our predecessors. We couldn't do our work if we didn't use their methods, results, and ideas. Few people would be interested in our results if we didn't indicate some relationship between them and what others have said and done before us."

This chapter guides you through the process of performing a literature review. The three major stages of a literature review that are delineated are searching the literature, reading the literature, and writing the literature review.

WHAT IS "THE LITERATURE"?

"The literature" consists of all written sources relevant to the topic you have selected. The published literature contains primary and secondary sources. A *primary source* is written by the person who originated, or is responsible for generating, the ideas published. In research publications, a primary source is written by the person or people who conducted the research. A primary theoretical source is written by the theorist who developed the theory or conceptual content.

A *secondary source* summarizes or quotes content from primary sources. Thus, authors of secondary sources paraphrase the works of researchers and theorists. The problem with a secondary source is that the author has interpreted the works of someone else, and this interpretation is influenced by that author's perception and bias. Sometimes errors and misinterpretations have been promulgated by authors using secondary sources rather than primary sources. You should use mostly primary sources to develop research proposals and reports. Secondary sources are used only if primary sources cannot be located or if a secondary source contains creative ideas or a unique organization of information not found in a primary source.

Two types of literature are used predominantly in the review of literature for research, theoretical and empirical. *Theoretical literature* consists of concept analyses, models, theories, and conceptual frameworks that support a selected research problem and purpose. *Empirical literature* comprises relevant studies in journals and books as well as unpublished studies, such as master's theses and doctoral dissertations. Other types of literature, such as descriptions of clinical situations, educational literature, and position papers, may be included in the discussion of background and significance of the research topic but because of their subjectivity often are not cited in the review of literature (Marchette, 1985; Pinch, 1995).

Integrative reviews are a type of secondary source that may be important to a review of the literature. Integrative reviews are conducted to identify, analyze, and synthesize the results from independent studies to determine the current knowledge (what is known and not known) in a particular area (Beyea & Nicoll, 1998; Ganong, 1987; Smith & Stullenbarger, 1991). Such a review contains a comprehensive list of references and summarizes empirical literature for selected topics (Cooper, 1984). An example is the *Annual Review of Nursing Research*, first published in 1983 by Werley and Fitzpatrick. The volumes of this publication, which continue to be published annually, contain excellent and thorough integrative reviews of research in the areas of nursing practice, nursing care delivery, nursing education, and the profession of nursing. Integrative reviews have also been published in a variety of clinical and nonclinical journals.

The *Online Journal of Nursing Synthesis*, published by Sigma Theta Tau, is limited to integrative reviews. The website *http://www.best4health.com/*, sponsored by a large number of nursing organizations, provides integrative reviews of research-based nursing interventions.

In some cases, an integrative review is built around one or more theories used in the field of research. Review articles are primary sources in terms of the author's synthesis of the literature; however, they are secondary sources in terms of the author's discussion of previous authors' works. To use this information, you need to turn to the primary source of each author's work. For some research problems, you will find policy papers, standards of practice, or proposed legislation that may be important to include as part of the literature review. Clinical papers may be important for addressing the background and significance of the problem, but they should not be included in the review of literature.

Auston and colleagues (1992) of The National Library of Medicine define a literature search as "a systematic and explicit approach to the identification, retrieval, and bibliographical management of independent studies (usually drawn from published sources) for the purpose of locating information on a topic, synthesizing conclusions, identifying areas for future study, and developing guidelines for clinical practice."

It is rarely, if ever, possible to identify every relevant source in the literature. The most extensive retrievals of literature are probably the funded literature review projects focused on defining evidence-based practice or developing clinical practice guidelines. In these projects, a literature review coordinator manages the literature review process. The project employs several full-time, experienced, professional librarians as literature searchers. For these projects, at least two preliminary computerized literature searches are performed; then a comprehensive search is conducted that may encompass material not included in electronic databases and unpublished sources; and finally, periodic searches are performed to update the material. The process requires at least 1 or 2 years of extensive work (Auston et al., 1992). When these extensive literature reviews are completed, the results are published so that you may have access to them and to the citations from the review, either on the World Wide Web (the Web) or in journal articles.

As a student or nurse researcher, your goal is to develop a search strategy designed to retrieve as much of the relevant literature as possible given the time and financial constraints of your study. Your literature review should be designed to address the following questions (Asian Institute of Technology, 2000; The Union Institute Research Engine, 1999):

- What is known about your topic?
- What is the chronology of the development of knowledge about your topic?
- What evidence is lacking, inconclusive, contradictory, or too limited?
- Is there a consensus or significant debate on issues? What are the various positions?
- What directions are indicated by the work of other researchers?
- What are the characteristics of the key concepts or variables?
- What are the relationships among the key concepts or variables?
- What are the existing theories in the field of research?
- Where are the inconsistencies or other shortcomings in the knowledge base?

- What views need to be (further) tested?
- Why should a research problem be (further) studied?
- What contribution can the present study be expected to make?
- What research designs or methods seem unsatisfactory?

TIME FRAME FOR A LITERATURE REVIEW

The time required to review the literature is influenced by the problem studied, sources available, and goals of the researcher. There is no set length of time for reviewing the literature, but there are guidelines for directing the review process. The narrower the focus of the study, the less time will be required to review the literature. The difficulty in identifying and locating sources and the number of sources to be located also influence the time involved.

If a researcher's goal is to conduct a study within a set time frame, the review of literature might have to be limited to meet the deadline. If a study is to be conducted within 1 year, the review of literature will probably take a minimum of a month but should not exceed 3 months. The intensity of the effort determines the time required to complete the review. Only through experience do researchers become knowledgeable about the time frame for a literature review. Novice researchers frequently underestimate the time needed for the review and ought to plan at least twice the amount of time originally projected.

If researchers attempted to read every source that is somewhat related to a selected problem, they would be well read but would probably never begin conducting their study. Some researchers, even after a thorough literature review, continue to believe that they do not know enough about their area of study, so they persist in their review; however, this ultimately becomes an excuse for not progressing with their research. The opposite of this situation is the researcher who wants to move rapidly through the review of literature to reach the "important part" of conducting the study. In both situations, the researcher has not been able to set realistic goals for conducting the literature review.

Students repeatedly ask, "How many articles should I have? How far back in years should I go to find relevant studies?" The answer to both those questions is an emphatic "It depends." You need to locate the key studies in the field of research. You need to identify the landmark or seminal studies done. *Seminal studies* are the first studies that prompted the initiation of the field of research. *Landmark studies* mark an important stage of development or a turning point in the field of research. Beyea and Nicoll (1998, p. 879) provide some good advice about knowing when you have sufficient sources. "Many people ask, 'How will I know when my literature search is complete?' On one hand, it never will be because new information constantly is being added to literature. Even so, it is important to know when to stop. From our experience, we found that research will reach an apparent saturation point. As you look at reference lists, you will realize that every article and every author is familiar to you. Or, you might see a pattern in the research and it will be evident when the search has reached its natural conclusion."

SEARCHING THE LITERATURE

The process of searching the literature has changed dramatically as the use of computers has increased. Gone are the days when researchers spent long hours (weeks, months, years!) in the library, methodically hunting through dusty card catalogues, searching for relevant journal articles in the red-bound volumes of *CINAHL* (*Cumulative Index to Nursing and Allied Health Literature*), with print so small that a magnifying glass was almost needed, pulling old bound journal volumes from the library shelves, making handwritten notes on yellow legal pads from the bound journal articles as they read them, and writing all the citation information on an index card for each of the references found. Index cards were then filed alphabetically for use when the paper was written. The literature available for review either was limited to that in the library or required travel to a larger library elsewhere. Although libraries are not the only resources at a university required for good research, good research tended to be limited to universities that had libraries with large holdings of books and journals, and good researchers migrated to these universities.

Today, good libraries provide access to large numbers of electronic databases that supply a broad scope of the available literature internationally, enabling library users not only to identify relevant sources quickly but also to print full-text versions of many of these sources immediately. Through the use of these databases, a large volume of references can be located quickly. Photocopies can be made from journals held by the library, and photocopies of other articles can often be obtained through Interlibrary Loan arrangements between your library and other libraries across the country. All libraries, public, private, college, and university, have Interlibrary Loan capabilities.

The most complex part of a literature review is identifying your material, not obtaining it. Increasingly, full-text copies of articles can be printed immediately from the Internet. These services, librarian consultations, database searching, Interlibrary Loan services, full-text article downloads, and more, are often available to faculty and student researchers, even those who live far from the university. We can link with the university library through the Internet, through direct modem connections to the library, and through e-mail. These resources are also available at many health care facilities and can be accessed by nurses employed there. Those without this access can purchase electronic facsimile (fax) copies of resources from some of the bibliographical search engines, although any library at which a researcher has borrowing privileges can use Interlibrary Loan. Because of these resources, the researcher can now spend more time reading and synthesizing and less time searching. The next section of the chapter guides you through the process of using these marvelous new strategies to obtain the relevant literature for your study.

DEVELOPING A SEARCH STRATEGY

Before you begin searching the literature, you must consider exactly what information you are seeking. A written plan of your search strategy saves you considerable time in this phase of your study. It helps you (1) avoid going back along paths you have already searched, (2) retrace your steps if need be, and (3) search new paths.

Your initial search should be based on the widest possible interpretation of your topic. This strategy enables you to get some vision of the extent of the relevant literature. As you see the results of the initial searches and begin reading the material, you will refine your topic, and then you can narrow the focus of your searches. Consider consulting with an information professional, such as a subject specialist librarian, to develop a literature search approach. More and more, such consultation can be performed via e-mail, so that communication occurs at both the researcher's and information professional's convenience. Many university libraries provide this consultation service without regard to the library user's affiliation to the university.

Select Databases To Search

A *bibliographical database* is a compilation of citations. The database may consist of citations relevant to a specific discipline or may be a broad collection of citations from a variety of disciplines. Databases can be divided into the following three distinct types:

Indexes and *abstracts* compile citations with subject headings and may include a paragraph or so about the citation.
Full-text reprint services may or may not include detailed subject analysis.
Citation search indexes link citations on the basis of the references at the end of articles.

The databases first used for literature searches were in printed form. They were card catalogues, abstract reviews, and indexes. In nursing, the most relevant print database is *CINAHL*, which contains citations of nursing literature published after 1955. The print version of *CINAHL* was fondly referred to by nursing scholars as "The Red Books" because all the editions were bound with red covers. The print version of *CINAHL* is still useful in searches when citations published prior to 1982 are needed or if computerized databases are not available. Another print database used by nurse researchers is the *Index Medicus* (*IM*), which was first published in 1879 and is the oldest health-related index. The *Index Medicus* includes some citations of nursing publications, with the number of nursing journals cited growing in recent years; however, *CINAHL* contains a more extensive listing of nursing publications and uses more nursing terminology as subject headings.

The earliest printed nursing index is the *Nursing Studies Index*, developed by Virginia Henderson, which consists of citations of nursing literature published from 1890 to 1959. The National Library of Medicine provides free access to several databases, including MEDLINE, the on-line equivalent of the *Index Medicus*, with access through Internet Grateful Med and PubMed software (available at *http://www.nlm.nih.gov/databases/freemedl.html*). Buenker (1999) offers instructions on using the Internet version of MEDLINE.

Electronic bibliographical databases began to be used by libraries at larger universities in the 1970s as the use of computers rapidly expanded. In the 1980s, the first end-user electronic bibliographical databases were provided on CD-ROMs, and updated versions were mailed to the library periodically. Currently, most libraries are using on-line bibliographical databases, in which the researcher can do the searches without needing librarian assistance. Most of the print databases are now available on line. Libraries subscribe to vendors who, for a fee, provide software, such as Silver Platter, OVID, and PaperChase, with which you can access multiple bibliographical databases.

Many government agencies that produce bibliographical databases, such as the National Library of Medicine, provide free access to them. However, vendors may distribute the same data, providing "value-added" enhancements with their search software.

Full-text databases of journal articles are now available for some journals. To have access to these databases, libraries must subscribe to the service. For a variety of reasons, including the cost of receipt and storage as well as convenience to library users, many libraries are discontinuing subscriptions to paper versions of journals and, instead, subscribing to services that provide access to electronic versions. This arrangement gives the user immediate access to articles that can be read on line, printed, or saved as a computer file, often whenever and wherever an affiliated user is located. As a result of these innovations, users now have more immediate access to a wide range of literature, including international sources.

Select Keywords

Keywords are the major concepts or variables that must be included in your search. To begin determining keywords, identify the concepts relevant to your study. Identify populations that are of particular interest in your area of study, particular interventions, measurement methods, or outcomes that are relevant.

In quantitative studies, information obtained from the review of literature influences the development of several steps in the research process; these steps are listed in Table 6–1. Search strategies should be designed to ensure that you obtain adequate information for each of the steps in Table 6–1. In most databases, subject headings and phrases can be used as well as single terms. Your problem and purpose statements give you some guidance in identifying relevant terms (see Chapter 5).

TABLE 6–1
PURPOSES OF THE LITERATURE REVIEW IN QUANTITATIVE RESEARCH

Clarify the research topic
Clarify the research problem
Verify the significance of the research problem
Specify the purpose of the study
Describe relevant studies
Describe relevant theories
Summarize current knowledge
Facilitate development of the framework
Specify research objectives, questions, or hypotheses
Develop definitions of major variables
Identify limitations and assumptions
Select a research design
Identify methods of measurement
Direct data collection and analysis
Interpret findings

You should then think of alternative terms (*synonyms*) that authors might use for each concept or variable you have identified. You may need to express your search using the exact words the authors have used in the literature you seek. Many bibliographical databases, such as *CINAHL*, have an article-specific subject analysis and provide formal subject headings for each article. These databases have a thesaurus that the researcher as well as anyone who reads the article can use as keyword search terms. By logging on to the database, you can access the thesaurus to select relevant terms. The formal subject terms included in the thesaurus may encompass a number of the terms that you have identified and allow you to expand your search to obtain more references or to focus your search to be more specific to your interest. This expansion or focus occurs because all citations with similar concepts have been grouped according to similar terms or concepts by someone who has already read the articles. For example, depending on the database, the researcher may not have to worry whether *teens, teenagers, youth, adolescents,* or *adolescence* must be searched individually or only one term needs to be identified. Frequently, word processing programs, dictionaries, and encyclopedias are helpful in identifying synonymous terms and subheadings. Some of the synonymous terms and subheadings for the research topic of postoperative experience are outlined in Table 6–2.

Truncating words can allow you to locate more citations related to that term. For example, authors might have used *intervene, intervenes, intervened, intervening, intervention,* or *intervenor.* To capture all of these terms, you can use a truncated term in your search (the form depends on the rule of the search engine being used), such as *interven, interven*,* or *interven$.* Do not truncate words to less than four letters; you will get far too many unwanted citations.

Pay attention to variant spellings. Consider irregular plurals, such as *woman* and *women.* You may need to know, for example, that *orthopedic* may also be spelled *orthopaedic.*

As you begin to examine the literature, you may find that certain authors are cited by many of the authors in the field. You may wish to use these commonly cited authors' names as search terms so that you are sure you are aware of all of their relevant publications. Recognize that some databases list authors only under first and middle initials, and others under full first names. Identifying and using citations to seminal studies in various citation indexes or full-text databases can lead you to other, more current works that have also used the seminal studies as references. You may also know of or discover particular journals that are key to your field of research. If so, you may wish to use a journal title as a search term.

Add your selected search terms to your written search plan. As you search, you may add other terms that you discover from the references you locate. For each search, record (1) the name of the database you used, (2) the date you performed the search, (3) the exact search strategy, (4) the number of articles found, and (5) the percentage of relevant articles. You can even develop a table to record this information from multiple search strategies. Save

TABLE 6–2
CLARIFYING A RESEARCH TOPIC

RESEARCH TOPIC	SYNONYMOUS TERMS	SUBHEADINGS
Postoperative experience	Postoperative care Postoperative recovery Postsurgical experience Surgical care Surgical recovery	Postoperative ambulation Postoperative attitude Postoperative complications Postoperative hospitalization Postoperative pain Postoperative teaching

the results of each search on your computer's hard disk or on a floppy disk for later reference; in your written search record, document the file name of the search results.

Use Reference Management Software

Reference management software can make tracking the references you have obtained through your searches considerably easier. You can use such software to conduct searches and to store the information on all search fields for each reference obtained in a search, including the abstract. Once you have done so, all of the needed citation information and the abstract are readily available to you electronically when you write the literature review. As you read the articles, you can also insert comments into the reference file about each one.

Reference management software has been developed to interface directly with the most commonly used word processing software to organize the reference information using whatever citation style you stipulate. You can insert citations into your paper with just a keystroke or two. The two most commonly used software packages, along with the websites with information about them, are as follows:

- ProCite *(http://www.isiresearchsoft.com/pc/PChome. html)*
- EndNote *(http://www.endnote.com/)*

You may download a trial version of either software package from the website and use the program to write one or two papers. In that way, you can judge each program's effectiveness in helping you track and cite references and decide whether to purchase it.

Locate Relevant Literature

Within each database, initiate your search by performing a separate search of each keyword you have identified. Search engines are unforgiving of misspellings, so watch your spelling carefully. Most databases allow you to indicate quickly where in the database records you wish to search for the

term—in the article titles, journal names, keywords, formal subject headings, or full texts of the articles. Citations are usually listed with the most recent ones first. You might be interested in examining the earliest citations.

Most databases provide abstracts of the articles in which the term is cited, allowing you to get some sense of their content, so you may judge whether the term is useful in relation to your selected topic. If you find it to be an important reference, save it to a file.

Do not try to examine all of the citations listed at this point. Look instead at the number of citations (or "hits") that the search found. In some cases, you may have obtained several thousand hits—far too many to examine. For example, in March 2000, a search of an on-line database using the keyword "coping" yielded 3926 hits. The keyword "social support" yielded 6195 hits.

After you have performed a search, save it as a file, record the number of citations, and proceed to the next keyword. When you have completed this activity, you will have some sense of the extent of available literature in your area of interest. At this point, you have the information you need to plan appropriately more complex searches.

PERFORMING COMPLEX SEARCHES

A *complex search* combines two or more concepts or synonyms in one search. You can also select specified areas or fields of a database record, such as "cited references" or "instrumentation," as a complex search. Selection of the concepts or synonyms to combine may be based on the results of your previous searches or performed for theoretical reasons. The method of performing more complex searches varies with the bibliographical database, so when you use a particular database for the first time, look for instructions and consider consulting with a librarian.

There are several ways to arrange terms in a database search phrase or phrases. The three most common ways are by using (1) Boolean, (2) locational, and (3) positional operators. *Operators* permit grouping of ideas, selection of places to search in a database record, and ways to show relationships within a database record, sentence, or paragraph. Examine the Help screen carefully to determine whether the operators you want to use are available and how they are used.

The *Boolean operators* are the three words AND, OR, and NOT. They are always in capital letters. The Boolean operators AND and NOT are used with your identified concepts. Use AND when you want to search for the presence of two or more terms in the same citation. Use NOT when you want to search for one idea but not another in the same citation. NOT is rarely used because it is too easy to lose good citations. The Boolean operator OR is most useful with synonymous terms or concepts. Use OR when you want to search for the presence of any of a group of terms in the same citation.

Locational operators identify terms in specific areas or fields of a record. These fields may be parts of the simple citation, such as the article title, author, and journal name, or may be from additional fields provided by the database, such as subject headings, abstracts, cited references, publication type notes, instruments used, and even the entire article. Common formats for locational searches use the database field codes. Each of the following examples shows two ways to perform the same type of search, depending on the specific database being used:

> Coping in ab *or* coping.ab.: Find the word *coping* in the abstract.
> Orem in rf *or* Orem.rf.: Find the name *Orem* in the cited references.
> ENABL in tx *or* ENABL.tx.: Find the program ENABL anywhere in the full text.

Positional operators are used to look for requested terms within certain distances of one another. Availability and phrasing of positional operators are very dependent on the database search software. Common positional operators are NEAR, WITH, and ADJ; they also are always entered in capital letters and may have numbers associated with them. A positional operator is most useful in records with a large amount of information, such as those with full-text articles attached, and is often used with locational operators, in either an implied

way or explicitly. For example, ADJ is an abbreviation for "adjacent"; it specifies that one term must be adjacent to another, in any order. ADJ2 commands that there must be no more than two intervening words between the search terms. NEAR usually defines the specific order of the terms; the command term1 NEAR1 term2 requires that the first term occur first and within 2 words of the second term. WITH often indicates that the terms must be within the same sentence, paragraph, or region (such as subject headings) of the record.

In highly textual records such as those with abstracts or entire articles, using truncation in keyword searches yield good results. Truncation symbols are also database defined and may have numbers associated with them. Common truncation symbols are: !, +, \$, *, ?, and #. They allow you to enter parts of words as the search phrase, so that the search engine locates all occurrences of that part of the word with additional letters attached. For example: Catheter\$ can retrieve *Catheter*, *catheters*, *catheterize*, *catheterization*, and so on. If the base of the term is very short, just a few letters, consider a limited truncation by using an associated number. For example: Pet\$1 can retrieve up to one character more, *pet* and *pets* but not petard.

Many of these various operators are quickly accessible in front of the database software, but others may require further exploration of the Help screens. Different search engines (software) may require different means of structuring your terms so that the software will perform the search in the way you conceive of it. For example, in *CINAHL* and using OVID software, you can performing searches for individual terms and then initiate a Boolean search by selecting the Combine option at the top of the screen. A new screen appears, listing the previous searches you have performed. You may select two or more of the previous searches to combine. For example, you might wish to combine the concepts "coping" and "social support." In March 2000, selecting the Combine AND option in *CINAHL* for the "coping" search and the "social support" search yielded 741 hits.

In some bibliographical databases, the term *and* is used to combine terms. In some databases, the word must be in uppercase. Sometimes quotation marks must be placed around the concepts—for example, "coping" and "social support." In others, just typing *coping* and *social support* will find the references you seek. Combining concepts in some databases is done by adding a plus sign (+) before each term you wish to include. The search terms would appear as follows: +coping +social support. There must be no space between the + and the term following it, but there must be a space after each term listed. These search methods find references in which both (all listed) terms appear in the same article.

In some databases, you can use the positional term NEAR to indicate that the two words you have selected must be near each other rather than just appear in the same article—for example, coping NEAR social support. The term OR can be used to expand a search. For example, you might wish to search with the phrase "intervention" OR "treatment"; in this case, if either term is used in an article or paper, it will be listed.

Searches for some topics may reveal that many hits are not useful because the search term you have selected also includes another term that is of no interest to you. For example, you may want to examine studies of coping but not those discussing coping in relation to support. To eliminate references with the term *support*, use as your search phrase "coping" NOT "support."

A number of other complex operations can be used to search databases, but the search methods described here will get you started. Look for instructions about search options in the database you are using. Some databases provide an advanced search option in which separate boxes are available for inclusion of multiple terms. For example, you might wish to include an author's last name, one or more key terms, and a journal title in a single search.

LIMITING YOUR SEARCH

You can use several strategies to limit your search if, after performing Boolean searches, you continue to get too many hits. The limits you can impose vary with the database. In *CINAHL,* for example, you may limit your search to English language articles. You can also limit the years of your search. For example, you might choose to limit the search to articles published in the last 10 years.

Searches can be limited to find only papers that are research, are reviews, are published in consumer health journals, include abstracts, or are available in full text.

When the combined search for "coping" and "social support," described in the last section, was limited to research papers in English, there were 393 hits. Limiting the search to research papers in English published between 1995 and 1999 yielded 161 hits. Limiting the search to research papers in English with full text available yielded 12 hits. Examining 393 hits is possible, and if you needed only the most recent studies, you might wish to examine only those 161 hits.

From the titles, you can select (by clicking the box to the left of the reference in the list of citations, OVID software) the hits that seem most relevant to your topic. You can then either print or save to a file the citations you have selected. Saving the citation to a file and then printing it with a word processing program takes considerably less paper than trying to print directly from the database. You may wish to select the full-text option for hits with full text available; you can then either print these papers or save them to files for printing later or reading later on the computer screen.

SELECTING SEARCH FIELDS

Search fields indicate the various pieces of information provided about an article by the bibliographical database. The fields vary with the bibliographical database. In *CINAHL,* by selecting Search Fields at the top of the search page, you can indicate search fields available in *CINAHL* you wish listed for the references you select. The following list explains the search fields available for this database:

Accession Number. The number assigned to the citation when it was entered into the CINAHL database.

Special Fields Contained. List of the special fields available for a particular citation. *Special fields* include abstracts and cited references.

Authors. Names of the authors, last name first, then initials of first names. Author names are in blue and underlined. The underlining indicates that clicking on the name will result in a search listing all of the citations in the database in which that individual is an author. This option allows you to identify other publications of authors who are central to building the body of knowledge about the topic you have elected to study.

Institution. The institution at which each author was affiliated at the time the article was published. This information might be useful if you wished to contact the author.

Title. Title of the article.

Source. Journal title, volume number, issue, page numbers, year, month, and number of references.

Abbreviated Source. Abbreviated version of the Journal title, volume number, issue, page numbers, year, month, and number of references.

Document Delivery. The National Library of Medicine (NLM) serial identifier number. This number is useful if you plan to request delivery of the document by fax, e-mail, or postal delivery. In many cases, there is a rather large fee for this service. Contact a library for Interlibrary Loan arrangements, which may be free or have a nominal cost.

Journal Subset. The categories to which the journal has been assigned. For example, the journal may be classified as a core nursing journal, a nursing journal, a peer-reviewed journal, or a USA journal.

Special Interest Category. The categories of specialization to which the journal has been assigned. For example, the journal may be classified in the category Oncologic Care.

CINAHL Subject Headings. The keywords from the CINAHL thesaurus that have been assigned to the article. These assignments have been made by professional indexers who have read the article. Examination of these subject headings in the references you have obtained in a search can suggest additional keywords for your keyword list.

Instrumentation. A list of the measurement instruments used in the study.

Abstract. An abstract of the study.

ISSN. The International Standard Serial Number, an identifier number for the journal.

Publication Type. The type of article. For example Journal Article, Research Journal Article, Dissertation. Also indicates the presence of tables, graphs, and charts.

Language. The language in which the article is written. In many cases, articles that are not in English have English abstracts.

Entry Month. The month in which the citation was entered in the CINAHL database.

Cited References. List of full references for all citations in the paper. These references can be valuable because you can use them to cross-check the completeness of your computer searches.

To accomplish a cross-check using the database's Cited References list, compare the list with the citations you have obtained from your searches. This is very easy to do if you have used reference management software. In many cases, you will find "treasures" you would have missed if you had relied only on the computer search. Some of the references may not be journals or books listed in the databases that you have searched and may provide clues to other databases containing additional useful sources. These references may also suggest new keywords for another computer search in the databases you have been using.

SEARCHING ELECTRONIC JOURNALS

A number of nursing journals have been developed that are published only in electronic form. Because of the high costs of publishing and distributing a printed journal, a publishing company risks losing money unless there is a very large market for the journal. Most of the electronic journals are targeted to specialty audiences that are relatively small. These journals may have more current information on your topic than you will find in traditional journals, because articles submitted by authors are reviewed and published within 3 to 4 months; for articles submitted to printed journals, the time from submission to publication is 1 to 2 years.

Many electronic journals have been established at universities by faculty members interested in a particular specialty area. In some cases, you may have to subscribe to the on-line journal to gain access to the articles. Some electronic journals are listed in available bibliographical databases, and you can access full-text articles from an electronic journal through the database. However, many electronic journals are not yet in the bibliographical databases or may not be in the database you are using. Ingenta *(http://www.ingenta.com/)* is a commercial website that allows you to search thousands of on-line journals from many disciplines.

To obtain relevant articles from an electronic journal, you need to locate the journal on the Internet and scan the titles of articles published. Many libraries have contracts with the vendors that enable their affiliated users to have off-campus access to some of these journals and databases. Some contracts require that nonaffiliated users may use the resources only within the library. Still other contracts require that all use of the resources must occur in the library or other specified building or terminal. A list of the current electronic nursing journals is available at the following Web addresses:

*http://www.nursefriendly.com/nursing/linksec-
tions/nursingjournals.htm*
*http://www.lib.umich.edu/hw/nursing/re-
sources.html*
http://www-sci.lib.uci.edu/HSG/Nursing.html#NN3
*http://www.nursing-portal.com/nursingjour-
nals.html*

Many libraries provide lists of the electronic journals available to their affiliated users. You should also examine the lists. If you are affiliated with the library, you may be able to obtain articles quite easily.

SEARCHING THE INTERNET/WORLD WIDE WEB

Although it is unlikely you will find studies relevant to your topic by searching the World Wide Web, you may find information relevant to the background, significance, framework, design, methods of measurement, and statistical procedures for your study.

One advantage of information obtained from the Web is that it is likely to be more current than material you find in books. One disadvantage is that the information is uneven in terms of accuracy. There is no screening process for information placed on the Web. Thus, you find a considerable amount of misinformation as well as some "gems" you might not find elsewhere. It is important to check the source of any information you obtain from the Web so that you can judge its validity.

A wide range of search engines are available for conducting Web searches. Search engines vary in (1) the approach used to search the Web, (2) the extent of Web coverage (most do not cover the entire Web, so you may need to use more than one engine), (3) the frequency with which they update the websites indexed by the search engine, and (4) ease of use. New search engines appear on the scene almost daily, so identifying the "best" search engine in this text is not particularly useful. Many university libraries provide a list of good search engines for your use.

Complex searches may be performed with search engines. The search methods vary with the search engine. Check the instructions for the search engine you are using. The following strategies are used by various engines to conduct complex searches:

■ Quotation marks
■ Brackets
■ NEAR (used to narrow the search to just those sites in which two words are close to each other on the page)
■ NOT *or* -
■ AND *or* +
■ OR (used when quotation marks or brackets are not used)

When you find a promising site, you can store its location in your web browser (called "Bookmarks" in Netscape and "Favorites" in Internet Explorer). Remember, however, that if you use a website as a reference in your bibliography, you will need to make note of the date you viewed it and the address (*URL*, Uniform Research Locator) it had when you viewed it, which are required for proper citation.

Storing a website's address in your browser allows you to return to the website easily to check information. Also, websites are frequently updated, and you can check for new information. Sometimes clicking on a *link* (underlined or highlighted name) on one website will send you to another website with helpful information. Following these links, referred to as *surfing the Web*, is an important part of a Web search. One problem you may encounter in surfing the Web is information overload; you find too much information and may need to be selective about what you retrieve.

Although both Internet Explorer and Netscape store a history of the websites you have visited as you move from one to another, it is wise to store their locations in your browser to avoid having to retrace your steps through the links. Also, websites are often changed or deleted, so you may wish to save a particularly useful Web page as a file. You may save the text, a graphic, or both from the Web. If space on your hard drive is limited, use a "zip" (file compression) program to store the file in a smaller form.

Metasearchers are relatively new approaches to searching the Web. These programs perform a search by using multiple search engines, enabling a single search to cover more of the Web. One disadvantage of metasearchers is that Boolean search methods cannot be reliably used with them (Kennedy, 1998, 1999). As of the writing of this chapter, our favorite metasearcher is Google, which can be found at *http://www.google.com*. Google uses an innovative strategy for searching that increases the number of hits on a topic.

READING AND CRITIQUING SOURCES

Reading and critiquing sources promotes understanding of the current knowledge of a research problem. It involves skimming, comprehending, analyzing, and synthesizing content from sources. An expertise in reading and critiquing sources is essential to the development of a high-quality literature review. Many projects require a review of the litera-

ture and a summary of current knowledge; examples are a project to use research findings in practice, a research proposal, and a research report. This section focuses mainly on reading skills, with a brief introduction to the critiquing process.

Skimming Sources

Skimming is quickly reviewing a source to gain a broad overview of its content. You would probably read the title, author's name, and an abstract or introduction for the source. Then you would read the major headings and sometimes one or two sentences under each heading. Finally, you would review the conclusion or summary. Skimming enables you to make a preliminary judgment about the value of a source and to determine whether it is a primary or secondary source. Secondary sources are reviewed and used to locate primary sources but frequently are not cited in a research proposal or report.

Comprehending Sources

Comprehending a source requires that you read all of it carefully. Focus on understanding major concepts and the logical flow of ideas within the source. Highlight the content you consider important; you might even want to record its ideas in the margins. Notes might be recorded on photocopies of articles, indicating where the information will be used in developing a research proposal.

The kind of information you highlight or note in the margins of a source depends on the type of study or source. The information highlighted on theoretical sources might include relevant concepts, definitions of those concepts, and relationships among them. The notes recorded in the margins of empirical literature might include relevant information about the researcher, such as (1) whether this is a critical or major researcher of a selected problem and (2) other studies this individual has conducted. For a research article, the research problem, purpose, framework, major variables, study design, sample size, data collection and analysis techniques, and findings are usually highlighted. You may wish to record quotations (including page numbers) that might be used in a review of literature section. The decision to paraphrase these quotes can be made later.

You might also record creative ideas about content that develop while you are reading a source. At this point, relevant categories are identified for sorting and organizing sources. These categories will ultimately serve as a guide for writing the review of literature section, and some may even be major headings in this section.

Analyzing Sources

Through *analysis,* you can determine the value of a source for a particular study. Analysis must take place in two stages. The first stage involves the critique of individual studies. The process of critiquing individual studies, including the steps of comprehension, comparison, analysis, evaluation, and conceptual clustering, is detailed in Chapter 26. During the critique, relevant content in sources is clearly identified, and sources are sorted into a sophisticated system of categories.

Pinch (1995) has developed a table format, which we have modified by adding two columns, that is useful in sorting information from studies into categories for analysis (see Table 6–3). Conducting an analysis of sources to be used in a research proposal requires some knowledge of the subject to be critiqued, some knowledge of the research process, and the ability to exercise judgment in evaluation (Fleming & Hayter, 1974; Pinch, 1995). However, the critique of individual studies is only the first step in developing an adequate review of the literature. Any written literature review that simply critiques individual studies paragraph by paragraph is inadequate.

The second stage of analysis involves making comparisons among studies. This analysis allows you to critique the existing body of knowledge in relation to the research problem. You will be able to determine (1) theoretical formulations that have been used to explain how the variables in the problem influence one another, (2) what methodologies have been used to study the problem, (3) the methodological flaws in previous studies, (4) what is known about the problem, and (5) what the most

critical gaps in the knowledge base are. The information gathered by using the table format shown in Table 6–3 can be useful in making these comparisons.

Various studies addressing a research problem have approached the examination of the problem from different perspectives. They may have organized the study from different theoretical perspectives, asked different questions related to the problem, selected different variables, used different designs. As Galvan (1999, p. 3) so wisely points out, "Due to the fact that empirical research provides only approximations and degrees of evidence on research problems that are necessarily limited in scope, creating a synthesis is like trying to put together a jigsaw puzzle, knowing in advance that most of the pieces are missing and that many of the available pieces are not fully formed." Sometimes, findings from different studies conflict, leaving understanding in that area unclear and pointing to the need for further research with improved methodologies. As Galvan (1999, p. 3) suggests, "you may soon find yourself acting like a juror, deliberating about which researchers seem to have the most cohesive and logical arguments, which ones have the strongest evidence and so on." O'Connor (1992) has developed a strategy for using graphing methods to visually indicate the linkage of studies. Lines are drawn from a study to all of the studies cited in it, using a time line to illustrate the development of ideas. This process is repeated until all the studies cited have been mapped.

Synthesizing Sources

Synthesis involves clarifying the meaning obtained from the source as a whole. Through synthesis, one can cluster and interrelate ideas from several sources to form a gestalt. Rather than using direct quotes from an author, you should paraphrase his or her ideas. *Paraphrasing* involves expressing the ideas clearly and in your own words. The meanings of these sources are then connected to the proposed study. Lastly, the meanings obtained from all sources are combined, or clustered, to determine the current knowledge of the research problem (Pinch, 1995). Synthesis is the basis for developing

TABLE 6–3

EXAMPLE OF LITERATURE REVIEW SUMMARY TABLE
(STRESS AND COPING IN CABG PATIENTS AND FAMILY MEMBERS)

SOURCE	PURPOSE/PROBLEM	SAMPLE	FRAMEWORK	CONCEPTS	DESIGN	INSTRUMENT(S)	RESULTS	IMPLICATIONS	COMMENTS
Acorn (1995)	Develop/eval education/support program for families of head-injured patients	19 family members of head-injured patients	Not specified	Coping Self-esteem Well-being	Pretest–posttest Quasi-experimental	Jalowiec Coping Scale; Rosenberg's Self-esteem Scale Life Satisfaction Index	Practical/experimental effects but not statistically significant	Community based Intervention does not necessarily lead to increase in coping	Short time frame Small sample Head injury families
Jalowiec (1981)	Compare stress of groups, and ID coping strategies used	25 ER patients and 25 hypertensive patients	Lazarus	Stress Coping	Comparative/descriptive	Modified Rahe's Stressful Life Events Quest. Jalowiec Coping Scale	Coping used: hope, control, problem-solving	Balance of strategies may be helpful	Not transplant Early Jalowiec patients
Twibell (1998)	Examine how family members used coping styles and effectiveness	59 family members	Not specified	Coping Needs	Exploratory/descriptive	Jalowiec Coping Scale	Effectiveness low Older used more than young	Interventions: discussion, flexible visiting; ID high-risk; diminish ineffective coping; share goals	ICU patients Family
Hanton (1998)	Examine stressors before heart transplantation via case study	1 child awaiting heart transplant	Lazarus & Folkman	Stress Appraisal Coping	Case study	Observation	Fatigue and financial concerns for parents	Evaluate and support family family coping skills Recognize that needs change Involve team	Little data on coping Child with/heart
LaMontagne, Pawlak (1990)	ID parents' stressors and coping strategies	30 parents of children in PICU	Lazarus	Stress Coping	Descriptive/exploratory	Semistructured interview Ways of Coping Quest	Combo of problem-solving and emotional Seeking social support	Clinicians can offer assistance and emotional support	PICU patients Parents
Voepel-Lewis et al. (1990)	ID stressors and coping strategies of family members of kidney transplant recipients after transplant	50 family members	Lazarus & Folkman	Stress Coping	Descriptive/exploratory	Kidney Transplant Quest	More stressors, more coping strategies used Self-controlling and problem-solving coping highest	Teaching plans Team support	Kidneys Family
Collins et al. (1996)	ID common stressors experienced by spouses of heart transplant candidates	85 heart transplant candidates	Lazarus & Folkman	Stress Appraisal	Comparative cross-sectional survey	Spouse Transplant Stressors Scale Jalowiec Coping Scale	High levels of spouse stress Fear of death worst	Could lead to interventions to reduce stress	Only spouses Heart transplant rather than liver Some patients not in ICU Coping scores not reported
Gilliss (1984)	Describe stressors of patient/spouses during/after CABG	41 couples	Not specified	Stress	Longitudinal descriptive	Semistructured interviews Impact of Event Scale	Need for info and emotional support	Develop educational program for families/expectations	CABG Coping not studied Spouses

Study	Purpose	Sample	Theory/Framework	Concept	Design	Instrument	Findings	Implications	Notes
Porter et al. (1991)	ID transplant patients' fears and concerns while waiting for organ	3 patients awaiting hearts	Not specified	Stress Coping	Retrospective case study	Interviews, open-ended and guided	Family and spiritual support important, Denial, humor, meeting with post-transplant patients	Larger, broader studies needed	Heart, Coping not focus, Small study, Patients
Nolan, Cupples et al. (1992)	Explore stress and coping strategies among families of pre–heart transplant patients	38 family members	T-Double ABCX Model of Family Adjustment	Stress Coping	Descriptive	Family Crisis Oriented Personal Scale, others	More coping strategies used than normal subjects, Problem solving	Coping strategies seen as effective in reducing stress	Heart, FCOPES, Families
Reider (1994)	Anxiety levels of family members and variables affecting them	75 family members	T-Double ABCX Model of Family Adjustment	Anxiety Stress	Descriptive	Brief Symptom Inventory FCOPES	Better coping = lower anxiety	ID coping patterns, Give info, Give family time with patient	General ICU patients, Family
Molter (1979)	ID needs of families, and whether being met	40 relatives of patients in critical condition	Crisis theory	Needs	Exploratory/descriptive	Structured interviews with Molter questions	Hope, caring, info	Info giving, Relatively well met	Needs survey, Nontransplant, Families
Daley (1984)	ID needs of family members of ICU patients and who can meet them	40 family members	Not specified (crisis noted)	Needs	Exploratory	Structured interview Molter survey	Relief of anxiety, Need for info, visiting	Team of dr/Rn, Info	Molter, Nontransplant, Coping not addressed, Family
Freichels (1991)	Compare family perceptions of needs over time	41 family members	Crisis theory, normalization theory	Needs	Exploratory longitudinal	Molter CCFNI	Hope, assurance high, Hope decreases over time	Generally consistent over time but lesser degree	ICU patients, Needs, Molter, Family
Kleinpell, Powers (1992)	ID needs of family members and whether being met	64 family members and 58 nurses	Family systems theory	Needs	Descriptive/comparative	Molter CCFNI	Info, hope, changes both important, Staff variable more important to families	Better staff role info to families	Needs, Molter, Family
Leske (1986)	ID/compare reported needs of families of ICU patients	55 family members of ICU patients	Crisis intervention theory	Needs	Comparative/descriptive	Molter survey, revised: CCFNI	Emotional needs high, Hope	Info and emotional support	Needs, continues, Molter, Families
Norris, Grove (1986)	ID perceptions of family and ICU nurses about family needs	20 family members, 20 nurses	Bertalanffy's General System Theory	Needs	Descriptive	Molter survey, revised	Hope, caring, info needs high for families, Nurses rate info over caring	Family focus for nursing interventions, Psychosocial	Molter, General ICU patients, Not coping, Family, nurses
Davis-Martin (1994)	Compare needs of families of long vs. short ICU stays	26 family members	Not specified	Needs	Descriptive, ex-post-facto	Molter survey	Needs similar, Info	Continue info and support strategies	Needs, Molter, SICU patients, Family
Weichler (1993)	ID info needs/concerns of caretakers of children after transplant	21 primary caretakers of children after transplant	Not specified	Stress Needs	Descriptive/exploratory	Semistructured questionnaire	Knowledge key to families	Nurses anticipating needs may decrease stress and increase coping	Mostly caucasian, Children, Post liver-renal transplant

Table continued on page 122

TABLE 6–3

EXAMPLE OF LITERATURE REVIEW SUMMARY TABLE CONTINUED

(STRESS AND COPING IN CABG PATIENTS AND FAMILY MEMBERS)

SOURCE	PURPOSE/PROBLEM	SAMPLE	FRAMEWORK	CONCEPTS	DESIGN	INSTRUMENT(S)	RESULTS	IMPLICATIONS	COMMENTS
Moser et al. (1993)	ID needs of patients and spouses following cardiac event	55 patient-spouse pairs	Not specified	Needs	Descriptive/comparative	Needs assessment instrument	Info needs differed Needs for info unmet by doctors, nurses	Better teaching	Cardiac patients/spouses
Carmody et al. (1991)	ID and rank the needs of families of patients undergoing oncology surgery	49 family members	Not specified	Needs	Exploratory/descriptive	Perioperative Family Needs Quest.	Info needs high priority	Info needs Keep informed about condition Designate info nurse	Oncology Coping not investigated Family
Kristenssenn-Hallstrom (1999)	Ways parents feel secure Degree of parental participation	224 parents of hospitalized children	Not specified	Security Participation	Nonrandom anonymous survey	Quest. developed for study	Parents wanted varied levels of participation	Role clarification might be helpful for parents	Parents of children, any illness Doesn't address coping specifically
Nyamathi, Jacoby et al. (1992)	Examine relationship of 6 factors of emotional/physical adjustment of spouses	100 spouses of critically ill adults	Comprehensive Health Seeking and Coping Paradigm	Adjustment Coping Personality Factors	Descriptive	Spousal Coping Instrument, revised	Emotional coping related to negative personality factors Problem coping with positive	Adjustment may be related to personality factors High-risk may be emotion-focused	Cardiac Spouses
Wainwright (1995)	Examine recovery/experiences of liver transplant patients	10 liver transplant patients	Grounded theory	Transformation Adjustment	Focused interviews	Topic guide	Family support important	Active teaching needed Support groups helpful	Small sample Patients, not families Liver transplant
Mishel, Murdaugh (1987)	Explore processes for handling uncertainty among families of heart transplant patients	20 family members of heart transplant patients	Grounded theory	Uncertainty Adaptation	Interviews	Open-ended question	Alteration in adaptation over time	High pyschosocial needs of families	Heart Little info on actual coping strategies Families

CABG, coronary artery bypass grafting; CCFNI, critical care family needs inventory; dr, doctor; ER, emergency room; eval, evaluate; ICU, intensive care unit; ID, identify; info, information; PICU, pediatric intensive care unit; Quest, Questionnaire; RN, Registered Nurse; SICU, surgical intensive care unit.
Modified, by graduate student Molly O'Brien, from Pinch, W. J. (1995). Synthesis: Implementing a complex process. *Nurse Educator, 20*(1), 34–40.
Note: Example provided to illustrate structure of table references not included in reference list.

the review of literature section for a research proposal, report, or utilization project.

Becker (1986) suggests that there is a drawback to reviewing the literature; it can "deform" the position you wish to take about the research topic and the direction further research should take.

Suppose there is real literature on your subject, the result of years of normal science or what, by extension, we could call normal scholarship. Everyone who works on the topic agrees on the kinds of questions to ask and the kinds of answers they will accept. If you want to write about the topic, or even use that subject matter as the material for a new topic, you will probably have to deal with the old way even though you think it quite foreign to your interests. If you take the old way too seriously, you can deform the argument you want to make, bend it out of shape in order to make it fit into the dominant approach. What I mean by bending your argument out of shape is this. What you want to say has a certain logic that flows from the chain of choices you made as you did the work. If the logic of your argument is the same as the logic of the dominant approach to the topic, you have no problem. But suppose it isn't. What you want to say starts from different premises, addresses different questions, recognizes a different kind of answer as appropriate. When you try to confront the dominant approach to this material, you start to translate your argument into its terms. Your argument will not make the kind of sense it made in its own terms; it will sound weak and disjointed and will appear ad hoc. It cannot look its best playing an opponent's game. And that phrasing puts the point badly, because what's involved is not a contest between approaches, after all, but a search for a good way to understand the world. The understanding you're trying to convey will lose its coherence if it is put in terms that grow out of a different understanding.

If, on the other hand, you translate the dominant argument into your terms, you will not give it a fair shake, for much the same reasons. When you translate from one way of analyzing a problem into another, there is a good chance that the approaches are, as Kuhn (1962) suggested, incommensurable. Insofar as they address different questions, the approaches have very little to do with one another. There is nothing to translate. They are simply not talking about the same things. . . . A serious scholar ought routinely to inspect competing ways of talking about the same subject matter. The feeling that you can't say what you mean in the language you are using will warn you that the literature is crowding you. . . . Use the literature, don't let it use you. (Becker, 1986 pp. 146–149)

WRITING THE REVIEW OF LITERATURE

A thorough, organized literature review facilitates the development of a research proposal. Students frequently ask how long the literature review should be. Unfortunately, there is no way for an instructor to answer this question. The length of the review varies considerably according to the extent of research that has been conducted in the area. In a relatively new area of research, you may find only two or three previous studies, whereas in an established field of research such as that of coping and social support, a vast quantity of literature exists.

Sorting Your Sources

Relevant sources (theoretical and empirical) are organized for inclusion in the different chapters of the research proposal. The sources to be included in the review of literature chapter are organized to reflect the current knowledge about the research problem. Those sources that provide background and significance for the study are included in the introduction chapter. Certain theoretical sources establish the framework for the study. Other relevant sources become the basis for defining research variables and identifying assumptions and limitations. Methodologically strong studies direct the development of the research design, guide the selection of instruments, influence data collection and analysis, and provide a basis for interpretation of findings. Usually, at this point, a researcher is beginning to get a complete picture of his or her study and is excited about its potential. The researcher commonly feels confident about his or her knowledge of the research problem and ability to make the study a reality.

Developing the Written Review

The purpose of the written literature review is to establish a context for your study. The literature review for a study has four major sections, (1) the introduction, (2) discussion of theoretical literature, (3) discussion of empirical literature, and (4) a summary.

INTRODUCTION

The introduction indicates the focus or purpose of the study, identifies the purpose of the literature review, and presents the organizational structure of the review. You should make clear in this section what you will and will not be covering. If you are taking a particular position or developing a logical argument for a particular perspective on the basis of the literature, make this position clear in the introduction. This section should be brief and should catch the interest of the reader (Galvan, 1999).

DISCUSSION OF THEORETICAL LITERATURE

The theoretical literature section contains concept analyses, models, theories, and conceptual frameworks that support the research purpose. Concepts, definitions of concepts, relationships among concepts, and assumptions are presented and analyzed to build a theoretical knowledge base for the study. This section of the literature review is sometimes used to present the framework for the study and may include a conceptual map that synthesizes the theoretical literature (see Chapter 7 for more detail on developing frameworks).

DISCUSSION OF EMPIRICAL LITERATURE

The presentation of empirical literature should be organized by concepts or organizing topics. Although in the past, for each study reviewed, the researcher was expected to present the purpose, sample size, design, and specific findings with a scholarly but brief critique of the study's strengths and weaknesses, this approach is expected less commonly now.

Currently, literature reviews tend to focus on synthesis of studies, with a critique of the strengths and weaknesses of the overall body of knowledge. This synthesis may be organized by concepts or variables that are the focus of the study. The findings from the studies should logically build on each other so that the reader can see how the body of knowledge in the research area evolved.

Evidence from multiple studies is pooled to reveal the current state of knowledge in relation to a particular concept or study focus (topic area). Conflicting findings and areas of uncertainty are explored. Similarities and differences in the studies should be explored. Gaps and areas needing more research are discussed. A summary of findings in the topic area is presented, along with inferences, generalizations, and conclusions you have drawn from your review of the literature. A *conclusion* is a statement about the state of knowledge in relation to the topic area. This should include a discussion of the strength of evidence available for each conclusion. You may feel a need to "stick to the facts" from the research and not venture forth with conclusions. However, after carefully reviewing the literature, you have become an expert in it, and you can justifiably state your views (Galvan, 1999).

Ethical issues must be considered in your presentation of sources (Gunter, 1981). The content from sources should be presented honestly, not distorted to support the selected problem. Researchers frequently read a study and wish that the author had studied a slightly different problem or that the study had been designed or conducted differently. However, they must recognize their own opinions and must be objective in presenting information.

The defects of a study need to be addressed, but it is not necessary to be highly critical of another researcher's work. The criticisms need to focus on the content that is in some way relevant to the proposed study and to be stated as possible or plausible explanations, so that they are more neutral and scholarly than negative and blaming.

Authors' works must be accurately documented so they receive credit for their publications. The reference list contains only those sources that have been cited in the development of the proposal or report.

SUMMARY

The summary consists of a concise presentation of the current knowledge base for the research problem. Other literature reviews conducted in relation to your field of research should be discussed. The gaps in the knowledge base are identified, with a discussion of how the proposed study will contribute to the development of knowledge in the defined field of research. A critique of the adequacy of methodologies used in the studies reviewed should be presented, along with recommendations for improving the methodologies in future studies (Galvan, 1999). The summary concludes with a statement of how your study will contribute to the body of knowledge in this field of research.

Checking References

All references used in the literature review should be carefully checked for accuracy and completeness. Anyone reviewing the literature has at some time been frustrated by inaccurate references in publications. Foreman and Kirchhoff (1987) studied the accuracy of references in 17 nursing journals; 65 of the inaccurate references were from clinical journals and 47 were from nonclinical journals. The errors were classified as major (preventing retrieval of the source) or minor (not preventing retrieval). Errors occurred more frequently in clinical journals (38.4%) than in nonclinical journals (21.3%). Clinical references also had a 4.5% incidence of major errors, whereas the nonclinical references had no major errors.

To prevent these errors, check all the citations within the text of your literature review and each citation in your reference list. Typing or keyboarding errors may result in inaccurate information. You may omit some information, planning to complete the reference later, and then forget to do so. The following reference citation errors are common in research studies:

- No citation is listed for a direct quotation.
- The citation for a direct quotation has the author's name and year, but no page number.
- The author's name is spelled differently in the text and in the reference list.
- The year of a citation is different in the text and in the reference list.
- The citation in the reference list is incomplete.
- A study is cited in the text for which there is no citation in the reference.
- A citation appears in the reference list for which there is no citation in the text.

In revising your text, you may rearrange or renumber citations, resulting in inaccuracies. Biancuzzo (1997) describes this sort of problem in one of her publications. "My own article (Biancuzzo, 1991) said '. . . although epidural anesthesia affects sensory neurons, motor neurons are not completely blocked.[16]' After publication, I was horrified to see that citation #16 was entitled "Maternal positions for childbirth: A historical review of nursing care practices." The correct citation should have been #15 entitled, "The influence of continuous epidural bupivacaine analgesia on the second stage of labor and method of delivery in nulliparous women." A similar problem can occur when you cite several publications written by the same author. In this case, it is easy to reference the right author but the wrong source.

To detect these easily made errors, check your references immediately prior to completing your paper. The most accurate check involves comparing each reference with the original journal article, or on-line with *CINAHL* or other bibliographical databases.

EXAMPLE OF A LITERATURE REVIEW

Parts of the literature review from an actual published study are presented here to reinforce the points that were addressed in this chapter. The study focuses on "behavioral analysis and nursing interventions for reducing disruptive behaviors of patients with dementia" (Boehm et al., 1995). Only selected content from this literature review is presented to demonstrate (1) the introduction, (2) organization of empirical and theoretical information according to the concepts of behavioral therapy, behavioral gerontology, and disruptive behaviors, and (3) the summary (Boehm et al., 1995, pp. 118–119).

• •

Introduction

"Behavioral gerontological research has successfully developed a number of effective behavioral interventions that have implications for nursing practice. (McCormick et al., 1988)"

Behavioral Therapy and Behavioral Gerontology

"The majority of the literature in behavioral gerontology is built on the conceptual underpinnings that 'behavior therapy includes interventions that attempt to change the frequency, intensity, duration, or location of a specific behavior or set of behaviors through systematic varying antecedent stimuli or consequential events.' (Hussian & Davis, 1985, p. 15)

"Behavioral analysis provides the basis for identification and development of behavioral interventions and is the process by which behavior is observed, documented, and analyzed from three perspectives. The three perspectives include (1) antecedent events that precede and serve as stimuli for the behavior, (2) small steps of behavior that comprise the whole behavior, and (3) consequences that follow the behavior. (Brigham, 1982)

"Behavior interventions have been used successfully to treat a variety of problems in elderly, institutionalized individuals (Vaccaro, 1990). The challenge in addressing behavioral problems of individuals with dementia, however, is that many of the successful behavioral interventions rely on memory and thus are not suitable for the patient with dementia (Carstensen & Erickson, 1986). Techniques must be developed to teach nurses to provide cues and consequences that may elicit desirable patient behavior instead of abusive behavior (Lewin & Lundervold, 1990). . . . One such tech-nique is behavioral modeling, which is the acquisition of behavior by observing other persons' behaviors and the consequences of their behaviors."

Disruptive Behaviors

"According to the 1989 National Nursing Home Survey (National Center for Health Statistics, 1989), 80% of nursing home patients required extra nursing care because of disruptive behaviors associated with dementia, such as Alzheimer's disease. Behavioral gerontology has directed considerable attention to such areas as depression, paranoia, pain, insomnia, incontinence, memory and cognition, alcohol abuse, anxiety, and social behavior, such as dependence."

Summary

"However, few behavioral researchers have used behavioral analysis techniques as a means of changing patients' disruptive behaviors (Fisher & Carstensen, 1990). Indeed, research evaluating behavioral analysis approaches for reducing such disquieting behaviors as wandering, inappropriate sexual behavior, and verbal and physical aggressive outbursts is needed by nurses and other caregivers for individuals with dementia (Carstensen & Erickson, 1986)."

▪ SUMMARY

Reviewing the existing literature related to your study is a critical step in the research process. This chapter guides you through the process of performing a literature review. The three major stages of a literature review delineated here are searching the literature, reading the literature, and writing the literature.

"The literature" is all written sources relevant to the topic you have selected. The published literature includes primary and secondary sources. A *primary source* is written by the person who originated or is responsible for generating the ideas published. In research publications, a primary source is written by the person(s) who conducted the research. A primary theoretical source is written by the theorist who developed the theory or conceptual content. A *secondary source* summarizes or quotes content from primary sources. You should use mostly primary sources to develop research proposals and reports.

Two types of literature are predominantly used in the review of literature for research, theoretical and empirical. *Theoretical literature* includes concept analyses, models, theories, and conceptual frameworks that support a selected research problem and purpose. *Empirical literature* includes relevant studies in journals and books as well as unpublished studies, such as master's theses and doctoral dissertations. Other types of literature, such as descriptions of clinical situations, educational literature, and position papers, may be included in the background and significant section of a paper but often are not cited in the review of relevant literature. Integrative reviews are a type of secondary source that may be important to a review of the literature. *Integrative reviews* are conducted to identify, analyze, and synthesize the results from independent studies to determine the current knowledge. These reviews contain a comprehensive list of references and summarize empirical literature for selected topics.

It is rarely, if ever, possible to identify every relevant source in the literature. As a student or nurse researcher, your goal is to develop a search strategy designed to retrieve as much of the relevant literature as possible given the time and financial constraints of your study. The time required to review the literature is influenced by the problem studied, the sources available, and the goals of the researcher.

The process of searching the literature has changed dramatically as the use of computers has increased. Through the use of electronic databases, a large volume of references can be located quickly. Before you begin searching the literature, develop a written plan of your search strategy. Select the bibliographical databases you plan to search. Select keywords for conducting your search. *Keywords* are the major concepts or variables that must be included in your search. Use reference management software to track the references you have obtained through your searches. Initiate your search by performing a separate search of each keyword you have identified. Then perform Boolean searches. A *Boolean* search combines two or more concepts in one search. There are several strategies you can use to limit your search if, after performing Boolean searches, you continue to get too many hits.

A number of new nursing journals have been developed that are published only in electronic form, because of the high costs of publishing a printed journal. To obtain relevant articles from such a journal, you need to locate the electronic journal on the Internet and scan the titles of articles published in it. Although it is unlikely you will find studies relevant to your topic by searching the World Wide Web, you may find information relevant to the background, significance, framework, design, methods of measurement, and statistical procedures for your study. One advantage of information obtained from the Web is that it is likely to be more current than material available in books. However, the Web contains a considerable amount of misinformation as well as some "gems." It is important to check the original source of any information you obtain from the Web so that you can judge its validity.

Reading and critiquing sources promotes understanding of the current knowledge of a research problem and involves skimming, comprehending, analyzing, and synthesizing content from sources. *Skimming* is a quick review of a source to gain a broad overview of the content. *Comprehending* a source requires that the entire source be read carefully. Through *analysis,* you can determine the value of a source for a particular study. The first stage involves the critique of individual studies, and the second stage, comparing studies. This analysis allows you to critique the existing body of knowledge in relation to the research problem. *Synthesis* involves clarifying the meaning obtained from a source as a whole.

A thorough, organized literature review facilitates the development of a research proposal. Relevant sources (theoretical and empirical) are organized for inclusion in the different chapters of the research proposal. The purpose of the written literature review is to establish a context for your study. The literature review for a study has four major sections: the introduction, discussion of theoretical literature, discussion of empirical literature, and a summary. The *introduction* indicates the focus or purpose of the study, identifies the purpose of the review, and presents the organization of the review. The *theoretical literature section* includes concept analyses, models, theories, and conceptual frameworks that support the research purpose. This section of the literature review is sometimes used to present the framework for the study and may contain a conceptual map that synthesizes the theoretical literature. The presentation of empirical literature should be organized by concepts or organizing topics. Currently, literature reviews tend to focus on synthesis of studies with a critique of the strengths and weaknesses of the overall body of knowledge. This synthesis may be organized by concepts or variables that are the focus of the study. The *summary* of a literature review contains a concise presentation of the current knowledge base for the research problem. It concludes with a statement about how the present study will contribute to the existing body of knowledge in this field of study. All references used in the literature review should be carefully checked for accuracy and completeness.

REFERENCES

American Psychological Association (APA). (1994). *Publication manual of the American Psychological Association* (4th ed.). Washington, D.C.: American Psychological Association.

Asian Institute of Technology, Center for Language and Educational Technology. *Writing and Research: The Literature Review* [On-line]. Available: *http://www.clet.ait.ac.th/EL21LIT.HTM/* [2/25/2000].

Auston, I, Cahn, M. A., Selden, C. R. (1992). *Literature search methods for the development of clinical practice guidelines.* National Library of Medicine, Office of Health Services Research Information [On-line]. Available: *http://www.nlm.nih. gov/nichsr.litsrch.html/* [2/25/2000].

Becker, H. S. (1986). Terrorized by the literature. In *Writing for social scientists: How to start and finish your thesis, book, or article*. Chicago: University of Chicago Press.

Beyea, S., & Nicoll, L. H. (1998). Writing an integrative review. *AORN Journal, 67*(4), 877–880.

Biancuzzo, M. (1991). Does the hands-and-knees posture help to rotate the occiput posterior fetus? *Birth, 18*(1), 40–47.

Biancuzzo, M. (1997). Checking references: Tips for reviewers. *Nurse Author & Editor, 7*(3), 1.

Boehm, S., Whall, A. L., Cosgrove, K. L., Locke, J. D., &

Schlenk, E. A. (1995). Behavioral analysis and nursing interventions for reducing disruptive behaviors of patients with dementia. *Applied Nursing Research, 8*(3), 118–122.

Brigham, T. (1982). Self-management: A radical behavioral perspective. In P. Karoly & F. H. Kanfer (Eds.), *Self-management and behavior change: From theory to practice* (pp. 32–59). New York: Pergamon.

Buenker, J. (1999). *Conducting a medical literature search: Accessing and using MEDLINE on the Internet/World Wide Web* [On-line]. Available: *http://alexia.lis.uiuc.edu/~buenker/web3.html*

Carstensen, L. L., & Erickson, R. J. (1986). Enhancing the social environments of elderly nursing home residents: Are high rates of interaction enough? *Journal of Applied Behavior Analysis, 19*(4), 349–355.

Cooper, H. M. (1984). *The integrative research review: A systematic approach.* Beverly Hills, CA: Sage.

Fisher, J. E., & Carstensen, L. L. (1990). Behavior management of the dementias. *Clinical Psychology Review, 10*(6), 611–629.

Fleming, J. W., & Hayter, J. (1974). Reading research reports critically. *Nursing Outlook, 22*(3), 172–175.

Foreman, M. D., & Kirchhoff, K. T. (1987). Accuracy of references in nursing journals. *Research in Nursing & Health, 10*(3), 177–183.

Galvan, J. L. (1999). Writing literature reviews. Los Angeles: Pyrczak.

Ganong, L. H. (1987). Integrative reviews of nursing research. *Research in Nursing & Health, 10*(1), 1–11.

Gunter, L. (1981). Literature review. In S. D. Krampitz & N. Pavlovich (Eds.), *Readings for nursing research* (pp. 11–16). St. Louis: Mosby.

Hussian, R. A., & Davis, R. L. (1985). *Responsive care: Behavioral interventions with elderly persons.* Champaign, IL: Research.

Kaplan, A. (1964). *The conduct of inquiry: Methodology for behavioral science.* New York: Chandler.

Kennedy, I. (1998). *How do I use the Web for research? Beginner* [On-line]. Available: *http://www.geocities.com/Athens/3238/begin.htm* [2/25/2000].

Kennedy, I. (1999). How do I use the Web for research? Intermediate [On-line]. Available: *http://www.geocities.com/Athens/3238/inter.htm* [2/26/2000].

Kuhn, T. (1962). *The structure of scientific revolutions* (2nd ed). Chicago: University of Chicago Press.

Lewin, L. M., & Lundervold, D. A. (1990). Behavioral analysis of separation—individuation conflict in the spouse of an Alzheimer's disease patient. *The Gerontologist, 30*(5), 703–705.

Marchette, L. (1985). Research: The literature review process. *Perioperative Nursing Quarterly, 1*(4), 69–76.

McCormick, K. A., Scheve, A. A., & Leahy, E. (1988). Nursing management of urinary incontinence in geriatric inpatients. *Nursing Clinics of North America, 23*(1), 231–264.

National Center for Health Statistics. (1989). *The national nursing home survey* (DHHS Publication No. PHS 8901758, Series 13, No. 97). Hyattsville, MD: Public Health Service.

O'Connor, S. E. (1992). Network theory—a systematic method for literature review. *Nurse Education Today, 12*(1), 44–50.

Pinch, W. J. (1995). Synthesis: Implementing a complex process. *Nurse Educator, 20*(1), 34–40.

Saba, V. K., Oatway, D. M., & Rieder, K. A. (1989). How to use nursing information sources. *Nursing Outlook, 37*(4), 189–195.

Smith, M. C., & Stullenbarger, E. (1991). A prototype for integrative review and meta-analysis for nursing research. *Journal of Advanced Nursing, 16*(11), 1272–1283.

The Union Institute Research Engine (1999). *What is a Literature Review?* [On-line]. Available: *http://www.tui.edu/Research/Resources/ResearchHelp/LitReviewLgPg.html* [2/25/00].

Vaccaro, F. J. (1990). Application of social skills training in a group of institutionalized aggressive elderly subjects. *Psychology and Aging, 5*(3), 369–378.

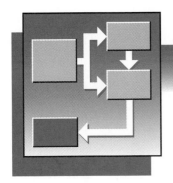

CHAPTER 7

FRAMEWORKS

A *framework* is the abstract, logical structure of meaning that guides the development of the study and enables the researcher to link the findings to nursing's body of knowledge. Frameworks are used in both quantitative and qualitative research. In quantitative studies, the framework is a testable theory that may emerge from a conceptual model or may be developed inductively from clinical observations. In qualitative research, the initial framework is a philosophy or world view; a theory consistent with the philosophy is developed as an outcome of the study.

Every study has a framework. The framework should be well integrated with the methodology, carefully structured, and clearly presented. This requirement applies whether the study is physiological or psychosocial. To critique studies for application in clinical practice or for use in further research, the reader must be able to identify and evaluate the framework. Each person's understanding of the meaning of study findings, which is based on the framework, determines how that person will use the findings. Thus, utilization is enhanced when readers understand the framework and can relate it to the findings for their use in nursing practice.

Unfortunately, in some studies, the ideas that compose the framework remain nebulous and vaguely expressed. The researcher holds in his or her mind the notion that the variables being studied are related in some fashion. In fact, the variables are selected because the researcher thinks there may be one or more important links among them. Other-

wise, why would the study be conducted? These ideas are the rudiments of a framework. In some rudimentary frameworks, the ideas may be expressed in the literature review; but then, the researcher stops without fully developing the ideas as a framework. Many studies have these implicit frameworks. Moody and colleagues (1988) found that 49% of nursing practice studies published between 1977 and 1986 had no identifiable theoretical perspective. According to Sarter (1988, p. 2), "nursing research shows an alarming absence of theoretical relevance."

There is, however, a growing expectation that frameworks be an integral part of nursing research and be introduced when the research process, critique, and utilization are taught to undergraduate nursing students. This knowledge can then later be expanded as the learner participates in the process of developing a framework while being taught to plan and implement studies. To facilitate development of the knowledge and skills needed to critique or develop a framework, this chapter explains relevant terms, describes framework development, and discusses the critique of frameworks.

DEFINITION OF TERMS

The first step in understanding theories and frameworks is to become familiar with the terms related to theoretical ideas and their application. These terms and the ways they are used come from the philosophy of science, the main concern of which is the nature of scientific knowledge (Feyera-

131

bend, 1975; Foucault, 1970; Frank, 1961; Gibbs, 1972; Hemple, 1966; Kaplan, 1964; Kerlinger, 1986; Kuhn, 1970; Laudan, 1977, 1981; Merton, 1968; Popper, 1968; Reynolds, 1971; Scheffler, 1967; Suppe, 1972; Suppe & Jacox, 1985). As nurses have studied philosophies of science, philosophies of nursing science are beginning to emerge. This is an exciting development in nursing. Because of differences of opinion in the philosophies of nursing science, however, some confusion exists in the nursing literature regarding the use of terms related to theory and research.

Nevertheless, a growing consensus is emerging in nursing about the terms that should be used and their meanings. These terms include *concept, relational statement, conceptual model, theory,* and *conceptual map.* The greatest confusion has involved differences in the use of the terms *theory* and *conceptual model.* Within philosophies of science, the term *theory* is used in a variety of ways that could include both specific theories and conceptual models (Suppe & Jacox, 1985). In philosophies of nursing science, however, *theory* tends to be defined narrowly and to be differentiated from *conceptual model.* The definitions used in this text reflect the predominant use of these terms in nursing.

Concept

A *concept* is a term that abstractly describes and names an object or phenomenon, thus providing it with a separate identity or meaning. An example of a concept is the term *anxiety.* At high levels of abstraction, concepts have very general meanings and are sometimes referred to as *constructs.* For example, a construct associated with the concept of anxiety might be "emotional responses."

At a more concrete level, terms are referred to as *variables* and are narrow in their definitions. A variable is more specific than a concept and implies that the term is defined so that it is measurable. The word *variable* implies that the numerical values associated with the term *vary* from one instance to another. A variable related to anxiety might be the extent of "palmar sweating" as measured by assigning numerical values to different amounts of palmar

sweat. The linkages among constructs, concepts, and variables are illustrated here:

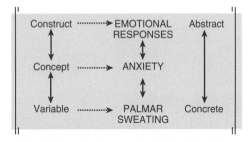

Defining concepts allows consistency in the way the term is used. A *conceptual definition* differs from the denotative (or dictionary) definition of a word. A conceptual definition (connotative meaning) is more comprehensive than a denotative definition, including associated meanings the word may have. For example, *fireplace* may connote hospitality and warm comfort. A conceptual definition can be established through concept synthesis, concept derivation, or concept analysis.

CONCEPT SYNTHESIS

In nursing, many phenomena have not yet been identified as discrete entities. The recognition and description of these phenomena are often critical to understanding the process and outcomes of nursing practice. The process of describing and naming a previously unrecognized concept is *concept synthesis.* In the discipline of medicine, Selye (1976) performed concept synthesis to identify and define the concept of stress. Before his work, stress as a phenomenon was unknown. Nursing studies often involve previously unrecognized and unnamed phenomena that need to be named and carefully defined. Concept synthesis is also important in the development of nursing theory (Walker & Avant, 1995).

CONCEPT DERIVATION

In some cases, the conceptual definition may be obtained from theories in other disciplines. Such a conceptual definition explains a phenomenon important to a nonnursing discipline. However, such a conceptual definition needs to be carefully evaluated to determine whether or not the concept has the same conceptual meaning within nursing. The conceptual definition may need to be modified so that it is meaningful within nursing and consistent with nursing thought (Walker & Avant, 1995). This process, referred to as *concept derivation*, may require a concept analysis that examines the use of the concept in nursing literature, compares the results with the existing conceptual definition, and if the two are different, modifies the definition to be consistent with nursing usage.

CONCEPT ANALYSIS

Concept analysis is a strategy through which a set of characteristics essential to the connotative meaning of a concept is identified. The procedure requires the reader to explore the various ways the term is used and to identify a set of characteristics that can be used to clarify the range of objects or ideas to which that concept may be applied. These characteristics are also used to distinguish the concept from similar concepts (Chinn & Kramer, 1995; Walker & Avant, 1995). A number of concept analyses have been published in the nursing literature. Concept analysis is a form of philosophical inquiry; an example of a concept analysis is provided in Chapter 23.

IMPORTANCE OF A CONCEPTUAL DEFINITION—AN EXAMPLE

The importance of a conceptual definition is illustrated in a study by Morse and colleagues (1990), who performed an analysis of published definitions of the concept of *caring* in a project funded by the National Center for Nursing Research. Although the concept of caring is central to the essence of nursing, efforts to define it have led to confusion rather than consensus. For example, it is difficult to separate meanings for *caring*, *care*, and *nursing care*. Caring may be an action, such as "taking care of," or a concern, such as "caring about." Caring may be viewed from the perspective of the nurse or of the patient. Research examining

caring in nursing practice is limited by the inadequacies in the conceptual definition of *caring*.

Morse and colleagues (1990) used content analysis to examine 35 authors' definitions of *caring*. The analysis included definitions of *caring* from three nursing theorists: Orem, Watson, and Leininger. Five categories of caring were identified, as follows: (1) caring as a human trait, (2) caring as a moral imperative, (3) caring as an affect, (4) caring as an interpersonal relationship, and (5) caring as a therapeutic intervention. In addition, two outcomes of caring were identified, (1) the subjective experience of the patient and (2) the physical response of the patient.

Morse and colleagues (1990) developed a model to illustrate the interrelationships among the categories discussed in the literature and identify the authors who had explored each category and each relationship (see Figure 7–1). The model looks really complex, but it is not. Each letter in the model refers to one of the authors listed at the bottom of the figure. These authors are identified in the reference list at the end of the chapter. If the letter is within a colored box, the specified author identified that element as essential to the conceptual meaning of caring. If the letter is alongside an arrow, the specified author suggested that the two elements linked by the arrow were related. Arrows with solid lines show that the author directly stated the relationship. Arrows with dotted lines indicate that the author implied the relationship without directly discussing it.

After examining this model, the researchers concluded that there was little consistency in the way *caring* was being defined by these authors. The following questions emerged from the analysis and must be considered in the development of a conceptual definition:

1. "Is caring a constant and uniform characteristic, or may caring be present in various degrees within individuals?" (Morse et al., 1990, p. 9)
2. Is caring an emotional state that can be depleted?
3. "Can caring be nontherapeutic? Can a nurse care too much?" (Morse et al., 1990, p. 10)

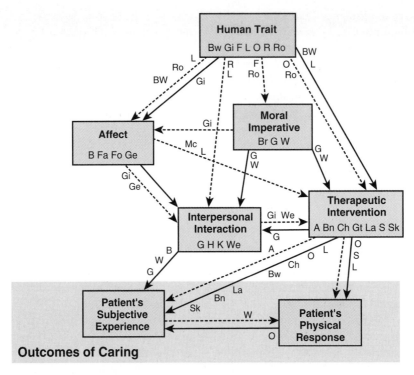

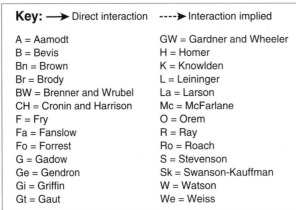

FIGURE 7–1 ▪ The interrelationship of five perspectives of caring. (Redrawn from *Advances in Nursing Science, 13*[1], 3, with permission of Aspen Publishers, Inc., © 1990.)

4. Can cure occur without caring? Can a nurse engage in safe practice without caring?
5. "What difference does caring make to the patient?" (Morse et al., 1990, p. 11)

These researchers concluded that, at the time of their analysis, a clear conceptual definition of *car-*

ing did not exist. In 1996, Amandah and Watson reviewed the literature on caring. They concluded that "caring is a complex phenomenon which lacks a clear definition and which can be conceptualized in a number of ways. Furthermore, there is no consensus about the place of caring in nursing" (Amandah & Watson, 1996, pp. 76–77).

Until *caring* is satisfactorily defined conceptually, measuring it will be difficult, because measurement depends on the conceptual definition. The inadequacy of the conceptual definition of caring impedes the development of studies examining caring in nursing practice.

Relational Statements

A *relational statement* declares that a relationship of some kind exists between or among two or more concepts (Walker & Avant, 1995). Relational statements are the core of the framework. Skills in expressing statements are essential for constructing an integrated framework that will, in turn, lead to a well-designed study. The statements expressed in a framework determine (1) the objective, question, or hypothesis formulated; (2) the design of the study; (3) the statistical analyses that will be performed; and (4) the type of findings that can be expected. Frameworks developed with inadequate expression of statements provide only a broad orientation for the study and do not guide the research process.

Understanding relational statements is essential also to the critique of frameworks. Evaluation of the links among the hypothesis, the design, and the framework is an essential part of critiquing a study. Judging whether the study was successful depends, in part, on identifying the statements in the framework and tracking their examination by the study.

CHARACTERISTICS OF RELATIONAL STATEMENTS

Relational statements describe the direction, shape, strength, symmetry, sequencing, probability of occurrence, necessity, and sufficiency of a relationship (Fawcett & Downs, 1986; Stember, 1986; Walker & Avant, 1995). One statement may have several of these characteristics; each characteristic is not exclusive of the others. Statements may be expressed in literary form (such as a sentence), in diagrammatic form (such as a map), or in mathematical form (such as an equation). Statements in nursing tend to be expressed primarily in literary and diagrammatic forms.

Direction

The *direction* of a relationship may be positive, negative, or unknown.

A *positive* linear relationship implies that as one concept changes (the value or amount of the concept increases or decreases), the second concept will also change in the same direction. For example, the literary statement "The risk of illness (A) increases as stress (B) increases" expresses a positive relationship. This positive relational statement could also be expressed as "The risk of illness decreases as stress decreases." Diagrammatically, this relationship could be depicted as follows:

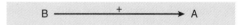

A *negative relationship* implies that as one concept changes, the other concept changes in the opposite direction. For example, the literary statement "As relaxation (A) increases, blood pressure (B) decreases" expresses a negative relationship. Diagrammatically, this relationship could be depicted as follows:

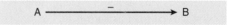

If a relationship is believed to exist but the nature of the relationship is *unclear,* the following diagram could be used to depict it:

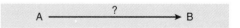

This last type of statement might be appropriate for discussing the relationship between coping and social support. We might say that there is evidence that a relationship exists between these two concepts but that studies examining that relationship have conflicting findings. Some researchers find coping to be positively related to social support, whereas others find that as social support increases, coping decreases. Thus, the nature of the relationship between coping and social support is uncertain. It is possible that the conflicting findings may be due to differences in the ways in which the two concepts have been defined and measured in various studies.

Shape

Most relationships are assumed to be linear, and statistical tests are conducted to look for linear relationships. In a *linear relationship,* the relationship between the two concepts remains consistent regardless of the values of each of the concepts. For example, if the value of A increases by 1 point each time the value of B increases by 1 point, the values continue to increase at the same rate whether the value is 2 or 200. The relationship can be illustrated by a straight line, as shown in Figure 7–2.

Relationships can be curvilinear or some other shape. In a *curvilinear relationship,* the relationship between two concepts varies according to the relative values of the concepts. The relationship between anxiety and learning is a good example of a curvilinear relationship. Very high or very low levels of anxiety are associated with low levels of learning, whereas moderate levels of anxiety are associated with high levels of learning (Fawcett & Downs, 1986). This type of relationship is illustrated by a curved line, as shown in Figure 7–3.

Strength

The *strength of a relationship* is the amount of variation explained by the relationship. Some of the variation in a concept, but not all, is associated with variation in another concept. The strength of a relationship is sometimes discussed using the term

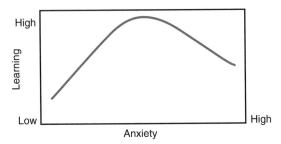

FIGURE 7–3 ■ Example of a curvilinear relationship.

effect size. The effect size explains how much "effect" variation in one concept has on variation in a second concept.

In some cases, a large portion or, in others, only a moderate or a small portion of the variation can be explained by the relationship. For example, one might examine the strength of the relationship between coping and compliance. Although a portion of the variance in a measure of compliance is associated with the measure of a person's coping ability, there is another portion of variation in the measure of compliance that cannot be explained by measuring how well a person copes. Conversely, only a portion of variation in a measure of a person's ability to cope can be explained by variation in a measure of his or her compliance. The portions of the two concepts that are associated are explained by the strength of the relationship.

Strength is usually determined by correlational analysis and is expressed mathematically by a correlation coefficient such as the following:

$$r = .35$$

The statistic r is the coefficient obtained by performing the statistical procedure Pearson's product moment correlation. A value of 0 would indicate no strength, whereas a +1 or a −1 would indicate the greatest strength, as indicated in the following diagram:

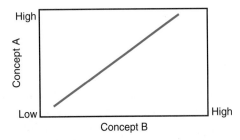

FIGURE 7–2 ■ Example of a linear relationship.

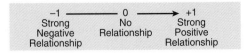

The + or − does not have an impact on strength. For example, $r = -.35$ is as strong as $r = +.35$. A weak relationship is usually considered one with an r value of .1 to .3; a moderate relationship one with an r value of .3 to .5; and a strong relationship one with an r value greater than .5. The greater the strength of a relationship, the easier it is to detect differences in groups being studied. This idea is explored further in the chapters on sampling, measurement, and data analysis.

Symmetry

Relationships may be symmetrical or asymmetrical. In an *asymmetrical relationship,* if A occurs (or changes), then B will occur (or change), but there may be no indication that if B occurs (or changes), A will occur (or change) (Fawcett & Downs, 1986). A previously cited example showed that when changes in relaxation level (A) occurred, changes in blood pressure (B) occurred. However, one cannot say that when changes in blood pressure occur, changes in relaxation levels occur. Therefore, the relationship is asymmetrical. An asymmetrical relationship may be diagrammed as follows:

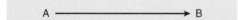

A *symmetrical relationship* is complex and actually contains two statements, such as "If A occurs (or changes), B will occur (or change); if B occurs (or changes), A will occur (or change)" (Fawcett & Downs, 1986). An example is the symmetrical relationship between the occurrences of cancer and impaired immunity. As the cancer increases, impaired immunity increases; as impaired immunity increases, cancer increases.

A symmetrical relationship may be diagrammed as follows:

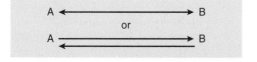

Sequencing

Time is the important factor in explaining the sequential nature of a relationship. If both concepts occur simultaneously, the relationship is *concurrent* (Fawcett & Downs, 1986). The relationship between relaxation (A) and blood pressure (B) may seem to be concurrent. If so, it would be expressed as follows:

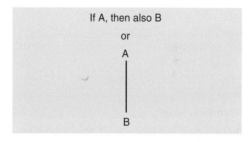

If one concept occurs later than the other, the relationship is *sequential.* If relaxation (A) was thought to occur first, and then blood pressure (B) decreased, the relationship is sequential. This relationship is expressed as follows:

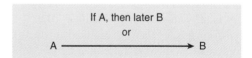

Probability of Occurrence

A relationship can be deterministic or probabilistic depending on the degree of certainty that it will occur. *Deterministic* (or *causal*) *relationships* are statements of what always occurs in a particular situation. A scientific law is one example of a deterministic relationship (Fawcett & Downs, 1986). It is expressed as follows:

If A, then always B

Another deterministic relationship describes what always happens if there are no interfering conditions. This is referred to as a *tendency statement.* A tendency statement might propose that an immobilized patient lying in a typical hospital bed (A) will always develop pressure sores (B) after 6 weeks if there are no interfering conditions. A tendency statement would be expressed in the following form:

If A, then always B
if there are no interfering conditions

A *probability statement* expresses the probability that something will happen in a given situation (Fawcett & Downs, 1986). This relationship is expressed as follows:

If A, then probably B

Probability statements are tested statistically to determine the extent of probability that B will occur in the event of A. For example, one could state that there is greater than a 50% probability that a patient who has an indwelling catheter for 1 week will experience a urinary bladder infection. This probability could be expressed mathematically as follows:

$$p > .50$$

The p is a symbol for probability. The $>$ is a symbol for "greater than." This mathematical statement asserts that there is more than a 50% probability that the relationship will occur.

Necessity

In a *necessary relationship,* one concept must occur for the second concept to occur. For example, one could propose that if sufficient fluids are administered (A), and only if sufficient fluids are administered, then the unconscious patient will remain hydrated (B). This is expressed as:

If A, and only if A, then B

In a *substitutable relationship,* a similar concept can be substituted for the first concept and the second concept will still occur. A substitutable relationship might propose that if tube feedings are

administered (A_1), or if hyperalimentation is administered (A_2), the unconscious patient can remain nourished (B). This relationship is expressed as follows:

If A_1, or if A_2, then B

Sufficiency

A *sufficient relationship* states that when the first concept occurs, the second concept will occur, regardless of the presence or absence of other factors (Fawcett & Downs, 1986). A statement could propose that if a patient is immobilized in bed longer than a week, bone calcium will be lost, regardless of anything else. This relationship is expressed as follows:

If A, then B, regardless of anything else

A *contingent relationship* will occur only if a third concept is present. For example, a statement might claim that if a person experiences a stressor (A), stress management (B) occurs, but only if effective coping strategies (C) are used. The third concept, in this case effective coping strategies, is referred to as an *intervening* (or *mediating*) *variable.* Intervening variables can affect the occurrence, strength, or direction of a relationship. A contingent relationship can be expressed as follows:

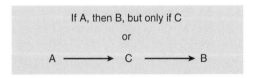

STATEMENT HIERARCHY

Statements about the same two conceptual ideas can be made at various levels of abstractness. The statements found in conceptual models (*general propositions*) are at a high level of abstraction. Statements found in theories (*specific propositions*) are at a moderate level of abstraction. *Hypotheses,* which are a form of statement, are at a low level of abstraction and are specific. As statements are expressed in a less abstract way, they become narrower in scope (Fawcett & Downs, 1986), as shown in following diagram:

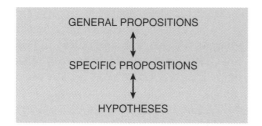

Statements at varying levels of abstraction that express relationships between or among the same conceptual ideas can be arranged in hierarchical form, from general to specific. Such an arrangement allows the reader to see the logical links among the various levels of abstraction. Statement sets link the relationships expressed in the framework with the hypotheses, research questions, or objectives that guide the methodology of the study.

Roy and Roberts (1981) developed statement sets related to Roy's nursing model that could be used in frameworks for research, as shown in the following excerpts.

● ●

General Proposition

"The magnitude of the internal and external stimuli will positively influence the magnitude of the physiological response of an intact system."

● ●

Specific Proposition

"The amount of mobility in the form of exercising positively influences the level of muscle integrity."

● ●

Hypothesis

"If the nurse helps the patient maintain muscle tone through proper exercising, the patient will experience fewer problems associated with immobility." (Roy & Roberts, 1981, p. 90) ■

Conceptual Models

A *conceptual model* is a set of highly abstract, related constructs that broadly explains phenomena of interest, expresses assumptions, and reflects a philosophical stance. A number of conceptual models have been developed in nursing. For example, Roy's (1984, 1988, 1990) model describes adaptation as the primary phenomenon of interest to nursing. This model identifies the constructs she considers essential to adaptation and how these constructs interact to produce adaptation. Orem (1995) considers self-care to be the phenomenon central to nursing. Her model explains how nurses facilitate the self-care of clients. Rogers (1970, 1980, 1983, 1986, 1988) regards human beings as the central phenomenon of interest to nursing, and her model is designed to explain the nature of human beings. A conceptual model may use the same or similar constructs as other models but define them in different ways. Thus, Roy, Orem, and Rogers may all use the construct *health* but define it in different ways.

Most disciplines have several conceptual models, each with a distinctive vocabulary. Fawcett and Downs (1986) identify 7 conceptual models in nursing: Johnson's behavioral system model (1980), King's open systems model (1981), Levine's conservation model (1973), Neuman's systems model (1989), Orem's self-care model (1995), Rogers's science of unitary human beings model (1970, 1980, 1983, 1986, 1988), and Roy's adaptation model (1984, 1988, 1990). Walker and Avant (1995) identify 19 conceptual models, which they refer to as *grand nursing theories* (see Table 7–1).

These conceptual models vary in their level of abstraction and the breadth of phenomena they explain. However, each provides a broad, overall picture, a gestalt of the phenomena they explain. It is not their purpose to provide detail or to be specific. These models are not directly testable through research and, thus, none can be used alone as the framework for a study (Fawcett & Downs, 1986; Walker & Avant, 1995). However, a framework could include a combination of a conceptual model and a theory.

TABLE 7-1
REPRESENTATIVE GRAND NURSING THEORIES

AUTHOR	DATE	PUBLICATION
Peplau	1952	Interpersonal Relations in Nursing
Orlando	1961	The Dynamic Nurse-Patient Relationship
Wiedenbach	1964	Clinical Nursing: A Helping Art
Henderson	1966	The Nature of Nursing
Levine	1967	The Four Conservation Principles of Nursing
Ujhely	1968	Determinants of the Nurse-Patient Relationship
Rogers	1970	An Introduction to the Theoretical Basis of Nursing
King	1971	Toward a Theory of Nursing
Orem	1971	Nursing: Concepts of Practice
Travelbee	1971	Interpersonal Aspects of Nursing
Neuman	1974	The Betty Neuman Health-Care Systems Model
Roy	1976	Introduction to Nursing: An Adaptation Model
Newman	1979	Toward a Theory of Health
Johnson	1980	The Behavioral System Model for Nursing
Parse	1981	Man-Living-Health
Erickson et al.	1983	Modeling & Role-Modeling
Leininger	1985	Transcultural Care Diversity and Universality
Watson	1985	Nursing: Human Science and Human Care
Newman	1986	Health as Expanding Consciousness

From Walker, L. O., & Avant, K. C. [1995]. *Strategies for theory construction in nursing* (p. 9). Norwalk, CT: Appleton & Lange.

Relatively few nursing studies have frameworks that include a conceptual nursing model. Moody and colleagues (1988), who examined nursing practice research from 1977 to 1986, found an increase in the number of studies using a nursing model as a framework from 8% in the first half of the decade under study to 13% in the second half. The most commonly used models were those of Orem, Rogers, and Roy. Silva (1986), who studied the extent to which five nursing models (those of Johnson, Roy, Orem, Rogers, and Newman) had been used as frameworks for nursing research, found 62 studies between 1952 and 1985 that had used these models. However, only 9 of these met her specified criterion of actually testing nursing theory; only in these 9 studies were statements extracted and tested by the study design.

An organized program of research is important for building a body of knowledge related to the phenomena explained by a particular conceptual model. This program of research is referred to as a *research tradition.* Development of a research tradition for a particular model requires the commitment of a group of scholars who are willing to dedicate their time and energy to this endeavor. Theories compatible with the model need to be developed. The research tradition for the conceptual model needs to be defined. The definition must incorporate (1) identification of acceptable strategies for developing and testing theory on the basis of the model, (2) definition of the phenomena to be studied, (3) establishment of priorities for testing theory statements, (4) development of research methods and measurement techniques, (5) description of data collection strategies, and (6) selection of acceptable approaches to data analyses.

Researchers conducting studies consistent with a particular tradition may be scattered across the country (or the world) but often maintain a network of communication about their work. In some cases, they hold annual conferences focused on the model to share research findings, explore theoretical ideas, and maintain network contacts. Conceptual models of nursing do not have well-established research traditions (Fawcett, 1995). However, research traditions are developing for some nursing models.

One example of a nursing model with an emerging research tradition is Orem's model of self-care. Orem's (1995) model focuses on the domain of nursing practice and on what nurses actually do when they practice nursing. She proposes that individuals generally know how to take care of themselves (*self-care*). If they are dependent in some way, as are children, the aged, or the handicapped, family members take on this responsibility (*dependent care*). If individuals are ill or have some defect (such as diabetes or a colostomy), these individuals or their family members acquire special skills to provide that care (*therapeutic self-care*). An individual's capacity to provide self-care is referred to as *self-care agency*. A *self-care deficit* occurs when self-care demand exceeds self-care agency.

Nursing care is provided only when there is a deficit in the self-care or dependent care that the individual and his or her family can provide (self-care deficit). In this case, the nurse or nurses develop a nursing system to provide the needed care. This system involves prescribing, designing, and providing the needed care. The goal of nursing care is to facilitate resumption of self-care by the person or family or both. There are three types of nursing systems: wholly compensatory, partly compensatory, and supportive-educative. The selection of one of these systems is based on the capacity of the person to perform self-care.

The notion of self-care as an important construct for nursing has drawn nurse researchers to Orem's work. Multiple studies have been performed to examine self-care in a variety of nursing situations (Bakker et al., 1995; Brugge, 1981; Davies, 1993; Frey & Denyes, 1989; Lasky & Eichelberger, 1985; McCaleb & Edgil, 1994; McDermitt, 1993; Moore, 1987a, 1987b, 1993; Rew, 1987; Saucier & Clark, 1993). The following instruments, consistent with Orem's model, have been developed:

- Exercise of Self-Care Agency Scale (Kearney & Fleischer, 1979; McBride, 1987; Riesch & Hauch, 1988)
- Self-Care Agency in Adolescents (Denyes, 1982)
- Self-Care Behavior Questionnaire (Dodd, 1984a)
- Self-Care Behavior Log (Dodd, 1984b, 1987)
- Perception of Self-Care Agency (Hanson & Bickel, 1985; Weaver, 1987)
- ADL Self-Care Scale (Gulick, 1987, 1988, 1989)
- Nurse Performance Evaluation Tool (Kostopoulos, 1988)
- Self-Care Agency Questionnaire (Bottorff, 1988)
- Nursing Care Role Orientation (Stemple, 1988)
- Mother's Performance of Self-Care Activities for Children (Moore & Gaffney, 1989)
- Children's Self-Care Performance Questionnaire (Moore, 1993)
- Bess's Measurement of Diabetes Self-Care Practices Scale (Bess, 1995)

- Maieutic Dimensions of Self-Care Agency (O'Connor, 1995)
- Self-Care of Older Persons Evaluation (Delasega, 1995)
- Self As Carer Inventory (Lukkarinen & Hentinen, 1997)
- Self-Care Management and Life-Quality Amongst Elderly (Lorenson, 1998)

Orem (1995) has developed three theories related to her model; they are the theory of self-care deficits, the theory of self-care, and the theory of nursing systems (also referred to as the general theory of nursing). Studies testing statements emerging from Orem's theories are appearing in the literature (Ailinger & Dear, 1997; Bess, 1995; Campbell & Soeken, 1999; Carroll, 1995; Cull, 1995; Hart, 1995; Hart & Foster, 1998; Jesek-Hale, 1994; Lee, 1999; Mapanga, 1994; McCaleb & Edgil, 1994; Moore & Mosher, 1997; Mosher & Moore, 1995; Robinson, 1995; Schoff-Baer et al., 1995; Villarreal, 1995; Wang, 1997; Wang & Fenske, 1996). Research methodologies acceptable for testing Orem's theories have not been specified. Orem did suggest that research be designed to examine the qualitative characteristics of self-care as well as its presence or absence. She also recommended studying the investigative and decision-making phases of self-care and the capability to engage in the production phase of self-care. Considerable work remains to be done in establishing a research tradition for Orem's model.

Theory

A theory is more narrow and specific than a conceptual model and is directly testable. A *theory* consists of an integrated set of defined concepts, existence statements, and relational statements that present a view of a phenomenon and can be used to describe, explain, predict, or control that phenomenon. Existence statements declare that a given concept exists or that a given relationship occurs. For example, an existence statement might claim that a condition referred to as *stress* exists and that there is a relationship between stress and health.

Relational statements clarify the type of relationship that exists between or among concepts. For example, a relational statement might propose that high levels of stress are related to declining levels of health. It is the statements of a theory that are tested through research, not the theory itself. Thus, identification of statements within theory is critical to the research endeavor and forms the basis of the framework of the study. The types of theory discussed here are scientific, substantive, and tentative.

SCIENTIFIC THEORY

The term *scientific theory* is restricted to a theory that has valid and reliable methods of measuring each concept and whose relational statements have been repeatedly tested through research and demonstrated to be valid. Scientific theories have *empirical generalizations*, statements that have been repeatedly tested and have not been disproved. There are no scientific theories within nursing. Scientific theories from other disciplines are commonly used within nursing practice. For example, most physiological theories are scientific in nature.

SUBSTANTIVE THEORY

Substantive theory is recognized within the discipline as useful for explaining important phenomena. Although there are few substantive theories within nursing, substantive theories developed within other disciplines are commonly used within nursing. The knowledge provided by a substantive theory may be in use in practice settings.

An example of a substantive theory is the theory of reasoned action (Ajzen & Fishbein, 1980; Fishbein & Ajzen, 1975), which proposes that a person's expectation that a particular behavior will lead to a given outcome increases his or her intention to perform the behavior. Intention has been found to be predictive of behavior. Blue (1995) has reviewed studies examining the capacity of this theory to predict engagement in exercise programs.

Substantive theories do not have the validity of a scientific theory. Some of the statements may have been tested and verified but others have not. In some cases, the statements in the theory may not have been clearly identified by the theorist or by those using the theory. Most theory testing has been performed by researchers in other disciplines. Few nursing studies actually test statements from substantive theory. Instead, in most cases, the substantive theory has been used rather shallowly to provide an overall orientation for the study. Concepts are defined for use in the framework and may be linked with the methods of measurement, but because statements are not extracted from the theory and used to develop research questions or hypotheses, the framework does not guide the research process.

Most substantive theories (or conceptual models) used in nursing research frameworks are from outside nursing (Walker & Avant, 1995). Moody and colleagues (1988) found that the largest group (49%) of nursing research frameworks were based on theoretical works from psychology. This group was followed by groups of studies with frameworks based on theoretical works from physiology and sociology. Theoretical works from other disciplines are an important source of nursing knowledge, but they need to be tested in nursing studies before being incorporated in nursing practice. Some researchers believe that substantive theories from other disciplines should be examined in terms of nursing theory (or the perspective of nursing) before being used in nursing practice.

TENTATIVE THEORY

A *tentative theory* is newly proposed, has had minimal exposure to critique by the discipline, and has undergone little testing. Tentative theories are developed to propose an integrated set of relationships among concepts that have not been satisfactorily addressed in a substantive theory. Because tentative theories are newly emerging and untested, they tend to be less well developed than substantive theories. Many tentative theories have short lives, but others may eventually be more extensively developed and validated through multiple studies.

Tentative theories may be developed from clinical insights, from elements of existing theories not previously related, or from conceptual models. One type of tentative theory of great importance in nursing today is intervention theories. These middle-range theories are developed to explain the dynamics of a patient problem and exactly how a specific nursing intervention is expected to change patient outcomes. Currently, these new theories are tentative, but some will likely become substantive in the future. These theories are discussed in detail in Chapter 13.

Tentative theories developed in nursing often contain concepts and relational statements derived from sociological, psychosocial, psychological, and physiological theories. In some cases, the framework may require that the nurse researcher merge concepts using theory from other sciences with concepts from nursing science theories. Figure 7–4 illustrates the merger of behavioral science variables and nursing science variables used in Benoliel's research (Wooldridge et al., 1983). In this figure, the solid lines indicate concepts and relationships taken from behavioral science theory. However, this theory was not sufficient to explain the phenomenon from a nursing practice perspective. Therefore, concepts and relationships from nursing practice theory were added to the behavioral science theory; these are indicated by dotted lines. Theory explaining reactions of family, health provider, and child were found in both nursing practice theory and behavioral science theory, as indicated by the use of both solid and dotted lines to illustrate these relationships.

Tentative theories in nursing often emerge from questions related to identified nursing problems or from the clinical insight that a relationship exists between or among elements important to desired outcomes. These situations tend to be concrete and require that the researcher express these concrete ideas in more abstract language. This issue is particularly difficult for the beginning researcher. The neophyte researcher's awareness of theoretical ideas related to the situation may be limited, or the researcher may perceive the situation in such concrete terms that even though the theories are known, he or she fails to make the link between the situation and available theory.

For example, one nurse, a novice researcher who worked in a newborn intensive care unit, was convinced from her clinical experiences that the frequency of visits to the newborn by the mother was related to the infant's weight gain. Her ideas could be diagrammed as follows:

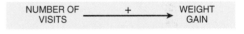

FIGURE 7–4 ■ Illustration of the merger of concepts using theory from other sciences with concepts from nursing science theories. (Redrawn from Wooldridge, P. J., Schmitt, M. J., Skipper, J. K., Jr., & Leonard, R. C. [1983]. *Behavioral science and nursing theory.* St. Louis: C. V. Mosby, p. 283.)

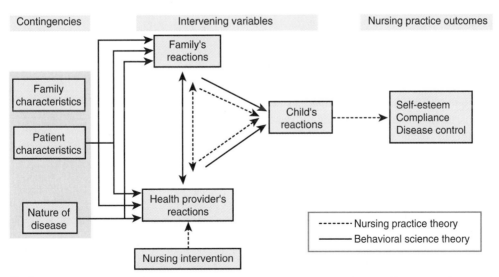

She wanted to study this relationship but was having difficulty expressing her ideas as a framework. Number of visits and weight gain are very concrete ideas. From the perspective of research, these ideas are variables. However, to develop a framework, the research must express the variables in a more abstract and general way as concepts. This novice researcher lacked the knowledge and skills needed to accomplish this task. She was "stuck" at a concrete level of viewing her problem.

Many students recognize that they are concrete thinkers and believe that they are incapable of moving beyond that very limited way of thinking. However, the capacity for abstract thinking is not an innate ability; it is a learned skill. Acquiring it simply requires that one invest the energy to obtain the knowledge and practice the skills.

Converting a concretely expressed term to a higher level of abstractness—from variable to concept—is a form of translation. Because the translation in this case is from a lower level of abstractness to a higher level (as shown in the following diagram), inductive reasoning is used.

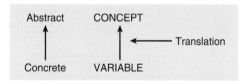

However, knowledge of equivalent terms at both the concrete and abstract levels is required to perform the translation. Conducting a literature search can be useful in identifying equivalent abstract terms. The search may be difficult if the novice researcher is blind to theoretical ideas presented in the literature and picks up only the concrete ideas.

Sometimes, probing questions facilitate the process of moving from concrete to more abstract thinking. For example, one could ask, "Why is it important that the mother visit?" "What happens when the mother visits?" Answering these questions may help label what happens when the mother

visits; existing theories have named this process *bonding* or *attachment*. There might be other names for it as well. The following diagram could be used to describe this process:

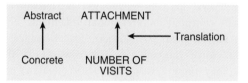

One can then ask, "What happens when the baby gains weight?" "Why is this important?" "How is it different from the baby who gains weight more slowly or fails to gain weight?" One name for this phenomenon is *growth*; another is *thriving*. There might be other ways the phenomenon could be described. The following diagram could be used to describe this process:

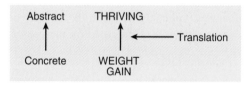

At this point, the novice nurse researcher is ready to search the literature more thoroughly. Theories related to bonding, attachment, growth, and thriving can be examined. The novice researcher may find literature that proposes a positive relationship between attachment and thriving. This relationship could be expressed as follows:

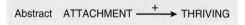

When the aforementioned ideas are linked, we have the beginning of a tentative theory. The diagram—really the beginning of a conceptual map—has the following appearance:

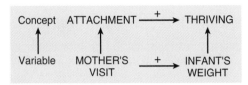

However, the ideas for a framework and a tentative theory are still incomplete. One needs to ask, "What other factors are important in influencing the relationship between mother's visits and infant's weight gain, between attachment and thriving?" Again, the literature can be consulted. Researchers in this field have examined elements relevant to this question. What concepts did they include? What relationships did they find? Are their findings consistent with the emerging framework? Clinically, what other elements seem to be associated with this phenomenon? Do the newly found concepts need to be included in the framework? While the researcher is pondering these questions, he or she can obtain conceptual definitions for *attachment* and *thriving* and statements expressing the relationship between the two concepts from the existing theories.

As the framework expressing a tentative theory takes shape, it is time to consider moving to an even higher level of abstraction, that of conceptual models. Is there a possible fit between a conceptual model in nursing and the tentative theory expressed in the developing framework? Can the study concepts be translated to the even more abstract constructs of a conceptual model? Are the study statements linked in any way with the broad statements of a conceptual model? If a conceptual nursing model is included in the framework, the links between the conceptual model and the tentative theory need to be made clear.

Conceptual Maps

One strategy for expressing a framework is a *conceptual map* that diagrams the interrelationships of the concepts and statements (Artinian, 1982; Fawcett & Downs, 1986; Moody, 1989; Newman, 1979; Silva, 1981). Figures 7–4 through 7–9 in this chapter are examples of conceptual maps. A conceptual map summarizes and integrates what is known about a phenomenon more succinctly and clearly than a literary explanation and allows one to grasp the gestalt of a phenomenon. A conceptual map should be supported by references from the literature (Artinian, 1982).

A conceptual map is developed to explain which concepts contribute to or partially cause an outcome. Conditions, both direct and indirect, that may produce the outcome are specified. The process in which factors must cumulatively interact over time in some sequence to have a causal effect is illustrated by a conceptual map. Conceptual maps vary in complexity and accuracy, depending on the available body of knowledge related to the phenomenon. Mapping is also useful in identifying gaps in the logic of the theory being used as a framework and reveals inconsistencies, incompleteness, and errors (Artinian, 1982).

Conceptual maps are useful beyond the study for which they were developed. A conceptual map may suggest hypotheses that can be tested in future studies. In addition, through map development, the researcher may gain insight about different situations in which the same process may be occurring. Publication of the map may stimulate the interest of other researchers, who may then use it in their own studies. Thus, a well-developed conceptual map may facilitate building a body of knowledge related to a particular theory. In addition to conceptual maps included as the framework for a study, more maps are being published that are outcomes of extensive reviews of the literature that are expressed as tentative theories.

THE STEPS OF CONSTRUCTING A STUDY FRAMEWORK

Developing a framework is one of the most important steps in the research process but, perhaps, also one of the most difficult. Examples of frameworks from the literature are helpful but not sufficient as a guide to framework development. The brief but impressive presentation of a framework in a published study often belies the careful, thoughtful work required to arrive at that point. Yet the neophyte researcher needs to learn how to perform that thoughtful work.

As the body of knowledge related to a phenomenon grows, the development of a framework to express the knowledge becomes easier. Therefore, frameworks for quasi-experimental and experimental studies, which should have a background of descriptive and correlational studies and perhaps some substantive theory, should be more easily and fully developed than those for descriptive studies. Descriptive studies often examine multiple factors to understand a phenomenon not previously well studied. Previous theoretical work related to the phenomenon may be tentative or nonexistent. Therefore, the framework may be less comprehensive. In qualitative studies, in which the framework development is an outcome of the study, even identification of concepts may not be clear at the beginning of the study, and statements will be synthesized from the data. The basis for the development of qualitative studies is more philosophical than theoretical.

A model for resilience by Woodgate (1999) is used here to illustrate the development of a framework. As you read through the extracts from this study, however, keep in mind that the nicely turned phrases in Woodgate's framework required much time, effort, thought, and reflection. They did not easily and miraculously appear in their present form. You are examining the finished framework and will not be able to see the process of thinking or the work involved as Woodgate developed her ideas.

To explain the process of framework development, a series of steps are identified and described. The steps are a way of introducing the reasoning used in developing a framework. The steps of the process are (1) selecting and defining concepts, (2) developing statements relating the concepts, (3) expressing the statements in hierarchical fashion, and (4) developing a conceptual map that expresses the framework. The steps presented are not usually performed in order. In reality, there is a move-

ment of the flow of thought from one step to another, back and forth, as ideas are developed and refined.

Selecting and Defining Concepts

Concepts are selected for a framework on the basis of their relevance to the phenomenon of concern. Thus, the problem statement, which describes the phenomenon of concern, is a rich source of concepts for the framework. If the researcher begins from a concrete clinical perspective, the ideas may be first identified as variables and then translated to concepts. Every major variable included in the study should be a reflection of a concept included in the framework. The framework may be modified as the rest of the study is developed. As the researcher gains additional insight into the phenomenon through a thorough search of theoretical, research, and clinical publications, additional relevant concepts may be identified or new relationships proposed. As these are incorporated into the framework, their implications for the study design also need to be considered.

Woodgate (1999, p. 36) defined the phenomenon of concern as "coping resources and individual competence and how families deal with specific crises that arise." The concepts Woodgate selected were stressors, vulnerability factors, protective factors, resilience, and maladaptation/adaptation.

Each concept included in a framework needs to be conceptually defined. When available and appropriate, conceptual definitions from existing theoretical works need to be used, with definitions quoted and sources cited. If theories that define the concept are not available, the researcher needs to develop the definition. Conceptual definitions may be available in the literature in the absence of theories that use the concept. For an example of the extraction of conceptual definitions from the literature, see Chapter 5 in *Understanding Nursing Research* (Burns & Grove, 1999).

One source of conceptual definitions is published concept analyses. Previous studies using the concept may also provide a conceptual definition. Another source of a conceptual definition is literature associated with instrument development related to the concept. Although the instrument itself is an operational definition of the concept, the author will often provide a conceptual definition on which the instrument development was based. The general literature can sometimes provide a conceptual definition. Although it may not have been as carefully thought out as the definitions in a theory or a concept analysis, this conceptual definition may reflect the only definition available in the discipline.

When acceptable conceptual definitions are not available, the researcher must perform concept synthesis or concept analysis to develop the definition. Various definitions of the concept from the literature must be presented to validate the conceptual definition the researcher selected for the study.

Woodgate (1999) provided the conceptual definitions in the following excerpts.

Resilience. "Haase (1997) defines resilience as the 'process of identifying or developing resources and strengths to flexibly manage stressors to gain a positive outcome, a sense of confidence, mastery, and self-esteem' (p. 20)." (Woodgate, 1999, p. 37)

Stressors. "Garmezy and Rutter (1983) refer to stressors as particular events or situations that evoke an emotional reaction." (Woodgate, 1999, p. 38)

Protective Factors. "Influences that modify, ameliorate, or alter a person's response to some environmental hazard that predisposes to a maladaptive outcome (Rutter, 1985). They provide resistance to stress and encourage outcomes that are marked by patterns of adaptation and competence (Kimchi & Schaffner, 1990; Rutter, 1987)." (Woodgate, 1999, p. 39)

Vulnerability Factors. "Modify the person's response to a risk situation. However, vulnerability factors act by intensifying the reaction to a stress factor that in ordinary circumstances will lead to a maladaptive outcome (Rutter, 1987)." (Woodgate, 1999, p. 39)

Adaptive/Maladaptive Outcomes. "Modification through the interaction of risk and protective factors of a person's response to the risk situation." (Woodgate, 1999, p. 40) ■

Developing Relational Statements

The next step in framework development is to link all of the concepts through relational statements. Whenever possible, relational statements must be obtained from theoretical works, and the sources cited. If such statements are unavailable, the researcher must propose the relationships. Evidence from the literature for the validity of each relational statement must be provided whenever available. This support needs to include a discussion of previous studies that have examined the proposed relationship and published observations from the clinical practice perspective.

The researcher developing a framework may have to extract statements that are embedded in the literary text of an existing theory. When you first begin extracting statements, the task can be overwhelming because every sentence in the text seems to be a relational statement. A little practice makes the task easier. The steps in the process of extracting statements are as follows:

1. Select a portion of a theory that discusses the relationships between or among two or three concepts.
2. Write down a single sentence from the theory that seems to be a relational statement.
3. Express it diagrammatically using the statement diagrams presented earlier in the chapter.
4. Move to the next statement, and express it diagrammatically.
5. Continue until all of the statements related to the selected concepts have been diagrammatically expressed.
6. Examine the linkages among the diagrammatic statements you have developed. The logic of what the theorist is saying will gradually become clearer.

This process is illustrated in greater detail in Chapter 5 of *Understanding Nursing Research* (Burns & Grove, 1999).

If statements relating the concepts of interest are

not available in the literature, *statement synthesis* is necessary. The researcher has to develop statements that propose specific relationships among the concepts being studied. Knowledge for use in statement synthesis may be obtained through clinical observation and integrative literature review (Walker & Avant, 1995).

In descriptive studies, theoretical statements related to the phenomenon may be sparse. In this case, developing a framework requires more synthesis and has a higher level of uncertainty. The statement set may include a statement that a relationship between A and B is proposed but the type of relationship is unknown. This statement may be followed by a research question based on this relationship rather than a hypothesis. For example, one might ask, "What is the nature of the relationship between A and B?" An objective might be to examine the nature of the relationship between A and B.

Woodgate (1999) offered the relational statements shown in the following excerpts, each of which is followed by a diagram of the relationship.

1. "The adolescent with cancer will experience multiple and varied events during the cancer illness trajectory. Whether such events become stressors for the adolescent depends on whether the adolescent perceives them to be events that cause emotional reactions." (Woodgate, 1999, p. 41)

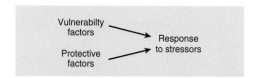

2. "How the adolescent responds to the stressors will vary and depends on the presence of vulnerability and protective factors." (Woodgate, 1999, p. 41)

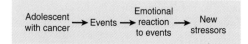

3. "These factors contribute to the degree of resilience in the adolescent or how the adolescent manages the stressors." (Woodgate, 1999, p. 41)

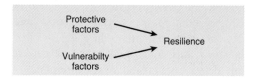

4. "Responses to the stressors will vary along a continuum of responses from maladaptive to adaptive." (Woodgate, 1999, p. 41)

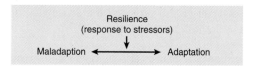

5. "The more resilient the adolescent is, the more likely the adolescent will be able to move towards adaptation." (Woodgate, 1999, p. 41)

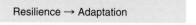

6. "How the adolescent responds to the stressor feeds directly back into the vulnerability and protective factors." (Woodgate, 1999, p. 41)

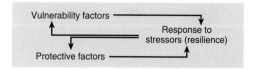

7. "The adolescent's response may also affect whether future events are perceived as stressful." (Woodgate, 1999, p. 41)

Response to stressor →
Perception of future events as stressful

8. "If circumstances change, then resilience will be altered" (Rutter, 1987; Woodgate, 1999, p. 41).

> Change in circumstances →
>   Change in resilience

Developing Hierarchical Statement Sets

A *hierarchical statement set* is composed of a specific proposition and a hypothesis or research question. If a conceptual model is included in the framework, the statement set may also include a general proposition. The proposition is listed first, with the hypothesis or research question immediately following. In some cases, more than one hypothesis may be related to a particular proposition. However, there must be a proposition for each hypothesis stated. This statement set indicates the link between the framework and the methodology.

Constructing a Conceptual Map

Conceptual maps are initiated early in the development of the framework, but refinement of the map will probably be one of the last steps accomplished. Before the map can be completed, the following information must be available:

1. A clear problem and purpose statement.
2. The concepts of interest, including conceptual definitions.
3. Results of an integrative review of the theoretical and empirical literature.
4. Relational statements linking the concepts, expressed literally and diagrammatically.
5. Identification and analysis of existing theories that address the relationships of interest.
6. Identification of existing conceptual models congruent with the developing framework.
7. Linking of proposed relationships with hypotheses, questions, or objectives (hierarchical statement sets).

Some nursing scholars believe that the map should be limited to those concepts included in the study (Fawcett & Downs, 1986). However, Artinian (1982) recommends that the map include all the concepts necessary to explain the phenomenon, plainly delineating that portion of the map to be studied. We agree with Artinian. It is important that the map be a full expression of the phenomenon of concern. This strategy is illustrated by Artinian's map of the conceptualization of the effects of role supplementation, presented in Figure 7–5. In this map, the scope of the study is enclosed by a gray box.

Developing your own concept map entails the following steps. First, arrange the concepts on the page in sequence of occurrence (or causal linkage) from left to right, with the concepts reflecting the outcomes located on the far right. Concepts that are elements of a more abstract construct can be placed in a frame or box. Sets of closely interrelated concepts can be linked by enclosing them in a frame or circle. Second, using arrows, link the concepts in a way consistent with the diagrammatic statements you have previously developed. For some studies, at some point on the map, the path of relationships may diverge, so that there are then two or more paths of concepts. The paths may converge at a later point. Every concept should be linked to at least one other concept. Third, examine the map for completeness by asking yourself the following questions:

- Are all the concepts that are included in the study on the map?
- Are all the concepts on the map defined?
- Does the map clearly portray the phenomenon?
- Does the map accurately reflect all the statements?
- Is there a statement for each of the linkages portrayed by the map? Is the sequence accurate?

Developing a well-constructed conceptual map requires repeated tries, but persistence pays off. You may need to go back and reexamine the statements identified. Are there some missing links? Are some of the links inaccurately expressed?

As the map takes shape and begins to seem right, show it to trusted colleagues. Can they follow your logic? Do they agree with your linkages? Can they identify missing elements? Can you explain the map to them? Seek out individuals who have experienced the phenomenon you are mapping. Does the process depicted seem valid to them? Find someone

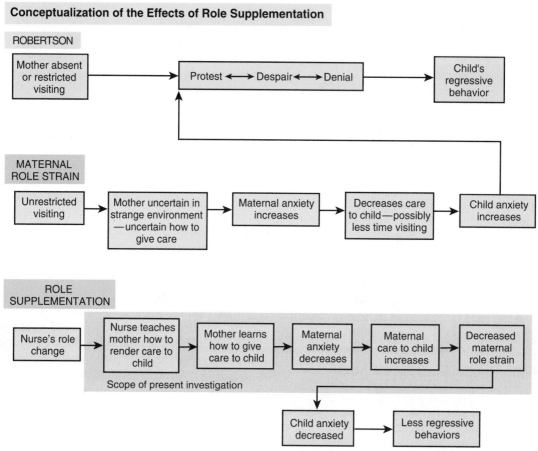

FIGURE 7–5 ■ Conceptual map outlining scope of present study: Conceptualization of the effects of role supplementation. (Redrawn from Artinian, B. M. [1982]. Conceptual mapping: Development of the strategy. *Western Journal of Nursing Research, 4*[4], 385. © 1982.)

more experienced than you in conceptual mapping to examine your map closely and critically.

Continue to revise your conceptual map until you achieve some degree of consensus with people you have consulted and you feel a sense of rightness about it. Examine Woodgate's conceptual map in Figure 7–6. Is it consistent with her concepts and statements? Does the process described seem valid to you?

Constructing a Study Framework From Substantive Theory

Developing a framework designed to test statements in a substantive theory requires that all con-

cepts in the framework be obtained from the substantive theory. These concepts must be defined as they are defined by the theorist. If the theorist has failed to define a concept, one should be developed that is consistent with the theorist's perspective. Operational definitions must be consistent with the conceptual definitions and should be accepted methods of measurement used for testing the selected theory. Statements (propositions) from the substantive theory must be identified. In a substantive theory, previous studies will have been conducted to test at least some of the relational statements. Findings from these studies must be discussed in the literature review or in the presentation of the framework in terms of evidence validating or refuting the

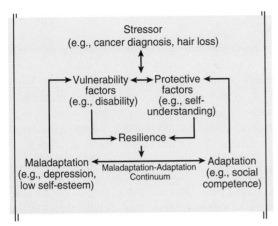

FIGURE 7–6 ▪ Resiliency model as applied to the adolescent cancer patient. (Redrawn from Woodgate, R. L. [1999]. Conceptual understanding of resilience in the adolescent with cancer: Part I. *Journal of Pediatric Oncology Nursing, 16*[1], 38.)

relational statements. Hypotheses for the present study must be designed to test one or more statements from the substantive theory.

The following excerpts, taken from a study by Stephenson (1999), illustrates a framework developed to test components of the Double ABCX Model of Family Adjustment and Adaptation. In this framework, relationships are expressed in an equation form.

Conceptual Framework and Empirical Research

"Concepts from the Double ABCX Model of Family Adjustment and Adaptation provided the framework for this study (McCubbin & Patterson, 1983, 1987) ([see Figure 7–7]). In the original ABCX Model (Hill, 1965) a family's course of adjustment and possible crisis (X) was influenced by the interaction of life events (stressors) and related hardships (a), family resources (b) and the family's perception of the event as threatening (c) (a + b + c = X). . . .

"Patterson and McCubbin (1983b) added other factors to form the Double ABCX model (pp. 21–36). First they added 'pile-up of demands' (A) to the stressor events (a). This 'pile-up of demands' (aA) referred to the cumulative effect over time of stressors and strains. Resources (b) were expanded to include family, personal, and community resources (bB). To the concept of perception (c), the Double ABCX model added redefinition (C). Coping became the central process involving the interaction of resources (bB) and perception (cC). Coping was defined as the ability to acquire and use the resources needed for family adaptation (Patterson & McCubbin, 1983a). Family coping was facilitated as families redefine a situation as a challenge, as an opportunity for growth or having special meaning

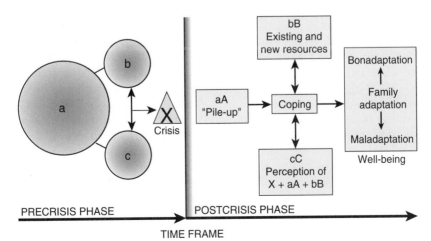

FIGURE 7–7 ▪ The Double ABCX Model of Family Adaptation. (Redrawn from Stephenson, C. [1999]. Well-being of families with healthy and technology-assisted infants in the home: A comparative study. *Journal of Pediatric Nursing, 14*[3], 165.)

(McCubbin & Figley, 1983; Patterson & McCubbin, 1983b). The interaction of stressors/strains, and coping influence family adaptation. Family adaptation (well-being) (Xx), the outcome variable, reflects the family's efforts to achieve a balance, whether positive (bon) or negative (maladaptation) (McCubbin & Thompson, 1987)." (Stephenson, 1999, p. 164–165)

• •

Empirical Research

Research Related to Family
Stressors/Strains (aA)

"Transition to parenthood is considered stressful for new parents (Dormire, Strauss & Clarke, 1989; Ventura, 1987; Umberson & Grove, 1989). Specific problems encountered by new parents include (1) physical stressors, including loss of sleep and extra work; (2) psychological stressors related to uncertainty about parenting competency and concerns for the infant; (3) strain in relationships within the family; (4) reduced social interaction; and (5) increased monetary cost (Miller & Myers-Walls, 1983; Sollie & Miller, 1980; Ventura, 1987). According to McCubbin and Patterson (1987), family stressors and the accompanying strain have a negative impact on family well-being. . . .

"Caring for a technology-assisted infant contributes additional stressors/strains. Most families experienced financial strain owing to increased out-of-pocket expenses (Andrews & Nielson, 1988; Fields, Rosenblatt, Polack, & Kaufman, 1991; Knecht, 1991; Nuttall, 1988; Quint, Chesterman, Crain, Winkleby & Boyce, 1990; Scharer & Dixon, 1989; Wasserman, 1984; Wills, 1983). In an outcome study by Wegener and Aday, family finance was a strong predictor of caregiver stress and impact on the family. . . .

"Equipment and monitoring problems were stressors to families because of false alarms, fear of not hearing the alarms, difficulties with leads, and restrictions imposed by monitoring (Black, Hersher, & Steinschneider, 1978; Fiser & Lyons, 1985; Nuttall, 1988; Wills, 1983). Limited monitoring instructions, difficulty with mobility of the equipment and lack of assistance were frustrating to parents (Andrews & Nielson, 1988; Black et al., 1978; DiMaggio & Sheetz, 1983; Fiser & Lyons, 1985; Nuttall, 1988;

Scharer & Dixon, 1989; Young, Creighton, & Sauve, 1988). . . .

"Vigilance and watchfulness in caring for the infant caused increased personal strain for family members (Stevens, 1990; Stevens, 1994; Young et al., 1988). Some parents reported that the increased responsibility of caring for the infant in the home required constant work, resulting in fatigue and loss of sleep (Andrews & Nielson, 1988; Black et al., 1978; Burr, Guyer, Todres, Abraham, & Chiodo, 1983; Hazlett, 1989; Lyman, Wurtele, & Wilson, 1985; Stevens, 1994, Wills, 1983). Some families expressed concern about their infants' health and future development including concerns about weight gain (Young et al., 1988), speech development, feeding, and possible infection (Wills, 1983; Nuttall, 1988). . . .

"Intrafamily stressors/strains included the lack of privacy, lack of adequate resources, and crowded living arrangements with extended family (Burr et al., 1983; Hazlett, 1989; Quint et al., 1990; Wegener & Aday, 1989; Wills, 1983). The additional infant care responsibilities, in some cases, affected the family relationships (Dean, 1986; Nuttall, 1988; Stengel, Echeveste, & Schmidt, 1985). Social isolation was reported owing to lack of respite care (Black et al., 1978; Burr et al., 1983; Cain, Kelly, & Shannon, 1980; Bendell, Culbertson, Shelton, & Carter, 1986; Dimaggio & Sheetz, 1983; Fiser & Lyons, 1985; Hazlett, 1989; Stevens, 1994; Wills, 1983; Young et al., 1988). . . .

"Families complained that the health care system was a source of strain. Some families received inconsistent medical care or conflicting information because of lack of a designated health care professional for case management (Fiser & Lyon, 1985; Nuttall, 1988; Scharer & Dixon, 1989; Wills, 1983). Parents thought that health care professionals minimized their ability to deal with the child, ignored them, or lacked the time to provide the needed help (Burr et al., 1983; Fiser & Lyon, 1985; Nuttall, 1988; Scharer & Dixon, 1989). Home care was limited for some owing to inadequate insurance, or lack of nurses knowledgeable in pediatric care (Andrews & Nielson, 1988; Hazlett, 1989). The distance from home to the medical center contributed to the strain of coordinating services (Hazlett, 1989; Nuttall, 1988). . . .

"Research has focused on describing the types of stressors/strains experienced by families with new infants. The research did indicate that families with technology-assisted infants had additional stressors/strains (Vohr, Chen, Coll, & Oh, 1988). However, research comparing levels of stressors/strains between families with healthy and technology-assisted infants was limited. McElroy, Steinschneider, & Weinstein (1986) found no significant difference between families with monitored and nonmonitored infants on recent life events. Studies with comparison groups did not explore other stressors/strains within the family that might influence well-being" (Stephenson, 1999, pp. 165–166).

Stephenson's study contained extensive sections discussing research related to family coping (bB + cC) and research related to family well-being (xX), which are not included here because of space limitations. In relation to family coping, Stephenson (1999, p. 167) indicated that "further investigation was needed in relating stressors/strains with coping and well-being and noting the differences and similarities between families." In relation to family well-being, Stephenson (1999, p. 168) indicated that "the research on well-being of families has been diverse, from focusing on parents' emotional and behavioral responses to focusing on parenting. Measurement that includes multiple components of well-being is limited. As a result, the focus of the current research was to use a more inclusive measure of family well-being." ■

Constructing a Study Framework on the Basis of a Conceptual Model

Although testing of extant nursing models is a critical need within nursing, few published studies have been designed for this purpose. One reason is the level of complexity required for such testing. Because conceptual models cannot be directly tested, a middle-range theory based on the conceptual model must be available (or must be developed as a tentative theory). The framework must include both the conceptual model and the middle-range

theory. Thus, the conceptual map for the study needs to illustrate relationships among the constructs of the model, the concepts of the middle-range theory, and the linkage between the concepts and relationships in the model and the concepts and relationships in the middle-range theory. Because of this complexity, in our opinion, the process should not be attempted by master's level students unless their research is being conducted collaboratively with doctorally prepared nurses. However, master's level students will be involved in critiquing published studies with such frameworks and applying them in practice situations.

A framework that includes a conceptual model has the following elements:

- Constructs from the conceptual model
- Definitions of constructs from the conceptual model
- Statements linking the constructs
- Concepts that represent portions of the selected constructs
- Conceptual definitions compatible with construct definitions
- Statements linking the concepts that express a tentative or substantive theory
- Selection of variables that represent portions of the concepts
- Operational definitions of the variables compatible with conceptual definitions
- Statement sets
- Conceptual map linking the constructs, concepts, and variables

In some cases, rather than beginning with the choice of a model, the development of the framework begins with identification of concepts relevant to a particular nursing problem. A theory related to the phenomenon of interest is identified or developed; and simultaneously or perhaps later, all or a portion of a conceptual model compatible with the researcher's interests is selected. The important issue is not where the development of the framework begins, but rather how well the various elements of the framework are logically linked together and how complete the end product is.

Lévesque and associates (1998) have identified a

tentative middle-range theory (model) derived from the Roy Adaptation Model and have provided empirical verification of the tentative theory. The following excerpts contain their description of the process of developing the theoretical model.

• •

"A group of nurse researchers, now known as the University of Montreal Research Team in Nursing Science (Montreal, Canada), has consolidated their efforts to work on a research program (Duquette, Ducharme, Ricard, Lévesque, & Bonin, 1996; Pepin et al., 1994) based on the Roy conceptual model of adaptation (Andrews & Roy, 1991). This program aims at further understanding a person's adaptation to various environmental stimuli, adaptative responses that influence adaptation (the person's biopsychological integrity), and nursing interventions that promote adaptation.

"As advocated by many scholars (Adam, 1987; Fawcett, 1991), the team believes in the importance of conducting research based on a conceptual model specific to the nursing discipline in order to contribute to the development of a coherent system of knowledge to guide nursing practice. A conceptual nursing model depicts concepts specific to nursing and describes general relationships between these concepts. Research based on an explicit conceptual model leads to the development of a theoretical model that would encompass precise relationships among concepts and interrelated propositions relevant to nursing science and practice. These propositions can then be empirically tested in order to validate the conceptual structure from which the theoretical model is derived (Fawcett, 1991). With time, such a research process should generate middle-range theories in nursing which can explain or predict nursing phenomena.

"In the context of the Montreal program, five longitudinal studies focusing on psychosocial factors associated with psychological adaptation were examined within the perspective of the Roy adaptation model (RAM). Four groups of subjects were considered in these studies: informal family caregivers of a demented relative at home, informal family caregivers of a psychiatrically ill relative at home at two periods (during a period of remission and during the crisis period requiring hospitalization of the ill relative), nurses as professional caregivers for elderly patients in geriatric institutions, and aged spouses in the community. These groups were selected on the basis of their vulnerability and the fact that they are at risk for health problems (Hare, Pratt, & Andrews, 1988; Schultz, Visintainer, & Williamson, 1990). . . ."

• •

Theoretical Model

Selection of the Conceptual Elements

"The five studies were initially guided by middle-range theories borrowed from other disciplines, such as psychology and sociology, compatible with the discipline of nursing. These middle-range theories focused on the relationships among the concepts of stress, social support, coping strategies, and psychological well-being. More specifically, the stress and coping theory of Lazarus and Folkman (1984) guided the three studies on informal family caregivers, while the theory proposed by Maddi and Kobasa (1984) and the family stress theory of McCubbin and Patterson (1983) guided the study of professional caregivers and that of aged spouses, respectively. (For details on these studies, see Ducharme, 1994; Duquette, Kérouac, Sandhu, Ducharme, and Saulnier, 1995; Lévesque, Cossette, and Lauren, 1995; Ricard, Fortin, and Bonin, 1995.)

"Given the theoretical commonalities across these studies, as well as the theoretical compatibility among the middle-range theories selected and the RAM, the current authors decided to analyze a posteriori these five studies within the perspective of the conceptual elements of the RAM. The conceptual elements selected for the elaboration of the theoretical model had to meet two criteria: They had to be considered in each study and correspond as closely as possible to the conceptual definitions of the RAM. This selection process led the research team to consider three elements of the RAM: environmental stimuli (focal and contextual), coping mechanisms, and adaptive/nonadaptive responses (for details, see Duquette, et al., 1996). [Table 7–2] presents correspondence between conceptual elements of the RAM and the studies' variables."

TABLE 7–2

CORRESPONDENCE BETWEEN CONCEPTUAL ELEMENTS OF THE ROY ADAPTATION MODEL AND FIVE STUDIES' VARIABLES

CONCEPTS FROM THE ROY MODEL	VARIABLES EXAMINED
Focal stimulus: an event that confronts the person's integrity directly and becomes the focus of attention for the person, who expends energy dealing with it in order to maintain or restore adaptation	Informal family caregiver studies: perceived feeling of being stressed or upset by the dysfunctional behaviors of the ill person Professional caregivers study: perceived feeling of being stressed or upset by the severe or terminal health Aged spouses study: perceived stress associated with situations occurring during the aging process
Contextual stimuli: factors (internal and external) that can act on the person's perception of the focal stimulus	Available or enacted social support Conflicts in the exchange of social support Gender
Coping mechanisms (cognator subsystem): information processing and judgment, which encompasses such activities as problem solving and decision making	Coping strategies
Self concept: the composite of beliefs and feelings that a person holds about himself or herself at a given time	Psychological distress

From Lévesque, L., Ricard, N., Ducharme, F., Duquette, A., & Bonin, J. (1998). Empirical verification of a theoretical model derived from the Roy Adaptation Model: Findings from five studies. *Nursing Science Quarterly*, *11*(1), 31–39.

Definition of the Conceptual Elements

"According to the RAM, the focal stimulus is an event that confronts the person's integrity directly. The event becomes the focus of attention for the person who expends energy dealing with it in order to maintain or restore adaptation. . . . The focal stimulus in the four caregivers studies was defined as the perceived feeling of being stressed or upset by the dysfunctional behaviors or the severe or terminal health problems of the ill person being cared for at home or in a geriatric setting. In the aged spouse study, the focal stimulus was the perceived stress associated with situations occurring during the aging process.

"According to the RAM, contextual stimuli were defined as factors (internal and external) which could act on the person's perception of the focal stimulus. In the five studies, available or enacted social support as well as conflicts in the exchange of social support were considered as contextual stimuli. Gender was also seen as a contextual stimulus since it is recognized as a determinant of men-

tal health (Nestmann & Schmerl, 1991), even if this stimulus cannot be modified by an intervention.

'Roy has conceptualized coping mechanisms as 'the complex controls within the person' (Roy & Andrews, 1991, p. 13) and has classified these mechanisms in two categories: the regulator subsystem acting through the neural-chemical-endocrine processes, and the cognator sub-system, which encompasses cognitive channels. Since the cognator sub-system cannot be empirically observed, indicators of two components of the cognator sub-system were considered: information processing and judgment, which 'encompasses such activities as problem solving and decision making' (Roy & Andrews, 1991, p. 14). In the five studies, coping strategies (the person's cognitive and behavioral efforts to deal with the focal stimulus of perceived stress) were considered indicators of the two components of the cognator sub-system.

"Lastly, level of psychological distress was selected as an indicator of adaptation in the self-concept mode. Though indicators of adaptation in other modes were selected, psychological distress was the only common indicator across the five studies." (Lévesque et al., 1988, pp. 31–33)

Propositions of the Theoretical Model
The authors then presented three propositions.

Proposition 1

"The three contextual stimuli (gender, conflicts, and available or enacted social support) will influence the focal stimulus of perceived stress. The theoretical literature on social support as well as empirical findings (for a review, see Gottlieb & Selby, 1989; Stewart, 1993) suggest that social support and conflicts in the exchange of support are often associated with perceived stress and psychological well-being. Although equivocal, some findings also reveal that women tend to report more perceived stress than men (Cook, 1988; Noh & Turner, 1987).

Hypothesis 1

"Conflicts in social support are positively linked to perceived stress, while available or enacted social support is negatively associated to perceived stress.

Hypothesis 2

"Women have a higher level of perceived stress than men.

Proposition 2

"The focal stimulus of perceived stress triggers coping strategies (indicators of coping mechanisms) in order to deal with stress. In the theoretical literature of the stress paradigm of coping and adaptation (e.g., that of Lazarus & Folkman, 1984), coping strategies are considered to be an individual's cognitive and behavioral response, activated by an event perceived as stressful (Wykle, Kahana, & Kowal, 1992). In other words, coping strategies refer to the cognitive and behavioral response made in order to manage specific demands that are perceived as taxing or exceeding the individual's avail-

able resources (Folkman et al., 1991). Many empirical studies have given credence to this theoretical perspective (Wykle et al., 1992).

Hypothesis 1

"There is a significant link between perceived stress and the use of coping strategies (either active, passive/avoidance, or both).

Proposition 3

"Coping strategies influence adaptation. As suggested in the literature (Moos, Cronkite, & Finney, 1990), two broad categories of coping strategies have been considered: active coping strategies (cognitive/behavioral attempts to actively manage a situation perceived as stressful) and passive/avoidance strategies (where effort to manage a stressful situation is lacking, or ignoring the situation is attempted). Some empirical findings propose that active coping strategies enhance psychological well-being, while passive/avoidance strategies tend to be related to a lower degree of well-being (Caslowitz, 1989; Edwards & Baglioni, 1993).

Hypothesis 1

"Active coping strategies are negatively linked with psychological distress, while passive/avoidance coping strategies are positively related to this outcome.

Empirical Verification

"An overview of the method used for empirical verification of the theoretical model will briefly be explained, followed by presentation of the results.

Samples
"In study 1, the convenience sample consisted of 265 informal primary caregivers living with a demented relative. In study 2, a convenience sample of 200 informal primary caregivers of a psychiatrically ill relative admitted to a psychiatric hospital (crisis period) were recruited, and in study 3, some of these caregivers (n = 163) were interviewed again when the ill person was back at home (remis-

sion period). The subjects of study 4 were professional caregivers (n = 1564 nurses) working in geriatric long-term hospitals and randomly selected through the Provincial Register of the Quebec Order of Nurses. In study 5, community-dwelling elderly couples (n = 135) were recruited through a multistage sampling strategy.

. . . .

Measurement

"The variables were measured using scales with established psychometric properties. Since subjects were all French-speaking, the French translation of some scales was done according to the back-translation method (Haccoun, 1987). Internal consistency tests (Cronbach's α) were performed with the current data for all the measures." (Lévesque, Ricard, Ducharme, Duquette, & Bonin, (1998, pp. 33–34).

Since each of the studies used different measures, the authors explain how the measures in each study are linked to the RAM concepts of focal stimulus, contextual stimulus, coping strategies, and adaptation in the self-concept mode.

. . . .

Statistical Analysis

"The model in [Figure 7–8] was tested in each study using structural equation analyses by means

of LISREL VIII (Jöreskog & Sörbom, 1993), designed to simultaneously estimate the paths of a model." (Lévesque, Ricard, Ducharme, Duquette, Bonin, 1998, p. 35) ■

This is a very complex statistical analysis; it is described in Chapter 20.

. . . .

Results

"For each of the five studies, the fit of the original model derived from the RAM [Figure 7–8] was not satisfactory according to the selected criteria. . . . These indexes suggested paths not previously hypothesized in the original model. . . . A synthesis of the common empirical links is presented in [Figure 7–9] . . . according to the expected paths of the original model derived from the RAM, the new paths found, and the total effects.

"**Expected Paths.** Of the six direct paths expected, three were supported in at least three studies (broken lines in [Figure 7–9]). One contextual stimulus, conflicts in the exchange of social support, had a direct and positive effect on the focal stimulus of perceived stress. Perceived stress is found to trigger passive/avoidance coping strategies. These strategies were directly and positively linked to psychological distress. The three expected paths not supported in at least three studies were those

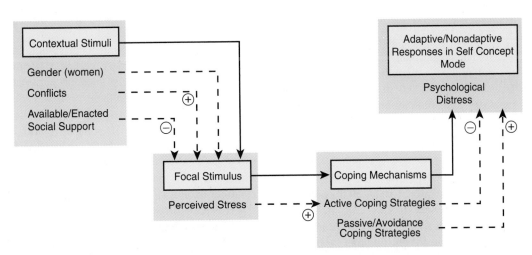

FIGURE 7–8 ■ Theoretical model and hypotheses derived from Roy's model. (Redrawn from Lévesque, L., Ricard, N., Ducharme, F., Duquette, A., & Bonin, J. P. [1998]. Empirical verification of a theoretical model derived from the Roy adaptation model: Findings from five studies. *Nursing Science Quarterly, 11*[1], 33.)

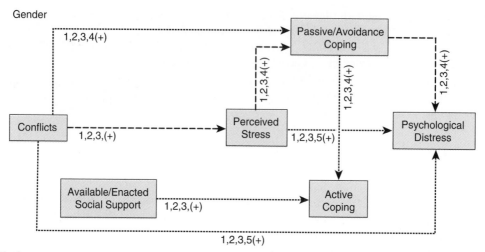

Figure 7–9 ■ Synthesis of significant linkages across at least three studies. (Redrawn from Lévesque, L., Ricard, N., Ducharme, F., Duquette, A, & Bonin, J. P. [1998]. Empirical verification of a theoretical model derived from the Roy adaptation model: Findings from five studies. *Nursing Science Quarterly, 11*[1], 36.)

between two contextual stimuli (gender and available or enacted social support) and the focal stimulus of perceived stress, and between active coping strategies and psychological distress.

"New Paths. There were five paths not hypothesized in the original model which were found to be significant in at least three studies (dotted lines in [Figure 7–9]). Three of these paths concern coping strategies. Available or enacted social support and passive/avoidance coping strategies had a direct and positive effect on active coping strategies, while conflicts had a direct and positive influence on passive/avoidance coping strategies. The other two paths not originally hypothesized concern the dependent variable. Conflicts in social support and perceived stress were directly and positively linked to psychological distress. . . .

. . . .

Discussion

"Based on one tenet of the RAM, one proposition of the theoretical model states that contextual stimuli influence the focal stimulus and, as a result, contextual stimuli can either indirectly promote or hinder adaptation. The current findings support this tenet only with regard to the contextual stimulus of conflicts in the exchange of social support. In the three studies of informal caregivers, conflicts were

found to have a direct and positive effect on the focal stimulus of perceived stress, which acted ultimately on adaptation (psychological distress). . . . Overall, the current findings underline the importance of considering the negative aspect of social support, not only the availability or the receipt of support. It seems relevant to shift away from the question of whether social support is a critical variable with regard to adaptation, and move toward a detailed examination of salient aspects of social support and ways in which different aspects play a role in the adaptation process.

"The proposition that the focal stimulus of perceived stress should trigger coping strategies was supported in the three studies of informal caregivers. However, no significant link was observed between the focal stimulus and coping strategies in the study on professional caregivers and that of aged spouses. In the study of aged spouses, any stimulus (focal or contextual) was related to coping strategies, and the current data do not allow a clear-cut explanation of this finding.

"The path between the active and the passive/avoidance coping strategies was not part of the original model. According to this unforeseen path, the passive/avoidance strategies trigger the active coping strategies. While no other similar observation was found in the literature, this finding indicates the need to further explore how these two typologies of coping strategies are interrelated. Given the actual results, the more that informal caregivers perceive the stressor as stressful, the greater the likelihood that the first coping responses are passive/avoidant. However, as previously mentioned, the use of passive/avoidance coping strategies leads to the use of active coping strategies. One possible explanation for this finding is that these caregivers may eventually realize that the passive/avoidance coping strategies are not that helpful in dealing with the perceived stress, and, therefore, they become more inclined to change these strategies or to add active ones to their coping repertoire. It has been observed that an initial reaction of avoidance to a situation, especially one that is stressful, is sometimes followed by a 'working through' process that prompts a person to consider active ways of coping (Holahan & Moos, 1994). . . .

"However, one should be cautious in considering these tentative explanations, since the path between passive/avoidance and active coping strategies, and all the other paths, has been observed using cross-sectional data. Statements regarding the paths are speculative and should be interpreted with caution. Empirical verification of the model using longitudinal data from the five studies has just been completed. This step in the research program should clarify the direction of the effect.

"The positive links between caregivers' passive/ avoidance coping strategies and psychological distress give ground to another tenet of the RAM, in which the cognator mechanisms are conceptualized as elements that can influence adaptation. However, the active coping strategies have no significant effect on psychological distress. . . .

"Lastly, the importance of the direct effect of perceived stress (the focal stimulus) on adaptation corroborates the vital role of perception as underlined in the RAM and as found by other investigators (Frederickson, Jackson, Strauman, & Strauman, 1991; Pollock, Frederickson, Carson, Massey, & Roy, 1994) working on a research program based on the RAM. However, in these studies, perception was not considered as a focal stimulus but part of the control process. . . . The results provide evidence that these concepts can be part of a middle-range theory of psychological adaptation. . . .

Overall, efforts should be devoted to developing measures that reflect as closely as possible the conceptual elements of the RAM. Lastly, it should be noted that the influence of contextual and focal stimuli and of coping strategies has been examined on only one mode of adaptation. Effects of these variables on the other three modes of adaptation are unknown.

"With regard to the development of the discipline of nursing, the ultimate long-term goal is to contribute to the development of a middle-range theory of psychological adaptation to guide nursing interventions. The development of this theoretical model of psychological adaptation is in its preliminary stages. The empirical verification of the model with longitudinal data from the five studies will shed light on the time precedence between and among variables. Moreover, in new projects within the Montreal research program, data are collected on other clinical populations, which will be used to acquire a certain level of generality, a characteristic of a middle-range theory. Development and evaluation of nursing interventions that focus on conflicts, perceived stress, and coping strategies are also under way. Together, theoretical and clinical inquiry will enable knowledge of adaptation to be embedded in nursing practice." (Lévesque et al., 1998, pp. 35–38) ■

THE CRITIQUE OF FRAMEWORKS: THEORETICAL SUBSTRUCTION

In the past, the common approach to critiquing a framework was to search for a statement by the author that the study was based on a particular theory. Strategies had not been developed for evaluating the extent to which the study was actually guided by the theory. This information was often not included in the published version of the study. In 1979, Hinshaw proposed using theoretical substruction as a strategy for evaluating study frameworks. However, the method proposed needed development. The process has been further refined by Dulock and Holzemer (1991) and now offers a viable approach to critiquing frameworks.

The term *substruction* is the opposite of construction and means "to take apart." With *theoretical substruction*, a framework of a published study is separated into component parts to evaluate (1) the logical consistency of the theoretical system and (2) the interaction of the framework with the study methodology. It essentially reverses the process described in this chapter. If components of the framework are inferred rather than clearly stated, the evaluator extracts those components and states them as clearly as possible. If a conceptual map is not presented, the evaluator may construct one.

Theoretical substruction needs to answer two questions, "Is the framework logically adequate?" and "Did the framework guide the methodology of the study?" Gaps and inconsistencies are identified. The conclusions of the study are evaluated in terms of whether they are logical, defensible, and congruent with the framework.

To perform theoretical substruction, an evaluator must extract the following elements from the published description of the framework:

- Concepts (and constructs if included)
- Conceptual definitions (and construct definitions if used)
- Operational definitions
- Conceptual sets linking constructs, concepts, and variables
- General propositions linking the constructs
- Specific propositions linking the concepts
- Hypotheses, research questions, or objectives
- Statement sets linking (a) general propositions, (b) specific propositions, and (b) hypotheses, questions, or objectives
- A conceptual map
- Sampling method and size
- Design
- Data analysis performed in relation to each hypothesis, question, or objective
- Findings related to each hypothesis, question, or objective
- Author's interpretation of findings in relation to the framework

The extracted information is used to analyze the logical structure of the framework and its link with the methodology. The following questions can be used to guide that analysis:

1. Is the framework based on a substantive theory or a tentative theory?

2. Was a conceptual model included in the framework?
3. Are the definitions of constructs consistent with the theorist's definitions?
4. Do the concepts reflect the constructs identified in the framework?
5. Do the variables reflect the concepts identified in the framework?
6. Are the conceptual definitions validated by references to the literature?
7. Are the operational definitions reflective of the conceptual definitions?
8. Are the reliability and validity of the operational definitions adequate?
9. Are the propositions logical and defensible?
10. Is evidence from the literature used to validate the propositions?
11. Are the hypotheses, questions, or objectives logically linked to the propositions?
12. Can diagrams of the propositions be linked to the conceptual map?
13. Is the conceptual map adequate to explain the phenomenon of concern?
14. Is the design appropriate to test the propositions?
15. Is the sample size adequate to avoid a Type II error? (Type II errors are discussed in Chapter 18.)
16. Are the data analyses appropriate for the hypotheses, questions, or objectives?
17. Are the findings for each hypothesis, question, or objective consistent with that proposed by the framework? If not, was the methodology adequate to test the hypothesis, question, or objective?
18. Were the findings interpreted by the author in terms of the framework?
19. Do the findings validate the framework?
20. Are the findings consistent with those of other studies using the same framework (or testing the same propositions)?

Critical reviews are now being published that examine studies related to selected areas of research. Theoretical substruction is being used to evaluate these studies. One example is Silva's (1986) examination of studies asserting to test nursing models. The use of substruction should strengthen frameworks appearing in published studies. In addition, it will assist in building a body of knowledge related to a specific theory that can then be applied to clinical practice situations with greater confidence. For further information on critiquing frameworks, see Chapter 26.

■ **SUMMARY**
. . . .

A *framework* is the abstract, logical structure of meaning that guides the development of the study and enables the researcher to link the findings to nursing's body of knowledge. Every study has a framework. The framework should be well integrated with the methodology, carefully structured, and clearly presented, whether the study is physiological or psychosocial. If a well-established theory is being tested, the framework is derived deductively from the theory. However, many theoretical ideas in nursing have not yet been formally expressed as theories. Nursing studies often emerge from questions related to identified nursing problems or from the clinical insight that a relationship exists between or among elements important to desired outcomes.

The first step in understanding theories and frameworks is to become familiar with the terms related to theoretical ideas and their application. A *concept* is a term that abstractly describes and names an object or phenomenon, thus providing it with a separate identity or meaning. A *relational statement* declares that a relationship of some kind exists between two or more concepts. Relational statements are the core of the framework; it is these statements that are tested through research. The type of statement expressed in a framework determines the design of the study, the statistical analysis that will be performed, and the type of findings that can be expected. Relational statements describe the direction, shape, strength, symmetry, sequencing, probability of occurrence, necessity, and sufficiency of a relationship.

Statements about the same two conceptual ideas can be made at various levels of abstractness. The statements found in conceptual models (*general propositions*) are at high levels of abstraction. Statements found in theories (*specific propositions*) are at a moderate level of abstraction. *Hypotheses*, which are a form of statement, are concrete and specific. As statements become more concrete, they become narrower in scope.

A *conceptual model* is a set of highly abstract, related constructs that broadly explains phenomena of interest, expresses assumptions, and reflects a philosophical stance. A *theory* is narrower and more specific than a conceptual model and is directly testable. A theory consists of an integrated set of defined concepts, existence statements, and relational statements that present a view of a phenomenon and can be used to describe, explain, predict, and control that phenomenon. A *scientific theory* has (1) valid and reliable methods of measuring each concept and (2) relational statements that have been repeatedly tested through research and demonstrated to be valid. A *substantive theory* has some recognition of its worth or meaning in the discipline and has been validated to some extent through research. A *tentative theory* is newly proposed, has had minimal exposure to critique by the discipline, and has undergone little testing.

One strategy for expressing a framework is a *conceptual map* that diagrams the interrelationships of the concepts and statements. A conceptual map succinctly summarizes and integrates what is known about a phenomenon and allows one to grasp the gestalt of the phenomenon.

Developing a framework is one of the most important steps in the research process. The steps of the process are (1) selecting and defining concepts, (2) developing statements relating the concepts, (3) expressing the statements in hierarchical fashion, and (4) developing a conceptual map. Developing a framework designed to test a substantive theory requires that all concepts and statements in the framework be obtained from the substantive theory. When conceptual models are used in a framework, the framework must also include a testable theory. The map for such a framework must also include both the model and theory.

Frameworks are evaluated through the use of *theoretical substruction*. The term *substruction* is the opposite of construction and means "to take apart." The evaluator separates the framework of a published study into its component parts to evaluate the logical consistency of the theoretical system and its interaction with the study methodology. This process provides a means of critiquing frameworks in published studies. The critique of frameworks strengthens their development and ultimate usefulness to practice.

● ●

REFERENCES

Adam, E. (1987). Nursing theory: What it is and what it is not. *Nursing Papers/Perspectives in Nursing, 19*(1), 5–14.

Ailinger, R. L., & Dear, M. R. (1997). An examination of the self-care needs of clients with rheumatoid arthritis [including commentary by N. Popovich]. *Rehabilitation Nursing, 22*(3), 135–140.

Ajzen, I., & Fishbein, M. (1980). *Understanding attitudes and predicting social behavior.* Englewood Cliffs, NJ: Prentice-Hall.

Amandah, L., & Watson, R. (1996). Caring research and concepts: A selected review of the literature. *Journal of Clinical Nursing, 5*(2), 71–77.

Andrews, H. A., & Roy, C. (1991). *The Roy adaptation model: The definitive statement.* Norwalk, CT: Appleton & Lange.

Andrews, M. M., & Nielson, D. W. (1988). Technology dependent children in the home. *Pediatric Nursing, 14*(2), 111–114, 151.

Artinian, B. (1982). Conceptual mapping: Development of the strategy. *Western Journal of Nursing Research, 4*(4), 379–393.

Bakker, R. H., Kastermans, M. C., & Dassen, T. W. N. (1995). An analysis of the nursing diagnosis Ineffective Management of Therapeutic Regimen compared to noncompliance and Orem's Self-Care Deficit Theory of Nursing. *Nursing Diagnosis, 6*(4), 161–166.

Bendell, R. D., Culbertson, J. L., Shelton, T. L., & Carter, B. D. (1986). Interrupted infantile apnea: Impact on early development, temperament and maternal stress. *Journal of Clinical Child Psychology, 15*(4), 304–310.

Benner, P., & Wrubel, J. (1989). *The primacy of caring: Stress and coping in health and illness.* Menlo Park, CA: Addison Wesley.

Bess, C. J. (1995). *Abilities and limitations of adult type II diabetic patients with integrating of self-care practices into their daily lives.* Unpublished doctoral dissertation, University of Alabama at Birmingham.

Bevis, E. O. (1981). Caring: A life force. In M. M. Leininger (Ed.), *Caring: An essential human need. Proceedings of Three National Caring Conferences* (pp. 49–60). Thorofare, NJ: Slack.

Black, L., Hersher, L., & Steinschneider, A. (1978). The impact of the apnea monitor in family life. *Pediatrics, 62*(5), 681–685.

Blue, C. L. (1995). The predictive capacity of the theory of reasoned action and the theory of planned behavior in exercise research: An integrated literature review. *Research in Nursing & Health, 18*(2), 105–121.

Bottorff, J. L. (1988). Assessing an instrument in a pilot project: The self-care agency questionnaire. *The Canadian Journal of Nursing Research, 20*(1), 7–16.

Brody, J. K. (1988). Virtue ethics, caring, and nursing. *Scholarly Inquiry in Nursing Practice, 2*(2), 31–42.

Brown, L. (1986). The experience of care: Patient perspectives. *Topics in Clinical Nursing, 8*(2), 56–62.

Brugge, P. (1981). The relationship between family as a social support system, health status, and exercise of self-care agency in the adult with a chronic illness. *Dissertation Abstracts International, 42,* 1704B. (University Microfilms No. 82–09, 277)

Burns, N., & Grove, S. (1999). *Understanding nursing research* (2nd ed). Philadelphia: W. B. Saunders.

Burr, G., Guyer, G., Todres, I., Abraham, B., & Chiodo, T. (1983). Home care for children on respirators. *The New England Journal of Medicine, 309*(21), 319–323.

Cain, L. P., Kelly, D. H., & Shannon, D. C. (1980). Parents' perceptions of the psychological and social impact of home monitoring. *Pediatrics, 66*(1), 37–41.

Campbell, J. C., & Soeken, K. L. (1999). Women's responses to battering: A test of the model. *Research in Nursing & Health, 22*(1), 49–58.

Carroll, D. L. (1995). The importance of self-efficacy expectations in elderly patients recovering from coronary artery bypass surgery. *Heart & Lung: Journal of Critical Care, 24*(1), 50–59.

Caslowitz, S. B. (1989). Burnout and coping strategies among hospital staff nurses. *Journal of Advanced Nursing, 14*(7), 553–558.

Chinn, P. L., & Kramer, M. K. (1995). *Theory and nursing: A systematic approach* (4th ed.). St. Louis: Mosby.

Cook, J. A. (1988). Who "mothers" the chronically mentally ill? *Family Relations, 37*(1), 42–49.

Cronin, S. N., & Harrison, B. (1988). Importance of nurse caring behaviors as perceived by patients after myocardial infarction. *Heart & Lung, 17*(4), 374–380.

Cull, V. V. (1995). *Exposure to violence and self-care practices of adolescents.* Unpublished doctoral dissertation, University of Alabama at Birmingham.

Davies, L. K. (1993). Comparison of dependent-care activities for well siblings of children with cystic fibrosis and well siblings in families without children with chronic illness. *Issues in Comprehensive Pediatric Nursing, 16*(2), 91–98.

Dean, P. G. (1986). Monitoring an apneic infant: Impact on the infant's mother. *Maternal-Child Nursing Journal, 15*(2), 65–76.

Delasega, C. (1995). SCOPE: A practical method for assessing the self-care status of elderly persons. *Rehabilitation Nursing Research, 4*(4), 128–135.

Denyes, M. J. (1982). Measurement of self-care agency in adolescents [Abstract]. *Nursing Research, 31*(1), 63.

DiMaggio, G., & Sheetz, A. (1983). The concerns of mothers caring for an infant on an apnea monitor. *MCN: American Journal of Maternal Child Nursing, 8*(3), 294–297.

Dodd, M. J. (1984a). Measuring informational intervention for chemotherapy knowledge and self-care behavior. *Research in Nursing & Health, 7*(1), 43–50.

Dodd, M. J. (1984b). Patterns of self-care in cancer patients receiving radiation therapy. *Oncology Nursing Forum, 10*(3), 23–27.

Dodd, M. J. (1987). Efficacy of proactive information on self-care in radiation therapy patients. *Heart & Lung, 16*(5), 538–544.

Dormire, S. L., Strauss, S. S., & Clarke, B. A. (1989). Social support and adaptation to the parent role in first-time adolescent mothers. *Journal of Obstetric, Gynecologic, and Neonatal Nursing, 18*(4), 327–337.

Ducharme, F. (1994). Conjugal support, coping behaviors, and psychological well-being of the elderly spouse: An empirical model. *Research on Aging, 16*(2), 167–190.

Dulock, H. L., & Holzemer, W. L. (1991). Substruction: Improving the linkage from theory to method. *Nursing Science Quarterly, 4*(2), 83–87.

Duquette, A., Ducharme, F., Ricard, N., Lévesque, L., & Bonin, J.-P. (1996). Élaboration d'un modèle théorique de déterminants de l'adaptation dérivé du modèle de Roy. *Recherche en Soins Infirmiers, 44*(3), 61–70.

Duquette, A., Kérouac, S., Sandhu, B. K., Ducharme, S., & Saulnier, P. (1995). Psychosocial determinants of burnout in geriatric nursing. *International Journal of Nursing Studies, 32*(5), 443–456.

Edwards, J. R., & Baglioni, A. J. (1993). The measurement of coping with stress: Construct validity of the Ways of Coping checklist and the Cybernetic Coping Scale. *Work and Stress, 7*(1), 17–31.

Fanslow, J. (1987). Compassionate nursing care: Is it a lost art? *Journal of Practical Nursing, 37*(2), 40–43.

Fawcett, J. (1991). Approaches to knowledge development in nursing. *The Canadian Journal of Nursing Research, 23*(4), 11–17.

Fawcett, J. (1995). *Analysis and evaluation of conceptual models of nursing* (3rd ed.). Philadelphia: F. A. Davis.

Fawcett, J., & Downs, F. (1986). *The relationship of theory and research.* Norwalk, CT: Appleton-Century-Crofts.

Feyerabend, P. (1975). *Against method.* London: Verso.

Fields, A. I., Rosenblatt, A., Pollack, M. M., & Kaufman, J. (1991). Home care cost-effectiveness for respiratory technology–dependent children. *American Journal of Diseases of Children, 145*(2), 729–733.

Fiser, D. H., & Lyons, L. (1985). Family acceptance of home apnea monitors. *American Journal of Medical Science, 290*(2), 52–55.

Fishbein, M., & Ajzen, I. (1975). *Belief, attitude, intention and behavior.* Boston: Addison-Wesley.

Folkman, S., Chesney, M., McKusick, L., Ironson, G., Johnson, D. S., & Coates, T. J. (1991). Translating coping theory into an intervention. In J. Elkenrode (Ed.), *The social context of coping* (pp. 239–260). New York: Plenum Press.

Forrest, D. (1989). The experience of caring. *Journal of Advanced Nursing, 14*(10), 815–823.

Foucault, M. (1970). *The order of things: An archaeology of the human sciences.* New York: Vintage.

Frank, P. (1961). The variety of reasons for the acceptance of scientific theories. In P. Frank (Ed.), *The validation of scientific theories* (pp. 13–25). New York: Collier.

Frederickson, K., Jackson, B. S., Strauman, T., & Strauman, J. (1991). Testing hypotheses derived from the Roy adaptation model. *Nursing Science Quarterly, 4*(4), 168–174.

Frey, M. A., & Denyes, M. J. (1989). Health and illness self-care in adolescents with IDDM: A test of Orem's theory. *Advances in Nursing Science, 12*(1), 67–75.

Fry, S. T. (1988). The ethic of caring: Can it survive in nursing? *Nursing Outlook, 36*(1), 48.

Gadow, S. A. (1985). Nurse and patient: The caring relationship. In A. N. Bishop & J. R. Scudder (Eds.), *Caring, curing, coping* (pp. 31–43). Birmingham, AL: University of Alabama.

Gardner, K. G., & Wheeler, E. C. (1981). The meaning of caring in the context of nursing. In M. M. Leininger (Ed.), *Caring: An essential human need. Proceedings of three national caring conferences* (pp. 69–82). Thorofare, NJ: Slack.

Garmezy, N., & Rutter, M. (1983). *Stress, coping, and development in children.* New York: McGraw-Hill.

Gaut, D. A. (1983). Development of a theoretically adequate description of caring. *Western Journal of Nursing Research, 5*(4), 313–324.

Gendron, D. (1988). *The expressive form of caring.* Toronto: University of Toronto.

Gibbs, J. (1972). *Sociological theory construction.* Hinsdale, IL: Dryden.

Gottlieb, B. H., & Selby, P. M. (1989). Social support and mental health: A review of the literature. National Health Research Development Program (NHRDP). Unpublished funded review, University of Guelph, Ontario, Canada.

Griffin, A. P. (1983). A philosophical analysis of caring in nursing. *Journal of Advanced Nursing, 8*(4), 289–295.

Gulick, E. E. (1987). Parsimony and model confirmation of the ADL self-care scale for multiple sclerosis persons. *Nursing Research, 36*(5), 278–283.

Gulick, E. E. (1988). The self-administered ADL scale for persons with multiple sclerosis. In C. Waltz & O. Strickland (Eds.), *The measurement of nursing outcomes* (Vol. 1, pp. 128–159). New York: Springer.

Gulick, E. E. (1989). Model confirmation of the MS-related symptom checklist. *Nursing Research, 38*(3), 147–153.

Haase, J. (1997). Hopeful teenagers with cancer: Living courage. *Reflections, 23*(1), 20.

Haccoun, R. R. (1987). Une nouvelle technique de vérification de l'équivalence de mésures psychologiques traduités. *Révue Québécoise de Psychologie, 8*(3), 30–39.

Hanson, B. R., & Bickel, L. (1985). Development and testing of the questionnaire on perception of self-care agency. In J. Riehl-Sisca (Ed.), *The science and art of self-care* (pp. 271–278). Norwalk, CT: Appleton-Century-Crofts.

Hare, J., Pratt, C. C., & Andrews, D. (1988). Predictors of burnout in professional and paraprofessional nurses working in hospital and nursing homes. *International Journal of Nursing Studies, 25*(2), 105–115.

Hart, M. A. (1995). Orem's Self-Care Deficit Theory: Research with pregnant women. *Nursing Science Quarterly, 8*(3), 120–126.

Hart, M. A., & Foster, S. N. (1998). Self-care agency in two groups of pregnant women. *Nursing Science Quarterly, 11*(4), 167–171.

Hazlett, D. E. (1989). A study of pediatric home ventilator management: Medical, psychosocial, and financial aspects. *Journal of Pediatric Nursing, 4*(4), 284–294.

Hemple, C. G. (1966). *Philosophy of natural science.* Englewood Cliffs, NJ: Prentice-Hall.

Hill, R. (1965). Generic features of families under stress. In J. J. Parad (Ed.), *Crisis intervention: Selected readings* (pp. 32–52). New York: Family Service Association of America.

Hinshaw, A. S. (1979). Theoretical substruction: An assessment process. *Western Journal of Nursing Research, 1*(4), 319–324.

Holahan, C. J., & Moos, R. H. (1987). The personal and contextual determinants of coping strategies. *Journal of Personalilty and Social Psychology, 52*(5), 946–955.

Holahan, C. J., & Moos, R. H. (1994). Life stressors and mental health: Advances in conceptualizing stress resistance. In W. R. Avison & I. H. Gotlib (Eds.), *Stress and mental health: Contemporary issues and prospects for the future.* New York: Plenum Press.

Horner, S. (1988). Intersubjective co-presence in a caring model. In *Caring and nursing explorations in the feminist perspectives.* Denver: School of Nursing, University of Colorado Health Sciences Center.

Jesek-Hale, S. R. (1994). *Self-care agency and self care in pregnant adolescents: A test of Orem's theory.* Unpublished doctoral dissertation, Rush University, College of Nursing.

Johnson, D. E. (1980). The behavioral system model for nursing. In J. P. Riehl & C. Roy (Eds.), *Conceptual models for nursing practice* (2nd ed., pp. 206–216). New York: Appleton-Century-Crofts.

Jöreskog, K., & Sörbom, D. (1993). *LISREL 8: Structural equation modeling with the Simplis command language.* Hillsdale, NJ: Lawrence Erlbaum.

Kaplan, A. (1964). *The conduct of inquiry.* San Francisco: Chandler.

Kearney, B., & Fleischer, B. (1979). Development of an instrument to measure exercise of self-care agency. *Research in Nursing & Health, 2*(1), 25–34.

Kerlinger, F. N. (1986). *Foundations of behavioral research* (3rd ed.). New York: Holt, Rinehart & Winston.

Kimchi, J., & Schaffner, B. (1990). Childhood protective factors and stress risk. In L. Arnold (Ed.), *Childhood stress* (pp. 475–500). New York: Wiley.

King, I. M. (1981). *A theory for nursing: Systems, concepts, process.* New York: Wiley.

Knecht, L. D. (1991). Home apnea monitoring: Mothers' mood states, family functioning and support systems. *Public Health Nursing, 8*(3), 1544–160.

Knowlden, V. (1988). Nurse caring as constructed knowledge. In *Caring and nursing explorations in the feminist perspectives.* Denver: School of Nursing, University of Colorado Health Sciences Center.

Kostopoulos, M. R. (1988). The reliability and validity of a nurse performance evaluation tool. In O. L. Strickland & C. F. Waltz (Eds.), *Measurement of nursing outcomes* (Vol. 2, pp. 77–95). New York: Springer.

Kuhn, T. (1970). *The structure of scientific revolutions* (2nd ed.). New York: Holt, Rinehart & Winston.

Larson, P. (1987). Comparison of cancer patients' and professional nurses' perceptions of important caring behaviors. *Heart & Lung, 16*(2), 187–193.

Lasky, P. A., & Eichelberger, K. M. (1985). Health-related views and self-care behaviors of young children. *Family Relations, 34*(1), 13–18.

Laudan, L. (1977). *Progress and its problems: Toward a theory of scientific growth.* Berkeley: University of California.

Laudan, L. (1981). A problem-solving approach to scientific progress. In I. Hacking (Ed.), *Scientific revolutions* (pp. 144–155). Fair Lawn, NJ: Oxford University.

Lazarus, R. S., & Folkman, S. (1984). *Stress, appraisal, and coping.* New York: Springer.

Lee, M. B. (1999). Power, self-care and health in women living in urban squatter settlements in Karach, Pakistan: A test of Orem's Theory. *Journal of Advanced Nursing, 30*(1), 248–259.

Leininger, M. (1979). *Transcultural nursing.* New York: Masson.

Leininger, M. M. (1981). *Caring: An essential human need. Proceedings of three national caring conferences.* Thorofare, NJ: Slack.

Leininger, M. M. (1984). *Care: The essence of nursing and health.* Thorofare, NJ: Slack.

Leininger, M. M. (1988). *Care: Discovery and uses in clinical and community nursing.* Thorofare, NJ: Slack.

Lévesque, L., Cossette, S., & Lauren, L. (1995). A multidimensional examination of psychological and social well-being of caregivers of a demented relative. *Research on Aging, 17*(3), 332–360.

Lévesque, L., Ricard, N., Ducharme, F., Duquette, A., & Bonin, J. (1998). Empirical verification of a theoretical model derived from the Roy Adaptation Model: Findings from five studies. *Nursing Science Quarterly, 11*(1), 31–39.

Levine, M. E. (1973). *Introduction to clinical nursing* (2nd ed.). Philadelphia: F. A. Davis.

Lorenson, M. (1998). Psychometric properties of self-care management and life-quality amongst elderly [including commentary by P. Draper and R. Watson, with author response]. *Clinical Effectiveness in Nursing, 2*(2), 78–85.

Lukkarinen, H., & Hentinen, M. (1997). Self-care agency and factors relating this agency among patients with coronary health disease. *International Journal of Nursing Studies, 34*(4), 295–304.

Lyman, R. D., Wurtele, S. K., & Wilson, D. R. (1985). Psychological effects on parents of home and hospital apnea monitoring. *Journal of Pediatric Psychology, 10*(4), 439–448.

Maddi, S. R., &. Kobasa, S. C. (1984). *The hardy executive: Health and stress.* Homewood, IL: Dow Jones Irving.

Mapanga, K. G. (1994). *The influence of family and friends' basic conditioning factors, and self-care agency on unmar-*

ried teenage primiparas' engagement in a contraceptive practice. Unpublished doctoral dissertation, Case Western Reserve University (Health Sciences), 1994.

McBride, S. (1987). Validation of an instrument to measure exercise of self-care agency. *Research in Nursing & Health, 10*(5), 311–316.

McCaleb, A., & Edgil, A. (1994). Self-concept and self-care practices of healthy adolescents. *Journal of Pediatric Nursing, 9*(4), 233–238.

McCubbin, H., & Patterson, J. (1983). The family stress process: The double ABCX model of adjustment and adaptation. *Marriage and Family Review, 6*(1–2), 7–37.

McCubbin, H. I., & Figley, C. R. (1983). Bridging normative and catastrophic family stress. In H. I. McCubbin & C. R. Figley (Eds.), *Stress and the family: Vol. 1. Coping with normative transition* (pp. 218–228). New York: Brunner/Mazel.

McCubbin, H. I., & Patterson, J. M. (1987). Family adaptation checklist. In H. McCubbin & A. Thompson (Eds.), *Family assessment inventories for research and practice*. Madison, WI: University of Wisconsin–Madison.

McCubbin, H., & Thompson, A. (1987). *Family assessment inventories for research and practice*. Madison, WI: University of Wisconsin–Madison.

McDermitt, M. A. N. (1993). Learned helplessness as an interacting variable with self-care agency: Testing a theoretical model. *Nursing Science Quarterly, 6*(1), 28–38.

McElroy, E., Steinschneider, A., & Weinstein, S. (1986). Emotional and health impact of home monitoring on mothers: A controlled prospective study. *Pediatrics, 78*(5), 780–786.

McFarlane, J. (1976). A charter for caring. *Journal of Advanced Nursing, 1*(3), 187–196.

Merton, R. K. (1968). *Social theory and social structure*. New York: Free Press.

Miller, B. C., & Myers-Walls, J. (1983). Parenthood: Stressors and coping strategies. In H. I. McCubbin & C. R. Figley (Eds.), *Stress and the family: Vol. I. Coping with normative transitions*. New York: Brunner/Mazel.

Moody, L. E. (1989). Building a conceptual map to guide research. *Florida Nursing Review, 4*(1), 1–5.

Moody, L. E., Wilson, M. E., Smyth, K., Schwartz, R., Tittle, M., & Van Cott, M. L. (1988). Analysis of a decade of nursing practice research: 1977–1986. *Nursing Research, 37*(6), 374–379.

Moore, J. B. (1987a). Determining the relationship of autonomy to self-care agency or locus of control in school-age children. *Maternal-Child Nursing Journal, 16*(1), 47–60.

Moore, J. B. (1987b). Effects of assertion training and first aid instruction on children's autonomy and self-care agency. *Research in Nursing & Health, 10*(2), 101–109.

Moore, J. B. (1993). Predictors of children's self-care performance: Testing the theory of self-care deficit. *Scholarly Inquiry for Nursing Practice: An International Journal, 7*(3), 199–217.

Moore, J. B., & Gaffney, K. F. (1989). Development of an instrument to measure mother's performance of self-care ac-

tivities for children. *Advances in Nursing Science, 12*(1), 76–84.

Moore, J. B., & Mosher, R. B. (1997). Adjustment responses of children and their mothers to cancer self-care and anxiety. *Oncology Nursing Forum, 24*(3), 519–525.

Moos, R. H., Cronkite, R. C., & Finney, J. W. (1990). *Health and Daily Living Form manual* (2nd ed.). Palo Alto, CA: Center of Health Care Evaluation, Stanford University Medical Center.

Morse, J. M., Solberg, S. M., Neander, W. L., Bottorff, J. L., & Johnson, J. L. (1990). Concepts of caring and caring as a concept. *Advances in Nursing Science, 13*(1), 1–14.

Mosher, R. B., & Moore, J. B. (1998). The relationship of self-concept and self-care in children with cancer. *Nursing Science Quarterly, 11*(3), 116–122.

Nestmann, L. S., & Schmerl, C. (1991). The lady is not for burning: The gender paradox in prevention and social support. In G. Albrecht, H.-U. Otto, S. Karstedt-Hemke, & K. Bollert (Eds.), *Social prevention and the social sciences* (pp. 217–234). Berlin: Walter de Gruyter.

Neuman, B. (1989). *The Neuman systems model*. Norwalk, CT: Appleton & Lange.

Newman, M. A. (1979). *Theory development in nursing*. Philadelphia: F. A. Davis.

Noh, S., & Turner, R. J. (1987). Living with psychiatric patients: Implications for the mental health of family members. *Social Science Medicine, 255*(3), 263–272.

Nuttall, P. (1988). Maternal responses to home apnea monitoring of infants. *Nursing Research, 37*(6), 3544–357.

O'Connor, N. A. (1995). *Maieutic dimensions of self-care in aging: Instrument development*. Unpublished doctoral dissertation, Wayne State University.

Orem, D. E. (1995). *Nursing: Concepts of practice* (5th ed.). New York: McGraw-Hill.

Patterson, J. M., & McCubbin, H. I. (1993a). The impact of family life events and changes on the health of a chronically ill child. *Family Relations: Journal of Applied Family & Child Studies, 32*(2), 255–264.

Patterson, J. M., & McCubbin, H. I. (1983b). Chronic illness: family stress and coping. In C. R. Figley, & H. I. McCubbin (Eds.), *Stress and the family: Vol. II. Coping with catastrophe* (pp. 21–36). New York: Brunner/Mazel.

Pepin, J., Ducharme, F., Kérouac, S., Lévesque, L., Ricard, N., & Duquette, A. (1994). Développement d'un programme de recherche basé sur une conception de la discipline infirmiére. *Canadian Journal of Nursing Research, 26*(1), 41–53.

Pollock, S. E., Frederickson, K., Carson, M. A., Massey, V. H., & Roy, C. (1994). Contributions to nursing science: Synthesis of findings from Adaptation Model research. *Scholarly Inquiry for Nursing Practice, 8*(4), 361–374.

Popper, K. (1968). *The logic of scientific discovery*. New York: Harper & Row.

Quint, R. D., Chesterman, E., Crain, L. S., Winkleby, M., & Boyce, W. T. (1990). Home care for ventilator-dependent children: psychosocial impact on the family. *American Journal of Diseases of Children, 144*(11), 1238–1241.

Ray, M. A. (1984). The development of a classification system of institutional caring. In M. M. Leininger (Ed.), *Care: The essence of nursing and health* (pp. 95–112). Thorofare, NJ: Slack.

Ray, M. A. (1987a). Health care economics and human caring in nursing: Why the moral conflict must be resolved. *Family and Community Health, 10*(1), 35–43.

Ray, M. A. (1987b). Technological caring: A new model in critical care. *Dimensions of Critical Care Nursing, 6*(3), 166–173.

Rew, L. (1987). The relationship between self-care behaviors and selected psychosocial variables in children with asthma. *Journal of Pediatric Nursing, 2*(5), 333–341.

Reynolds, P. D. (1971). *A primer in theory construction.* Indianapolis, IN: Bobbs-Merrill.

Ricard, N., Fortin, F., & Bonin, J. P. (1995). *Fardeau subjectif et état de santé d'aidants naturels de personnes atteintes de troubles mentaux en situation de crise at de rémission.* Rapport soumis au Conseil Québécois de la Recherche Sociale. Université de Montréal, Faculté des Sciences Infirmiéres.

Riesch, S. K., & Hauch, M. R. (1988). The exercise of self-care agency: An analysis of construct and discriminant validity. *Research in Nursing & Health, 11*(4), 245–255.

Roach, M. S. (1987). *The human act of caring: A blueprint for health professions.* Toronto: Canadian Hospital Association.

Robinson, M. K. (1995). *Determinants of functional status in chronically ill adults.* Unpublished doctoral dissertation, University of Alabama at Birmingham.

Rogers, M. E. (1970). *An introduction to the theoretical basis of nursing.* Philadelphia: F. A. Davis.

Rogers, M. E. (1980). Nursing: A science of unitary man. In J. P. Riehl & C. Roy (Eds.), *Conceptual models for nursing practice* (2nd ed., pp. 329–337). Norwalk, CT: Appleton-Century-Crofts.

Rogers, M. E. (1983). A paradigm for nursing. In I. W. Clements & F. B. Roberts (Eds.), *Family health: A theoretical approach to nursing care* (pp. 219–227). New York: Wiley.

Rogers, M. (1986). Science of unitary human beings. In V. M. Malinski (Ed.), *Explorations on Martha Rogers' science of unitary human beings* (pp. 3–8). Norwalk, CT: Appleton-Century-Crofts.

Rogers, M. E. (1988). Nursing science and art: A prospective. *Nursing Science Quarterly, 1*(3), 99–102.

Roy, C. (1984). *Introduction to nursing: An adaptation model* (2nd ed.). Englewood Cliffs, NJ: Prentice-Hall.

Roy, C. (1988). An explication of the philosophical assumptions of the Roy adaptation model. *Nursing Science Quarterly, 1*(1), 26–34.

Roy, C. (1990). Response to dialogue on a theoretical issue: Strengthening the Roy Adaptation Model through conceptual clarification. *Nursing Science Quarterly, 3*(2), 64–66.

Roy, C., & Andrews, H. A. (1991). *The Roy Adaptation Model: The definitive statement.* Norwalk, CT: Appleton & Lange.

Roy, C., & Roberts, S. L. (1981). *Theory construction in nursing: An adaptation model.* Englewood Cliffs, NJ: Prentice-Hall.

Rutter, M. (1985). Resilience in the face of adversity: Protective factors and resistance to psychiatric disorder. *British Journal of Psychiatry, 147*, 598–611.

Rutter, M. (1987). Psychosocial resilience and protective mechanisms. *American Journal of Orthopsychiatry, 57*(3), 316–331.

Sarter, B. (1988). *The stream of becoming: A study of Martha Rogers's theory.* New York: National League for Nursing.

Saucier, C. P., & Clark, L. M. (1993). The relationship between self-care and metabolic control in children with insulin-dependent diabetes mellitus. *Diabetes Education, 19*(2), 133–135.

Scharer, K., & Dixon, D. M. (1989). Managing chronic illness: Parents with a ventilator-dependent child. *Journal of Pediatric Nursing, 4*(4), 236–247.

Scheffler, I. (1967). *Science and subjectivity.* Indianapolis, IN: Bobbs-Merrill.

Schoff-Baer, D., Fisher, L., & Gregory, C. (1995). Dependent care, caregiver burden, hardiness and self-care agency of caregivers. *Cancer Nursing, 18*(4), 299–305.

Schultz, R., Visintainer, P., & Williamson, G. M. (1990). Psychiatric and physical morbidity effects of caregiving. *Journal of Gerontology, 45*(5), 181–191.

Seyle, H. (1976). *The stress of life.* New York: McGraw-Hill.

Silva, M. C. (1981). Selection of a theoretical framework. In S. D. Krampitz & N. Pavlovich (Eds.), *Readings for nursing research* (pp. 17–28). St. Louis: C. V. Mosby.

Silva, M. C. (1986). Research testing nursing theory: State of the art. *Advances in Nursing Science, 9*(1), 1–11.

Sollie, D. L., & Miller, B. C. (1980). The transition to parenthood: A critical time for building family strengths. In J. Stennett, B. Chesser, J. DeFrain, & P. Knaub (Eds.), *Family strengths: Positive model for family life.* Lincoln, NB: University of Nebraska Press.

Stember, M. L. (1986). Model building as a strategy for theory development. In P. L. Chinn (Ed.), *Nursing research methodology: Issues and implementation* (pp. 103–119). Rockville, MD: Aspen.

Stemple, J. (1988). Measuring nursing care role orientation. In O. L. Strickland & C. F. Waltz (Eds.), *Measurement of nursing outcomes* (Vol. 2, pp. 19–31). New York: Springer.

Stengel, J. C., Echeveste, D. W., & Schmidt, G. C. (1985). Problems identified by registered nurse students in families with apnea-monitored infants. *Family & Community Health, 8*(3), 52–61.

Stephenson, C. (1999). Well-being of families with healthy and technology-assisted infants in the home: A comparative study. *Journal of Pediatric Nursing, 14*(3), 164–176.

Stevens, M. S. (1990). A comparison of mothers' and fathers' perception of caring for an infant requiring home cardiorespiratory monitoring. *Issues in Comprehensive Pediatric Nursing, 13*(2), 81–95.

Stevens, M. S. (1994). Parents coping with infant requiring home cardiorespiratory monitoring. *Journal of Pediatric Nursing, 9*(1), 2–12.

Stevenson, J. (1990). Quantitative care research: Review of content, process and product. In J. Stevenson & T. Tripp-Reimer (Eds.), *Knowledge about care and caring: State of the art and future development* (pp. 97–118). Kansas City, KS: American Academy of Nursing.

Stewart, M. J. (1993). *Integrating social support in nursing.* Newbury Park, CA: Sage.

Suppe, F. (1972). What's wrong with the received view on the structure of scientific theories? *Philosophy of Science, 39*(1), 1–19.

Suppe, F., & Jacox, A. K. (1985). Philosophy of science and the development of nursing theory. In H. H. Werley & J. J. Fitzpatrick (Eds.), *Annual review of nursing research* (Vol. 3, pp. 241–267). New York: Springer.

Swanson-Kauffman, K. M. (1986). Caring in the instance of unexpected early pregnancy loss. *Topics in Clinical Nursing, 8*(2), 37–46.

Swanson-Kauffman, K. M. (1988). Caring needs of women who miscarried. In M. M. Leininger (Ed.), *Care: Discovery and uses in clinical and community nursing* (pp. 55–70). Detroit: Wayne State University.

Tulman, L., & Fawcett, J. (1990). A framework for studying functional status after diagnosis of breast cancer. *Cancer Nursing, 13*(2), 98.

Umberson, D., & Grove, W. R. (1989). Parenthood and psychological well-being. *Journal of Family Issues, 10*(4), 440–462.

Ventura, J. N. (1987). The stresses of parenthood reexamined. *Family Relations: Journal of Applied Family & Child Studies, 36*(1), 26–29.

Villarreal, A. M. (1995). Mexican-American cultural meanings, expressions, self-care and dependent-care actions associated with experiences of pain. *Research in Nursing & Health, 18*(5), 427–436.

Vohr, B. R., Chen, A., Coll, C. G., & Oh, W. (1988). Mothers of preterm and full-term infants on home apnea monitors. *American Journal of Diseases in Children, 142*(2), 229–231.

Walker, L. O., & Avant, K. C. (1995). *Strategies for theory construction in nursing* (3rd ed.). Norwalk, CT: Appleton & Lange.

Wang, C. (1997). The cross-cultural applicability of Orem's conceptual framework. *Journal of Cultural Diversity, 4*(2), 44–48.

Wang, C., & Fenske, M. M. (1996). Self-care of adults with non-insulin-dependent diabetes mellitus: Influences of family and friends. *Diabetes Educator, 22*(5), 465–470.

Wasserman, A. L. (1984). A prospective study of the impact of home monitoring on the family. *Pediatrics, 74*(3), 323–329.

Watson, J. (1988). *Nursing: Human science and human care. A theory of nursing.* New York: National League for Nursing.

Weaver, M. T. (1987). Perceived self-care agency: A LISREL factor analysis of Bickel and Hanson's questionnaire. *Nursing Research, 36*(6), 381–387.

Wegener, D. H., Aday, L. A. (1989). Home care for ventilator-assisted children: Predicting family stress. *Pediatric Nursing, 15*(4), 371–376.

Weiss, C. J. (1988). Model to discover, validate, and use care in nursing. In M. M. Leininger (Ed.), *Care: Discovery and uses in clinical and community nursing* (pp. 139–150). Detroit: Wayne State University.

Wills, J. M. (1983). Concerns and need of mothers providing home care for children with tracheostomies. *Maternal-Child Nursing Journal, 12*(3), 89–107.

Woodgate, R. L. (1999). Conceptual understanding of resilience in the adolescent with cancer: Part I. *Journal of Pediatric Oncology Nursing, 16*(1), 35–43.

Wooldridge, P. J., Schmitt, M. J., Skipper, J. K., Jr., & Leonard, R. C. (1983). *Behavioral science and nursing theory.* St. Louis: C. V. Mosby.

Wykle, M. L., Kahana, E., & Kowal, J. (1992). *Stress and health among the elderly.* New York: Springer.

Young, L. Y., Creighton, D. E., & Sauve, R. S. (1988). The needs of families of infants discharged home with continuous oxygen therapy. *Journal of Obstetric, Gynecologic, and Neonatal Nursing, 17*(3), 187–193.

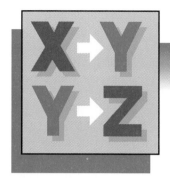

CHAPTER 8

OBJECTIVES, QUESTIONS, AND HYPOTHESES

Research objectives, questions, or hypotheses are formulated to bridge the gap between the more abstractly stated research problem and purpose and the detailed design and plan for data collection and analysis. Objectives, questions, and hypotheses delineate the research variables, the relationships among the variables, and, often, the population to be studied.

Research variables are concepts at various levels of abstraction that are measured, manipulated, or controlled in a study. Concrete concepts, such as temperature, weight, and blood pressure, are referred to as *variables* in a study; abstract concepts, such as creativity, empathy, and social support, are sometimes referred to as *research concepts*. Variables and concepts are conceptually defined, based on the study framework, and either measured or manipulated in research.

This chapter focuses on formulating research objectives, questions, and hypotheses, with an emphasis on testing different types of hypotheses. The process for selecting objectives, questions, or hypotheses to direct a study is addressed. The chapter concludes with a discussion of variables and direction for conceptually and operationally defining variables for a study.

FORMULATING RESEARCH OBJECTIVES

Research objectives are clear, concise, declarative statements that are expressed in the present tense.

For clarity, an objective usually focuses on one or two variables (or concepts) and indicates whether the variables are to be *identified* or *described*. Sometimes, their focus is to identify relationships or associations among variables (*relational*) or to determine *differences* between groups regarding selected variables.

Possible formats for developing objectives are as follows, with the type of objective identified in parentheses:

1. To identify the elements or characteristics of variable X in a specified population. (Identification)
2. To describe the existence of variable X in a specified population. (Description)
3. To determine the difference between group 1 and group 2 regarding variable X in a specified population. (Difference)
4. To determine or identify the relationship between variable X and variable Y in a specified population. (Relational)
5. To determine whether certain independent variables are predictive of a dependent variable. (Prediction)

Objectives are developed from the research problem and purpose, and they clarify the variables (or concepts) and population to be studied. Excerpts from a descriptive study by Brown (1997) demonstrate the logical flow from research problem and purpose to research objectives.

Research Problem

"In the United States, cardiovascular disorders cause more deaths among adults than all other diseases combined. Approximately one third of all deaths in the United States are caused by ischemic heart disease, and of these, one half result from an acute myocardial infarction (AMI). Today, there is a new population at risk for the development of cardiovascular disease, the cocaine user. The use of cocaine as a recreational drug by young adults has increased markedly since the early 1980s and has resulted in a significant increase in hospital emergency room admissions, mortality, and morbidity. Traditionally, only case studies, animal studies, and small samples of patients with AMI attributed to cocaine use have been reported. Little is known about chest pain syndromes after cocaine use, the patient's clinical symptomatology in the emergency department, or the risk factor profile of the cocaine user." (Brown, 1997, p. 136)

Research Purpose

"The purpose of this study was to examine the incidence of chest pain and cocaine use in 18–40 year-old persons who were seen in a public inner city emergency department." (Brown, 1997, p. 136)

Research Objectives

The objectives of this study were "(1) to describe the incidence of cocaine use in 18–40 year-old persons seen in a hospital emergency department with complaints of chest pain, and (2) to determine if there is a relationship among demographics, physiological, diagnostic, and patient history data associated with chest pain and cocaine use." (Brown, 1997, p. 136) ■

As shown in the example, the problem provides a basis for the purpose, and the objectives evolve from the purpose and clearly indicate the focus or goal of the study. The focus of the first objective was *description* of the incidence of cocaine use (research variable) in 18- to 40-year-old persons with complaints of chest pain (populations) seen in a hospital emergency department (setting). The sec-

ond objective focused on the *examination of relationships* among selected variables that constitute the risk factor profile of a cocaine user (demographics, physiological, diagnostic, and patient history data) and the incidence of chest pain with cocaine use.

The findings from this study identified the following risk factor profile for a cocaine user: (1) an average age of 29 years, (2) history of tobacco use and drug abuse, (3) presentation to emergency room (ER) between 12:00 PM and 5:00 AM, (3) complaint of "tight chest pain" confined to chest, sternum, and arm, (4) occurrence of symptoms usually 7.5 hours after cocaine use, and (5) electrocardiogram changes indicative of localized injury and damage to the anterolateral region of the myocardium. This study furnished significant information to direct the diagnosis and treatment of chest pain in the ER.

The objectives in some studies are complex and include several variables. For example, Kemp and associates (1990) conducted a predictive correlational study to examine factors that contribute to pressure ulcers in surgical patients and identified the following objectives to direct their study.

"1. To determine whether there was a relationship between (a) time on the operating table, (b) proportion of diastolic hypotensive episodes during surgery (diastolic blood pressure <60 mm Hg), (c) age, (d) preoperative albumin levels, (e) preoperative total protein levels, and (f) preoperative Braden scores, and the development of pressure ulcers.

"2. To determine how time on the operating table, proportion of diastolic hypotensive episodes during surgery, age, preoperative albumin and total protein levels, and preoperative Braden scores could be combined to best predict the development of pressure ulcers." (Kemp et al., 1990, p. 295)

The first objective focused on the *relationships* of six variables to pressure ulcer development. The second objective was concerned with *prediction* of the development of pressure ulcers (dependent variable) using the independent variables time on the operating table, proportion of diastolic hypotensive episodes during surgery, age, preoperative albumin and total protein levels, and preoperative Braden scores.

Kemp and associates (1990) found that age, time on the operating table, and extracorporeal circulation were the most useful in identifying patients at risk for development of pressure ulcers during elective surgery. The relationships identified in this study could be developed into hypotheses that predict the independent variables that contribute to pressure ulcer development and that could be tested in future studies. These study findings also provided direction for the development and testing of interventions to prevent pressure ulcers during surgery.

FORMULATING RESEARCH QUESTIONS

A *research question* is a concise, interrogative statement that is worded in the present tense and includes one or more variables (or concepts). The foci of research questions are (1) *description* of the variable or variables, (2) determination of *differences* between two or more groups regarding selected variables, (3) examination of relationships among variables (*relational*), and (4) use of independent variables to *predict* a dependent variable.

The possible formats for research questions are as follows, with the focus for each shown in parentheses:

1. How is variable *X* described in a specified population? (Description)
2. What is the perception of variable *X* in a specified population? (Description)
3. Is there a difference between group 1 and group 2 regarding variable *X?* (Difference)
4. Is variable *X* related to variables *Y* and *Z* in a specified population? (Relational)
5. What is the relationship between variables *X* and *Y* in a specified population? (Relational)
6. Are independent variables *W, X,* and *Y* useful in predicting dependent variable Z? (Prediction)

Wilson (1999) conducted a study of parental preparation of children for a routine physical examination. She developed research questions to direct this comparative descriptive study. The flow from research problem and purpose to research questions is demonstrated in the following excerpts from her study.

....

Research Problem

"The review of the literature indicates that preparation of the child for health care encounters is necessary to decrease the child's anxiety, fears, and uncooperative behaviors (Manion, 1990). Preparation is also necessary in establishing a positive relationship between the child and health care professionals, which may benefit the child in any future encounters within the health care system. Preparation for the annual routine physical examination, which has stressful elements, has not been studied in as much depth as other less common health care encounters. This is an area that requires further investigation because the physical examination is a recurring state-mandated event in the lives of school children and, in addition, portions of the physical examination are performed during visits for acute illness episodes." (Wilson, 1999, p. 330)

....

Research Purpose

"The purpose of this study was to ascertain the methods (discussion/reading/play/other) and level of discussion used by patients/caretakers in readying their children for routine physical examinations." (Wilson, 1999, p. 330)

Research Questions

"1. What methods do parents/caretakers use in preparing their children for the six selected events (take temperature, look in ears, look at the throat, listen to the heart, feel stomach, and give a shot) of a routine physical examination?
2. Does the method of preparation differ depending on the age of the child (preschool versus school-age)?
3. Does the method of preparation differ depending on the gender of the child (male versus female)?
4. What are the levels of discussion used by parents in preparing their children for routine physical examinations?" (Wilson, 1999, p. 330) ■

Question 1 focused on *description* of the methods for preparing children for their examination. Questions 2 and 3 focused on examining *differences* in preparation methods between preschool and school-aged children and between genders. The last question focused on *description* of the discussion used to prepare children for an examination.

The findings indicated that parents lacked the information to prepare their children for routine physical examinations and that they were more likely to prepare their preschooler than their school-aged child for the exam. Wilson (1999) linked her study findings to practice by providing "General Guidelines for Preparation of Children for Routine Physical Examinations" that would be useful in primary care practice.

The research questions formulated for quantitative and qualitative studies have many similarities. However, the questions directing qualitative studies are commonly broader in focus and include concepts that are more complex and abstract than those of quantitative studies. The phenomenology study by Beck (1998), from which the following excerpts are taken, can help nurses recognize panic disorder during the postpartum period.

. . . .

Research Problem

"Panic disorder is estimated to affect 1.5% of the population of the United States. Initial onset of panic disorder during the postpartum period was reported by Metz, Sichel, and Goff (1988). Yet to be investigated is the effect of panic disorder on the quality of life of new mothers as they struggle to cope with new demands.

. . . .

"Metz and colleagues (1988) urge clinicians to differentiate between postpartum depression and postpartum panic disorder. Postpartum depression has been used as a catchall phrase for many postpartum emotional symptoms. Mothers may be misdiagnosed with postpartum depression when in actuality they are suffering from postpartum onset of panic disorder. Each of these mood disorders has its own constellation of symptoms, unique potential for disrupting the newly formed family unit, and each requires different treatments." (Beck, 1998, p. 131)

. . . .

Research Purpose

"The purpose of this study was to describe the meaning of women's experiences with panic during the postpartum period." (Beck, 1998, p. 131)

. . . .

Research Questions

"The research question was: What is the essential structure of the experience of panic in mothers who developed the onset of panic disorder after delivery?" (Beck, 1998, p. 131). ■

The study question focused on *description* of the complex experience of panic in mothers after delivery. Beck (1998) identified six themes that are descriptive of postpartum onset panic disorder. These themes help advanced practice nurses in the diagnosis and treatment of panic disorder in this population.

FORMULATING HYPOTHESES

A *hypothesis* is the formal statement of the expected relationship or relationships between two or more variables in a specified population. The hypothesis translates the problem and purpose into a clear explanation or prediction of the expected results or outcomes of the study. This section describes the purpose, sources, and types of hypotheses and the process for developing and testing hypotheses in studies.

Purpose of Hypotheses

The purpose of a hypothesis is similar to that of research objectives and questions. A hypothesis (1) specifies the variables to be manipulated or measured, (2) identifies the population to be examined, (3) indicates the type of research, and (4) directs the conduct of the study. Hypotheses also influence the study design, sampling technique, data collection and analysis methods, and the interpretation of findings. Hypotheses differ from objectives and questions by predicting the outcomes of a study, and the research findings indicate rejection, nonrejection, support, or nonsupport of each hypothesis.

Hypothesis testing is a means of generating knowledge through the testing of theoretical statements or relationships that have been identified in previous research, proposed by theorists, or observed in practice. In addition, hypotheses are developed to direct the testing of new treatments and are often viewed as tools for uncovering ideas rather than as ends in themselves (Beveridge, 1950).

Sources of Hypotheses

Hypotheses are generated by observing phenomena or problems in the real world, analyzing theory, and reviewing the literature. Many hypotheses originate from real-life experiences. Clinicians and researchers observe events in the world and identify relationships among these events (theorizing), which are the basis for formulating hypotheses. For example, clinicians notice that the hospitalized patient who complains the most receives the most pain medicine. The relationship identified is a prediction about events in the world that has potential for empirical testing. Theory to support this relationship could be identified through a literature review.

Fagerhaugh and Strauss (1977) developed a theory of pain management by identifying the following relationship: "As expressions of pain increase, pain management increases." This theory was developed through the use of grounded theory research but requires additional testing to determine its usefulness in describing pain expression and management in a variety of practice situations. On the basis

of theory and clinical observation, the following hypothesis might be formulated: "The more frequently a hospitalized patient complains of pain, the more often doses of analgesic medications are administered."

Some hypotheses are initially generated from relationships expressed in a theory, when the intent of the researcher is to test a theory (Chinn & Kramer, 1999). When a theory is being tested, the propositions (relationships) expressed in the theory are used to generate hypotheses. For example, Jennings-Dozier (1999) tested the theory of planned behavior (TPB) in predicting the intentions of African American and Latina women to obtain a Papanicolauou (Pap) smear. Figure 8–1 illustrates a model of the TPB developed by Ajzen (1985). This model includes direct and indirect relationships among the concepts, as indicated in the following propositions. The following propositions are the basis for the generation of the study hypotheses:

1. External variables (age, education, income, and acculturation) have a direct effect on behavioral beliefs, normative beliefs, and control beliefs.
2. Behavioral beliefs have a direct effect on attitude; normative beliefs have a direct effect on subjective norm; and control beliefs have a direct effect on perceived behavioral control.
3. Attitude, subjective norm, and perceived behavioral control have a direct effect on intention.
4. Intention has a direct effect on behavior.
5. External variables have an indirect effect on attitude, subjective norm, and perceived control.

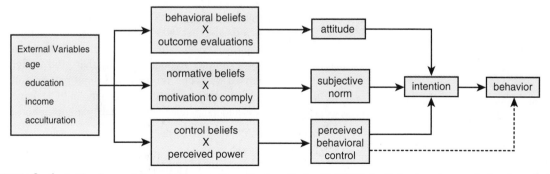

FIGURE 8–1 ■ The theory of planned behavior. (From Jennings-Dozier, K. [1999]. Predicting intentions to obtain a Papanicolaou (Pap) smear among African American and Latina women: Testing the theory of planned behavior. *Nursing Research, 48*[4], 200.)

6. External variables have an indirect effect on intention.
7. Behavioral beliefs, normative beliefs, and control beliefs have an indirect effect on intention.

The first hypothesis for Jennings-Dozier's study was as follows.

. . . .

"Belief-based measures of attitude, subjective norm, and perceived behavioral control would have (a) an indirect effect on intention to obtain a Pap smear and (b) a direct effect on the direct measures of attitude, subjective norm, and perceived behavior control, respectively, which in turn would have (c) direct effects on the intention of African American and Latina women to obtain a Pap smear" (Jennings-Dozier, 1999, p. 199). ■

The seven propositions from TPB, listed previously, can be linked to this study hypothesis in the following way:

Part (a) of the hypothesis tests proposition 7.

Part (b) of the hypothesis tests proposition 2.

Part (c) of the hypothesis tests proposition 3.

Jennings-Dozier's second hypothesis was as follows.

. . . .

"External variables (age, level of education, level of income, and level of acculturation for Latinas) would have (a) a direct effect on the belief-based measures of attitude, subjective norm, and perceived behavioral control; (b) an indirect effect on the direct measures of attitude, subjective norms, and perceived behavioral control; and (c) an indirect effect on the intention of African American and Latina women to obtain a Pap smear." (Jennings-Dozier, 1999, pp. 199–200) ■

The seven propositions from TPB can be linked to the second study hypothesis in the following way:

Part (a) of the hypothesis tests proposition 1.

Part (b) of the hypothesis tests proposition 5.

Part (c) tests proposition 6.

The hypotheses of this study were formulated to test the propositions from TPB. The study findings indicated that attitude and perceived behavior control were predictors of intentions to obtain a Pap smear but that the subjective norms were not. Thus, the study supported some of the relationships in the TPB but not others (Jennings-Dozier, 1999). Further research is needed to determine the effectiveness of the TPB to explain health promotion and illness prevention intentions and behaviors.

Hypotheses can also be generated by reviewing the literature and synthesizing findings from different studies. For example, Anderson and colleagues (1999) synthesized the findings from several studies focused on the outcomes of coronary artery bypass graft (CABG) surgery and formulated the following hypotheses to direct their study.

"1. CABG patients who stay 1 day in ICU begin ambulation in an inpatient cardiac rehabilitation program earlier than patients who stay 2 days in ICU.
"2. CABG patients who stay 1 day in ICU have a shorter postoperative hospitalization than patients who stay 2 days in ICU." (Anderson et al., 1999, p. 169).

The results of this study supported the first hypothesis because patients who stayed 1 day in the ICU had significantly earlier ambulation than those staying 2 days in the ICU. The second hypothesis was not supported because there was no significant difference in postoperative length of stay between patients who stayed 1 day and those who stayed 2 days in the ICU. These mixed findings indicate the need for replication of this study and further research in this problem area. You might revise the hypothesis that was tested by Anderson and colleagues (1999) and focus on a different variable. For example, hypothesis 1 of that study might be revised to focus on patient symptoms, as follows: "CABG patients who stay 1 day in ICU have less reported pain and anxiety than patients who stay 2 days in ICU."

Types of Hypotheses

Different types of relationships and numbers of variables are identified in hypotheses. Studies might have one, three, five, or more hypotheses, depending on the complexity of the study. The type of hypothesis developed is based on the problem and purpose of the study. Hypotheses can be described by examining them in terms of the following four categories: (1) associative versus causal, (2) simple versus complex, (3) directional versus nondirectional, and (4) null versus research.

ASSOCIATIVE VERSUS CAUSAL HYPOTHESES

The relationships identified in hypotheses are associative or causal. An *associative* relationship identifies variables that occur or exist together in the real world (Reynolds, 1971). In an associative relationship, when one variable changes, the other variable changes.

A format for expressing an associative hypothesis follows:

1. Variable X is related to variable Y in a specified population. (Predicts a relationship.)
2. Variable X increases as variable Y increases in a specified population. (Predicts a positive relationship.)
3. Variable X decreases as variable Y decreases in a specified population. (Predicts a positive relationship.)
4. Variable X increases as variable Y decreases in a specified population. (Predicts a negative or inverse relationship.)
5. Variable X decreases as variable Y increases in a specified population. (Predicts a negative or inverse relationship.)

Georges and Heitkemper (1994) examined the relationship between "dietary fiber and distressing gastrointestinal (GI) symptoms in midlife women" and formulated the following associative hypotheses to direct their study.

"II. An inverse relationship exists between fiber intake and symptom reports in this group.
III. A positive relationship exists between caffeine/alcohol intake and symptom reports in this group." (Georges & Heitkemper, 1994, p. 357)

Hypothesis II presents a negative or inverse relationship, indicating that a decrease in fiber intake (X) is associated with an increase in GI symptom reports (Y). A diagram of this relationship follows:

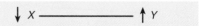

Hypothesis III presents a positive relationship, indicating that an increase in caffeine/alcohol intake (X) is associated with an increase in GI symptom reports (Y) or a decrease in caffeine intake or alcohol intake or both (X) is associated with a decrease in GI symptom reports (Y). A diagram of these two relationships follows:

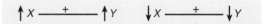

Causal relationships identify a cause-and-effect interaction between two or more variables, which are referred to as independent and dependent variables. The *independent variable* (intervention, treatment, or experimental variable) is manipulated by the researcher to cause an effect on the dependent variable. The *dependent variable* (outcome or criterion variable) is measured to examine the effect created by the independent variable.

A format for stating a causal hypothesis is as follows: The subjects exposed to the independent variable demonstrate greater change as measured by the dependent variable than the subjects not exposed to the independent variable.

Parker and associates (1999) tested an intervention to prevent further abuse to pregnant women and formulated the following causal hypothesis: Women in the experimental group that received empowerment intervention plus group counseling report less abuse in the 12 months after pregnancy than women in the experimental group receiving the empowerment intervention only or the comparison group. In this hypothesis, pregnant women are the population; the two independent variables are empowerment intervention (X_1) and group counseling

(X_2); and the dependent variable is abuse (Y). The arrow in the following diagram indicates that the independent variables (X_1 and X_2) cause an effect on the dependent variable (Y).

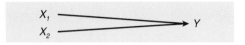

SIMPLE VERSUS COMPLEX HYPOTHESES

A *simple hypothesis* states the relationship (associative or causal) between two variables. One format for stating a simple associative hypothesis is: Variable X is related to variable Y. A simple causal hypothesis identifies the relationship between one independent variable and one dependent variable.

A *complex hypothesis* predicts the relationship (associative or causal) among three or more variables. A complex associative hypothesis would indicate the relationships among variables, where variables X, Y, and Z are interrelated. In complex causal hypotheses, relationships are predicted between two (or more) independent variables, two (or more) dependent variables, or two (or) more independent or dependent variables.

For example, Harris and colleagues (1998) studied an intervention for changing high-risk HIV (human immunodeficiency virus) behaviors of African American drug-dependent women; their hypothesis was worded as follows.

· ·

"A peer counseling and leadership training (PCLT) program administered to methadone-dependent, African American women: (a) improves their level of self-esteem; (b) lowers their level of depression; (c) increases their self-reported number of safer sex practices; and (d) increases their self-reported level of participation in AIDS-related community action." (Harris et al., 1998, p. 241) ■

This complex hypothesis has one independent variable, PCLT program (X), and four dependent variables, level of self-esteem (Y_1), level of depression (Y_2), number of safer sex practices (Y_3), and

level of participation in AIDS-related community action (Y_4). A diagram of this hypothesis follows:

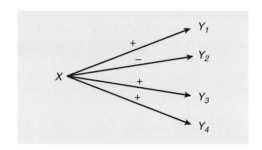

The findings of this study supported part of the hypothesis and indicated that the PCLT program was effective in producing three of the four outcomes (decreased depression, increased number of safer sexual behaviors, and higher level of participation in community action related to AIDS. Often, in real-life situations, multiple variables cause an event or an intervention results in multiple outcomes. Therefore, complex rather than simple causal hypotheses are often more representative of nursing practice.

Some studies include both simple and complex hypotheses. Chang (1999) conducted a quasi-experimental study of the effectiveness of a cognitive-behavioral (CB) intervention for homebound caregivers of persons with dementia. Table 8–1 includes the study's hypotheses, which are labeled as simple or complex according to the number of independent and dependent variables in each hypothesis. These hypotheses might have been more reflective of the population studied rather than of the sample if they had been expressed in the present tense (*reports*) rather than the modal form (*would report*). This idea is expanded in the section on developing hypotheses.

NONDIRECTIONAL VERSUS DIRECTIONAL HYPOTHESES

A *nondirectional hypothesis* states that a relationship exists but does not predict the nature of the relationship. If the direction of the relationship be-

TABLE 8–1
SIMPLE AND COMPLEX HYPOTHESES

	INDEPENDENT VARIABLES	DEPENDENT VARIABLES
Complex Hypotheses		
"Caregivers within the cognitive-behavioral (C-B) group would report less burden, more satisfaction, less anxiety, and less depression over time (at baseline, 4 weeks, 8 weeks, and 12 weeks)" (Chang, 1999, p. 175).	Cognitive-Behavioral Intervention	Burden, satisfaction, anxiety, depression
"Caregivers within the attention-only (A-O) group would report an increase in burden, decrease in satisfaction, and increase in anxiety, and more depression over time" (Chang, 1999, p. 175).	Attention Only	Burden, satisfaction, anxiety, depression
Simple Hypotheses		
"Caregivers in the C-B group would show a significant increase in the use of a problem-focused coping strategy over time" (Chang, 1999, p. 175).	Cognitive-Behavioral Intervention	Problem-focused coping strategy
"Persons with dementia in the C-B group would show significant improvement in their functional status over time" (Chang, 1999, p. 175).	Cognitive-Behavioral Intervention	Functional status

ing studied is not clear in clinical practice or the theoretical or empirical literature, the researcher has no clear indication of the nature of the relationship. Under these circumstances, nondirectional hypotheses are developed, such as those developed by Jirovec and Kasno (1990) to direct their study, as shown in the following excerpt.

"1. Elderly nursing home residents' self-appraisals of their self-care abilities are related to the basic conditioning factors of sex, sociocultural orientation, health, and family influences.

2. Elderly nursing home residents' self-appraisals of their self-care abilities are related to their perceptions of the nursing home environment." (Jirovec & Kasno, 1990, p. 304)

The first hypothesis is complex (five variables), associative, and nondirectional. The second hypothesis is simple (two variables), associative, and nondirectional. Both hypotheses state that a relationship exists but do not indicate the direction of the relationship.

A *directional hypothesis* states the nature of the relationship between two or more variables. These hypotheses are developed from theoretical statements, findings of previous studies, and clinical experience. As the knowledge on which a study is based increases, the researcher is able to make a prediction about the direction of a relationship between the variables being studied. The use of such terms as *less, more, increase, decrease, greater,* and *smaller* indicate the directions of relationships in hypotheses. Directional hypotheses can be associative or causal and simple or complex.

Keats and associates (1999) hypothesized that leisure-time physical activity throughout the cancer experience is related to the best psychosocial well-being in adolescents after a cancer diagnosis. This simple, associative, directional hypothesis was supported by the study findings, indicating the importance of leisure-time physical activities in promoting well-being during the treatment of cancer.

A *causal hypothesis* predicts the effect of an independent variable on a dependent variable, specifying the direction of the relationship. Thus, all causal hypotheses are directional. For example, Taylor (1999) examined the effectiveness of an intervention, Premenstrual Syndrome Symptom Management Program (PMS-SMP), in the treatment of PMS. The following complex, causal hypothesis was used to direct this study.

. . . .

"Women completing the PMS-SMP would have reduced perimenstrual symptom severity, reduced personal demands (distress, anxiety, and depression), increased personal resources (self-esteem and well-being), and increased health behaviors maintained overtime." (Taylor, 1999, p. 498) ■

The study findings supported this hypothesis and indicated that a nonpharmacological intervention (PMS-SMP) (independent variable) can be effective in reducing perimenstrual symptom severity and personal distress and improving personal resources (dependent variables) for women experiencing severe premenstrual syndrome.

NULL VERSUS RESEARCH HYPOTHESES

The *null hypothesis* (H_0), also referred to as a *statistical hypothesis*, is used for statistical testing and interpretation of statistical outcomes. Even if the null hypothesis is not stated, it is implied, because it is the converse of the research hypothesis (Kerlinger, 1986). A null hypothesis can be simple or complex, associative or causal. An associative null hypothesis states: There is no relationship between the variables. An example of a simple associative null hypothesis is: "There is no relationship between the number of experiences performing a developmental assessment skill and learning of the skill, as measured by clinical performance test scores" (Koniak, 1985, p. 85).

A causal null hypothesis might be stated in the following format:

1. There is no effect of one variable on another.
2. There is no difference between the experimental group exposed to the independent variable and the control group as measured by the dependent variable.

Fahs and Kinney (1991, p. 204) developed the following complex null hypothesis to direct their study: "There is no difference in the occurrence of a bruise at injection site with low-dose heparin therapy when administered in three different subcutaneous sites" (the sites were the abdomen, thigh, and arm). They found that there was no statistically significant difference in bruising at 60 and 72 hours after injection among the three sites. Thus, this null hypothesis was supported.

A *research hypothesis* is the alternative hypothesis $(H_1$ or $H_A)$ to the null. The research hypothesis states that there is a relationship between two or more variables and can be simple or complex, nondirectional or directional, and associative or causal. Researchers have different beliefs about when to state a research hypothesis or a null hypothesis. Some researchers state the null hypothesis because it is more easily interpreted on the basis of the results of statistical analyses. The null hypothesis is also used when the researcher believes there is no relationship between two variables and when there is inadequate theoretical or empirical information to state a research hypothesis (Kerlinger, 1986).

A research hypothesis is used to make a prediction about the existence or direction of a relationship between variables. The prediction in a research hypothesis needs to be based on theoretical statements, previous research findings, or clinical experience. Jadack and colleagues (1995) "examined gender differences in knowledge about HIV, the reported incidence of risky sexual behavior, and comfort with safer sexual practices among young adults" and formulated both research and null hypotheses. In the following excerpt from their study, hypotheses (a) and (b) are simple null hypotheses, and hypotheses (c) and (d) are complex, nondirectional, associative research hypotheses.

. . . .

"(a) There will be no difference between men and women in knowledge about HIV transmission routes (sexual, needle sharing, casual); (b) there will be no difference between men and women in knowledge about the effectiveness of measures to prevent sexual transmission of HIV; (c) men and women will differ with respect to reported frequency and type of behaviors that could lead to the transmission of HIV; and (d) men and women will differ with respect to reported level of comfort and safer sexual practices." (Jadack et al., 1995, p. 315) ■

Developing Hypotheses

Developing hypotheses requires inductive and deductive thinking. Most people have a predominant way of thinking and will use that thinking pattern in developing hypotheses. *Inductive* thinkers have a tendency to focus on relationships that are observed in clinical practice, and they synthesize these observations to formulate a general statement about the relationships observed (Chinn & Kramer, 1999). For example, inductive thinkers might note that elderly patients who are not instructed about the reasons for early postoperative ambulation make no effort to get out of bed. *Deductive* thinkers examine more abstract statements from theories or previous research and then formulate a hypothesis for study. Deductive thinkers might translate a statement such as "people who receive instruction in self-care are more responsible in caring for themselves" into a hypothesis.

Research development requires both inductive and deductive thinking. The inductive thinker must link the relational statement or hypothesis that was developed from clinical observations with a theoretical framework to improve the usefulness of the study findings, which requires deductive thinking. The deductive thinker must use inductive thinking to determine whether the relationship of events in clinical practice is accurately predicted by the proposition from a theory. Without this real-world experience, the selection of subjects and the identification of ways to measure the variables would be unclear. Thus, hypothesis development requires both inductive and deductive thinking. An example hypothesis for potential study is: "Elderly patients who receive self-care instruction on activity ambulate earlier and have a shorter hospital stay after surgery than elderly patients who receive no self-care instruction."

In formulating a hypothesis, a researcher has several decisions to make. These decisions are directed by the problem studied and by the expertise and preference of the researcher. The researcher must decide whether the problem to be studied is best investigated with the use of simple or complex hypotheses. Complex hypotheses frequently require complex methodology, and the outcomes may be difficult to interpret. Some beginning researchers prefer the clarity of simple hypotheses.

The research problem and purpose determine whether an associative or causal relationship is to be studied. Testing a hypothesis that states a causal relationship requires expertise in implementing a treatment and controlling extraneous variables. Another decision the researcher must make involves the formulation of a research or a null hypothesis. This decision must be made according to what the researcher believes is the most accurate prediction of the relationship between the variables.

A hypothesis that is clearly and concisely stated gives the greatest direction for conducting a study. For clarity, hypotheses are expressed as declarative statements written in the present tense. Thus, hypotheses need to be written without the phrase "There *will be* no relationship . . . ," because the future tense refers to the sample being studied. Hypotheses are statements of relationships about populations, not about study samples. According to mathematical theory related to generalization, one cannot generalize to the future (Kerlinger, 1986).

Hypotheses are clearer without the phrase "There is no *significant* difference . . . ," because the level of significance is only a statistical technique applied to sample data (Armstrong, 1981). In addition, hypotheses should not identify methodological points, such as techniques of sampling, measurement, and data analysis (Kerlinger, 1986). Therefore, statements such as "*measured by,*" "in a *random sample* of," or "*using ANOVA* (analysis of variance)" are not appropriate.

Thus, hypotheses are not limited to the variables, methodology, and sample identified for one study. Hypotheses need to reflect the variables (or concepts) and population outlined in the research problem and purpose. A well-formulated hypothesis clearly identifies the relationship between the variables to be studied. There is no set number for how many hypotheses are needed to direct a study, but the number formulated is usually reflective of the researcher's expertise and the complexity of the problem studied. However, most studies contain one to five hypotheses, and the relationships identified in these hypotheses set the limits for a study.

Testing Hypotheses

A hypothesis's value is ultimately derived from whether or not it can be tested in the real world. A *testable hypothesis* is one that contains variables that can be measured or manipulated in the world, such as the one developed by Corff and associates (1995) and shown in the following exerpts from and descriptions of the study.

• •

Research Purpose

The purpose was to determine the "effectiveness of facilitated tucking, a nonpharmacological nursing intervention, as a comfort measure in modulating preterm neonates' physiologic and behavioral responses to minor pain." (Corff et al., 1995, p. 143)

• •

Hypothesis

The hypothesis for this prospective study was that "preterm neonates would have less variation in heart rate, oxygen saturation, and sleep state (shorter crying and sleep disruption time and less fluctuation in sleep states) in response to the painful stimulus of a heelstick with facilitated tucking than without." (Corff et al., p. 144)

Independent Variable—Facilitate Tucking

Conceptual Definition. A nonpharmacological comfort measure that involves the motoric containment of an infant's arms and legs.

Operational Definition. The infant's arms and legs are contained in "a flexed, midline position close to the infant's trunk with the infant in a side-lying or supine position." (Corff et al., 1995, p. 144) (See Figure 8–2.)

Dependent Variables—Heart Rate and Oxygen Saturation

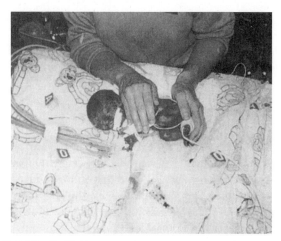

FIGURE 8–2 ■ Facilitated tucking of a premature infant. (From Corff, K. E., Seideman, R., Venkataraman, P. S., et al. [1995]. Facilitated tucking: A nonpharmacological comfort measure for pain in preterm neonates. *JOGNN, 24*[2], 144.

Conceptual Definition. Physiological responses that are influenced by painful stimuli.

Operational Definition. Heart rate and oxygen saturation per pulse oximetry "were recorded visually and were graphed using a System VI Air Shields Infant Monitor with Data Logger." (Corff et al., 1995, p. 145)

Dependent Variable—Sleep State

Conceptual Definition. The behavioral responses crying, sleep disruption time, and fluctuation in sleep state, which are influenced by painful stimuli.

Operational Definition. "Sleep states were recorded by one of two observers who reached 90% reliability in reading sleep states, as defined in the Neonatal Individualized Developmental Care and Assessment Program. Sleep states are defined as state 1 = deep sleep; state 2 = light sleep; state 3 = drowsiness; state 4 = awake, alert; state 5 = aroused, fussy; and state 6 = crying. Sleep states were recorded during a 12-minute baseline period, the heelstick period, and a 15-minute post-stick period for both control and experimental trials." (Corff et al., 1995, p. 145)

Hypotheses are evaluated with statistical analyses. If the hypothesis states an associative relationship, then correlational analyses, such as Spearman rank order correlation or Pearson's correlation, are conducted to determine the existence, type, and degree of the relationship between the variables studied.

A hypothesis that states a causal relationship is analyzed through the use of statistics that examine differences, such as Mann-Whitney U, t-test, and analysis of variance (ANOVA). It is the null hypothesis (stated or implied) that is tested. The intent is to determine whether the independent variable had a significant effect on the dependent variable. The level of significance, alpha (α) = .05, .01, .001, is set after the generation of causal hypotheses. Further discussion about selecting statistical tests and a level of significance for testing hypotheses can be found in Chapter 18.

The results obtained from testing a hypothesis are described with the use of certain terminology. Hypotheses are not proven true or false by the findings from research. Hypotheses are statements of relationships or differences in populations; the findings from one study do not prove a hypothesis. Even after a series of studies, the word *proven* is not used in scientific language because of the tentative nature of science. Research hypotheses are described as being *supported* or *not supported* in a study. When a null hypothesis is tested, it is either rejected or accepted. Accepting the null hypothesis indicates that no relationship or effect was found among the variables. Rejecting the null hypothesis indicates the possibility that a relationship or difference exists.

In the previously described study by Corff and associates (1995, p. 145) study, the hypothesis identified a causal relationship between facilitated tucking and heart rate, oxygen saturation, and sleep state. The results "suggest that facilitated tucking is an effective comfort measure in attenuating preterm neonates' physiologic and behavioral responses to minor painful stimuli. Significantly improved homeostasis and stability were demonstrated within the parameters of heart rate, sleep state changes, crying time, and sleep disruption" but not with oxygen saturation. Thus, the causal relationships between facilitated tucking, heart rate, and sleep state were

supported by the findings, but the causal relationship between facilitated tucking and oxygen saturation was not supported.

SELECTING OBJECTIVES, QUESTIONS, OR HYPOTHESES FOR QUANTITATIVE OR QUALITATIVE RESEARCH

Selecting objectives, questions, or hypotheses for a study is often based on (1) the number and quality of relevant studies conducted on a selected problem (existing knowledge base), (2) the framework of the study, (3) the expertise and preference of the researcher, and (4) the type of study to be conducted (quantitative or qualitative). Commonly, if minimal or no research has been conducted on a problem, investigators state objectives or questions, because inadequate knowledge is available to formulate hypotheses. The framework for a study indicates whether the intent is to develop or to test theory. Objectives and questions are usually stated to guide theory development, and the focus of a hypothesis is to test theory.

Researcher expertise and preference can also influence the selection of objectives, questions, or hypotheses to direct a study. Moody and colleagues (1988) analyzed the focus of nursing practice research from 1977 to 1986 and found that 16% of the studies had research questions and 31% contained hypotheses. The number of nursing studies containing hypotheses continues to grow, and there appears to be a "trend away from descriptive and fact-finding studies toward efforts to establish relationships between variables and to test hypotheses" (Brown et al., 1984, p. 31). The greater use of hypotheses to direct research could indicate the growth of knowledge in selected problem areas and the increasing sophistication of nurse researchers. However, Brown and associates (1984) noted that only 51% of the studies they reviewed contained explicitly stated hypotheses; and the other studies had implicit or implied hypotheses. The explicit statement of hypotheses is important to provide clear direction for the conduct of a study and the use of the findings in practice.

The objectives, questions, or hypotheses designated for study frequently indicate a pattern that the researcher uses in conducting investigations. Problems can be investigated in a variety of ways; some researchers start at the core of a problem and work their way outward. Other investigators study a problem from the outside edge and work to the core (Kaplan, 1964). Each study needs to logically build on the other, as the researcher establishes a pattern for studying a problem area that will affect the quality and quantity of the knowledge generated in that area.

Researchers select objectives, questions, or hypotheses according to the type of study to be conducted. Objectives and questions are typically stated when the intent of the study is to identify or describe characteristics of variables or to examine relationships among variables or both. Thus, objectives or questions are often formulated to direct qualitative and selected quantitative (descriptive and correlational) studies (see Table 8–2). However, some experienced researchers can clearly focus and develop a study without using objectives or questions. In these studies, a research purpose directs the research process.

In some qualitative research, only a problem and purpose are used to direct the study. The specification of objectives or questions might limit the scope of the study and the methods of data collection and analysis. Discovery is important in qualitative research, and sometimes the "research questions may be unclear, the objectives ambiguous and the final outcome uncertain. Hypotheses and detailed accounts of precise research strategies are not necessary nor desirable in a well constructed qualitative design" (Aamodt, 1983, p. 399).

Researchers often develop hypotheses when the relationships or results of a study can be anticipated or predicted. Hypotheses are typically used in quantitative research to direct predictive correlational, quasi-experimental, and experimental studies.

DEFINING RESEARCH VARIABLES

The research purpose and objectives, questions, and hypotheses identify the variables or concepts to be examined in a study. Variables are qualities, properties, or characteristics of persons, things, or situations that change or vary. In research, variables are characterized by degrees, amounts, and differences. Variables are also concepts of various levels of abstraction that are concisely defined to facilitate their measurement or manipulation within a study (Kaplan, 1964; Moody, 1990).

The concepts examined in research can be concrete and directly measurable in the real world, such as heart rate, hemoglobin, and lung tidal volume. These concrete concepts are usually referred to as *variables* in a study. Other concepts, such as anxiety, coping, and pain are more abstract and are indirectly observable in the real world (Fawcett & Downs, 1986). Thus, the properties of these concepts are inferred from a combination of measurements. For example, one can infer the properties of anxiety by combining information obtained from (1) observing the signs and symptoms of anxiety (frequent movement and verbalization of anxiety), (2) examining completed questionnaires or scales (A-state and trait anxiety scales), and (3) measuring physiological responses (galvanic skin response). The concept of anxiety might be represented by the variables "reported anxiety" or "perceived level of anxiety."

In many qualitative studies and in some quantitative studies (descriptive and correlational), the focus is abstract concepts, such as grieving, caring, and health promotion. Researchers identify the elements of the study as *concepts*, not variables. In the phe-

---

TABLE 8–2
SELECTING OBJECTIVES, QUESTIONS, OR HYPOTHESES FOR DIFFERENT TYPES OF RESEARCH

TYPES OF RESEARCH	USE OF OBJECTIVES, QUESTIONS, OR HYPOTHESES?
Qualitative research	Objectives, questions, or none
Quantitative research	
Descriptive studies	Objectives, questions, or none
Correlational studies	Objectives, questions, hypotheses, or none
Quasi-experimental studies	Questions or hypotheses
Experimental studies	Hypotheses

nomenological study previously described, Beck (1998) investigated the concept of panic experienced by women during their postpartum period. *Panic* was defined according to the Diagnostic and Statistical Manual of Mental Disorders (DSM-IV) (American Psychological Association [APA}, 1994, p. 397) as: "The presence of recurrent, unexpected panic attacks followed by at least 1 month of persistent concern about having another panic attack, worry about the possible implications or consequences of the panic attacks, or a significant behavioral change related to the attacks." Beck's (1998) study expanded this definition of *panic* for new mothers to include the following indicators: hysterical crying, distortion regarding time, and painful feelings in the head. This clarification of the signs and symptoms of panic will promote accurate diagnosis of panic disorder in postpartum women.

Types of Variables

Variables have been classified into a variety of types to explain their use in research. Some variables are manipulated; others are controlled. Some variables are identified but not measured; others are measured with refined measurement devices. The types of variables presented in this section are independent, dependent, research, extraneous, demographic, moderator, and mediator.

INDEPENDENT AND DEPENDENT VARIABLES

The relationship between independent variables and dependent variables is the basis for formulating hypotheses for correlational, quasi-experimental, and experimental studies. An *independent variable* is a stimulus or activity that is manipulated or varied by the researcher to create an effect on the dependent variable. The independent variable is also called an *intervention*, *treatment*, or *experimental variable*.

A *dependent variable* is the response, behavior, or outcome that the researcher wants to predict or explain. Changes in the dependent variable are presumed to be caused by the independent variable. The dependent variable can also be called an *effect variable* or a *criterion measure* (Kerlinger, 1986).

The hypothesis developed by Parker and associates (1999), introduced earlier in the chapter, stated that pregnant women who received the empowerment intervention and group counseling would have less abuse in the 12 months following pregnancy than women in the group receiving empowerment intervention only or the comparison group. One independent variable was the empowerment intervention, which was based on the McFarlane and Parker (1994) abuse prevention protocol. The other independent variable, group counseling, consisted of three sessions of counseling and information at a local shelter to strengthen the empowerment intervention. The dependent variable was abuse, which was measured in frequency by the *Index of Spouse Abuse (ISA) Scale* and in severity by the *Severity of Violence Against Women Scales (SVAWS)*. The study findings indicated that women in both experimental groups reported significantly less abuse than those in the comparison group, but there was no significant difference between the two experimental groups. Thus, the hypothesis was partially supported, and additional research is needed to address the problem of abuse in pregnant women.

RESEARCH VARIABLES OR CONCEPTS

Qualitative studies and some quantitative (descriptive and correlational) studies involve the investigation of research variables or concepts. Research variables or concepts are the qualities, properties, or characteristics identified in the research purpose and objectives or questions that are observed or measured in a study. They are used when the intent of the study is to observe or measure variables as they exist in a natural setting without the implementation of a treatment. Thus, no independent variables are manipulated, and no cause-and-effect relationships are examined.

Olson (1995) investigated the relationships between a nurse's empathy and selected patient outcomes. This study yielded a greater understanding of the concepts of nurse empathy and patient outcomes by examining the following research variables: nurse-expressed empathy, patient-perceived empathy, and patient distress. These variables are conceptually and operationally defined later in this chapter.

EXTRANEOUS VARIABLES

Extraneous variables exist in all studies and can affect the measurement of study variables and the relationships among them. Extraneous variables are of primary concern in quantitative studies, because they can interfere with obtaining a clear understanding of the relational or causal dynamics within the studies. Extraneous variables are classified as (1) recognized or unrecognized and (2) controlled or uncontrolled.

The extraneous variables that are not recognized until the study is in process or are recognized before the study is initiated but cannot be controlled are referred to as *confounding variables.* Sometimes these variables can be measured during the study and controlled statistically during analysis. However, in other cases, measurement of a confounding variable is not possible and the variable thus hinders the interpretation of findings. Such extraneous variables must be identified as areas of study weakness in the discussion section of a research report. As control decreases in quasi-experimental and experimental studies, the potential influence of confounding variables increases.

Researchers attempt to recognize and control as many extraneous variables as possible in quasi-experimental and experimental studies, and specific designs have been developed to control the influence of such variables (see Chapter 11). Corff and associates (1995) controlled some of the extraneous variables in their study, previously described, by using inclusion and exclusion criteria for sample selection, as the following excerpt describes.

· ·

"Inclusion criteria included neonates of 25–35 weeks gestational age at birth, appropriate for gestational age, 36 weeks or less postconceptual age, and less than 22 days postnatal age at time of testing. Exclusion criteria included neonates with chromosomal or genetic anomalies; significant central nervous system abnormalities (congenital or acquired, including grade II or greater intraventricular hemorrhage); Apgar scores of less than 5 at 5 min-

utes; congenital heart disease; dysmorphic syndrome; and infants receiving paralytic, analgesic, or sedating medications." (Corff et al., 1995, p. 144) ■

These researchers also disqualified six infants to control extraneous variables that might have influenced the implementation of the treatment or measurement of the dependent variables. The infants were disqualified "because of changes in their physiologic or respiratory status ($n = 3$), infiltrated intravenous site as a source of additional pain ($n = 1$), or transfer out of NICU ($n = 2$) between the first and second observations" (Corff et al., 1995, p. 144).

Environmental variables are a type of extraneous variable that make up the setting in which the study is conducted. Examples are climate, home, health care system, community setting, and governmental organizations. If a researcher is studying humans in an uncontrolled or natural setting, it is impossible and undesirable to control all the environmental variables. In qualitative and some quantitative (descriptive and correlational) studies, little or no attempt is made to control environmental variables. The intent is to study subjects in their natural environment without controlling or altering it. The environmental variables in quasi-experimental and experimental research can be controlled through the use of a laboratory setting or a specially constructed research unit in a hospital.

In intervention effectiveness research, the extraneous variables are referred to as context variables. *Context variables* are those factors that could influence the implementation of an intervention and, thus, the outcomes of the study or could directly influence the study outcomes (Sidani & Braden, 1998). These contextual or extraneous factors include social, environmental, setting, and individual variables that can influence the intervention and study outcomes.

For a study to yield the best understanding of an intervention and its usefulness to practice, the study design must provide for examination of relevant contextual variables and link them to the study interventions and outcomes. Thus, rather than controlling or preventing the influence of extraneous variables as do quasi-experimental and experimental

	TABLE 8–3				
	MEANS AND STANDARD DEVIATIONS OF SOCIODEMOGRAPHIC				
	VARIABLES OF COGNITIVE-BEHAVIORAL (COGNITIVE-BEHAVIORS				
	INTERVENTION) AND ATTENTION-ONLY GROUPS AT BASELINE				

	COGNITIVE-BEHAVIORAL ($n = 34$)		**ATTENTION-ONLY** ($n = 31$)		
VARIABLES	**M**	**SD**	**M**	**SD**	**Sig**
Caregivers					
Age	64.51	13.16	68.73	10.64	NS
Education	14.31	2.61	13.40	2.77	NS
Income Category*	3.04	1.91	2.23	1.48	NS
Global health	1.41	0.67	1.34	0.81	NS
Number of Yrs Caregiving	3.55	2.58	3.15	2.98	NS
Number of roles	1.38	0.57	1.51	0.85	NS
Time for self	3.71	2.63	3.29	4.70	NS
Person with Dementia					
Age	78.63	7.50	78.67	9.23	NS
Pt. Education	12.89	3.81	13.76	5.17	NS

*Household home category: 0 = less than $10,000; 1 = $10,001 to 20,000; 2 = $20,001 to 30,000; 3 = $30,001 to 40,000; 4 = $40,001 to 50,000; 5 = $50,001 to 60,000; 6 = Over $60,000

M, mean; NS, not significant; Pt., patient; SD, standard deviation.

From Chang, B. L. (1999). Cognitive-behavioral intervention for homebound caregivers of persons with dementia. *Nursing Research, 48*[3], p. 175.)

research, intervention effectiveness research focuses on studying them. Identifying and studying the effects of contextual (extraneous) variables greatly increases the complexity of a study but also improves the accuracy of the findings for practice. Intervention effectiveness research is the focus of Chapter 13.

DEMOGRAPHIC VARIABLES

Demographic variables are characteristics or attributes of the subject that are collected to describe the sample. Some common demographic variables examined in nursing research are age, gender, ethnicity, educational level, income, job classification, length of hospital stay, and medical diagnosis. Demographic variables are selected by the researcher on the basis of experience and previous research; however, age, gender, and ethnicity are essential demographic variables to examine in a study. These demographics are essential to describing the sample and determining the population for generalization of the findings. More research is

needed to improve health care for elderly, women, and minorities, and studies of these individuals often receive priority by funding agencies.

To obtain data on demographic variables, subjects are asked to complete a demographic or information sheet. When a study is completed, the demographic information is analyzed to provide a picture of the sample, which is called the *sample characteristics.* Sample characteristics are presented in a table or discussed in the narrative of the research report or both. Chang (1999), in the study of cognitive-behavioral intervention for homebound caregivers of persons with dementia, presented the demographic results for both the caregiver and the person with dementia receiving care for the two study groups (cognitive-behavioral intervention or experimental group and the attention-only or comparison group) in a table (see Table 8–3). Chang (1999, p. 175) also provided demographic results for the caregivers in the narrative, as follows: The caregivers were female and "the majority of subjects were spouses (88.6%) with a mean age of 66.5 years and a mean education of 14 years. Caregivers were predominantly married (86.2%), with 12.6% widowed, and predominantly Caucasian Americans of European background (79.1%), or African-American (16.3%)."

MODERATOR AND MEDIATOR VARIABLES

Moderator and mediator variables are examined in intervention effectiveness research to improve the understanding of the effect of the intervention on practice-related outcomes. A *moderator variable* occurs with the intervention (independent variable) and alters the causal relationship between the intervention and the outcomes. Moderator variables include characteristics of the subjects and of the person implementing the intervention. *Mediator variables* bring about the effects of the intervention after it has occurred and, thus, influence the outcomes of the study (Sidani & Braden, 1998).

The theoretical model that provides the framework for the study usually identifies the relevant moderator and mediator variables to be examined in the study. The design is developed to examine not only the independent (intervention) and dependent (outcomes) variables of the study but also the moderator, mediator, and context variables (see Chapter 13 for a detailed discussion and examples of these types of variables).

OPERATIONALIZING VARIABLES OR CONCEPTS

Operationalizing a variable or concept involves developing conceptual and operational definitions. A *conceptual definition* provides the theoretical meaning of a concept or variable (Fawcett & Downs, 1986) and is derived from a theorist's definition of that concept or is developed through concept analysis. The study framework, which includes concepts and their definitions, provides a basis for conceptually defining the variables. Hargreaves and Lander (1989, p. 159) studied the "effects of transcutaneous electrical nerve simulation (TENS) on incisional pain." The analgesic effects of the TENS (independent variable) was conceptually defined through the use of gate-control theory, as shown in the following excerpt.

Conceptual Definition of TENS. "TENS is thought to activate the large diameter, myelinated A-beta fibers which have a low threshold for electrical stimulation. The increased activity in these fibers would serve to decrease the transmission of painful stimuli through the small diameter A-delta and C fibers (Hargreaves & Lander 1989, p. 159).

This conceptual definition links the TENS variable to the concepts and relationships in the gate-control theory developed by Melzack and Wall (1984). It also provides a basis for formulating an operational definition.

An *operational definition* is derived from a set of procedures or progressive acts that a researcher performs either to implement a treatment (independent variable) or to receive sensory impressions (such as sounds or visual or tactile impressions) that measure the existence or the degree of existence of the dependent variable (Reynolds, 1971). Operational definitions need to be independent of time and setting, so that variables can be investigated at different times and in different settings through the use of the same operational definitions. An operational definition is developed so that a variable can be manipulated (independent variable) or measured (dependent variable) in a concrete situation, and the knowledge gained from studying the variable improves the understanding of the theoretical concept that the variable represents. Hargreaves and Lander (1989) operationalized the TENS as follows.

Operational Definition of TENS. "Piece of equipment with a portable GRASS SD9 stimulator (Grass Instrument Co., Quincy, MA) and two prejelled, sterile surface electrodes 3 cm in diameter (Myo-Trode II, No. 410)." (Hargreaves & Lander, 1989, p. 160)

The variables in quasi-experimental and experimental research are narrow and specific in focus and are capable of being quantified (converted to numbers) or manipulated through the use of specified steps. In addition, the variables are objectively defined to reduce researcher bias.

The concepts or variables in descriptive and correlational studies are usually more abstract and broadly defined than the variables in quasi-experimental studies. Olson (1995) conducted a correlational study to examine the relationships among three research variables, nurse-expressed empathy, patient-perceived empathy, and patient distress. The researcher developed three hypotheses indicating various relationships between them, as described in the following excerpt.

. . . .

There are "(a) . . . negative relationships between nurse-expressed empathy and measures of patient distress, (b) . . . negative relationships between patient-perceived empathy and measures of patient distress, and (c) . . . positive relationships between measures of nurse-expressed empathy and patient-perceived empathy." (Olson, 1995, p. 318) ■

These three variables were then conceptually and operationally defined as follows.

Variable—Nurse-Expressed Empathy

Conceptual Definition. "Understanding what a patient is saying and feeling, then communicating this understanding verbally to the patient." (Olson, 1995, p. 318)

Operational Definition. Nurse-expressed empathy was measured using two instruments, the Behavioral Test of Interpersonal Skills (BTIS) and the Staff-Patient Interaction Response Scale (SPIRS).

Variable—Patient-Perceived Empathy

Conceptual Definition. "The patient's feeling of being understood and accepted by the nurse." (Olson, 1995, p. 318)

Operational Definition. Patient-perceived empathy was measured with one instrument, the Barrett-Lennard Relationship Inventory (BLRI).

Variable—Patient Distress

Conceptual Definition. "A negative emotional state." (Olson, 1995, p. 318)

Operational Definition. Patient distress was measured with two instruments, Profile of Mood States Inventory (POMS) and Multiple Affect Adjective Check List (MAACL).

Some researchers believe that the concepts in qualitative studies do not require operational definitions because sensitizing or experiencing the real situation rather than operationalizing the concepts is

most important (Benoliel, 1984). Operational definitions are thought to limit the focus of the investigation so that a phenomenon, such as pain, or a characteristic of a culture, such as the health practices, is not completely experienced or understood from the investigation. In other qualitative studies, the phenomena being examined are not named until the data analysis step. Thus, some concepts may not be identified or defined until late in the study.

■ SUMMARY
. . . .

Research objectives, questions, or hypotheses are formulated to bridge the gap between the more abstractly stated research problem and purpose and the detailed design and plan for data collection and analysis. *Research objectives* are clear, concise, declarative statements that are expressed in the present tense. For clarity, an objective usually focuses on one or two variables (or concepts) and indicates whether the variables are to be identified or described. Sometimes, the foci of objectives include identifying relationships among variables and determining differences between two groups regarding selected variables.

A *research question* is a concise, interrogative statement that is worded in the present tense and consists of one or more variables (or concepts). The foci of questions are descriptions of variables, examination of relationships among variables, and determination of differences between two or more groups regarding selected variables.

A *hypothesis* is the formal statement of the expected relationship or relationships between two or more variables in a specified population. The hypothesis translates the research problem and purpose into a clear explanation or prediction of the expected results or outcomes of the study. Researchers generate hypotheses by observing phenomena or problems in the real world, analyzing theory, and reviewing the literature. Hypotheses can be described in terms of four categories: (1) associative versus causal, (2) simple versus complex, (3) nondirectional versus directional, and (4) null versus research. A hypothesis is developed with the use of inductive and deductive reasoning and is expressed as a declarative statement in the present tense. Testable hypotheses contain variables that can be measured or manipulated, and the hypotheses are evaluated by means of statistical analyses.

Selecting objectives, questions, or hypotheses for a study is based on (1) the number and quality of relevant studies conducted on a selected problem (existing knowledge base), (2) the framework of the study, (3) the expertise and preference of the researcher, and (4) the type of study to be conducted (quantitative or qualitative). The research purpose and objectives, questions, and hypotheses identify the variables to be examined in a study. Variables are concepts of various levels of abstraction that are measured, manipulated, or controlled in a study. The concepts examined in research can be concrete and directly measurable in the real world, such as heart rate, hemoglobin, and lung tidal volume. These concrete concepts are usually referred to as variables in a study. Other concepts, such as anxiety, coping, and pain, are more abstract and are indirectly observable in the world.

Variables are qualities, properties, or characteristics of persons, things, or situations that change or vary. The types of variables discussed in this chapter are independent, dependent, research, extraneous, demographic, moderator, and mediator. An independent variable is a stimulus or intervention that is manipulated or varied by the researcher to create an effect on the dependent variable. A dependent variable is the response, behavior, or outcome that the researcher wants to predict or explain. *Research variables* or concepts are the qualities, properties, or characteristics that are observed or measured in a study.

Extraneous variables exist in all studies and can affect the measurement of study variables and the relationships among them. These variables are of primary concern in quantitative studies, because they can interfere with obtaining a clear understanding of the relational or causal dynamics within these studies. *Environmental variables* are a type of extraneous variable that make up the setting where the study is conducted. In intervention effectiveness research, extraneous variables are referred to as *context variables* and are examined as part of the design of the study to improve the understanding of their impact on the intervention and outcomes of the study. *Demographic variables* are characteristics or attributes of the subjects that are collected to describe the sample. These variables are collected through the use of a demographic or information sheet, and the data are analyzed to provide a picture of the sample, or sample characteristics. *Moderator and mediator variables* are studied in intervention effectiveness research to obtain a complete understanding of the complex relationship between the intervention and the outcomes of the study.

The variables or concepts in a study require conceptual and operational definitions. *A conceptual definition* provides the theoretical meaning of a concept or variable and is derived from a theorist's definition of the concept or is developed through concept analysis. The study framework, which includes concepts and their definitions, provides a basis for conceptually defining the variables. The conceptual definition provides a basis for formulating an operational definition. *An operational definition* is derived from a set of procedures or progressive acts that a researcher performs either to manipulate an independent variable or to measure the existence or degree of existence of the dependent variable. Operational definitions need to be independent of time and setting, so that variables can be investigated at different times and in different settings with the use of the same definitions. Operational definitions in quasi-experimental and experimental studies are specific and precisely developed. In qualitative studies, the definitions of concepts are fairly abstract and broad so that the scope of the investigation is not limited.

● ●

REFERENCES

Aamodt, A. M. (1983). Problems in doing nursing research: Developing a criteria for evaluating qualitative research. *Western Journal of Nursing Research, 5*(4), 398–402.

Ajzen, I. (1985). From intention to action: A theory of planned behavior. In J. Kuhl & J. Beckmann (Eds.), *Action control: From cognition to behavior* (pp. 11–39). New York: Springer.

American Psychological Association (1994). Diagnostic and statistical manual of mental disorders (4th ed.). Washington, D. C.: Author.

Anderson, B., Higgins, L., & Rozmus, C. (1999). Critical pathways: Application to selected patient outcomes following coronary artery bypass graft. *Applied Nursing Research, 12*(4), 168–174.

Armstrong, R. L. (1981). Hypothesis formulation. In S. D. Krampitz & N. Pavlovich (Eds.), *Readings for nursing research* (pp. 29–39). St. Louis: Mosby.

Beck, C. T. (1998). Postpartum onset of panic disorder. *Image— The Journal of Nursing scholarship, 30*(2), 131–135.

Benoliel, Q. (1984). Advancing nursing science: Qualitative approaches. *Western Journal of Nursing Research, 6*(3), 1–8.

Beveridge, W. B. (1950). *The art of scientific investigation.* New York: Vintage Books.

Brown, J. S., Tanner, C. A., & Padrick, K. P. (1984). Nursing's search for scientific knowledge. *Nursing Research, 33*(1), 26–32.

Brown, S. C. (1997). Chest pain and cocaine use in 18 to 40-year-old persons: A retrospective study. *Applied Nursing Research, 10*(3), 136–142.

Chang, B. L. (1999). Cognitive-behavioral intervention for homebound caregivers of persons with dementia. *Nursing Research, 48*(3), 173–182.

Chinn, P. L., & Kramer, M. K. (1999). *Theory and nursing: Integrated knowledge development* (5th ed.). St. Louis: Mosby.

Corff, K. E., Seideman, R., Venkataraman, P. S., Lutes, L., & Yates, B. (1995). Facilitated tucking: A nonpharmacological comfort measure for pain in preterm neonates. *Journal of Obstetric, Gynecologic, and Neonatal Nursing, 24*(2), 143–147.

Fagerhaugh, S. Y., & Strauss, A. (1977). *Politics of pain management.* Menlo Park, CA: Addison-Wesley.

Fahs, P. S., & Kinney, M. R. (1991). The abdomen, thigh, and arm as sites for subcutaneous sodium heparin injections. *Nursing Research, 40*(4), 204–207.

Fawcett, J., & Downs, F. S. (1986). *The relationship of theory and research.* Norwalk, CT: Appleton-Century-Crofts.

Georges, J. M., & Heitkemper, M. M. (1994). Dietary fiber and distressing gastrointestinal symptoms in midlife women. *Nursing Research, 43*(6), 357–361.

Hargreaves, A., & Lander, J. (1989). Use of transcutaneous electrical nerve stimulation for postoperative pain. *Nursing Research, 38*(3), 159–161.

Harris, R. M., Bausell, R. B., Scott, D. E., Hetherington, S. E., & Kavanagh, K. H. (1998). An intervention for changing high-risk HIV behaviors of African American drug-dependent women. *Research in Nursing & Health, 21*(3), 239–250.

Jadack, R. A., Hyde, J. S., & Keller, M. L. (1995). Gender and knowledge about HIV, risky sexual behavior, and safer sex practices. *Research in Nursing & Health, 18*(4), 313–324.

Jennings-Dozier, K. (1999). Predicting intentions to obtain a Pap smear among African American and Latina women: Testing the theory of planned behavior. *Nursing Research, 48*(4), 198–205.

Jirovec, M. M., & Kasno, J. (1990). Self-care agency as a function of patient-environmental factors among nursing home residents. *Research in Nursing & Health, 13*(5), 303–309.

Kaplan, A. (1964). *The conduct of inquiry: Methodology for behavioral science.* New York: Harper & Row.

Keats, M. R., Courneya, K. S., Danielsen, S., & Whitsett, S. F. (1999). Leisure-time physical activity and psychosocial well-being in adolescents after cancer diagnosis. *Journal of Pediatric Oncology Nursing, 16*(4), 180–188.

Kemp, M. G., Keithley, J. K., Smith, D. W., & Morreale, B. (1990). Factors that contribute to pressure sores in surgical patients. *Research in Nursing & Health, 13*(5), 293–301.

Kerlinger, F. N. (1986). *Foundations of behavioral research* (3rd ed.). New York: Holt, Rinehart & Winston.

Koniak, D. (1985). Autotutorial and lecture-demonstration instruction: A comparative analysis of the effects upon students' learning of a developmental assessment skill. *Western Journal of Nursing Research, 7*(1), 80–100.

Manion, J. (1990). Preparing children for hospitalization, procedures, or surgery. In M. Craft & J. Denehy (Eds.), *Nursing interventions for infants and children.* Philadelphia: W. B. Saunders.

McFarlane, J., & Parker, B. (1994). *Abuse during pregnancy: A protocol for prevention and intervention.* New York: National March of Dimes Birth Defects Foundation.

Melzack, R., & Wall, P. D. (1984). *The challenge of pain.* Suffolk, Great Britain: Chaucer Press.

Metz, A., Sichel, D., & Goff, D. (1988). Postpartum panic disorder. *Journal of Clinical Psychiatry, 49*(7), 278–279.

Moody, L. E. (1990). *Advancing nursing science through research* (Vol. 1). Newbury Park, CA: Sage.

Moody, L. E., Wilson, M. E., Smyth, K., Schwartz, R., Tittle, M., & Van Cott, M. L. (1988). Analysis of a decade of nursing practice research: 1977–1986. *Nursing Research, 37*(6), 374–379.

Olson, J. K. (1995). Relationships between nurse-expressed empathy, patient-perceived empathy and patient distress. *Image—The Journal of Nursing Scholarship, 27*(4), 317–322.

Parker, B., McFarlane, J., Soeken, K., Silva, C., & Reel, S. (1999). Testing an intervention to prevent further abuse to pregnant women. *Research in Nursing & Health, 22*(1), 59–66.

Reynolds, P. D. (1971). *A primer in theory construction.* Indianapolis, IN: Bobbs-Merrill.

Sidani, S., & Braden, C. J. (1998). *Evaluating nursing interventions: A theory-driven approach.* Thousand Oaks, CA: Sage.

Taylor, D. (1999). Effectiveness of professional–peer group treatment: Symptom management for women with PMS. *Research in Nursing & Health, 22*(6), 496–511.

Wilson, C. J. (1999). Parental preparation of children for routine physical examinations. *Journal of Pediatric Nursing, 14*(5), 329–335.

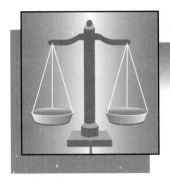

CHAPTER 9
....

ETHICS AND RESEARCH

The conduct of nursing research requires not only expertise and diligence but also honesty and integrity. Conducting research ethically starts with the identification of the study topic and continues through the publication of the study. Over the years, ethical codes and regulations have been developed to provide guidelines for (1) the selection of the study purpose, design, methods of measurement, and subjects; (2) the collection and analysis of data; (3) the interpretation of results; and (4) the presentation and publication of the study. Promoting ethical research is still a significant concern, because a few published studies contain evidence that subjects' rights were violated during the performance of the studies (Beecher, 1966; Nelson-Marten & Rich, 1999).

An ethical problem that received greater attention in the 1980s and 1990s is scientific or research misconduct (Hawley & Jeffers, 1992; Rankin & Esteves, 1997). *Research misconduct* involves practices such as (1) the fabrication, falsification, or forging of data; (2) dishonest manipulation of the design or methods; and (3) plagiarism (Powledge, 1999). Misconduct has occurred during the performance, reporting, and publication of research, with "one half of the top 50 research institutions in the United States having had fraud investigations" (Chop & Silva, 1991, p. 166). Thus, many disciplines, including nursing, are concerned about the quality of their research-generated knowledge base (Rankin & Esteves, 1997).

Ethical research is essential to generate sound knowledge for practice, but what does the ethical conduct of research involve? This is a question that has been debated for many years by researchers, politicians, philosophers, lawyers, and even research subjects. The debate about ethics and research continues, probably because of the complexity of human rights issues; the focus of research in new, challenging arenas of technology and genetics; the complex ethical codes and regulations governing research; and the variety of interpretations of these codes and regulations.

Even though the phenomenon of the ethical conduct of research defies precise delineation, certain historical events, ethical codes, and regulations presented in the chapter provide guidance for nurse researchers. The chapter also discusses the following ethical actions essential in research: (1) protecting the rights of human subjects, (2) balancing benefits and risks in a study, (3) obtaining informed consent, and (4) submitting a research proposal for institutional review. The chapter concludes with a consideration of two timely ethical issues in research, research misconduct and the use of animals in studies.

HISTORICAL EVENTS AFFECTING THE DEVELOPMENT OF ETHICAL CODES AND REGULATIONS

Since the 1940s, the ethical conduct of research has received greater attention because of the mistreatment of human subjects. Four experimental projects have been highly publicized for their unethical treatment of subjects: (1) Nazi medical experiments, (2) the Tuskegee Syphilis Study, (3) the Willowbrook study, and (4) the Jewish Chronic Disease Hospital study. Although these were biomedical studies and the primary investigators were physicians, there is evidence that nurses were aware of the research, identified potential research subjects, delivered treatments to the subjects, and served as data collectors in these projects. The four projects demonstrate the importance of ethical conduct for anyone reviewing, participating in, and conducting nursing or biomedical research. They also influenced the formulation of ethical codes and regulations to direct the conduct of research today.

Nazi Medical Experiments

From 1933 to 1945, atrocious, unethical activities were implemented by the Third Reich in Europe (Steinfels & Levine, 1976). The programs of the Nazi regime consisted of sterilization, euthanasia, and numerous medical experiments to produce a population of racially pure Germans, or Aryans, who were destined to rule the world. The Nazis encouraged population growth among the Aryans ("good Nazis") and sterilized people they regarded as racial enemies, such as the Jews. They also practiced what they called "euthanasia," which involved killing various groups of people whom they considered racially impure, such as the insane, deformed, and senile. In addition, numerous medical experiments were conducted on prisoners of war as well as racially "valueless" persons who had been confined to concentration camps.

The medical experiments involved exposing subjects to high altitudes, freezing temperatures, malaria, poisons, spotted fever (typhus), and untested drugs and operations, usually without any form of anesthesia (Steinfels & Levine, 1976). For example, in the hypothermia studies, subjects were immersed in bath temperatures ranging from 2 to 12°C. The researchers noted that "immersion in water 5°C is tolerated by clothed men for 40 to 60 minutes, whereas raising the water temperature to 15°C increases the period of tolerance to four to five hours" (Berger, 1990, p. 1436). These medical experiments were conducted not only to generate knowledge about human beings but also to destroy certain groups of people. Extensive examination of the rec-

ords from some of the studies showed that they were poorly conceived and conducted. Thus, they generated little if any useful scientific knowledge.

The Nazi experiments violated numerous rights of human research subjects. The selection of subjects for the studies was racially based, demonstrating an unfair selection process. The subjects also had no opportunity to refuse participation; they were prisoners who were coerced or forced to participate. Subjects were frequently killed during, or sustained permanent physical, mental, and social damage as a result of, the experiments (Levine, 1986; Steinfels & Levine, 1976). These studies were not conducted by a few isolated scientists and physicians; they were "the product of coordinated policymaking and planning at high governmental, military, and Nazi Party levels, conducted as an integral part of the total war effort" (Nuremberg Code, 1949, p. 425).

Nuremberg Code

The people involved in the Nazi experiments were brought to trial before the Nuremberg Tribunals, which publicized these unethical activities. The mistreatment of human subjects in these studies led to the development of the *Nuremberg Code* in 1949. This ethical code of conduct contains rules, some general, others specific, that were developed to guide investigators in conducting research ethically. The code contains guidelines for (1) voluntary consent; (2) withdrawal of subjects from studies; (3) protection of subjects from physical and mental suffering, injury, disability, and death; and (4) the balance of benefits and risks in a study (see Table 9–1). The Nuremberg Code was formulated mainly to direct the conduct of biomedical research; however, the rules it contains are essential to the conduct of research in other sciences, such as nursing, psychology, and sociology.

Declaration of Helsinki

The Nuremberg Code provided the basis for the development of the Declaration of Helsinki, which was adopted in 1964 and amended in 1975, 1983, and 1989 by the World Medical Association. The

TABLE 9–1
THE NUREMBERG CODE

1. The voluntary consent of the human subject is absolutely essential.

2. The experiment should be such as to yield fruitful results for the good of society, unprocurable by other methods or means of study, and not random and unnecessary in nature.

3. The experiment should be so designed and based on the results of animal experimentation and a knowledge of the natural history of the disease or other problem under study that the anticipated results will justify the performance of the experiment.

4. The experiment should be so conducted as to avoid all unnecessary physical and mental suffering and injury.

5. No experiment should be conducted where there is a priori reason to believe that death or disabling injury will occur, except, perhaps, in those experiments where the experimental physicians also serve as subjects.

6. The degree of risk to be taken should never exceed that determined by the humanitarian importance of the problem to be solved by the experiment.

7. Proper preparations should be made and adequate facilities provided to protect the experimental subject against even remote possibilities of injury, disability, or death.

8. The experiment should be conducted only by scientifically qualified persons. The highest degree of skill and care should be required through all stages of the experiment of those who conduct or engage in the experiment.

9. During the course of the experiment the human subject should be at liberty to bring the experiment to an end if he has reached the physical or mental state where continuation of the experiment seems to him to be impossible.

10. During the course of the experiment the scientist in charge must be prepared to terminate the experiment at any stage, if he has probable cause to believe, in the exercise of the good faith, superior skill, and careful judgment required of him, that a continuation of the experiment is likely to result in injury, disability, or death to the experimental subject.

From The Nuremberg Code. (1949). In R. J. Levine (Ed.), *Ethics and regulation of clinical research* (2nd ed., pp. 425–426). Baltimore-Munich: Urban & Schwarzenberg.

Declaration of Helsinki differentiated therapeutic research from nontherapeutic research. *Therapeutic research* gives the patient an opportunity to receive an experimental treatment that might have beneficial results. *Nontherapeutic research* is conducted to generate knowledge for a discipline, and the results

from the study might benefit future patients but will probably not benefit those acting as research subjects. The Declaration requires that (1) greater care be exercised to protect subjects from harm in nontherapeutic research, (2) there be strong, independent justification for exposing a healthy volunteer to substantial risk of harm just to gain new scientific information, and (3) the investigator protect the life and health of the research subject (Declaration of Helsinki, 1986). The Declaration of Helsinki was adopted by most institutions in which clinical research is conducted. However, neither this document nor the Nuremberg Code has prevented some investigators from conducting unethical research (Beecher, 1966).

Tuskegee Syphilis Study

In 1932, the U.S. Public Health Service (USPHS) initiated a study of syphilis in black men in the small, rural town of Tuskegee, Alabama (Brandt, 1978; Rothman, 1982). The study, which continued for 40 years, was conducted to determine the natural course of syphilis in the adult black man. The research subjects were organized into two groups: One group consisted of 400 men who had untreated syphilis, and the second group of 200 men without syphilis, who served as a control group. Many of the subjects who consented to participate in the study were not informed about the purpose and procedures of the research. Some individuals were unaware that they were subjects in a study.

By 1936, it was apparent that the men with syphilis developed more complications than the control group. Ten years later, the death rate of the group with syphilis was twice as high as that for the control group. The subjects were examined periodically but did not receive treatment for syphilis, even after penicillin was determined to be an effective treatment for the disease in the 1940s (Levine, 1986). Information about an effective treatment for syphilis was withheld from the subjects, and deliberate steps were taken to keep them from receiving treatment (Brandt, 1978).

Published reports of the Tuskegee Syphilis Study first started appearing in 1936, and additional papers were published every 4 to 6 years. No effort was made to stop the study; in fact, in 1969, the U.S. Centers for Disease Control (CDC) decided that it should continue. Numerous individuals were involved in conducting this study, including "three generations of doctors serving in the venereal disease division of the USPHS, numerous officials at the Tuskegee Institute and its affiliated hospital, hundreds of doctors in the Macon County and Alabama medical societies, and numerous foundation officials at the Rosenwald Fund and the Milbank Memorial Fund" (Rothman, 1982, p. 5).

In 1972, an account of the study published in the *Washington Star* sparked public outrage. Only then did the U.S. Department of Health, Education, and Welfare (DHEW) stop the study. The Tuskegee Syphilis Study was investigated and found to be ethically unjustified, but its racial implications were never addressed (Brandt, 1978). There are still many unanswered questions about this study, such as "Where were the checks and balances in the government and health care systems that should have prevented this unethical study from continuing for 40 years?" "Why was an effective treatment withheld from the subjects for several years?" "Why was public outrage the only effective means of halting the study?"

Willowbrook Study

From the mid-1950s to the early 1970s, research on hepatitis was conducted by Dr. Saul Krugman at Willowbrook, an institution for the mentally retarded (Rothman, 1982). The subjects, all children, were "deliberately infected with the hepatitis virus; early subjects were fed extracts of stool from infected individuals and later subjects received injections of more purified virus preparations" (Levine, 1986, p. 70). During the 20-year study, Willowbrook closed its doors to new inmates because of overcrowded conditions. However, the research ward continued to admit new inmates. To gain their child's admission to the institution, the parents were forced to give permission for the child to be a subject in the study.

From the late 1950s to early 1970s, Krugman's research team published several articles describing the study protocol and findings. In 1966, the Wil-

lowbrook study was cited by Beecher in a *New England Journal of Medicine* article as an example of unethical research. The investigators defended injection of the children with the virus by citing their own belief that most of the children would have acquired the infection upon admission to the institution. The investigators also stressed the benefits the subjects received, which were a cleaner environment, better supervision, and a higher nurse-patient ratio on the research ward (Rothman, 1982). Despite the controversy, this unethical study continued until the early 1970s.

Jewish Chronic Disease Hospital Study

Another highly publicized example of unethical research was a study conducted at the Jewish Chronic Disease Hospital in the 1960s. Its purpose was to determine the patients' rejection responses to live cancer cells. Twenty-two patients were injected with a suspension containing live cancer cells that had been generated from human cancer tissue (Hershey & Miller, 1976; Levine, 1986).

The rights of the patients were not protected, because they were not informed that they were taking part in research or that the injections they received were live cancer cells. In addition, the study was never presented to the research committee of the Jewish Chronic Disease Hospital for review; even the physicians caring for the patients were unaware that the study was being conducted. The physician directing the research was an employee of the Sloan-Kettering Institute for Cancer Research, and there was no indication that this institution had conducted a review of the research project (Hershey & Miller, 1976). The research project was conducted without the informed consent of the subjects and without institutional review and had the potential to cause the human subjects injury, disability, and even death.

Other Unethical Studies

In 1966, Henry Beecher published a now classic article describing 22 of the 50 examples of unethical or questionably ethical studies that he had identified in the published literature. The examples, which included the Willowbrook and Jewish Chronic Disease Hospital studies, indicated a variety of ethical problems that were relatively widespread. Consent was mentioned in only 2 of the 50 studies, and many of the investigators had unnecessarily risked the health and lives of their subjects. Beecher (1966, p. 1356) believed that many of the abuses in the research were due to "thoughtlessness and carelessness, not a willful disregard of patients' rights." These studies reinforce the importance of conscientious institutional review and ethical researcher conduct.

U.S. Department of Health, Education, and Welfare Regulations

The continued conduct of harmful, unethical research made additional controls necessary. In 1973, the DHEW published its first set of regulations on the protection of human subjects. By May 1974, clinical researchers were presented with stiff regulations for research involving humans. The DHEW published additional regulations to protect persons having limited capacities to consent, such as the ill, mentally impaired, and dying (Levine, 1986).

In the 1970s, researchers went from having to follow a few vague regulations to needing to follow almost overwhelming guidelines that controlled the research they conducted. All research involving human subjects had to undergo full institutional review. Nursing studies, which commonly involved minimal risks to human subjects, required complete review. Institutional review improved the protection of human subjects; reviewing all studies, however, without regard for the degree of risk involved, overwhelmed the review process and greatly prolonged the time required for a study to be approved.

National Commission for the Protection of Human Subjects of Biomedical and Behavioral Research

Because the issue of protecting human subjects in research was far from resolved by the DHEW regulations, the National Commission for the Protection of Human Subjects of Biomedical and Behavioral Research (1978) was formed. This commission was established by the National Research Act (Public Law 93-348) passed in 1974. The goals of the commission were (1) to identify the basic ethical principles that should underlie the conduct of biomedical and behavioral research involving human subjects and (2) to develop guidelines based on these principles.

The commission developed *The Belmont Report,* which identified three ethical principles as relevant to the conduct of research involving human subjects: the principles of respect for persons, beneficence, and justice. The *principle of respect for persons* holds that persons have the right to self-determination and the freedom to participate or not participate in research. The *principle of beneficence* requires the researcher to do good and "above all, do no harm." The *principle of justice* holds that human subjects should be treated fairly. The commission developed ethical research guidelines based on these three principles and made recommendations to the U.S. Department of Health and Human Services (USDHHS) in the form of *The Belmont Report.* It was dissolved in 1978 (National Commission, 1978).

The USDHHS developed a set of regulations in response to the commission's recommendations in 1981 and revised them in 1983 and 1991. The 1991 regulations, which provide direction for the protection of human subjects in current research, are codified as Title 45, Part 46 of the *Code of Federal Regulations* (CFR), Protection of Human Subjects (45 CFR 46). These regulations provide direction for (1) protection of human subjects in research, (2) documentation of informed consent, and (3) implementation of the institutional review board (IRB) process (USDHHS, 1991). These regulations are available on-line at *http://helix.nih.gov:8001/ohsr/mpa/45cfr46.php3* and are interpreted by the Office of Human Subjects Research (OHSR). The OHSR operates within the National Institutes of Health (NIH), an agency within DHHS (NIH OHSR, 1991). The OHSR promotes the protection of human subjects' rights in research and other responsibilities, which are detailed on their website at *http://helix.nih.gov:8001/ohsr.*

PROTECTION OF HUMAN RIGHTS

Human rights are claims and demands that have been justified in the eyes of an individual or by the consensus of a group of individuals. Having rights is necessary for the self-respect, dignity, and health of an individual (Sasson & Nelson, 1971). Researchers and reviewers of research have an ethical responsibility to recognize and protect the rights of human research subjects. The human rights that require protection in research are the (1) right to self-determination, (2) right to privacy, (3) right to anonymity and confidentiality, (4) right to fair treatment, and (5) protection from discomfort and harm (American Nurses Association [ANA], 1985a, 1985b; American Psychological Association [APA], 1982).

Right to Self-Determination

The *right to self-determination* is based on the ethical principle of respect for persons. This principles holds that because humans are capable of self-determination or controlling their own destiny, they should be treated as autonomous agents, who have the freedom to conduct their lives as they choose without external controls. Researchers treat prospective subjects as autonomous agents by informing them about a proposed study and allowing them to voluntarily choose to participate or not. In addition, subjects have the right to withdraw from a study at any time without a penalty (Levine, 1986).

VIOLATION OF THE RIGHT TO SELF-DETERMINATION

A subject's right to self-determination can be violated through the use of (1) coercion, (2) covert data collection, and (3) deception. *Coercion* occurs when an overt threat of harm or excessive reward is intentionally presented by one person to another to obtain compliance (National Commission, 1978). Some subjects are coerced to participate in research because they fear that they will suffer harm or discomfort if they do not participate. For example, some patients believe that their medical or nursing care will be negatively affected if they do not agree

to be research subjects. Sometimes students feel forced to participate in research to protect their grades or prevent negative relationships with the faculty conducting the research. Other subjects are coerced to participate in studies because they believe that they cannot refuse the excessive rewards offered, such as large sums of money, special privileges, and jobs.

An individual's right to self-determination can also be violated if he or she becomes a research subject without realizing it. Some researchers have exposed persons to experimental treatments without their knowledge, a prime example being the Jewish Chronic Disease Hospital study. Most of the patients and their physicians were unaware of the study. The subjects were informed that they were receiving an injection of cells but the word *cancer* was omitted (Beecher, 1966). With *covert data collection,* subjects are unaware that research data are being collected because the investigator develops "descriptions of natural phenomena using information that is provided as a matter of normal activity" (Reynolds, 1979, p. 76). This type of data collection has more commonly been used by psychologists to describe human behavior in a variety of situations, but it has also been used by nursing and other disciplines (APA, 1982). Covert data collection is considered acceptable in some situations but not when research deals with sensitive aspects of a subject's behavior, such as illegal conduct, sexual behavior, or drug and alcohol use (USDHHS, 1991). If covert data collection is used, subjects must be informed of the research activities and the findings at the end of the study.

The use of deception in research can also violate a subject's right to self-determination. *Deception* is the actual misinforming of subjects for research purposes (Kelman, 1967). A classic example of deception is the Milgram (1963) study, in which the subjects were to administer electric shocks to another person. During the study, the subjects thought that they were giving the shocks to another person, but the person was really a professional actor who pretended to feel the shocks. Some subjects experienced severe mental tension, almost to the point of collapse, because of their participation in this study. The use of deception is not uncommon in social and psychological research, but it is a controversial research activity (Kelman, 1967). Nurse researchers considering the use of deception in their studies should examine the ethical and methodological implications of this activity as well as its implications for the future of nursing research.

PERSONS WITH DIMINISHED AUTONOMY

Some persons have diminished autonomy or are vulnerable and less advantaged because of legal or mental incompetence, terminal illness, or confinement to an institution (Levine, 1986; Watson, 1982). These persons require additional protection of their right to self-determination, because they have a decreased ability, or an inability, to give informed consent. In addition, these persons are vulnerable to coercion and deception. Researchers must provide justification for the use of subjects with diminished autonomy, and the need for justification increases as the subjects' risk and vulnerability increase (Levine, 1986). However, in many situations, the knowledge needed to improve nursing care to vulnerable populations can be gained only by studying them.

Legally and Mentally Incompetent Subjects

Children (minors), the mentally impaired, and unconscious patients are legally or mentally incompetent to give informed consent. These individuals lack the ability to comprehend information about a study and to make decisions regarding participation in or withdrawal from the study. They have a range of vulnerability from minimal to absolute. The use of persons with diminished autonomy as research subjects is more acceptable if (1) the research is therapeutic so that the subjects have the potential to benefit from the experimental process (Watson, 1982), (2) the researcher is willing to use both vulnerable and nonvulnerable individuals as subjects, and (3) the risk is minimized and the consent process is strictly followed to secure the rights of the prospective subjects (Levine, 1986).

Children. The laws defining the minor status of a child are statutory and vary from state to state. Often a child's competency to consent is governed

by age, with incompetence being nonrefutable up to age 7 years (Broome, 1999; Thompson, 1987). Thus, a child younger than 7 years is not believed to be mature enough to give assent or consent to research. By age 7, however, a child is capable of concrete operations of thought and can give meaningful assent to participate as a subject in studies (Thompson, 1987). With advancing age and maturity, a child should have a stronger role in the consent process.

The federal regulations require "soliciting the assent of the children (when capable) and the permission of their parents or guardians" (NIH OHSR, 1991, 45 CFR Section 46.404). "*Assent* means a child's affirmative agreement to participate in research. *Permission* means the agreement of parent(s) or guardian to the participation of their child or ward in research" (NIH OHSR, 1991, 45 CFR Section 46.402). Using children as research subjects is also influenced by the therapeutic nature of the research and the risks versus the benefits. Thompson (1987) developed a guide for obtaining informed consent that is based on the child's level of competence, the therapeutic nature of the research, and the risks versus the benefits (see Table 9–2). Children who are experiencing a developmental delay, cognitive deficit, emotional disorder, or physical illness must be considered individually (Broome, 1999; Broome & Stieglitz, 1992).

A child 7 years or older with normal cognitive development can provide assent, and the process for obtaining the assent is included in the research proposal. The child must be given information on the study purpose, expectations, and the benefit-risk ratio (discussed later). Videotapes, written materials, demonstrations, diagrams, role-modeling, and peer discussions are methods for communicating study information. The child also needs an opportunity to sign an assent form and to have a copy of this form. An example assent form is presented in Table 9–3. During the study, the child must be given the opportunity to ask questions and to withdraw from the study if he or she desires (Broome, 1999).

In addition to the assent of the child, researchers must obtain permission from the child's parent or guardian for the child's participation. In studies of minimal risk, permission from one parent is usually

TABLE 9–2
GUIDE TO OBTAINING INFORMED CONSENT, BASED ON THE RELATIONSHIP BETWEEN A CHILD'S LEVEL OF COMPETENCE, THE THERAPEUTIC NATURE OF THE RESEARCH, AND RISK VERSUS BENEFIT

	NONTHERAPEUTIC		THERAPEUTIC	
	MMR-LB	MR-LB	MR-HB	MMR-HB
Child, incompetent (generally 0–6 yr)				
Parents' consent	Necessary	Necessary	Sufficient*	Sufficient
Child's assent	Optional†	Optional†	Optional	Optional
Child, relatively competent (7 yr and older)				
Parents' consent	Necessary	Necessary	Sufficient‡	Recommended
Child's assent	Necessary	Necessary	Sufficient§	Sufficient

Key: MMR, more than minimal risk; MR, minimal risk; LB, low benefit; HB, high benefit.

*A parent's refusal can be superseded by the principle that a parent has no power to forbid the saving of a child's life.

†Children making "deliberate objection" would be precluded from participation by most researchers.

‡In cases not involving the privacy rights of a "mature minor."

§In cases involving the privacy rights of a "mature minor."

From Thompson, P. J. (1987). Protection of the rights of children as subjects for research. *Journal of Pediatric Nursing, 2*(6), 397.

sufficient for the research to be conducted. For research that involves more than minimal risk and has no prospect of direct benefit to the individual subject, however, "permission is to be obtained from the parents; both parents must give their permission unless one parent is deceased, unknown, incompetent, or not reasonably available, or when only one parent has legal responsibility for the care and custody of the child" (NIH OHSR, 1991, 45 CFR Section 46.408b).

Adults. Because of mental illness, cognitive impairment, or a comatose state, certain adults are incompetent and incapable of giving informed consent. Persons are said to be incompetent if, in the judgment of a qualified clinician, they have attributes that ordinarily provide the grounds for designating incompetence (Levine, 1986). Incompetence can be temporary (e.g., inebriation), permanent (e.g., advanced senile dementia), or subjective or transitory (e.g., behavior or symptoms of psychosis).

If an individual is judged incompetent and incapable of consent, the researcher must seek approval from the prospective subject and his or her legally authorized representative. A "legally authorized representative means an individual or judicial or other body authorized under applicable law to consent on behalf of a prospective subject to the subject's participation in the procedure(s) involved in the research" (NIH OHSR, 1991, 45 CFR Section 46.102). However, individuals can be judged incompetent and can still assent to participate in certain minimal-risk research if they have the ability to understand what they are being asked to do, to make reasonably free choices, and to communicate their choices clearly and unambiguously (Levine, 1986).

To and Chan (2000) conducted a study to examine the effectiveness of a progressive muscle relaxation program in reducing the aggressive behaviors of mentally handicapped patients. Because these patients were incompetent to give informed consent, the researchers followed a detailed process for obtaining their assent and their parents' or guardians' permission for participation in the study. The following excerpt from their study provides direction for researchers about protecting the rights of persons with diminished autonomy.

TABLE 9–3
SAMPLE ASSENT FORM FOR CHILDREN AGED 6 TO 12 YEARS: PAIN INTERVENTIONS FOR CHILDREN WITH CANCER

Oral explanation

I am a nurse who would like to know if relaxation, special ways of breathing, and using your mind to think pleasant things help children like you to feel less afraid and feel less hurt when the doctor has to do a bone marrow aspiration or spinal tap. Today, and the next 5 times you and your parent come to the clinic, I would like for you to answer some questions about the things in the clinic that scare you. I would also like for you to tell me about how much pain you felt during the bone marrow or spinal tap. In addition, I would like to videotape (take pictures of) you and your mom and/or dad during the tests. The second time you visit the clinic I would like to meet with you and teach you special ways to relax, breathe, and use your mind to imagine pleasant things. You can use the special imagining and breathing then during your visits to the clinic. I would ask you and your parent to practice the things I teach you at home between your visits to the clinic. At any time you could change your mind and not be in the study anymore.

To child

1. I want to learn special ways to relax, breathe, and imagine.
2. I want to answer questions about things children may be afraid of when they come to clinic.
3. I want to tell you how much pain I feel during the tests I have.
4. I will let you videotape me while the doctor does the tests (bone marrow and spinal taps).

If the child says YES, have him/her put an "X" here. _____

If the child says NO, have him/her put an "X" here. _____

Date: _____

Child's signature _____

Broome, M. E. (1999). Consent (assent) for research with pediatric patients. *Seminars in Oncology Nursing, 15*(2), p. 101.

. . . .

Consent for Study

"Before the study, informed consent that described the purpose of the study, potential risk/benefits, right to confidentiality, and right to withdrawal, were distributed and explained to all subjects and their parents/guardians. Because of the subjects' limited cognitive abilities, it was believed that comprehension of the informed consent might pose some difficulty. Therefore, special care and effort were taken to ensure the subjects' understanding of the information in the document. For example, the researchers played a tape about the muscle relaxation training and asked the subjects whether they wanted to learn the exercises. Moreover, all subjects were told that the training would help them to decrease their aggressive behaviors. They were told that the training would enable them to learn new behavior that could be useful when they were unhappy. After a detailed explanation, all subjects showed an understanding of the study. Written consent was gained from the subjects (assent) and subjects' parents/guardians (permission)." (To & Chan, 2000, p. 41) ■

A growing number of people have become permanently incompetent from the advanced stages of senile dementia of the Alzheimer type (SDAT). A minimum of 60% of nursing home residents have this condition (Floyd, 1988). Most long-term care settings have no IRB for research, and the families or guardians of patients in such settings are reluctant to give consent for the patients' participation in research. Nursing research is needed to establish methods of comforting and caring for individuals with SDAT. Floyd (1988) recommended the development of IRBs in long-term care settings and the use of client advocates to assist in the consent process. Levine (1986) identified two approaches that families, guardians, researchers, or IRBs might use when making decisions on behalf of these incompetent individuals: (1) best interest standard and (2) substituted judgment standard. The *best interest standard* involves doing what is best for the individual on the basis of a balancing of risks and benefits. The *substituted judgment standard* is concerned with determining the course of action that incompetent individuals would take if they were capable of making a choice.

Terminally Ill Subjects

When conducting research on terminally ill subjects, the investigator should determine (1) who will benefit from the research and (2) whether it is ethical to conduct research on individuals who might not benefit from the study. Participating in research could have greater risks and minimal or no benefits for these subjects. In addition, the dying subject's condition could affect the study results and lead the researcher to misinterpret the results (Watson, 1982). For example, patients with cancer have become an overstudied population, in whom "it is not unusual for the majority of bloods, bone marrows, lumbar punctures, and biopsies to be conducted for purposes of research, to fulfill protocol requirements" (Strauman & Cotanch, 1988, p. 666).

Many ethical questions have been raised regarding the conduct of research on children with human immunodeficiency virus (HIV) (Twomey, 1994). Biomedical research projects can easily compromise the care of these individuals, posing ethical dilemmas for nurses. More and more nurses will be responsible for ensuring ethical standards in research as they participate in institutional review of research and serve as patient advocates in the clinical setting (Carico & Harrison, 1990; Davis, 1989; McGrath, 1995).

Some terminally ill individuals are willing subjects because they believe that participating in research is a way to contribute to society before they die. Others want to take part in research because they believe that the experimental process will benefit them. Many people infected with HIV or with acquired immunodeficiency syndrome (AIDS) want to participate in AIDS research to gain access to experimental drugs and hospitalized care. However, researchers are concerned because these individuals often do not comply with the research protocol (Arras, 1990). This is a serious dilemma for researchers studying a population with any type of terminal illness, because they must consider the rights of the subjects and must be responsible for conducting high-quality research.

Subjects Confined to Institutions

Hospitalized patients have diminished autonomy because they are ill and are confined in settings that are controlled by health care personnel (Levine, 1986). Some hospitalized patients feel obliged to be research subjects because they want to assist a particular practitioner (nurse or physician) with his or her research. Others feel coerced to participate because they fear that their care will be adversely affected if they refuse. Nurses conducting research with hospitalized patients must make every effort to protect these subjects from feeling coercion.

In the past, prisoners have experienced diminished autonomy in research projects because of their confinement. They might feel coerced to participate in research because they fear harm if they refuse or because they desire the benefits of early release, special treatment, or monetary gain. Prisoners were frequently used for drug studies in which there were no health-related benefits and there was possible harm for them (Levine, 1986). Federal regulations regarding research involving prisoners require that "the risks involved in the research are commensurate with risks that would be accepted by nonprisoner volunteers and procedures for the selection of subjects within the prison are fair to all prisoners and immune from arbitrary intervention by prison authorities or prisoners" (NIH OHSR, 1991, 45 CFR Section 46.305). Researchers must evaluate each prospective subject's capacity for self-determination and protect subjects with diminished autonomy.

Right to Privacy

Privacy is the right an individual has to determine the time, extent, and general circumstances under which personal information will be shared with or withheld from others. Such information consists of one's attitudes, beliefs, behaviors, opinions, and records. The research subject's privacy is protected if the subject is informed and consents to participate in a study and voluntarily shares private information with a researcher (Levine, 1986).

INVASION OF PRIVACY

An *invasion of privacy* occurs when private information is shared without an individual's knowledge or against his or her will. Invading an individual's privacy might cause loss of dignity, friendships, or employment or might create feelings of anxiety, guilt, embarrassment, or shame. Research subjects experience an invasion of privacy most commonly during the data collection process. For example, invasive questions might be asked during an interview, such as "Are you an illegitimate child?" "Were you an abused child?" "What are your sexual activities?" or "Do you use drugs?" Some researchers have gathered data from subjects without their knowledge by taping conversations, observing through one-way mirrors, and using hidden cameras and microphones. Such a situation, because subjects have no knowledge that their words and actions are being shared with a researcher, is an invasion of privacy (Kelman, 1977).

The invasion of subjects' right to privacy brought about the Privacy Act of 1974. As a result of this act, data collection methods are to be scrutinized to protect subjects' privacy, and data cannot be gathered from subjects without their knowledge. Individuals also have the right to access their records and to prevent access by others to their records (Kelman, 1977). One of the reasons for the Privacy Act was the improvements in technology that made it possible to collect and rapidly disseminate data without the knowledge or control of the subject.

Right to Autonomy and Confidentiality

On the basis of the right to privacy, the research subject has the right to anonymity and the right to assume that the data collected will be kept confidential. Complete *anonymity* exists if the subject's identity cannot be linked, even by the researcher, with his or her individual responses (ANA, 1985b; Sasson & Nelson, 1971). In most studies, researchers know the identity of their subjects and promise that their identity will be kept anonymous from others.

Confidentiality is the researcher's management of private information shared by a subject that must not be shared with others without the authorization of the subject. Confidentiality is grounded in the following premises:

- Individuals can share personal information to the extent they wish and are entitled to have secrets.
- One can choose with whom to share personal information.
- People who accept information in confidence have an obligation to maintain confidentiality.
- Professionals, such as researchers, have a "duty to maintain confidentiality that goes beyond ordinary loyalty" (Levine, 1986, p. 164).

BREACH OF CONFIDENTIALITY

A *breach of confidentiality* can occur when a researcher, by accident or direct action, allows an unauthorized person to gain access to the raw data of a study. Confidentiality can also be breached in the reporting or publication of a study when a subject's identity is accidentally revealed, violating the subject's right to anonymity (Ramos, 1989). Breaches of confidentiality can harm subjects psychologically and socially as well as destroy the trust they had in the researcher. Breaches of confidentiality can be especially harmful to a research subject if they involve (1) religious preferences, (2) sexual practices, (3) employment, (4) racial prejudices, (5) drug use, (6) child abuse, and (7) personal attributes, such as intelligence, honesty, and courage.

Some nurse researchers have encountered health care professionals who believe that they should have access to information about the patients in the hospital and will request to see the data the researchers have collected. Sometimes, family members or close friends would like to see the data collected on specific subjects. Sharing research data in these circumstances is a breach of confidentiality. When requesting permission to conduct a study, the nurse researcher should tell health care professionals, family members, and others in the setting that the raw data will not be shared. The research report, including a summary of the data and findings from the study, might be shared with health care providers, family members, and other interested parties.

MAINTAINING CONFIDENTIALITY

Researchers have a responsibility to protect the anonymity of subjects and to maintain the confidentiality of data collected during a study. The anonymity of subjects can be protected by giving each subject a code number. The researcher keeps a master list of the subjects' names and their code numbers in a locked place; for example, subject Mary Jones might be assigned the code number "001." All instruments and forms completed by Mary and data collected by the researcher about her during the study will be identified with the "001" code number, not her name. The master list of subjects' names and code numbers is best kept separate from the data collected to protect subjects' anonymity. Signed consent forms should not be stapled to instruments or other data collection tools; such a practice would make it easy for unauthorized persons to readily identify the subjects and their responses. Consent forms are often stored with the master list of subjects' names and code numbers. The data collected should be entered in the computer with the use of code numbers for identification. The original data collection tools should then be locked in a secure place.

The anonymity of subjects can also be protected by having them generate their own identification codes (Damrosch, 1986). With this approach, each subject generates an individual code from personal information, such as the first letter of a mother's name, the first letter of a father's name, the number of brothers, the number of sisters, and middle initial. Thus, the code would be composed of three letters and two numbers, such as "BD21M." This code would be identified on each form that the subject completes. The subject's identity would be anonymous even for the researcher, who would know only the subject's code. If the data collected are highly sensitive, researchers might want to use this type of coding system.

The data collected should undergo group analysis so that an individual cannot be identified by his or her responses. If the subjects are divided into groups for data analysis and there is only one subject in a group, that subject's data should be combined with that of another group, or the data should be deleted. In writing the research report, the investigator should report the findings so that an individual or group of individuals cannot be identified by their responses.

Maintaining confidentiality is often more difficult in qualitative research than in quantitative research. The nature of qualitative research requires that the "investigator must be close enough to understand the depth of the question under study, and must present enough direct quotes and detailed description to answer the question" (Ramos, 1989, p. 60). The small number of subjects used in a qualitative study and the depth of detail gathered on each subject make it difficult to disguise the subject's iden-

tity. Ford and Reutter (1990) recommend that to maintain confidentiality, the researcher (1) use pseudonyms instead of the participants' names and (2) distort certain details in the subjects' stories while leaving the contents unchanged. Researchers must respect subjects' privacy as they decide how much detail and editing of private information are necessary to publish a study (Robley, 1995).

Researchers should also take precautions during data collection to maintain confidentiality. The interviews conducted with subjects are frequently taped and later transcribed, so the subject's name should not be mentioned on the tape. Subjects have the right to know whether anyone other than the researcher will be transcribing information from the interview. In addition, subjects should be informed on an ongoing basis that they have the right to withhold information (Ford & Reutter, 1990; Robley, 1995).

Right to Fair Treatment

The *right to fair treatment* is based on the ethical principle of justice. This principle holds that each person should be treated fairly and should receive what he or she is due or owed. In research, the selection of subjects and their treatment during the course of a study should be fair.

FAIR SELECTION OF SUBJECTS

In the past, injustice in subject selection has resulted from social, cultural, racial, and sexual biases in society. For many years, research was conducted on categories of individuals who were thought to be especially suitable as research subjects, such as the poor, charity patients, prisoners, slaves, peasants, dying persons, and others who were considered undesirable (Reynolds, 1972, 1979). Researchers often treated these subjects carelessly and had little regard for the harm and discomfort they experienced. The Nazi medical experiments, Tuskegee Syphilis Study, and Willowbrook study all exemplify unfair subject selection and treatment.

The selection of a population to study and the specific subjects to study should be fair; and the risks and benefits of a study should be fairly distributed on the basis of the subject's efforts, needs, and rights. Subjects should be selected for reasons directly related to the problem being studied and not for "their easy availability, their compromised position, or their manipulability" (National Commission, 1978, p. 10).

Another concern with subject selection is that some researchers select certain people as subjects because they like them and want them to receive the specific benefits of a study. Other researchers have been swayed by power or money to make certain individuals subjects so that they can receive potentially beneficial treatments. Random selection of subjects can eliminate some of the researcher's biases that might influence subject selection.

A current concern in the conduct of research is finding an adequate number of appropriate subjects to take part in certain studies. As a solution to this problem, some biomedical researchers have offered physicians finder's fees for identifying research subjects. For example, investigators studying patients with lung cancer would give a physician a fee for every patient with lung cancer the physician referred to them. The ethics of this practice are questionable, because the physician is receiving money for the referral. Are the rights of the patient being protected? Researchers who are using finders' fees should include such information in their proposal, and the institutional human rights review committees must make a decision regarding this practice. Some agencies, such as Massachusetts General Hospital, have reviewed the pros and cons of using finders' fees to obtain research subjects and have decided against the practice (Lind, 1990).

FAIR TREATMENT OF SUBJECTS

Researchers and subjects should have a specific agreement about what the subject's participation involves and what the role of the researcher will be (APA, 1982). While conducting a study, the researcher should treat the subjects fairly and respect that agreement. If the data collection requires appointments with the subjects, the researcher should be on time for each appointment and should terminate the data collection process at the agreed-upon time. The activities or procedures that the subject is to perform should not be changed without the subject's consent.

The benefits promised the subjects should be provided. For example, if a subject is promised a copy of the study findings, he or she should receive one when the study is completed. In addition, subjects who participate in studies should receive equal benefits, regardless of age, race, and socioeconomic level. Treating subjects fairly often facilitates the data collection process and decreases subjects' withdrawal from a study.

Right to Protection from Discomfort and Harm

The right to *protection from discomfort and harm* is based on the ethical principle of beneficence, which holds that one should do good and, above all, do no harm. According to this principle, members of society should take an active role in preventing discomfort and harm and promoting good in the world around them (Frankena, 1973). Therefore, researchers should conduct their studies to protect subjects from discomfort and harm and try to bring about the greatest possible balance of benefits in comparison with harm.

Discomfort and harm can be physiological, emotional, social, and economic in nature. Reynolds (1972) identified the following five categories of studies, which are based on levels of discomfort and harm: (1) no anticipated effects, (2) temporary discomfort, (3) unusual levels of temporary discomfort, (4) risk of permanent damage, and (5) certainty of permanent damage. Each level is defined in the following discussion.

NO ANTICIPATED EFFECTS

In some studies, no positive or negative effects are expected for the subjects. For example, studies that involve reviewing patients' records, students' files, pathology reports, or other documents have no anticipated effects on the subjects. In these types of studies, the researcher does not interact directly with the research subjects. Even in these situations, however, there is a potential risk of invading a subject's privacy.

TEMPORARY DISCOMFORT

Studies that cause temporary discomfort are described as minimal-risk studies, in which the discomfort encountered is similar to what the subject would experience in his or her daily life and ceases with the termination of the experiment. Many nursing studies require the completion of questionnaires or participation in interviews, which usually involve minimal risk for the subjects. The physical discomforts might be fatigue, headache, or muscle tension. The emotional and social risks might entail the anxiety or embarrassment associated with responding to certain questions. The economic risks might consist of the time spent participating in the study or travel costs to the study site. Participation in many nursing studies is considered a mere inconvenience for the subject, with no foreseeable risks or harm.

Most clinical nursing studies examining the impact of a treatment involve minimal risk. For example, a study might involve examining the effects of exercise on the blood glucose levels of diabetics. During the study, the subjects would be asked to test their blood glucose level one extra time per day. There is discomfort when the blood is drawn, and a potential risk of physical changes that might occur with exercise. The subjects might also experience anxiety and fear in association with the additional blood testing, and the testing could be an added expense. The diabetic subjects in this study would experience similar discomforts in their daily lives, and the discomforts would cease with the termination of the study.

UNUSUAL LEVELS OF TEMPORARY DISCOMFORT

In studies that involve unusual levels of temporary discomfort, the subjects commonly experience discomfort both during the study and after its termination. For example, subjects might experience prolonged muscle weakness, joint pain, and dizziness after participating in a study that required them to be confined to bed for 10 days to determine the effects of immobility. Studies that require subjects to experience failure, extreme fear, or threats to their identity or to act in unnatural ways involve unusual levels of temporary discomfort. In some qualitative studies, subjects are asked questions that reopen old emotional "wounds" or involve reliving traumatic events (Ford & Reutter, 1990). For example, asking subjects to describe their rape experience could precipitate feelings of extreme fear, anger, and sadness. In these types of studies, investigators should be vigilant about assessing the subjects' discomfort and should refer them for appropriate professional intervention as necessary.

RISK OF PERMANENT DAMAGE

Subjects participating in some studies have the potential to suffer permanent damage; this potential is more common in biomedical research than in nursing research. For example, medical studies of new drugs and surgical procedures have the potential to cause subjects permanent physical damage. Some topics investigated by nurses have the potential to damage subjects permanently, both emotionally and socially. Studies examining sensitive information, such as sexual behavior, child abuse, or drug use, can be risky for subjects. These types of studies have the potential to cause permanent damage to a subject's personality or reputation. There are also potential economic risks, such as reduced job performance or loss of employment.

CERTAINTY OF PERMANENT DAMAGE

In some research, such as the Nazi medical experiments and the Tuskegee Syphilis Study, the subjects experience permanent damage. Conducting research that will permanently damage subjects is highly questionable, regardless of the benefits that will be gained. Frequently, the benefits gained are for other people but not for the subjects. Studies causing permanent damage to subjects violate the fifth principle of the Nuremberg Code (1949, p. 426), which states, "No experiment should be conducted where there is an a priori reason to believe that death or disabling injury will occur except, perhaps, in those experiments where the experimental physicians (or other health professionals) also serve as subjects."

BALANCING BENEFITS AND RISKS FOR A STUDY

Researchers and reviewers of research must examine the balance of benefits and risks in a study. To determine this balance or benefit-risk ratio, the researcher must (1) predict the outcome of a study, (2) assess the actual and potential benefits and risks on the basis of this outcome, and then (3) maximize the benefits and minimize the risks (see Figure 9–1). The outcome of a study is predicted on the basis of previous research, clinical experience, and theory.

Assessment of Benefits

The probability and magnitude of a study's potential benefits must be assessed. A *research benefit* is defined as something of health-related, psychosocial, or other value to an individual research subject, or something that will contribute to the acquisition of generalizable knowledge. Money and other compensations for participation in research are not benefits but, rather, are remuneration for research-related inconveniences (NIH OHSR, 1991, 45 CFR Section 46.102). In most proposals, the research benefits are described for the individual subjects, the subjects' families, and society. Frequently, opti-

mistic researchers tend to overestimate these benefits (Levine, 1986).

Reviewers of research must be cautious in examining study benefits and balancing the benefits with risks. An important benefit of research is the development and refinement of knowledge, which can affect the individual subject; more importantly, however, this knowledge can have a forceful influence on a discipline and members of society.

The type of research conducted, whether therapeutic or nontherapeutic, affects the potential benefits for the subjects. In therapeutic nursing research, the individual subject has the potential to benefit from the procedures, such as skin care, range of motion, and touch, and other nursing interventions, that are implemented in the study. The benefits might include improvement in the subject's physical condition, which could facilitate emotional and social benefits. In addition, the knowledge generated from the research might expand the subjects' and their families' understanding of health.

The conduct of nontherapeutic nursing research does not benefit the subject directly but is important to generate and refine nursing knowledge. By participating in research, subjects have the potential to increase their understanding of the research process and an opportunity to know the findings from a particular study.

Assessment of Risks

Researchers must assess the type, severity, and number of risks the subjects experience or might experience by participating in a study. The risks involved depend on the purpose of the study and the procedures used to conduct it. Risks can be physical, emotional, social, and economic in nature and can range from no risk or mere inconvenience to the risk of permanent damage (Levine, 1986; Reynolds, 1972). Studies can have actual (known) risks and potential risks for subjects. In a study of the effects of prolonged bed rest, for example, an actual risk would be muscle weakness and the potential risks would include severe muscle cramps or lower extremity thrombophlebitis. Some studies have actual or potential risks for the sub-

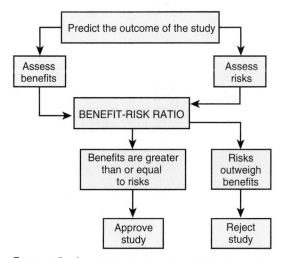

FIGURE 9–1 ■ Balancing benefits and risks for a study.

jects' families and society. The researcher must try to determine the likelihood of the risks and must take precautions to protect the rights of subjects when implementing the research.

Benefit-Risk Ratio

The *benefit-risk ratio* is determined on the basis of the maximized benefits and the minimized risks. The researcher attempts to maximize the benefits and minimize the risks by making changes in the study purpose or procedures or both. If the risks cannot be eliminated or further minimized, the researcher should be able to justify their existence (Levine, 1986). If the risks outweigh the benefits, the study should be revised, or a new study developed. If the benefits equal or outweigh the risks, the researcher can justify conducting the study and it will probably be approved by an IRB (see Figure 9–1).

Say, for example, that you want to balance the benefits and risks of a study that would examine the effect of an exercise and diet program on the participants' serum lipid values (serum cholesterol, low-density lipoprotein [LDL], and high-density lipoprotein [HDL]) and cardiovascular (CV) risk level. The benefits to the participants are exercise and diet instruction and information about their serum lipid values and CV risk level at the start of the program and 1 year later. The potential benefits are improved serum lipid values, lowered CV risk level, and better exercise and dietary habits. The risks consist of the discomfort of having blood specimens drawn twice for serum lipid measurements and the time spent participating in the study (Bruce & Grove, 1994). These discomforts are temporary, are no more than what the subject would experience in his or her daily life, and would cease with the termination of the study. The subjects' time participating in the study can be minimized through organization and precise scheduling of research activities. When you examine the ratio of benefits to risks, you find that (1) the benefits are greater in number and importance than the risks and (2) the risks are temporary and can be minimized. Thus, you could justify conducting this study, and it would receive approval from the IRB.

The obligation to balance the benefits and risks of studies is the responsibility of the researcher, professionals, and society. The researcher must balance the benefits and risks of a particular study and protect the subjects from harm during it. Professionals must participate on IRBs to ensure the conduct of ethical research. Society must be concerned with the benefits and risks of the entire enterprise of research and with the protection of all human research subjects from harm.

OBTAINING INFORMED CONSENT

Obtaining *informed consent* from human subjects is essential for the conduct of ethical research (Brent, 1990; Nusbaum & Chenitz, 1990; Rosse & Krebs, 1999). *Informing* is the transmission of essential ideas and content from the investigator to the prospective subject. *Consent* is the prospective subject's agreement to participate in a study as a subject, which is reached after assimilation of essential information. Prospective subjects, to the degree that they are capable, should have the opportunity to choose whether or not to participate in research. The phenomenon of informed consent was formally defined in the first principle of the Nuremberg Code as follows:

The voluntary consent of the human subject is absolutely essential. . . . This means that the person involved should have *legal capacity* to give consent; should be so situated as to be able to exercise *free power of choice,* without the intervention of any element of force, fraud, deceit, duress, over-reaching or other ulterior form of constraint or coercion; and should have *sufficient knowledge* and *comprehension* of the elements of the subject matter involved as to enable him to make an understanding and enlightened decision. (Nuremberg Code, 1949, p. 425)

This definition of informed consent provided a basis for the discussion of consent in all subsequent codes and regulations and has general acceptance in the research community (Levine, 1986). As indicated in the definition, informed consent consists of four elements: (1) disclosure of essential information, (2) comprehension, (3) competency, and (4) voluntarism. This section describes the elements of informed consent and the methods of documenting consent.

Information Essential for Consent

Informed consent requires the researcher to disclose specific information to each prospective subject. The following information is identified by the *Code of Federal Regulations, Part 46: Protection of Human Subjects*, to be essential for informed consent in research (NIH OHSR, 1991; federal regulations are available on-line at *http://helix.nih.gov: 8001/ohsr/mpa/45cfr46.php3*).

Introduction of Research Activities. The introduction of the research consists of a designation that this activity is a study, the purpose of the study, and an explanation of study procedures. Each prospective subject is given "a statement that the study involves research" and the individual is being asked to participate as a subject (NIH OHSR, 1991, 45 CFR Section 46.116a). In clinical nursing research, the patient, serving as a subject, must know which nursing activities are research activities and which are routine nursing interventions.

The researcher must also provide "an explanation of the purposes of the research and the expected duration of the subject's participation" (NIH OHSR, 1991, 45 CFR Section 46.116a). The purposes of some qualitative studies are broad, so additional information regarding the study goals might be supplied during the study (Ford & Reutter, 1990; Ramos, 1989). If at any point the prospective subjects disagree with the researcher's goals or the intent of the study, they can decline participation.

Prospective subjects receive a complete "description of the procedures to be followed and identification of any procedures which are experimental in the study" (NIH OHSR, 1991, 45 CFR Section 46.116a). Thus, the investigator describes the research variables and the procedures or mechanisms that will be used to observe, examine, manipulate, or measure these variables. In addition, the prospective subjects are informed about when the study procedures will be implemented, how many times, and in what setting.

Description of Risks and Discomforts. Prospective subjects are informed of any "reasonably foreseeable risks or discomforts" (physical, emotional, social, or economic) that might result from the study (NIH OHSR, 1991, 45 CFR Section 46.116a). The investigator then indicates how the risks of the study have been or will be minimized. If the study involves greater than minimal risk, the researcher usually encourages the prospective subjects to consult another person regarding their participation. A trusted advisor, such as a friend, family member, or another nurse, could serve as a consultant (Levine, 1986; Rosse & Krebs, 1999).

Description of Benefits. The investigator also describes "any benefits to the subject or to others which may reasonably be expected from the research" (NIH OHSR, 1991, 45 CFR Section 46.116a). The study might benefit the current subjects or might generate knowledge that will influence patient care in the future.

Disclosure of Alternatives. The investigator must disclose the "appropriate, alternative procedures or courses of treatment, if any, that might be advantageous to the subject" (NIH OHSR, 1991, 45 CFR Section 46.116a). For example, the researchers of the Tuskegee Syphilis Study should have informed the subjects with syphilis that penicillin was an effective treatment for their disease.

Assurance of Anonymity and Confidentiality. Prospective subjects must be given a "statement describing the extent, if any, to which confidentiality of records identifying the subject will be maintained" (NIH OHSR, 1991, 45 CFR Section 46.116a). Thus, subjects must know that their responses and the information obtained from their records during a study will be kept confidential. They also must be assured that their identity will remain anonymous in presentations, reports, and publications of the study.

Compensation for Participation in Research. For research involving more than minimal risks, the prospective subjects must be given an explanation as to whether any compensation or medical treatments or both are available if injury occurs. If medical treatments are available, the type and extent of the treatments are described. When appropriate, the prospective subject is informed as to whether "the particular treatment or procedure may involve risks to the subject (or to the embryo or fetus, if the subject is or may become pregnant) which are currently unforeseeable" (NIH OHSR, 1991, 45 CFR Section 46.116b).

Offer to Answer Questions. The researcher offers to answer any questions that are raised by the prospective subjects. Prospective subjects are provided an "explanation of whom to contact for answers to pertinent questions about the research and research subjects' rights, and whom to contact in the event of a research-related injury" (NIH OHSR, 1991, 45 CFR Section 46.116a) as well as a mechanism for contacting that person.

Noncoercive Disclaimer. A *noncoercive disclaimer* is "a statement that participation is voluntary, refusal to participate will involve no penalty or loss of benefits to which the subject is otherwise entitled" (NIH OHSR, 1991, 45 CFR Section 46.116a). This statement can facilitate a relationship between prospective subjects and the investigator, especially if the relationship has a potential for coercion.

Option to Withdraw. Subjects "may discontinue participation (withdraw from a study) at any time without penalty or loss of benefits" (NIH OHSR, 1991, 45 CFR Section 46.116a). However, researchers do have the right to ask subjects if they think that they will be able to complete the study, to decrease the number of subjects withdrawing early.

There may be circumstances "under which the subject's participation may be terminated by the investigator without regard to the subject's consent" (NIH OHSR, 1991, 45 CFR Section 46.116b). For example, if a particular treatment becomes potentially dangerous to a subject, the researcher has an obligation to discontinue the subject's participation in the study. Thus, prospective subjects are told under what circumstances they might be withdrawn from a study. The researcher also makes a general statement about the circumstances that could lead to the termination of the entire project (Levine, 1986).

Consent to Incomplete Disclosure. In some studies, subjects are not completely informed of the study purpose, because that knowledge would alter the subjects' actions. However, prospective subjects must know that certain information is being withheld deliberately. The researcher ensures that there are no undisclosed risks to the subjects that are more than minimal, and the subjects' questions regarding the study are answered truthfully.

Subjects who are exposed to nondisclosure of information must know when and how they will be debriefed about the study. The researcher *debriefs* the subjects by informing them of the actual purpose of the study and the results that were obtained. If the subjects experience adverse effects related to the study, the researcher ought to make every attempt to reconcile the effects.

Comprehension of Consent Information

Informed consent implies not only the imparting of information by the researcher but also the comprehension of that information by the subject. Studies performed to determine subjects' levels of comprehension after they received the essential information for consent have found the comprehension to be frequently low (Levine, 1986). Researchers must take the time to teach prospective subjects about a study. The amount of information to be taught depends on the subjects' knowledge of research and the specific research project proposed. The purpose, benefits, and risks of the study must be presented clearly in the consent document.

The federal regulations require that the information given to the "subject or the representative shall be in language understandable to the subject or representative" (NIH OHSR, 1991, 45 CFR Section 46.116). Thus, the consent information must be written and verbalized in lay terminology, not professional jargon, and must be presented without the use of loaded or biased terms that might coerce a subject into participating in a study. Meade (1999) identified the following tips for promoting the comprehension of a consent document by potential research subjects:

- Introduce the purpose of the study early in the consent form.
- Outline the study treatment with specificity and conciseness.

- Convey the elements of informed consent in an organized fashion.
- Define technical terms, and be consistent in the use of terminology.
- Use clear terminology and avoid professional jargon.
- Develop the document using headings, upper and lower case letters, and spacing to make it easy to read.
- Use headings for major elements in the consent form, such as "Purpose," "Benefits," and "Risks."
- Use a readable font, that is, a minimum of a size 12–14 for text and size 16–18 for the headers.
- Address the subject directly, using phrases such as, "You are being asked to take part in this study . . . ."
- Estimate the reading level of the document with the use of a computerized readability formula, and revise it to achieve no higher than an eighth grade reading level.

Meade (1999) used these tips to simplify a paragraph from an example consent form, as shown in Table 9–4.

Once the consent document is developed, it should be pilot tested with patients who are comparable to the proposed subjects for the study. These patients can give feedback on the ease of reading, clarity, and understandability of the consent document. The document can then be revised as needed on the basis of the feedback. Using these guidelines can facilitate the development of a high-quality consent document that can be comprehended by the study subjects.

In qualitative research, the subjects might comprehend their participation in a study at the beginning, but unexpected events or consequences might occur during the study to obscure that understanding. These events might precipitate a change in the focus of the research and the type of participation by the subjects. Thus, informed consent is an ongo-

---

TABLE 9–4
SIMPLIFICATION OF CONSENT DOCUMENT

ORIGINAL CONSENT DOCUMENT	REVISED SIMPLIFIED CONSENT DOCUMENT
Example A*: Side effects of the marrow infusion are uncommon and consist primarily of an unusual taste from the preservative, occasional nausea and vomiting, and, rarely, fever and chills. In addition, your chest may feel tight for a while, but that will pass.	*Example A*:* **Side effects of getting stem cells:** ■ An unusual or funny taste in your mouth ■ Mild nausea and vomiting ■ Fever and chills (rarely) ■ Tightness in chest (rarely)
Example B†: The standard approach to treating breast cancer is to give several "cycles" (repeated doses at regularly specified intervals) of a combination of two or more chemotherapy drugs (drugs that kill cancer cells). Recent information suggests that it may be more beneficial to give several cycles of one drug followed by several cycles of another drug. Some researchers think that the second approach may kill more cells that are resistant to chemotherapy. The approach being tested in this study is to administer four cycles of standard chemotherapy (doxorubicin/cyclophosphamide) followed by four cycles of the drug paclitaxel. Researchers hope to show that cancer cells resistant to the doxorubicin/cyclophosphamide chemotherapy may be sensitive to paclitaxel. This may then result in prolonged patient survival and result in a decrease in the number of patients experiencing a recurrence.	*Example B†:* **Why is this study being done?** The purpose of this research study is to find out whether adding the drug Taxol (paclitaxel) to a commonly used chemotherapy is better than the commonly used chemotherapy by itself at preventing your cancer from coming back. The study also will see what side effects there are from adding Taxol to the commonly used chemotherapy. Taxol has been found to be effective in treating patients with advanced breast cancer. In this study, we want to see whether Taxol will help to treat patients with early stage breast cancer and whether the side effects seem to be worth the possible benefit.

*Standard doses versus myeloablative therapy for previously untreated symptomatic multiple myeloma. Phase III. SWOG 9321.
†A randomized trial evaluating the worth of paclitaxel (Taxol) following doxorubicin (Adriamycin)/cyclophosphamide (Cytoxan) in breast cancer.
NCI Model Document Sub-Group: Comprehensive Working Group on Informed Consent, 1998.
From Broome, M. E. (1999). Consent (assent) for research with pediatric patients. *Seminars in Oncology Nursing, 15*(2), p. 130.

ing, evolving process in qualitative research. The researcher must renegotiate the subjects' consent and determine their comprehension of that consent as changes occur in the study. Continually informing and determining the comprehension of subjects establishes trust between the researcher and subjects and promotes ethical, high-quality study outcomes (Munhall, 1999).

ASSESSMENT OF SUBJECTS' COMPREHENSION

The researcher can take steps to determine the prospective subjects' level of comprehension. Silva (1985) studied the comprehension of information for informed consent by spouses of surgical patients and found that 72 of the 75 spouses had adequate comprehension of the consent information. The subjects' comprehension of consent information was assessed using the following questions: "(1) What is the purpose of this study? (2) What risks are involved in the study procedures? (3) What does your participation in this study involve? (4) Approximately how long will your participation in this study take? (5) When can you withdraw from this study? (6) How will your name be associated with the study data? (7) With whom will the study information be shared? and (8) What direct personal benefit will come to you as a result of participating in this study?" (Silva, 1985, p. 121)

Comprehension of consent information becomes more difficult in complex, high-risk studies. In some high-risk studies, the prospective subjects are tested on consent information, and they do not become subjects unless they pass the tests (Hershey & Miller, 1976).

Competency to Give Consent

Autonomous individuals, who are capable of understanding and weighing the benefits and risks of a proposed study, are competent to give consent. The competence of the subject is often determined by the researcher (Douglas & Larson, 1986). Persons with diminished autonomy due to legal or mental incompetence, terminal illness, or confinement to an institution might not be legally competent to consent to participate in research (see the earlier discussion of the right to self-determination). However, the researcher makes every effort to present the consent information at a level potential subjects can understand, so they can assent to the research. In addition, the researcher presents the essential information for consent to the legally authorized representative, such as the parents or guardian, of the prospective subject (Levine, 1986).

Voluntary Consent

Voluntary consent means that the prospective subject has decided to take part in a study of his or her own volition without coercion or any undue influence (Douglas & Larson, 1986). Voluntary consent is obtained after the prospective subject has been given essential information about the study and has shown comprehension of this information. Some researchers, because of their authority, expertise, or power, have the potential to coerce subjects into participating in research. Researchers must make sure that their persuasion of prospective subjects does not become coercion. Thus, the rewards offered in a study ought to be congruent with the risks taken by the subjects.

Documentation of Informed Consent

The documentation of informed consent depends on (1) the level of risk involved in the study and (2) the discretion of the researcher and those reviewing the study. Most studies require a written consent form, although in some studies, the consent form is waived.

WRITTEN CONSENT WAIVED

The requirements for written consent may be waived in research that "presents no more than minimal risk of harm to subjects and involves no procedures for which written consent is normally required outside of the research context" (NIH OHSR, 1991, 45 CFR Section 46.117c). For example, researchers using questionnaires to collect relatively harmless data would not need to obtain a signed consent form from the subjects. The subject's completion of the questionnaire may serve as consent. The top of the questionnaire might contain a statement such as "Your completion of this questionnaire indicates your consent to participate in this study."

Written consent is also waived in a situation when "the only record linking the subject and the research would be the consent document and the principal risk would be potential harm resulting from a breach of confidentiality. Each subject will be asked whether the subject wants documentation linking the subject with the research, and the subject's wishes will govern" (NIH OHSR, 1991, 45 CFR Section 46.117c). Thus, in this situation, subjects are given the option to sign or not sign a consent form that links them to the research. The four elements of consent—disclosure, comprehension, competency, and voluntariness—are essential in all studies whether written consent is waived or required.

WRITTEN CONSENT DOCUMENTS

Short Form Written Consent Document

The *short form* consent document includes the following statement: "The elements of informed consent required by Section 46.116 [see the section on information essential for consent] have been presented orally to the subject or the subject's legally authorized representative" (NIH OHSR, 1991, 45 CFR Section 46.117a). The researcher must develop a written summary of what is to be said to the subject in the oral presentation, and the summary must be approved by an IRB. When the oral presentation is made to the subject or to the subject's representative, a witness is required. The subject or representative must sign the short form consent document. "The witness shall sign both the short form and a copy of the summary, and the person actually obtaining consent shall sign a copy of the summary" (NIH OHSR, 1991, 45 CFR Section 46.117a). Copies of the summary and short form are given to the subject and the witness; the original documents are retained by the researcher. The researcher must keep these documents for 3 years.

The short form written consent documents might be used in studies that present minimal or moderate risk to the subjects.

The Formal Written Consent Document

The written consent document includes the elements of informed consent required by the federal regulations (see the previous section on information essential for consent). In addition, a consent form might include other information required by the institution where the study is to be conducted or by the agency funding the study. A sample *consent form* is presented in Figure 9–2 with descriptors of the essential consent information. The consent form can be read by the subject or read to the subject by the researcher; however, it is wise also to explain the study to the subject. The form is signed by the subject and is witnessed by the investigator or research assistant collecting the data. This type of consent can be used for any type of study from minimal to high-risk. All persons signing the consent form must receive a copy of it, which include the subject, researcher, and any witnesses. The original consent form is kept by the researcher for 3 years.

Studies that involve subjects with diminished autonomy require a written consent form. If these prospective subjects have some comprehension of the study and agree to participate as subjects, they must sign the consent form. However, the form also must be signed by the subject's legally authorized representative. The representative indicates his or her relationship with the subject under the signature (see Figure 9–2).

The written consent form used in a high-risk study often contains the signatures of two witnesses, (1) the researcher and (2) an additional person. The additional person signing as a witness must observe the informed consent process and must not be otherwise connected with the study (Hershey & Miller, 1976). The best witnesses are research subject advocates or patient advocates who are employed in the institution.

Sometimes nurses are asked to sign a consent form as a witness for a biomedical study. They must know the study purpose and procedures and

Study title: The Needs of Family Members of Critically Ill Adults
Investigator: Linda L. Norris, R.N.

Ms. Norris is a registered nurse studying the emotional and social needs of family members of patients in the Intensive Care Units (**research purpose**). Although the study will not benefit you directly, it will provide information that might enable nurses to identify family members' needs and to assist family members with those needs (**potential benefits**).

The study and its procedures have been approved by the appropriate people and review boards at The University of Texas at Arlington and X hospital (**IRB approval**). The study procedures involve no foreseeable risks or harm to you or your family (**potential risks**). The procedures include: (1) responding to a questionnaire about the needs of family members of critically ill patients and (2) completing a demographic data sheet (**explanation of procedures**). Participation in this study will take approximately 20 minutes (**time commitment**). You are free to ask any questions about the study or about being a subject and you may call Ms. Norris at (999) 999-9999 (work) or (999) 999-9999 (home) if you have further questions (**offer to answer questions**).

Your participation in this study is voluntary; you are under no obligation to participate (**voluntary consent**). You have the right to withdraw at any time and the care of your family member and your relationship with the health care team will not be affected (**option to withdraw**).

The study data will be coded so they will not be linked to your name. Your identity will not be revealed while the study is being conducted or when the study is reported or published. All study data will be collected by Ms. Norris, stored in a secure place, and not shared with any other person without your permission (**assurance of anonymity and confidentiality**).

I have read this consent form and voluntarily consent to participate in this study.

(If Appropriate)

_____   _____
Subject's Signature   Date   Legal Representative   Date

I have explained this study to the above subject and have sought his/her understanding for informed consent

_____
Investigator's Signature   Date

FIGURE 9–2 ■ Sample consent form.

the subject's comprehension of the study before signing the form (Carico & Harrison, 1990; Chamorro & Appelbaum, 1988). The role of the witness is more important in the consent process if the prospective subject is in awe of the investigator and does not feel free to question the procedures of the study.

TAPE-RECORDING OR VIDEOTAPING THE CONSENT PROCESS

A researcher might elect to tape-record or videotape the consent process. These methods document what was said to the prospective subject and record the subject's questions and the investigator's answers. Tape-recording and videotaping are time consuming and costly, however, and are not appropriate for studies of minimal or moderate risk. If a study is considered high risk, complete documentation of the consent process with a tape might be wise to protect the subjects and the researcher. Both the researcher and the subject would retain a copy of the tape recording or videotape.

DOCUMENTING CONSENT RATES

Informed consent can be documented in a variety of ways, as previously discussed. Researchers must report the way informed consent was obtained and must document the consent rates. *Consent rate* is a percentage determined by the number of people willing to participate divided by the total number approached. If the consent rate is low, several people refused to participate in the study, which limits the generalizability of the results. Low consent rates can also indicate biased results, because only certain people are willing to participate in the study. A 1994 survey of research articles found that only 41% of the studies reported their consent rate. Of those reporting a consent rate, the mean consent rate was 72%, with rate being higher for clinical than for nonclinical studies (Douglas et al., 1994).

Schaefer and Moos (1996), who studied the effects of work stressors and work climate on job morale and functioning of long-term care staff, provided the following information about the consent rate and informed consent process for their study.

. . . .

"Of the 695 staff who met the study criteria, 84% (585) agreed to participate, and 74% (435) completed the inventories. . . .

"Staff were screened and recruited both by personal contact at work and by telephone at home. A cover letter, the inventories, and a consent form were mailed to staff members who agreed to participate. To ensure confidentiality, staff returned the inventories and signed consent forms in separate postage-paid envelopes." (Schaefer & Moos, 1996, pp. 65–66) ■

In this study, the consent rate was 84%, and informed consent was documented with a formal consent form. However, although 84% of the staff approached about the study consented to participate in it, only 74% of the potential subjects actually did so.

INSTITUTIONAL REVIEW

In *institutional review,* a study is examined for ethical concerns by a committee of the researcher's peers. The first federal policy statement on protection of human subjects by institutional review was issued by the USPHS in 1966. The statement required that research involving human subjects must be reviewed by a committee of peers or associates to confirm that (1) the rights and welfare of the individuals involved were protected, (2) the appropriate methods were used to secure informed consent, and (3) the potential benefits of the investigation were greater than the risks (Levine, 1986).

In 1974, DHEW passed the National Research Act, which required that all research involving human subjects undergo institutional review. The DHHS reviewed and revised these guidelines in 1981, 1983, and 1991. The regulations describe the membership, functions, and operations of an institutional review board. An *institutional review board* (IRB) is a committee that reviews research to ensure that the investigator is conducting the research ethically. Universities, hospital corporations, and many managed care centers have IRBs to promote the conduct of ethical research and protect the rights of prospective subjects at their institutions.

Each IRB has at least five members of varying background (cultural, economic, educational, gender, racial) to promote complete and adequate review of research that is commonly conducted in an institution. The members must have sufficient experience and expertise to review research and must not have conflicting interest related to the research conducted in the institution. The IRB also must include other members whose primary concern is nonscientific, such as an ethicist, lawyer, or minister. At least one of the members ought to be someone who is not affiliated with the institution (NIH OHSR, 1991, 45 CFR Section 46.107a–f). The IRBs in hospitals are often composed of physicians, lawyers, scientists, clergy, community lay persons, and, more recently, nurses (Chamorro & Appelbaum, 1988).

Levels of Reviews Conducted by Institutional Review Boards

The functions and operations of an IRB involve the review of research at three different levels: (1) exempt from review, (2) expedited review, and (3) complete review. The level of the review required for each study is decided by the IRB chairperson or committee or both, not by the researcher.

Studies are usually *exempt* from review if they pose no apparent risks for the research subjects. The studies that are usually considered exempt from review by the federal regulations are identified in Table 9–5. Nursing studies that have no foreseeable risks or are a mere inconvenience for subjects are usually identified as exempt from review by the chairperson of the IRB committee.

TABLE 9–5
RESEARCH QUALIFYING FOR EXEMPTION FROM REVIEW

Unless otherwise required by department or agency heads, research activities in which the only involvement of human subjects will be in one or more of the following categories are exempt from review.

(1) Research conducted in established or commonly accepted educational settings, involving normal educational practices, such as (i) research on regular and special education instructional strategies, or (ii) research on the effectiveness of or the comparison among instructional techniques, curricula, or classroom management methods.

(2) Research involving the use of educational tests (cognitive, diagnostic, aptitude, achievement), survey procedures, interview procedures or observation of public behavior, unless:

(i) information obtained is recorded in such a manner that human subjects can be identified, directly or through identifiers linked to the subjects; and (ii) any disclosure of the human subjects' responses outside the research could reasonably place the subjects at risk of criminal or civil liability or be damaging to the subjects' financial standing, employability, or reputation.

(3) Research involving the use of educational tests (cognitive, diagnostic, aptitude, achievement), survey procedures, interview procedures, or observation of public behavior that is not exempt under paragraph (b)(2) of this section, if:

(i) the human subjects are elected or appointed public officials or candidates for public office; or (ii) Federal statute(s) require(s) without exception that the confidentiality of the personally identifiable information will be maintained throughout the research and thereafter.

(4) Research involving the collection or study of existing data, documents, records, pathological specimens, or diagnostic specimens, if these sources are publicly available or if the information is recorded by the investigator in such a manner that subjects cannot be identified, directly or through identifiers linked to the subjects.

(5) Research and demonstration projects which are conducted by or subject to the approval of Department or Agency heads, and which are designed to study, evaluate, or otherwise examine:

(i) Public benefit or service programs; (ii) procedures for obtaining benefits or services under those programs; (iii) possible changes in or alternatives to those programs or procedures; or (iv) possible changes in methods or levels of payment for benefits or services under those programs.

(6) Taste and food quality evaluation and consumer acceptance studies, (i) if wholesome foods without additives are consumed or (ii) if a food is consumed that contains a food ingredient at or below the level and for a use found to be safe, or agricultural chemical or environmental contaminant at or below the level found to be safe, by the Food and Drug Administration or approved by the Environmental Protection Agency or the Food Safety and Inspection Service of the U.S. Department of Agriculture.

From National Institutes of Health, Office of Human Subjects Research. (1991). Protection of human subjects. *Code of Federal Regulations,* Title 45 Public Welfare, Part 46.

Excerpted from *Federal Register* of June 18, 1991 [DHHS, 1991, Section 46.101b]. Available on-line: http://helix.nih.gov.8001/chb/mpa/45cfr46.php3.

Studies that have some risks, which are viewed as minimal, are expedited in the review process. *Minimal risk* means "that the risks of harm anticipated in the proposed research are not greater, considering probability and magnitude, than those ordinarily encountered in daily life or during the performance of routine physical or psychological examinations or tests" (NIH OHSR, 1991, 45 CFR Section 46.102i).

Expedited review procedures can also be used to review minor changes in previously approved research (NIH OHSR, 1991, 45 CFR Section 46.110b). Under *expedited review* procedures, "the review may be carried out by the IRB chairperson or by one or more experienced reviewers designated by the chairperson from among members of the IRB. In reviewing the research, the reviewers may exercise all of the authorities of the IRB except disapproval of the research. A research activity may be disapproved only after review in accordance with the nonexpedited procedure" (NIH OHSR, 1991, 45 CFR Section 46.110b). Table 9–6 identifies research that usually qualifies for expedited review.

Studies that have greater than minimal risks must receive a complete review by an IRB. To obtain IRB approval, researchers must ensure that (1) risks to subjects are minimized, (2) risks to subjects are reasonable in relation to anticipated benefits, (3) selection of subjects is equitable, (4) informed consent will be sought from each prospective subject or the subject's legally authorized representative, (5) informed consent will be appropriately documented, (6) the research plan makes adequate provision for monitoring data collection for subjects' safety, and (7) adequate provisions are made to protect the privacy of subjects and to maintain the confidentiality of data (NIH OHSR, 1991, 45 CFR Section 46.111a). The process of seeking approval from a research review committee to conduct a study is described in Chapter 28.

Published studies often indicate that the research project was approved by an IRB. For example Mahon and colleagues (2000) studied the positive and negative outcomes of anger in early adolescence and identified the IRB approval and consent process for their study, as described in the following excerpt. The subjects in this study were boys and girls 12 to 14 years old; such subjects can assent to

TABLE 9-6
RESEARCH QUALIFYING FOR EXPEDITED INSTITUTIONAL REVIEW BOARD REVIEW

Expedited review (by committee chairpersons or designated members) for the following research involving no more than minimal risk is authorized:

1. Collection of: hair and nail clippings, in a nondisfiguring manner; deciduous teeth and permanent teeth if patient care indicates a need for extraction.
2. Collection of excreta and external secretions including sweat, uncannulated saliva, placenta removed at delivery, and amniotic fluid at the time of rupture of the membrane prior to or during labor.
3. Recording of data from subjects 18 years of age or older using noninvasive procedures routinely employed in clinical practice. This includes the use of physical sensors that are applied either to the surface of the body or at a distance and do not involve input of matter or significant amounts of energy into the subject or an invasion of the subject's privacy. It also includes such procedures as weighing, testing sensory acuity, electrocardiography, electroencephalography, thermography, detection of naturally occurring radioactivity, diagnostic echography, and electroretinography. It does not include exposure to electromagnetic radiation outside the visible range (for example, x-rays, microwaves).
4. Collection of blood samples by venipuncture, in amounts not exceeding 450 milliliters in an eight-week period and no more than two times per week, from subjects 18 years of age or older and who are in good health and not pregnant.
5. Collection of both supra- and subgingival dental plaque and calculus, provided the procedure is not more invasive than routine prophylactic scaling of the teeth and the process is accomplished in accordance with accepted prophylactic techniques.
6. Voice recordings made for research purposes such as investigations of speech defects.
7. Moderate exercise by health volunteers.
8. The study of existing data, documents, records, pathological specimens, or diagnostic specimens.
9. Research on individual or group behavior or characteristics of individual, such as studies of perception, cognition, game theory, or test development, where the investigator does not manipulate subjects' behavior and research will not involve stress to subjects.
10. Research on drugs or devices for which an investigational new drug exemption or an investigational device exemption is not required.

From National Institutes of Health, Office of Human Subjects Research. (1991). Protection of human subjects. *Code of Federal Regulations,* Title 45 Public Welfare, Part 46.
Excerpted from *Federal Register* of June 18, 1991 [DHHS, 1991, Section 46.110]. (Additional regulations that apply to research involving fetuses, pregnant women, human in vitro fertilization, and prisoners are available in the *Federal Register,* 1991, paA 46.) Available on-line: http://helix.nih.gov.8001/ohrs/mpa/45cfr46.php3

subjects were adolescents with diminished autonomy, a full review by an IRB probably would have been required.

● ●

"After approval to conduct the study was granted by the university Institutional Review Board, access was gained to an urban middle school. The principal and seventh and eighth grade teachers reviewed and approved the instrument packets for appropriateness of content and reading levels for seventh and eighth graders, except for those in special education classes.

"One week prior to testing, all seventh and eighth graders who were not in special education classes received a packet containing an explanation about the study and a consent form for their parents. On the testing date one week later, students who had parental consent and gave informed consent (assent) as well participated in the study." (Mahon et al., 2000, pp. 20–21) ■

Proposed Reform of Institutional Review Boards

In the 1990s, concerns were expressed about the quality of the research reviews conducted by IRBs in a variety of educational and clinical facilities. The Office of the Inspector General, at USDHHS, began a review of IRBs and noted that their effectiveness was in jeopardy. A report issued in June of 1998 pointed to the need for reform of the IRBs because of the following problems:

(1) IRBs face major changes in the research environment as research becomes more commercialized, as research becomes more multicentered, as the number of proposals increases, and as consumer demand for access to research increases; (2) IRBs review too much, too quickly, and with too little expertise; (3) IRBs provide minimal training for investigators and board members; and (4) neither review boards nor the DHHS devote much time or emphasis to evaluation of effectiveness. (Nelson-Marten & Rich, 1999, p. 87)

The review of IRBs is continuing, with a plan to identify and implement relevant reforms. Since 1998, federal regulators have become much more involved in monitoring the activities of institutional

participate in research, but permission for participation must be obtained from their parents or guardians. This study had minimal risks, but because the

IRBs and researchers. The regulators have imposed an unprecedented number of suspensions of institutional research projects involving human subjects. The institutions were cited for not following mandatory federal guidelines to safeguard the safety and dignity of the human subjects. The federal regulators believed that the institutions were putting human subjects at risk, and the research institutions believed that the regulators were overreaching in their enforcement of IRB rules. These issues will be a focus in the future, because millions of dollars of research funds from NIH and pharmaceutical companies are at stake (Brainard, 2000).

RESEARCH MISCONDUCT

The goal of research is to generate sound scientific knowledge, which is possible only through the honest conduct, reporting, and publication of studies. During the 1980s, however, a number of fraudulent studies were conducted and then were published in prestigious scientific journals.

An example of scientific misconduct was evident in the publications of Dr. Robert Slutsky, a heart specialist at the University of California, San Diego, School of Medicine. He resigned in 1986 when confronted with inconsistencies in his research publications. His publications contained "statistical anomalies that raised the question of data fabrication" (Friedman, 1990, p. 1416). In 6 years, Slutsky published 161 articles, and at one time, he was completing an article every 10 days. Eighteen of the articles were found to be fraudulent and have retraction notations, and 60 articles were judged to be questionable (Friedman, 1990; Henderson, 1990).

Stephen Breuning, a psychologist at the University of Pittsburgh, engaged in deceptive and misleading practices in reporting his research on retarded children. He used his fraudulent research to obtain more than $300,000 in federal grants. In 1988, he was criminally charged with research fraud, pleaded guilty, was fined $20,000, and was sentenced to up to 10 years in prison (Chop & Silva, 1991; Garfield & Welljams-Dorof, 1990; Leino-Kilpi & Tuomaala, 1989).

In 1989, two new federal agencies were organized for the reporting and investigation of scientific misconduct. The Office of Research Integrity Review (ORIR) was established to manage scientific misconduct by grant recipients. The Office of Research Integrity (ORI) supervises the implementation of the rules and regulations related to scientific misconduct and manages any investigations (USDHHS, 1989; Hawley & Jeffers, 1992). The investigations by these federal agencies revealed a variety of fraudulent behaviors. In some situations, the fraudulent studies were never conducted, and the data and results were fabricated by the researchers. In other cases, the findings were consciously distorted, or the works of other researchers were plagiarized. Some of the common types of scientific misconduct are presented in Table 9–7 (Larson, 1989).

Proposed Policy for Research

Scientific misconduct continued to be a major concern in the 1990s, with evidence of fabrication of research results, falsification of steps of the research process, and plagiarism in research presentations and publications. In 1993, the ORI was formed to protect the integrity of the USPHS's extramural and intramural research programs. The ex-

TABLE 9–7 DISHONESTY IN RESEARCH	
TYPE	**DESCRIPTION**
Fabrication, falsification, or forging	Deliberate invention of nonexistent information
Manipulation of design or methods	Intentional planning of the study design or data collection methods so that the results will be biased toward the research hypothesis
Selective retaining or manipulation of data	Choosing only data that are consistent with the research hypothesis and discarding the rest
Plagiarism	Intentional representation of the work or ideas of others as one's own, or rewording one's own work to produce a new paper based on the same data; abuse of confidentiality of information from others
Irresponsible collaboration	Failure to participate appropriately in an investigative team or fulfill responsibilities as a coauthor

Reprinted from Larson, E. (1989). Maintaining quality in clinical research and evaluation: When corrective action is necessary. *Journal of Nursing Care Quality, 3*(4), 30, © 1989, Aspen Publishers.

tramural program provides funding to research institutions, and the intramural program provides funding for research conducted within the federal government. The current functions of the ORI are as follows (U.S. Department of Health and Human Services, Office of Research Integrity [USDHHS ORI], 2000):

- Develop and promulgate policies, procedures, rules, and regulations aimed at preventing, monitoring, and imposing administrative actions concerning misconduct and protecting whistle blowers from retaliation
- Administer an assurance program
- Review completed investigations conducted by applicant or awardee institutions
- Provide on-site technical assistance to institutions during inquiries and investigations when requested
- Review institutional findings and recommend administrative actions to the Assistant Secretary of Health, who makes the final decisions regarding misconduct, subject to appeal
- Present misconduct findings in administrative hearings before the DHHS Departmental Appeals Board (DAB)
- Promote scientific integrity through a variety of educational programs and activities

In 1996, a review and revision of the existing scientific misconduct policy were initiated to (1) develop a uniform research misconduct policy across the agencies of the federal government, (2) establish a policy that addresses behavior that has the potential to affect the integrity of the research record, and (3) develop a procedure to safeguard the handling of allegations of research misconduct. The revision took 3 years, and the proposed policy on research misconduct was published on the World Wide Web for comment until December 13, 1999 (*http://ori/ dhhs.gov/fedreg101499.htm*). This policy is expected to have been finalized late in 2000.

The revised policy on scientific misconduct contains the following definitions:

Research misconduct is defined as fabrication, falsification, or plagiarism in proposing, performing, or reviewing research, or in reporting research results. *Fabrication* is making up results and recording or reporting them. *Falsification* is manipulating research materials,

equipment, or processes, or changing or omitting data or results such that the research is not accurately represented in the research record. *Plagiarism* is the appropriation of another person's ideas, processes, results, or words without giving appropriate credit, including those obtained through confidential review of others' research proposals and manuscripts. Research misconduct does not include honest error or honest differences of opinion. (USDHHS ORI, 1999)

The policy holds that to be classified as research misconduct, an act must meet the following criteria: (1) the act involves a significant departure from the acceptable practice of the scientific community for maintaining the integrity of the research record; (2) the act was committed intentionally; and (3) the allegation can be proved by a preponderance of evidence.

The policy also addresses the responsibilities of federal agencies and research institutions in maintaining the integrity of the research process. Guidelines are provided to assist agencies and research institutions to develop fair and timely procedures for responding to allegations of research misconduct. The administrative actions taken in a situation depend on the seriousness of the misconduct. The actions available include, "but are not limited to, letters of reprimand; the imposition of special certification or assurance requirements to ensure compliance with applicable regulations or terms of an award; suspension or termination of an active award; or suspension and debarment" (USDHHS ORI, 1999). If criminal violations are suspected, the agency is to refer the situation to the appropriate criminal investigative body.

Editors of journals have a major role in monitoring and preventing research misconduct in the published literature. Friedman (1990) identified criteria for classifying a publication as fraudulent, questionable, or valid. According to these criteria, research articles were classified as "*fraudulent* if there was documentation or testimony from coauthors that the publication did not reflect what had actually been done" (Friedman, 1990, p. 1416). Articles were considered *questionable* if no coauthor could produce the original data or if no coauthor had personally observed or performed each phase of the research or participated in the research publication. A research article was considered *valid* "if some coauthor had personally performed or participated in each aspect of the research and publication" (Friedman, 1990, p. 1416).

Preventing the publication of fraudulent research requires the efforts of authors, coauthors, reviewers, and editors (Hansen & Hansen, 1995; Hawley & Jeffers, 1992; Relman, 1990). Authors who are primary investigators for research projects must be responsible in their conduct, reporting, and publication of research. Coauthors and coworkers should question and, if necessary, challenge the integrity of a researcher's claims. Sometimes, well-known scientists have been added to a research publication as coauthors to give it credibility. Individuals should not be listed as coauthors unless they were actively involved in the conduct and publication of the research.

Peer reviewers have a key role in determining the quality and publishability of a manuscript. They are considered experts in the field, and their role is to examine research for inconsistencies and inaccuracies. Editors must monitor the peer review process and must be cautious about publishing manuscripts that are at all questionable. Editors also need procedures for responding to allegations of research misconduct (Friedman, 1990). They must decide what actions to take if the journal contains an article that has proved to be fraudulent. Usually, fraudulent publications require retraction notations and are not to be cited by authors in future publications. Pfeifer and Snodgrass (1990), however, studied the continued citation of retracted, invalid scientific literature; they found that articles commonly continued to cite retracted articles in U.S. publications and even more so in the literature of other countries.

The publication of fraudulent research is a major concern in medicine and a growing concern in nursing. The smaller pool of funds available for research and the greater emphasis on research publications could lead to an higher incidence of fraudulent publications.

The proposed policy on research misconduct to protect the integrity of the research record will address many of the current concerns; (USDHHS ORI, 1999): it will

■ Provide a definition of research misconduct
■ Designate responsibilities and actions related to research misconduct

■ Identify mechanisms to distribute the policy to scientists
■ Designate the membership of investigating committees
■ Identify the administrative actions for acts of research misconduct
■ Develop a process for notifying funding agencies and journals of acts of research misconduct
■ Provide for public disclosure of the incidents of scientific misconduct

Each researcher is responsible for monitoring the integrity of his or her research protocols, results, and publications. In addition, nursing professionals must foster a spirit of intellectual inquiry, mentor prospective scientists regarding the norms for good science, and stress quality, not quantity, in publications (Wocial, 1995).

ANIMALS AS RESEARCH SUBJECTS

The use of animals as research subjects is a controversial issue of growing concern to nurse researchers. A small but increasing number of nurse scientists are conducting physiological studies that require the use of animals. Many scientists, especially physicians, believe that the current animal rights movement could threaten the future of health research. Animal rights groups are active in antiresearch campaigns and are backed by massive resources, with a treasury that was estimated at $50 million in 1988 (Pardes et al., 1991). Some of the animal rights groups are trying to raise the consciousness of researchers and society to ensure that animals are used wisely in the conduct of research and treated humanely.

Other animal rights groups have tried to frighten the public with sometimes distorted stories about inhumane treatment of animals in research. Some of the activist leaders have made broad comparisons between human life and animal life. For example, a major animal rights group called People for the Ethical Treatment of Animals (PETA) has stated, "There is no rational basis for separating out the human animal. A rat is a pig is a dog is a boy. They're all mammals." (Pardes et al., 1991, p. 1641). Some of these activists have now progressed to violence, using "physical attacks, including real bombs, arson, and vandalism" (Pardes et al., 1991, p. 1642). Even more damage is being done to research through lawsuits that have blocked the conduct of research and the development of new research centers. "Medical schools are now spending over $15 million annually for security, public education, and other efforts to defend research" (Pardes et al., 1991, p. 1642).

Two important questions must be addressed: "Should animals be used as subjects in research?" and "If animals are used in research, what mechanisms ensure that they are treated humanely?" In regard to the first question, the type of research project developed influences the selection of subjects. Animals are just one of a variety of types of subjects used in research; others are human beings, plants, and computer data sets. If possible, most researchers use nonanimal subjects, because they are generally less expensive. In studies that are low risk, which most nursing studies are, human beings are commonly used as subjects.

Some studies, however, require the use of animals to answer the research question. "In practice, the selection of an animal subject means that the scientific, political, and legal arguments for using a particular animal species outweigh the scientific, cultural, and ethical arguments against its uses" (Thomas et al., 1988, p. 1630). Approximately 17 to 22 million animals are used in research each year, and 90% of them are rodents, with the combined percentage of dogs and cats being only 1% to 2% (Pardes et al., 1991).

Because animals are deemed valuable subjects for selected research projects, the second question, concerning their humane treatment, must also be answered. At least five separate types of regulations exist to protect research animals from mistreatment. The federal government, state governments, independent accreditation organization, professional societies, and individual institutions work to ensure that research animals are used only when necessary and only under humane conditions (Thomas et al., 1988). At the federal level, animal research is conducted according to the guidelines of USPHS Policy on Humane Care and Use of Laboratory Animals, which was adopted in 1986 and reprinted essentially unchanged in 1996 (National Institutes of Health, Office for Protection from Research Risks

[NIH OPRR, 1996; available on-line at *http://grants.nih.gov/grants/olaw/olaw.htm*).

The USPHS Policy on Humane Care and Use of Laboratory Animals defines *animal* as any live, vertebrate animal used or intended for use in research, research training, experimentation, or biological testing or for related purposes. Any institution proposing research involving animals must have a written Animal Welfare Assurance statement acceptable to the USPHS that documents compliance with the USPHS policy. Every assurance statement is evaluated by the NIH's Office for Protection from Research Risks (OPRR) to determine the adequacy of the institution's proposed program for the care and use of animals in activities conducted or supported by the USPHS (NIH OPRR, 1996).

Institutions' assurance statement about compliance with the USPHS Policy have promoted the humane care and treatment of animals in research. In addition, more than 700 institutions conducting health-related research have sought accreditation by the American Association for Accreditation of Laboratory Animal Care (AAALAC), which was developed to ensure the humane treatment of animals in research (Pardes et al., 1991). In conducting research, each investigator must carefully select the type of subject needed; and if animals are used as subjects, they require humane treatment.

■ SUMMARY

The conduct of nursing research requires not only expertise and diligence but also honesty and integrity. The ethical conduct of research starts with the identification of the study topic and continues through the publication of the study. Ethical research is essential to generate sound knowledge for practice, but what does the ethical conduct of research involve? This is a question that has been debated for many years by researchers, politicians, philosophers, lawyers, and even research subjects. The debate about ethics and research continues, probably because of (1) the complexity of human rights issues, (2) the focus of research in new, challenging arenas of technology and genetics, (3) the complex ethical codes and regulations governing research, and (4) the variety of interpretations of these codes and regulations.

Even though the phenomenon of the ethical conduct of research defies precise delineation, certain historical events, ethical codes, and regulations provide guidelines for nurse researchers. Two historical documents that have had a strong impact on the conduct of research are the Nuremberg Code and the Declaration of Helsinki. More recently, the U.S. Department of Health and Human Services (USDHHS) (1981, 1983, 1991) has promulgated regulations that direct the ethical conduct of research. These regulations include (1) general requirements for informed consent, (2) documentation of informed consent, (3) institutional review board (IRB) review of research, (4) exempt and expedited review procedures for certain kinds of research, and (5) criteria for IRB approval of research.

Conducting research ethically requires protection of the human rights of subjects. *Human rights* are claims and demands that have been justified in the eyes of an individual or by the consensus of a group of individuals. The human rights that require protection in research are (1) self-determination, (2) privacy, (3) anonymity and confidentiality, (4) fair treatment, and (5) protection from discomfort and harm.

The rights of the research subjects can be protected by balancing benefits and risks of a study, securing informed consent, and submitting the research for institutional review. To balance the benefits and risks of a study, the type, level, and number of risks are examined, and the potential benefits are identified. If possible, the risks must be minimized and the benefits maximized to achieve the best possible benefit-risk ratio. *Informed consent* involves the transmission of essential information, comprehension of that information, competency to give consent, and voluntary consent of the prospective subject. The guidelines for seeking consent from subjects and for institutional review are described. In institutional review, a study is examined for ethical concerns by a committee of peers called an institutional review board (IRB). The IRB conducts three levels of review—exempt, expedited, and complete.

A serious ethical problem of the 1980s and 1990s was the conduct, reporting, and publication of fraudulent research. Researchers have fabricated data and research results for publication, distorted or incorrectly reported research findings, or mismanaged the implementation of study protocols. Authors, coauthors, reviewers of research, and editors of journals must take an active role to decrease the incidence of fraudulent publications. All disciplines have a responsibility to protect the integrity of scientific knowledge. A Federal Policy on Research Misconduct to Protect the Integrity of the Research Record has been proposed, with probable approval anticipated in 2000. This policy defines and provides guidance for managing acts of research misconduct.

Another current ethical concern in research is the use of animals as subjects. Some animal rights groups, by means of their antiresearch campaigns, are threatening the future of health research. Two important questions are addressed: "Should animals be used as research subjects?" and "If animals are used in research, what mechanisms ensure that they are treated humanely?" The U.S. Public Health Service Policy on Humane Care and Use of Laboratory Animals provides direction for the conduct of research with animals as subjects.

* *

REFERENCES

American Nurses Association. (1985a). *Code for nurses with interpretive statements.* Kansas City, MO: Author.

American Nurses Association. (1985b). *Human rights guidelines for nurses in clinical and other research* (Document No. D-46 5M). Kansas City, MO: Author.

American Psychological Association. (1982). *Ethical principles in the conduct of research with human participants.* Washington, D.C.: Author.

Arras, J. D. (1990). Noncompliance in AIDS research. *Hastings Center Report, 20*(5), 24–32.

Beecher, H. K. (1966). Ethics and clinical research. *New England Journal of Medicine, 274*(24), 1354–1360.

Berger, R. L. (1990). Nazi science: The Dachau hypothermia experiments. *New England Journal of Medicine, 322*(20), 1435–1440.

Brainard, J. (2000, February 4.). Government & politics: Spate of suspensions of academic research spurs questions about federal strategy. *The Chronicle of Higher Education, XLVI* (22), A29–A32.

Brandt, A. M. (1978). Racism and research: The case of the

Tuskegee syphilis study. *Hastings Center Report, 8*(6), 21–29.

Brent, N. J. (1990). Legal issues in research: Informed consent. *Journal of Neuroscience Nursing, 22*(3), 189–191.

Broome, M. E. (1999). Consent (assent) for research with pediatric patients. *Seminars in Oncology Nursing, 15*(2), 96–103.

Broome, M. E., & Stieglitz, K. A. (1992). The consent process and children. *Research in Nursing & Health, 15*(2), 147–152.

Bruce, S. L, & Grove, S. K. (1994). The effect of a coronary artery risk evaluation program on serum lipid values and cardiovascular risk levels. *Applied Nursing Research, 7*(2), 67–74.

Carico, J. M., & Harrison, E. R. (1990). Ethical considerations for nurses in biomedical research. *Journal of Neuroscience Nursing, 22*(3), 160–163.

Chamorro, T., & Appelbaum, J. (1988). Informed consent: Nursing issues and ethical dilemmas. *Oncology Nursing Forum, 15*(6), 803–808.

Chop, R. M., & Silva, M. C. (1991). Scientific fraud: Definitions, policies, and implications for nursing research. *Journal of Professional Nursing, 7*(3), 166–171.

Damrosch, S. P. (1986). Ensuring anonymity by use of subject-generated identification codes. *Research in Nursing & Health, 9*(1), 61–63.

Davis, A. J. (1989). Informed consent process in research protocols: Dilemmas for clinical nurses. *Western Journal of Nursing Research, 11*(4), 448–457.

Declaration of Helsinki. (1986). In R. J. Levine (Ed.), *Ethics and regulations of clinical research* (2nd ed., pp. 427–429). Baltimore-Munich: Urban & Schwarzenberg.

Douglas, S., Briones, J., & Chronister, C. (1994). The incidence of reporting consent rates in nursing research articles. *Image–The Journal of Nursing Scholarship, 26*(1), 35–40.

Douglas, S., & Larson, E. (1986). There's more to informed consent than information. *Focus on Critical Care, 13*(2), 43–47.

Floyd, J. (1988). Research and informed consent: The dilemma of the cognitively impaired client. *Journal of Psychosocial Nursing and Mental Health Services, 26*(3), 13–21.

Ford, J. S., & Reutter, L. I. (1990). Ethical dilemmas associated with small samples. *Journal of Advanced Nursing, 15*(2), 187–191.

Frankena, W. K. (1973). *Ethics* (2nd ed.). Englewood Cliffs, NJ: Prentice-Hall.

Friedman, P. J. (1990). Correcting the literature following fraudulent publication. *JAMA, 263*(10), 1416–1419.

Garfield, E., & Welljams-Dorof, A. (1990). The impact of fraudulent research on the scientific literature: The Stephen E. Breuning case. *JAMA, 263*(10), 1424–1426.

Hansen, B. C., & Hansen, K. D. (1995). Academic and scientific misconduct: Issues for nursing educators. *Journal of Professional Nursing, 11*(1), 31–39.

Hawley, D. J., & Jeffers, J. M. (1992). Scientific misconduct as a dilemma for nursing. *Image—The Journal of Nursing Scholarship, 24*(1), 51–55.

Henderson, J. (1990, March). When scientists fake it. *American Way,* pp. 56–101.

Hershey, N., & Miller, R. D. (1976). *Human experimentation and the law.* Germantown, MD: Aspen.

Kelman, H. C. (1967). Human use of human subjects: The problem of deception in social psychological experiments. *Psychological Bulletin, 67*(1), 1–11.

Kelman, H. C. (1977). Privacy and research with human beings. *Journal of Social Issues, 33*(3), 169–195.

Larson, E. (1989). Maintaining quality in clinical research and evaluation: When corrective action is necessary. *Journal of Nursing Quality Assurance, 3*(4), 28–35.

Leino-Kilpi, H., & Tuomaala, U. (1989). Research ethics and nursing science: An empirical example. *Journal of Advanced Nursing, 14*(6), 451–458.

Levine, R. J. (1986). *Ethics and regulation of clinical research* (2nd ed.). Baltimore-Munich: Urban & Schwarzenberg.

Lind, S. E. (1990). Sounding board: Finder's fees for research subjects. *New England Journal of Medicine, 323*(3), 192–195.

Mahon, N. E., Yarcheski, A., & Yarcheski, T. J. (2000). Positive and negative outcomes of anger in early adolescents. *Research in Nursing & Health, 23*(1), 17–24.

McGrath, P. (1995). It's OK to say no! A discussion of ethical issues arising from informed consent to chemotherapy. *Cancer Nursing, 18*(2), 97–103.

Meade, C. D. (1999). Improving understanding of the informed consent process and document. *Seminars in Oncology Nursing, 15*(2), 124–137.

Milgram, S. (1963). Behavioral study of obedience. *Journal of Abnormal and Social Psychology, 67*(4), 371–378.

Munhall, P. L. (1999). Ethical considerations in qualitative research. In P. L. Munhall & C. O. Boyd (Eds.), *Nursing research: A qualitative perspective* (2nd Ed.). New York: National League for Nursing.

National Commission for the Protection of Human Subjects of Biomedical and Behavioral Research. (1978). *Belmont report: Ethical principles and guidelines for research involving human subjects* (DHEW Publication No. [05] 78–0012). Washington, D.C.: U.S. Government Printing Office.

National Institutes of Health, Office for Protection from Research Risks. (1996). *Public health service policy on humane care and use of laboratory animals* [On-line]. Available: *http://grants.nih.gov/grants/oprr/phspol.htm* {2/20/2000].

National Institutes of Health, Office of Human Subjects Research. (1991). Protection of human subjects. *Code of Federal Regulations,* Title 45 Public Welfare, Part 46 [On-line]. Available: *http://helix.nih.gov:8001/ohrs/mpa/45cfr46.php3* [2/19/2000].

Nelson-Marten, P., & Rich, B. A. (1999). A historical perspective of informed consent in clinical practice and research. *Seminars in Oncology Nursing, 15*(2), 81–88.

Nuremberg Code. (1986). In R. J. Levine (Ed.), *Ethics and regulation of clinical research* (2nd ed., pp. 425–426). Baltimore-Munich: Urban & Schwarzenberg.

Nusbaum, J. G., & Chenitz, W. C. (1990). A grounded theory study of the informed consent process for pharmacologic research. *Western Journal of Nursing Research, 12*(2), 215–228.

Pardes, H., West, A., & Pincus, H. A. (1991). Physicians and the animal-rights movement. *New England Journal of Medicine, 324*(23), 1640–1643.

Pfeifer, M. P., & Snodgrass, G. L. (1990). The continued use of retracted, invalid scientific literature. *JAMA, 263*(10), 1420–1423.

Powledge, T. M. (1999). *Ain't misbehavin': Addressing wrongdoing in research* [On-line]. Available: *http://www.biomednet.com/hmsbeagle/67/notes/adapt* [2/26/1999].

Ramos, M. C. (1989). Some ethical implications of qualitative research. *Research in Nursing & Health, 12*(1), 57–63.

Rankin, M., & Esteves, M. D. (1997). Perceptions of scientific misconduct in nursing. *Nursing Research, 46*(5), 270–275.

Relman, A. S. (1990). Publishing biomedical research: Roles and responsibilities. *Hastings Center Report, 20*(5), 23–27.

Reynolds, P. D. (1972). On the protection of human subjects and social science. *International Social Science Journal, 24*(4), 693–719.

Reynolds, P. D. (1979). *Ethical dilemmas and social science research.* San Francisco, CA: Jossey-Bass.

Robley, L. R. (1995). The ethics of qualitative nursing research. *Journal of Professional Nursing, 11*(1), 45–48.

Rosse, P. A., & Krebs, L. U. (1999). The nurse's role in the informed consent process. *Seminars in Oncology Nursing, 15*(2), 116–123.

Rothman, D. J. (1982). Were Tuskegee and Willowbrook "studies in nature"? *Hastings Center Report, 12*(2), 5–7.

Sasson, R., & Nelson, T. M. (1971). The human experimental subject in context. In J. Jung (Ed.), *The experimenter's dilemma* (pp. 265–296). New York: Harper & Row.

Schaefer, J. A., & Moos, R. H. (1996). Effects of work stressors and work climate on long-term care staff's job morale and functioning. *Research in Nursing & Health, 19*(1), 63–73.

Silva, M. C. (1985). Comprehension of information for informed consent by spouses of surgical patients. *Research in Nursing & Health, 8*(2), 117–124.

Steinfels, P., & Levine, C. (1976). Biomedical ethics and the shadow of Naziism. *Hastings Center Report, 6*(4), 1–20.

Strauman, J. J., & Cotanch, P. H. (1988). Oncology nurse research issues: Overstudied populations. *Oncology Nursing Forum, 15*(5), 665–667.

Thomas, J. A., Hamm, T. E., Perkins, P. L., Raffin, T. A., & Stanford University Medical Center Committee on Ethics. (1988). Animal research at Stanford University: Principles, policies and practices. *New England Journal of Medicine, 318*(24), 1630–1632.

Thompson, P. J. (1987). Protection of the rights of children as subjects for research. *Journal of Pediatric Nursing, 2*(6), 392–399.

To, M. Y. F., & Chan, S. (2000). Evaluating the effectiveness of progressive muscle relaxation in reducing the aggressive behaviors of mentally handicapped patients. *Archives of Psychiatric Nursing, 14*(1), 39–46.

Twomey, J. G. (1994). Investigating pediatric HIV research ethics in the field. *Western Journal of Nursing Research, 16*(4), 404–413.

U.S. Department of Health and Human Services. (1981, January 26). Final regulations amending basic HHS policy for the protection of human research subjects. *Code of Federal Regulations,* Title 45 Public Welfare, Part 46.

U.S. Department of Health and Human Services. (1983, March 8). Protection of human subjects. *Code of Federal Regulations,* Title 45 Public Welfare, Part 46.

U.S. Department of Health and Human Services. (1989). Final rule: Responsibilities of awardee and applicant institutions for dealing with and reporting possible misconduct in science. *Federal Register, 54,* 32446–32451.

U.S. Department of Health and Human Services. (1991, June 18). Protection of human subjects. *Code of Federal Regulations,* Title 45 Public Welfare, Part 46.

U.S. Department of Health and Human Services, Office of Research Integrity (1999). Proposed federal policy on research misconduct to protect the integrity of the research record. *Federal Register* [On-line]. Available: *http://ori.dhhs.gov/fedreg101499.htm.* [3/19/2000].

U.S. Department of Health and Human Services, Office of Research Integrity (2000). *Introduction to the ORI* [On-line]. Available: *http://ori.dhhs.gov/.* [3/20/2000].

Watson, A. B. (1982). Informed consent of special subjects. *Nursing Research, 31*(1), 43–47.

Wocial, L. D. (1995). The role of mentors in promoting integrity and preventing scientific misconduct in nursing research. *Journal of Professional Nursing, 11*(5), 276–280.

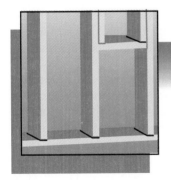

CHAPTER 10

UNDERSTANDING RESEARCH DESIGN

research design is a blueprint for conducting the study that maximizes control over factors that could interfere with the validity of the findings. The research design guides the researcher in planning and implementing the study in a way that is most likely to achieve the intended goal. The control provided by the design increases the probability that the study results are accurate reflections of reality. Skill in selecting and implementing research design is important to improving the quality of the study and, thus, the usefulness of the findings. Being able to identify the study design and to evaluate the threats to validity of findings due to design flaws is an important part of critiquing studies.

The term *research design* is used in two ways. Some consider research design to be the entire strategy for the study, from identification of the problem to final plans for data collection. Others limit design to clearly defined structures within which the study is implemented. In this text, the first definition refers to the *research methodology* and the second is a definition of the *research design*.

The design of a study is the end-result of a series of decisions made by the researcher concerning how the study will be implemented. The design is closely associated with the framework of the study and guides planning for implementation of the study. As a blueprint, the design is not specific to a particular study. It is, rather, a broad pattern or guide that can be applied to many studies. Just as the blueprint for a house must be individualized to

the specific house being built, so the design must be made specific to a study. Using the problem statement, framework, research questions, and clearly defined variables, the researcher can map out the design to achieve a detailed research plan for data collection and analysis. This research plan specifically directs the implementation of the study. Developing a research plan is discussed in Chapter 17.

Elements central to the study design include the presence or absence of a treatment, the number of groups in the sample, the number and timing of measurements to be performed, the sampling method, the time frame for data collection, planned comparisons, and control of extraneous variables. Finding answers to the following questions leads to development of the design:

1. Is the primary purpose of the study to describe variables and groups within the study situation, to examine relationships, or to examine causality within the study situation?
2. Will a treatment be used?
3. If so, will the treatment be controlled by the researcher?
4. Will the sample be pretested before the treatment?
5. Will the sample be randomly selected?
6. Will the sample be studied as a single group or divided into groups?
7. How many groups will there be?
8. What will be the size of each group?
9. Will there be a control group?
10. Will groups be randomly assigned?

11. Will there be repeated measures of variables?
12. Will the data be collected cross-sectionally or over time?
13. Have extraneous variables been identified?
14. Are data being collected on extraneous variables?
15. What strategies are being used to control for extraneous variables?
16. What strategies are being used for comparison of variables or groups?
17. Will data be collected at a single site or at multiple sites?

Developing a design for a study requires consideration of multiple details such as the foregoing. The more carefully thought out these details are, the stronger the design. These questions are important because of their link to the logic on which research design is based. To give you the information necessary to understand and answer the foregoing questions, this chapter discusses (1) the concepts important to design, (2) design validity, (3) the elements of a good design, (4) participatory research, and (5) triangulation, a relatively recent approach to research design.

CONCEPTS IMPORTANT TO DESIGN

Many terms used in discussing research design have special meanings within this context. An understanding of the meaning of these concepts is critical to understanding the purpose of a specific design. Some of the major concepts used in relation to design are causality, bias, manipulation, control, and validity.

Causality

The first assumptions one must make in examining *causality* are that things have causes and that causes lead to effects. Some of the ideas related to causation emerged from the logical positivist philosophical tradition. Hume, a positivist, proposed that the following three conditions must be met to establish causality: (1) there must be a strong correlation between the proposed cause and the effect, (2) the proposed cause must precede the effect in time, and

(3) the cause has to be present whenever the effect occurs. Cause, according to Hume, is not directly observable but must be inferred (Cook & Campbell, 1979).

A philosophical group known as essentialists proposed that two concepts must be considered in determining causality, necessary and sufficient. The proposed cause must be *necessary* for the effect to occur. (The effect cannot occur unless the cause first occurs.) The proposed cause must also be *sufficient* (requiring no other factors) for the effect to occur. This leaves no room for a variable that may sometimes, but not always, serve as the cause of an effect.

John Stuart Mill, another philosopher, added a third idea related to causation. He suggested that, in addition to the preceding criteria for causation, there must be no alternative explanations for why a change in one variable seems to lead to a change in a second variable (Cook & Campbell, 1979).

Causes are frequently expressed within the propositions of a theory. Testing the accuracy of these theoretical statements indicates the usefulness of the theory. A theoretical understanding of causation is considered important because it improves the ability to predict and, in some cases, to control events in the real world. The purpose of an experimental design is to examine cause and effect. The independent variable in a study is expected to be the cause, and the dependent variable is expected to reflect the effect of the independent variable.

Multicausality

Multicausality, the recognition that a number of interrelating variables can be involved in causing a particular effect, is a more recent idea related to causality. Because of the complexity of causal relationships, a theory is unlikely to identify every variable involved in causing a particular phenomenon. A study is unlikely to include every component influencing a particular change or effect.

Cook and Campbell (1979) have suggested three levels of causal assertions that one must consider in establishing causality. *Molar* causal laws relate to large and complex objects. *Intermediate mediation* considers causal factors operating between molar and micro levels. *Micromediation* examines causal connections at the level of small particles, such as atoms. Cook and Campbell (1979) use the example of turning on a light switch, which causes the light to come on (molar). An electrician would tend to explain the cause of the light coming on in terms of wires and electrical current (intermediate mediation). However, the physicist would explain the cause of the light coming on in terms of ions, atoms, and subparticles (micromediation).

The essentialists' ideas of necessary and sufficient do not hold up well when one views a phenomenon from the perspective of multiple causation. The light switch may not be necessary to turn on the light if the insulation has worn off the electrical wires. Additionally, the light will not come on even though the switch is turned on if the light bulb is burned out. Although this is a rather concrete example, it is easy to relate to common situations in nursing.

Very few phenomena in nursing can be clearly reduced to a single cause and a single effect. However, the greater the proportion of causal factors that can be identified and explored, the clearer the understanding of the phenomenon. This greater understanding improves the ability to predict and control. For example, currently, nurses have only a limited understanding of patients' preoperative attitudes, knowledge, and behaviors and their effects on postoperative attitudes and behaviors. Nurses assume that high preoperative anxiety leads to less healthy postoperative responses and that providing information before surgery improves healthy responses in the postoperative period. Many nursing studies have examined this particular phenomenon. However, the causal factors involved are complex and have not been clearly delineated. This lack of knowledge limits the effectiveness of nursing actions in facilitating the healthiest response to the surgical experience.

Probability

The original criteria for causation required that a variable should cause an identified effect each time the cause occurred. Although this criterion may apply in the basic sciences, such as chemistry or physics, it is unlikely to apply in the health sciences or social sciences. Because of the complexity of the nursing field, nurses deal in probabilities. *Probability* addresses relative, rather than absolute, causality. From the perspective of probability, a cause will not produce a specific effect each time that particular cause occurs.

Reasoning changes when one thinks in terms of probabilities. The researcher investigates the probability of an effect's occurring under specific circumstances. Rather than seeking to prove that A causes B, a researcher would state that if A occurs, there is a 50% probability that B will occur.

The reasoning behind probability is more in keeping with the complexity of multicausality. In the previously described example about preoperative attitudes and postoperative outcomes, nurses could seek to predict the probability of unhealthy postoperative patient outcomes when preoperative anxiety levels are high.

Causality and Nursing Philosophy

Traditional theories of prediction and control are built on theories of causality. The first research designs were also based on causality theory. Nursing science must be built within a philosophical framework of multicausality and probability. The strict senses of single causality and of "necessary and sufficient" are not in keeping with the progressively complex, holistic philosophy of nursing. Acquiring an understanding of multicausality and increasing the probability of being able to predict and control the occurrence of an effect will require an understanding of both wholes and parts.

Nursing knowledge for practice requires understanding of molar, intermediate mediational, and micromediational aspects of a particular phenomenon. A variety of differing approaches, reflecting both qualitative and quantitative, descriptive and experimental research are necessary to develop a knowledge base for nursing. Explanation and causality have been seen by some as different and perhaps opposing forms of knowledge. Nevertheless, the nurse must join these forms of knowledge, sometimes within the design of a single study, to acquire the knowledge needed for nursing practice.

Bias

The term *bias* means to slant away from the true or expected. A biased opinion has failed to include both sides of the question. Cutting fabric on the bias means to cut across the grain of the woven fabric. A biased witness is one who is strongly for or against one side of the situation. A biased scale is one that does not provide a valid measure.

Bias is of great concern in research because of the potential effect on the meaning of the study findings. Any component of the study that deviates or causes a deviation from true measure leads to distorted findings. Many factors related to research can be biased—the researcher, the measurement tools, the individual subjects, the sample, the data, and the statistics. Thus, an important concern in designing a study is to identify possible sources of bias and eliminate or avoid them. If they cannot be avoided, the study must be designed to control these sources of bias. Designs, in fact, are developed to reduce the possibilities of bias.

Manipulation

In nursing, *manipulation* tends to have a negative connotation and is associated with one person underhandedly causing another person to behave in a desired way. To *manipulate* means to move around or to control the movement of, such as manipulating a syringe. In research, manipulation is used in experimental or quasi-experimental research and is sometimes called the *treatment*. Thus, in a study on preoperative care, preoperative teaching might be manipulated so that one group receives the treatment and another does not. In a study on oral care, the frequency of care might be manipulated.

In nursing research, when experimental designs are used to explore causal relationships, the nurse must be free to manipulate the variables under study. If the freedom to manipulate a variable (e.g., pain control measures) is under the control of someone else, a bias is introduced into the study. In qualitative, descriptive, and correlational studies, no attempt is made to manipulate variables. Instead, the purpose is to describe a situation as it exists.

Control

Control means having the power to direct or manipulate factors to achieve a desired outcome. The idea of control is very important in research, particularly in experimental and quasi-experimental studies. The greater the amount of control the researcher has of the study situation, the more credible the study findings. The purpose of research designs is to maximize control factors in the study situation.

STUDY VALIDITY

Study validity, a measure of the truth or accuracy of a claim, is an important concern throughout the research process. Questions of validity refer back to the propositions from which the study was developed. Thus, validity is an examination of the approximate truth or falsity of the propositions (Cook & Campbell, 1979). Is the theoretical proposition an accurate reflection of reality? Was the study designed well enough to provide a valid test of the proposition? Validity is a complex idea that is important to the researcher and to those who read the study report and consider using the findings in their practice. Critical analysis of research involves being able to think through threats to validity that have occurred and make judgments about how seriously these threats affect the integrity of the findings. Validity provides a major basis for making decisions about which findings are useful for patient care.

Cook and Campbell (1979) have described four types of validity: statistical conclusion validity, internal validity, construct validity, and external validity. When conducting a study, the researcher is confronted with major decisions about the four types of validity. To make decisions about validity, the researcher must address a variety of questions, such as the following:

1. Is there a relationship between the two variables? (statistical conclusion validity)
2. Given that there is a relationship, is it plausibly causal from one operational variable to the other, or would the same relationship have been obtained in the absence of any treatment of any kind? (internal validity)

3. Given that the relationship is plausibly causal and is reasonably known to be from one variable to another, what are the particular cause-and-effect constructs involved in the relationship? (construct validity)
4. Given that there is probably a causal relationship from construct A to construct B, how generalizable is this relationship across persons, settings, and times? (external validity) (Cook & Campbell, 1979, p. 39)

Statistical Conclusion Validity

The first step in inferring cause is to determine whether the independent and dependent variables are related. The determination of a relationship (*covariation*) is made through statistical analysis. *Statistical conclusion validity* is concerned with whether the conclusions about relationships or differences drawn from statistical analysis are an accurate reflection of the real world.

The second step is to identify differences between groups. However, there are reasons why false conclusions can be drawn about the presence or absence of a relationship or difference. The reasons for the false conclusions are called *threats to statistical conclusion validity*. These threats are described here.

LOW STATISTICAL POWER

Low statistical power increases the probability of concluding that there is no significant difference between samples when actually there is a difference (Type II error). A Type II error is most likely to occur when the sample size is small or when the power of the statistical test to determine differences is low. The concept of statistical power and strategies to improve it are discussed in Chapters 14 and 18.

VIOLATED ASSUMPTIONS OF STATISTICAL TESTS

Most statistical tests have assumptions about the data being used, such as that the data are interval data, that the sample was randomly obtained, or that there is a normal distribution of scores to be analyzed. If these assumptions are violated, the statistical analysis may provide inaccurate results. The assumptions of each statistical test are provided in Chapters 20, 21, and 22.

FISHING AND THE ERROR RATE PROBLEM

A serious concern in research is incorrectly concluding that a relationship or difference exists when it does not (Type I error). The risk of Type I error increases when the researcher conducts multiple statistical analyses of relationships or differences; this procedure is referred to as *fishing*. When fishing is used, a given portion of the analyses show significant relationships or differences simply by chance. For example, the *t* test is commonly used to make multiple statistical comparisons of mean differences in a single sample. This procedure increases the risk of a Type I error because some of the differences found in the sample occurred by chance and are not actually present in the population. Multivariate statistical techniques have been developed to deal with this error rate problem (Goodwin, 1984). Fishing and error rate problems are discussed in Chapter 18.

THE RELIABILITY OF MEASURES

The technique of measuring variables must be reliable if true differences are to be found. A measure is reliable if it gives the same result each time the same situation or factor is measured. For example, a thermometer would be reliable if it showed the same reading when tested repeatedly on the same patient. If a scale is used to measure anxiety, it should give the same score if repeatedly given to the same person in a short time (unless, of course, repeatedly taking the same test causes anxiety to increase or decrease).

THE RELIABILITY OF TREATMENT IMPLEMENTATION

If the method of administering a research treatment varies from one person to another, the chance of detecting a true difference decreases. The lack of standardization in administering the treatment must be controlled during the planning phase by ensuring that the treatment will be provided in exactly the same way each time it is administered.

RANDOM IRRELEVANCIES IN THE EXPERIMENTAL SETTING

Environmental (extraneous) variables in complex field settings can influence scores on the dependent variable. These variables increase the difficulty of detecting differences. Consider the activities occurring on a nursing unit. The numbers and variety of staff, patients, crises, and work patterns merge into a complex arena for the implementation of a study. Any of the dynamics of the unit can influence manipulation of the independent variable or measurement of the dependent variable.

RANDOM HETEROGENEITY OF RESPONDENTS

Subjects in a treatment group can differ in ways that are correlated with the dependent variable. This difference can have an influence on the outcome of the treatment and prevent detection of a true relationship between the treatment and the dependent variable. For example, subjects may vary in response to preoperative attempts to lower anxiety because of unique characteristics associated with differing levels of anxiety.

Internal Validity

Internal validity is the extent to which the effects detected in the study are a true reflection of reality rather than the result of extraneous variables. Although internal validity should be a concern in all studies, it is addressed more commonly in relation to studies examining causality than in other studies. In studies examining causality, the researcher must determine whether the independent and dependent variables may have been caused by a third, often unmeasured, variable (an *extraneous variable*). The possibility of an alternative explanation of cause is sometimes referred to as a *rival hypothesis*. Any study can contain threats to internal validity, and these validity threats can lead to a false-positive or false-negative conclusion. The following question must be considered: Is there another reasonable

(valid) explanation (rival hypothesis) for the finding other than that proposed by the researcher? Threats to internal validity are described here.

HISTORY

History is an event that is not related to the planned study but that occurs during the time of the study. History could influence the responses of subjects to the treatment.

MATURATION

In research, *maturation* is defined as growing older, wiser, stronger, hungrier, more tired, or more experienced during the study. Such unplanned and unrecognized changes can influence the findings of the study.

TESTING

Sometimes, the effect being measured can be due to the number of times the subject's responses have been tested. The subject may remember earlier, inaccurate responses that can be modified, thus altering the outcome of the study. The test itself may influence the subject to change attitudes or increase the subject's knowledge.

INSTRUMENTATION

Effects can be due to changes in measurement instruments between the pretest and the posttest rather than a result of the treatment. For example, a scale that was accurate when the study began (pretest) could now show subjects to weigh 2 lb less than they actually weigh (posttest). Instrumentation is also involved when people serving as observers or data collectors become more experienced between the pretest and the posttest, thus altering in some way the data they collect.

STATISTICAL REGRESSION

Statistical regression is the movement or regression of extreme scores toward the mean in studies using a pretest–posttest design. The process involved in statistical regression is difficult to understand. When a test or scale is used to measure a variable, some subjects achieve very high or very low scores. In some studies, subjects are selected to be included in a particular group because their scores on a pretest are high or low. A treatment is then performed, and a posttest is administered. However, with no treatment, subjects who initially achieve very high or very low scores tend to have more moderate scores when retested. Their scores regress toward the mean. The treatment did not necessarily cause the change. If the pretest scores were low, the posttest may show statistically significant differences (higher scores) from the pretest, leading to the conclusion that the treatment caused the change (Type I error). If the pretest scores were high, the posttest scores would tend to be lower (because of a tendency to regress toward the mean) even with no treatment. In this situation, the researcher may mistakenly conclude that the treatment caused no change (Type II error).

SELECTION

Selection addresses the process by which subjects are chosen to take part in a study and how subjects are grouped within a study. A selection threat is more likely to occur in studies in which randomization is not possible. In some studies, people selected for the study may differ in some important way from people not selected for the study. In other studies, the threat is due to differences in subjects selected for study groups. For example, people assigned to the control group could be different in some important way from people assigned to the experimental group. This difference in selection could cause the two groups to react differently to the treatment; in this case, the treatment would not have caused the differences in group responses.

MORTALITY

The mortality threat is due to subjects who drop out of a study before completion. Mortality becomes a threat when (1) those who drop out of a study are a different type of person from those who remain in the study or (2) there is a difference between the kinds of people who drop out of the experimental group and the people who drop out of the control group.

INTERACTIONS WITH SELECTION

The aforementioned threats can interact with selection to further complicate the validity of the study. The threats most likely to interact with selection are history, maturation, and instrumentation. For example, if a control group selected for the study has a different history from that of the experimental group responses to the treatment may be due to this interaction rather than to the treatment.

AMBIGUITY ABOUT THE DIRECTION OF CAUSAL INFLUENCE

Ambiguity about the direction of a causal influence occurs most frequently in correlational studies that address causality. In a study in which variables are measured simultaneously and only once, it may be impossible to determine whether A caused B, B caused A, or the two variables interact in a noncausal way.

DIFFUSION OR IMITATION OF TREATMENTS

The control group may gain access to the treatment intended for the experimental group (diffusion) or a similar treatment available from another source (imitation). For example, suppose a study examined the effect of teaching specific information to hypertensive patients as a treatment and then measured the effect of the teaching on blood pressure readings and adherence to treatment protocols. Suppose that the control group patients communicated with the experimental patients and the teaching information was shared. The control group patients' responses to the outcome measures may show no differences from those of the experimental group even though the teaching actually did make a difference (Type II error).

COMPENSATORY EQUALIZATION OF TREATMENTS

When the experimental group receives a treatment that is seen as desirable, such as a new treatment for acquired immunodeficiency syndrome, administrative people and other health professionals may not tolerate the difference and may insist that the control group also receive the treatment. The researcher therefore no longer has a control group and cannot document the effectiveness of the treatment through the study. In health care, both giving and withholding treatment have ethical implications.

COMPENSATORY RIVALRY BY RESPONDENTS RECEIVING LESS DESIRABLE TREATMENTS

In some studies, the design and plan of the study are publicly known. The control group subjects then know the expected difference between their group and the experimental group and may attempt to reduce or reverse the difference. This phenomenon may have occurred in the national hospice study funded by the Health Care Financing Administration and conducted by Brown University (Greer et al., 1983). In this study, 26 hospices were temporarily reimbursed through Medicare while a comparison of the care between hospices and hospitals was examined. The study made national headlines and was widely discussed in Congress. Health policy decisions related to reimbursement of hospice care hinged on the findings of the study. The study found no significant differences in care between the two groups, although there were cost differentials. In addition to a selection threat (hospitals providing poor care to dying cancer patients were unlikely to agree to participate in the study), health care professionals in the hospitals selected may have been determined to counter the criticism that the care they provided was poor in quality. The rivalry in this situation could have influenced the outcomes of the study and, thus, threatened its validity.

RESENTFUL DEMORALIZATION OF RESPONDENTS RECEIVING LESS DESIRABLE TREATMENTS

If control group subjects believe that they are receiving less desirable treatment, they may react by withdrawing, giving up, or becoming angry. Changes in behavior resulting from this reaction rather than from the treatment can lead to differences that cannot be attributed to the treatment.

Construct Validity

Construct validity examines the fit between the conceptual definitions and operational definitions of variables. Theoretical constructs or concepts are defined within the framework (conceptual definitions). These conceptual definitions provide the basis for the development of operational definitions of the variables. Operational definitions (methods of measurement) must validly reflect the theoretical constructs. (Theoretical constructs are discussed in Chapter 7; conceptual and operational definitions of concepts and variables are discussed in Chapter 8.)

Is use of the measure a valid inference about the construct? Examination of construct validity determines whether the instrument actually measures the theoretical construct it purports to measure. The process of developing construct validity for an instrument often requires years of scientific work. When selecting methods of measurement, the researcher must determine previous development of instrument construct validity. (Instrument construct validity is discussed in Chapter 15.) The threats to construct validity are related both to previous instrument development and to the development of measurement techniques as part of the methodology of a particular study. Threats to construct validity are described here.

INADEQUATE PREOPERATIONAL EXPLICATION OF CONSTRUCTS

Measurement of a construct stems logically from a concept analysis of the construct, either by the theorist who developed the construct or by the researcher. The conceptual definition should emerge from the concept analysis, and the method of measurement (operational definition) should clearly reflect both. A deficiency in the conceptual or operational definition leads to low construct validity.

MONO-OPERATION BIAS

Mono-operation bias occurs when only one method of measurement is used to measure a construct. When only one method of measurement is used, fewer dimensions of the construct are measured. Construct validity is greatly improved if the researcher uses more than one instrument. For example, if anxiety were a dependent variable, more than one measure of anxiety could be used. More than one measurement of the dependent variable can often be accomplished with little increase in time, effort, or cost.

MONOMETHOD BIAS

In *monomethod bias*, the researcher uses more than one measure of a variable but all the measures use the same method of recording. Attitude measures, for example, may all be paper and pencil scales. Attitudes that are personal and private, however, may not be detected through the use of paper and pencil tools. Paper and pencil tools may be influenced by feelings of nonaccountability for responses, acquiescence, or social desirability. For example, construct validity would be improved if anxiety were measured by a paper and pencil test, verbal messages of anxiety, the galvanic skin response, and observer recording of incidence and frequency of behaviors that have been validly linked with anxiety.

HYPOTHESIS—GUESSING WITHIN EXPERIMENTAL CONDITIONS

Many subjects within a study can guess the hypotheses of the researcher. The validity concern is related to behavioral changes that may occur in the subjects as a consequence of knowing the hypothesis. The extent to which this issue modifies study findings is not currently known.

EVALUATION APPREHENSION

Subjects wish to be seen in a favorable light by researchers. They want to be seen as competent and psychologically healthy. Their responses in the experiment may be due to this desire rather than the effects of the independent variable.

EXPERIMENTER EXPECTANCIES (ROSENTHAL EFFECT)

The expectancies of the researcher can bias the data. For example, if a researcher expects a particular intervention to be effective in pain relief, the data he or she collects may reflect this expectation. If another researcher who does not believe the intervention would be effective had collected the data, results could have been different. The extent to which this effect actually influences studies is not known. Because of this concern, some researchers are not involved in the data collection process. In other studies, data collectors do not know which subjects are assigned to treatment and control groups.

Another way to control this threat is to design the study so that data collectors differ in expectations. If the sample size is large enough, comparisons could be made in data collected by the different data collectors. Failing to determine a difference in the data collected by the two data collection groups would give evidence of construct validity.

CONFOUNDING CONSTRUCTS AND LEVELS OF CONSTRUCTS

When developing the methodology of a study, the researcher makes decisions about the intensity of a variable that will be measured or provided as a treatment. The intensity of the variable measured influences the level of the construct that will be reflected in the study. These decisions can affect validity, because the method of measuring the variable influences the outcome of the study and the understanding of the constructs in the study framework.

For example, the researcher might find that variable A does not affect variable B when, in fact, it does, but either not at the level of A that was manipulated or not at the level of B that was measured. This issue is a particular problem when A is not linearly related to B or when the effect being studied is weak. Control of this threat involves including several levels of A in the design and measuring many levels of B. For example, in a study in which A is preoperative teaching and B is anxiety, (1) the instrument being used to measure anxiety measures only high levels of anxiety or (2) the preoperative teaching is provided for 15 minutes but 30 minutes or an hour of teaching is required to cause significant changes in anxiety.

In some cases, there is confounding of variables,

which leads to mistaken conclusions. Few measures of a construct are pure measures. Rather, a selected method of measuring a construct can measure a portion of the construct and also other related constructs. Thus, the measure can lead to confusing results, because the variable measured does not provide an accurate reflection of the construct.

INTERACTION OF DIFFERENT TREATMENTS

The interaction of different treatments is a threat to construct validity if subjects receive more than one treatment in a study. For example, a study might examine the effectiveness of pain relief measures, and subjects might receive medication, massage, and distraction and relaxation strategies. In this case, each one of the treatments interacts with the others, and the effect of any single treatment on pain relief would be impossible to extract. The findings of the study could not be generalized to any situation in which patients did not receive all four pain treatments.

INTERACTION OF TESTING AND TREATMENT

In some studies, pretesting the subject is thought to modify the effect of the treatment. In this case, the findings can be generalized only to subjects who have been pretested. Although there is some evidence that pretest sensitivity does not have the extent of impact that was once feared, it must be considered in examining the validity of the study. One design, the Solomon Four-Group Design (discussed in Chapter 11) tests this threat to validity. Repeated posttests can also lead to an interaction of testing and treatment.

RESTRICTED GENERALIZABILITY ACROSS CONSTRUCTS

When designing studies, the researcher must consider the impact of the findings on constructs other than those originally conceived in the problem statement. Often, including another measure or two enables the generalization of the findings to clinical settings and the translation back to theoretical dimensions to be much broader.

External Validity

External validity is concerned with the extent to which study findings can be generalized beyond the sample used in the study. With the most serious threat, the findings would be meaningful only for the group being studied. To some extent, the significance of the study depends on the number of types of people and situations to which the findings can be applied. Sometimes, the factors influencing external validity are subtle and may not be reported in research papers; however, the researcher must be responsible for these factors. Generalization is usually more narrow for a single study than for multiple replications of a study using different samples, perhaps from different populations in different settings. The threats to the ability to generalize the findings (external validity) in terms of study design are described here.

INTERACTION OF SELECTION AND TREATMENT

Seeking subjects who are willing to participate in a study can be difficult, particularly if the study requires extensive amounts of time or other investments by subjects. If a large number of the persons approached to participate in a study decline to participate, the sample actually selected tends to be limited in ways that might not be evident at first glance. Only the researcher knows the subjects well. Subjects might tend to be volunteers, "do-gooders," or those with nothing better to do. In this case, generalizing the findings to all members of a population, such as all nurses, all hospitalized patients, or all persons experiencing diabetes, is not easy to justify.

The study must be planned to limit the investment demands on subjects to improve participation. The number of persons who were approached and refused to participate in the study must be reported so that threats to external validity can be judged. As the percentage of those who decline to participate increases, external validity decreases. Sufficient data must be collected on the subjects to allow the researcher to be familiar with the characteristics of subjects and, to the extent possible, the characteristics of those who decline to participate. Handwritten notes of verbal remarks made by those who decline and observations of behavior, dress, or other significant factors can be useful in determining selection differences.

INTERACTION OF SETTING AND TREATMENT

Bias exists in types of settings and organizations that agree to participate in studies. This bias has been particularly evident in nursing studies. For example, some hospitals welcome nursing studies and encourage employed nurses to conduct studies. Others are resistant to the conduct of nursing research. These two types of hospitals may be different in important ways; thus, there might be an interaction of setting and treatment that limits the generalizability of the findings. The researcher must consider this factor when making statements about the population to which the findings can be generalized.

INTERACTION OF HISTORY AND TREATMENT

The circumstances in which a study was conducted (history) influence the treatment and, thus, the generalizability of the findings. Logically, one can never generalize to the future; however, replication of the study during various periods gives further strength to the usefulness of findings over time. In critiquing studies, one must always consider the period of history during which the study was conducted and the effect of nursing practice and societal events during that period on the reported findings.

ELEMENTS OF A GOOD DESIGN

The purpose of design is to set up a situation that maximizes the possibilities of obtaining accurate responses to objectives, questions, or hypotheses. The design selected must be (1) appropriate to the purpose of the study, (2) feasible given realistic constraints, and (3) effective in reducing threats to validity. In most studies, comparisons are the basis of obtaining valid answers. A good design provides the subjects, the setting, and the protocol within which those comparisons can be clearly examined. The comparisons may focus on differences or relationships or both. The study may require that comparisons be made between or among individuals, groups, or variables. A comparison may also be made of measures taken before a treatment (pretest) and measures taken after a treatment (posttest). After these comparisons have been made, the sample values are compared with statistical tables reflecting population values. In some cases, the study may involve comparing group values with population values.

Designs were developed to reduce threats to the validity of the comparisons. However, some designs are more effective in reducing threats than others. In some cases, it may be necessary to modify the design to reduce a particular threat. Before selecting a design, the researcher must identify the threats to validity that are most likely to occur in a particular study.

Strategies for reducing threats to validity are sometimes addressed in terms of control. Selecting a design involves decisions related to control of the environment, sample, treatment, and measurement. Increasing control (to reduce threats to validity) requires that the researcher carefully think through every facet of the design.

Controlling the Environment

The study environment has a major effect on research outcomes. An uncontrolled environment introduces many extraneous variables into the study situation. Therefore, the study design may include strategies for controlling that environment. In many studies, it is important that the environment be consistent for all subjects. Elements in the environment that may influence the application of a treatment or the measurement of variables must be identified and, when possible, controlled.

Controlling Equivalence of Subjects and Groups

When comparisons are made, it is assumed that the individual units of the comparison are relatively equivalent except for the variables being measured. The researcher does not want to be comparing "apples and oranges." To establish equivalence, the researcher defines sampling criteria. Deviation from this equivalence is a threat to validity. Deviation occurs when sampling criteria have not been adequately defined or when unidentified extraneous variables increase variation in the group.

The most effective strategy for achieving equivalence is random sampling followed by random assignment to groups. However, this strategy does not guarantee equivalence. Even when randomization has been used, the researcher must examine the extent of equivalence by measuring and comparing characteristics for which the groups must be equivalent. This comparison is usually reported in the description of the sample.

Contrary to the aforementioned need for equivalence, groups must be as different as possible in relation to the research variables. Small differences or relationships are more difficult to distinguish than large differences. These differences are often addressed in terms of effect size. Although sample size plays an important role, effect size is maximized by a good design. Effect size is greatest when variance within groups is small.

CONTROL GROUPS

If the study involves an experimental treatment, the design usually calls for a comparison of outcome measures for individuals who receive the experimental treatment with outcome measures for those who do not receive the experimental treatment. This comparison requires a *control group,* subjects who do not receive the experimental treatment.

One threat to validity is the lack of equivalence between the experimental and control groups. This threat is best controlled by random assignment to groups. Another strategy used in some designs is for the subjects to serve as their own controls. With this design strategy, pretest and posttest measures are taken of the subjects in the absence of a treatment as well as before and after the treatment. In this case, the timing of measures must be comparable between control and treatment conditions.

Controlling the Treatment

In a well-designed experimental study, the researcher has complete control of any treatment pro-

vided. The first step in achieving control is to make a detailed description of the treatment. The next step is to use strategies to ensure consistency in implementing the treatment. Consistency may involve elements of the treatment such as equipment, time, intensity, sequencing, and staff skill.

Variations in the treatment reduce the effect size. It is likely that subjects who receive less optimal applications of the treatment will have a smaller response, resulting in more variance in posttest measures for the experimental group. To avoid this problem, the treatment is administered to each subject exactly the same way. This consideration requires the researcher to think carefully through every element of the treatment to reduce variation wherever possible.

For example, if information is being provided as part of the treatment, some researchers videotape the information, present it to each subject in the same environment, and attempt to decrease variation in the experience of the subject before and during the viewing of the videotape. Variations include elements such as time of day, mood, anxiety, experience of pain, interactions with others, and amount of time spent waiting.

In many nursing studies, the researcher does not have complete control of the treatment. It may be costly to control the treatment carefully, it may be difficult to persuade staff to be consistent in the treatment, or the time required to implement a carefully controlled treatment may seem prohibitive. In some cases, the researcher may be studying causal outcomes of an event occurring naturally in the environment.

Regardless of the reason for the researcher's decision, internal validity is reduced when the treatment is inconsistently applied. The risk of a Type II error is higher owing to greater variance and a smaller effect size. Thus, studies with uncontrolled treatments need larger samples to reduce the risk of a Type II error. External validity may be improved if the treatment is studied as it typically occurs clinically. If a statistically significant difference is not found with such a study, it may be the case that, as the treatment is typically applied clinically, it does not have an important effect on patient outcomes. The question would still arise as to whether a difference might have been found if the treatment had been consistently applied.

COUNTERBALANCING

In some studies, each subject receives several different treatments (e.g., relaxation, distraction, or visual imagery) or various levels of the same treatment (e.g., different doses of a drug or varying lengths of relaxation time). Sometimes the application of one treatment can influence the response to later treatments, a phenomenon referred to as a *carryover effect*. If a carryover effect is known to occur, it is not advisable to use this design strategy for the study. However, even when no carryover effect is known, the researcher may choose to take precautions against the possibility that this effect will influence outcomes. In one such precaution, known as *counterbalancing*, the various treatments are administered in random order rather than being provided consistently in the same sequence.

Controlling Measurement

Measurements play a key role in the validity of a study. Measures must have documented validity and reliability. When measurement is crude or inconsistent, variance within groups is high, and it is more difficult to detect differences or relationships among groups. Thus, the study does not provide a valid test of the hypotheses. Validity is enhanced by consistent implementation of measurements. For example, each subject must receive the same instructions about completing scales. Data collectors must be trained and observed for consistency. Designs define the timing of measures (e.g., pretest, posttest). Sometimes, the design calls for multiple measures over time. The researcher must specify the points in time during which measures will be taken. The research report must include a rationale for the timing of measures.

Controlling Extraneous Variables

When designing the study, the researcher must identify variables not included in the design (extraneous variables) that could explain some of the variance in measurement of the study variables. In a good design, the effect of these variables on variance is controlled. Extraneous variables that are commonly encountered in nursing studies are age, education, gender, social class, severity of illness, level of health, functional status, and attitudes. For a specific study, the researcher must think carefully through the variables that could have an impact on that study.

Design strategies used to control extraneous variables include random sampling, random assignment to groups, selecting subjects that are homogeneous in terms of a particular extraneous variable, selecting a heterogeneous sample, blocking, stratification, matching subjects between groups in relation to a particular variable, and statistical control. Table 10–1 summarizes some nursing studies and the various strategies they have used to control extraneous variables.

RANDOM SAMPLING

Random sampling increases the probability that subjects with various levels of an extraneous variable are included and are randomly dispersed throughout the groups within the study. This strategy is particularly important for controlling unidentified extraneous variables. Whenever possible, however, extraneous variables must be identified, measured, and reported in the description of the sample.

RANDOM ASSIGNMENT

Random assignment enhances the probability that subjects with various levels of extraneous variables are equally dispersed in treatment and control groups. Whenever possible, however, this dispersion must be evaluated rather than assumed.

HOMOGENEITY

Homogeneity is a more extreme form of equivalence in which the researcher limits the subjects to only one level of an extraneous variable to reduce its impact on the study findings. To use this strategy, the researcher must have previously identified

TABLE 10–1
STUDIES USING CONTROL STRATEGIES FOR EXTRANEOUS VARIABLES

AIM	DESIGN STRATEGIES	EXTRANEOUS VARIABLE	CONTROL METHOD

To examine the effects of standardized rest periods on the sleep-wake states of preterm infants who were convalescing (Holditch-Davis et al., 1995)	Random assignment
	Controlled treatment
	  Feeding schedule
	  Nap schedule
	  Bed darkened for nap
	
	  Nap disturbed only for urgent care
	  Checked every 15 min
	  Awakened gently
	  Trained observers
		Gestational age
		Race
		Sex
		Body size
		Multiple birth
		Chronological age on admission
		
		>40 weeks gestational age
		Major congenital anomalies
		Terminal condition
			Matching
			Matching
			Matching
			Matching
			Matching
			Matching
			Exclusion
			
			Exclusion
			Exclusion
			Exclusion

To compare the effects of a low-technology environment of care based on a nurse-managed care delivery system (special care unit environment) with the traditional high-technology intensive care unit environment based on a primary nursing care delivery system (Rudy et al., 1995)	Random assignment using biased coin format Controlled treatment	Acuity of illness	Homogeneity
To determine the effect of exercise on subcutaneous tissue oxygen tension (Whitney et al., 1995)	Convenience sample Repeated measures	Gender Smoking behavior Ambient temperature Humidity Fitness	Homogeneity Homogeneity Homogeneity Homogeneity Heterogeneity
Evaluate the effect of feeding a high-calorie diet on food and caloric intake and body weight of tumor-bearing rats (Fredriksdottir & McCarthy, 1995)	Random assignment Experimental and control groups Controlled treatment Repeated measures	Type of rat Tumor type Gender Initial weight Light-dark cycle	Homogeneity Homogeneity Homogeneity Matching Homogeneity
To compare the individual and combined effects of jaw relaxation and music on the sensory and affective components of pain after the first postoperative ambulation (Good, 1995)	Random assignment Four treatment groups, including control Tape used to explain each treatment, practice by patient, coaching, and mastery Assessment of mastery	Protocol for pain medication Preoperative anxiety Preambulatory sensation and distress	Homogeneity Statistical control Statistical control
To determine the impact over time on the cognitive and behavioral functioning of the care recipient with dementia from a home-based intervention program of active cognitive stimulation implemented by the family caregiver (Quayhagen et al., 1995)	Random assignment Treatment group, placebo group, control group Repeated measures Caregiver training for 12 weekly in-home sessions for treatment group Return demonstrations by caregivers Caregiver-recorded weekly log of successes or problems Data collectors blinded to treatment group assignment	Stage of Alzheimer's disease Cognitive impairment Gender	Homogeneity Stratification Statistical control

TABLE 10–1 Continued
STUDIES USING CONTROL STRATEGIES FOR EXTRANEOUS VARIABLES

AIM	DESIGN STRATEGIES	EXTRANEOUS VARIABLE	CONTROL METHOD
Comparing the effectiveness of (a) a combination of mutual goal setting and the operant behavioral management techniques of prompting, shaping, and positive reinforcement, (b) mutual goal setting alone, and (c) usual nursing care in fostering morning self-care behaviors in dependent nursing home residents (Blair, 1995)	Random assignment of nursing homes Staff training Reacquisition-of-skills phase of 6 weeks, during which staff helped subjects overcome self-care deficits 16-week phase during which staff helped subjects maintain gains in self-care	Reliance on staff to perform morning self-care Judgment by staff of capability to do tasks without assistance Cognitive intactness	Homogeneity Homogeneity Homogeneity

To examine nongenetic influences of obesity on the lipid profile and systolic and diastolic blood pressure (cross-sectionally) during two phases of development—the school-age years and adolescence—and (longitudinally) in the transition between these two developmental phases (Hayman et al., 1995)	Longitudinal design with cross-sectional elements random assignment for risk factor assessment
	Assignment of school-aged twin to heavy or light group based on measure of obesity
	Assignment of adolescent twin to heavy or light group based on change in obesity
		Genetic influences on
		  Obesity
		  Gender
		  Age
			
			Matching (twins)
			Heterogeneity
			Stratification

the extraneous variables. Using this strategy, the researcher might choose to include subjects with only one level of an extraneous variable in the study. For example, only subjects between the ages of 20 and 30 years may be included, or only male subjects. The study may include only breast cancer patients who have been diagnosed within 1 month, are at a particular stage of disease, and are receiving a specific treatment for cancer. The difficulty with this strategy is that it limits generalization to the types of subjects included in the study. Findings could not justifiably be generalized to types of people excluded from the study.

HETEROGENEITY

In studies in which random sampling is not used, the researcher may attempt to obtain subjects with a wide variety of characteristics (or who are *heterogeneous*) to reduce the risk of biases. With the use of this strategy, subjects may be sought from multiple diverse sources. The strategy is designed to increase generalizability. Characteristics of the sample must be described in the research report.

BLOCKING

In *blocking,* the researcher includes subjects with various levels of an extraneous variable in the sample but controls the numbers of subjects at each level of the variable and their random assignment to groups within the study. Designs using blocking are referred to as *randomized block designs.* The extraneous variable is then used as an independent variable in the data analysis. Therefore, the extraneous variable must be included in the framework and the study hypotheses.

Using this strategy, the researcher might randomly assign equal numbers of subjects in three age categories (younger than 18 years, 18 to 60 years, and older than 60 years) to each group in the study. The researcher could use blocking for several extraneous variables. For example, the study might be blocked in relation to both age and ethnic background (African American, Hispanic, white, and Asian). An example of this approach is summarized in Table 10–2.

During data analysis for the randomized block design, each cell in the analysis is treated as a group. Therefore, the cell size for each group and

TABLE 10-2 EXAMPLE OF BLOCKING USING AGE AND ETHNIC BACKGROUND				
AGE	**ETHNIC GROUP**		**EXPERIMENTAL**	**CONTROL**
Younger than 18 years $n = 160$	African American	$n = 40$	$n = 20$	$n = 20$
	Hispanic	$n = 40$	$n = 20$	$n = 20$
	Caucasian	$n = 40$	$n = 20$	$n = 20$
	Asian	$n = 40$	$n = 20$	$n = 20$
19 to 60 years $n = 160$	African American	$n = 40$	$n = 20$	$n = 20$
	Hispanic	$n = 40$	$n = 20$	$n = 20$
	Caucasian	$n = 40$	$n = 20$	$n = 20$
	Asian	$n = 40$	$n = 20$	$n = 20$
Older than 60 years $n = 160$	African American	$n = 40$	$n = 20$	$n = 20$
	Hispanic	$n = 40$	$n = 20$	$n = 20$
	Caucasian	$n = 40$	$n = 20$	$n = 20$
	Asian	$n = 40$	$n = 20$	$n = 20$

the effect size must be evaluated to ensure adequate power to detect differences. A minimum of 20 subjects per group is recommended. The example described for Table 10-2 would require a minimal sample of 480 subjects.

STRATIFICATION

Stratification involves the distribution of subjects throughout the sample, using sampling techniques similar to those used in blocking, but the purpose of the procedure is even distribution throughout the sample. The extraneous variable is not included in analysis of the data. Distribution of the extraneous variable is included in the description of the sample.

MATCHING

Because of the importance of ensuring that subjects in the control group are equivalent to subjects in the experimental group, some studies are designed to match subjects in the two groups. *Matching* is used when a subject in the experimental group is randomly selected and then a subject similar in relation to important extraneous variables is randomly selected for the control group. Clearly, the pool of available subjects would have to be large to accomplish this goal. In quasi-experimental studies, matching may be performed without randomization.

STATISTICAL CONTROL

In some studies, it is not considered feasible to control extraneous variables through the design. However, the researcher recognizes the possible impact of extraneous variables on variance and effect size. Therefore, measures are obtained for the identified extraneous variables. Data analysis strategies that have the capacity to remove (*partial out*) the variance explained by the extraneous variable are performed before the analysis of differences or relationships between or among the variables of interest in the study. One statistical procedure commonly used for this purpose is analysis of covariance, described in Chapter 22. Although statistical control seems to be a quick and easy solution to the problem of extraneous variables, its results are not as satisfactory as those of the various methods of design control.

PARTICIPATORY RESEARCH

Participatory research is a strategy designed to include representatives of the community under study as members of the research team. It allows members of the community to have a voice in the way the study is conducted and the means that will be used to disseminate the results. The strategy also serves as a check on the researchers' biases and makes the scientific community directly accountable to the client communities. Commonly, issues related to imbalances in power between the researchers and the community representatives must be addressed.

In vulnerable populations, suspicion of researchers is prevalent. Many people fear being misused. Establishing and maintaining trust is the ongoing key to success. In a participatory research project, the people being studied form a partnership with the researchers and are involved in all phases of the research process. Questions of immediate concern to the community may be added to the research program. Through dialogue, the researchers often gain new insights into the problem under study as well as interventions that might be effective in addressing the problem. Change is one of the primary purposes of the project (Henderson, 1995; Seng, 1998).

Participatory research strategies were originally developed by Friere, a Brazilian scholar whose ideas are described in Chapter 4. The methods used to promote social change are those of critical social theory. Participatory studies include a variety of designs, some qualitative, some quantitative, and some a triangulated mix of strategies. Some of the strategies that might be used in a participatory research project are described in more detail in Chapter 13. Although this method is not commonly used in nursing studies, Zachariah and Lundeen (1997) describe some of the participatory research strategies they used in their study.

TRIANGULATION

There has been much controversy among researchers about the relative validity of various approaches to research. Designing quantitative experimental studies with rigorous controls may provide strong internal validity but questionable or limited external validity. Qualitative studies may have strong external validity but questionable internal validity. A single approach to measuring a concept may be inadequate to justify a claim that it is a valid measure of a theoretical concept. Testing a single theory may leave the results open to the challenge of rival hypotheses from other theories.

Researchers have been exploring alternative design strategies that might increase the overall validity of studies. The strategy generating the most interest is triangulation. First used by Campbell and Fiske in 1959, *triangulation* is the combined use of two or more theories, methods, data sources, investigators, or analysis methods in the study of the same phenomenon. Denzin (1989) identified the following four types of triangulation: (1) data triangulation, (2) investigator triangulation, (3) theoretical triangulation, and (4) methodological triangulation. Kimchi and colleagues (1991) have suggested a fifth type, analysis triangulation. *Multiple triangulation* is the combination of more than one of these types.

Data Triangulation

Data triangulation involves the collection of data from multiple sources for the same study. For the collection to be considered triangulation, the data must all have the same foci. The intent is to obtain diverse views of the phenomenon under study for purposes of validation (Kimchi et al., 1991). These data sources provide an opportunity to examine how an event is experienced by different individuals, groups of people, or communities; at different times; or in different settings (Mitchell, 1986).

Longitudinal studies are not a form of triangulation because their purpose is to identify change. When time is triangulated, the purpose is validation of the congruence of the phenomenon over time. For a multisite study to be triangulated, data from the settings must be cross-validated for multisite consistency. When person triangulation is used, data from individuals might be compared for consistency with data obtained from groups. The intent is to use data from one source to validate data from another source (Kimchi et al., 1991).

Investigator Triangulation

In *investigator triangulation,* two or more investigators with diverse research training backgrounds examine the same phenomenon (Mitchell, 1986).

For example, a qualitative researcher and a quantitative researcher might cooperatively design and conduct a study of interest to both. Kimchi and colleagues (1991, p. 365) hold that investigator triangulation has occurred when "(a) each investigator has a prominent role in the study, (b) the expertise of each investigator is different, and (c) the expertise (disciplinary bias) of each investigator is evident in the study." The use of investigator triangulation removes the potential for bias that may occur in a single-investigator study (Denzin, 1989; Duffy, 1987). Kimchi and colleagues (1991) suggest that investigator triangulation is difficult to discern from published reports. They advise that, in the future, authors claim that they have performed investigator triangulation and describe how it was achieved in their study.

Theoretical Triangulation

Theoretical triangulation is the use of all the theoretical interpretations "that could conceivably be applied to a given area" (Denzin, 1989, p. 241) as the framework for a study. Using this strategy, the researcher critically examines various theoretical points of view for utility and power. Competing hypotheses are developed on the basis of the different theoretical perspectives and are tested using the same data set. Greater confidence can then be placed in the accepted hypotheses because they have been pitted against rival hypotheses (Denzin, 1989; Mitchell, 1986). This is a tougher test of existing theory in a field of study because alternative theories are examined rather than a single test of a proposition or propositions from one theory. Theoretical triangulation can lead to the development of more powerful substantive theories that have some scientific validation. Denzin (1989) recommends the following steps to achieve theoretical triangulation:

1. A comprehensive list of all possible interpretations in a given area is constructed. This will involve bringing a variety of theoretical perspectives to bear upon the phenomena at hand (including interactionism, phenomenology, Marxism, feminist theory, semiotics, cultural studies, and so on).
2. The actual research is conducted, and empirical materials are collected.

3. The multiple theoretical frameworks enumerated in Step 1 are focused on the empirical materials.
4. Those interpretations that do not bear on the materials are discarded or set aside.
5. Those interpretations that map and make sense of the phenomena are assembled into an interpretive framework that addresses all of the empirical materials.
6. A reformulated interpretive system is stated based at all points on the empirical materials just examined and interpreted. (Denzin, 1989, p. 241)

Currently, few nursing studies meet Denzin's criteria for theoretical triangulation, although some frameworks for nursing studies are developed to compare propositions from more than one theory. For example, Yarcheski and associates (1999) conducted an empirical test of alternative theories of anger in early adolescents.

Methodological Triangulation

Methodological triangulation is the use of two or more research methods in a single study (Mitchell, 1986). The difference can be at the level of design or of data collection. Methodological triangulation, the most common type of triangulation, is frequently used in the examination of complex concepts. Complex concepts of interest in nursing include caring, hope in terminal illness, coping with chronic illness, and promotion of health.

There are two different types of methodological triangulation, (1) within-method triangulation and (2) across-method triangulation (Denzin, 1989). *Within-method triangulation*, the simpler form, is used when the phenomenon being studied is multidimensional. For example, two or three different quantitative instruments might be used to measure the same phenomenon. Conversely, two or more qualitative methods might be used. Examples of different data collection methods are questionnaires, physiological instruments, scales, interviews, and observation techniques. *Across-method* or *between-method triangulation* involves combining research strategies from two or more research traditions in the same study. For example, methods from qualitative research and quantitative research might be used in the same study (Duffy, 1987; Mitchell, 1986; Morse, 1991; Porter, 1989). From these research traditions, different types of designs, methods of measurement, data collection processes, or data analysis techniques might be used to examine a phenomenon to try to achieve convergent validity.

Mitchell (1986, pp. 22–23) identified the following four principles that should be applied with methodological triangulation: "(1) the research question must be clearly focused; (2) the strengths and weaknesses of each chosen method must complement each other; (3) the methods must be selected according to their relevance to the phenomenon being studied; and (4) the methodological approach must be monitored throughout the study to make sure the first three principles are followed."

Analysis Triangulation

In *analysis triangulation,* the same data set is analyzed with the use of two or more differing analyses techniques. The purpose is to evaluate the similarity of findings. The intent is to provide a means of cross-validating the findings (Kimchi et al., 1991).

Pros and Cons of Triangulation

It is possible that triangulation will be the research trend of the future. However, before jumping on this bandwagon, we would be prudent to consider the implications of using these strategies. There is concern that triangulation will be used in studies for which it is not appropriate. An additional concern is that the popularization of the method will generate a number of triangulated studies that have been poorly conducted. Sohier (1988, p. 740) points out that "multiple methods will not compensate for poor design or sloppy research. Ill-conceived measures will compound error rather than reduce it. Unclear questions will not become clearer."

The suggestion that qualitative and quantitative methods be included in the same study has generated considerable controversy in the nursing research community (Clarke & Yaros, 1988; Mitchell, 1986; Morse, 1991; Phillips, 1988a, 1988b). Myers and Haase (1989) believe that the integration of these two research approaches is inevitable and es-

sential. Clarke and Yaros (1988) suggest that combining methods is the first step in the development of new methodologies, which are greatly needed to investigate nursing phenomena. Hogan and DeSantis (1991) believe that triangulation of qualitative and quantitative methods will lead to the development of substantive theory. Phillips (1988a, 1988b) holds the position that the two methods are incompatible because they are based on different world views. If a single investigator attempted to use both methods in one study, he or she would have to interpret the meaning of the data from two different philosophical perspectives. Because researchers tend to acquire their research training within a particular research tradition, attempts to incorporate another research tradition may be poorly achieved. As Sandelowski (1995, p. 569) states, "a misplaced ecumenicism, definitional drift, and conceptual misappropriation are evident in discussions of triangulation, which has become a technique for everything."

Mitchell (1986) identifies a number of problems that may be encountered by investigators using this method. These strategies require many observations and result in large volumes of data for analysis. The investigator must have the ability and the desire to deal with complex design, measurement, and analysis issues with limited resources. Mitchell (1986) identifies the following issues that the investigator must consider during the data analysis:

- How to combine numerical (quantitative) data and linguistic or textual (qualitative) data
- How to interpret divergent results from numerical data and linguistic data
- What to do with overlapping concepts that emerge from the data and are not clearly differentiated from one another
- Whether and how to weight data sources
- Whether each different method used should be considered equally sensitive and weighted equally

Myers and Haase (1989) provide guidelines that they believe are necessary when one is merging qualitative and quantitative methods. Their guidelines, which follow, are based on the assumption that at least two investigators (one qualitative and one quantitative) are involved in any study combining these two methods.

1. The world is viewed as a whole, an interactive system with patterns of information exchange between subsystems or levels of reality.
2. Both subjective and objective data are recognized as legitimate avenues for gaining understanding.
3. Both atomistic and holistic thinking are used in design and analysis.
4. The concept of research "participant" includes not only those who are the subjects of the methodology but also those who administer or operate the methodology.
5. Maximally conflicting points of view are sought with provision for systematic and controlled confrontation. Respectful, honest, open confrontation on points of view between investigators is essential. Here, conflict is seen as a positive value because it offers potential for expanding questioning and consequent understanding. Confrontation occurs between co-investigators with differing expertise who recognize that both approaches are equally valid and vulnerable. Ability to consider participants' views which may differ from the investigator's perspective is equally important. (Myers & Haase, 1989, p. 300)

Morse (1991) believes that qualitative and quantitative methods cannot be equally weighted in a research project. The project either (1) is theoretically driven by qualitative methods and incorporates a complementary quantitative component or (2) is theoretically driven by the quantitative method and incorporates a complementary qualitative component. However, each method used must be complete in itself and must meet appropriate criteria for rigor. For example, if qualitative interviews are conducted, "the interviews should be continued until saturation is reached, and the content analysis conducted inductively, rather than forcing the data into some preconceived categories to fit the quantitative study or to prove a point" (Morse, 1991, p. 121).

Morse (1991) also holds that the greatest threat to validity of methodological triangulation is not philosophical incompatibility but the use of inadequate or inappropriate samples. The quantitative requirement for large, randomly selected samples is inconsistent with the qualitative requirement that subjects be selected according to how well they represent the phenomena of interest, and sample selection ceases when saturation of data is reached. Morse (1991) does not consider it necessary, however, for the two approaches to use the same samples for the study. In all aspects of a methodologically triangulated study, Morse (1991) believes, strategies must be implemented to maintain the validity for each method. Overall, Morse supports the use of methodological triangulation, believing that it "will strengthen research results and contribute to theory and knowledge development." (Morse, 1991, p. 122)

Duffy holds that triangulation, "when used appropriately, combines different methods in a variety of ways to produce richer and more insightful analyses of complex phenomena than can be achieved by either method separately." (Duffy, 1987, p. 133) Coward (1990) opines that the combining of qualitative and quantitative methods will increase support for validity. "Construct validity is enhanced when results are stable across multiple measures of a concept. Statistical conclusion validity is enhanced when results are stable across many data sets and methods of analysis. Internal validity is enhanced when results are stable across many potential threats to causal inference. External validity is supported when results are stable across multiple settings, populations and times" (Coward, 1990, p. 166).

Sandelowski recommends that "the concept of triangulation ought to be reserved for designating a technique for conformation employed within paradigms in which convergent and consensual validity are valued and in which it is deemed appropriate to use information from one source to corroborate another. Whether triangulation or not, the purpose, method of execution, and assumptions informing any research combinations should be clearly delineated." (Sandelowski, 1995, p. 573)

■ SUMMARY

Research design is a blueprint for the conduct of a study that maximizes control over factors that could interfere with the desired outcomes from studies. The design of a study is the end-result of a series of decisions made by the researcher about how the study will be implemented. Elements central to the study design are the presence or absence of a treatment, number of groups in the sample, number and timing of measurements to be performed, sampling method, the time frame for data collection, planned comparisons, and control of extraneous variables.

Selecting a design requires an understanding of certain concepts: causality, bias, manipulation, control, and validity. In *causality*, there is an assumption that things have causes and that causes lead to effects. Nursing science must be built within a philosophical framework of multicausality and probability. *Multicausality* is the recognition that a number of interrelating variables can be involved in causing a particular effect. *Probability* deals with the likelihood that a specific effect will occur after a particular cause occurs. *Bias* is of great concern in research because of the potential effect on the meaning of the study findings. Any component of the study that deviates or causes a deviation from true measure leads to distorted findings. *Manipulation* means to move around or to control the movement, such as the manipulation of the independent variable. If the freedom to manipulate a variable is under the control of someone other than the researcher, a bias is introduced into the study. *Control* means having the power to direct or manipulate factors to achieve a desired outcome. The greater the amount of control of the researcher over the study situation, the more credible the study findings.

Validity is a measure of the truth or accuracy of a claim. When conducting a study, the researcher is confronted with major decisions regarding four types of study validity: statistical conclusion validity, internal validity, construct validity, and external validity. *Statistical conclusion validity* is concerned with whether the conclusions about relationships drawn from statistical analysis are an accurate reflection of the real world. However, there are reasons why false conclusions can be drawn about the presence or absence of a relationship; these are called *threats* to statistical conclusion validity. *Internal validity* is the extent to which the effects detected in the study are a true reflection of reality, rather than being a result of the effects of extraneous variables. Any study can have threats to internal validity, and these validity threats can lead to a false-positive or false-negative conclusion.

Construct validity examines the fit between the conceptual definitions and operational definitions of variables. The threats to construct validity are related to both previous instrument development and the development of measurement techniques as part of the methodology of a particular study. *External validity* is concerned with the extent to which study findings can be generalized beyond the sample used in the study. The most serious threat would lead to the findings being meaningful only for the group being studied.

The purpose of design is to set up a situation that maximizes the possibilities of obtaining valid answers to research questions or hypotheses. The design selected must be (1) appropriate to the purpose of the study, (2) feasible given realistic constraints, and (3) effective in reducing threats to validity. In most studies, comparisons are the basis of obtaining valid answers. A good design provides the subjects, the setting, and the protocol within which these comparisons can be clearly examined. Designs were developed to reduce threats to the validity of the comparisons. However, some designs are more effective in reducing threats than others. Selecting a design involves decisions related to control of the environment, the sample, the treatment, and measurement.

An uncontrolled environment introduces many extraneous variables into the study situation. The study design may include strategies for controlling that environment. When comparisons are made, the assumption is that the individual units of the comparison are relatively equivalent except for the variables being measured. To establish equivalence, sampling criteria are defined. Deviation occurs when sampling criteria have not been adequately defined or when unidentified extraneous variables result in deviation in parts of the sample. The most effective strategy for achieving equivalence is random sampling followed by random assignment to groups. If the study includes a treatment, the design usually calls for a comparison of outcome measures of individuals who receive the treatment with those who do not receive the treatment. This comparison requires a *control group*, subjects who do not receive the treatment. One threat to validity is the lack of equivalence between the experimental and the control groups.

In a well-designed experimental study, the researcher has complete control of any treatment provided. The first step in achieving control is a detailed description of the treatment. The next step is to use strategies to ensure consistency in implementing the treatment. When the subject will receive several different treatments or various levels of the same treatment, *counterbalancing* is used, meaning that the various treatments are administered in random order. Designs define the timing of measures (e.g., pretest, posttest). Sometimes, the design calls for multiple measures over time.

In designing the study, the researcher must identify variables not included in the design (*extraneous variables*) that could explain some of the variance in measurement of the study variables. In a good design, the effect of these variables on variance is controlled. Design strategies used to control extraneous variables include random sampling, random assignment to groups, selecting subjects who are homogeneous in terms of a particular extraneous variable, selecting a heterogeneous sample, blocking, stratification, matching subjects between groups in relation to a particular variable, and statistical control.

Researchers have been exploring alternative design strategies that might increase the overall validity of studies. The strategy generating the most interest recently is triangulation. *Triangulation* is the combined use of two or more theories, methods, data sources, investigators, or analysis methods in the study of the same phenomenon. Five types of triangulation have been identified: data triangulation, investigator triangulation, theoretical triangulation, methodological triangulation, and analysis triangulation.

There is concern that triangulation will be used in studies for which it is not appropriate. An additional concern is that the popularization of the method will generate a number of triangulated studies that have been poorly conducted. The suggestion that qualitative and quantitative methods be included in the same study has sparked considerable controversy in the nursing research community. Some hold that the two methods are incompatible because they are based on different world views. Because researchers tend to acquire their research training within a particular research tradition, their

attempts to incorporate another research tradition may be poorly achieved. A number of problems may be encountered by investigators using this method. Other researchers believe that combining the two methods holds great promise for strengthening research results and contributing to theory and knowledge development.

• •

REFERENCES

Blair, C. E. (1995). Combining behavior management and mutual goal setting to reduce physical dependency in nursing home residents. *Nursing Research, 44*(3), 160–165.

Campbell, D. T., & Fiske, D. W. (1959). Convergent and discriminant validation by the multitrait-multimethod matrix. *Psychological Bulletin, 56*(2), 81–105.

Clarke, P. N., & Yaros, P. S. (1988). Research blenders: Commentary and response. *Nursing Science Quarterly, 1*(4), 147–149.

Cook, T. D., & Campbell, D. T. (1979). *Quasi-experimentation: Design and analysis issues for field settings.* Chicago: Rand McNally.

Coward, D. D. (1990). Critical multiplism: A research strategy for nursing science. *Image—The Journal of Nursing Scholarship, 22*(3), 163–167.

Denzin, N. K. (1989). *The research act: A theoretical introduction to sociological methods* (3rd ed.). New York: McGraw-Hill.

Dodd, M., Dibble, S., & Thomas, M. (1992). Outpatient chemotherapy: Patients' and family members' concerns and coping strategies. *Public Health Nursing, 9*(1), 37–44.

Dodd, M., Thomas, M., & Dibble, S. (1991). Self care for patients experiencing cancer chemotherapy side effects: A concern for home care nurses. *Home Healthcare, 9*(6), 21–26.

Duffy, M. E. (1987). Methodological triangulation: A vehicle for merging quantitative and qualitative research methods. *Image—The Journal of Nursing Scholarship, 19*(3), 130–133.

Fredriksdottir, N., & McCarthy, D. O. (1995). The effect of caloric density of food on energy intake and body weight in tumor-bearing rats. *Research in Nursing & Health, 18*(4), 357–363.

Good, M. (1995). A comparison of the effects of jaw relaxation and music on postoperative pain. *Nursing Research, 44*(1), 52–57.

Goodwin, L. D. (1984). Increasing efficiency and precision of data analysis: Multivariate vs. univariate statistical techniques. *Nursing Research, 33*(4), 247–249.

Greer, D. S., Mor, V., Sherwood, S., Morris, J. M., & Birnbaum, H. (1983). National hospice study analysis plan. *Journal of Chronic Disease, 36*(11), 737–780.

Hayman, L. L., Meininger, J. C., Coates, P. M., & Gallagher, P.

R. (1995). Nongenetic influences of obesity on risk factors for cardiovascular disease during two phases of development. *Nursing Research, 44*(5), 277–283.

Henderson, D. J. (1995). Consciousness raising in participatory research: Method and methodology for emancipatory nursing inquiry. *Advances in Nursing Science, 17*(3), 58–69.

Hogan, N., & DeSantis, L. (1991). Development of substantive theory in nursing. *Nursing Education Today, 11*(3), 167–171.

Holditch-Davis, D., Barham, L. N., O'Hale, A., & Tucker, B. (1995). Effect of standard rest periods on convalescent pre-term infants. *Journal of Gynecologic and Neonatal Nursing, 24*(5), 424–432.

Kimchi, J., Polivka, B., & Stevenson, J. S. (1991). Triangulation: Operational definitions. *Nursing Research, 40*(6), 364–366.

Lewis, F., Wood, H., & Ellison, E. (1989). [Family impact study: The impact of cancer on the family.] Unpublished preliminary analysis report.

Mitchell, E. S. (1986). Multiple triangulation: A methodology for nursing science. *Advances in Nursing Science, 8*(3), 18–26.

Morse, J. M. (1991). Approaches to qualitative-quantitative methodological triangulation. *Nursing Research, 40*(1), 120–123.

Myers, S. T., & Haase, J. E. (1989). Guidelines for integration of quantitative and qualitative approaches. *Nursing Research, 38*(5), 299–301.

Phillips, J. R. (1988a). Research issues: Research blenders. *Nursing Science Quarterly, 1*(1), 4–5.

Phillips, J. R. (1988b). Dialogue on research issues: Diggers of deeper holes. *Nursing Science Quarterly, 1*(4), 149–151.

Porter, E. J. (1989). The qualitative-quantitative dualism. *Image—The Journal of Nursing Scholarship, 21*(2), 98–102.

Quayhagen, M. P., Quayhagen, M., Corbeil, R. R., Roth, P. A., & Rodgers, J. A. (1995). A dyadic remediation program for care recipients with dementia. *Nursing Research, 44*(3), 153–159.

Rudy, E. B., Daly, B. J., Douglas, S., Montenegro, H. D., Song, R., & Dyer, M. A. (1995). Patient outcomes for the chronically critically ill: Special care unit versus intensive care unit. *Nursing Research, 44*(6), 324–331.

Sandelowski, M. (1995). Triangles and crystals: On the geometry of qualitative research. *Research in Nursing & Health, 18*(6), 569–574.

Seng, J. S. (1998). Praxis as a conceptual framework for participatory research in nursing. *Advances in Nursing Science, 20*(4), 37–48.

Sohier, R. (1988). Multiple triangulation and contemporary nursing research. *Western Journal of Nursing Research, 10*(6), 732–742.

Whitney, J. D., Stotts, N. A., & Goodson, W. H. III. (1995). Effects of dynamic exercise on subcutaneous oxygen tension and temperature. *Research in Nursing & Health, 18*(2), 97–104.

Yarcheski, A., Mahon, M. E., & Yarcheski, T. J. (1999). An empirical test of alternate theories of anger in early adolescents. *Nursing Research, 48*(6), 317–323.

Zachariah, R., & Lundeen, S. P. (1997). Research and practice in an academic community nursing center. *Image—The Journal of Nursing Scholarship, 29*(3), 255–260.

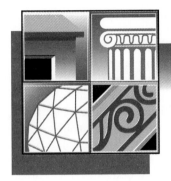

CHAPTER 11
. . . .

SELECTING A RESEARCH DESIGN

The purpose of a design is to achieve greater control and thus improve the validity of the study in examining the research problem. Determining the appropriate research design for a study requires the integration of many elements. The individual critiquing a nursing study is confronted with a similar dilemma. Many published studies do not identify the design used in the study. Identifying the design may require putting together bits of information from various parts of the research report. The questions given at the beginning of Chapter 10 will help you select a design or identify the design of a study for a critique.

This chapter describes the designs most commonly used in nursing research, using the categories described in Chapter 3—descriptive, correlational, quasi-experimental, and experimental. Descriptive and correlational designs examine variables in natural environments and do not include researcher-designed treatments. Quasi-experimental and experimental designs examine the effects of an intervention by comparing differences between groups that have received the intervention and those that have not received the intervention. As you review each design, note the threats to validity controlled by the design, keeping in mind that uncontrolled threats in the design you choose may weaken the validity of your study. Table 11–1 lists the designs discussed in this chapter. After the descriptions of the designs, a series of decision trees are provided to assist the researcher in the selection of the appropriate design or the reader in the identification of the design used in a published study.

Designs have been developed by researchers to meet unique research needs as they emerged. The first experimental designs were developed in the 1930s by Sir Ronald A. Fisher (1935) and published in a book entitled *The Design of Experiments*. However, most work on design has been conducted since the 1970s (Abdellah & Levine, 1979; Anderson & McLean, 1974; Cook & Campbell, 1979; Cox, 1958; Trochim, 1986). During this time, designs have become much more sophisticated and varied. There is no universal standard for categorizing designs. Names of designs change as they are discussed by various authors. Researchers sometimes merge elements of several designs to meet the research needs of a particular study. From these developments, new designs sometimes emerge.

Originally, only experimental designs were considered of value. In addition, many believe that the only setting in which an experiment can be conducted is a laboratory, in which much stricter controls can be maintained than in a field or natural setting. This approach is appropriate for the natural sciences but not for the social sciences. From the social sciences have emerged additional quantitative designs (descriptive, correlational, and quasi-experimental) and qualitative designs.

At present, nurse researchers are using designs developed in other disciplines, such as psychology, that meet the needs of that discipline. Will these designs be effective in adding to nursing's knowledge base? These designs are a useful starting point, but nurse scientists must go beyond these

TABLE 11–1
RESEARCH DESIGNS

Descriptive designs
  Typical descriptive study design
  Comparative descriptive design
  Time dimensional designs
    Longitudinal designs
    Cross-sectional designs
    Trend designs
    Event-partitioning designs
  Case study design
Correlational designs
  Descriptive correlational design
  Predictive design
  Model-testing designs
Quasi-experimental designs
  Nonequivalent control group designs
    The one-group posttest–only design
    The posttest–only design with nonequivalent groups
    The one-group pretest–posttest design
    The untreated control group design with pretest and posttest
    The removed-treatment design with pretest and posttest
    The reversed-treatment nonequivalent control group design
      with pretest and posttest
  Interrupted time-series designs
    Simple interrupted time series
    Interrupted time series with a nonequivalent no-treatment
      control group time series
    Interrupted time series with multiple replications
Experimental study designs
  Pretest–posttest control group design
  Posttest–only control group design
  Randomized block design
  Factorial designs
  Nested designs
  Crossover or counterbalanced designs
  Randomized clinical trials

designs to develop designs that will more appropriately meet the needs of nursing's knowledge base. To go beyond the current designs, nurse scientists must have a working knowledge of available designs and of the logic on which they are based. Designs created to meet nursing needs should be congruent with nursing philosophy. They must provide a means to examine dimensions of nursing within a holistic framework and must allow examination of nursing dimensions over time. Designs must be developed that can seek answers to important nursing questions rather than answering only questions that can be examined by existing designs.

Innovative design strategies are beginning to appear within nursing research. One example is the intervention research design described in Chapter 13. Developing designs to study the outcomes of nursing actions is also important. This emerging field of research in nursing is described in Chapter 12. The use of time-series analysis strategies (described later in the chapter) holds great promise for examining important dimensions of nursing. Nurse researchers must see themselves as credible scientists to dare to develop new design strategies that facilitate examination of little-understood aspects of nursing. Developing a new design requires careful consideration of possible threats to validity and ways to diminish them. It also requires a willingness to risk the temporary failures that are always inherent in the development of something new.

DESCRIPTIVE STUDY DESIGNS

Descriptive studies (see Table 11–1) are designed to gain more information about characteristics within a particular field of study. Their purpose is to provide a picture of situations as they naturally happen. In many aspects of nursing, there is a need for a clearer delineation of the phenomenon before causality can be examined. A descriptive design may be used for the purpose of developing theory, identifying problems with current practice, justifying current practice, making judgments, or determining what others in similar situations are doing (Waltz & Bausell, 1981). No manipulation of variables is involved. Dependent and independent variables should not be used within a descriptive design, because the design involves no attempt to establish causality.

Descriptive designs vary in levels of complexity. Some contain only two variables, whereas others may have multiple variables. The relationships among variables are identified to obtain an overall picture of the phenomenon being examined, but examination of types and degrees of relationships is not the primary purpose of a descriptive study. Protection against bias in a descriptive design is achieved through (1) linkages between conceptual and operational definitions of variables, (2) sample selection and size, (3) the use of valid and reliable instruments, and (4) data collection procedures that achieve some environmental control.

Typical Descriptive Study Design

The most commonly used descriptive design is presented in Figure 11–1. The design is used to examine characteristics of a single sample. It involves identification of a phenomenon of interest and of the variables within the phenomenon, development of conceptual and operational definitions of the variables, and description of the variables. The description of the variables leads to an interpretation of the theoretical meaning of the findings and provides knowledge of the variables and the study population that can be used for future research in the area.

Very few studies use a typical descriptive design; however, many contain descriptive components. An example of a descriptive design is Mimnaugh and colleagues' (1999) study of sensations experienced during removal of tubes in acute postoperative patients. The following excerpt describes the design of their study.

. . . .

"The major purpose of this study was to determine the types and intensity of sensations that patients experience when chest tubes (CTs) and Jackson-Pratt (JP) abdominal tubes are removed. A convenience sample of 62 hospitalized subjects, 31 with CTs and 31 with JP tubes, participated. Each subject was interviewed after tube removal. Sensations were identified, and intensity of sensation was marked on a 100-mm Visual Analogue Scale." (Mimnaugh et al., 1999, p. 78)

. . . .

"The following research questions were addressed:

1. What sensations do patients experience when abdominal JP tubes are removed?
2. What sensations do patients experience when CTs are removed?
3. What is the intensity of the sensations patients experience when abdominal and chest tubes are removed?
4. What factors affect the perception and intensity of sensations that are experienced?
5. What types of information are patients commonly given before tube removal?
6. What types of information do patients indicate that they would like to receive before removal of abdominal or chest tubes?" (Mimnaugh et al., 1999, p. 79) ■

Comparative Descriptive Design

The *comparative descriptive design* (see Figure 11–2) examines and describes differences in variables in two or more groups that occur naturally in the setting. Descriptive statistics and inferential statistical analyses may be used to examine differences between or among groups. Commonly, the results

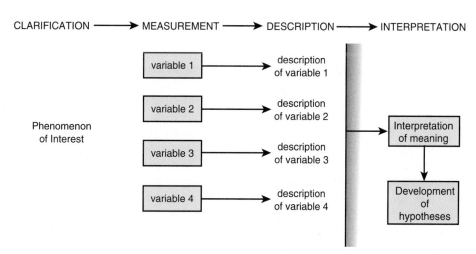

CLARIFICATION ⟶ MEASUREMENT ⟶ DESCRIPTION ⟶ INTERPRETATION

FIGURE 11–1 ■ Descriptive study design.

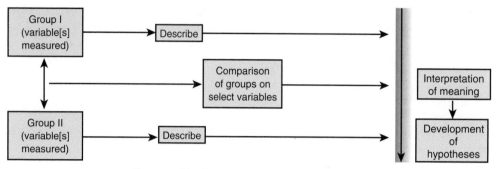

FIGURE 11–2 ▪ Comparative descriptive design.

obtained from these analyses are not generalized to a population. An example of this design is the study by Williams and associates (1999) of fatigue in mothers of infants discharged home with apnea monitors. The following extract describes the study.

· ·

"A comparative study was done to determine differences in caregiver fatigue between two groups of mothers of preterm infants at baseline, in the hospital (Time 1), 1 week postdischarge (Time 2), and 1 month postdischarge (Time 3). Group 1 infants were discharged home on apnea monitors (AM) (n = 28), and Group 2 infants were not on apnea monitors (nonAM) (n = 46)." (Williams et al., 1999, p. 69) ▪

Time Dimensional Designs

Time dimensional designs were developed within the discipline of epidemiology, in which the occurrence and distribution of disease among populations are studied. These designs examine sequences and patterns of change, growth, or trends over time. The dimension of time, then, becomes an important factor. Within the field of epidemiology, the samples in time dimensional studies are called *cohorts*. Originally, cohorts were age categories; however, the concept has been expanded to apply to groups distinguished by many other variables. Other means of classifying populations that have relevance in relation to time are time of diagnosis, point of entry

into a treatment protocol, point of entry into a new lifestyle, and age at which the subject started smoking. An understanding of temporal sequencing is an important prerequisite to examining causality between variables. Thus, the results of these designs lead to the development of hypotheses and are often forerunners of experimental designs.

Epidemiological studies that use time dimensional designs are developed to determine the risk factors or causal factors of illness states. Cause determined in this manner is called *inferred causality*. The best-known studies in this area are those on smoking and cancer. Because of the strength of studies that have undergone multiple repetitions, the causal link is strong. The strategy is not as powerful as experimental designs in supporting causality; however, in this situation, as in many others, one can never ethically conduct a true experiment.

Epidemiologists use two strategies to examine a situation over time, retrospective studies and prospective studies. The norm in epidemiological studies is to use *cohorts* to refer to groups of subjects in prospective studies, but the term is generally not used in retrospective studies. In *retrospective* studies, both the proposed cause and the proposed effect have already occurred. For example, the subjects could have a specific type of cancer, and the researcher could be searching for commonalities among subjects that may have led to the development of that type of cancer. In a *prospective* study, causes may have occurred, but the proposed effect has not.

The Framingham study is the best-known example of a prospective study (U.S. Department of Health and Human Services, 1968). In this study, members of a community were monitored for 20 years by researchers who examined variables such as dietary patterns, exercise, weight, and blood lipid levels. As the subjects experienced illnesses, such as heart disease, hypertension, or lung disease, their illnesses could be related to previously identified variables.

Prospective studies are considered more powerful than retrospective studies in inferring causality, because it can be demonstrated that the risk factors occurred before the illness and are positively related to the illness. Both designs are important for use in nursing studies, because a person's responses to health situations are patterns that developed long before the health situation occurred (Newman, 1986). These patterns then influence responses to nursing interventions.

Several designs are used to conduct time dimensional studies: longitudinal, cross-sectional, trend, and treatment partitioning.

LONGITUDINAL DESIGNS

Longitudinal designs examine changes in the same subjects over an extended period. This design is sometimes called a *panel design* (see Figure 11–3). Longitudinal designs are expensive and require a long period of researcher and subject commitment. The area to be studied, the variables, and their measurement must be clearly identified before data collection begins. Measurement must be carefully planned and implemented because the measures will be used repeatedly over time. If children are being studied, the measures must be valid for all the ages being studied. The researcher must be familiar with how the construct being measured is patterned over time, and clear rationale must be given for the points of time selected for measurement. There is often a bias in selection of subjects because of the requirement for a long-term commitment. In addition, loss of subjects (mortality) can be high and can decrease the validity of findings.

Power analysis must be calculated according to the number of subjects expected to complete the study, not the number recruited initially. The researcher must invest considerable energy in developing effective strategies to maintain the sample; some strategies for this purpose are discussed in Chapter 10. The period during which subjects will be recruited into the study must be carefully planned, and a time line depicting data collection points for each subject must be developed to enable planning for the numbers and availability of data collectors. If this issue is not carefully thought out, data collectors may be confronted with the need to continue to recruit new subjects while they are attempting to collect data scheduled for subjects recruited earlier. The researcher must also decide whether all data from a particular subject will be collected by a single data collector or whether a different data collector will be used at each point to ensure that data are collected blindly.

Because of the large volumes of data acquired in a longitudinal study, careful attention must be given to strategies for managing the data. The repetition of measures requires that data analysis be carefully thought through. Analyses commonly used are repeated measures analyses of variance, multivariate analyses of variance (MANOVA), regression analysis, cluster analysis, and time-series analysis (Barnard et al., 1987).

An example of a longitudinal design is the study by Martinson and colleagues (1999), "Comparison of Chinese and Caucasian Families Caregiving to Children with Cancer at Home." An abstract of that study follows.

FIGURE 11–3 ■ Longitudinal design.

Time 1	Time 2	Time 3	Time 4	Time..*n*
measure variables	measure variables	measure variables	measure variables	measure variables
Sample 1	Sample 1	Sample 1	Sample 1	Sample 1

"An exploratory, longitudinal design was used to compare the caregiving patterns and practices that occur within the family in Chinese and matched Caucasian families who have a child newly diagnosed with cancer. Both quantitative and qualitative methods were used to collect and analyze the data. . . . A total of 18 families participated in the study. Group A consisted of 19 Chinese families having a child newly diagnosed with cancer. Two of the Chinese children could not be matched during the span of the study. Group B consisted of eight Caucasian families having a child matched for diagnosis, age, and sex with a child in group A. Five Chinese families from Taiwan and five from Mainland China participated. . . . Data were collected at three points: (1) as soon as the Chinese child living in North American was diagnosed and the interview arrangements were able to be made, (2) after remission or 4–6 months after diagnosis, and (3) 1 year after diagnosis." (Martinson et al., 1999, pp. 101–103) ■

CROSS-SECTIONAL DESIGNS

Cross-sectional designs are used to examine groups of subjects in various stages of development simultaneously (see Figure 11–4). The assumption is that the stages are part of a process that will progress over time. Selecting subjects at various points in the process provides important information about the totality of the process, even though the same subjects are not monitored through the entire process. The processes of development selected for the study might be related to age, position in an educational system, growth pattern, or stages of maturation or personal growth (if they could be clearly enough defined to develop criteria for inclusion within differentiated groups). Subjects are then categorized by group, and data on the selected variables are collected at a single point in time.

For example, one might wish to study grief reactions at various periods after the death of a spouse. With a cross-sectional design, a group of individuals whose spouse had died 1 week ago could be tested, another whose loss was 6 months ago, another 1 year, another 2 years, and another 5 years.

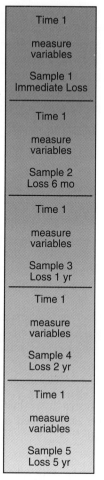

FIGURE 11–4 ■ Cross-sectional study design.

All these groups could be studied during one period, but a pattern of grief reactions over a 5-year period could be described. The design is not as strong as the longitudinal design but allows some understanding of the phenomenon over time when time allowed for the study is limited.

Aaronson and Kingry (1988) describe a strategy for mixing cross-sectional data and longitudinal data to maximize the strengths of both designs. In their study of health behavior and beliefs during pregnancy, data were collected cross-sectionally on subjects, subjects were asked to recall previous attitudes, and a small portion of the sample were followed longitudinally to validate the cross-sectional findings.

Doering and colleagues (1999) conducted a cross-sectional study entitled "Evidence of Time-Dependent Autonomic Reinnervation after Heart Transplantation." The following excerpt describes the design of their study.

· ·

"A sample of 33 orthotopic heart transplant recipient volunteers from an urban, university-affiliated tertiary care center and 16 healthy normal control volunteers matched to the age and sex of transplant recipients were enrolled in the study. Of the transplant recipients, 16 were less than 5 months posttransplant (early transplant group) and 17 were more than 1 year posttransplant (late transplant group)." (Doering et al., 1999, p. 310)

· ·

"Handgrip and deep breathing tests, passive 80E head-up tilt, and heart rate (HR) responsiveness of 33 transplant recipients . . . were compared with those of 16 age- and sex-matched control participants." (Doering et al, 1999, p. 308) ■

TREND DESIGNS

Trend designs examine changes in the general population in relation to a particular phenomenon (see Figure 11–5). Different samples of subjects are selected from the same population at preset intervals of time, and at each selected time, data are collected from that particular sample. The researcher must be able to justify generalizing from the samples to the population under study. Analysis involves strategies to predict future trends from examination of past trends. An example of this design

is the study by Wilbur and associates (1990) of the career trends of master's-prepared family nurse practitioners. They described their design as follows.

· ·

"The study consisted of FNPs [family nurse practitioners] who had completed graduate studies between 1974 and 1984. . . . A structured survey questionnaire was used to obtain information on employment, NP practice, professional, and demographic variables. . . . A second questionnaire was used to structure the past employment and demographic variables. . . . The subjects were asked to recall employment information for a maximum of four jobs held since graduation. . . . To identify and compare career trends, the decision was made to group graduating classes into three cohorts representing the early, intermediate, and recent graduates. To identify career trends, the role characteristics of both the first job held following graduation and the present job were examined." (Wilbur et al., 1990, pp. 71–72) ■

EVENT-PARTITIONING DESIGNS

A merger of the cross-sectional or longitudinal and trend designs, the *event-partitioning design*, is used in some cases to increase sample size and to avoid the effects of history on the validity of findings. Cook and Campbell (1979) refer to these as cohort designs with *treatment partitioning* (see Figures 11–6 and 11–7). The term *treatment* is used loosely here to mean a key event that is thought to lead to change. In a descriptive study, the researcher would not cause or manipulate the key event but rather would clearly define it so that when it occurred naturally, it would be recognized.

Time 1	Time 2	Time 3	Time 4	Time..n	
measure variables	measure variables	measure variables	measure variables	measure variables	⟶ PREDICTION
Sample 1	Sample 2	Sample 3	Sample 4	....n	

FIGURE 11–5 ■ Trend study design.

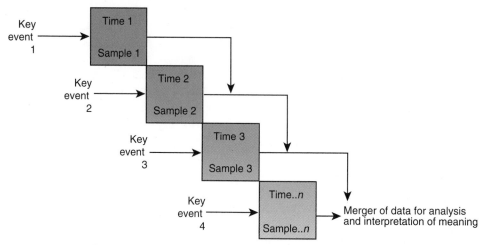

FIGURE 11−6 ■ Cross-sectional study with treatment partitioning.

For example, the event-partitioning design could be used to study subjects who have completed programs to stop smoking. Smoking behaviors and incidence of smoking-related diseases might be measured at intervals of 1 year for a 5-year period. However, the number of subjects available at one time might be insufficient for adequate analysis of findings. Therefore, subjects from several programs offered at different times could be used. Data would be examined in terms of the relative time since the subjects' completion of the stop-smoking program,

not the absolute length of time. Data would be assumed to be comparable, and a larger sample size would be available for analysis of changes over time.

An example of this design is Lepczyk and associates' (1990) study on the timing of preoperative patient teaching. The following excerpt describes the study design.

. . . .

"The convenience sample was selected from a population of patients who presented themselves for preoperative classes before coronary artery by-

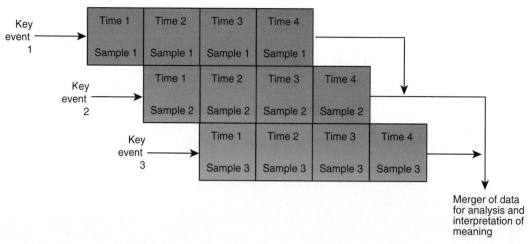

FIGURE 11−7 ■ Longitudinal design with treatment partitioning.

pass surgery at two large metropolitan hospitals. Group 1 (from one hospital, $n = 32$) received teaching 2–7 days prior to hospital admission. Group 2 (from the other hospital, $n = 42$) received teaching on the afternoon of hospital admission. Seventy-four patients consented to participate. Data were collected over 8 months." (Lepczyk et al., 1990, p. 302) ▪

Case Study Design

The *case study design* involves an intensive exploration of a single unit of study, such as a person, family, group, community, or institution, or a very small number of subjects who are examined intensively. Although the number of subjects tends to be small, the number of variables involved is usually large. In fact, it is important to examine all variables that might have an impact on the situation being studied.

Case studies were commonly used in nursing research in the 1970s but appear in the literature less frequently today. Well-designed case studies are good sources of descriptive information and can be used as evidence for or against theories. Sterling and McNally (1992) recommend single-subject case studies for examining process-based nursing practice. The strategy allows the researcher to investigate daily observations and interventions that are a common aspect of nursing practice. Case studies are also commonly used in qualitative studies (Sandelowski, 1996). There are even experimental designs for single case studies (Barlow & Hersen, 1984). A variety of sources of information can be collected on each concept of interest through the use of different data collection methods. This approach allows detailed study of all aspects of a single case. Such a strategy can greatly expand the understanding of the phenomenon under study.

Case studies are also useful in demonstrating the effectiveness of specific therapeutic techniques. In fact, the reporting of a case study can be the vehicle by which the technique is introduced to other practitioners. The case study design also has potential for revealing important findings that can generate new hypotheses for testing. Thus, the case study can lead to the design of large sample studies to examine factors identified through the case study.

The design of a case study depends on the circumstances of the case but usually includes an element of time. History and previous behavior patterns are usually explored in detail. As the case study proceeds, the researcher may become aware of components important to the phenomenon being examined that were not originally built into the study. A case study is likely to have both quantitative and qualitative elements, and these components must be incorporated into the study design. Large volumes of data are generally obtained during a case study. Organizing the findings of a case study into a coherent whole is a difficult but critical component of the study. Generalization of study findings in the statistical sense is not appropriate; however, generalizing the findings to theory is appropriate and important (Barnard et al., 1987; Crombie & Davies, 1996; Gray, 1998; Yin, 1984).

An example of this design is Lewis's (1995) study, "One Year in the Life of a Woman with Premenstrual Syndrome: A Case Study." An abstract of that study follows.

· ·

"Over the course of 1 year (13 menstrual cycles), data were collected on a daily basis using Likert-scale ratings of symptom presence and severity, as well as narrative journal entries. The participant was a 37-year-old healthy woman (mean cycle length = 26.7 days, $SD \pm 1.8$) with prospectively screened well-defined premenstrual syndrome (PMS), not on hormones or other drugs, and without a psychiatric history. Using the autocorrelation function (ACF), there was evidence for a statistically significant predictive cycle-to-cycle symptom pattern (ACF $r = .49$, $p < .05$; Bartlett Band range of significance $= \pm .13$). Cycle-phase-dependent coexistence of symptoms was noted, along with particular narrative themes, most dramatically exemplified by the theme of death. For this subject, the findings provided evidence for predictive symptom patterns and an effect of symptom presence on her interpretation of her environment and herself." (Lewis, 1995, p. 111) ▪

Surveys

The term *survey* is used in two ways within scientific thought. It is used in a broad sense to mean any descriptive or correlational study; in this sense, *survey* tends to mean nonexperimental. In a narrower sense, *survey* is used to describe a technique of data collection in which questionnaires (collected by mail or in person) or personal interviews are used to gather data about an identified population.

Surveys, in the narrower definition, are used to gather data that can be acquired through self-report. Because of this limitation in data, some researchers view surveys as rather shallow and as contributing in a limited way to scientific knowledge. This belief has led to a bias in the scientific community against survey research. In this context, the term *survey* is used derisively. However, surveys can be an extremely important source of data. In this text, the term survey is used to designate a data collection technique, not a design. Surveys can be used within many designs, including descriptive, correlational, and quasi-experimental studies.

CORRELATIONAL STUDIES

Correlational studies examine relationships among variables. The examination can occur at several levels. The researcher can seek to describe a relationship, predict relationships among variables, or test the relationships proposed by a theoretical proposition. In any correlational study, a representative sample must be selected for the study, a sample reflecting the full range of scores possible on the variables being measured. In correlational designs, a large variance in the variable scores is necessary to determine the existence of a relationship. Therefore, correlational designs are unlike experimental designs, in which variance in variable scores is controlled (limited).

In correlational designs, if the range of scores is truncated, the obtained correlation will be artificially depressed. *Truncated* means that the lowest scores and the highest scores either are not measured or are condensed and merged with less extreme scores. For example, if an attitude scale were scored from a low score of 1 to a high score of 50, truncated scores might indicate only scores in the range 10 to 40. More extreme scores would be combined with scores within the designated range. If truncation is performed, the researcher may not find a correlation when the variables are actually correlated.

Neophyte researchers tend to make two serious errors with correlational studies. First, they often attempt to establish causality by correlation, reasoning that if two variables are related, one must cause the other. Second, they confuse studies in which differences are examined with studies in which relationships are examined. Although the existence of a difference assumes the existence of a relationship, the design and statistical analysis of studies examining differences are different from those examining relationships. In a study examining two or more groups in terms of one or more variables, the researcher is exploring differences between groups as reflected in scores on the identified variables. In a study examining a single group in terms of two or more variables, the researcher is exploring relationships between variables. In a correlational study, the relationship examined is that between two or more research variables within an identified situation.

Descriptive Correlational Design

The purpose of a descriptive correlational design is to examine the relationships that exist in a situation. Using this design facilitates the identification of many interrelationships in a situation in a short time. Descriptive correlational studies are also used to develop hypotheses for later studies (see Figure 11–8).

A descriptive correlational study may examine variables in a situation that has already occurred or in a currently occurring situation. No attempt is made to control or manipulate the situation. As with descriptive studies, variables must be clearly identified and defined. An example of a descriptive correlational design is the study by Johnson and colleagues (1999) that examined the relationships among attitudes, beliefs, knowledge, and values related to adolescent sexuality and sexually transmitted diseases. An abstract of their study follows.

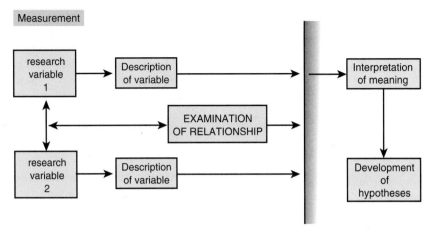

FIGURE 11–8 ■ Descriptive correlational design.

• •

"This study described rural adolescents' attitudes, beliefs, knowledge, and values with regard to sexuality and sexually transmitted diseases (STDs). Rotter's Social Learning Theory (1954) provided the theoretical framework for this descriptive, correlational design. The convenience sample consisted of 170 students from one rural high school." (Johnson et al., 1999, p. 177) ■

Predictive Design

Predictive designs are developed to predict the value of one variable on the basis of values obtained from another variable or variables. Prediction is one approach to examining causal relationships between variables. Because causal phenomena are being examined, the terms *dependent* and *independent* are used to describe the variables. One variable is classified as the dependent variable, and all other variables are classified as independent variables.

The aim of a predictive design is to predict the level of the dependent variable from the indepen-

dent variables (see Figure 11–9). Independent variables most effective in prediction are highly correlated with the dependent variable but not highly correlated with other independent variables used in the study. Predictive designs require the development of a theory-based mathematical hypothesis proposing the variables that are expected to predict the dependent variable effectively. The hypothesis is then tested with regression analysis.

Jennings-Dozier (1999) conducted a predictive correlational study to predict intentions to obtain a Papanicolaou (Pap) smear among African American and Latina women. The study was designed as a test of the Theory of Planned Behavior. The following abstract describes this study.

• •

"A correlational design was used, and a convenience sample of 108 African American and 96 Latina adult women were recruited from urban community-based agencies located in a large mid-Atlantic metropolitan area. . . . Direct relationships between attitude and perceived behavioral

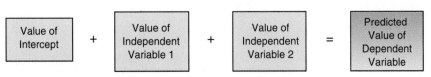

FIGURE 11–9 ■ Predictive design.

control and intention to obtain an annual Pap smear were found for African American and Latina women. The subjective norm did not significantly predict intention. . . . [T]he study findings did not support the empirical adequacy of the Theory of Planned Behavior for either of the ethnic groups." (Jennings-Dozier, 1999, p. 395) ■

Model-Testing Designs

Some studies are designed specifically to test the accuracy of a hypothesized causal model. The design requires that all variables relevant to the model be measured. A large, heterogeneous sample is required. All the paths expressing relationships between concepts are identified, and a conceptual map is developed (see Figure 11–10). The analysis determines whether or not the data are consistent with the model. In some studies, data from some subjects are set aside and not included in the initial path analysis. These data are used to test the fit of the paths defined by the initial analysis in another data set.

Variables are classified into three categories, exogenous variables, endogenous variables, and residual variables. *Exogenous variables* are within the theoretical model but are caused by factors outside of this model. *Endogenous variables* are those whose variation is explained within the theoretical model. Exogenous variables influence the variation of endogenous variables. *Residual variables* indicate the effect of unmeasured variables not included in the model. These variables explain some of the variance found in the data but not the variance within the model (Mason-Hawkes & Holm, 1989).

In Figure 11–10, the illustration of a model-testing design, paths are drawn to demonstrate directions of cause and effect. The arrows (paths) from the exogenous variables 1, 2, and 3 lead to the endogenous variable 4, indicating that variable 4 is theoretically proposed to be caused by variables 1, 2, and 3. The arrow (path) from endogenous variable 4 to endogenous variable 5 indicates that variable 4 causes variable 5.

The researcher measures exogenous and endogenous variables by collecting data from the experimental subjects and analyzes the accuracy of the proposed paths. Initially, these analysis procedures were performed with a series of regression analyses. Now, statistical procedures have been developed specifically for path analysis using the computer programs LISREL and EQS; these programs are described in Chapter 20. Path coefficients are calculated that indicate the effect that one variable has

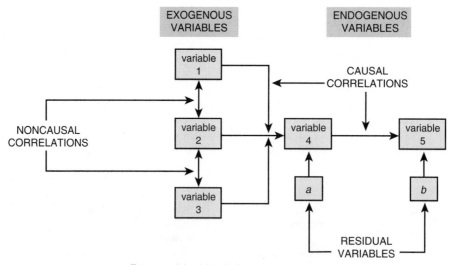

Figure 11–10 ■ Model testing design.

on another. The amount of variance explained by the model as well as the fit between the path coefficients and the theoretical model indicates the accuracy of the theory. Variance that is not accounted for in the statistical analysis is attributed to residual variables (variables *a* and *b*) not included in the analyses (Mason-Hawkes & Holm, 1989).

An example of this design is Hagerty and Willams's (1999) study, "The Effects of Sense of Belonging, Social Support, Conflict, and Loneliness on Depression." The following abstract describes the study.

· ·

"A sample of clients with major depressive disorder and students in a midwestern community college participated in the study by completing questionnaires. Path analysis showed significant direct paths as postulated, with 64% of the variance of depression explained by the variables in the model. Social support had only an indirect effect on depression, and this finding supported the buffer theory of social support. Sense of belonging was a better predictor of depression." (Hagerty & Williams, 1999, p. 215) ■

QUASI-EXPERIMENTAL STUDY DESIGNS

The purpose of quasi-experimental and experimental designs is to examine causality. The power of the design to accomplish this purpose depends on the extent to which the actual effects of the experimental treatment (the independent variable) can be detected by measurement of the dependent variable. Obtaining an understanding of the true effects of an experimental treatment requires action to control threats to the validity of the findings. Threats to validity are controlled through selection of subjects, control of the environment, manipulation of the treatment, and reliable and valid measurement of the dependent variables.

Experimental designs, with their strict control of variance, are the most powerful method of examining causality. For many reasons, both ethical and practical, however, experimental designs cannot always be used in social science research. Quasi-experimental designs were developed to provide al-

ternative means of examining causality in situations not conducive to experimental controls. Quasi-experimental designs were first described as a group by Campbell and Stanley in 1963, when only experimental designs were considered of any worth. Cook and Campbell expanded this description in 1979. Quasi-experimental designs facilitate the search for knowledge and examination of causality in situations in which complete control is not possible. These designs have been developed to control as many threats to validity as possible in a situation in which at least one of the three components of true experimental design (random sampling, control groups, and manipulation of the treatment) is lacking.

There are differences of opinion in nursing about the classification of a particular study as quasi-experimental or experimental. The experimental designs emerged from a logical positivist perspective with the purpose of determining cause and effect. The focus is on determining differences between groups using statistical analyses on the basis of decision theory (see Chapter 18 for an explanation of decision theory). The true experimental design (from a logical positivist view) requires the use of random sampling to obtain subjects, random assignment to control and experimental groups, rigorous control of the treatment, and designs that controlled threats to validity.

A less rigorous type of experimental design, referred to as *comparative experimental design*, is being used by some researchers in both nursing and medicine for clinical situations in which the expectation of random sampling is difficult if not impossible to achieve. These studies use convenience samples with random assignment to groups. For example, clinical trials do not use randomly obtained samples but tend to be considered experimental in nature. The rationale for classifying such studies as experimental is that they have internal validity if the two groups are comparable on variables important to the study even though there are biases in the original sample. However, threats to statistical conclusion validity and threats to external validity by the nonrandom sample are not addressed by these designs. Threats to external validity have not, in the past, been considered a serious concern because they affect not the claim that the treatment caused a difference but rather the ability to generalize the findings. The importance of external validity, although discounted in the past, is taking on greater importance in the current political and health policy climate. See Chapter 12 on outcomes research for a discussion of concerns related to the validity of clinical trials.

Random Assignment to Groups

Random assignment is a procedure used to assign subjects to treatment or control groups randomly. Random assignment is most commonly used in nursing and medicine to assign subjects obtained through convenience sampling methods to groups for purposes of comparison. Random assignment used without random sampling is purported to decrease the risk of bias in the selection of groups. However, a meta-analysis by Ottenbacher (1992), examining the effect of random assignment versus nonrandom assignment on outcomes, failed to reveal significant differences in these two sampling techniques. He suggests that previous assumptions about design strategies should be empirically tested.

Traditional approaches to random assignment involve using a random numbers table or flipping an unbiased coin to determine group assignment. However, these procedures can lead to unequal group sizes and, thus, a decrease in power. Hjelm-Karlsson (1991) suggests using what is referred to as a *biased coin design* to randomly assign subjects to groups. With this technique, selection of the group to which a particular subject will be assigned is biased in favor of groups that have smaller sample sizes at the point of the assignment of that subject. This strategy is particularly useful when assignment is being made to more than two groups. Calculations for the sequencing of assignment to groups can be completed before initiation of data collection, thus freeing the researcher for other activities during this critical period. Hjelm-Karlsson (1991) suggests using cards to make group assignments. The subject numbers and random group assignments are written on cards. As each subject agrees to participate in the study, the next card is drawn from the stack, indicating that subject's number and group assignment.

Stout and colleagues (1994) suggest a similar strategy they refer to as *urn randomization*, which they describe as follows:

"One would begin the study with two urns, each urn containing a red marble and a blue marble. There is one urn for each level of the stratifying variable; that is, in this example there is an urn for severely ill patients and another urn for the less severe patients. When a subject is ready for randomization, we determine whether or not he/she is severely ill and consult the corresponding urn. From this urn (say, for the severely ill group) we randomly select one marble and note its color. If the marble is red we assign the patient to Treatment A. Then we drop that marble back into the urn *and put a blue marble into the urn as well*. This leaves the 'severely ill' urn with one red and two blue marbles. The next time a severely ill patient shows up, the probability that he/she will be assigned to Group B will be 2/3 rather than 2, thus biasing the selection process toward balance. A similar procedure is followed every time a severely ill subject presents for randomization. After each subject is assigned, the marble chosen from the urn is replaced together with a marble of the opposite color. The urn for the less severely ill group is not affected. If a low-severity patient presents for the study, that patient's probability of assignment to either treatment is not affected by the assignment of patients in the other stratum. To some extent, urn randomization can be tailored to maximize balancing or to maximize randomization." (Stout et al., 1994, p. 72). ■

These authors also provide strategies for balancing several variables simultaneously during random assignment.

Chang (1999) used random assignment in her study of a cognitive-behavioral intervention for homebound caregivers of people with dementia. She describes her sampling procedure as follows.

"Objective: To examine the effects of an 8-week cognitive-behavioral (C-B) intervention tailored to the specific deficits of persons with dementia (PWDs) on selected outcomes for homebound care-

givers and the functional status of the PWD."
(Chang, 1999, p. 173)

• •

"Method: The design was a two-group randomized trial with measures taken at baseline, 4 weeks, 8 weeks, and 12 weeks." (Chang, 1999, p. 173).

• •

"Procedure: Caregiving dyads were randomly assigned to C-B or A-O groups." (Chang, 1999, p. 175) ■

Each of the quasi-experimental designs described in this section involves threats to validity owing to constraints in controlling variance. Some achieve greater amounts of control than others. When choosing designs, the researcher selects the design that offers the greatest amount of control possible within the study situation. Even the first designs described in this section, which have very low power in terms of establishing causality, can provide useful information on which to design later studies.

Nonequivalent Control Group Designs

A *nonequivalent control group* is one in which the control group is not selected by random means. Some groups are more nonequivalent than others, and some quasi-experimental designs involve using groups (control and treatment) that have evolved naturally rather than being developed randomly. These groups cannot be considered equivalent because the individuals in the control group may be different from individuals in the treatment group. Individuals have selected the group in which they are included rather than being selected by the researcher. Thus, selection becomes a threat to validity.

The approach to statistical analysis is problematic in quasi-experimental designs. Although many researchers use the same approaches to analysis as are used for experimental studies, the selection bias inherent in nonequivalent control groups makes this practice questionable. Reichardt (1979) recommends using multiple statistical analyses to examine the data from various perspectives and to compare levels of significance obtained from each analysis. The researcher must carefully assess the potential threats to validity in interpreting statistical results, because statistical analysis cannot control for threats to validity. The following sections describe examples of nonequivalent control group design.

THE ONE-GROUP POSTTEST-ONLY DESIGN

The one-group posttest-only design is referred to as *pre-experimental* rather than quasi-experimental because of its weaknesses and the numerous threats to validity. It is inadequate for making causal inferences (see Figure 11–11). Usually in this design, no attempt is made to control the selection of subjects who receive the treatment (the experimental group). Generalization of findings beyond those tested is difficult to justify. The group is not pretested; therefore, there is no direct way to measure change. The researcher cannot claim that posttest scores were a consequence (effect) of the treatment if scores before the treatment are unknown. Because there is no control group, one does not know whether groups not receiving the treatment would have similar scores on the dependent variable. The one-group posttest-only design is commonly used by the inexperienced researcher to evaluate a treatment program or a nursing intervention.

Cook and Campbell (1979) suggest situations in which the one-group posttest-only design can be appropriate and adequate for inferring causality. For example, the design could be used to determine that a single factory's use of vinyl chloride is causing an increase in the rate of neighborhood and employee cancers. The incidence of cancer in the community at large is known. The fact that vinyl chloride causes cancer and the types of cancer caused by it are also known. These norms would then take the place of the pretest and the control group. Thus, to use this design intelligently, one must know a great deal about the causal factors interacting within the situation.

THE POSTTEST-ONLY DESIGN WITH NONEQUIVALENT GROUPS

Although the posttest-only design with nonequivalent groups offers an improvement on the previous design, because of the addition of a nonequi-

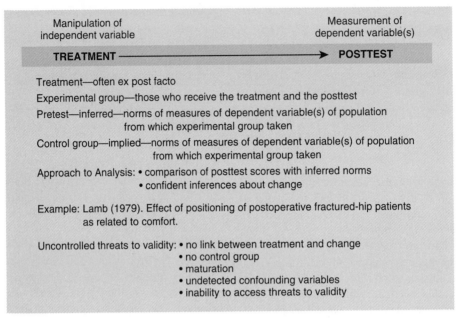

FIGURE 11–11 ■ One-group posttest–only design.

valent control group, it is still referred to as *pre-experimental* (see Figure 11–12). The addition of a nonequivalent control group can lead to a false confidence in the validity of the findings. Selection threats are a problem with both groups. The lack of a pretest remains a serious impediment to defining change. Differences in posttest scores between groups may be caused by the treatment or by differential selection processes.

THE ONE-GROUP PRETEST–POSTTEST DESIGN

Another pre-experimental design, the one-group pretest–posttest design, is one of the more commonly used designs but has such serious weaknesses that findings are often uninterpretable (see Figure 11–13). Pretest scores cannot adequately serve the same function as a control group. Events can occur between the pretest and posttest that alter responses to the posttest. These events then serve as alternative hypotheses to the proposal that the change in posttest scores is due to the treatment. Posttest scores might be altered by (1) maturation processes, (2) administration of the pretest, and (3) changes in instrumentation. Additionally, sub-

jects in many studies using this design are selected on the basis of high or low scores on the pretest. Thus, there is an additional threat that changes in the posttest may be due to regression toward the mean. The addition of a nonequivalent control group, as described in the next design, can greatly strengthen the validity of the findings.

THE UNTREATED CONTROL GROUP DESIGN WITH PRETEST AND POSTTEST

The pretest-posttest design with an untreated or placebo group is most commonly used in social science research (see Figure 11–14). This quasi-experimental design is the first design discussed here that is generally interpretable. The uncontrolled threats to validity are primarily due to the absence of randomization and, in some studies, the inability of the researcher to manipulate the treatment. The effects of these threats on interpreting study findings are discussed in detail by Cook and Campbell (1979).

Variations in this design include the use of (1) proxy pretest measures (a different pretest that correlates with the posttest), (2) separate pretest and

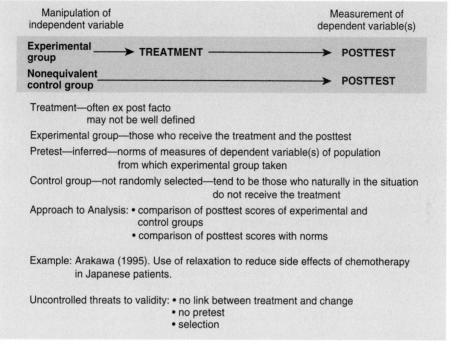

Manipulation of
independent variable

Measurement of
dependent variable(s)

Experimental group ——→ TREATMENT ————————————→ POSTTEST

Nonequivalent control group ————————————————————→ POSTTEST

Treatment—often ex post facto
      may not be well defined

Experimental group—those who receive the treatment and the posttest

Pretest—inferred—norms of measures of dependent variable(s) of population
      from which experimental group taken

Control group—not randomly selected—tend to be those who naturally in the situation
      do not receive the treatment

Approach to Analysis: • comparison of posttest scores of experimental and
      control groups
      • comparison of posttest scores with norms

Example: Arakawa (1995). Use of relaxation to reduce side effects of chemotherapy
      in Japanese patients.

Uncontrolled threats to validity: • no link between treatment and change
      • no pretest
      • selection

FIGURE 11–12 ■ Posttest–only design with nonequivalent groups.

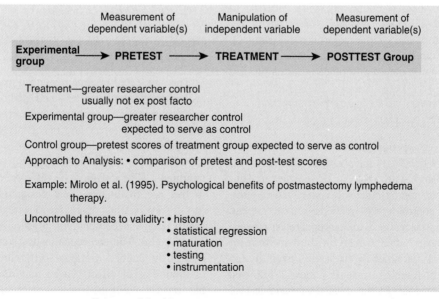

Measurement of
dependent variable(s)

Manipulation of
independent variable

Measurement of
dependent variable(s)

Experimental group ——→ PRETEST ——→ TREATMENT ——→ POSTTEST Group

Treatment—greater researcher control
      usually not ex post facto

Experimental group—greater researcher control
      expected to serve as control

Control group—pretest scores of treatment group expected to serve as control

Approach to Analysis: • comparison of pretest and post-test scores

Example: Mirolo et al. (1995). Psychological benefits of postmastectomy lymphedema
      therapy.

Uncontrolled threats to validity: • history
      • statistical regression
      • maturation
      • testing
      • instrumentation

FIGURE 11–13 ■ One-group pretest–posttest design.

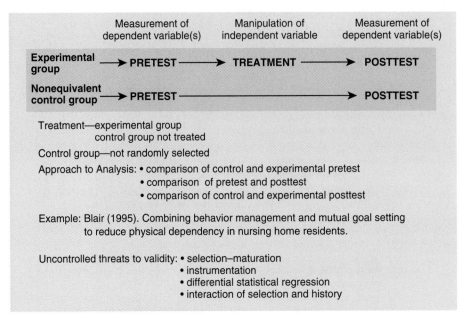

FIGURE 11–14 ■ Untreated control group design with pretest and posttest.

posttest samples, and (3) pretest measures at more than one time interval. The first two variations weaken the design, but the last variation greatly strengthens it.

In some studies, the placebo treatment consists of the usual treatment provided in the clinical setting. Because there is commonly wide variation in usual treatment among patients, this strategy reduces the effect size of the experimental treatment, increases the variance, and decreases the possibility of obtaining a significant difference between groups.

THE REMOVED-TREATMENT DESIGN WITH PRETEST AND POSTTEST

In some cases, gaining access to even a nonequivalent control group is not possible. The removed-treatment design with pretest and posttest creates conditions that approximate the conceptual requirements of a control group receiving no treatment. The design is basically a one-group pretest-posttest design. However, after a delay, a third measure of the dependent variable is taken, followed by an interval in which the treatment is removed, followed by a fourth measure of the dependent variable (see Figure 11–15). The periods between measures must

be equivalent. In nursing situations, the ethics of removing an effective treatment must be considered. Even if doing so is ethically acceptable, the response of subjects to the removal may make interpreting changes difficult.

THE REVERSED-TREATMENT NONEQUIVALENT CONTROL GROUP DESIGN WITH PRETEST AND POSTTEST

The reversed-treatment nonequivalent control group design with pretest and posttest introduces two independent variables—one expected to produce a positive effect and one expected to produce a negative effect (see Figure 11–16). There are two experimental groups, each exposed to one of the treatments. The design tests differences in response to the two treatments. This design is more useful for theory testing than the no-treatment control group design because of its high construct validity of the cause. The theoretical causal variable must be rigorously defined to allow differential predictions of directions of effect. To be maximally interpretable, the following two groups must be added: (1) a placebo control group in which the treatment is not

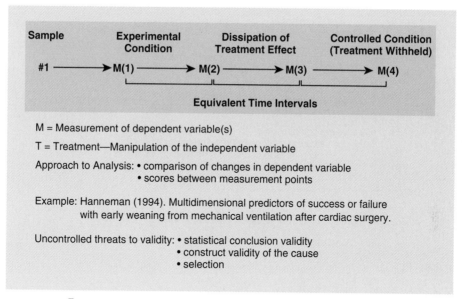

FIGURE 11–15 ■ Removed-treatment design with pretest and posttest.

expected to affect the dependent variable and (2) a no-treatment control group to provide a baseline.

Interrupted Time-Series Designs

The *interrupted time-series design* is similar to descriptive time designs except that a treatment is applied at some point in the observations. Time-series analyses have some advantages over other quasi-experimental designs. First, repeated pretest observations can assess trends in maturation before the treatment. Second, the repeated pretest observations allow measures of trends in scores before the treatment, decreasing the risk of statistical regression, which would lead to misinterpretation of findings. If records are kept of events that could influence subjects in the study, the researcher can determine whether historical factors that could modify responses to the treatment were in operation between the last pretest and the first posttest.

Some threats, however, are particularly problematic in time-series designs. Record-keeping procedures and definitions of constructs used for data collection tend to change over time. Thus, maintaining consistency can be a problem. The treatment can result in attrition so that the sample before

treatment may be different in important ways from the posttreatment group. Seasonal variation or other cyclical influences can be interpreted as treatment effects. Therefore, identifying cyclical patterns that may be occurring and controlling for them are critical to the analysis of study findings.

McCain and McCleary (1979) suggest the use of the ARIMA (autoregressive integrated moving average) statistical model (see Chapter 20) to analyze time-series data. ARIMA is a relatively new model that has some distinct advantages over regression analysis techniques. For adequate statistical analysis, at least 50 measurement points are needed; however, Cook and Campbell (1979) believe that even small numbers of measurement points can provide better information than that obtained in cross-sectional studies. The numbers of measures shown in the designs illustrated here (Figures 11–17 through 11–19) are limited by space and are not meant to suggest limiting measures to the numbers shown.

SIMPLE INTERRUPTED TIME SERIES

The simple interrupted time series is similar to the descriptive study, with the addition of a treatment that occurs or is applied at a given point in time (see Figure 11–17). The treatment, which in

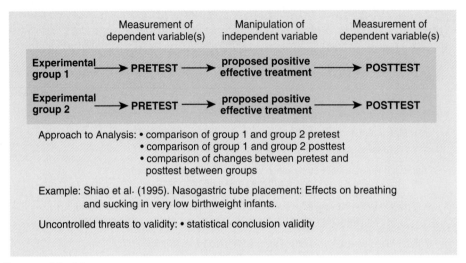

FIGURE 11–16 ■ The reversed-treatment nonequivalent control group design with pretest and posttest.

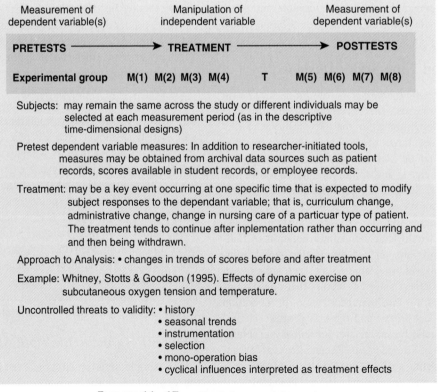

FIGURE 11–17 ■ Simple interrupted time series.

some cases is not completely under the control of the researcher, must be clearly defined. The use of multiple methods to measure the dependent variable greatly strengthens the design. Threats that are well controlled by this design are maturation and statistical regression.

INTERRUPTED TIME SERIES WITH A NONEQUIVALENT NO-TREATMENT CONTROL GROUP TIME SERIES

The addition of a control group to the interrupted time-series design greatly strengthens the validity of the findings. The control group allows examination of differences in trends between groups after the treatment and of the persistence of treatment effects over time (see Figure 11–18). Although the treatment may continue (e.g., a change in nursing man-

agement practices or patient teaching strategies), the initial response to the change may differ from later responses.

INTERRUPTED TIME SERIES WITH MULTIPLE REPLICATIONS

The interrupted time series with multiple replications is a powerful design for inferring causality (see Figure 11–19). It requires greater researcher control than is usually possible in social science research outside closed institutional settings, such as laboratories or research units. The studies that led to the adoption of behavior modification techniques used this design. For significant differences to be interpretable, the pretest and posttest scores must be in different directions. Within this design, treatments can be modified through substitution of one

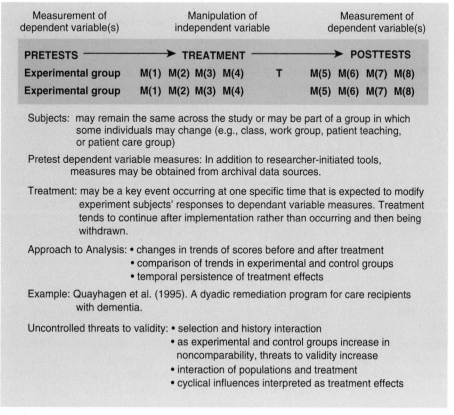

FIGURE 11–18 ■ Interrupted time series with a nonequivalent no-treatment control group time series.

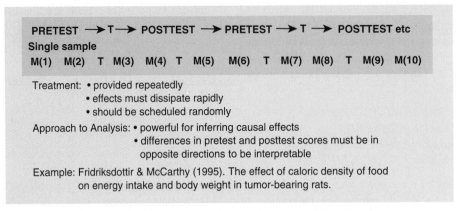

FIGURE 11–19 ▪ Interrupted time series with multiple replications.

EXPERIMENTAL STUDY DESIGNS

treatment for another or combining of two treatments and examination of interaction effects.

Experimental designs are set up to provide the greatest amount of control possible to examine causality more closely. To examine cause, one must eliminate all factors influencing the dependent variable other than the cause (independent variable) being studied. Other factors are eliminated by controlling them. The study is designed to prevent any other element from intruding into observation of the specific cause and effect that the researcher wishes to examine.

The three essential elements of experimental research are (1) randomization, (2) researcher-controlled manipulation of the independent variable, and (3) researcher control of the experimental situation, including a control or comparison group. Experimental designs exert much effort to control variance. Sample criteria are explicit, the independent variable is provided in a precisely defined way, the dependent variables are carefully operationalized, and the situation in which the study is conducted is rigidly controlled to prevent the interference of unstudied factors from modifying the dynamics of the process being studied.

The Classic Experimental Design

The original or classic experimental design is still the most commonly used experimental design (see Figure 11–20). There are two randomized groups, one receiving the experimental treatment and one receiving no treatment, a placebo treatment, or the usual treatment. Comparison of pretest scores allows evaluation of the effectiveness of randomization in providing equivalent groups. The treatment is under the control of the researcher. The dependent variable is measured twice, before and after the manipulation of the independent variable. As with all well-designed studies, the dependent and independent variables are conceptually linked, conceptually defined, and operationalized. Instruments used to measure the dependent variable clearly reflect the conceptual meaning of the variable and have good evidence of reliability and validity. Often, more than one means of measuring the dependent variable is advisable to avoid mono-operation and mono-method biases.

Most other experimental designs are variations of the classic experimental design. Multiple groups (both experimental and control) can be used to great advantage in the pretest-posttest design and the posttest-only design. For example, one control group could receive no treatment and another control group could receive a placebo treatment. Multiple experimental groups could receive varying lev-

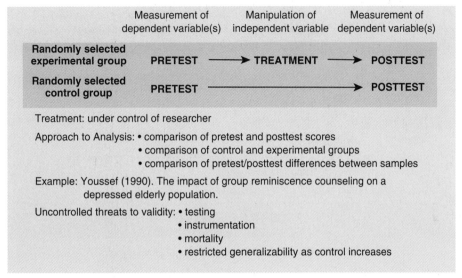

	Measurement of dependent variable(s)	Manipulation of independent variable	Measurement of dependent variable(s)
Randomly selected experimental group	PRETEST	⟶ TREATMENT ⟶	POSTTEST
Randomly selected control group	PRETEST	⟶	POSTTEST

Treatment: under control of researcher

Approach to Analysis: • comparison of pretest and posttest scores
• comparison of control and experimental groups
• comparison of pretest/posttest differences between samples

Example: Youssef (1990). The impact of group reminiscence counseling on a depressed elderly population.

Uncontrolled threats to validity: • testing
• instrumentation
• mortality
• restricted generalizability as control increases

FIGURE 11–20 ■ Pretest–posttest control group design.

els of the treatments, such as differing frequency, intensity, or duration of nursing care measures. These additions greatly increase the generalizability of the study findings.

Posttest-only Control Group Design

In some studies, the dependent variable cannot be measured before the treatment. For example, before the beginning of treatment, it is not possible to make meaningful measurements of the responses to interventions designed to control nausea from chemotherapy or postoperative pain. Additionally, in some cases, subjects' responses to the posttest can be due, in part, to learning from or subjective reaction to the pretest (*pretest sensitization*). If this issue is a concern in a specific study, the pretest may be eliminated and a posttest-only control group design can be used (see Figure 11–21). However, this elimination prevents the use of many powerful statistical analysis techniques within the study. Additionally, the effectiveness of randomization in obtaining equivalent experimental and control groups cannot be evaluated in terms of the study variables. Nevertheless, the groups can be evaluated in terms of sample characteristics and other relevant variables.

Randomized Block Design

The *randomized block design* uses the two-group pretest-posttest pattern or the two-group posttest pattern with one addition, a blocking variable. The blocking variable, if uncontrolled, is expected to confound the findings of the study. To prevent confounding of the findings, the subjects are rank-ordered in relation to the blocking variable.

For example, if effectiveness of a nursing intervention to relieve postchemotherapy nausea were the independent variable in a study, severity of nausea could confound the findings. Subjects would be ranked according to severity of nausea. The two subjects with the most severe nausea would be identified and randomly assigned, one to the experimental group and one to the control group. The two subjects next in rank would then be identified and randomly assigned. The pattern would be followed until the entire sample was randomly assigned as matched pairs. This procedure ensures that the experimental group and the control group are equal in relation to the potentially confounding variable.

The effect of blocking can also be accomplished statistically (through the use of analysis of covariance) without categorizing the confounding variable

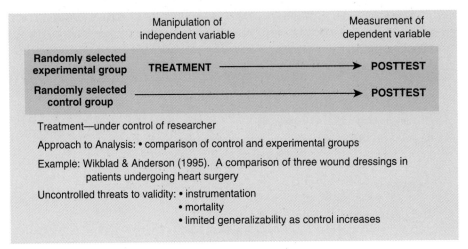

FIGURE 11–21 ■ Posttest–only control group design.

into discrete components. However, for this analysis to be accurate, one must be careful not to violate the assumptions of the statistical procedure (Spector, 1981). An example of this design is McCurren and associates' (1999) study testing an intervention strategy for depression among nursing home elders. The following excerpt describes the study design.

· ·

"A randomized block design was used; i.e., subjects were first categorized in blocks according to initial Geriatric Depression Scale (GDS) score (mildly or severely depressed) and then randomly assigned to either the experimental or the control group." (McCurren et al., 1999, p. 13) ■

Factorial Designs

In a *factorial design*, two or more different characteristics, treatments, or events are independently varied within a single study. This design is a logical approach to examining multiple causality. The simplest arrangement is one in which two treatments or factors are involved and, within each factor, two levels are manipulated (for example, the presence or absence of the treatment); this is referred to as a *2 × 2 factorial design*. This design is illustrated in Figure 11–22, in the two independent variables are relaxation and distraction as means of pain relief.

A 2 × 2 factorial design produces a study with four cells (A through D). Each cell must contain an equivalent number of subjects. Cells B and C allow examination of each intervention separately. Cell D subjects receive no treatment and serve as a control group. Cell A allows examination of the interaction between the two independent variables. This design can be used, as in the randomized block design, to control for confounding variables. The confounding variable is included as an independent variable, and interactions between it and the other independent variable are examined (Spector, 1981).

Extensions of the factorial design to more than two levels of variables are referred to as M × N factorial designs. Within this design, independent variables can have any number of levels within

Level of Relaxation	Level of Distraction	
	Distraction	No Distraction
Relaxation	A	B
No Relaxation	C	D

FIGURE 11–22 ■ Example of factorial design.

practical limits. Note that a 3 × 3 design involves 9 cells and requires a much larger sample size. A 4 × 4 design would require 16 cells. A 4 × 4 design would allow relaxation to be provided at four levels of intensity, such as no relaxation, relaxation for 10 minutes twice a day, relaxation for 15 minutes three times a day, and relaxation for 20 minutes four times a day. Distraction would be provided at similar levels.

Factorial designs are not limited to two independent variables; however, interpretation of larger numbers becomes more complex and requires greater knowledge of statistical analysis. Factorial designs do allow the examination of theoretically proposed interrelationships between multiple independent variables. However, very large samples are required.

An example of factorial design is the study by Henker and associates (1995), which evaluated four methods of warming intravenous fluids (IVF). An excerpt from that study follows.

• •

"The methods of warming IVF and the control were evaluated with a 5 × 5 factorial experimental design. Each method of warming and the control were evaluated at each flow rate and replicated two times, yielding three measurements for each warming method at each rate." (Henker et al., 1995, p. 386) ▪

Nested Designs

In some experimental situations, the researcher wishes to consider the effect of variables that are found only at some levels of the independent variables being studied. Variables found only at certain levels of the independent variable are called *nested variables*. Possible nested variables are gender, race, socioeconomic status, and education. A nested variable may also be the patients who are cared for on specific nursing units or at different hospitals; the statistical analysis in this case would be conducted as though the unit or hospital were the subject rather than the individual patient. Figure 11–23 illustrates the nested design. In actual practice, nursing units used in this manner would have to be much larger in number than those illustrated, because each unit would be considered a subject and would be randomly assigned to a treatment.

The following excerpt from Harris and Hyman's (1984) study, "Clean vs. Sterile Tracheotomy Care and Level of Pulmonary Infection," is an example of this design.

• •

"The purpose of this research was to determine if clean tracheotomy care was more effective than sterile as measured by levels of postoperative pulmonary infection. Ten hospitals with large Head and Neck/ENT services were selected as data collection sites. . . . To increase external validity, possible unique effects associated with hospitals were controlled by use of a nested design—hospital nested within treatment procedure. . . . At these centers a minimum of 15 tracheostomy patient charts were reviewed pre- and postoperatively for clinical and laboratory data related to infection. Patient level of infection was defined using the Weighted Level of Pulmonary Infection Tool, which was constructed for this study." (Harris & Hyman, 1984, pp. 80–83) ▪

Crossover or Counterbalanced Designs

In some studies, more than one treatment is administered to each subject. The treatments are provided sequentially rather than concurrently. Comparisons are then made of the effects of the different treatments on the same subject. For example, two different methods known to achieve relaxation might be used as the two treatments. One difficulty encountered in this type of study is that exposure to one treatment may result in effects (called *carryover effects*) that persist and influence responses of the subject to later treatments. Also, subjects can improve as they become more familiar with the experimental protocol, which is called a *practice effect*. They may become tired or bored with the study, which is called a *fatigue effect*. The direct interaction of one treatment with another, such as the use of two drugs, can confound differences in the two treatments.

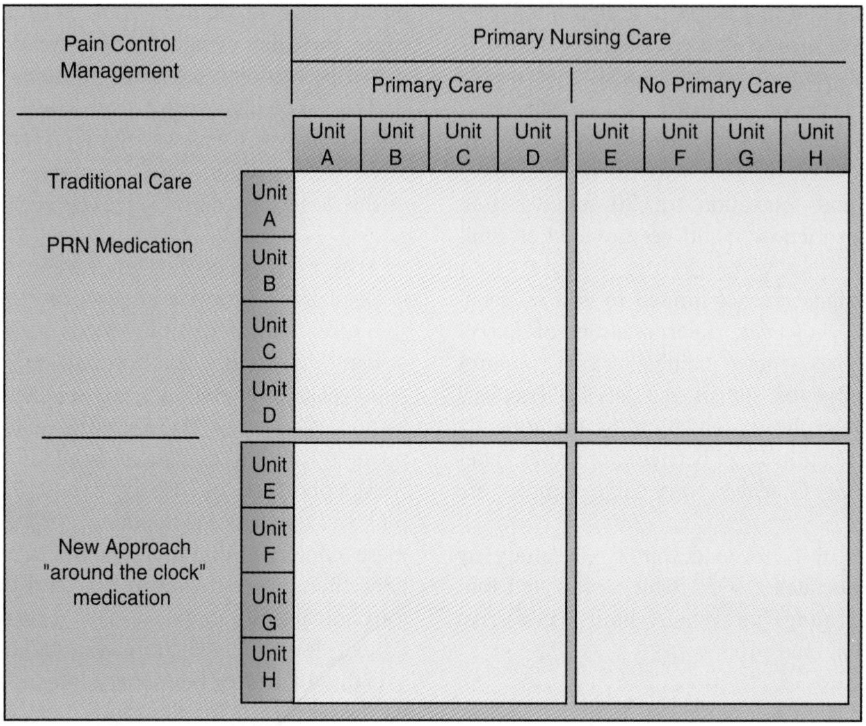

Pain Control Management		Primary Nursing Care							
		Primary Care				No Primary Care			
		Unit A	Unit B	Unit C	Unit D	Unit E	Unit F	Unit G	Unit H
Traditional Care	Unit A								
	Unit B								
PRN Medication	Unit C								
	Unit D								
New Approach "around the clock" medication	Unit E								
	Unit F								
	Unit G								
	Unit H								

FIGURE 11–23 ■ Design using nesting.

Crossover, or *counterbalancing,* is a strategy designed to guard against possible erroneous conclusions resulting from carryover effects. With counterbalancing, subjects are randomly assigned to a specific sequencing of treatment conditions. This approach distributes the carryover effects equally throughout all the conditions of the study, thus canceling them out. To prevent an effect related to time, the same amount of time must be allotted to each treatment, and the crossover point must be related to time, not to the condition of the subject.

In addition, the design must allow for an adequate interval between treatments to dissipate the effects of the first treatment; this is referred to as a *washout period.* For example, the design would specify that each treatment would last 6 days and that on the eighth day, each subject would cross over to the alternative treatment after a 2-day washout period.

The researcher also must be alert to the possibil-ity that changes may be due to factors such as disease progression, the healing process, or the effects of treatment of the disease rather than the study treatment. The process of counterbalancing can become complicated when more than two treatments are involved. Counterbalancing is effective only if the carryover effect is essentially the same from treatment A to treatment B as it is from treatment B to treatment A. If one treatment is more fatiguing than the other or more likely to modify response to the other treatment, counterbalancing will not be effective. The crossover design controls the variance in the study and thus allows the sample size to be smaller. The sample size required to detect a significant effect is considerably smaller because the subjects serve as their own controls. Because the data collection period is longer, however, the rate of subject dropout may increase (Beck, 1989).

An example of this design is Legault and Goulet's (1995) study comparing kangaroo and traditional methods of removing preterm infants from incubators. An excerpt of the study follows.

· ·

"The intervention was use of the kangaroo or traditional method of maintaining body temperature of preterm infants. The dependent variables were physiologic parameters (skin temperature, heart rate, respiratory rate, and oxygen saturation) measured five times with each method. Mother's satisfaction was measured at the end of each testing period and mother's preference at the end of the experiment. The kangaroo method produced less variation in oxygen saturation and longer duration of testing, and it was preferred by most of the mothers." (Legault & Goulet, 1995, p. 501) ■

Randomized Clinical Trials

Randomized clinical trials have been used in medicine since 1945. Wooding (1994) describes the strategies that were used to introduce new medical therapies before that time:

· ·

"Until very recently, the genesis and use of new treatments came about by means having little to do with the scientific method. For millennia, the majority of therapies appear to have evolved by one of three methods: accidental discovery of treatments with unmistakable efficacy; the use of hypotheses alone, without any experimentation; or the utilization of experimentation without controls, randomization, blinding . . ., or adequate sample sizes. Treatments originating by one of the latter two routes frequently persisted for a very long time despite a lack of unbiased evidence of their efficacy. Bloodletting, purging, and the use of homeopathic dosages of drugs are examples. Failure of a treatment in any particular case was usually attributed by its practitioners to its misuse, to poor diagnosis, or to complicating factors." (Wooding, 1994, p. 26) ■

The methodology for a clinical trial uses strategies for medical research (Meinert & Tonascia, 1986; Piantadosi, 1997; Pocock, 1996; Whitehead, 1992; Wooding, 1994). The Phase I, II, III and IV clinical trial categories were developed specifically for testing experimental drug therapy. *Phase I*, the initial testing of a new drug, focuses on determining the best drug dose and identifying safety effects. *Phase II* trials seek preliminary evidence of efficacy and side effects of the drug dose determined by the Phase I trial. Phase I and Phase II trials do not include control groups or randomization and therefore could not be classified as experimental. They are more similar to pilot studies (Whitehead, 1992).

Phase III trials are comparative definitive studies in which the new drug's effects are compared with those of the drug considered standard therapy. Phase III trials are sometimes referred to as "full scale definitive clinical trials," suggesting that a decision is made on the basis of the findings as to whether the experimental drug is more effective than standard treatment. In some Phase III clinical trials, the sample size is not determined before initiation of data collection. Rather, data are analyzed at intervals to test for significant differences between groups. If a significant difference is found, data collection may be discontinued. Otherwise, the data collection will continue and retesting is initiated after accrual of additional subjects (Meinert & Tonascia, 1986; Whitehead, 1992). Phase IV trials occur after regulatory approval of the drug, are designed to follow patients over time to identify uncommon side effects and test marketing strategies, and do not include a control group or randomization (Piantadosi, 1997; Wooding, 1994).

Piantadosi (1997) recommends redefining these stages to be broader and applicable to more types of trials. He recommends using the following terminology: early development, middle development, comparative studies, and late development. The purpose of *early development* trials would be to develop and test the treatment mechanism (thus, they could also be called *TM trials*). *Middle development* studies would focus on clinical outcomes and treatment "tolerability." Tolerability would have three components: feasibility, safety, and efficacy; thus, Piantadosi (1997) refers to middle development studies as safety and efficacy or *SE trials*. In this phase, the researcher would estimate the probability that patients would benefit from the treatment (or experience side effects from it). Performance criteria such as success rate might be used.

Comparative studies or *late development* trials, according to Piantadosi (1997), would have defined clinical end points and would address comparative treatment efficacy (so could be called *CTE trials*). These studies would include a concurrent control group that receives the standard treatment and an experimental group that receives the experimental treatment. *Late development* studies would be designed to identify uncommon side effects, interactions with other treatments, or unusual complications. They would be developed as expanded safety or *ES trials*.

Elwood (1998) suggests that clinical trial methodology could be used for prevention intervention studies as well as testing treatments. Murray (1998) proposes methods of randomizing groups rather than subjects in prevention studies and explores issues related to community-based trials such as sample mortality.

Until recently, the term *clinical trial* has not been used to describe studies conducted in nursing research. The clinical trial is perceived by many to be the "Cadillac" of designs. (There are serious criticisms of the clinical trial, however; they are discussed in Chapter 12.) If the clinical trial is to be used in nursing, the methodology should be redefined to fit the knowledge-building needs of nursing. Sidani and Braden (1998) have made a start in this direction by proposing such a methodology, which is described in Chapter 13. Criteria for defining a study as a clinical trial as opposed to referring to it as an experimental study have not been clarified in the nursing literature.

Meinert & Tonascia (1986) defines a clinical trial as follows:

· ·

"[A] planned experiment designed to assess the efficacy of a treatment in man by comparing the outcomes in a group of patients treated with the test treatment with those observed in a comparable group of patients receiving a control treatment, where patients in both groups are enrolled, treated, and followed over the same time period. The groups may be established through randomization or some other method of assignment. The outcome measure may be death, a nonfatal clinical event, or a laboratory test. The period of observation may be short or long depending on the outcome measure." (Meinert & Tonascia, 1986, p. 3) ■

Conceptually, the term *clinical trial*, as it is used in the nursing literature, seems to be associated with a Phase III trial and has the following expectations:

1. The study is designed to be a definitive test of the hypothesis that the intervention causes the defined effects.
2. Previous studies have provided evidence that the intervention causes the desired outcome.
3. The intervention is clearly defined and a protocol has been established for its clinical application.
4. The study is conducted in a clinical setting, not in a laboratory.
5. The design meets the criteria of an experimental study.
6. Subjects are drawn from a reference population through the use of clearly defined criteria. Baseline states are comparable in all groups included in the study. Selected subjects are then randomly assigned to treatment and control groups; thus the term *randomized clinical trial*.
7. Subjects are accrued individually over time as they enter the clinical area, are identified as meeting the study criteria, and agree to participate in the study.
8. The study has high internal validity. The design is rigorous and involves a high level of control of potential sources of bias that will rule out possible alternative causes of the effect. The design may include blinding or double-blinding to accomplish this purpose. *Blinding* means that either the patient or those providing care to the patient are unaware of whether the patient is in the experimental group or the control group. *Double-blinding* means that neither the patient nor the caregivers are aware of the group assignment of the patient.
9. The treatment is equal and consistently applied to all subjects in the experimental group.
10. Dependent variables are measured consistently.
11. The proposed study has been externally reviewed by expert researchers who have approved the design.

12. The study has received external funding sufficient to allow a rigorous design with a sample size adequate to provide a definitive test of the intervention.
13. If the clinical trial results indicate a significant effect of the intervention, the evidence is sufficient to warrant application of the findings in clinical practice.
14. The intervention is defined in sufficient detail so that clinical application can be achieved.

Clinical trials may be carried out simultaneously in multiple geographical locations to increase sample size and resources and to obtain a more representative sample (Meinert & Tonascia, 1986). In this case, the primary researcher must coordinate activities at all the sites. Meinert & Tonascia (1986) indicates that the costs per patient per year of study are less for multicenter studies than for single-center trials. The researcher using this technique must confront several problems. Coordination of a project of this type requires much time and effort. Keeping up with subjects is critical but may be difficult. Communication with and cooperation of staff assisting with the study in the various geographical locations are essential but sometimes difficult. The researcher may encounter attempts to ignore the protocol and provide traditional care (Fetter et al., 1989; Tyzenhouse, 1981). Meinert & Tonascia (1986) recommends the development of a coordinating center for multisite clinical trials that will be responsible for receiving, editing, processing, analyzing, and storing data generated in the study.

The use of the clinical trial is growing in nursing research. Brooten and colleagues (1986) conducted a clinical trial of early hospital discharge and home follow-up of very low birth weight infants. Burgess and associates (1987) performed a clinical trial of cardiac rehabilitation. Later studies defined in the literature as clinical trials are those by Clarke (1999), deMoissac and Jensen (1998), Griebel and associates (1998), Ippoliti and Neumann (1998), Rawl and colleagues (1998), and Turner and associates (1998).

An example of a clinical trial in nursing is the study by Gilliss and Kulkin (1991), who described the administrative management of a clinical trial

designed to examine nursing strategies for improving recovery from cardiac surgery. The study was funded by the National Center for Nursing Research. Baseline data were collected on individual health, psychological status, self-efficacy, family functioning, and coping. These variables were also used as outcome measures. A model of the design is illustrated in Figure 11–24. Gilliss and Kulkin's (1991) description of their study follows.

....

"Improving Recovery from Cardiac Surgery, or the Family Heart Study, was a randomized clinical trial of in-hospital and postdischarge nursing interventions designed to improve individual and family recovery from cardiac surgery. Eligible patients were between 25 and 75 years of age, spoke English, were scheduled for CABG [coronary artery bypass graft] or valve repair, were available for telephone contact for 6 months, and had a consenting partner who would care for them in early recovery. Subjects who experienced postsurgical complications of significance were excluded after surgery. All pairs inducted into the study were assigned to experimental or control status using a block randomization scheme. Patients received "standard care" (Intervention 1) at the two study hospitals. This involved viewing a slide-tape presentation ("Move into Action") on cardiac risk reduction prepared by the Santa Clara (California) Heart Association. Experimental patient/caregiver pairs received additional education and counseling (Intervention 2) prior to discharge. This included an original slide-tape presentation ("Working Together for Recovery") that was patterned after the American Heart Association tapes and educated the pairs about common psychological and relationship responses to recovery from surgery. Following the viewing, each pair met with a study nurse to discuss the applicability of the slide-tape content to their particular situation.

....

"Finally, experimental patients and caregivers were contacted at 1, 2, 3, 4, 6, and 8 weeks after discharge by graduate nurse researcher assistants for outcall telephone monitoring and recovery coaching (Intervention 3). These calls followed a semistructured guide and were intended to rein-

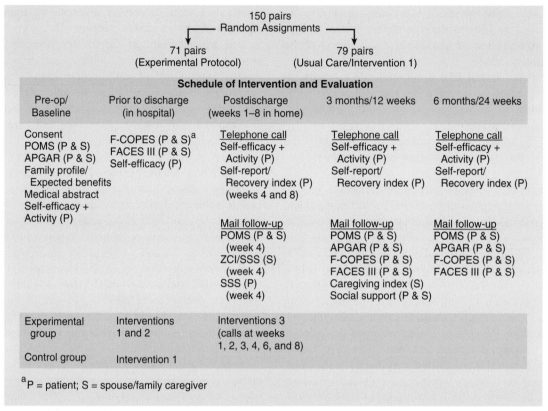

Figure 11–24 ■ Design model for clinical trial. (From Gilliss, C. L., & Kulkin, I. L. [1991]). Monitoring nursing interventions and data collection in a randomized clinical trial. *Western Journal of Nursing Research, 13*(3), 416–422.

force hospital-based education programs, detect early complications and drug effects, answer questions, and offer support for recovery; however, an overriding aim was to offer personalized nursing care." (Gilliss & Kulkin, 1991, pp. 416–417) ■

STUDIES THAT DO NOT USE TRADITIONAL RESEARCH DESIGNS

In some approaches to research, the research designs described in this chapter cannot be used. These studies tend to be in highly specialized areas that require unique design strategies to accomplish their purposes. Designs for primary prevention and health promotion, secondary analysis, meta-analysis, and methodological studies are described here.

Primary Prevention and Health Promotion Studies

Studying primary prevention and health promotion involves applying a treatment of primary prevention (the cause) and then attempting to measure the effect (an event that does not occur if the treatment was effective). *Primary prevention* studies, then, attempt to measure things that do not happen. One cannot select a sample to study, apply a treatment, and then measure an effect. The sample must be the community. The design involves examining changes in the community, and the variables are called *indicators*. A change in an identified indicator is inferred to be a consequence of the effectiveness of the prevention program (treatment).

Specific indicators would depend on the focus of

prevention. For example, the indicators identified by the National Institution on Drug Abuse are (1) changes in drug-related perceptions, attitudes, knowledge, and action; (2) changes in prevalence and incidence of drug use as well as drug-related mortality or morbidity, or both; (3) institutional policy or programs, or both; (4) involvement of youth or parent, or both, in the community; and (5) accident rates (French & Kaufman, 1981). Because one indicator alone would be insufficient to infer effect, multiple indicators and statistical analyses appropriate for these indicators must be used.

Van Rossum and colleagues (1991) describe the design of a study to determine the effect of preventive home visits to the elderly by public health nurses. The goals of the visits were to increase independence of the elderly and prevent or postpone institutional care. Outcome measures, or indicators, used in the study were perceived state of health, well-being, functional state, mental state, use of health care services, institutionalization, and mortality. A parallel group randomized trial was used. Subjects were limited to people 75 to 84 years of age. A questionnaire and letter were sent to all individuals of this age group living in Weert, a town in The Netherlands with a population of 60,000. The response rate was 85%, and 92% of those responding agreed to participate. Those already receiving home nursing care were excluded. A sample of 600 subjects was randomly selected through the use of a computer from the possible pool of 1285 questionnaire respondents.

To control for extraneous variables, the participants were stratified by the following four variables before being randomly assigned to groups: (1) gender, (2) composition of household, (3) perceived state of health, and (4) social class. Subjects were then randomly assigned to treatment and control groups within each stratum, again with the use of a computer. Those receiving the treatment were randomly assigned to a public health nurse. Subjects were monitored for 3 years. Those receiving public health nursing visits were visited every 3 months by the same public health nurse. The nurse could be contacted daily, and additional visits were made when needed. Control group subjects received no visits but had access to all traditional health care services.

Secondary Analysis

Secondary analysis design involves studying data previously collected in another study. Data are reexamined with the use of different organizations of the data and different statistical analyses from those previously used. The design involves analyzing data to validate the reported findings, examining dimensions previously unexamined, or redirecting the focus of the data to allow comparison with data from other studies (Gleit & Graham, 1989). As data sets accumulate from the research programs of groups of faculty, secondary analyses can be expected to increase. This approach allows the investigators to examine questions related to the data that were not originally posed. These data sets may provide opportunities for junior faculty members or graduate students to become involved in a research program.

Of concern in secondary analyses of data is the tendency of some researchers to write as many papers as possible from the planned analyses of a study to increase the number of their publications—a strategy referred to as "salami slicing." Researchers performing secondary analyses should always identify the original source of data and the previous publications emerging from the analysis of that data set. Aaronson (1994) points out the problem with this practice, as follows:

• •

"Fundamentally, each paper written from the same study or the same dataset must make a distinct and significant scientific contribution. Presumably this is not only the major overriding criterion used by reviewers, but also the author's intent when writing the paper. When a particular paper is one of several from the same study, project, or dataset, the author's responsibility to identify the source of the data is that much greater. To lead readers to think a report is from a new study or a different dataset than that used in the authors' previous work is dishonest, particularly if the second paper purports to substantiate findings of the first one. . . . Apart from the overriding concern about 'milking the data,' the most common objection to multiple articles from a single study is concern about the age of the data. . . . Concerns in nursing about the number of papers generated from a single study may reflect the emerging status of secondary analysis as a legitimate approach to nursing research. . . .

"All of the reasons offered for using secondary analysis—answering new questions with existing data, applying new methods to answer old questions, the real exigencies of cost and feasibility—serve equally to justify the continued use of data collected years ago, by the original investigator of a large project, as well as by others. . . . The issue remains one of sound science. The question that must be asked is: Does this particular paper make a meaningful and distinct contribution to the scientific literature?" (Aaronson, 1994, pp. 61–62) ▪

An example of secondary analysis is Lauver and Tak's (1995) study, "Optimism and Coping with a Breast Cancer Symptom." An excerpt from this study follows.

• •

"This cross-sectional study was a part of a larger investigation to explain care seeking for breast cancer symptoms. Complementary findings have been described elsewhere (Lauver, 1992, 1994). Data were collected in a breast surgery clinic of an urban hospital that provided care for the medically indigent. Participants were seeking evaluation for self-identified breast cancer symptoms, such as a lump or discharge. Eligible participants were older than 18 years of age, had no personal history of cancer, and could communicate in English." (Lauver & Tak, 1995, p. 203) ▪

Meta-Analysis Designs

Meta-analysis design involves merging findings from many studies that have examined the same phenomenon. The design uses specific statistical analyses to determine the overall findings from a combined examination of reports of statistical findings of each study. The statistical values used include the means and standard deviations for each group in the study. One of the outcomes of a meta-analysis is the estimation of a population effect size for the topic under study. Because studies seldom have exactly the same focus, conclusions are never absolute but do give some sense of unity to knowledge within that area (O'Flynn, 1982).

One problem consistently encountered in meta-analyses is that the studies being examined are inconsistent in design quality. However, researchers conducting meta-analyses have not been successful in identifying a generally acceptable means to measure the research quality of studies. Brown (1991) proposed a research quality scoring method to accomplish this important task. Another problem encountered by researchers performing meta-analyses is that basic research information is often missing from research reports. Calculating effect sizes requires means and standard deviations in each study for both experimental and control groups. In addition, the beginning sample size must be reported as well as the sample size at the time of the posttest. Often, the treatment has been poorly described, making it difficult to determine the most effective treatments (Brown, 1991).

An example of a meta-analysis is Brown and Grimes's (1995) meta-analysis of nurse practitioners and nurse midwives in primary care, an abstract of which follows.

• •

"This meta-analysis was an evaluation of patient outcomes of nurse practitioners (NPs) and nurse midwives (NMs), compared with those of physicians, in primary care. The sample included 38 NP and 15 NM studies. Thirty-three outcomes were analyzed. In studies that employed randomization to provider, greater patient compliance with treatment recommendations was shown with NPs than with physicians. In studies that controlled for patient risk in ways other than randomization, patient satisfaction and resolution of pathological conditions were greater for NP patients. NPs were equivalent to MDs on most other variables in controlled studies. In studies that controlled for patient risk, NMs used less technology and analgesia than did physicians in intrapartum care of obstetric patients. NMs

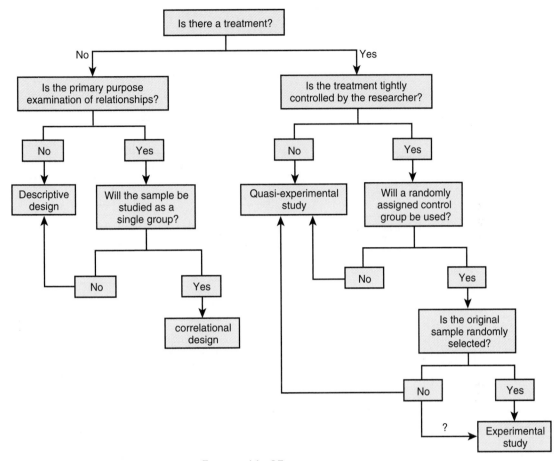

FIGURE 11–25 ■ Type of study.

achieved neonatal outcomes equivalent to those of physicians. Limitations in data from primary studies precluded answering questions of why and under what conditions these outcomes apply and whether these services are cost-effective." (Brown & Grimes, 1995, p. 332) ■

Methodological Designs

Methodological designs are used to develop the validity and reliability of instruments to measure constructs used as variables in research. The process is lengthy and complex. The average length of researcher time required to develop a research tool to

the point of appropriate use in a study is 5 years. An example of this design is Ludington-Hoe and Kasper's (1995) study, "A Physiologic Method for Monitoring Premature Infants." The abstract from that study follows.

. . . .

"Instrumentation capable of handling 12 continuous hours of nine-channel real-time physiologic data sampled at 10 Hz was needed to test within and between subject variability and preterm infant responses to skin-to-skin contact with the mother. A review of basic electrical components, electrical principles related to physiologic monitoring, and electrophysiology concepts generic to physiologic

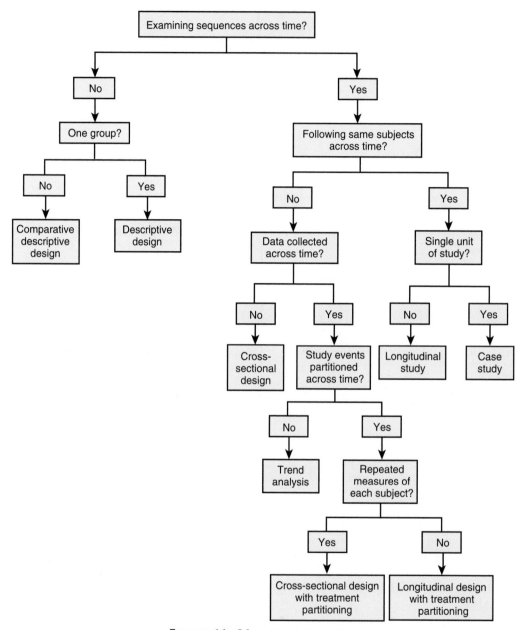

FIGURE 11–26 ■ Descriptive studies.

monitoring is presented. The development, specification and applications of a new instrument to monitor premature infant cardiorespiratory adaptations are discussed." (Ludington-Hoe & Kasper, 1995, p. 13) ■

DECISION TREES FOR SELECTING RESEARCH DESIGNS

Selecting a research design involves following paths of logical reasoning. A calculating mind is

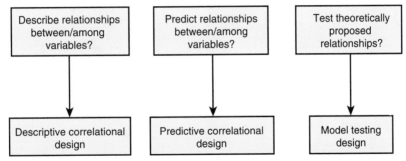

FIGURE 11–27 ■ Correlational studies.

needed to explore all the possible consequences of using a particular design in a study. In some ways, selecting a design is like thinking through the moves in a chess game. One must carefully think through the consequences of each option. The research design organizes all the components of the study in a way that is most likely to lead to valid answers to the questions that have been posed.

To help you select the most appropriate design, a series of decision trees have been provided here. The first decision tree, Figure 11–25, helps identify the type of study being conducted. The next four decision trees (see Figures 11–26 through 11–29) assist in the selection of specific designs for each of the types of studies. The selection of a design is not a rigid, rule-guided task. The researcher has considerable flexibility in choosing a design. The pathways within the decision trees are not absolute and are to be used as guides.

■ SUMMARY

Designs have been developed by researchers to meet unique research needs as they emerge. At present, nursing research is using designs developed by other disciplines. These designs are a useful starting point, but nurse scientists must go beyond them to develop designs that will more appropriately meet the needs of nursing's knowledge base.

Descriptive studies are designed to gain more information about variables within a particular field of study. Their purpose is to provide a picture of situations as they naturally happen. No manipulation of variables is involved. Descriptive designs vary in levels of complexity. Some contain only two variables, whereas others may include multiple variables. The relationships between variables are identified to obtain an overall picture of the phenomenon being examined. Protection against bias is achieved through conceptual and operational definitions of variables, sample selection and size, valid and reliable instruments, and data collection procedures that achieve some environmental control.

Correlational studies examine relationships between variables. This examination can occur at several levels. The researcher can seek to describe a relationship, predict relationships among variables, or test the relationships proposed by a theoretical proposition. In correlational designs, a large variance in the variable scores is necessary to determine the existence of a relationship. Researchers tend to make two serious errors with correlational studies. First, they often attempt to establish causality by correlation, reasoning that if two variables are related, one must cause the other. Second, they confuse studies in which differences are examined with studies in which relationships are examined.

The purpose of *quasi-experimental* and *experimental* designs is to examine causality. The power of the design to accomplish this purpose depends on the degree to which the actual effects of the experimental treatment (the independent variable) can be detected by measurement of the dependent variable. Obtaining an understanding of the true effects of an experimental treatment requires action to control threats to the validity of the findings. Threats to validity are controlled through selection

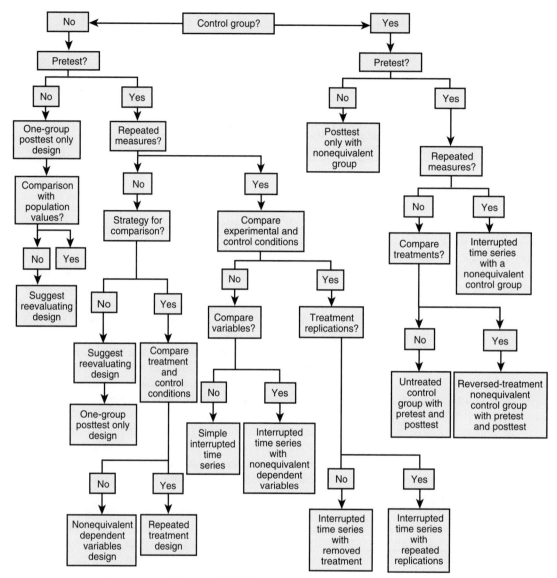

FIGURE 11–28 ■ Quasi-experimental studies.

of subjects, manipulation of the treatment, and reliable measurement of variables. Experimental designs with their strict control of variance are the most powerful method of examining causality. Quasi-experimental designs were developed to provide alternate means for examining causality in situations not conducive to experimental controls. Experimental designs are set up to provide the greatest

amount of control possible to examine causality more closely. To examine cause, one must eliminate all factors influencing the dependent variable other than the cause (independent variable) being studied. Other factors are eliminated by controlling them. The three essential elements of experimental research are (1) randomization, (2) researcher-controlled manipulation of the independent variable,

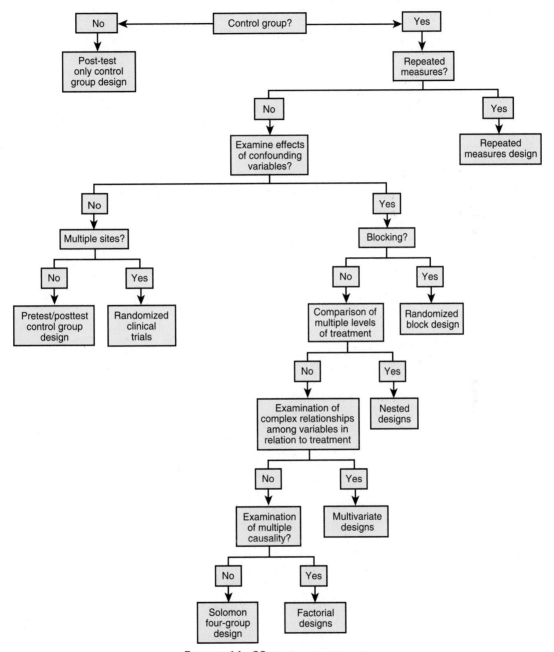

FIGURE 11–29 ■ Experimental studies.

and (3) researcher control of the experimental situation, including a control or comparison group.

Studies in highly specialized areas require unique design strategies to accomplish their purposes.

Studying *primary prevention* and *health promotion* involves applying a treatment of primary prevention (the cause) and then attempting to measure the effect (an event that does not occur if the treatment was effective). The design involves examining changes in the community, and the variables are called indicators. *Secondary analysis* is the study of data previously collected in another study. Data are re-examined using different organizations of the data and different statistical analyses from those previously used. *Meta-analysis* is the merging of findings from many studies that have examined the same phenomenon. Specific statistical analyses are used to determine the overall findings from joint examination of reported statistical findings. *Methodological studies* are designed to develop the validity and reliability of instruments to measure constructs used as variables in research. The average length of researcher time required to develop a research tool to the point of appropriate use in a study is 5 years.

• •

REFERENCES

Aaronson, L. S. (1994). Milking data or meeting commitments: How many papers from one study? *Nursing Research, 43*(1), 60–62.

Aaronson, L. S., & Kingry, M. J. (1988). A mixed method approach for using cross-sectional data for longitudinal inferences. *Nursing Research, 37*(3), 187–198.

Abdellah, F. G., & Levine, E. (1979). *Better patient care through nursing research.* New York: Macmillan.

Anderson, V. L., & McLean, R. A. (1974). *Design of experiments: A realistic approach.* New York: Marcel Dekker.

Arakawa, S. (1995). Use of relaxation to reduce side effects of chemotherapy in Japanese patients. *Cancer Nursing, 18*(1), 60–66.

Barlow, D. H., & Hersen, M. (1984). *Single case experimental designs: Strategies for studying behavior change.* New York: Pergamon.

Barnard, K. E., Magyary, D. L., Booth, C. L., & Eyres, S. J. (1987). Longitudinal designs: Considerations and applications to nursing research. *Recent Advances in Nursing, 17,* 37–64.

Beck, S. L. (1989). The crossover design in clinical nursing research. *Nursing Research, 38*(5), 291–293.

Blair, C. E. (1995). Combining behavior management and mutual goal setting to reduce physical dependency in nursing home residents. *Nursing Research, 44*(3), 160–165.

Brooten, D., Kuman, S., Brown, L. P., Butts, P., Finkler, S. A., Bakewell-Sachs, S., Gibbons, A., & Delivoria-Papadopoulos, M. (1986). A randomized clinical trial of early hospital discharge and home follow-up of very-low-birth-weight infants. *New England Journal of Medicine, 315*(15), 934–939.

Brown, S. A. (1991). Measurement of quality of primary studies for meta-analysis. *Nursing Research, 40*(6), 352–355.

Brown, S. A., & Grimes, D. E. (1995). A meta-analysis of nurse practitioners and nurse midwives in primary care. *Nursing Research, 44*(6), 332–339.

Burgess, A. W., Lerner, D. J., D'Agostino, R. B., Vokonas, P. S., Hartman, C. R., & Gaccione, P. (1987). A randomized control trial of cardiac rehabilitation. *Social Science and Medicine, 24*(4), 359–370.

Campbell, D. T., & Stanley, J. C. (1963). *Experimental and quasi-experimental designs for research.* Chicago: Rand McNally.

Chang, B. L. (1999). Cognitive-behavioral intervention for home-bound caregivers of persons with dementia. *Nursing Research, 48*(3), 173–182.

Clarke, D. A. (1999). Advancing my health care practice in aromatherapy. *Australian Journal of Holistic Nursing, 6*(1), 32–38.

Cook, T. D., & Campbell, D. T. (1979). *Quasi-experimentation: Design and analysis issues for field settings.* Chicago: Rand McNally.

Cox, D. R. (1958). *Planning of experiments.* New York: Wiley.

Crombie, I. K., & Davies, H. T. O. (1996). *Research in health care: Design, conduct and interpretation of health services research.* New York: Wiley.

deMoissac, D., & Jensen, L. (1998). Changing IV administration sets: Is 48 versus 24 hours safe for neutropenic patients with cancer? *Oncology Nursing Forum, 25*(5), 907–913.

Doering, L. V., Dracup, K., Moser, D. K., Czer, L. S. C., & Peter, C. T. (1999). Evidence of time-dependent autonomic reinnervation after heart transplantation. *Nursing Research, 48*(6), 308–316.

Elwood, J. M. (1998). *Critical appraisal of epidemiological studies and clinical trials.* New York: Oxford University Press.

Fetter, M. S., Fettham, S. L., D'Apolito, K., Chaze, B. A., Fink, A., Frink, B. B., Hougart, M. K., & Rushton, C. H. (1989). Randomized clinical trials: Issues for researchers. *Nursing Research, 38*(2), 117-120.

Fisher, R. A. (1935). *The design of experiments.* New York: Hafner.

French, J. F., & Kaufman, N. J. (1981). *Handbook for prevention evaluation: Prevention evaluation guidelines.* Rockville, MD: National Institute on Drug Abuse.

Fridriksdottir, M., & McCarthy, D. O. (1995). The effect of caloric density of food on energy intake and body weight in tumor-bearing rats. *Research in Nursing & Health, 18*(4), 357–363.

Gilliss, C. L., & Kulkin, I. L. (1991). Monitoring nursing interventions and data collection in a randomized clinical trial. *Western Journal of Nursing Research, 13*(3), 416–422.

Gleit, C., & Graham, B. (1989). Secondary data analysis: A valuable resource. *Nursing Research, 38*(6), 380–381.

Gray, M. (1998). Introducing single case study research design: An overview. *Nurse Researcher, 5*(4), 15–24.

Griebel, B, Wewers, M. E., & Baker, C. A. (1998). The effectiveness of a nurse-managed minimal smoking-cessation intervention among hospitalized patients with cancer. *Oncology Nursing Forum, 25*(5), 897–902.

Hagerty, B. M., & Williams, R. A. (1999). The effects of sense of belonging, social support, conflict, and loneliness on depression. *Nursing Research, 48*(4), 215–219.

Hanneman, S. K. G. (1994). Multidimensional predictors of success or failure with early weaning from mechanical ventilation after cardiac surgery. *Nursing Research, 43*(1), 4–10.

Harris, R. B., & Hyman, R. B. (1984). Clean vs. sterile tracheotomy care and level of pulmonary infection. *Nursing Research, 33*(2), 80–85.

Henker, R., Bernardo, L. M., O'Connor, K., & Sereika, S. (1995). Evaluation of four methods of warming intravenous fluids. *Journal of Emergency Nursing, 21*(5), 385–390.

Hjelm-Karlsson, K. (1991). Using the biased coin design for randomization in health care research. *Western Journal of Nursing Research, 13*(2), 284–288.

Ippoliti, C., & Neumann, J. (1998). Octreotide in the management of diarrhea induced by graft versus host disease. *Oncology Nursing Forum, 25*(5), 873–878.

Jennings-Dozier, K. (1999). Predicting intentions to obtain a Pap smear among African American and Latina women: Testing the Theory of Planned Behavior. *Nursing Research, 48*(4), 198–205.

Johnson, L. S., Rozmus, C., & Edmisson, K. (1999). Adolescent sexuality and sexually transmitted diseases: Attitudes, beliefs, knowledge, and values. *Journal of Pediatric Nursing, 14*(3), 177–185.

Lamb, K. (1979). Effect of positioning of postoperative fractured-hip patients as related to comfort. *Nursing Research, 28*(5), 291–294.

Lauver, D. (1992, October). *Promoting prompt care seeking for breast cancer symptoms in Caucasian and African-American women.* Paper presented at University of Illinois Conference: Reframing Women's Health: Multidisciplinary Research and Practice, Chicago, IL.

Lauver, D. (1994). Care-seeking behavior with breast cancer symptoms in Caucasian and African-American women. *Research in Nursing & Health, 17*(6), 421–431.

Lauver, D., & Tak, Y. (1995). Optimism and coping with a breast cancer symptom. *Nursing Research, 44*(4), 202–207.

Legault, M., & Goulet, C. (1995). Comparison of kangaroo and traditional methods of removing preterm infants from incubators. *Journal of Gynecologic and Neonatal Nursing, 24*(6), 501–506.

Lepczyk, M., Raleigh, E. H., & Rowley, C. (1990). Timing of preoperative patient teaching. *Journal of Advanced Nursing, 15*(3), 300–306.

Lewis, L. L. (1995). One year in the life of a woman with premenstrual syndrome: A case study. *Nursing Research, 44*(2), 111–116.

Ludington-Hoe, S., & Kasper, C. E. (1995). A physiologic method for monitoring premature infants. *Journal of Nursing Measurement, 3*(1), 13–29.

Martinson, I. M., Leavitt, M., Liu, C., Armstrong, V., Hornberger, L., Zhang, J., & Han, X. (1999). Comparison of Chinese and Caucasian families caregiving to children with cancer at home: Part I. *Journal of Pediatric Nursing, 14*(2), 99–109.

Mason-Hawkes, J., & Holm, K. (1989). Causal modeling: A comparison of path analysis and LISREL. *Nursing Research, 38*(5), 312–314.

McCain, L. J., & McCleary, R. (1979). The statistical analysis of the simple interrupted time-series quasi-experiment. In T. D. Cook & D. T. Campbell (Eds.), *Quasi-experimentation: Design and analysis issues for field settings* (pp. 233–293). Chicago: Rand McNally.

McCurren, C., Dowe, D., Ratle, D., & Looney, S. (1999). Depression among nursing home elders: Testing an intervention. *Applied Nursing Research, 12*(4), 185–195.

Meinert, C. L., & Tonascia, S. (1986). *Clinical trials: Design, conduct, and analysis.* New York: Oxford University Press.

Mimnaugh, L., Winegar, M., Mabrey, Y., & Davis, J. E. (1999). Sensations experienced during removal of tubes in acute postoperative patients. *Applied Nursing Research, 12*(2), 78–85.

Mirolo, B. R., Bunce, I. H., Chapman, M., Olsen, T., Eliadis, P., Hennessy, J. M., Ward, L. C., & Jones, L. C. (1995). Psychosocial benefits of postmastectomy lymphedema therapy. *Cancer Nursing, 18*(3), 197–205.

Murray, D. M. (1998). *Design and analysis of group-randomized trials.* New York: Oxford University Press.

Newman, M. A. (1986). *Health as expanding consciousness.* St. Louis: Mosby.

O'Flynn, A. I. (1982). Meta-analysis. *Nursing Research, 31*(5), 314–316.

Ottenbacher, K. (1992). Impact of random assignment on study outcome: An empirical examination. *Controlled Clinical Trials, 13*(1), 50–61.

Piantadosi, S. (1997). *Clinical trials: A methodologic perspective.* New York: Wiley.

Pocock, S. J. (1996). *Clinical trials: A practical approach.* New York: Wiley.

Quayhagen, M. P., Quayhagen, M., Corbeil, R. R., Roth, P. A., & Rodgers, J. A. (1995). A dyadic remediation program for care recipients with dementia. *Nursing Research, 44*(3), 153–159.

Rawl, S. M., Easton, K. L., Kwiatkowski, S., Zemen, D., & Burczyk, B. (1998). Effectiveness of a nurse-managed follow-up program for rehabilitation patients after discharge. *Rehabilitation Nursing, 23*(4), 204–209.

Reichardt, C. S. (1979). The statistical analysis of data from nonequivalent group designs. In T. D. Cook & D. T. Campbell (Eds.), *Quasi-experimentation: Design and analysis issues for field settings* (pp. 147–206). Chicago: Rand McNally.

Rotter, J. B. (1954). *Social learning and clinical psychology.* New York: Prentice-Hall.

Sandelowski, M. (1996). One is the liveliest number: The case orientation of qualitative research. *Research in Nursing & Health, 19*(6), 525–529.

Shiao, S. P. K., Youngblut, J. M., Anderson, G. C., DiFiore, J. M., & Martin, R. J. (1995). Nasogastric tube placement: Effects on breathing and sucking in very-low-birth-weight infants. *Nursing Research, 44*(2), 82–88.

Sidani, S. & Braden, C. J. (1998). *Evaluating nursing interventions: A theory-driven approach.* Thousand Oaks: Sage.

Spector, P. E. (1981). *Research designs.* Beverly Hills, CA: Sage.

Sterling, Y. M., & McNally, J. A. (1992). Single-subject research for nursing practice. *Clinical Nurse Specialist, 6*(1), 21–26.

Stewart, B. J., & Archbold, P. G. (1992). Nursing intervention studies require outcome measures that are sensitive to change, part 1. *Research in Nursing & Health, 15*(6), 477–481.

Stout, R. L., Wirtz, P. W., Carbonari, J. P., & Del Boca, F. K. (1994). Ensuring balanced distribution of prognostic factors in treatment outcome research. *Journal of Studies in Alcoholism, 12*(Suppl.), 70–75.

Trochim, W. M. K. (1986). *Advances in quasi-experimental design and analysis.* San Francisco: Jossey-Bass.

Turner, J. G., Clark, A. J., Gauthier, D. K., & Williams, M. (1998). The effect of therapeutic touch on pain and anxiety in burns patients. *Journal of Advanced Nursing, 28*(1), 10–20.

Tyzenhouse, P. S. (1981). Technical notes: The nursing clinical trial. *Western Journal of Nursing Research, 3*(1), 102–109.

U. S. Department of Health and Human Services (1968). *The Framingham Study: An epidemiological investigation of cardiovascular disease* (USDHHS Publication No. RC667F813). Bethesda, MD: Author.

Van Rossum, E. V., Frederiks, C., Philipsen, H., Lierop, J. K., Mantel, A., Portengen, J., & Knipschild, P. (1991). Design of a Dutch study to test preventive home visits to the elderly. *Nursing Research, 40*(3), 185–188.

Waltz, C. F., & Bausell, R. B. (1981). *Nursing research: Design, statistics and computer analysis.* Philadelphia: F. A. Davis.

Whitehead, J. (1992). *The design and analysis of sequential clinical trials.* New York: Ellis Horwood.

Whitney, J. D., Stotts, N. A., & Goodson, W. H., III. (1995). Effects of dynamic exercise on subcutaneous oxygen tension and temperature. *Research in Nursing & Health, 18*(2), 97–104.

Wikblad, K., & Anderson, B. (1995). A comparison of three wound dressings in patients undergoing heart surgery. *Nursing Research, 44*(5), 312–316.

Wilbur, J., Zoeller, L. H., Talashek, M., & Sullivan, J. A. (1990). Career trends of master's-prepared family nurse practitioners. *Journal of the American Academy of Nurse Practitioners, 2*(2), 69–78.

Williams, P. D., Press, A., Williams, A. R., Piamjariyakul, U., Keeter, L. M., Schultz, J., & Hunter, K. (1999). Fatigue in mothers of infants discharged to the home on apnea monitors. *Applied Nursing Research, 12*(2), 69–77.

Wooding, W. M. (1994). *Planning pharmaceutical clinical trials: Basic statistical principles.* New York: Wiley.

Yin, R. (1984). *Case study research: Design and methods.* Applied Social Research Methods Series, Vol. 5. Beverly Hills, CA: Sage.

Youssef, F. A. (1990). The impact of group reminiscence counseling on a depressed elderly population. *Nurse Practitioner, 15*(4), 32–38.

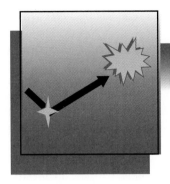

CHAPTER 12

OUTCOMES RESEARCH

A new paradigm for research, *outcomes research,* focuses on the end-results of patient care. The momentum propelling outcomes research comes from policymakers, insurers, and the public. There is a growing demand that providers justify interventions and systems of care in terms of improved patient lives and that costs of care be considered in the evaluation of treatment outcomes (Hinshaw, 1992). The strategies used in outcomes research are, to some extent, a departure from the accepted scientific methodology for health care research, and they incorporate evaluation methods, epidemiology, and economic theory.

This chapter consists of a brief history of endeavors to examine outcomes, outcomes research and nursing practice, the theoretical basis of outcomes research, and methodologies used in outcomes research. A broad base of literature from a variety of disciplines was used to develop the content for this chapter, in keeping with the multidisciplinary perspective of outcomes research.

A BRIEF HISTORY OF OUTCOMES RESEARCH

Prominent Figures in History

Sir William Petty (1623–1687) was the first physician to question the effectiveness of medical care (at least, in writing). Sir Petty was also a professor at Oxford and an economist. He is considered by many to be the father of economics and epidemiology. He influenced public policy through his writing and challenged the Royal College of Physicians by asking the following questions about the medical practice of the time:

• •

"Whether they [Englishmen] take as much medicine and remedies as the like number of men of other societyes.

"Whether of 1,000 patients to the best physicians, aged of any decad, there do not dye as many as out [of] the inhabitants of places where there dwell no physicians.

"Whether of 100 sick of acute diseases who use physicians, as many dye and [in] misery, as where no art is used, or only chance." (Petty, as cited in White, 1993, p. 12) ▪

In the 18th century, French statisticians developed methods of examining the effectiveness of medical interventions. These statistical methods were applied by a French physician, Louis (1787–1872), to clinical data. Using his *numerical method,* Louis demonstrated the uselessness and often harmfulness of bloodletting. The following excerpt from his writing illustrates his approach to examining medical practice:

• •

"In any epidemic . . . let us suppose 500 of the sick, *taken indiscriminately,* to be subjected to one kind of treatment, and 500 others, taken in the same manner, to be treated in a different mode; if the mortality is greater among the first, than among the second, must we not conclude that the treatment was less appropriate or less efficacious in the first class, than in the second? . . . [I]t is impossible to appreciate each case with mathematical exactness, and it is precisely on this account that enumeration becomes necessary; by so doing the errors (which are inevitable) being the same in both groups of patients subjected to different treatment, mutually compensate each other, and they may be disregarded without sensibly affecting the exactness of the results." (Louis, as cited in White, 1993, p. 12) ■

Louis's approach angered the physicians of his period, who believed that their own personal experience was sufficient to provide understanding of origins, diagnosis, treatment, and outcomes of disease. However, he continued to teach his medical students to appraise the effectiveness of their practice critically. A number of American physicians traveled to Paris for postgraduate studies with Louis, among them Oliver Wendell Holmes (1809–1894), who later made himself unpopular with practicing physicians in America with his observations on the causes of puerperal fever (White, 1993).

Semmelweiss, a Viennese physician of the 18th century, used hospital records to show that women in labor who were assisted by midwives had lower mortality rates than those attended by physicians in hospital wards. After prolonged efforts, he was able to identify the specific cause and to demonstrate an effective prophylaxis (rigorous hand-washing). Many physicians scoffed at his ideas, which were not widely applied to medical practice for some time (Johnson & Granger, 1994).

Florence Nightingale (1823–1910), nurse, statistician, administrator, and health policy advocate, was also among the first to conduct outcomes studies. She developed the first uniform hospital discharge data set and used the data to link mortality rates with diagnoses and treatments. Nightingale was a pioneer in statistical analysis who used graphical representations of her results to demonstrate that patient care outcomes could be changed. She was astute in disseminating her findings to those who formulated health policy, distributing them widely to members of Parliament, the government, and the army. She enraged the military and civilian medical establishment of her day, and it was several decades before the medical community

began to apply her ideas (Mahrenholz, 1991; White, 1993).

Early in the 20th century, Ernest A. Codman, a Boston surgeon, proposed a method of evaluating the effectiveness of care based on an examination of the patient 1 year after surgery or discharge from a hospital. He believed that this process would speed up the time required for physicians to determine whether a particular operative procedure was worthwhile, ineffective, or even harmful. He also proposed that the information be used to identify the types of errors physicians made and to serve as a basis for promotion in hospitals and medical schools. Results of the patient examinations could be recorded on end-result cards, which could then be used by patients in choosing where to obtain medical care. Codman asked questions such as "What was the patient's problem?" "Did the doctors diagnose it in time?" "Did the patient get entirely well?" "If not, why not?" "Was it the fault of the surgeon, the disease, or the patient?" and "What could be done to prevent similar failures in the future?" (Altman, 1993; Bloom, 1990; Neuhauser, 1990).

Codman's ideas were very unpopular at Harvard, where he taught, and at Massachusetts General Hospital, where he practiced. He was roundly attacked by his colleagues and, under pressure, had to leave his position. He established his own private hospital, where he implemented his proposed end-result cards. However, because of intense competition from the Boston medical establishment, he lost money and had to close the hospital. His ideas lay fallow for three decades before being reconsidered. Ultimately, his ideas were the basis for the formation of the Joint Commission for the Accreditation of Healthcare Organizations (JCAHO).

Efforts of the Health Care Financing Administration (HCFA) and the New York State Health Department in the early 1990s sparked an even greater controversy than Codman had, by using a variation of his end-result cards to publish a ranking of outcomes of doctors and hospitals performing cardiac surgery in New York. Newspapers obtained information for this ranking—in spite of obstructionist efforts by physicians and hospitals—by appealing to the courts through the use of the Freedom of Information Act (Altman, 1993; Bloom, 1990; Neuhauser, 1990; White, 1993).

The Agency for Health Services Research

In 1959, two National Institutes of Health study sections, the Hospital and Medical Facilities Study Section and the Nursing Study Section, met to discuss concerns about the adequacy and appropriateness of medical care, patient care, and hospital and medical facilities. As a result of their dialogue, a Health Services Research Study Section was initiated. This study section eventually became the Agency for Health Services Research (AHSR). With small amounts of funding from Congress, the AHSR continued to study the effectiveness of health services, primarily supporting the research of economists, epidemiologists, and health policy analysts (White, 1993). Two projects that were to have the greatest impact were small area analyses and the Medical Outcomes Study (MOS).

SMALL AREA ANALYSES

In the 1970s, an epidemiologist named Wennberg began a series of studies examining small area variations in medical practice across towns and counties. He found a wide variation in the tonsillectomy rate from one town to another in the New England area that could not be explained by differences such as health status, insurance, and demographics. These findings were replicated for a variety of medical procedures. Investigators began a search for the underlying causes of such variation and their implications for health status (O'Connor et al., 1993; Wennberg et al., 1993). Studies also revealed that many procedures, such as coronary artery bypass, were being performed on patients who did not have appropriate clinical indications for such surgery (Power et al., 1994).

THE MEDICAL OUTCOMES STUDY

The MOS was the first large-scale study to examine factors influencing patient outcomes. The study was designed to identify elements of physician care associated with favorable patient outcomes. The conceptual framework for the MOS is shown in Figure 12–1. Variations in use of resources and in physician technical and interpersonal styles were examined (Greenfield, et al., 1992; Kelly et al., 1994; Riesenberg & Glass, 1989; Stewart et al., 1989). However, Kelly and colleagues (1994) complained that the MOS failed to control for the effects of nursing interventions, staffing patterns, and nursing practice delivery models on medical outcomes. Coordination of care, counseling, and referrals, activities more commonly performed by nurses than physicians, were considered in the MOS to be components of medical practice.

The Agency for Health Care Policy and Research

The Agency for Health Care Policy and Research (AHCPR), created in 1989 by Congress, replaced the AHSR. The congressional mandate for AHCPR was "to carry out research, demonstrations, guideline development, training, and dissemination activities with respect to health care services and systems of information regarding the following areas: the effectiveness, efficiency, quality, and outcomes of health services; clinical practice, including primary care; health care technologies, facilities, and equipment; health care costs, productivity, and market forces; health promotion and disease prevention; health statistics and epidemiology; and medical liability" (Gray, 1992, p. 40). A National Advisory Council for Health Care Policy, Research, and Evaluation was also established by Congress. The Council was required to include (1) health care researchers, (2) health professionals (specifically including nurses), (3) individuals from business, law, ethics, economics, and public policy, and (4) individuals representing the interests of consumers. The budget for outcomes research increased to $1.9 million in 1988, $5.9 million in 1989, and $37.5 million in 1990.

With a growing budget and strong political support, proponents of AHCPR were becoming a powerful force demanding change in health care be-

Structure of Care	Process of Care	Outcomes
System characteristics • Organization • Specialty mix • Financial incentives • Workload • Access/convenience	**Technical style** • Visits • Medications • Referrals • Test ordering • Hospitalizations • Expenditures • Continuity of care • Coordination	**Clinical end points** • Symptoms and signs • Laboratory values • Death
Provider characteristics • Age • Gender • Specialty training • Economic incentives • Beliefs/attitudes • Preferences • Job satisfaction	**Interpersonal style** • Interpersonal manner • Patient participation • Counseling • Communication level	**Functional status** • Physical • Mental • Social • Role
Patient characteristics • Age • Gender • Diagnosis/condition • Severity • Comorbid conditions • Health habits • Beliefs/attitudes • Preferences		**General well-being** • Health perceptions • Energy/fatigue • Pain • Life satisfaction
		Satisfaction with care • Access • Convenience • Financial coverage • Quality • General

FIGURE 12–1 ■ The MOS conceptual framework. (From American Medical Association. [1989]. *Journal of the American Medical Association, 262,* 925–930. Copyrighted 1989, American Medical Association.)

cause of the demand for health care reform that existed throughout the government and among the public. However, there was much controversy about the role of AHCPR. For example, orthopedic surgeons were upset about the guidelines for the treatment of back pain. AHCPR was under attack by powerful forces and was in danger of being eliminated or having a greatly reduced budget. In the 1997 fiscal year budget, AHCPR funding was cut by $35 million. The intimidation of agencies and or researchers by special-interest groups has serious implications for both scientists and society. Fardon, Garfin, and Saal, in a letter to *The New England Journal of Medicine* (1997, pp. 1315–1316) express concern about this problem.

••••••••••••••••••••••••••••••••

"Harassment of researchers and funding agencies is a substantial disincentive to pursuing certain research on medical care or health risks. In effect, special-interest groups with money and power want to define acceptable questions and shape the range of acceptable answers. Eliminating public, peer-reviewed funding would slow the production of objective knowledge, force investigators to seek funding that may not be free of conflict of interest, and leave patients, physicians, and insurers without essential scientific evidence. University faculty members are governed by financial conflict-of-interest rules intended to prevent them from conducting research in which they or their relatives might have a financial stake. Thus, the elimination of public research support and the intimidation of independent investigators are inimical to larger social interests. Professional societies, universities, and the government need to weigh in quickly and heavily against strategies and specific cases of intimidation and vengeful budget cuts. . . . Inquiry may be warranted concerning the extent to which special-interest groups block or delay the publication of unwanted findings. Journals may need to make a special effort to avoid relying on otherwise highly qualified reviewers and editorialists who have financial conflicts of interests, especially consultants to firms whose products receive negative evaluations. Journals may also need to set up defenses against potential threats of withholding advertising. . . . When funding agencies come under attack from groups with narrow interests, prompt and unambiguous responses from universities and professional organizations are needed. Self-interested attacks must be pointed out to politicians, who may otherwise be unable to distinguish self-interested parties from disinterested ones. This is especially true when organizations adopt misleading names, (Deyo et al., 1977, pp. 1176–1180) as in the case involving spinal-fusion surgery." ▪

The AHCPR operated without authorization from 1995 until December 6, 1999, receiving operating funds through congressional appropriations. The reauthorization act changed the name of AHCPR to the Agency for Healthcare Research and Quality (AHRQ). AHRQ is designated as a scientific research agency. The term *policy* was removed from the agency name to avoid the perception that the agency determined federal health care policies and regulations. The word *quality* was added to the agency's name, establishing AHRQ as the lead federal agency on quality of care research, with a new responsibility to coordinate all federal quality improvement efforts and health services research. The new legislation eliminated the requirement that the AHRQ support the development of clinical practice guidelines, a program that ended in 1996. However, AHRQ will still support these efforts through its 12 Evidence-based Practice Centers and the dissemination of evidence-based guidelines through its National Guideline Clearinghouse. Congress voted $205 million for the AHRQ in Fiscal Year 2000.

The new legislation defines the AHRQ's mission as follows:

▪ Meet the information needs of its customers— patients and clinicians, health system leaders, and policymakers—so that they can make more informed healthcare decisions.
▪ Build the evidence base for what works and doesn't work in healthcare and develop the infor-

mation, tools, and strategies that decisionmakers can use to make good decisions and provide high-quality healthcare based on evidence.
▪ Develop scientific knowledge in these areas but will not mandate guidelines or standards for measuring quality. (Agency for Health Care Research and Quality, 1999, pp. 2–3).

Before all of the previously described brouhaha, AHCPR had initiated several major research efforts to examine medical outcomes. Two of the most significant, which are described here, are the Medical Treatment Effectiveness Program (MEDTEP), and a component of MEDTEP referred to as Patient Outcomes Research Teams (PORTs) (Greene et al., 1994).

THE MEDICAL TREATMENT EFFECTIVENESS PROGRAM

MEDTEP was established by Congress in 1989 to be implemented by AHCPR. The purpose of the program was to improve the effectiveness and appropriateness of medical practice. The term *medical* was used by Congress when the program was mandated. However, it was broadly interpreted to include health care in general, particularly—from our perspective—nursing care. The program was charged to develop and disseminate scientific information about the effects of health care services and procedures on patients' survival, health status, functional capacity, and quality of life, a remarkable shift from the narrow focus of traditional medical research. The three research areas funded through this program were (1) patient outcomes research (PORTs), (2) database development, and (3) research on effective methods of disseminating the information gathered. In 1993, studies were implemented to examine the effects of pharmaceuticals on patient outcomes, and $19 million was provided to establish Research Centers on Minority Populations (Clinton, 1993).

PATIENT OUTCOMES RESEARCH TEAM PROJECTS

PORTs are large-scale, multifaceted, and multidisciplinary projects mandated by Congress to "identify and analyze the outcomes and costs of current alternative practice patterns in order to determine the best treatment strategy and to develop and test methods for reducing inappropriate variations" (U.S. Congress, 1994, p. 67). The PORTs are required to "conduct literature reviews and synthesis; analyze practice variations and associated patient outcomes, using available data augmented by primary data collection where desired; disseminate research findings; and evaluate the effects of dissemination" (U.S. Congress, 1994, p. 67).

Questions that might be addressed by PORTs include "Do patients benefit from the care provided?" "What treatments work best?" "Has the patient's functional status improved?" "According to whose viewpoint?" and "Are health care resources well spent?" (Tanenbaum, 1994; Wood, 1990). PORTs have studied outcomes of treatment for hip fracture repair and osteoarthritis, prevention of low-birth-weight and its sequelae in minority and high-risk women, total knee replacements, therapies for benign prostatic hypertrophy and localized prostate cancer, pneumonia, back pain, biliary tract disease, ischemic heart disease, schizophrenia, stroke prevention, acute myocardial infarction, cataracts, childbirth, and diabetes (Goldberg & Cummings, 1994). Smaller projects have examined the management of peripheral vascular disease, cerebral vascular disease, hip disease, colon cancer, gallbladder disease, and coronary artery disease (Wood, 1990).

A major task of PORTs is to disseminate their findings and change the practice of health care providers to improve patient outcomes. A framework for dissemination has been developed that identifies the audiences for disseminated products, the media involved, and the strategies that foster assimilation and adoption of information (Goldberg, et al., 1994). A Cost of Care Workgroup, consisting of a representative from each PORT, was convened with the following four goals: (1) to determine the best methods for estimating the cost of certain conditions using claims data, (2) to evaluate methods for estimating the cost of care using billing information and patient interview data, (3) to examine methods for determining the indirect cost of care, and (4) to evaluate methods for comparing the cost of care internationally (Lave et al., 1994).

Clinical guideline panels were developed to incorporate available evidence on health outcomes into sets of recommendations concerning appropriate management strategies for patients with the studied conditions (Wennberg et al., 1993). This information is being widely disseminated to providers and to patients. Current guidelines can be obtained on the World Wide Web at the following Internet address: *http:/www.guideline.gov/*

Example: Guidelines for Management of Heart Failure

The process used in a PORT guideline panel is illustrated by two papers by Hadorn and Baker (1994) and Hadorn and associates (1994) that describe the development of heart failure guidelines. This project was led by two cochairpeople, one a cardiologist and the other a doctorally prepared nurse. The decision about which health care outcomes are important and relevant in the development of clinical practice guidelines and the evaluation of patient response to treatment is critical. Rather than using biochemical, physiological, anatomical, or histological outcomes, this team focused on clinical outcomes, such as reduced mortality, improved physical functioning, and lessened symptoms, to study patients experiencing heart failure. Contrary to the practice in most medical studies, patient self-reports played an important role in determining symptoms and functional status in this study.

Clinical algorithms were used to develop practice guidelines. *Algorithms* are flow diagrams with branching-logic pathways, allowing carefully defined criteria to be used to develop appropriate management strategies, as illustrated in Figure 12–2. Developing the algorithms helped the Guideline Panel identify key clinical decision points, organize the guideline, and make specific recommendations (Hadorn & Baker, 1994).

The focus of outcomes research has been medical practice, perhaps because the greatest problems in health care—from the perspective of both cost and quality—are seen as related to the actions of physicians (Wennberg, 1990). According to O'Connor and colleagues (1993, p. 45), "the individual clinician rarely knows with certainty the quality of care that he or she is providing." Unlike

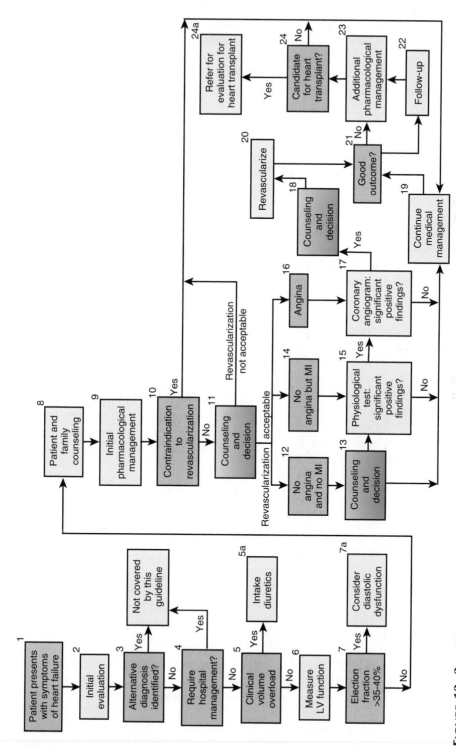

FIGURE 12–2 ■ Management algorithm for patients with heart failure. LV = left ventricle, MI = myocardial infarction. (From Hadorn, D. C., & Baker, D. [1994]. Development of the AHCPR-sponsored heart failure guideline: Methodological and procedural issues. *Joint Commission Journal of Quality Improvement, 20*[10], 543.)

nurses, the practicing physician rarely has opportunities to compare his or her practice patterns with those of other clinicians. In addition, the existing evidence of the effect medical practice has on patients is of such poor quality that it is impossible to determine the most desirable approaches to care.

OUTCOMES RESEARCH AND NURSING PRACTICE

Outcomes studies provide rich opportunities to build a stronger scientific underpinning for nursing practice (Rettig, 1990). "Nursing needs to be able to explain the impact of care provided by its practitioners through measures of outcomes of patient care that reflect nursing practice" (Moritz, 1991, p. 113). We need to know how nurses make decisions. Most clinical judgment research focuses on medical practice and examines diagnostic judgments. Outcomes studies by nurses examining nursing practice are in a very preliminary stage. Patient satisfaction surveys have been used for many years in nursing, but the link to specific nursing care is vague. Nurses have conducted quality assurance or quality improvement studies, primarily in hospital settings, and critical pathways and care maps have stimulated interest in studying related outcomes.

Nurse case management lends itself well to evaluation with an outcomes research focus. We need to know how case management is implemented in an organization, the roles of case managers, how high-risk patients are identified, who is most likely to benefit from case management, and the effect of case management on the quality of patient care and costs (Lamb, 1992; Marschke & Nolan, 1993). Issel (1995) designed an approach to evaluating obstetrical case management programs, which is illustrated in Table 12–1.

Nurse practitioners, an emerging force in the primary health care arena, need to be proactive in defining the uniqueness of the interventions they provide and in documenting their effectiveness. A flurry of studies in the 1970s documented the effectiveness of nurse practitioner outcomes compared with those of physicians. Few studies have been conducted since that time to define nursing practitioner interventions or to examine the outcomes of nurse practitioner practice. Nurse practitioners, as a

group, are as yet uncommitted to examining the outcomes of their practice. Given what is happening to reimbursement for medical interventions, this attitude seems, at the least, shortsighted. Molde and Diers (1985) recommend studies examining questions related to outcomes of advanced nurse practitioner practice, such as the following:

. . . .

"What explains when hypertensive patients cared for by nurse practitioners have better controlled blood pressures than those cared for by physicians (Ramsey, McKenzie, & Fish, 1982); why the suicide rate dropped in a jail staffed with nurse practitioners (Hastings et al., 1980), and how nurse practitioners are more effective in helping patients lose weight, keep appointments, and comply with recommendations (Watkins & Wagner, 1982). Clearly the style of practice that has evolved in nurse practitioner work is different than that of physicians. This style of practice needs to be described." (Molde & Diers, 1985, p. 362) ■

Sidani and Irvine (1999) have developed a conceptual framework that can be used for evaluating the nursing practitioner role in acute care settings.

Community health is an area of practice that is expected to greatly expand in the future. Mittelmark and associates (1993) point out:

. . . .

"[I]t is clear that a community turns first to its medical leaders when questions about new health promotion programs arise. Very little is known about the potential for community change that rests with primary care providers who are not physicians. In many communities, nurse practitioners, physician assistants, chiropractors, podiatrists, dietitians, and others are in daily contact with patients and many are leaders of community organizations. . . . Most if not all of these professions are attracted to the idea that prevention is integral to primary care." (Mittelmark et al, 1993) ■

Nursing must take the lead in conducting studies to examine the outcomes of programs designed to protect or improve the health of the community.

Hospitals are a major target of outcomes research, and yet the outcomes are attributed either to the hospital as a whole or to physicians. Nursing practice in the hospital setting is invisible as a force

TABLE 12–1
HEALTH OUTCOMES CATEGORIES AND SUGGESTED IMPACT INDICATORS FOR OBSTETRICAL CASE MANAGEMENT PROGRAMS

OUTCOME CATEGORY	PREPREGNANCY ANTECEDENTS	BASELINE AT ENTRY TO CASE MANAGEMENT	OUTCOMES AT DELIVERY	POSTPARTUM OUTCOMES
Physical status and morbidity	Race, age		Type of delivery	
	Prepregnancy weight Height	Accurate weight Height Nutritional status	Gestational weight gain	Weight of mother
				Nutritional status of mother
	Medical history Obstetrical history	Morbidity	Maternal morbidity	Maternal morbidity Using birth control method of choice
			Weeks' gestation at delivery Birth weight Newborn morbidity	Nutritional status of infant Weight of infant Infant morbidity
Psychological, behavioral, and developmental	History of substance abuse	Substance abuse		Substance abuse
		Social support network Depression or anxiety Smoking pattern Readiness for parenthood	Depression or anxiety Smoking pattern Readiness for parenthood Independently sought needed services Attachment to infant Satisfaction with care	Social support network Depression Smoking pattern Parenting confidence
				Parent-infant interactions Satisfaction with care
Knowledge	Educational level	Self-care behavior Nutritional behavior Labor and delivery knowledge	Self-care behavior	Self-care behavior Nutritional behavior
			Breast-feeding Infant-care behavior	Breast-feeding Infant-care behavior Growth and development knowledge Family planning knowledge Knowledge of community resources
Family and role functioning	Occupation	Working status		Working status
		Marital status Family functioning History of domestic violence Size and composition of family	Participation of significant others during pregnancy	Marital status Family functioning History of domestic violence
		Income	Infant caretaking	Infant caretaking
Utilization and cost		Health insurance type	Length of stay for mother Length of stay for infant	
	Previous health services utilization		Number/type of health services utilized during pregnancy	Number/type of health services utilized
	Previous social services		Number/type of social services utilized during pregnancy	Number/type of social services utilized

From Issel, L. M. (1995). Evaluating case management programs. *Maternal-Child Nursing, 20*(2), 67–70, 72–74.

influencing patient outcomes (Clark & Lang, 1992; Kelly et al., 1994). In any practice setting, the physician sees the patient for only a fraction of the total time in which care is being provided and generally does not personally deliver the medical interventions that he or she prescribes. In addition, not all health care is related to medical diagnosis and treatment (Kelly et al., 1994). Other providers (e.g., nurses, pharmacists, therapists, social workers) affect treatment through their interventions and styles of care delivery. When outcomes of care involving multiple disciplines are being studied, attributing outcomes to a single provider is not appropriate and raises questions about the validity and reliability of the research findings. Hegyvary (1992) suggests that each group of practitioners define and measure their actions and the intended results, and then integrate those disparate views. The interdependence of health care providers in producing health outcomes must be recognized (Holzemer, 1990; Kelly et al., 1994). The momentum to make this happen must come from within nursing. We cannot rely on some benevolent force to do this for us.

In 1992, the National Center for Nursing Research (NCNR) sponsored the Conference on Patient Outcomes Research: Examining the Effectiveness of Nursing Practice. In the keynote speech, Hinshaw, then director of NCNR, made the following suggestions:

· ·

"From a nursing perspective, particular clinical conditions need to be identified that are more specific to nursing's focus on prevention, health promotion, symptom management, and the amelioration of the effects of acute and chronic illnesses. We are all familiar with clinical conditions that are central to our practice, such as skin integrity, pain, urinary incontinence, nausea and vomiting, nutritional deficits, confusion, restricted mobility, depression, fatigue, and illness-related stress. It will be particularly important in our research programs that we begin to both define and refine the patient outcomes specific to interventions focused on such clinical conditions." (Hinshaw, 1992, p. 9) ■

Examining the impact of nursing on overall hospital outcomes will require inclusion of nursing data in the large databases used to analyze outcomes. The cost of adding new variables to these databases is high. Nursing is competing with the voices of others who wish to add variables. Currently, adding nursing variables is considered a low priority. We must make our voice heard.

NCNR, now the National Institute for Nursing Research (NINR), developed a partnership with AHCPR to fund outcomes studies of importance to nursing. Calls for proposals jointly supported by AHCPR and NINR are being announced each year. These calls for proposals can be found in NINR's home page on the World Wide Web at the following Internet address: *http://www.nih.gov/ninr/*

EVIDENCE-BASED PRACTICE

Evidence-based practice, which shifts the provision of health care away from opinion, past practice, and precedent toward a more scientific basis, is increasingly required of the clinician and the health care facility. This new approach to making judgments about clinical practice renders outdated knowledge and personal opinions unacceptable as justification for clinical decisions. In many practice areas, however, there is no critical mass of scientific knowledge that can be drawn upon for this purpose. Clinicians must rely on the best evidence available to justify their practice until further evidence can be accrued (Alison, 1997).

At this point, the target of demands for evidence-based practice has been the physician. However, for the goals of evidence-based practice to be met, a culture of practice must be developed in which all clinicians from every discipline are expected to justify their practices from the best evidence currently available. Alison (1997) remarks that this process will initiate a shift in professional boundaries and knowledge bases. Thus, it is important for nursing to be included in this shift in practice. Alison (1997) also suggests, however, that a clinician cannot be held accountable for evidence-based practice until the following three conditions are met:

1. Clinicians from the discipline influence patient outcomes.
2. Clinicians from the discipline assume full responsibility for their practice.
3. The discipline has a body of scientific knowledge that the clinician contributes to and uses for practice.

Although nurses know from experience that they influence patient outcomes, scientific evidence of this influence is scanty. Nurse practitioners have considerable control over their practice, but control over practice of nurses working within health care facilities such as hospitals must be mediated through other, more powerful groups. Outcomes research methods will be an important means to document the effect that nursing practice has on patient outcomes and to build the scientific base for evidence-based practice in nursing. This evidence, as it builds, will drive the control that nursing has over practice (Alison, 1997). Evidence-based practice websites for nurse researchers are available at the following Internet address: *http://www.nursing.uc. edu/nrm/duffy11799.htm*

THE THEORETICAL BASIS OF OUTCOMES RESEARCH

The theory on which outcomes research is based emerged from evaluation research. The theorist Avedis Donabedian, MD, PhD (1987), proposed a theory of quality health care and the process of evaluating it. Quality is the overriding construct of the theory, although Donabedian never defines this concept (Mark, 1995). The cube shown in Figure 12–3 is used to explain the elements of quality health care. The three dimensions of the cube are health, subjects of care, and providers of care. The concept *health* has many aspects; three are shown on the cube: physical-physiological function, psychological function, and social function. Donabedian (1987, p. 4) proposes that "the manner in which we conceive of health and of our responsibility for it, makes a fundamental difference to the concept of quality and, as a result, to the methods that we use to assess and assure the quality of care."

The concept *subjects of care* has two primary aspects: patient and person. A *patient* is defined as someone who has already gained access to some care, and a *person* as someone who may or may not have gained access to care. Each of these concepts is further categorized by the concepts *individual* and *aggregate*. Within patient, the aggregate is a case load; within person, the aggregate is a target population or a community.

The concept *providers of care* shows levels of aggregation and organization of providers. The first level is the individual practitioner. At this level, no consideration is given to anyone else who might be involved in the care of a subject of care, whether individual or aggregate. As the levels progress, providers of care include several practitioners, who might be of the same profession or different professions and "who may be providing care concurrently, as individuals, or jointly, as a team" (Donabedian, 1987, p. 5). At higher levels of aggregation, the provider of care is institutions, programs, or the health care system as a whole.

Donabedian theorizes that the dimensions of health are defined by the subjects of care, not by the providers of care, and are based on "what consumers expect, want, or are willing to accept" (Donabedian, 1987, p. 5). Thus, practitioners cannot unilaterally enlarge the definition of *health* to include other aspects; this action requires social consensus that "the scope of professional competence and responsibility embraces these areas of function" (Donabedian, 1987, p. 5). Donabedian indicates, however, that providers of care may make efforts to persuade subjects of care to expand their definition of the dimensions of health.

The *primordial cell* of Donabedian's framework is the physical-physiological function of the individual patient being cared for by the individual practitioner. Examining quality at this level is relatively simple. As one moves outward to include more of the cubical structure, the notions of quality and its assessment become increasingly difficult. When more than one practitioner is involved, both individual and joint contributions to quality must be evaluated. Concepts such as coordination and teamwork must be conceptually and operationally defined. When a person is the subject of care, an important attribute is access. When an aggregate is the subject of care, an important attribute is resource allocation. Access and resource allocation are interrelated, because they each define who gets care, the kind of care received, and how much care is received.

As more elements of the cube are included, conflicts among competing objectives emerge. The chief conflict is between the practitioner's responsibilities to the individual and to the aggregate. The practitioner is expected to have an exclusive com-

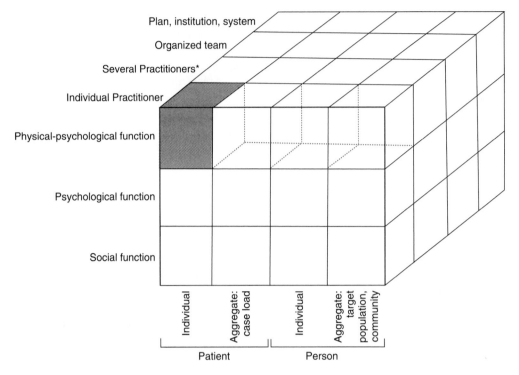

FIGURE 12–3 ■ Level and scope of concern as factors in the definition of quality. (From Donabedian, A. [1987]. Some basic issues in evaluating the quality of health care. In L. K. Rinke [Ed.], *Outcome measures in home care* [Vol. 1, pp. 3–28]. New York: National League for Nursing.)

mitment to each patient, and yet, the aggregate demands a commitment to the well-being of the society, leading to ethical dilemmas for the practitioner. Spending more time with an individual patient decreases access for other patients. Society's demand to reduce costs for an overall financing program may require raising costs to the individual. From an examination of the cube, logic would suggest that one could build up quality beginning with the primordial cell and increase by increments with the assumption that each increment would contribute positively to a greater total quality. However, the conflicts among competing objectives may preclude this possibility and lead instead to moral dilemmas.

Loegering and colleagues (1994) modified Donabedian's levels to include the patient and family and the community as providers of care as well as recipi-

ents of care. They suggest that access to care is one dimension of the provision of care by the community. Figure 12–4 is a model of their modifications.

Donabedian (1987) identifies three objects of evaluation in appraising quality: structure, process, and outcome. A complete quality assessment program requires the simultaneous use of all three concepts and an examination of the relationships among the three. However, researchers have had little success in accomplishing this theoretical goal. Studies designed to examine all three concepts would require sufficiently large samples of various structures, each with the various processes being compared and large samples of subjects who have experienced the outcomes of those processes. The funding and the cooperation necessary to accomplish this goal are not yet available.

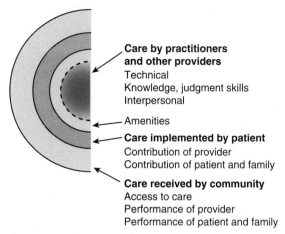

**Care by practitioners
and other providers**
Technical
Knowledge, judgment skills
Interpersonal

Amenities

Care implemented by patient
Contribution of provider
Contribution of patient and family

Care received by community
Access to care
Performance of provider
Performance of patient and family

FIGURE 12–4 ■ Various levels at which the quality of health care can be assessed. (From Donabedian, A. [1988]. The quality of care: How can it be assessed? *Journal of the American Medical Association, 260*[12], 1744. © 1988, American Medical Association.)

Evaluating Outcomes

The goal of outcomes research is the evaluation of outcomes as defined by Donabedian. However, this goal is not as simplistic as it might immediately appear. Donabedian's theory requires that identified outcomes be clearly linked with the process that caused the outcome. To accomplish this linking, the researcher must define the process and justify the causal links with the selected outcomes. The identification of desirable outcomes requires dialogue between the subjects of care and the providers of care. Although the providers of care may delineate what is achievable, the subjects of care must clarify what is desirable. The outcomes must also be relevant to the goals of the health professionals, the health care system of which the professionals are a part, and society.

Outcomes are time dependent. Some outcomes may not be apparent for a long period after the process that is purported to cause them, whereas others may be apparent immediately. Some outcomes are temporary and others are permanent. Thus, the selection of an appropriate time frame for determining the selected outcomes must be established.

A final obstacle to outcomes evaluation is one of attribution. This requires assigning the place and degree of responsibility for the outcomes observed. A particular is often influenced by a multiplicity of factors. Lewis (1995) points out that health care represents only one dimension of a complex situation. Patient factors, such as compliance, predisposition to disease, age, propensity to use resources, high-risk behaviors (e.g., smoking), and lifestyle, must also be taken into account. Environmental factors such as air quality, public policies related to smoking, and occupational hazards must also be included. Responsibility for outcomes may be distributed among providers, patients, employers, insurers, and the community.

There is as yet little scientific basis for judging the precise relationship between each factor and the selected outcome. Many of the influencing factors may be outside the jurisdiction or influence of the health care system or of the providers within it. One solution to this problem is to define a set of proximate outcomes specific to the condition for which care is being provided. Critical pathways and care maps may be useful in defining at least proximate outcomes.

Evaluating Process

The process of clinical management has been, for most health professionals, an art rather than a science. Understanding the process sufficiently to study it must begin with much careful reflection, dialogue, and observation. There are multiple components of clinical management, many of which have not yet been clearly defined or tested. Bergmark and Oscarsson (1991, pp. 139–140) suggest the following questions as important to consider in evaluation process: (1) "What constitutes the 'therapeutic agent'?" (2) "Do practitioners actually do what they say they do?" (3) "Do practitioners always know what they do?" Current outcomes studies are using process variables that are easy to identify. Answers to questions such as those posed by Bergmark and Oscarsson are more difficult to define and will initially require observation, interviews, and the use of qualitative research methodologies. Three components of process of particular interest to Donabedian are standards of care, practice styles, and costs of care.

STANDARDS OF CARE

A *standard of care* is a norm on which quality of care is judged. Clinical guidelines, critical paths, and care maps define standards of care. According to Donabedian, a practitioner has legitimate responsibility to apply available knowledge in the management of a dysfunctional state. This management consists of (1) the identification or diagnosis of the dysfunction, (2) the decision whether or not to intervene, (3) the choice of intervention objectives, (4) the choice of methods and techniques to achieve the objectives, and (5) the skillful execution of the selected techniques.

Donabedian recommends the development of criteria to be used as a basis for judging the quality of care. These criteria may take the form of clinical guidelines or care maps based on prior validation of the contribution of the care to outcomes. The clinical guidelines published by AHCPR establish norms on which the validity of clinical management can be judged. However, the core of the problem, from Donabedian's perspective, is clinical judgment. Analysis of the process of making diagnoses and therapeutic decisions is critical to the evaluation of the quality of care. The emergence of decision trees and algorithms is a response to Donabedian's concerns and provides a means of evaluating the adequacy of clinical judgments.

PRACTICE STYLES

The style of practice is another dimension of the process of care that influences quality; however, it is problematic to judge what constitutes "goodness" in style and to provide justification for the decisions. Problem-solving styles identified by Donabedian are (1) routine approaches to care versus flexibility, (2) parsimony versus redundancy, (3) variations in degree of tolerance of uncertainty, (4) propensity to take risks, and (5) preference for Type I errors versus Type II errors. There are also diverse styles of interpersonal relationships.

Lowenberg (1994) has initiated a research program to examine practice styles of nurses. She has identified five dimensions of the nurse-patient relationship: affectivity, specificity, status differential, placebo salience, and trust. Previous nursing research in this area has focused on affectivity.

COSTS OF CARE

A third dimension of the examination of quality of care is cost. There are cost consequences to maintaining a specified level of quality of care. Providing more and better care is likely to increase costs but is also likely to produce savings. Economic benefits can be obtained by preventing illness, preventing complications, maintaining a higher quality of life, or prolonging productive life.

A related issue is who bears the costs of care. Some measures purported to reduce costs have instead simply shifted costs to another party. For example, a hospital might reduce its costs by discharging a particular type of patient early, but total costs could increase if the necessary community-based health care raised costs above those incurred by keeping the patient hospitalized longer. In this case, the third-party provider could experience higher costs. In many cases, the costs are shifted from the health care system to the family as out-of-pocket costs. Studies examining changes in costs of care must consider total costs.

Evaluating Structure

Structures of care are the elements of organization and administration that guide the processes of care. The first step in evaluating structure is to identify and describe the elements of the structure. Various administration and management theories could be used to identify the elements of structure to be studied. These elements might be leadership, tolerance of innovativeness, organizational hierarchy, decision-making processes, distribution of power, financial management, and administrative decision-making processes.

The second step is to evaluate the impact of various structure elements on the process of care and upon outcomes. This evaluation requires comparing different structures that provide the same processes of care. In the evaluation of structures, the unit of measure is the structure. The evaluation requires access to a sufficiently large sample of like structures with similar processes and outcomes, which can then be compared with a sample of another structure providing the same processes and outcomes. For example, one might compare various structures providing primary health care, such as the private physician office, the health maintenance organization (HMO), the rural health clinic, the community-oriented primary care clinic, and the nurse-managed center. One might examine surgical care provided within the structures of a private outpatient surgical clinic, a private hospital, a county hospital, and a teaching hospital associated with a health science center. Within each of these examples the focus of study would be the impact of structure on processes of care and outcomes of care.

A number of frameworks for research have emerged from Donabedian's theory. Each begins with Donabedian's basic concepts, adds more detail, and organizes the concepts somewhat differently. For examples, see Figures 12–5 through 12–8.

METHODOLOGIES FOR OUTCOMES STUDIES

A research tradition for the outcomes paradigm is still emerging. A *research tradition* defines acceptable research methodologies. The lack of an established set of methodologies should encourage greater creativity in seeking new strategies for studying the phenomena of concern. Small single studies using untried methodologies may be useful. Research teams need to develop research programs with a planned sequence of studies focused on a particular outcome concern. The PORTs are beginning to define a research process for conducting programs of funded outcomes studies. These pro-

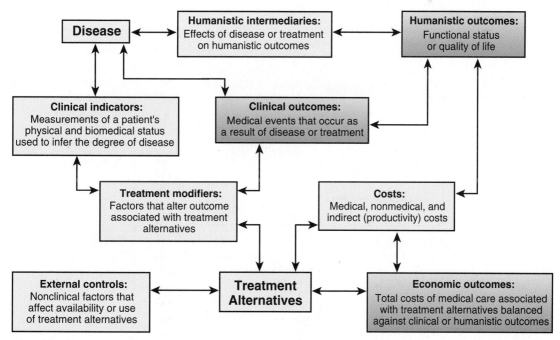

FIGURE 12–5 ■ The conceptual model: Economic, clinical, and humanistic outcome (ECHO) model. (From Kozma, C. M., Reeder, C. E., & Schulz, R. M. [1993]. Economic, clinical, and humanistic outcomes: A planning model for pharmacoeconomic research. *Clinical Therapeutics, 15*[6], 1125.)

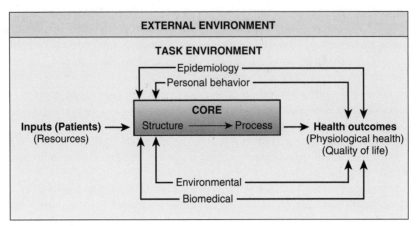

Figure 12–6 ▪ A systems perspective of health services research. (From Anderson, R. M., Davidson, P. L., & Ganz, P. A. [1994]. Symbiotic relationships of quality of life, health services research and other health research. *Quality of Life Research, 3*[5], 367.)

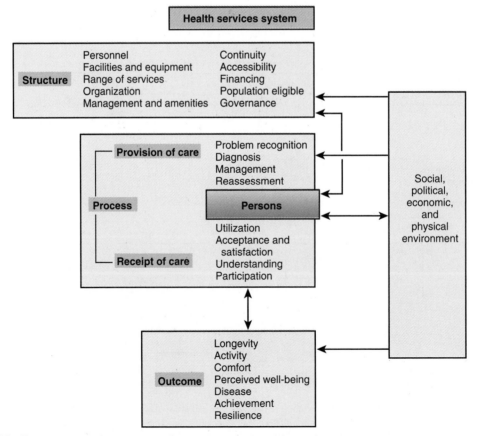

Figure 12–7 ▪ The health services system. (From Vivier, P. M., Bernier, J. A., & Starfield, B. [1994]. Current approaches to measuring health outcomes in pediatric research. *Current Opinions in Pediatrics, 6*[5], 531.)

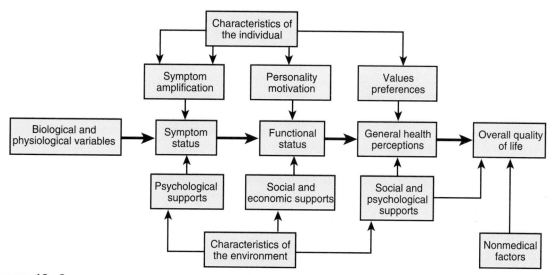

FIGURE 12−8 ■ Relationships among measures of patient outcome in a health-related quality-of-life conceptual model. (From Wilson, I. B., & Cleary, P. D. [1995]. Linking clinical variables with health-related quality of life: A conceptual model of patient outcomes. *Journal of the American Medical Association, 273*[1], 60. Copyright 1995, the American Medical Association.)

grams are complex and may consist of multiple studies using a variety of research strategies whose findings must be merged during the formulation of conclusions.

Although implementing a research program as extensive as a PORT would be unrealistic without the funding a PORT receives, ideas for developing outcomes research programs on a smaller scale may be generated through an examination of these plans. The following steps were constructed combining PORT plans proposed by Freund and colleagues (1990), Sledge (1993), and Turk and Rudy (1994).

1. Perform a critical review of the published literature or a meta-analysis.
2. Conduct large database analyses on the basis of the results of the critical literature review.
3. Identify outcomes measures for use in the study, and evaluate their sensitivity to change.
4. Identify variables that might affect the outcomes.
5. Achieve consensus on definitions for all variables to be used in the research program.
6. Develop assessment instruments or techniques.
7. Conduct patient surveys or focus groups to gain information on outcomes, such as level of func-

tional status and perceived pain, and on how these outcomes may improve or regress over time.

8. Determine patterns of care (Who provides care at what points of time for what purposes?).
9. Perform a cohort analysis: Monitor a cohort of patients, some of whom will receive one treatment and others of whom will not receive the treatment, to assess changes in outcomes over time. Use a telephone survey at selected intervals to gather information. Evaluate the proportion of patients who improve as well as the group mean differences.
10. Determine, through follow-up studies, differences in patient selection or interventions that are associated with different outcomes. Evaluate the durability of change by conducting sufficiently long follow-up. Determine the percentage of patients dropping out of groups receiving different treatments and, when possible, determine their reasons for dropping out.
11. Determine the clinical significance of improvement as well as the statistical significance.
12. Determine the cost-benefit and cost-effectiveness of the treatments under evaluation.
13. Use decision analyses to synthesize information

about patients' outcomes and preferences for various types of outcomes.

14. Disseminate information to both patients and health care providers about which individuals would and which would not benefit from the procedure.
15. Conduct a clinical trial to evaluate the effects of the intervention.
16. Incorporate findings into treatment guidelines.
17. Modify provider and patient behavior so that proven, effective treatment is given to those who are most likely to benefit.

The PORTs have recognized the need to allow diversity in research strategies, measures, and analyses to facilitate methodological advances (Fowler et al., 1994). Creative flexibility is often necessary to develop ways to answer new questions. Finding ways to determine the impact of a condition on a person's life is difficult. Interpreting results can also be problematic, because clinical significance is considered as important as statistical significance. This issue requires a judgment by the research team as to what constitutes clinical significance in their particular area of study.

The following section describes some of the sampling issues, research strategies, measurements, and statistical approaches being used by researchers in outcomes studies. The descriptions provided are not sufficient to guide the researcher in using the approaches described but rather provide a broad overview of a variety of methodologies being used. For additional information, refer to the citations in each section. Outcomes studies cross a variety of disciplines, thus the emerging methodologies are being enriched by a cross-pollination of ideas, some of which may be new to nursing research.

Samples and Sampling

The preferred methods of obtaining samples are different in outcomes studies; random sampling is not considered desirable and is seldom used. Heterogeneous, rather than homogeneous, samples are obtained. Rather than using sampling criteria that restrict subjects included in the study to decrease possible biases and that reduce the variance and

increase the possibility of identifying a statistically significant difference, outcomes researchers seek large heterogeneous samples that reflect, as much as possible, all patients who would be receiving care in the real world. Samples, then, must include, for example, patients with various comorbidities and patients with varying levels of health status. In addition, persons must be identified who do not receive treatment for their condition. Devising ways to evaluate the representativeness of such samples is problematic. Developing strategies to locate untreated individuals and include them in follow-up studies will be a challenge.

Traditional researchers and statisticians argue that when patients are not selected randomly, biases and confounding variables are more likely to occur and that this issue is a particular problem when the sample size is small. In nonexperimental studies, variation is likely to be greater, resulting in a higher risk of a Type II error. Traditional analysts consider nonrandomized studies to be based on observational data and therefore not to be credible (Orchard, 1994). Using this argument, traditionalists claim that the findings of most outcomes studies are not valid and should not be used as a basis to establish guidelines for clinical practice or to build a body of knowledge.

LARGE DATABASES AS SAMPLE SOURCES

One source of samples used for outcomes studies is large databases. Two broad categories of databases emerge from patient care encounters, clinical databases and administrative databases, as illustrated by Figure 12–9. Clinical databases were created by providers such as hospitals, HMOs, and health care professionals. The clinical data are generated either as a result of routine documentation of care or in relation to a research protocol. Some databases are data registries that have been developed to gather data related to a particular disease, such as cancer (Lee & Goldman, 1989). With the use of a clinical database, it is possible to link observations made by many practitioners over long periods. Links can be made between the process of care and outcomes (Mitchell et al., 1994; Moses, 1995).

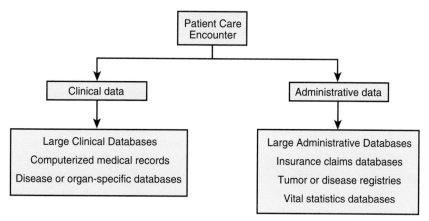

FIGURE 12–9 ■ Types of databases emanating from patient care encounters. (From Lange, L. L., & Jacox, A. [1993]. Using large databases in nursing and health policy research. *Journal of Professional Nursing, 9*[4], 204.)

Administrative databases are created by insurance companies, government agencies, and others not directly involved in providing patient care. Administrative databases have standardized sets of data for enormous numbers of patients and providers (Deyo et al., 1994; McDonald & Hui, 1991). An example is the Medicare database managed by the HCFA. These large databases can be used to determine the incidence or prevalence of disease, geographic variations in medical care utilization, characteristics of medical care, outcomes of care, and complementarity with clinical trials. Wray and colleagues (1995) caution, however, that analyses should be restricted to outcomes specific to a particular subgroup of patients, rather than one adverse outcome of all disease states.

There are problems with the quality of data in the large databases. The data have been gathered and entered by hundreds of individuals in a variety of settings. There are few quality checks on the data, and within the same data sets, records may have different lengths and structures. Missing data are common. Sampling and measurement errors are inherent in all large databases. *Sampling error* is a result of the way in which cases are selected for inclusion in the database; *measurement error* emerges from problems related to the operational definition of concepts. Thus, reliability and validity of the data are a concern (Davis, 1990; Lange & Jacox, 1993).

Large databases are used in outcomes studies to examine patient care outcomes. The outcomes that can be examined are limited to those recorded in the database and, thus, tend to be rather general. Existing databases can be used for analyses such as (1) assessment of nursing care delivery models, (2) variation in nursing practices, or (3) evaluation of patients' risk of hospital-acquired infection, hospital-acquired pressure ulcer, or falls. Lange and Jacox (1993) identify the following important health policy questions related to nursing that should be examined through the use of large databases:

1. What is standard nursing practice in various settings?
2. What is the relationship between variations in nursing practice and patient outcomes?
3. What are the effects of different nursing staff mixes on patient outcomes and costs?
4. What are the total costs for episodes of treatment of specific conditions, and what part of those are attributable to nursing care?
5. Who is being reimbursed for nursing care delivery? (Lange & Jacox, 1993, p. 207)

To examine these questions, nurses must develop the statistical and methodological skills needed for working with large databases. Large databases contain patient and institutional information from huge numbers of patients. They exist in computer-readable form, require special statistical methods and computer techniques, and can be used by researchers who were not involved in the creation of the database.

Regrettably, nursing data are noticeably missing from these large databases and, thus, from funded health policy studies using them. A nursing minimum data set has been repeatedly recommended for inclusion in these databases (Werley et al., 1991; Werley & Lang, 1988; Zielstorff et al., 1993). This minimum data set would comprise a set of variables necessary and sufficient to describe an episode of illness or the care given by a provider. The American Nurses' Association (ANA) has mandated the formation of a Steering Committee on Databases to Support Clinical Nursing Practice. The Committee has recognized the following four nursing classification schemes for use in national databases (McCormick et al., 1994):

- The North American Nursing Diagnosis Association (NANDA) classification
- The Omaha System: Applications for Community Health Nursing classification
- The Home Health Care Classification, developed by Saba and colleagues (1997)
- The Nursing Interventions Classification (NIC).

According to McNeil (1993), the following information which must be available to allow evaluation or monitoring of individual patient care: (1) information about the patient, such as disease severity, comorbidity, and types of outcomes, (2) processes of care provided, (3) patient status over time, and (4) follow-up information. Because of the absence of this information, current databases are inadequate to allow judgments about the appropriateness of individual patient care.

A research team at The University of Iowa is currently developing the Nursing Sensitive Outcome Classification (NOC), which establishes the first comprehensive standardized language for measuring and communicating patient outcomes that are influenced by nursing care (Johnson & Maas, 1997, 1998; Maas et al., 1996). NOC is being tested in several clinical sites (Moorhead et al., 1998).

Timm and Behrenbeck (1998) described their work in a NOC test site to evaluate the clinical usefulness and comprehensiveness of NOC. This test site is a tertiary care facility that uses an elec-tronic medical record (EMR) in their outpatient and inpatient settings. One factor critical to acceptance of a facility as a test site was a strong commitment from nursing at the facility to using a standardized nursing language. The facility had incorporated NANDA and NIC into their Computer Information System (CIS). Thus, the information system staff and the nurses practicing at the facility were familiar with the use of these classification systems. Informatics Nurse Specialists at the facility coordinated the NOC implementation. Informatics Nurse Specialists are playing an important role in implementing and coordinating the use of nursing classification systems in large health care facilities. This work will enable nursing studies that heretofore have not been possible.

Temple (1990, p. 211) expressed the following concerns regarding the use of large data sets rather than controlled trials to assess effectiveness of treatments: "We have traveled this route before with uncontrolled observations. It has always been hoped, and has often been asserted, that uncontrolled databases can be adjusted in some way that will allow valid comparisons of treatments. I know of no systematic attempt to document this." Outcomes researchers counter these criticisms by pointing out that experimental studies lack external validity and are not useful for application in clinical settings. They claim that the findings of clinical trials are not being used by clinicians because they are not representative of the patients seeking care.

Research Strategies for Outcomes Studies

Outcomes research programs usually consist of studies with a mix of strategies carried out sequentially. Although these strategies could be referred to as designs, for some the term *design* as used in Chapters 10 and 11 is inconsistent with the use of the term here. Research strategies for outcomes studies have emerged from a variety of disciplines, and innovative new strategies continue to appear in the literature. Strategies for outcomes studies tend to have less control than traditional research designs and cannot be as easily categorized. The research strategies for outcomes studies described in this section are only a sampling from the literature; they are consensus knowledge building, practice pattern profiling, prospective cohort studies, retrospective cohort studies, population-based studies, clinical decision analysis, study of the effectiveness of interdisciplinary teams, geographical analyses, economic studies, ethical studies, and defining and testing of interventions.

CONSENSUS KNOWLEDGE BUILDING

Consensus knowledge building is usually performed by a multidisciplinary group representing a variety of constituencies. Initially, an extensive international search of the literature on the topic of concern, including unpublished studies, studies in progress, dissertations, and theses, is conducted. Several separate reviews may be performed, focusing on specific questions about the outcomes of care, diagnosis, prevention, or prognosis. Because meta-analytic methods often cannot be applied to the literature pertinent to PORTs, systematic approaches to critique and synthesis have been developed to identify relevant studies and gather and analyze data abstracted from the studies (Powe et al., 1994).

The results are dispersed to researchers and clinical experts in the field, who are asked to carefully examine the material and then participate in a consensus conference. The consensus conference yields clinical guidelines, which are published and widely distributed to clinicians. The clinical guidelines are also used as practice norms to study process and outcomes in that field. Gaps in the knowledge base are identified and research priorities determined by the consensus group.

Preliminary steps in this process might include conducting extensive integrative reviews and seeking consensus from a multidisciplinary research team and locally available clinicians. A review could be accomplished by establishing a World Wide Web site and conducting dialogue with experts via the Internet. The review could be published in Sigma Theta Tau's online journal, *Knowledge Synthesis in Nursing,* and then dialogue related to the review could be conducted over the Internet.

The Delphi method has also been used to seek consensus (Vermeulen et al., 1995).

PRACTICE PATTERN PROFILING

Practice pattern profiling is an epidemiological technique that focuses on patterns of care rather than individual occurrences of care. Large database analysis is used to identify a provider's pattern of practice and compare it with that of similar providers or with an accepted standard of practice. The technique has been used to determine overutilization and underutilization of services, to determine costs associated with a particular provider's care, to uncover problems related to efficiency and quality of care, and to assess provider performance. The provider being profiled could be an individual practitioner, a group of practitioners, or a health care organization, such as a hospital or HMO.

The provider's pattern is expressed as a rate aggregated over time for a defined population of patients under the provider's care. For example, the analysis might examine the number of sigmoidoscopy claims filed per 100 Medicare patients seen by the provider in a given year. Analyses might examine (1) whether diabetic patients have had at least one annual serum glucose test and have received an ophthalmology examination or (2) the frequency of flu shots, Papanicolaou smears, and mammograms for various target populations (Lasker et al., 1992; McNeil et al., 1992).

Profiling can be used when the data contain hierarchical groupings: Patients could be grouped by nurse, nurses by unit, and units by larger organizations. The analysis uses regression equations to examine the relationship of an outcome to the characteristics of the various groupings. To be effective, the analysis must include data on the different sources of variability that might contribute to a given outcome.

The structure of the analysis reflects the structure of the data. For example, patient characteristics could be data on disease severity, comorbidity, emergent status, behavioral characteristics, socioeconomic status, and demographics. Nurse characteristics might consists of level of education, specialty status, years of practice, age, gender, and certifications. Unit characteristics could comprise number of beds, nursing management style used on the unit, ratio of patients to nurses, and the proportion of staff who are Registered Nurses (RNs) (McNeil et al., 1992).

Profiles are designed to generate some type of action, such as to inform the provider that his or her rates are too high or too low compared with the norm. By examining aggregate patterns of practice, profiling can be used to compare the care provided by different organizations or received by different populations of patients. Critical pathways or care maps can then be used to determine the proportion of patients who diverged from the pathway for a particular nurse, group of nurses, or group of nursing units. Profiling can be used for quality improvement, assessment of provider performance, and utilization review.

Methods of improving outcomes are not addressed by profiling, although this process can identify problem areas. It can be used to determine how and by whom performance should be changed to improve outcomes. Profiling can also identify outliers, allowing more detailed examination of these individuals.

The databases currently being used for profiling are not ideal, because they were developed for other purposes. Outcomes that can be examined are limited to broad outcomes, such as morbidity and mortality, complications, readmissions, and frequency of utilization of various services (Lasker et al., 1992; McNeil et al., 1992). Table 12–2 lists examples of the large database measures that might be used in profiling.

PROSPECTIVE COHORT STUDIES

A *prospective cohort study* is an epidemiological study in which a group of people are identified who are at risk for experiencing a particular event. Sample sizes for these studies often must be very large, particularly if only a small portion of the at-risk group will experience the event. The entire group is followed over time to determine the point at which the event occurs, variables associated with the

event, and outcomes for those who experienced the event compared with those who did not.

The Harvard Nurses Health Study, which is still being conducted, is an example of a prospective cohort study. This study recruited 100,000 nurses to determine the long-term consequences of the use of birth control pills. Nurses are sent a questionnaire every 2 years to gather data about their health and health behaviors. The study has now been in progress for more than 20 years. Multiple studies have been reported in the literature that have used the large data set yielded by the Harvard study. Prospective cohort nursing studies could be conducted on a smaller scale on other populations, such as patients identified as being at high risk for the development of pressure ulcers.

RETROSPECTIVE COHORT STUDIES

A *retrospective cohort study* is an epidemiological study in which a group of people are identified who have experienced a particular event. This is a common research technique used by epidemiology to study occupational exposure to chemicals. Events of interest to nursing that could be studied in this manner include a procedure, an episode of care, a nursing intervention, and a diagnosis. Nurses might use a retrospective cohort study to follow a cohort of women who had received a mastectomy for breast cancer or of patients in whom a urinary bladder catheter was placed during and after surgery. The cohort is evaluated after the event to determine the occurrence of changes in health status, usually the development of a particular disease or death. Nurses might be interested in the pattern of recovery after an event or, in the case of catheterization, the incidence of bladder infections in the months after surgery.

On the basis of the study findings, epidemiologists calculate relative risk of the identified change in health for the group. For example, if death were the occurrence of interest, the expected number of deaths would be determined. The observed number of deaths divided by the expected number of deaths and multiplied by 100 yields a *standardized mortality ratio* (SMR), which is regarded as a measure of

TABLE 12-2
EXAMPLES OF LARGE DATABASE MEASURES USED IN PROFILING

QUALITY OF CARE ISSUE	MEASURES	EXAMPLE	CRITERIA
Access	Proportion of population receiving care during the year, classified by age and sex	% of children under age 2 seen for at least one well-care visit	National
		% of children seen in emergency rooms for any reason, for trauma, and for medical problems	Trends
Preventive	Proportion of population in specific age and sex groups receiving recommended tests or procedures	% of children by group having recommended immunizations in previous year	National recommendation
		% of women age 50 and over having mammography in past year	National recommendation
		% of deliveries with prenatal care beginning in first trimester	National recommendation
Diagnosis	% of population diagnosed (and under care) for specific chronic conditions by age and sex	% of adults diagnosed at one or more visits as having essential hypertension by age and sex	Epidemiologic data on prevalence of hypertension
Treatment	Medications Average number of new prescriptions per person per year	Average number of new prescriptions for antibiotics per person per year	Trends and comparison data
	Surgery Rate of surgical procedures per year; total, inpatient, and ambulatory (if applicable)	Cesarean section rate for all deliveries	Trends and comparison data
Outcomes	Hospital readmissions within 3 months of discharge	% of readmissions for same condition	Comparison data and trends
		% of readmissions identifying a complication	

Table reproduced in part from Steinwachs, D. M., Weiner, J. P., & Shapiro, S. (1989). Management information systems and quality. In N. Goldfield and D. B. Nash. (Eds.), *Providing quality care: The challenge to clinicians* (pp. 160–180). Philadelphia: ACP.

the relative risk of the studied group to die of a particular condition. In nursing studies, patients might be followed over time after discharge from a health care facility (Swaen & Meijers, 1988).

In retrospective studies, researchers commonly ask patients to recall information relevant to their previous health status. This information is often used to determine the amount of change occurring before and after an intervention. Recall can easily be distorted, however, misleading researchers, and, thus, should be used with caution. Herrmann (1995) identified three sources of distortion in recall, as follows: (1) the question posed to the subject may

be conceived or expressed incorrectly, (2) the recall process may be in error, and (3) the research design used to measure recall can result in the recall's appearing to be different from what actually occurred. Herrmann (1995, p. AS90) also identified four bases of recall:

Direct recall: the subject "accesses the memory without having to think or search memory," resulting in correct information.

Indirect recall: the subject "accesses the memory after thinking or searching memory," resulting in correct information.

Limited recall: "access to the memory does not occur but information that suggests the contents of the memory is accessed," resulting in an educated guess.

No recall: "neither the memory nor information relevant to the memory may be accessed," resulting in a wild guess.

POPULATION-BASED STUDIES

Population-based studies are also important in outcomes research. Conditions must be studied in the context of the community rather than of the medical system. With this method, all cases of a condition occurring in the defined population are included, rather than only patients treated at a particular health care facility, because the latter could introduce a selection bias. Efforts might be made to include individuals with the condition who had not received treatment.

Community-based norms of tests and survey instruments obtained in this manner provide a clearer picture of the range of values than the limited spectrum of patients seen in specialty clinics. Estimates of instrument sensitivity and specificity are more accurate. This method is useful in enabling the understanding of the natural history of a condition or of the long-term risks and benefits of a particular intervention (Guess et al., 1995).

CLINICAL DECISION ANALYSIS

Clinical decision analysis is a systematic method of describing clinical problems, identifying possible diagnostic and management courses of action, assessing the probability and value of various outcomes, and then calculating the optimal course of action. Decision analysis is based on the following four assumptions: (1) decisions can be quantified, (2) all possible courses of action can be identified and evaluated, (3) the different values of outcomes, viewed from the perspective of the physician, patient, payer, and administrator, can be examined, and (4) the analysis allows selection of an optimal course of therapy.

To perform the analysis, the researchers must define the boundaries of the clinical in terms of a logical sequence of events over time. All the possible courses of action are then determined. These courses of action are usually represented in a decision tree consisting of a starting point, available alternatives, probable events, and outcomes. Next, the goals and objectives of problem resolution are defined. The probability of occurrence of each path of the decision tree is calculated. For each potential path, there is an outcome. Each outcome is assigned a value. These values may be expressed in terms of money, morbidity incidents, quality-of-life measures, or length of stay. A simplified decision tree for breech delivery in obstetrics is shown in Figure 12–10. An optimal course of action is identified according to which decision maximizes the chances of the most desirable outcomes (Crane, 1988; Keeler, 1994; Sonnenberg et al., 1994).

Nursing decisions have not reached the point of definition to allow decision analyses, and little is known about how nurses make decisions regarding their nursing practice (Greiner, 1994).

Studies analyzing clinical decisions have primarily used questionnaires and interviews. However,

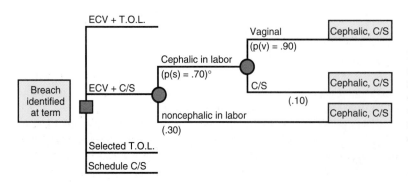

FIGURE 12–10 ■ Simplified decision tree for breech delivery. (Numbers in parentheses refer to estimated probability of event.) (From Keeler, E. B. [1994]. Decision analysis and cost-effectiveness analysis in women's health care. *Clinical Obstetrics and Gynecology, 37*[1], 208.)

determining the clinical decisions of practitioners is not an easy task. Much of patient care involves the clinician and the patient alone. The underlying theories of care and the processes of care are hidden from view. Thus, it is difficult for clinicians to compare their approaches to care. Among physicians, care delivered by other physicians is rarely observed (O'Connor et al., 1993). Studies have found that physicians have difficulty recalling their decisions and providing rationales for them (Chaput de Saintonge & Hattersley, 1985; Kirwan et al., 1986).

Chaput de Saintonge and associates (1988) propose a strategy for analyzing clinical decisions using "paper patients." The techniques seem to parallel the decisions made by clinicians in the clinical setting. In their study, 10 common clinical variables used to evaluate the status of patients with rheumatoid arthritis were collected at two points on 30 patients participating in a clinical trial, at the time of entry and 1 year later. Twenty of the patients were duplicated throughout the table to check the consistency of responses, making 50 responses in all. The variables were presented to rheumatologists on a single sheet of paper labeled "before" and "after a year." Physicians were asked to indicate the extent of change in each patient's condition using a visual analogue scale (VAS) with the ends labeled "greatest possible deterioration" and "greatest possible improvement." They were also asked whether they considered the change clinically important. Then they were asked to indicate the relative importance of each variable, rating the variables on a scale of 1 to 100.

Regression analyses were performed in which the VAS values were used as the dependent variable. With increasing VAS values, judgments of clinical importance changed from "not important" to "important." This change occurred over a 5-mm length of the scale or less. (VAS scales are traditionally 100 mm in length.) The researchers designated the midpoint of this transition zone as the "threshold value of clinical importance." Consistency of responses was tested through the use of the Spearman rank correlation to compare responses to the duplicate cases. The researchers then developed a consensus model by weighing each physician's responses on the basis of the Spearman coefficient.

The VAS scores were multiplied by the Spearman coefficient. These VAS scores were then used as the dependent variable in another regression analysis. This method is useful in identifying the variables important in the making of clinical decisions and the consistency with which practitioners make their decisions.

STUDY OF THE EFFECTIVENESS OF INTERDISCIPLINARY TEAMS

According to Schmitt and colleagues (1988, p. 753), *interdisciplinary teams* have the following characteristics: "(1) multiple health disciplines are involved in the care of the same patients, (2) the disciplines encompass a diversity of dissimilar knowledge and skills required by the patients, (3) the plan of care reflects an integrated set of goals shared by the providers of care, and (4) the team members share information and coordinate their services through a systematic communication process." Part of the communication process consists of regularly scheduled face-to-face meetings. The assumption is that collaborative team approaches provide more effective care than nonteam approaches or than noncollaborative multidisciplinary approaches (parallel care).

Interdisciplinary teams are becoming more common as health care changes. Examples are hospice care teams, home health teams, and psychiatric care teams. Studying the effectiveness of interdisciplinary teams is difficult, however. The characteristics that makes team care more effective have not been identified. Studies usually focus on the evaluation of a single team rather than conducting comparison studies. The outcomes of team care are also multidimensional, requiring the use of multiple dependent variables.

Evaluation studies examining team care often examine only posttreatment data without baseline data. If groups are compared, there is no evidence that the groups were similar in terms of important variables before the intervention. Involvement of family members with the team has not been examined. Clearly, this is an important focus of research requiring more rigorous designs than have previously been used.

GEOGRAPHICAL ANALYSES

Geographical analyses are used to examine variations in health status, health services, patterns of care, or patterns of use by geographical area and are sometimes referred to as *small area analyses*. Variations may be associated with sociodemographic, economic, medical, cultural, or behavioral characteristics. Locality-specific factors of a health care system, such as capacity, access, and convenience, may play a role in explaining variations. The social setting, environment, living conditions, and community may also be important factors.

The interactions between the characteristics of a locality and of its inhabitants are complex. The characteristics of the total community may transcend the characteristics of individuals within the community and may influence subgroup behavior. High education levels in the community are commonly associated with greater access to information and receptiveness to ideas from outside the community.

Regression analyses are commonly used to develop models using all the risk factors and the characteristics of the community. Results are often displayed through the use of maps (Kieffer et al., 1992). After the analysis, the researcher must determine whether differences in rates are due to chance alone and whether high rates are too high. From a more theoretical perspective, the researcher must then explain the geographic variation uncovered by the analysis (Volinn et al., 1994).

Geographical information systems (GISs) can provide an important tool for performing geographic analyses. A GIS uses relational databases to facilitate processing of spatial information. The software tools in a GIS can be used for mapping, data summaries, and analysis of spatial relationships. GISs have the capability of modeling data flows so that the effect of proposed changes in interventions applied to individuals or communities on outcomes can be modeled (Auffrey, 1998).

ECONOMIC STUDIES

Many of the problems studied in health services research address concerns related to the efficient use of scarce resources and, thus, to economics. Health economists are concerned with the costs and benefits of alternative treatments or ways of identifying the most efficient means of care. The economist's definition of *efficiency* is the least cost method of achieving a desired end with the maximum benefit to be obtained from available resources. If available resources must be shared with other programs or other types of patients, an economic study can determine whether changing the distribution of resources will increase total benefit or welfare.

To determine the efficiency of a treatment, the economist conducts a *cost-effectiveness analysis*. This technique uses a single measure of outcomes, and all other factors are expressed in monetary terms as net cost per unit of output (Ludbrook, 1990). Cost-effectiveness analyses compare different ways of accomplishing a clinical goal, such as diagnosing a condition, treating an illness, or providing a service. The alternative approaches are compared in terms of costs and benefits. The purpose is to identify the strategy that provides the most value for the money. There are always tradeoffs between costs and benefits (Oster, 1988). Stone (1998) describes the methodology for performing a cost-effectiveness analysis.

It is time for nurses to take a more active role in conducting cost-effectiveness research. Nurses are well-positioned to evaluate health care practices and have the incentive to conduct the studies. Nursing practice is seldom a subject of cost-effectiveness analyses. The knowledge gained from this effort could enable nurses to refine their practice, substituting interventions that maximize nurses' time to the best advantage, in terms of the patient's health, for interventions that offer less gain (Siegel, 1998).

As Lieu and Newman (1998) point out:

• •

"'[C]ost effective' does not necessary mean 'cost-saving' (Doubilet, Weinstein, & McNeil, 1986). Many health interventions, even preventive ones, do not save money (Tengs et al., 1995). Rather, a service should be called cost-effective if its benefits are judged worth the costs. Recently, a consensus panel supported by the National Institutes of Health published recommendations that define standards for conducting cost-effectiveness analysis (Gold,

Siegel, Russell, & Weinstein, 1996). Cost-effectiveness analysis is only one of several methods that can be used for the economic evaluation of health services (Drummond, Stoddart, and Torrance, 1987). Although these methods are useful, an intervention cannot be cost-effective without being effective." (Lieu & Newman, 1998) ■

To examine overall benefits, a *cost-benefit analysis* is performed. With this method, the costs and benefits of alternative ways of using resources are assessed in monetary terms, and the use that produces the greatest net benefit is chosen. The costs included in an economic study are defined in exact ways. The actual costs associated with an activity, not prices, must be used. Cost is not the same as price. In most cases, price is greater than cost. *Costs* are a measure of the actual use of resources rather than the price charged. Charges are a poor reflection of actual costs. Costs that might be included in a cost-benefit analysis are costs to the provider, costs to third-party payers (e.g., insurance), out-of-pocket costs, and opportunity costs.

Out-of-pocket costs are those expenses incurred by the patient or family or both that are not reimbursable by the insurance company; they include costs of buying supplies, dressings, medications, and special food, transportation expenses, and unreimbursable care expenses.

Opportunity costs are lost opportunities that the patient, family member, or others experience. For example, a family member might have been able to earn more money if he or she had not had to stay home to care for the patient. The child might have been able to advance her education if she had not had to drop out of school for a semester to care for a parent. A husband might have been able to take a better job if the family could have moved to another town rather than stay in place to enable a member to receive specific medical care.

Opportunity costs are often not included in the consideration of overall costs. This omission results in an underestimation of costs and an overestimation of benefit. For example, one can demonstrate that caring for an acutely ill patient at home is cost-effective if one does not consider out-of-pocket costs and opportunity costs. However, the total

costs of providing the care, regardless of who pays or who receives the money, must be included. In performing such a study, it is important to state whose costs are being considered and who is to weigh the benefits against the consequences.

Allred and colleagues (1998) critiqued the seven nursing studies between 1992 and 1996 in which cost-effectiveness analyses were performed. They found these studies to be equivalent in quality to those from other disciplines. They concluded that more emphasis must be placed on cost-effectiveness analyses in nursing research, and they provided guidelines for conducting these studies.

Stone (1998) has described the recommended guidelines for journal reports of cost-effectiveness analyses. Cost-effectiveness studies should be used as aids in decision making rather than as the end decision. If a cost-effectiveness study is conducted to inform those who make resource allocation decisions, a standard reference case should be presented to allow the decision makers to compare a proposed new health intervention with existing practice.

ETHICAL STUDIES

Outcomes studies often result in the development of policies for the allocation of scarce resources. Ethicists take the position that moral principles, such as justice, must be considered as constraints on the use of costs and benefits to choose treatments in terms of maximizing the benefit per unit cost. Value commitments are inherent in choices about research methods and about the selection and interpretation of outcome variables, and these commitments should be acknowledged by researchers. "The choices researchers make should be documented and the reasons for those choices should be given explicitly in publications and presentations so that readers and other users of the information are enabled and expected to bear more responsibility for interpreting and applying the findings appropriately" (Lynn & Virnig, 1995). Veatch (1993) proposes that analysis of the implications of rationing decisions in terms of the principles of justice and autonomy will provide more acceptable criteria than outcomes predictors alone. As an example, Veatch performs an ethical analysis of the use of outcome predictors in decisions related to early withdrawal of life support. Ethical studies should play an important role in outcomes programs of research.

Measurement Methods

The selection of appropriate outcome variables is critical to the success of a study (Bernstein & Hilborne, 1993). As in any study, evidence of validity and reliability of the methods of measurement must be evaluated. Outcomes selected for nursing studies should be those most consistent with nursing practice and theory (Harris & Warren, 1995). In some studies, rather than selecting the final outcome of care, which may not occur for months or years, measures of intermediate end points are used. *Intermediate end points* are events or markers that act as precursors to the final outcome. It is important, however, to document the validity of the intermediate end point in predicting the outcome (Freedman & Schatzkin, 1992). A selection of outcome measures that have been used in published studies are listed in Table 12–3. In early outcomes studies, researchers selected outcome measures that could be easily obtained, rather than those most desirable for outcomes studies.

Characteristics important to evaluate in the selection methods of measuring outcomes are identified in Table 12–4. In evaluating a particular outcome measure, the researcher should consult the literature for previous studies that have used that particular method of measurement, including the publication describing development of the method of measurement. Information related to the measurement can be organized into a table such as Table 12–5, allowing easy comparison of several methods of measuring a particular outcome.

Outcomes researchers are moving away from classic measurement theory as a means of evaluating the reliability of measurement methods. They are interested in identifying change in measures over time in a subject, and instruments developed through the use of measurement theory are often not sensitive to these changes. The magnitude of change that can be detected is also important to determine. In addition, measures may detect change within a particular range of values but may not be sensitive to changes outside that range. The sensi-

TABLE 12–3
EXAMPLES OF MEASURES COMMONLY USED IN OUTCOME STUDIES

Patient Characteristics

Age
Beliefs/attitudes
Comorbid conditions
Diagnosis/condition
Gender
Health habits
Laboratory values
Medical care utilization
Medications
Preferences
Prognosis
Resource use
Severity of illness
Symptoms and signs
Understanding of a condition

Provider Personal Characteristics

Age
Beliefs/attitudes
Economic incentives
Gender
Job satisfaction
Preferences
Specialty training

Provider Technical Style

Continuity of care
Coordination
Expenditures
Hospitalizations
Medications
Referrals
Test ordering
Visits

Provider Interpersonal Style

Communication level
Counseling
Interpersonal manner
Patient participation

Institutional Characteristics

Avoidable deaths
Cancellation of an ambulatory procedure on the day of the procedure
Cases in which a discrepancy between initial and final radiology reports required an adjustment in patient management
Cesarean sections
Costs
Council on Teaching Hospitals membership
Fetal death rate
Hospital-acquired infections
Iatrogenic problems
Incidence of complications
Inpatient mortality
Neonatal mortality
Number of technological services available

TABLE 12–3
EXAMPLES OF MEASURES COMMONLY USED IN OUTCOME STUDIES *Continued*

Patients in the emergency department more than 6 hours
Patients leaving the emergency department prior to completion of treatment
Patient satisfaction
Access
Convenience
Organization
Specialty mix
Financial incentives
Percentage of board-certified physicians
Perinatal death rate
Perinatal mortality rate
Perioperative death rate
Postneonatal mortality rate
Presence of discharge planning services
Provider mix
Ratio of registered nurses to beds
Readmission rates
Risk adjustment
Service mix
Surgical wound infections
Unplanned admissions after ambulatory procedures
Unplanned readmissions
Unplanned returns to a special care unit
Unplanned returns to the operating room
Unplanned returns to the emergency department within 72 hours
Whether patients were dead or alive at the end of the hospital stay
Nursing workload

Community Outcomes
Immunization rate
Incidence of infectious diseases (e.g., measles)
Infant mortality rate
Neonatal mortality rate

Process Characteristics
Appropriateness of care
Posthospital care
Time

Functional Status
Amount of assistance needed
Disability
Behavioral functioning
Task performance
    Speed
    Pain
    Confidence
Dependence
Quality of performance
Functional changes in advanced dementia
Handicap
  Social roles
  Social expectations
Impairment
  Range of motion

Strength
Endurance
Pain
Productive activity
  Gainful employment
  Homemaking
  School or training
  Volunteer services
  Leisure activities
Skill indicators
  Self-care
  Mobility
  Social behavior
  Communication
  Vocational activity
  Homemaking

Physiological Outcomes
Asthma symptoms
Complications
Health status
Survival

Social Outcomes
School absence rates
Social support
Social investment
Status indicators
  Employment
  Income
  Education
Family role
Living arrangements

Quality of Life
Health-related quality of life
Quality-adjusted life years (QALYs) quality of life

General Well-Being
Energy/fatigue
Health perceptions
Life satisfaction
Living arrangements at discharge
Pain

Behavioral Outcomes
Activity pattern indicators
  Percentage of time spent out of the residence
  Time in travel
  Diversity of activities
  Time spent in inactivity
  Time spent in passive recreation
Breast-feeding after hospital discharge
Self-report of health behavior
Weight change

Mental Health Outcomes
Increased screening and early detection efforts
Reductions in the incidence or prevalence of diagnosable emotional and behavioral disorders
Reductions in the need for mental health services

TABLE 12-4
Characteristics of Outcomes Assessment Instruments

CHARACTERISTIC	CONSIDERATIONS IN PATIENT OUTCOMES EVALUATION	REFERENCE

Applicability	Consider purpose of instruments
	  Discriminate between subjects at a point in time
	  Predict future outcomes
	  Evaluate changes within subjects over time
	  Screen for problems
	  Provide case-mix adjustment
	  Assess quality of care
	Consider whether
	  Norms are established for clinical population of interest
	  Instrument format is compatible with assessment approach (e.g., observer rated vs. self-administered)
	  Setting in which instrument was developed
		Deyo & Carter, 1992
		Stewart et al., 1989
		Guyatt, Walter, & Norman, 1987
		Feinstein, Josephy, & Wells, 1986
		Deyo, 1984

Practicality (clinical utility)	The instrument:
	  Includes outcomes important to the patient
	  Is short and easy to administer (low respondent burden)
	  Questions are easy to understand and acceptable to patients and interviewers
	  Scores reflect condition severity, condition-specific features, and discriminate those with condition from those without
	  Is easily scored and scores are readily understandable
	  Level of measurement allows a change score to be determined
	  Provides information that is clinically useful
	  Performance or capacity based
	  Includes patient rating of magnitude of effort and support needed for performance of physical tasks
		Leidy, 1991
		Nelson, Landgraf, Hays, Wasson, & Kirk, 1990
		Stewart et al., 1989
		Lohr, 1988
		Bombardier & Tugwell, 1987
		Feinstein et al., 1986
		Kirshner & Guyatt, 1985
		Deyo, 1984

Comprehensiveness	Generic measures are designed to summarize a spectrum of concepts applied to different impairments, illness, patients, and populations Disease-specific measures are designed to assess specific patients with specific conditions or diagnoses Dimensions of the instrument; a core set of physical, mental, and role functions desirable	Nelson et al., 1990 Patrick & Deyo, 1989 Deyo, 1984
Reliability	Can be influenced by day-to-day variations in patients, differences between observers, items in the scale, mode of administration This is the critical determinant of usefulness of an instrument designed for discriminative purpose	Nelson et al., 1990 Spitzer, 1987 Guyatt et al., 1987 Deyo, 1984
Validity	No consensus of what are scientifically admissible criteria for many indices No "goal standard" exists for establishing criterion validity for many indices	Spitzer, 1987 Deyo, 1984
Responsiveness	Not yet indexed for virtually any evaluative measures Coarse scale rating may not detect changes Aggregated scores may obscure changes in subscales Useful for determining sample size and statistical power Reliable instruments are likely to be responsive but reliability not adequate as sole index of consistent results over time Consider detail in scaling As baseline variability of score changes within stable subjects, may need larger treatment effects to demonstrate efficacy Consider temporal relationship between intervention and outcome	Stewart & Archbold, 1992 Leidy, 1991 Jaeschke, Singer, & Guyatt, 1989 Guyatt et al., 1989 Bombardier & Tugwell, 1987 Guyatt et al., 1987 Deyo & Centor, 1986 Deyo, 1984

From Harris, M. R., & Warren, J. J. (1995). Patient outcomes: Assessment issues for the CNS. *Clinical Nurse Specialist, 9*(2), 82.

TABLE 12-5
CHARACTERISTICS OF THE KATZ ADL SCALE, A PROPOSED OUTCOME INSTRUMENT

CHARACTERISTIC	REFERENCE
Applicability	Katz et al., 1970
Purpose is to objectively evaluate results of treatment in chronically ill and aging populations	
Predicts service utilization in elderly population	Wiener et al., 1990
Used in case-mix adjustments	Fries, 1990
Scale discriminates well on disability in elderly population, norms easily referenced	Spector, 1990
Ratings judgment based on direct observation and caregiver reports, known differences in observed vs. reported ratings	Spector, 1990 Burns, 1992
Practicality	Katz et al., 1970
Brief, 6 items with 3 levels of dependency	
Can be used by clinicians and non-clinicians	Spector, 1990
Measures performance (not ability)	Katz et al., 1970
Aggregate score represents increasing level of dependency	Spector, 1990
Comprehensiveness	Katz et al., 1970
Includes bathing, dressing, toileting, transfer, continence, and eating	
Does not explain etiology of level of performance	Kane & Bayer, 1991
Generic measure (not disease-specific)	
Reliability	Kane & Bayer, 1991
Performance may be influenced by motivational, social, and environmental factors	
High internal consistency reported	Spector, 1990
Validity	Spector, 1990
Content and construct validity assessments are acceptable	
Responsiveness	
No published reports that quantify relationship of scale change to minimal clinically important change	

From Harris, M. R., & Warren, J. J. (1995). Patient outcomes: Assessment issues for the CNS. *Clinical Nurse Specialist, 9*(2), 85.

tivity to change of many commonly used outcome measures has not been examined (Deyo & Carter, 1992; Felson et al., 1990). Studies must be conducted specifically to determine the sensitivity of measures before they are used in outcomes studies.

As the sensitivity of a measure increases, statistical power increases, allowing smaller sample sizes to detect significant differences.

Creative methods of collecting data on instruments for large outcomes studies must be explored. In a busy office or clinic setting, the typical strategy of having clerks or other staff administer questionnaires or scales to patients is time intensive and costly and may result in lost data. Greist and colleagues (1997) recommend using the computer and the telephone to collect such data. Computers containing the instrument can be placed in locations convenient to patients, so the instrument can be completed with a minimum of staff involvement.

Another option is telephone interviews using the computer. The traditional telephone interview using interviewers to ask questions is costly. However, the same interactive voice response (IVR) technology used in voice mail can be used in telephone interviewing by computer. IVR allows the patient to respond to yes-no and multiple-choice questions by pressing numbers on the keypad or by saying "yes" or "no" or a number from 0 to 9. Patients can record answers in their own voices.

Measuring the frequency and nature of care activities of various staff has been problematic in studies of the process of care. Strategies commonly used are chart review, time and motion studies, work sampling, and retrospective recall. None of these is a satisfactory indicator of the actual care that occurs (Hale et al., 1997). Holmes and associates (1997) recommend the use of barcode methodology to measure service inputs. The barcodes capture what care is provided, for whom, by whom, and at what time. Barcoded service sheets and a portable barcode reader are used with an accompanying database management system.

THE ANALYSIS OF MEASUREMENT RELIABILITY

Estimating the reliability of outcome measures through the use of classic measurement theory may be problematic. The traditional concept of measurement reliability was developed to evaluate quantities that were not expected to change over time in an individual. This assessment of reliability is irrelevant or only partially relevant to assessing the suitability or precision of measures selected because of their sensitivity to change within the individual over time. Traditional evaluations of measurement methods assume that any change in group values is a result of variation between individuals. Patient change, however, results in changes within the individual. With traditional measurement theory analysis, a measure that did not vary between individuals would have zero (or poor) reliability. This measure, however, may be an excellent measure of change over time if individuals change on that measure (even if group averages do not change much). Thus, it is inappropriate to assess the reliability of difference scores according to the internal consistency of measures (Collins & Johnston, 1995).

In some outcomes studies, measures obtained from individuals are used as indicators of characteristics of a group. The data from the measures are aggregated to reflect the group. In this case, the researcher must assess the extent to which the responses represent the group. Although the group mean is usually expected to serve this purpose, it may not adequately represent the group. Verran and colleagues (1992) describe techniques that can be employed to examine the psychometric properties of instruments used to describe group level phenomenon. Items of the instrument should be assessed for content validity to determine how well they measure group level concepts. Reliability and validity must be assessed at the aggregated level rather than the individual level.

Commonly, multiple outcomes measures are used in outcomes studies. Researchers wish to evaluate all relevant effects of care. However, quantity of measures is not necessarily evidence of the quality of the measures. The measures most relevant to the treatment should be selected. Measures selected should not be closely correlated. Interpreting the results of studies in which multiple outcomes have been used can be problematic. For example, Felson and colleagues (1990, p. 141) ask "which is the better therapy, the one that shows a change in 6 outcome measures out of 12 tested or the one that shows a change in 4 of the 12 measures? What if the 4 that demonstrate change with one therapy are not the same as the 6 that show a change in another therapy?" If multiple comparisons are made, it is important to make statistical adjustments for them; the risk of a Type I error is greater when multiple comparisons are made.

Some researchers recommend combining various measures into a single summary score (DesHarnais et al., 1991; Felson et al., 1990). However, such global composite measures have not been widely used. The various measures used in such an index may not be equally weighted and may be difficult to combine. Also, the composite index value may not be readily interpretable by clinicians.

The focus of most measures developed for outcomes studies has been the individual patient. However, a number of organizations are now developing measures of the quality of performance of systems of care. In 1990, the Consortium Research on Indicators of System Performance (CRISP) project began to develop indicators of the quality of performance of integrated delivery systems. From the perspective of CRISP, the success of a health system is associated with its ability to decrease the number of episodes of diseases in the population. Therefore, the impact of the delivery system on the community is considered an important measure of performance. CRISP has developed a number of indicators now in use by consortium members, who pay to participate in the studies (Bergman, 1994).

The JCAHO is also applying outcomes data to quality management efforts in hospitals using the IMSystem (Information Management System) (McCormick, 1990; Nadzim et al., 1993). The National Committee for Quality Assurance, the organization that accredits managed care plans, has developed a tool (HEDIS) for comparing managed care plans. Comparisons involve more than 60 measures, including patient satisfaction, quality of care, and financial stability (Guadagnoli & McNeil, 1994). Researchers at the Henry Ford Health Systems' Center for Health System Studies in Detroit have evolved 80 performance indicators to evaluate health systems (Anderson, 1991).

The ANA (1995) has generated a Nursing Care Report Card for Acute Care. Their model, identifying concepts critical to quality acute care and illustrating the relationships among them, is shown in Figure 12–11. The Acute Care Nursing Quality Indicators developed through this project are listed in Figure 12–12. Pilot studies have been conducted

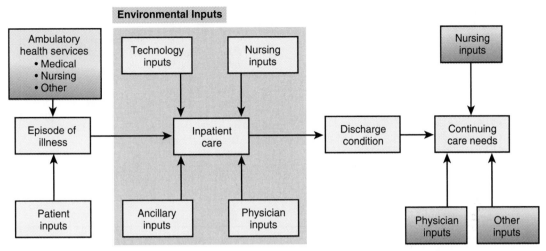

FIGURE 12-11 ■ Framework for ANA Report Card. (From American Nurses Association [1995]. *Nursing report card for acute care.* Washington, D.C.: ANA, with permission.)

using the indicators (Robinson & Finch, 1997). Problems with use of the indicators and consistency of measurement among facilities were identified. Strategies for improving consistency in measurement have been developed, and a second phase of study was implemented late in 1995.

Statistical Methods for Outcomes Studies

Although outcomes researchers test for statistical significance of their findings, this is not considered sufficient to judge the findings as important. The focus of their attention is on the clinical significance of study findings (see Chapter 18 for more information on clinical significance). In analyzing data, outcomes researchers have moved away from statistical analyses that use the mean to test for group differences. They place greater importance on analyzing change scores and use exploratory methods of examining the data to identify outliers.

THE ANALYSIS OF CHANGE

With the focus on outcomes studies has come a renewed interest in methods of analyzing change. Gottman and Rushe (1993) reported that the first book addressing change in research, *Problems in Measuring Change* edited by Harris (1967), is the basis for most current approaches to analyzing change. Since then, a number of new ideas have emerged regarding the analysis of change (e.g., in studies by Collins & Horn, 1991; Rovine & Von Eye, 1991; Von Eye, 1990a, 1990b). However, many researchers are unfamiliar with these new ideas and continue to base their reasoning on Harris's 1967 book. Gottman and Rushe (1993) suggest that many beliefs related to the analysis of change are based on little more than the following fallacies:

Fallacy 1: In change, regression toward the mean is an unavoidable law of nature.
Fallacy 2: The difference score between premeasurement and postmeasurement is unreliable.
Fallacy 3: Analysis of covariance (ANCOVA, or related methods such as path analysis) is the way to analyze change.
Fallacy 4: Two points (pretest and posttest) are adequate for the study of change.
Fallacy 5: The correlation between change and initial level is always negative.

The method of analysis of change is also being questioned by outcomes researchers. Collins and Johnston (1995) suggest that the recommended analysis method of regressing pretest scores on outcome scores and basing the analysis of change on

Patient-focused Outcome Indicators

- Mortality rate
- Length of stay
- Adverse incidents
  - Adverse incident rate (total)
  - Medication error rate
  - Patient injury rate
- Complications
  - Total complication rate
  - Decubitus ulcer rate
  - Nosocomial infection rate (total)
  - Nosocomial urinary tract infecton rate
  - Nosocomial pneumonia rate
  - Nosocomial surgical wound infection rate

- Patient/family satisfaction with nursing care
  - Patient willingness to recommend hospital to others/use hospital again
- Patient adherence to discharge plan
  - Readmission rates
  - Emergency room visits post discharge
  - Unscheduled physician visits post-discharge
  - Patient knowledge of disease/condition and care requirements

Process of Care Indicators

- Nurse satisfaction
- Assessment and implementation of patient care requirements
- Assessment of patient care requirements
- Development of a nursing care plan
- Accurate and timely execution of therapeutic interventions and procedures
- Documentation of nursing diagnoses, therapeutic objectives, and care given
- Pain management
- Maintenance of skin integrity

- Patient education
- Discharge planning
- Assurance of patient safety
  - Overall assurance of patient safety
  - Appropriate use of restraints (all)
  - Appropriate use of pharmaceutical restraints
  - Appropriate use of physical restraints
- Responsiveness to unplanned patient care needs

Structure of Care Indicators—Nurse Staffing Patterns

- Ratio of total nursing staff to patients
  - RN/patient ratio
  - LPN/patient ratio
  - Unlicensed workers/patient ratio
- Ratio of RNs to total nursing staff
  - RN staff experience
  - RN staff education (i.e., MSNs, BSNs)

- Total nursing care hours provided per patient (case mix, acuity adjusted)
  - RN hours per patient
  - LPN hours per patient
  - unlicensed worker hours per patient
- Staff continuity
  - Use of agency nurses
  - Use of float nurses
  - Unsafe assignment rate
  - Nurse staff turnover rates
  - FT/PT RN ratio
- RN overtime
- Nursing staff injury rate

FIGURE 12–12 ■ Acute care nursing quality indicators. (From American Nurses Association. [1995]. *Nursing report card for acute care.* Washington, D.C.: American Nurses Association.)

residual change scores is overly conservative and tends to understate the extent of real change. There are serious questions about the conceptual meaning of these residual change scores.

For some outcomes, the changes may be nonlinear or may go up and down rather than always increasing. Thus, it is as important to uncover patterns of change as it is to test for statistical differences over time. Some changes may occur in relation to stages of recovery or improvement. These changes may occur over weeks, months, or even years. A more complete picture of the process of recovery can be obtained by examining the process in greater detail and over a broader range. With this approach, a recovery curve can be developed, which provides a model of the recovery process and can then be tested (Collins & Johnston, 1995; Ottenbacher et al., 1995).

THE ANALYSIS OF IMPROVEMENT

In addition to reporting the mean improvement score for all patients treated, it is important to report what percentage of patients improve. Do all patients improve slightly, or is there a divergence among patients, with some improving greatly and others not improving at all? This divergence may best be illustrated by plotting the data. Researchers studying a particular treatment or approach to care might develop a standard or index of varying degrees of improvement that might occur. The index would allow better comparisons of the effectiveness of various treatments. Characteristics of patients who experience varying degrees of improvement should be described, and outliers should be carefully examined. This step requires that the study design include baseline measures of patient status, such as demographic characteristics, functional status, and disease severity measures. Analysis of improvement will allow better judgments of the appropriate use of various treatments (Felson et al., 1990).

VARIANCE ANALYSIS

Variance analysis is used to track individual and group variance from a specific critical pathway. The goal is to decrease preventable variance in process, thus helping patients and their families achieve optimal outcomes. Some of the variance is due to comorbidities. Keeping a patient with comorbidities on the desired pathway may require utilization of more resources early in their care. Thus, it is important to track both variance and comorbidities. Studies examining variations from pathways may facilitate the tailoring of existing critical pathways for specific comorbidities.

Variance analysis can also be used to identify at-risk patients who might benefit from the services of a case manager. Variance analysis tracking is ex-

pressed through the use of graphics, and the expected pathway is plotted on the graph. The care providers plot deviations (negative variance) on the graph, allowing immediate comparison with the expected pathway. Deviations may be related to the patient, the system, or the provider (Tidwell, 1993).

THE LONGITUDINAL GUTTMAN SIMPLEX MODEL

The longitudinal Guttman simplex (LGS) model is an extension of the Guttman scale that involves times as well as items and persons. For example, an LGS model of mobility might involve the following items:

M1: moving unassisted from bed to chair
M2: moving unassisted from bed to another room
M3: moving unassisted up stairs

Table 12–6 shows hypothetical data collected with this measure on three patients at three periods, showing a pattern of improving ability over time (Collins & Johnston, 1995).

TABLE 12–6
SAMPLE DATA USING LONGITUDINAL GUTTMAN SCALE

| | FUNCTIONAL ITEMS | | |
	M1	M2	M3
Patient A			
Time 1	Fail	Fail	Fail
Time 2	Pass	Fail	Fail
Time 3	Pass	Pass	Fail
Patient B			
Time 1	Fail	Fail	Fail
Time 2	Pass	Pass	Fail
Time 3	Pass	Pass	Fail
Patient C			
Time 1	Pass	Fail	Fail
Time 2	Pass	Pass	Fail
Time 3	Pass	Pass	Pass

M1, moving unassisted from bed to chair; M2, moving unassisted from bed to another room; M3, moving unassisted up stairs.
From Collins, L. M., & Johnston, M. V. (1995). Analysis of stage-sequential change in rehabilitation research. *American Journal of Physical Medicine and Rehabilitation, 74*(2), 167.

LATENT TRANSITION ANALYSIS

Latent transition analysis (LTA) is used in situations in which stages or categories of recovery have been defined and transitions between stages can be identified. To use the analysis method, the researchers assign each member of the population in a single category or stage for a given point of time. However, stage membership changes over time. The analysis tests stage membership to provide a realistic picture of development. Collins and Johnston (1995) describe an example of this type of analysis with a hypothetical model of recovery from functional neglect after stroke, in the following excerpt:

• •

"Let's assume that we can define a study subpopulation displaying four latent stages or types of functional neglect: sensory limitations (S), cognitive limitations (C), both (S and C) or patients may recover and adapt to the point that they are functional (F). . . . Membership in each category is inferred from several clinical symptoms or test items, which supposedly go together but in fact may not for some patients. The items have some error and are imperfect indicators of true (latent) stage membership. Our objective is to estimate in which category a patient probably falls at any point in time and the probability of movement between stages over time, conditional on previous stage membership. . . . Suppose we use a large number of times periodically to monitor progress, testing the same group of patients at multiple points in time. We record which items the patient passes and which the patient does not." (Collins & Johnston, 1995, p. 47) ■

After the use of a computerized program designed to perform LTA analysis, the results of the study were obtained; they are shown in Table 12–7. Only two points of time are shown here, although the program can handle up to five points in time.

The first line of the table contains the estimate of the proportion of patients in each of the four stages at Time 1. In this example, 30% of the sample had both S and C limitations, 30% had S limitations, and 40% had C limitations, and none was functional. At Time 2, the proportion in each functional limitation appears to have declined, except sensory limitations, which is unchanged, and 27% are now

TABLE 12–7
A HYPOTHETICAL LATENT TRANSITION MODEL OF RECOVERY FROM NEGLECT FOLLOWING STROKE

	LATENT STATUS			
	F	C	S	S and C
Total Marginal Proportions				
Time 1 proportions	0.0	0.40	0.30	0.30
Time 2 proportions	0.27	0.25	0.30	0.18

TIME 1 LATENT STATUS	TIME 2 LATENT STATUS			
	F*	C	S	S and C
Time 1 to Time 2 Transition				
Proportions within Rows				
Functional (F)	0	0	0	0
Cognitive limitation (C)	0.46	0.54	0.0	0.0
Sensory limitation (S)	0.30	0.0	0.70	0.0
S and C	0.0	0.10	0.30	0.60

* No patients were functional at time 1.
From Collins, L. M., & Johnston, M. V. (1995). Analysis of stage-sequential change in rehabilitation research. *American Journal of Physical Medicine and Rehabilitation*, 74(2), 168.

in the functional stage. The bottom half of the table is a matrix of transition probabilities that reveals patterns of change. Of patients who started with S, 30% improved; however, the overall percentage at S remained the same because 30% of the patients who started at S and C moved to the S category. Of patients who initially had C problems alone, 46% moved to the functional category.

A third set of quantities estimated by the full LTA model but not shown in the table are the relationships between items and stage memberships. This relationship indicates the probability that when a subject moves from one category to another, each item will also change to reflect the new stage membership. Thus, this relationship is a determination of the effectiveness of the test items or clinical symptoms as indicators of stage membership.

MULTILEVEL ANALYSIS

Multilevel analysis is used in epidemiology to study how environmental factors (aggregate-level characteristics) and individual attributes and behaviors (individual-level characteristics) interact to influence individual-level health behaviors and disease risks. For example, the risk that an adolescent will start smoking is associated with the following variables: (1) attributes of the child (e.g., self-esteem, academic achievement, refusal skills), (2) attributes of the child's family (e.g., parental attitudes toward smoking, smoking behavior of parents), (3) general characteristics of the community (e.g., ease of minors' access to cigarettes, school policies regarding smoking, city smoking ordinances, social norms of students toward smoking), and (4) general social factors (e.g., geographic region, economic policies that influence the price of cigarettes). The researchers might ask, "Does smoking status covary with the level of restriction of smoking in public places after we have controlled for the individual-level variables that influence smoking risks?" (Von Korff et al., 1992).

DISSEMINATING OUTCOMES RESEARCH FINDINGS

Including plans for the dissemination of findings as a component of a program of research is a new idea within nursing if one considers the process of dissemination to be more than publishing the results in professional journals. The costs associated with dissemination are not included in funding for nursing studies beyond those of publication of the research findings. As discussed in Unit III of this text, strategies for the dissemination of research findings tend to be performed by groups other than the original researchers. The transfer of knowledge from nurse researchers to nurse clinicians has been, for the most part, ineffective.

Nursing, as a discipline, has not yet addressed the various constituencies for nursing research knowledge. A research team conducting a program of outcomes research must identify their constituencies. These should include (1) the clinicians, who will apply the knowledge to practice, (2) the public, who may make health care decisions on the basis of the information, (3) health care institutions, which must evaluate care in their facilities on the basis of the information, (4) health policymakers, who may set standards on the basis of the information, and

(5) researchers, who may use the information in designing new studies. Disseminating information to these various constituencies through presentations at meetings and publications in a wide diversity of journals and magazines, as well as release of the information to the news media, requires careful planning. Mattson and Donovan (1994) suggest that dissemination involves strategies for debunking myths, addressing issues related to feasibility, communicating effectively, and identifying opinion leaders.

■ SUMMARY

Outcomes research was developed to examine the end-results of patient care. The momentum propelling outcomes research today is coming from policymakers, insurers, and the public. The scientific approaches used in outcomes studies differ in some important ways from those used in traditional research. These differences have led traditional researchers and statisticians to criticize the credibility of outcomes research. Outcomes researchers counter these criticisms by saying that experimental studies lack external validity and are not useful for application in clinical settings.

A number of health care providers throughout history have attempted to examine the outcomes of patient care. Their efforts were not well received by the medical community. Because of growing concerns about the quality of medical care, the Agency for Health Services Research (AHSR) was established in 1959. This agency supported small area analyses that examined variations in medical practice across towns and counties. The first large-scale study of patient outcomes, the Medical Outcomes Study (MOS), was funded through this agency.

In 1989, the Agency for Health Care Policy and Research (AHCPR) replaced the AHSR and, with much greater funding, was mandated to conduct studies of patient outcomes of health care. Large-scale, multifaceted, multidisciplinary projects called Patient Outcomes Research Teams (PORTs) were designed to address this mandate. The focus of outcomes research has been medical practice. However, nursing must become involved in examining the outcomes of nursing practice in hospital settings, in managed care, and in community settings such as provision of primary health care by nurse practitioners.

The theory on which outcomes research is based was developed by Donabedian (1987). Quality is the overriding construct of the theory, although Donabedian never defines this concept. The three major concepts of the theory are health, subjects of care, and providers of care. Donabedian identifies three objects of evaluation in appraising quality: structure, process, and outcome. The goal of outcomes research is the evaluation of outcomes as defined by Donabedian, whose theory requires that identified outcomes be clearly linked with the process that caused the outcome. Three components of process are of interest to Donabedian: standards of care, practice styles, and costs of care. Structures of care are the elements of organization and administration that guide the processes of care.

Because outcomes research is relatively new, methods are still being developed to provide answers to the questions posed. However, a research process for conducting outcomes studies is being defined. Outcomes research programs are complex and may consist of multiple studies using a variety of designs whose findings must be merged in the process of forming conclusions. Outcome designs tend to have less control than traditional research designs and, except for the clinical trial, seldom use random samples; rather, they use large representative samples. Outcomes selected for nursing studies should be those most consistent with nursing practice and theory. The researcher must consider the measure's sensitivity to change and the magnitude of change that can be detected. Multiple outcome measures are commonly used in outcomes studies. Although the focus of most measures developed for outcomes studies has been the individual patient, a number of organizations are now evolving measures of the quality of performance of systems of care.

Statistical approaches used in outcomes studies include new approaches to examining measurement reliability, strategies to analyze change, and the analysis of improvement. A variety of techniques have been developed to address the analysis needs of outcomes researchers, including ways to use structural equation modeling, the longitudinal Gutt-man simplex model, latent transition analysis, variance analysis, profiling, multilevel analysis, and geographic analyses. Strategies must be developed in nursing to disseminate the findings from outcomes studies to the various constituencies needing the information.

● ●

REFERENCES

Alison, K. (1997). Using evidence to demonstrate the value of nursing. *Nursing Standard, 11*(28), 34–39.

Allred, C. A., Arford, P. H., Mauldin, P. D., & Goodwin, L. K. (1998). Cost-effectiveness analysis in the nursing literature, 1992–1996. *Image—The Journal of Nursing Scholarship, 30*(3), 235–242.

Altman, L. K. (1993). Bringing the news to the public: The role of the media. *Annals of the New York Academy of Sciences, 703,* 200–209.

American Nurses' Association. (1995). *Nursing report card for acute care.* Washington, D. C.: American Nurses' Publishing.

Anderson, H. J. (1991). Sizing up systems: Researchers to test performance measures. *Hospitals, 65*(20), 33–34.

Auffrey, C. (1998). Geographic information systems as a tool for community health research and practice. *Nursing Research Methods* [Online]. Available: *http://www.nursing.uc.edu/nrm/AUFFREY51598.htm*

Bergman, R. (1994). Are my outcomes better than yours? *Hospital Health Network, 68*(15), 113–116.

Bergmark, A., & Oscarsson, L. (1991). Does anybody really know what they are doing? Some comments related to methodology of treatment service research. *British Journal of Addiction, 86*(2), 139–142.

Bernstein, S. J., & Hilborne, L. H. (1993). Clinical indicators: The road to quality care? *Joint Commission Journal on Quality Improvement, 19*(11), 501–509.

Bloom, B. S. (1990). Does it work? The outcomes of medical interventions. *International Journal of Technology Assessment in Health Care, 6*(2), 326–332.

Bombardier, C., & Tugwell, P. (1987). Methodological considerations in functional assessment. *Journal of Rheumatology, 14*(Suppl. 15), 7–10.

Burns, R. B., Moskowitz, M. A., Ash, A., Kane, R. L., Finch, M. D., & Bak, S. M. (1992). Self-report *versus* medical record functional status. *Medical Care, 30*(Suppl. 5), MS85–MS95.

Chaput de Saintonge, D. M., & Hattersley, L. A. (1985). Antibiotics for otitis media: Can we help doctors agree? *Family Practice, 2*(4), 205–212.

Chaput de Saintonge, D. M., Kirway, J. R., Evans, S. J., & Crane, G. J. (1988). How can we design trials to detect clinically important changes in disease severity? *British Journal of Clinical Pharmacology, 26*(4), 355–362.

Clark, J., & Lang, N. (1992). Nursing's next advance: An internal classification for nursing practice. *International Nursing Review, 39*(4), 109–111, 128.

Clinton, J. J. (1993). Financing medical effectiveness research: Role of the agency for health care policy and research. *Annals of the New York Academy of Sciences, 703,* 295–297.

Collins, L. M., & Horn, J. L. (1991). *Best methods for the analysis of change: Recent advances, unanswered questions, future directions.* Washington, D. C.: American Psychological Association.

Collins, L. M., & Johnston, M. V. (1995). Analysis of stage-sequential change in rehabilitation research. *American Journal of Physical Medicine and Rehabilitation, 74*(2), 163–170.

Crane, V. S. (1988). Economic aspects of clinical decision making: Applications of clinical decision analysis. *American Journal of Hospital Pharmacy, 45*(3), 548–553.

Davis, K. (1990). Use of data registries to evaluate medical procedures: Coronary artery surgery study and the balloon valvuloplasty registry. *International Journal of Technology Assessment in Health Care, 6*(2), 203–210.

DesHarnais, S., McMahon, L. F., Jr., & Wroblewski, R. (1991). Measuring outcomes of hospital care using multiple risk-adjusted indexes. *HSR: Health Services Research, 26*(4), 425–445.

Deyo, R. A. (1984). Measuring functional outcomes in therapeutic trials for chronic disease. *Controlled Clinical Trials, 5*(3), 223–240.

Deyo, R. A., & Carter, W. B. (1992). Strategies for improving and expanding the application of health status measures in clinical settings. *Medical Care, 30*(5), MS176–MS186.

Deyo, R. A., & Centor, R. M. (1986). Assessing the responsiveness of functional scales to clinical change: An analogy to diagnostic test performance. *Journal of Chronic Disease, 39*(11), 897–906.

Deyo, R. A., Psaty, B. M., Simon, G., Wagner, E. H., Omenn, G. S. (1997). The messenger under attack—intimidation of researchers by special interest groups. *New England Journal of Medicine, 336*(16), 1176–1180.

Deyo, R. A., Taylor, V. M., Diehr, P., Conrad, D., Cherkin, D. C., Ciol, M., & Kreuter, W. (1994). Analysis of automated administrative and survey databases to study patterns and outcomes of care. *Spine, 19*(18S), 2083S–2091S.

Donabedian, A. (1987). Some basic issues in evaluating the quality of health care. In L. T. Rinke (Ed.), *Outcome measures in home care* (Vol. I, pp. 3–28). New York: National League for Nursing. (Original work published 1976)

Doubilet, P., Weinstein, M. C., & McNeil, B. H. (1986). Use and misuse of the term "cost effective" in medicine. *The New England Journal of Medicine, 314*(4), 253–255.

Drummond, M. F., Stoddart, G. L. & Torrance, G. W. (1987). Method for the economic evaluation of health care programs. New York: Oxford University Press.

Fardon, D. F., Garfin, S. R. & Saal, J. A. (1997). Intimidation of researchers by special interest groups [letter; comment]. *The New England Journal of Medicine, 337*(18), 1315–1316.

Feinstein, A. R., Josephy, B. R., & Wells, C. K. (1986). Scientific and clinical problems in indexes of functional disability. *Annals of Internal Medicine, 105*(3), 413–420.

Felson, D. T., Anderson, J. J., & Meenan, R. F. (1990). Time for changes in the design, analysis, and reporting of rheumatoid arthritis clinical trials. *Arthritis and Rheumatism, 33*(1), 140–149.

Fowler, F. J., Jr., Cleary, P. D., Magaziner, J., Patrick, D. L., & Benjamin, K. L. (1994). Methodological issues in measuring patient-reported outcomes: The agenda of the work group on outcomes assessment. *Medical Care, 32*(7 Suppl.), JS65–JS76.

Freedman, L. S., & Schatzkin, A. (1992). Sample size for studying intermediate endpoints within intervention trials or observational studies. *American Journal of Epidemiology, 136*(9), 1148–1159.

Freund, D. A., Dittus, R. S., Fitzgerald, J., & Heck, D. (1990). Assessing and improving outcomes: Total knee replacement. *HSR: Health Services Research, 25*(5), 723–726.

Fries, B. E. (1990). Comparing case-mix systems for nursing home payment. *Health Care Financing Review, 11*(4), 103–119.

Gold, M. R., Siegel, J. E., Russell, L. B., & Weinstein, M. C. (ed.). (1996). *Cost-effectiveness in health and medicine.* New York: Oxford University Press.

Goldberg, H. I., & Cummings, M. A. (1994). Conducting medical effectiveness research: A report from the Inter-PORT work groups. *Medical Care, 32*(7 Suppl.), JS1–JS12.

Goldberg, H. I., Cummings, M. A., Steinberg, E. P., Ricci, E. M., Shannon, T., Soumerai, S. B., Mittman, B. S., Eisenberg, J., Heck, D. A., Kaplan, S., Kenzora, J. E., Vargus, A. M., Mulley, A. G., Jr., & Rimer, B. K. (1994). Deliberations on the dissemination of PORT products: Translating research findings into improved patient outcomes. *Medical Care, 32*(7 Suppl.), JS90–JS110.

Gottman, J. M., & Rushe, R. H. (1993). The analysis of change: Issues, fallacies, and new ideas. *Journal of Consulting and Clinical Psychology, 61*(6), 907–910.

Gray, B. H. (1992). The legislative battle over health services research. *Health Affairs, 11*(4), 38–66.

Greene, R., Bondy, P. K., & Maklan, C. W. (1994). The national medical effectiveness research initiative. *Diabetes Care, 17*(Suppl. 1), 45–49.

Greenfield, S., Nelson, E. C., Zubkoff, M., Manning, W., Rogers, W., Kravitz, R. L., Keller, A., Tarlov, A. R., & Ware, J. E., Jr. (1992). Variations in resource utilization among medical specialties and systems of care: Results from the Medical Outcomes study. *JAMA, 267*(12), 1624–1630.

Greiner, J. E. (1994). Microlevel documentation: Relational database for critical path development. *Seminars for Nurse Managers, 2*(2), 72–78.

Greist, J. H., Jefferson, J. W., Wenzel, K. W., Kobak, K. A., Bailey, T. M., Katzelnich, D. J., Hagerson, S. J., & Dottl, S. L. (1997). The telephone assessment program: Efficient patient monitoring and clinician feedback. *M. D. Computing, 14*(5), 382–387.

Guadagnoli, E., & McNeil, B. J. (1994). Outcomes research: Hope for the future or the latest rage? *Inquiry, 31*(1), 14–24.

Guess, H. A., Jacobsen, S. J., Girman, C. J., Oesterling, J. E., Chute, C. G., Panser, L. A., & Lieber, M. M. (1995). The role of community-based longitudinal studies in evaluating treatment effects: Example: Benign prostatic hyperplasia. *Medical Care, 33*(4 Suppl.), AS26–AS35.

Guyatt, G., Walter, S., & Norman, G. (1987). Measuring change over time: Assessing the usefulness of evaluative instruments. *Journal of Chronic Disease, 40*(2), 171–178.

Hadorn, D., Baker, D., Dracup, K., & Pitt, B. (1994). Making judgments about treatment effectiveness based on health outcomes: Theoretical and practical issues. *Joint Commission Journal of Quality Improvement, 20*(10), 547–554.

Hadorn, D. C., & Baker, D. (1994). Development of the AHCPR-sponsored heart failure guideline: Methodologic and procedural issues. *Joint Commission Journal of Quality Improvement, 20*(10), 539–547.

Hale, C. A., Thomas, L. H., Bond, S., & Todd, C. (1997). The nursing record as a research tool to identify nursing interventions. *Journal of Clinical Nursing, 6*(3), 207–214.

Harris, C. W. (Ed.). (1967). *Problems in measuring change.* Madison: University of Wisconsin Press.

Harris, M. R., & Warren, J. J. (1995). Patient outcomes: Assessment issues for the CNS. *Clinical Nurse Specialist, 9*(2), 82–86.

Hastings, G. E., Vick, L., Lee, G., Sasmor, L., Natiello, T. A., & Sanders, J. H. (1980). Nurse practitioners in a jailhouse clinic. *Medical Care, 18*(7), 731–744.

Hegyvary, S. T. (1992). Outcomes research: Integrating nursing practice into the world view. In *Patient Outcomes Research: Examining the Effectiveness of Nursing Practice: Proceedings of a Conference Sponsored by the National Center for Nursing Research, September 11–13, 1991* (NIH Publication No. 93–3411). Washington, D.C.: U.S. Department of Health and Human Services, Public Health Services, National Institutes of Health.

Herrmann, D. (1995). Reporting current, past, and changed health status: What we know about distortion. *Medical Care, 33*(4 Suppl.), AS89–AS94.

Hinshaw, A. S. (1992). Welcome: Patient outcome research conference. In *Patient Outcomes Research: Examining the Effectiveness of Nursing Practice: Proceedings of a Conference Sponsored by the National Center for Nursing Research, September 11–13, 1991* (NIH Publication No. 93–3411). Washington, D.C.: U.S. Department of Health and Human Services, Public Health Services, National Institutes of Health.

Holmes, D., Teresi, J., Lindeman, D. A., & Glandon, G. L. (1997). Measurement of personal care inputs in chronic care settings. *Journal of Mental Health and Aging, 3*(1), 119–127.

Holzemer, W. (1990). Quality and cost of nursing care. *Nursing and Health Care, 11*(8), 412–415.

Issel, L. M. (1995). Evaluating case management programs. *Maternal-Child Nursing, 20*(2), 67–70, 72–74.

Jaeschke, R., Singer, J., & Guyatt, G. H. (1989). Measurement of health status: Ascertaining the minimal clinically important difference. *Controlled Clinical Trials, 10*(4), 407–415.

Johnson, M., & Maas, M. (1997). *Iowa Outcomes Project: Nursing Outcomes Classification (NOC).* St. Louis: Mosby.

Johnson, M., & Maas, M. (1998). The Nursing Outcomes Classification. *Journal of Nursing Care Quality, 12*(5), 9–20, 85–87.

Johnston, M. V., & Granger, C. V. (1994). Outcomes research in medical rehabilitation: A primer and introduction to a series. *American Journal of Physical and Medical Rehabilitation, 73*(4), 296–303.

Kane, R. A., & Bayer, A. J. (1991). Assessment of functional status. In M. S. J. Pathy (Ed.), *Principles and practices of geriatric medicine* (2nd ed., pp. 265–277). New York: John Wiley & Sons Ltd.

Katz, S., Downs, T. D., Cash, H. R., & Grotz, R. C. (1970). Progress in the development of the Index of ADL. *The Gerontologist* (Spring), 20–30.

Keeler, E. B. (1994). Decision analysis and cost-effectiveness analysis in women's health care. *Clinical Obstetrics and Gynecology, 37*(1), 207–215.

Kelly, K. C., Huber, D. G., Johnson, M., McCloskey, J. C., & Maas, M. (1994). The Medical Outcomes Study: A nursing perspective. *Journal of Professional Nursing, 10*(4), 209–216.

Kieffer, E., Alexander, G. R., & Mor, J. (1992). Area-level predictors of use of prenatal care in diverse populations. *Public Health Reports, 107*(6), 653–658.

Kirshner, B., & Guyatt, G. (1985). A methodological framework for assessing health indices. *Journal of Chronic Diseases, 38*(1), 27–36.

Kirwan, J. R., Chaput de Saintonge, D. M., Joyce, C. R. B., Holmes, J., & Currey, H. L. F. (1986). Inability of rheumatologists to describe their true policies for assessing rheumatoid arthritis. *Annals of Rheumatic Diseases, 45,* 156–161.

Lamb, G. S. (1992). Conceptual and methodological issues in nurse case management research. *Advances in Nursing Science, 15*(2), 16–24.

Lange, L. L., & Jacox, A. (1993). Using large data bases in nursing and health policy research. *Journal of Professional Nursing, 9*(4), 204–211.

Lasker, R. D., Shapiro, D. W., & Tucker, A. M. (1992). Realizing the potential of practice pattern profiling. *Inquiry, 29*(3), 287–297.

Lave, J. R., Pashos, C. L., Anderson, G. F., Brailer, D., Bubloz, T., Conrad, D., Freund, D. A., Fox, S. H., Keeler, E., Lipscomb, J., Luft, H. S., & Provenzano, G. (1994). Costing medical care: Using Medicare administrative data. *Medical Care, 32*(7), JS77–JS89.

Lee, T. H., & Goldman, L. (1989). Development and analysis of observational data bases. *Journal of the American College of Cardiology, 14*(3, Suppl. A), 44A–47A.

Leidy, N. K. (1991). Survey measures of functional ability and disability of pulmonary patients. In B. L. Metzger (Ed.), *Synthesis conference on altered functioning: Impairment and disability* (pp. 52–79). Indianapolis, IN: Nursing Center Press of Sigma Theta Tau International.

Lewis, B. E. (1995). HMO outcomes research: Lessons from the field. *Journal of Ambulatory Care Management, 18*(1), 47–55.

Lieu, T. A., & Newman, T. B. (1998). Issues in studying the effectiveness of health services for children: Improving the quality of healthcare for children: An agenda for research. *HSR: Health Services Research, 4*(33), 1041.

Loegering, L., Reiter, R. C., & Gambone, J. C. (1994). Measuring the quality of health care. *Clinical Obstetrics and Gynecology, 37*(1), 122–136.

Lohr, K. N. (1988). Outcome measurement: Concepts and questions. *Inquiry, 25*(1), 37–50.

Lowenberg, J. S. (1994). The nurse-patient relationship reconsidered: An expanded research agenda. *Scholarly Inquiry for Nursing Practice: An International Journal, 8*(2), 167–190.

Ludbrook, A. (1990). Using economic appraisal in health services research. *Health Bulletin, 48*(2), 81–90.

Lynn, J., & Virnig, B. A. (1995). Assessing the significance of treatment effects: Comments from the perspective of ethics. *Medical Care, 33*(4), AS292–AS298.

Maas, M. L., Johnson, M., & Moorhead, S. (1996). Classifying nursing-sensitive patient outcomes. *Image—The Journal of Nursing Scholarship, 28*(4), 295–301.

Mahrenholz, D. M. (1991). Outcomes research and nurses. *Nursing Connections, 4*(1), 58–61.

Mark, B. A. (1995). The black box of patient outcomes research. *Image—The Journal of Nursing Scholarship,*(1), 42.

Marschke, P., & Nolan, M. T. (1993). Research related to case management. *Nursing Administration Quarterly, 17*(3), 16–21.

Mattson, M. E., & Donovan, D. M. (1994). Clinical applications: The transition from research to practice. *Journal of Studies on Alcohol, 12*(Suppl.), 163–166.

McCormick, B. (1990). Outcomes in action: The JCAHO's clinical indicators. *Hospitals, 64*(19), 34–38.

McCormick, L. A., Lang, N., Zielstorff, R., Milholland, K., Saba, V., & Jacox, A. (1994). Toward standard classification schemes for nursing language: Recommendations of the American Nurses Association Steering Committee on Databases to Support Clinical Nursing Practice. *Journal of the Medical Informatics Association, 1*(6), 421–427.

McDonald, C. J., & Hui, S. L. (1991). The analysis of humongous databases: Problems and promises. *Statistics in Medicine, 10*(4), 511–518.

McNeil, B. (1993). Use of claims data to monitor patients over time: Acute myocardial infarction as a case study. *Annals of the New York Academy of Sciences, 703,* 63–73.

McNeil, B. J., Pedersen, S. H., & Gatsonis, C. (1992). Current issues in profiling quality of care. *Inquiry, 29*(3), 298–307.

Mitchell, J. B., Bubolz, T., Pail, J. E., Pashos, C. L., Escarce, J. J., Muhlbaier, L. H., Weisman, J. M., Young, W. W., Epstein, R. S., & Javitt, J. C. (1994). Using Medicare claims for outcomes research. *Medical Care, 32*(7 Suppl.), JS38–JS51.

Mittelmark, M. B., Hunt, M. K., Heath, G. W., & Schmid, T. L. (1993). Realistic outcomes: Lessons from community-based research and demonstration programs for the prevention of cardiovascular diseases. *Journal of Public Health Policy, 14*(4), 437–462.

Molde, S., & Diers, D. (1985). Nurse practitioner research: Selected literature review and research agenda. *Nursing Research, 34*(6), 362–367.

Moorhead, S., Clarke, M., Willits, M., & Tomsha, K. A. (1998). Nursing Outcomes Classification implementation projects across the care continuum. *Journal of Nursing Care Quality, 12*(5), 52–63.

Moritz, P. (1991). Innovative nursing practice models and patient outcomes. *Nursing Outlook, 39*(3), 111–114.

Moses, L. E. (1995). Measuring effects without randomized trials? Options, problems, challenges. *Medical Care, 33*(4), AS8–AS14.

Nadzim, D. M., Turpin, R., Hanold, L. S., & White, R. E. (1993). Data-driven performance improvement in health care: The Joint Commission's Indicator Measurement System (IMSystem). *The Joint Commission Journal on Quality Improvement, 19*(11), 492–500.

Nelson, E. C., Landgraf, J. M., Hays, R. D., Wasson, J. H., & Kirk, J. W. (1990). The functional status of patients: How can it be measured in physicians' offices? *Medical Care, 28*(12), 1111–1126.

Neuhauser, D. (1990). Ernest Amory Codman, M.D., and end results of medical care. *International Journal of Technology Assessment in Health Care, 6*(2), 307–325.

O'Connor, G. T., Plume, S. K., & Wennberg, J. E. (1993). Regional organization for outcomes research. *Annals of the New York Academy of Sciences, 703,* 44–51.

Orchard, C. (1994). Comparing healthcare outcomes. *British Medical Journal, 308*(6942), 1493–1496.

Oster, G. (1988). Economic aspects of clinical decision making: Applications in patient care. *American Journal of Hospital Pharmacy, 45*(3), 543–547.

Ottenbacher, K. J., Johnson, M. B., & Hojem, M. (1995). The significance of clinical change and clinical change of significance: Issues and methods. *American Journal of Occupational Therapy, 42*(3), 156–163.

Patrick, D. L., & Deyo, R. A. (1989). Generic and disease-specific measures in assessing health status and quality of life. *Medical Care, 27*(3 Suppl.), S217–S232.

Powe, N. R., Turner, J. A., Maklan, C. W., & Ersek, M. (1994). Alternative methods for formal literature review and meta-analysis in AHCPR Patient Outcomes Research Teams. *Medical Care, 32*(7), JS22–JS37.

Power, E. J., Tunis, S. R., & Wagner, J. L. (1994). Technology assessment and public health. *Annual Review of Public Health, 15,* 561–579.

Prior, D. B., & DeLong, E. R. (1994). Programmed Outcome Research Teams (PORTs) and implications for clinical practice. *The American Journal of Cardiology, 73*(6), 34B–38B.

Ramsey, J. A., McKenzie, J. K., & Fish, D. G. (1982). Physicians and nurse practitioners: Do they provide equivalent health care? *American Journal of Public Health, 72*(1), 55–57.

Rettig, R. (1990). History, development, and importance to nursing of outcomes research. *Journal of Nursing Quality Assurance, 5*(2), 13–17.

Riesenberg, D., & Glass, R. M. (1989). The Medical Outcomes Study. *JAMA, 262*(7), 943.

Robinson, J. O., & Finch, D. (1997). Elements for a report care: One institution's experience moving from theory to trial. Communicating health–care quality. *Journal of Nursing Care Quality, 11*(6), 14–25.

Rovine, M. J., & Von Eye, A. (1991). *Applied computational statistics in longitudinal research.* San Diego, CA: Academic Press.

Saba V. K. (1997). An innovative home health care classification (HHCC) system. In MJ Rantz, et al. *Classification of nursing diagnosis.* Proceedings of the 12th Conference of the North American Nursing Diagnosis Association. Glendale, CA: Cinahl Information Systems, pp. 13–15.

Schmitt, M. H., Farrell, M. P., & Heinemann, G. D. (1988). Conceptual and methodological problems in studying the effects of interdisciplinary geriatric teams. *The Gerontologist, 28*(6), 753–764.

Sidani, S., & Irvine, D. (1999). A conceptual framework for evaluating the nurse practitioner role in acute care settings. *Journal of Advanced Nursing, 30*(1), 58–66.

Siegel, J. E. (1998). Cost-effectiveness analysis and nursing research—Is there a fit? *Image—The Journal of Nursing Scholarship, 30*(3), 221–222.

Sledge, C. B. (1993). Why do outcomes research? *Orthopedics, 16*(10), 1093–1096.

Sonnenberg, F. A., Roberts, M. S., Tsevat, J., Wong, J. B., Barry, M., & Kent, D. L. (1994). Toward a peer review process for medical decision analysis models. *Medical Care, 32*(7), JS52–JS64.

Spector, W. D. (1990). Functional disability scales. In B. Spilker (Ed.), *Quality of life assessments in clinical trials* (pp. 115–129). New York: Raven Press.

Spitzer, W. O. (1987). State of science 1986: Quality of life and functional status as target variables for research. *Journal of Chronic Disease, 40*(6), 465–471.

Stewart, A. L., Greenfield, S., Hays, R. D., Wells, K., Rogers, W. H., Berry, S. D., McGlynn, E. A., & Ware, J. E. (1989). Functional status and well-being of patients with chronic conditions. *JAMA, 262*(7), 907–913.

Stewart, B. J., & Archbold, P. G. (1992). Nursing intervention studies require outcome measures that are sensitive to change: Part 2. *Research in Nursing & Health, 16*(1), 77–81.

Stone, D. W. (1998). Methods for conducting and reporting cost-effectiveness analysis in nursing. *Image—The Journal of Nursing Scholarship, 30*(3), 229–234.

Swaen, G. M. H., & Meijers, J. M. M. (1988). Influence of design characteristics on the outcomes of retrospective cohort studies. *British Journal of Industrial Medicine, 45*(9), 624–629.

Tanenbaum, S. J. (1994). Knowing and acting in medical practice: The epistemological politics of outcomes research. *Journal of Health Politics, Policy and Law, 19*(1), 27–44.

Temple, R. (1990). Problems in the use of large data sets to assess effectiveness. *International Journal of Technology Assessment in Health Care, 6*(2), 211–219.

Tengs, T. O., Adams, M. E., Pliskin, J. S., Safran, D. G., Siegel, J. E., Weinstein, M. C., & Graham, J. D. (1995). Five hundred life-saving interventions and their cost-effectiveness. *Risk Analysis, 15*(3), 369–390.

Tidwell, S. L. (1993). A graphic tool for tracking variance & comorbidities in cardiac surgery case management. *Progress in Cardiovascular Nursing, 8*(2), 6–19.

Timm, J. A., & Behrenbeck, J. G. (1998). Implementing the Nursing Outcomes Classification in a clinical information system in a tertiary care setting. *Journal of Nursing Care Quality, 12*(5), 64–72.

Turk, D. C., & Rudy, T. E. (1994). Methods for evaluating treatment outcomes: Ways to overcome potential obstacles. *Spine, 19*(15), 1759–1763.

U.S. Congress, Office of Technology Assessment. (1994). *Identifying health technologies that work: Searching for evidence* (Publication No. OTA-H-608). Washington, D. C.: U.S. Government Printing Office.

Veatch, R. M. (1993). Justice and outcomes research: The ethical limits. *The Journal of Clinical Ethics, 4*(3), 258–261.

Vermeulen, L. C., Jr., Ratko, T. A., Erstad, B. L., Brecher, M. E., & Matuszewski, K. A. (1995). A paradigm for consensus: The University Hospital Consortium Guidelines for the use of albumin, nonprotein colloid, and crystalloid solutions. *Archives of Internal Medicine, 155*(4), 373–379.

Verran, J. A., Mark, B. A., & Lamb, G. (1992). Psychometric examination of instruments using aggregated data. *Research in Nursing & Health, 15*(3), 237–240.

Volinn, E., Diehr, P., Ciol, M. A., & Loeser, J. D. (1994). Why does geographic variation in health care practices matter (And seven questions to ask in evaluating studies on geographic variation)? *Spine, 19*(18S), 2092S–2100S.

Von Eye, A. (Ed.). (1990a). *Statistical methods in longitudinal research: Volume I: Principles and structuring change.* Boston: Academic Press.

Von Eye, A. (Ed.). (1990b). *Statistical methods in longitudinal research: Volume II: Time series and categorical longitudinal data.* Boston: Academic Press.

Von Korff, M., Koepsell, T., Curry, S., & Diehr, P. (1992). Multi-level analysis in epidemiologic research on health behaviors and outcomes. *American Journal of Epidemiology, 135*(10), 1077–1082.

Watkins, L., & Wagner, E. (1982). Nurse practitioner and physician adherence to standing orders: Criteria for consultation or referral. *American Journal of Public Health, 72*(1), 55–57.

Wennberg, J. E. (1990). Outcomes research, cost containment, and the fear of health care rationing. *The New England Journal of Medicine, 323*(17), 1202–1204.

Wennberg, J. E., Barry, M. J., Fowler, F. J., & Mulley, A. (1993). Outcomes Research, PORTs, and health care reform. *Annals of the New York Academy of Sciences, 703,* 52–62.

Werley, H., Devine, E., Zorn, C., Ryan, P., & Westra, B. (1991). The nursing minimum data set: Abstraction tool for standardized, comparable, essential data. *American Journal of Public Health, 81*(4), 421–426.

Werley, H., & Lang, N. (1988). *Identification of the nursing minimum data set.* New York: Springer.

White, K. L. (1993). Health care research: Old wine in new bottles. *The Pharos of Alpha Omega Alpha Honor Medical Society, 56*(3), 12–16.

Wiener, J. M., Hanley, R. J., Clark, R., & Van Norstrand, J. F. (1990). Measuring the activities of daily living: Comparisons across national surveys. *Journal of Gerontology, 45*(6), S229–S237.

Wilson, I. B., & Cleary, P. D. (1995). Linking clinical variables with health-related quality of life: A conceptual model of patient outcomes. *JAMA, 273*(1), 60.

Wood, L. W. (1990). Medical treatment effectiveness research. *Journal of Occupational Medicine, 32*(12), 1173–1174.

Wray, N. P., Ashton, C. M., Kuykendall, D. H., Petersen, N. J., Souchek, J., & Hollingsworth, J. C. (1995). Selecting disease-outcome pairs for monitoring the quality of hospital care. *Medical Care, 33*(1), 75–89.

Zielstorff, R., Hudgings, C., Grobe, S., & the National Commission on Nursing Implementation Project (NCNIP) Task Force on Nursing Information Systems. (1993). *Next generation nursing information systems: Essential characteristics for professional practice.* Washington, D. C.: American Nurses' Association.

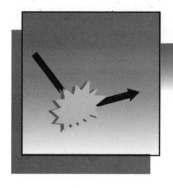

CHAPTER 13

INTERVENTION RESEARCH

This chapter describes a revolutionary new approach to intervention research that holds great promise for designing and testing nursing interventions. The approach is very new, and you are unlikely to find many published studies using the techniques. The current approach to testing interventions, the "true experiment," is being seriously questioned by an growing number of scholars, because modifications in the original design have decreased its validity (Adelman, 1986; Bergmark & Oscarsson, 1991; Chen, 1990; Egan et al., 1992; Fawcett et al., 1994; Lipsey, 1993; Nolan & Grant, 1993; Rothman & Thomas, 1994; Scott & Sechrest, 1989; Sechrest et al., 1983; Sidani & Braden, 1998; Yeaton & Sechrest, 1981). The presentation of the new methodology for designing and testing interventions in this chapter is heavily based on two decisive books that reflect this new approach, Sidani and Braden's (1998) *Evaluating Nursing Interventions: A Theory Driven Approach* and Rothman and Thomas's (1994) *Framework For Intervention Research,* and on the works of scholars on which these books are based.

The chapter content defines the term *nursing intervention*, discusses problems with the "true experiment," provides an overview of intervention research, and describes the process of conducting intervention research—which consists of planning the project, gathering information, developing an intervention theory, designing the intervention, establishing an observation system, testing the intervention, collecting and analyzing data, and disseminating results. Examples of the steps of the process are provided from published studies.

WHAT ARE NURSING INTERVENTIONS?

Nursing interventions are defined as "deliberative cognitive, physical, or verbal activities performed with, or on behalf of, individuals and their families [that] are directed toward accomplishing particular therapeutic objectives relative to individuals' health and well-being" (Grobe, 1996, p. 50). We would expand this definition to include nursing interventions that are performed with, or on behalf of, communities. Sidani and Braden (1998, p. 8) define interventions as "treatments, therapies, procedures, or actions implemented by health professionals to and with clients, in a particular situation, to move the clients' condition toward desired health outcomes that are beneficial to the clients."

A nursing intervention can be defined in terms of (1) a single act (e.g., changing the position of a patient), (2) a series of actions at a given point in time (e.g., management by an intensive care nurse of an abrupt increase in the intracranial pressure of a patient with brain injury, responding to the grief of a family whose loved one has died), (3) a series of actions over time (e.g., implementing a protocol for the management of a newly diagnosed diabetic patient by a primary care nurse practitioner, management of a chronically depressed patient), or (4) a series of acts performed collaboratively with other professionals (e.g., implementing a clinical pathway, conducting a program to reduce smoking in a community). Rather than targeting patients, some interventions target health care providers (e.g., a continuing education program), the setting (e.g., a change in staffing pattern), or the care delivery (e.g., a change in the structure of care).

Currently, nursing interventions tend to be viewed as discrete actions. For example, "Position the limb with sandbags." "Raise the head of the bed 30 degrees." and "Explore the need for attention with the patient." There is little conceptualization of how these discrete actions fit together (McCloskey & Bulechek, 1992). Interventions must be described more broadly as all of the actions required to address a particular problem (Abraham et al., 1992).

Some of the purposes of interventions are risk reduction, prevention, treatment or resolution of a health-related problem or symptom, management of a problem or symptom, and prevention of complications associated with a problem. Some interventions have multiple purposes or multiple outcomes or both. Desired outcomes vary with the purpose and might include continued absence of a problem, resolution of a problem, successful management of a problem, or absence of complications (Sidani & Braden, 1998).

The terminology and operationalization of a nursing intervention varies with the clinical setting and among individual nurses. Each nurse may describe a particular intervention differently. Nursing intervention vocabulary varies in different settings, such as intensive care, home care, extended care, and primary care. There is little consistency in the performance of an intervention. An intervention is often applied differently each time by a single nurse and is even less consistently applied by different nurses. There is lack of clarity in how an intervention should be implemented. Even in published nursing studies, descriptions of interventions tested lack the specificity and clarity given to describing the methods of measurement used in a study (Egan et al., 1992).

The problem with definition and operationalization of nursing interventions is illustrated by the work of Schmelzer and Wright (1993a, 1993b), gastroenterology nurses who, in 1993, began a series of studies examining the procedure for administering an enema. They found no research in nursing or medical literature that tested the effectiveness of various enema procedures. There is no scientific evidence to justify the use of various procedures for administering enemas. The amount of solution, temperature of solution, speed of administration, content of the solution (soap suds, normal saline, water?), positioning of the patient, measurement of expected outcomes, or possible complications are based on tradition and have no scientific basis.

For their first study, Schmelzer and Wright (1996) conducted telephone interviews with nurses across the country, trying to identify nursing practice patterns in the methods used to administer enemas. They found none. They developed a protocol for administering enemas and pilot-tested it on hospitalized patients awaiting liver transplantation. In their subsequent study, using a sample of liver transplant patients, these researchers tested for differences in effect of different enema solutions (Schmelzer et al., 2000). Currently, Schmelzer (1999–2001) is conducting a study funded by the National Institute for Nursing Research to compare the effects of three enema solutions on the bowel mucosa. Well subjects are paid $100 for each of three enemas, after which a small biopsy specimen is collected.

The strategy taken by these researchers must be used to test the effectiveness of many current nursing interventions. What methods should be used for this testing, however? The "true experiment," quasi-experimental studies, or the new intervention research methods? The "gold standard" has been the "true experiment."

PROBLEMS WITH THE TRUE EXPERIMENT

Clark (1998) points out that the true experiment is based on a logical-positivist approach to research, an atheoretical strategy that focuses on discovering laws through the accumulation of facts. Few nurse researchers hold to the logical-positivist perspective. The logical-positivist approach is not consistent with nursing philosophy or with the theory-based approach through which nursing is building its body of knowledge.

Traditionally, adherence to rigid rules was required to define a study as a true experiment

(Fisher, 1935). These rules were (1) random sampling from individuals representative of the population, (2) equivalence of groups, (3) complete control of the treatment by the researcher, (4) a control group that receives no treatment or a placebo treatment, (5) control of the environment in which the study is conducted, and (6) precise measurement of hypothesized outcomes. True experiments are powerful in demonstrating the validity of the cause. However, the method is easier to apply in studying corn (as Fisher did) than when studying humans (as we do).

Studying humans requires modifications in the true experiment that have weakened the power of the design and threatened its validity. Because of requirements related to the use of human subjects and problems related to access to sufficient numbers of subjects, random sampling has been abandoned by most health care researchers. This change has decreased representativeness of the sample. Subjects in "true experiments" (e.g., clinical trials) are increasingly unlike the target population. Compared with the patients in a typical clinical practice, subjects selected for experimental studies are less likely to include, for example, individuals who have comorbidities, who are being cared for by a primary care provider, who are not receiving treatment, who are in a managed care program or health maintenance organization (HMO), who receive Medicare benefits, who are uninsured, undereducated, or poor, or who are members of minority groups. Treatments affect various groups differently and for some groups have no effect. Knowing how various groups are affected has become increasingly important with the advent of managed care (Orchid, 1994). Equivalence of groups, a critical element of the experimental design, continues to be addressed through random assignment. In analyzing data from clinical trials, however, Ottenbacher (1992) found random assignment ineffective in making groups more equivalent.

Complete control of the intervention is a problem in many experimental studies. Often clinicians, unskilled staff, or family members, rather than the researchers, apply the intervention. It is sometimes difficult to determine the extent to which (or even whether) a subject received the defined experimental treatment. Sometimes the intervention must be modified to meet the needs of particular subjects, a practice problematic to the assumptions of the experimental design. Comparison groups are often given the usual treatment, but the "usual treatment" is seldom defined. In most cases, there is wide variation in usual treatment that makes valid comparisons with the treatment group problematic and increases the risk of a Type II error.

Dependent variables selected to test the intervention sometimes do not reflect actual outcomes. In many clinical situations, the desired outcomes of an intervention occur a considerable time after the intervention, making their measurement during a reasonable period (in a funded study) difficult, if not impossible. Intermediate outcomes may be substituted, with the assumption that end outcomes can be inferred from intermediate outcomes, a questionable assumption in many cases (Orchid, 1994).

'True experiments,' as they were originally designed, are the most effective way to determine validity of the cause; modifications make them less valid. Using quasi-experimental designs creates more threats to internal validity. Statistical conclusion validity is threatened by a number of problems related to the newly defined "true experiment," the most important of which is the absence of a random sample. External validity is threatened by problems with representativeness.

To what extent can one deviate from the original definition of a true experiment and be justified in using the term to refer to one's study? To what extent can quasi-experimental studies justifiably replace the true experiment as a means to validate the effectiveness of an intervention? Does an atheoretical, modified true experiment provide sufficient evidence to justify implementing an intervention in clinical practice?

With the growing demand for evidence-based practice, it is essential that nursing interventions be clearly defined and tested for effectiveness, including those that have become part of nursing through history, tradition, or trial-and-error, and that new interventions be designed and tested to address unresolved nursing problems (Abraham et al., 1992).

What strategies, however, do we use to accomplish this?

INTERVENTION RESEARCH

Intervention research is a revolutionary new methodology that holds great promise as a more effective way of testing interventions. Intervention research shifts the focus from causal connection to causal explanation. In *causal connection*, the focus of a study is to provide evidence that the intervention causes the outcome. In *causal explanation*, in addition to demonstrating that the intervention causes the outcome, the researcher must provide scientific evidence to explain why the intervention causes changes in outcomes, how it does so, or both. Causal explanation is theory based. Thus, research focused on causal explanation is guided by theory, and the findings are expressed theoretically. A broad base of methodologies, including qualitative ones, is used to examine the effectiveness of the intervention (Rothman & Thomas, 1994; Sidani & Braden, 1998).

It is becoming increasingly clear that the design and testing of a nursing intervention require an extensive program of research rather than a single well-designed study (Rothman & Thomas, 1994; Sidani & Braden, 1998). It is also clear that a larger portion of nursing studies must be focused on designing and testing interventions.

THE PROCESS OF INTERVENTION RESEARCH

The process of intervention research described here was derived from strategies currently being used in a variety of disciplines, including evaluation research and the design and development approach used in engineering. The process begins with an extensive search for relevant information that is applied to the development of an intervention theory. The intervention theory guides the design and development of an intervention, which is then extensively tested, refined, and retested. When the intervention is sufficiently refined and evidence of effectiveness has been obtained, field testing is used to ensure that the intervention can be effectively implemented in clinical settings. Results of field tests are used to further refine the intervention to improve clinical application. An observation system is developed for use throughout the design and development process, allowing the researchers to observe events related to the intervention naturalistically and to perform analyses of these observations. Efforts to disseminate the newly refined intervention are extensive and are planned as an integral part of the research program.

Project Planning

Because an intervention research project comprises multiple studies conducted over a period of years, careful planning is advised in advance of initiating the project. Some of the issues that must be decided initially are (1) who will be included in the project team, (2) how the team will function, and (3) whether or not to use participatory research methods, which stipulate the inclusion of stakeholders and key informants as members of the project team.

FORMING A PROJECT TEAM

Because of the nature of intervention research, it may be advisable to gather a multidisciplinary project team to facilitate distribution of the work and a broader generation of ideas. Because both quantitative data and qualitative data will be gathered during the research program, the team should include members experienced in various qualitative and quantitative data collection and analyses approaches. Including a team member with marketing expertise will be beneficial, because the final step of the project will be to market the intervention. Teams will be enhanced by the inclusion of undergraduate, master's, and doctoral nursing students.

Recruiting colleagues located in other areas of the country or the world for the research team can add an important dimension, permitting multisite evaluation studies. Strategies to achieve this goal include (1) contacting researchers with similar interests, (2) attending specialty conferences related to the research area, during which dialogue with researchers can lead to extending an invitation to participate in the project, (3) inviting colleagues to join the project after presentations at a professional meeting, (4) developing a project Internet website that invites participation by other researchers, and (5) developing or participating in an Internet mailing list (listserv) related to the topic. The process of developing a team is dynamic rather than static, with changes occurring as development of the research program continues.

THE WORK OF THE PROJECT TEAM

There is almost always a core group in a project team that carries on most of the work and facilitates maintenance of group activities and task achievement. However, the addition of other people who can contribute in lesser ways can benefit the project. For example, it may be useful to establish liaison groups from the clinical facilities in which the intervention will be studied. In some cases, the addition of other advisory groups can be helpful.

The initial focus of the team is to clarify the problem. In analyzing identified problems, the team should answer the questions listed in Table 13–1. Considering these questions may provide new insights, leading to a redefinition of the problem, and may enable the design of a more effective intervention. Sidani and Braden (1998) caution the project team to be alert to the risk of making a Type III error. A *Type III error* is the risk of asking the wrong question—a question that does not address the problem of concern. This error is most likely to occur when a thorough analysis of the problem is not conducted and, thus, the researchers have a fuzzy or inaccurate understanding of the problem for which a solution is needed. The solution, then, does not fit the problem. A study conducted on the basis of a Type III error provides the right answer to the wrong question, leading to the incorrect conclusion that the newly designed intervention will resolve the problem.

Once the problem to be examined by the project is clarified, the goals and objectives of the project must be established. Project team tasks include gathering information, developing an intervention theory, designing the intervention, establishing an observation system, testing the intervention, collect-

TABLE 13–1
PROBLEM ANALYSIS QUESTIONS

1. For whom is the situation a problem?
2. What are the negative consequences of the problem for the affected individuals?
3. What are the negative consequences of the problem for the community (health care providers, system, or agency)?
4. Who (if anyone) benefits from conditions as they are now?
5. How do they benefit?
6. Who should share the responsibility for "solving" the problem?
7. What behaviors (of whom) must be changed for patients to consider the problem solved?
8. What conditions must be changed to establish or support needed change?
9. What is an acceptable level of change?
10. At what level should the problem be addressed?
11. Is this a multilevel problem requiring action at a variety of levels of change?
12. Is it feasible (technically, financially, politically) to make changes at each identified level?
13. What behaviors (of whom) need to change for providers to consider the problem solved?
14. Who are stakeholders?
15. What does each stakeholder have invested in the status quo?
16. Who might support change?
17. Who might function as champion?

Questions 1 through 12 adapted from Fawcett S. B., Suarez-Belcazar, Y., Belcazar F. E., White, G. W., Paine, A. L., Blanchard, K. A., & Embree, M. G. (1994). Conducting intervention research—the design and development process. In J. Rothman & E. J. Thomas (Eds.), *Intervention research: Design and development for human service* (pp. 25–54). New York: Haworth Press.

ing and analyzing data, and disseminating the intervention. Seeking funding for the various studies of the project will be an ongoing effort.

USING PARTICIPATORY RESEARCH METHODS

A *participatory research strategy*, which involves including representatives from all groups that will be affected by the change (*stakeholders*) as collaborators, is recommended by some supporters of intervention research. This strategy facilitates broad-based support for the new intervention from the target population, the professional community, and the general public. Disadvantaged groups are recommended as stakeholders in interventions that would or should affect members of that group (Fawcett et al., 1994). Table 13–2 lists examples of stakeholder groups.

TABLE 13–2
EXAMPLES OF STAKEHOLDER GROUPS

Clinical nurses
Physicians
Pharmacists
Administrators
Other allied health professionals
Third party payers
Chaplains
Representatives of the target population
Families living in poverty
Residents of low-income groups
Ethnic groups
Groups for whom English is a second language
People with poor access to care
People not currently receiving care
Institutionalized psychiatric patients
Patients of public health services
Representatives of rural communities
Youth
People with physical disabilities

The selection of *key informants* is also recommended, unless the researchers are currently practicing in the setting or settings in which the intervention will be implemented (Fawcett et al., 1994). Key informants can help researchers become familiar with settings. Whether the setting is a clinical agency or an element of the community, key informants can explain local ways to researchers and help them gain access to the settings. Interactions with key informants can also assist researchers in identifying what the researchers can offer to the setting and how to articulate the benefits of the project to groups or organizations. Key informants in stakeholder groups, such as "natural leaders," advocates, and service providers, can furnish information useful for determining and addressing the concerns or needs of these groups as the intervention project is being planned (Fawcett et al., 1994).

If a participatory research approach is used, the project team consists of the researchers, stakeholders, and key informants. At the initial meeting, members of the team familiar with the process of intervention research should be asked to explain the process to the team. A team discussion of the problem and possible solutions is then conducted. One rule of team meetings should be that team members will avoid imposing their views of the problem or its solution on the group but, rather, will attempt to understand issues of importance to others on the project team. Consensus is used to arrive at decisions. All members of the team will be involved in activities such as reviewing and integrating literature and other information gathered, developing the intervention theory, designing studies, interpreting results, and disseminating findings (Fawcett et al., 1994).

Gathering Information

An extensive search for information related to the project is conducted. This gathering of information is considerably more extensive than the traditional literature review. A wide variety of methods is used to gather information. These include the methods listed in Table 13–3, which are used to obtain in-depth information on the topics listed in Table 13–4. Of particular importance is gathering sources of information about the intervention. In designing a study, it is important not to "reinvent the wheel." Therefore, the researchers must do what others have done to address the problem.

TABLE 13–3
METHODS USED FOR INFORMATION GATHERING

Integrative reviews of the literature
News media
Consumer publications
Position papers
Standards or guidelines
Meta-analyses
Introspection related to personal experience
Observation
Case studies
Qualitative studies
Focus groups
Consensus conferences
Concept analyses
Foundational studies
Health policy analyses
Ethical analyses
Health services research
Retrospective chart reviews
Outcomes studies
Descriptive and correlational studies, including regression analyses and path analyses
Q-sorts
Delphi studies
Methodological studies to develop or validate methods of measurement

TABLE 13–4
Topics for Information Gathering

The Problem

Nature of the problem (actual or potential)
Manifestations
Causative factors
Level of severity
Variation in different patient populations
Variation in different conditions

The Intervention

How people who have actually experienced the problem have
addressed it
Previous interventions designed to address the problem
Unsuccessful interventions
Value to target population
Sensitivity to cultural diversity
Biases or prejudices
Processes underlying the intervention effects
Intervention actions
  Components
  Mode of delivery
  Strength of dosage
    Amount
    Frequency
    Duration

Mediating Processes

Patient characteristics
Setting characteristics
Intervener characteristics

Expected Outcomes

Contextual factors
Environmental factors
Patient characteristics
Provider factors
Health care system factors

Potential sources of information about interventions for the problem of concern are listed in Table 13–5 and discussed here. During the exploration of each source of information, the queries listed in Table 13–6 should be addressed. Information gathered from all sources requires careful analysis and synthesis. Undergraduate, master's, and doctoral nursing students as well as clinicians, working with the project team, could play a major role in the gathering and synthesis of information.

TAXONOMIES

An *intervention taxonomy* is an organized categorization of all interventions performed by nurses.

A number of classifications of nursing interventions have been developed: The Nursing Diagnosis Taxonomy (Warren & Hoskins, 1995), Home Health Care Classifications (Saba, 1995), the Omaha System (Martin & Scheet, 1995), the Nursing Interventions Classification (NIC) (Bulechek & McCloskey, 1999; Bulechek et al., 1995), and the Nursing Intervention Lexicon and Taxonomy (NILT) (Grobe, 1996). Grobe (1996, p. 50) suggests that "theoretically, a validated taxonomy that describes and categorizes nursing interventions can represent the essence of nursing knowledge about care phenomena and their relationship to one another and to the overall concept of care." Although taxonomies may contain brief definitions of interventions, they do not provide sufficient detail to allow one to implement the intervention. Also, the actions identified in taxonomies may be too discrete for testing and may not be linked to resolution of a particular patient problem (Sidani & Braden, 1998).

DATABASES

Some health care agencies now have databases storing information about patient care activities. These databases can be used for secondary analyses examining many of the topics listed in Table 13–3. For example, a group of 17 home health care agen-

TABLE 13–5
Sources of Information About Interventions

Nursing intervention taxonomies
Computerized databases containing data on nursing interventions
Nursing textbooks
State-of-the-art journal articles on nursing interventions
Previous intervention studies (theses, dissertations, publications)
Clinical guidelines: *http://www.guidelines.gov*
Critical pathways
Intervention protocols
Best Practices Network: *http://www.best4health.org*
Interviews with patients who have experienced the problem and
related interventions
Interviews with providers who have addressed the problem
Interviews with researchers who have tested previous interventions
Probing of personal experiences
Observations of care provided to patients with the problem
Consumer groups who are stakeholders, e.g., Gilda Clubs, Reach
for Recovery

TABLE 13–6
QUERIES RELEVANT TO ALL SOURCES

1. Are there existing interventions or practices that have been successful?
2. What made a particular practice effective?
3. Are there existing interventions or practices that were unsuccessful?
4. What caused them to fail?
5. Which events appeared to be critical to success (or failure)?
6. What conditions (e.g., organizational features, patient characteristics, broader environmental factors) may have been critical to success (or failure)?
7. What specific procedures were used in the practice?
8. Was information provided to patients or change agents about how and under what conditions to act?
9. Were modeling, role-playing, practice, feedback, or other training procedures used?
10. What positive consequences, such as rewards or incentives, and negative consequences, such as penalties or disincentives, helped establish and maintain desired changes?
11. What environmental barriers, policies, or regulations were removed to make it easier for the changes to occur?
12. What proportion of people experiencing a specific cluster of symptoms were diagnosed (correctly or not) as having a particular diagnosis, and of this group, who received what treatment?
13. Should a treatment or procedure have been performed?
14. Did persons with a particular diagnosis receive appropriate treatment?
15. What proportion of people with the cluster of symptoms received no treatment?

Adapted from Fawcett S. B., Suarez-Belcazar, Y., Belcazar F. E., White, G. W., Paine, A. L., Blanchard, K. A., & Embree, M. G. (1994). Conducting intervention research—the design and development process. In J. Rothman & E. J. Thomas (Eds.), *Intervention research: Design and development for human service* (pp. 25–54). New York: Haworth Press; and Kase & Lune (1992).

cies in Tarrant County, Texas, arranged to jointly establish a joint patient care database. All the home care nurses were provided with laptops linked to the database. They entered data related to their patient care visits into the database and were able to access information about a patient while in the patient's home. The central database site employed nurses with master's degrees and a statistician as well as computer technicians. Reports from the database were generated and sent to the individual nursing homes. Data could be pooled for analysis purposes. It was possible to query the database for information on patients receiving a particular intervention. Information related to patient characteristics, the timing of the intervention in relation to the emer-

gence of the problem, costs, outcomes, and characteristics of the intervener could be obtained.

TEXTBOOKS

Textbooks often provide little or no instruction on how the interventions listed should be implemented. If they provide any information, it is usually in the form of a long list of nursing actions that should be taken in a particular patient situation. The lists given for the same patient situation vary with the textbook (McCloskey & Bulechek, 1992). One exception is a textbook by Bulechek and McCloskey (1999) entitled *Nursing Interventions: Essential Nursing Treatments* (1999), which is organized by the NIC taxonomy and provides detailed descriptions of nursing interventions with a known research base.

STATE-OF-THE ART JOURNAL ARTICLES

Articles delineating state-of-the-art care in relation to particular patient care situations are appearing in nursing journals. Such an article is generally the result of an extensive review of the literature and may be a good source of information when available. The article often contains a discussion of the problem and elements of an intervention theory and proposes strategies for future research. References cited in such articles can often add valuable information to that obtained by computer search. Letters to the editor sections of practice journals are also good sources of information about strategies being used by clinicians.

PREVIOUS STUDIES

Previous studies are also an important source of information about the intervention. A previous study usually discusses the problem, describes the intervention procedure, presents measurement methods for variables, offers approaches to design and analysis, gives information that can be used to determine effect size, and discusses problems related to the intervention or the research methodology. Examination of previous studies should include theses and dissertations that may not be published. A search for other unpublished studies may yield valuable information. Use of nursing listservs on the World Wide Web can be an effective way to seek unpublished studies. As with state-of-the-art journals, references from previous studies often yields sources not previously identified through computer searches.

CLINICAL GUIDELINES

Clinical guidelines have been developed for patient care situations by the Agency for Health Care Policy and Research (AHCPR) and other organizations. These guidelines are available on the Internet at *http://www.guidelines.gov* and discussed in Chapter 27. Clinical guidelines define the standard of care for particular patient situations, are interdisciplinary, and are based on an extensive review of the literature focused on findings from previous studies. Although these guidelines are not specific to nursing, elements of the guidelines specify nursing actions.

CRITICAL OR CLINICAL PATHWAYS

Health care agencies often develop critical or clinical pathways that define the expected care activities and the expected outcomes of the care in specific patient care situations. Critical pathways may be developed through the use of findings from previous research, analyses of agency databases, and clinical experiences of the practitioners in the agency. Some agencies consider their critical pathways to be proprietary information, limiting the possibilities of testing them and publishing the results. However, written documentation related to the pathway or interaction with committee members involved in developing the pathway can be useful in specifying the problem, defining the intervention, and obtaining information related to moderator or mediator variables (see later discussion) and outcomes.

BEST PRACTICES NETWORK

The website Best Practices Network (available at: *http://www.best4health.org*) provides recent news about clinical interventions and encourages clinicians to send descriptions of innovative care strategies they have devised. Practices with a sound re-

search base are described. This site is also a good source of information on unpublished intervention strategies being used by clinicians.

PROVIDER INTERVIEWS

Clinicians are an important source of information about the intervention. They have first-hand experience in implementing interventions for the patient problem. They are more familiar than most with the nuances and variations of the situation. Their knowledge often is not sought and seldom is available in journal articles. Information from these sources about unsuccessful practices is particularly valuable (Fawcett et al., 1994).

RESEARCHER INTERVIEWS

Interviews with researchers who have developed and/or tested previous interventions for the problem of concern can provide excellent information to guide the development and testing of a new intervention. Obtaining information from such interviews can often help the project team avoid repeating mistakes in designing the intervention or in the development of the methodology for testing it. Researchers may be contacted by phone, e-mail, or letter. In some cases, it may be important to make a site visit for an interview (Fawcett, et al, 1994).

PATIENT INTERVIEWS

Patients who have experienced the problem under study can provide valuable information often not available from other sources. They offer a completely different perspective from that of providers. Patients or their family members or both may have used interventions not documented in the literature and may have insights about what is needed that may not have been considered previously (Fawcett et al., 1994).

PROBING OF PERSONAL EXPERIENCE

Because of the sparsity of information in the literature on nursing interventions, the researchers may have to rely heavily on a personal knowledge base emerging from expertise in clinical practice.

This knowledge can be elicited through introspection and dialogue with colleagues.

OBSERVATIONS OF PATIENT CARE

Observations of patient care are essential in determining the dynamics of the process of patient care, because in many cases, the care activities are so familiar to clinicians that, in describing it, they leave out components important to the overall process. These observations will be components of the observation system described later in the chapter.

Developing An Intervention Theory

The knowledge obtained through a synthesis of collected information is used to develop a middle-range intervention theory. An intervention theory is explanatory and combines characteristics of descriptive, middle-range theories and prescriptive, practice theories. A *descriptive theory* describes the causal processes occurring. A *prescriptive theory* specifies what must be done to achieve the desired effects, including (1) the components, intensity, and duration required, (2) the human and material resources needed, and (3) the procedures to be followed to produce the desired outcomes.

An intervention theory is also action oriented, providing guidance on how to design, test, and implement the intervention. The intervention theory should contain conceptual definitions, propositions, hypotheses, and any empirical generalizations available from previous studies (Chen, 1990; Chen & Rossi, 1989; Finney & Moos, 1989; Rothman & Thomas, 1994; Sidani & Braden, 1998). The theory will be further refined during the design and development process. Master's and doctoral nursing students, working in collaboration with faculty researchers or with the project team, can provide valuable input for the development of the intervention theory by (1) conducting literature reviews and synthesis, (2) developing class papers related to the intervention theory, (3) conducting class discussions about the intervention theory, which are then communicated to the project team, or (4) meeting with the project team to participate in discussions during development of the intervention theory.

An intervention theory must include a careful description of the problem to be addressed by the intervention, the intervening actions that must be implemented to address the problem, moderator variables that might change the impact of the intervention, mediator variables that might alter the effect of the intervention, and expected outcomes of the intervention. Components of an intervention theory are listed in Table 13–7. Further detail about developing each intervention theory element is provided in the following discussion.

THE PROBLEM

The problem that the intervention theory addresses might be one of alterations in function or of inadequacies in functioning that have the potential of resulting in dysfunction. The problem might also be expressed as a nursing diagnosis. The theoretical description of the problem must include a discussion of the causal dynamics of the problem and how the problem is manifested. The causal processes through which the intervention is expected to affect the problem should be addressed. Variations of the problem in different populations and in different conditions must be clarified. The following excerpt, from a study by Powe and Weinrich (1999) of an intervention designed to reduce cancer fatalism among rural elders, is an example description of the problem that an intervention theory addresses.

• •

"Although the incidence of colorectal cancer has declined among Caucasians, the rates have remained constant among African Americans (American Cancer Society [ACS], 1998). Furthermore, African Americans are 30% more likely to die of cancer than Caucasians (ACS). Detection of colorectal cancer in the early, asymptomatic stages is crucial in reducing mortality. Five-year survival rates approach 93% when the cancer is found early and treated in its localized stages, but they are less than 7% when distant metastases are present at diagnosis (ACS). The incidence of colorectal cancer increases with age (ACS; Griffith, 1993; Hansen, 1995; U.S. Preventive Services Task Force, 1996), and colorectal cancer mortality rates are especially high among rural, socioeconomically disadvantaged African American elders (ACS; U.S. Department of

TABLE 13–7
ELEMENTS OF INTERVENTION THEORY

Problem
  Nature of the problem
  Manifestations
  Causative factors
  Level of severity
  Variation in different patient populations
  Variation in different conditions

Critical Inputs
  Activities to be performed
  Procedures to be followed
  Amounts of the intervention elements (intensity)
  Frequency of the intervention
  Duration of the intervention

Mediating Processes
  Stages of change that occur after the intervention
  Mediating variables that bring about treatment effects
  Hypothesized relations among mediating variables

Expected Outcomes
  Aspects of health status affected
    Physical
    Mental
    Social
    Spiritual
  Timing and pattern of changes
  Hypothesized interrelationships among outcomes

Extraneous Factors
  Contextual factors
  Environmental factors
  Patient characteristics

Treatment Delivery System Resources
  Setting
  Equipment
  Intervener characteristics

Health and Human Services [USDHHS], Public Health Service, 1990). However, these elders are less likely than other Americans to participate in colorectal cancer screening programs (Powe, 1995a; 1995b; Underwood, Hoskins, Cummins, Morris, & Williams, 1994; Weinrich, Weinrich, Boyd, Atwood, & Cervanka, 1992).

". . . ACS currently recommends fecal-occult blood testing (FOBT) annually after age 50. . . . Many factors can influence participation in colorectal cancer screening. Barriers to screening that are known to confront rural, socioeconomically disadvantaged African American elders include cancer fatalism, lack of knowledge of cancer, poverty, and poor access to care (Martin & Henry, 1989; Olsen & Frank-Stromborg, 1993; Powe, 1995b, 1995c, 1997; Underwood & Hoskins, 1994; Weinrich, Weinrich, Boyd, Atwood, et al., 1992).

"Despite awareness of these barriers, successful strategies to increase participation in cancer screening have not been forthcoming. Use of multidimensional interventions that provide information about colorectal cancer in a manner that is culturally sensitive and culturally appropriate for rural, socioeconomically disadvantaged African American elders has been suggested. In particular, interventions must address fatalism, which is believed to be the result of a complex psychological cycle characterized by perceptions of hopelessness, worthlessness, meaninglessness, powerlessness, and social despair (Freeman, 1989; West, Aiken & Todd, 1993). Fatalism has the potential to affect every aspect of the human experience (West, Aiken & Todd, 1993). Cancer fatalism, defined as the belief that death is inevitable when cancer is present, can be viewed as a situational manifestation of fatalism in which the individual becomes entrapped in a cycle of late cancer diagnosis, limited treatment options, and death. Cancer fatalism is most prevalent among African American females, and people with low incomes and low educational levels (Freeman, 1989); Powe, 1995a, 1995b; Underwood & Hoskins, 1994). Fatalistic people are less likely to participate in FOBT (Powe, 1995b).

"Spirituality may provide the cultural foundation to effectively address fatalistic perceptions. Many rural, socioeconomically disadvantaged African American elders exhibit overwhelming spirituality (Powe, 1997). They find meaning through an organized body of thought, experience, and faith concerning the fundamental problems of existence (Emblem, 1992; Reed, 1992). Spirituality is believed to provide a source of meaning and connection to God as well as hope in the face of seemingly overwhelming circumstances (Dombeck & Karl, 1987; Dwyer, Clarke, & Miller, 1990; Emblem, 1992; Scandrett, 1994). Spirituality may be actualized through visits with clergy, interactions with family and friends, personal prayer, and the verbalization of beliefs. These activities play a crucial role in enhancing hope, coping abilities, and positive health beliefs, healthcare behaviors, and healthcare outcomes (Lincoln & Mamiya, 1990; Lloyd, Mc-Connell, & Zahorik, 1994; Reed (1992); Scandrett (1994); Thomas, 1994). Including these aspects of spirituality in an intervention may effectively decrease cancer fatalism.

"Interventions used to increase participation of rural, socioeconomically disadvantaged African American elders in FOBT also must address lack of knowledge of cancer, low literacy, poor vision, and hearing impairments that are prevalent among this population (Hoskins & Rose, 1989; Powe, 1997; Powe & Johnson, 1995; Rosella, Regan-Kubinski, & Albrecht, 1994). Rural, socioeconomically disadvantaged African American elders have less knowledge of colorectal cancer than other Americans (Weinrich, Weinrich, Boyd, Atwood, et al., 1992), and elders with less knowledge have been found to be more fatalistic (Powe, 1995c, 1997) and less likely to participate in FOBT (Powe, 1995b; Weinrich, Weinrich, Boyd, Atwood, et al., 1992)." (Powe & Weinrich, 1999, pp. 583–584) ■

THE INTERVENTION

The theoretical presentation of the intervention must specify what actions, procedures, and intervention strength are required to produce the desired effects. For example, in Powe and Weinrich's (1999) study, if fecal occult blood testing (FOBT) were free, what actions would be required to produce the desired effects? Causal interactions among various elements of the intervention must be explored.

Strong interventions contain large amounts of the elements constituting the intervention. *Strength* of intervention is defined in terms of amount, frequency, and duration. *Intensity* defines the amount of each activity that must be given and the frequency with which each activity is implemented. *Duration* is the total length of time the intervention is to be implemented (Scott & Sechrest, 1989; Sechrest et al., 1983; Sidani & Braden, 1998; Yeaton & Sechrest, 1981). For example, if the intervention were mouth care for stomatitis, (controlling for severity, white blood count, and day in the treatment cycle) strength would be (1) the amount or concentration of mouth solution used, (2) the frequency with which the

mouth care was given, and (3) the number of days (duration) that the mouth care was provided.

Some interventions are relatively simple, and others may be very complex. The *complexity* of the intervention is determined by the type and number of activities to be performed. Complex, multicomponent interventions may require multiple, highly skilled interveners. The effect of moderator variables (see later discussion) on the effectiveness of the intervention must be explored. The theoretical presentation given here guides the operational development of the intervention design.

The intervention designed by Powe and Weinrich (1999) included free transportation to a senior citizen center, free FOBT, and a video presentation described as follows.

· ·

"The intervention group participants viewed a 20-minute videotape titled Telling the Story . . . To Live Is God's Will. A critical element in videotaped interventions is video modeling, or demonstrating the desired behavior, attitudes, and cognitive effects (Meade, 1996). Therefore, the majority of the participants in the video were African American, and the intervention incorporated the study population's language, dress, food preferences, customs, traditions, attitudes, values, and spiritual belief systems (Landrine & Klonoff, 1994; Rosella et al, 1994).

"Telling the Story . . . To Live Is God's Will includes an introduction, three scenes, and a concluding segment. Segments are connected with narration and gospel music. Scene one depicts a dynamic interaction between two elderly women (Ruth and Naomi) in a senior citizen center. Their discussion centers around Naomi's previous participation in colorectal cancer screening, the diagnosis of her colorectal cancer in its early stages, her survival of the cancer, and her encouragement to Ruth to participate in FOBT. Scene one is designed to provide an overview of colorectal cancer and cancer screening and to portray survival after a diagnosis of cancer. Scene two portrays the interaction of Ruth, her husband, and their minister. The discussion allows Ruth and her husband to express their fears of cancer and cancer screening to the minister. The minister alleviates these fears by discussing the importance of caring for one's health from a scriptural perspective. The scene concludes with Ruth, her husband, and the minister agreeing to attend a colorectal cancer screening program. Scene three depicts Ruth, her husband, the minister, and others at a question-and-answer session in which a nurse discusses colorectal cancer and scriptural support for health care and encourages FOBT among the group. The nurse models completion of the FOBT using peanut butter and allows Ruth a return demonstration. This scene is designed to reinforce the information given earlier about colorectal cancer, portray the minister's support for colorectal cancer screening as an acceptable option, and models the appropriate techniques for completing the FOBT kits." (Powe & Weinrich, 1999, p. 585) ■

MODERATOR VARIABLES

A moderator variable is, in effect, a separate independent variable affecting outcomes. A *moderator variable* alters the causal relationship between the intervention and the outcomes. The moderator effect occurs simultaneously with the intervention effect. A moderator variable also may interact with elements of the intervention to alter the direction or strength of changes caused by the intervention. Thus, a moderator variable could cause the intervention to have a negative rather than a positive effect or to have a less powerful effect on outcomes. Moderator variables could also increase the maximum effectiveness of the treatment. An understanding of the causal links between moderator variables and the intervention is critical to implementing an effective intervention in various patient care situations. Moderator variables may be characteristics of patients or of interveners or may be situational (Baron & Kenny, 1986; Lindley & Walker, 1993).

One of the most familiar moderators is the effect of stress on learning from the intervention of patient education. The causal relationship in this case can be modeled as follows:

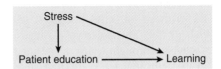

The level of stress occurring at the time of the patient education can change the effect of the education. In very low stress, the patient may not experience a need to know what is being taught, and thus, learning is reduced. High stress at the time of the patient education interferes with the patient's ability to incorporate and apply the information provided by the patient education and thus reduces learning. Moderate stress at the time of patient education maximizes the effect of the intervention.

The level of stress also has a direct effect (as an independent variable) on learning. The relationship of stress in this case could be modeled as follows:

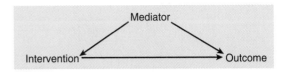

MEDIATOR VARIABLES AND PROCESSES

A *mediator variable* brings about treatment effects after the treatment has occurred. The effectiveness of the treatment process relies on mediator variables. The intervention may have a direct effect on the outcomes, a direct effect on the mediator or mediators, and an indirect effect on outcomes through the mediator variables. The relationship could be modeled as follows:

```
                    Mediator

Intervention ─────────────────► Outcome
```

In other cases, the effect of the intervention occurs only through its effect on the mediator, as follows:

```
Intervention        Mediator        Outcome
```

The expected outcomes of an intervention are the result of a transformational process that occurs as a series of changes in participants and mediator variables after initiation of the intervention. The series of changes are referred to *as mediating processes*. For any intervention, a number of mediating processes may ensue that lead to the outcomes. Although broadly the intervention causes the outcomes, defining the mediating processes explains exactly how the intervention causes the outcomes.

To understand each mediating process, the causal processes must be dissected to identify hypothesized relations among the mediator variables that result in the outcomes. Because the same variable can function as a mediator in some situations and a moderator in other situations, it is important for the intervention theory to specify the mediator-moderator role of the different variables important to the understanding of the phenomenon of interest. The stages of change through which a participant progresses in the transition to the desired state can be expressed in the map of the intervention theory (Baron & Kenny, 1986; Lindley & Walker, 1993; Sidani & Braden, 1998).

In the cancer fatalism study by Powe and Weinrich (1999), the intervention consisted of free transportation, free FOBT, and a spirituality-focused educational program presented by video. The desired outcome was the use of FOBT to screen for colorectal cancer. The researchers listed four barriers to achieving this outcome: cancer fatalism, lack of knowledge of cancer, poverty, and poor access to care. The free FOBT and free transportation addressed the barriers of poverty and poor access to care. The educational component provided information about colon cancer and screening, and the spirituality component targeted cancer fatalism. Information about colon cancer and screening alone has not been effective in raising the number of African American women who use FOBT to screen for colorectal cancer. The mediator variables in the intervention theory were (1) spirituality, (2) cancer fatalism, (3) hope, (4) coping, (5) positive health beliefs, (6) health care behaviors, (7) poverty, and (8) poor access to care. They are illustrated in the map in Figure 13–1.

EXPECTED OUTCOMES

Outcomes are determined by the problem and purpose of the intervention and are the various effects of the intervention. They reflect the changes that occur as a consequence of the intervention. Outcomes may be physical, mental, social, spiritual, or any combination of these types. The timing and pattern of changes must also be specified. *Timing* is the point in time after the intervention that a change is expected to occur. Some changes occur immediately after an intervention, whereas others may not appear for some time. Mediators are referred to in

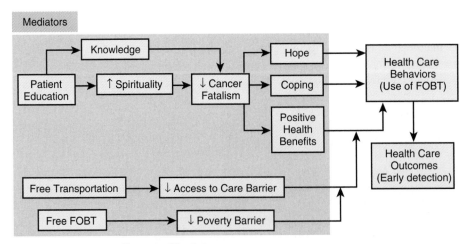

FIGURE 13–1 ■ Map of an intervention theory.

some studies as *intermediate outcomes*. Hypothesized interrelationships among the outcomes must be indicated in the theory.

In Powe and Weinrich's (1999) study, the only outcome measured was increased use of FOBT. In their intervention theory, however, these researchers proposed that the mediators of decreased fatalism, hope, coping, and positive health beliefs resulting from the intervention would be sustained and would continue to generate positive health care behaviors. This proposition could be tested through follow-up longitudinal studies.

EXTRANEOUS FACTORS

Extraneous factors are elements of the environment or characteristics of the patient that significantly affect the problem, the treatment process, or the outcomes. Unlike mediator variables, extraneous factors tend not to be well understood and often are unidentifiable before initiation of a study. They are seldom included in explanations of the causal links between intervention and outcomes. Thus, they are extraneous to existing theoretical explanations of cause. They are sometimes referred to as *confounding variables*. If the researcher recognizes their potential effect, extraneous factors may be held constant (not allowed to vary) or measured so that they can be statistically controlled during analysis. Careful analyses may indicate that some variables defined as extraneous are actually moderator or mediator variables (Sidani & Braden, 1998).

In Powe and Weinrich's (1999) study, an important confounding variable might have been previous experience with cancer in a subject's family. Only one subject in Powe and Weinrich's study reported a family member with colorectal cancer, so the effect of this potentially confounding variable could not be examined.

PATIENT CHARACTERISTICS

Researchers are increasingly attending to the influence of individual characteristics on the patients' response to illness or to treatment. Sidani and Braden (1998, p. 64) point out that "client characteristics may affect the clients' general susceptibility to illness; the nature and extent of the presenting prob-

lem; the design and selection of interventions; the clients' beliefs, values, and preferences for treatments; and the clients' response to illness and to treatment." Patient characteristics also affect the extent to which the patient becomes involved in health-promoting lifestyles.

Patient characteristics of importance to a particular intervention can be identified (1) during the information gathering period, (2) through pilot studies designed to test the intervention, and (3) through the established observation system. The intervention theory must identify and categorize patient characteristics that have the potential of influencing response to the treatment (Frank-Stromborg et al., 1990; Johnson et al., 1993). The researcher must identify or develop methods to measure patient characteristics relevant to the intervention using the observation system. Patient characteristics that have been identified by researchers as influencing the response to illness or the treatment are listed in Table 13–8. In Powe and Weinrich's (1999) study, previous experiences with cancer would be an important patient characteristic.

ENVIRONMENTAL FACTORS

An intervention "occurs in a sociocultural, economic, political, and organizational context, any part of which may affect both the processes and the outcomes, usually in ways we little understand" (Hegyvary, 1992, p. 21). Environmental factors identified in Powe and Weinrich's (1999) study were African American culture, rural residence, and poverty. Two environmental factors of particular importance to the problem, the intervention, and the outcomes in many intervention theories are intervener characteristics and setting characteristics.

Intervener Characteristics

Interveners are individuals who are involved in the delivery of the study intervention. They are usually health care professionals functioning in the role of clinicians or researchers. In some cases, however, the intervener may be a family member, a neighbor, the patient, or an unskilled staff person employed within the treatment delivery system. The personal and professional characteristics of interveners affect

TABLE 13–8
PATIENT CHARACTERISTICS

Personal characteristics	Demographic characteristics (age, gender, education, ethnicity)
	Personality traits
	Emotional status
	Cognitive processes
	Beliefs and attitudes
	Values
	Resourcefulness
	Sense of mastery
	Perceived self-competence
	Lifestyle
	Learning style preference
	Behavior
	Cognitive processes
	Cultural norms
	Affect
	  Anxiety
	  Depression

Illness or health-related characteristics	Physiological and physical functioning Biological characteristics Psychosocial functioning Individual's definition of health Value for health Beliefs about health and illness Severity of illness Stage of illness Perceived symptom burden Functional status Ability to perform activities of daily living Number of symptoms experienced
Available resources	Social support Employment Health care cost coverage Income Coping strategies

interpersonal and technical aspects related to implementation of the intervention. Thus, it is important to identify important intervener characteristics in the intervention theory. The researchers must develop measurement methods to gather data on the interveners for the observation system. Table 13–9 lists some of the personal and professional intervener characteristics identified by Sidani and Braden (1998) that might modify the implementation of an intervention. In Powe and Weinrich's (1999) study, intervener characteristics that might modify implementation of the intervention are age, gender, ethnicity, familiarity with the community, language use, dress, attitudes, values, spiritual belief systems, and previous interactions with the participants.

Setting Characteristics

The setting in which the intervention will be delivered has a potential influence on the expected intervention outcomes. For example, variation in the clinical activities performed by the staff nurses in different settings can affect outcomes. The setting can serve as a moderator variable either by facilitating or impeding implementation of the intervention or by muting or intensifying intervention effects (Conrad & Conrad, 1994). In addition, the setting may modify the way the intervention is implemented. Such influences can be threats to the external validity of conclusions and cannot be ignored.

TABLE 13–9
INTERVENER CHARACTERISTICS

Personal characteristics	Age Gender Ethnicity Communication skills Demeanor Friendliness Courtesy Sensitivity Being gentle and understanding Tone of voice Body language Appearance Attractiveness Neatness Method of presentation Maturity Emotional well-being Perceptual and cognitive style Expectancies Economic incentives
Professional competencies	Skills needed to implement intervention Educational background Discipline Specialty training Level of competence or expertise Beliefs and attitudes toward health and health care Preferences for treatment modalities Manual dexterity Job satisfaction

The setting of Powe and Weinrich's (1999) study was a senior citizen center. The setting was familiar to study participants, who attended the center daily and were given lunch there. They were also acquainted with other participants. In their intervention theory, Powe and Weinrich set forth the expectation that the familiarity and comfortableness of the setting for participants would enhance their response to the intervention.

Other aspects of the setting that must be addressed by the intervention theory are the resources needed to carry out the activities of the intervention. Resources include (1) equipment, (2) space for the intervention, (3) the availability of adequately educated professional interveners with the experience needed to provide the intervention, (4) adequate support staff, (5) a political-social environment that facilitates implementation of the intervention, and (6) access to telephones and computers (Sidani & Braden, 1998). Table 13–10 lists some of the setting characteristics identified by Sidani and Braden (1998).

TABLE 13–10
SETTING CHARACTERISTICS

Personal features	Access to participants
	Convenience to participants
	Availability of equipment
	Physical layout and attractiveness
	Noise level
	Ambient temperature
	Light
	Comfort of furniture
	Provision for privacy
	Room interior design or decoration
	Familiarity to participants
	General ambience
Psychosocial features	Organizational culture
	Norms and policies
	Standards and protocols of care
	Composition of interdisciplinary health care team
	Differences in skill mix of providers
	Number of providers
	Type of institution
	Geographical context
	Staff satisfaction
	Stress levels of staff
	Leadership style
	Professional practice model

The Health Care System

In today's health care arena, factors related to the system of care within which the intervention is provided may play an important role in the effectiveness of the intervention. The system of care may be a managed care system, an HMO, a home health care system, a nursing home corporation, the community, a primary care provider's office, a public health clinic in the community, or the patient's home. In some cases, the patient may be the community, and a group of committed citizens may be the health care system of interest.

DEVELOPING A CONCEPTUAL MAP OF THE INTERVENTION THEORY

The researcher should develop a map illustrating the elements of the intervention and the causal links among them. Elements must be clearly defined, and causal links explained. The map should show all causal pathways described in the intervention theory, including moderator and mediator variables. Testable propositions emerging from the theory must be listed.

Although Powe and Weinrich (1999) did not develop a map expressing an intervention theory, the map shown in Figure 13–1 was constructed from the discussion of elements of the intervention theory and causal links in their paper.

Designing the Intervention

During the design period, and guided by the intervention theory, the project team specifies the procedural elements of the intervention and develops an observation system (Fawcett et al., 1994). The intervention may be (1) a strategy, (2) a technique, (3) a program, (4) informational or training materials, (5) environmental design variables, (6) a motivational system, or (7) a new or modified policy. The intervention must be specified in sufficient detail to allow its consistent implementation by interveners.

During the design process, the intervention will emerge in stages, as it is repeatedly tested, redesigned, and retested. Training materials and programs for interveners also must be developed and repeatedly tested and revised. Design criteria are established to evaluate the implementation of the intervention and outcomes.

In addition to detailed development of the intervention, operational development of the design guided by the theory should include the following activities:

- Define the target population
- List acceptable strategies for selecting a sample
- Identify subgroups that might show differential effects of the intervention
- Specify essential characteristics of interveners
- Determine study variables
- Indicate appropriate measures of variables
- Specify the appropriate time or times to measure outcomes
- Indicate what analyses to perform and what rela-

tionships to test on the basis of the relationships among the treatment and the moderator, mediator, and outcome variables specified by the intervention theory

Ulbrich (1999) describes a detailed and carefully thought out development of an intervention theory of exercise as self-care, for which she then proposes an intervention design. The following summary and extracts from her study illustrate the theory and the proposed intervention design.

● ●

Intervention Theory

A map of Ulbrich's theory is shown in Figure 13–2. The central concept of the theory is exercise.

"Exercise as a health behavior is a purposeful physical activity of a type, intensity, and duration needed to reach a moderate level of exertion and

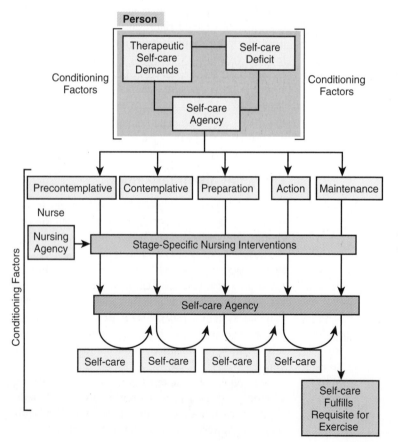

FIGURE 13–2 ■ Ulbrich's theory. (From Ulbrich, S. L. [1999]. Nursing practice theory of exercise as self-care. *Journal of Nursing Scholarship, 31*[1], 69.)

improve some aspect of health or well-being. The activity of exercise must be goal directed and consciously chosen, not accidental or random. Exercise results from the relationship among the type, intensity, and duration of activity. While all exercise is physical activity, not all physical activity is exercise. The degree or amount of physical activity required in order for an activity to be exercise is determined by the level of exertion resulting from energy and oxygen consumption. At least a moderate level of exertion must be reached for an activity to be considered exercise. Exercise is ultimately done to improve some aspect of health, the objective state of bodily and mental functioning, or well-being, a person's subjective perceptions of one's current condition of existence (Orem, 1995).

"The antecedents of exercise, those elements that must occur before exercise can occur, are a person, time, energy, oxygen, a conducive environment, physical capabilities, knowledge, motivation, intention, and a decision to exercise. Contextual factors are characteristics of people and their sociocultural or physical environments that have been shown to influence exercise behavior, such as attitude, self-efficacy, age, health, social support, and knowledge.

"The consequences of exercise are numerous and depend on the specific exercise behavior and the frequency that it is performed. The goal of this model is to prevent cardiovascular disease (CVD) and improve cardiovascular fitness as a consequence of exercise. Clinical evidence is clear and there is professional consensus that exercise reduces the risk of CVD by: reducing blood pressure, reducing resting heart rate, improving cardiovascular fitness, improving peripheral and coronary circulation, improving lipoprotein profiles, improving blood glucose control in diabetics, and weight loss and control (American College of Sports Medicine [ACMS], 1995; U.S Department of Health and Human Services [DHHS], 1996).

"In Orem's Self-Care Deficit Nursing Theory, self-care is defined as, 'learned goal-oriented activity of individuals (the) behavior that exists in concrete life situations directed by people to self or the environment to regulate factors that affect their own development and functioning in the interests of life,

health, and well-being' (Orem, 1995, p. 435). Exercise would be considered self-care because it is a purposeful action done by people in the interests of life, health, and well-being. People have a self-care demand for exercise because it is an action that should be done by the individual over time to promote life, health, and well-being. Self-care agency is the ability of mature people to identify factors that must be controlled to meet self-care demands, to develop a plan of self-care, and perform self-care to meet their requisites (Orem, 1995). . . .

"The transtheoretical model is based on the belief that people progress through specific stages of change (SOC) as they reduce high-risk behaviors or adopt health promotional behaviors. Progression through SOC reflects the temporal dimension in which change occurs (Prochaska & Marcus, 1994). These stages are precontemplation (not thinking about changing), contemplation (seriously thinking about changing but not doing it yet), preparation (intending, deciding, and preparing for change but not actually or consistently performing the new behavior), action (the first 6 months of overtly performing a behavior), and maintenance (regular practice of a behavior after the first 6 months). . . . Most interventions currently used to promote exercise behavior are designed for people in the preparation stage and are not effective because only a small percentage of people are in that stage. The majority of people are in the precontemplative and contemplative stages. In the transtheoretical model interventions are designed for each stage of change using the processes of change and decisional balance factors most likely to influence a person's behavior or decision making in that stage. People are expected to progress through one stage per month until maintenance is achieved. Interventions can include any combination of stage-based self-help manuals, counseling, pamphlets, personal phone calls, computer reports and programs, and mailed literature." (Ulbrich, 1999, pp. 67–68)

Target Population

"This practice theory was developed for adults at risk for CVD, one of the most prevalent conditions in the U.S. population. CVD is any chronic progressive disease of the heart and blood vessels (AHA,

1997). . . . To identify members of this population, a classification system was developed using range definitions of Orem's basic conditioning factors, therapeutic self-care demands, self-care limitations, and nursing systems. These elements not only define the population but they also provide information about factors that affect the self-care and nursing agency in meeting the self-care requisite for exercise. The target population is adults between the ages of 18 and 65 years." (Ulbrich, 1999, p. 68)

Sample Selection

"Subjects include those that need exercise and are willing to participate. . . . Potential subjects are assessed for potential risk factors. . . . The person's SOC is determined. . . . A person is identified as at risk for CVD by using a risk-factor questionnaire and an activity recall measure. The reported activity or exercise would have been compared to the self-care requisite for exercise to reduce CVD risk. If this self-care demand were greater than the person's self-care agency, an exercise self-care deficit would exist." (Ulbrich, 1999, p. 69)

"No racial, religious, socioeconomic, or gender group is excluded. To be at increased risk for CVD and have a self-care deficit, their risk factors must include (a) physical activity that does not meet the requisite for cardiorespiratory health and (b) at least one other risk factor. However, these people do not have previously diagnosed CVD, major signs and symptoms suggestive of CVD, or any other illness in which exercise is not physically possible or contraindicated (ACSM, 1995). The patterns of living vary from living independently or with spouses and children. Developmentally these people range from early adulthood to early retirement." (Ulbrich, 1999, p. 68)

Subgroups

No subgroups were identified.

Essential Characteristics of Interveners

"These situations require nurses to have special knowledge and skill in order to provide nursing care to people (Orem, 1995). Knowledge of the practice theory, Orem's theory, the transtheoretical model, the population, and exercise is an essential part of nursing agency needed to promote exercise as self-care. Because exercise requires volitional control, consciousness, and some physical capabilities, nurse actions to promote exercise as self-care could only be done in partial and supportive-educative nursing systems." (Ulbrich, 1999, p. 67)

Intervention

"The nurse, in a supportive educative system, enters into a relationship with a person that needs [the intervention] and is willing to participate. Mutual goal setting occurs. Ideally, the aim is to progress through one stage each month until the self-care demand for exercise is met. The nurse acts using nursing self-care agency to implement stage-specific nursing interventions. These enhance the person's self-care agency and basic conditioning factors. In time, the person progresses to the SOC as determined by reassessment, and new nursing interventions are implemented. This process can continue until the maintenance stage is reached and the self-care requisite for exercise is fulfilled." (Ulrich, 1999, p. 69)

Variables

"The processes of change, decisional balance factors, self-efficacy, and other basic conditioning factors should be assessed to determine their influence on the person's exercise self-care agency and self-care demands. . . . Outcomes measures for this practice theory are changes in exercise behavior and changes in stage of change for exercise and self-efficacy for exercise." (Ulbrich, 1999, p. 69)

Measures

"Stage of change, self-efficacy, and processes of change can be determined using the stages-of-change, or stage of exercise-adoption instrument (Marcus, Selby, Niaura, & Rossi, 1992), processes-of-change measure (Marcus, Rossi, Selby, Niaura, & Abrams, 1992), and self-efficacy measure (Marcus, Selby, Niaura, & Rossi, 1992). The tools in existence have proven helpful, reliable, and valid in some studies but measurement of exercise behavior is difficult. Therefore, measurement tools should be selected with care." (Ulbrich, 1999, p. 69)

Times to Measure Outcomes

Outcomes are assessed monthly until the self-care requisite for exercise is fulfilled.

Statistical Analyses

Statistical analyses were not discussed. ■

Establishing an Observation System

The use of an observation system is a novel idea in nursing intervention research. However, it is one of the important strengths of intervention research. The observation system is designed and implemented before any changes are made in the patient care situation. An *observation system* allows the researchers to (1) observe events related to the phenomenon naturalistically, (2) discover the extent of the problem, (3) observe the intervention being implemented, and (4) detect effects of the intervention. Patients affected by the problem under study can help identify behaviors and environmental conditions that must be observed. Observations should be made also of patient characteristics, intervener characteristics, setting characteristics, dynamics of the health care system, and use of resources (Fawcett et al., 1994; Sidani & Braden, 1998). Possible elements of the observation system are listed in Table 13–11.

Observations lead to insights about what must be changed by the intervention or changed in the system so that the intervention can be effective. The observation system also serves as a means of feedback for refining early prototypes of the intervention and, thus, is closely tied to designing and pilottesting the intervention. Behavioral events that are elements of the intervention or that are components of the environment that could affect the effectiveness of the intervention must be defined and observed. The observation activities provide information important to specifying the procedural elements of the intervention. Procedural elements that are important to observe include (1) use of information, (2) use of skills, (3) training, (4) environmental

TABLE 13–11
ELEMENTS OF OBSERVATION SYSTEM

Before the Intervention
  Characteristics of the problem
  Patient characteristics
    Characteristics of patients with the problem who receive the intervention
    Characteristics of patients with the problem who do not receive the intervention
  Intervention characteristics
    Elements of intervention
    Intensity of intervention
    Duration of intervention
  Use of the intervention
  Intervener characteristics
    Professional and personal characteristics
  Setting characteristics
    Resources used, e.g., equipment and supplies
    Physical layout
    Staff
    Organizational support
    Events occurring during the study that affected the intervention

During the Intervention
  Problem characteristics
  Patient characteristics
    Who were the target population?
    How many participants were recruited?
    How many who were approached refused to participate?
    What reasons did they give for refusal?
    What were the characteristics of the participants?
    What were the characteristics of those who refused to participate?
    How do those who accepted and those who refused compare with the target population?
  Intervention characteristics
    Elements of intervention
    Intensity of intervention
    Duration of intervention
  Intervener characteristics
    Professional and personal characteristics
    Were training sessions provided?
    Content of training sessions
    What interveners attended training sessions?
    How did interveners handle participants?
    Did more than one intervener care for a participant?
  Setting characteristics
    Administrative arrangements made
    Events occurring during intervention that might affect implementation
    Type of equipment used
    Was the same type of equipment used for all participants?

After the Intervention
  Process of outcomes

change strategies, (5) policy changes or enforcement strategies used, and (6) reinforcement and punishment procedures (Fawcett et al., 1994; Sidani & Braden, 1998).

Nursing students at all levels of education could participate in the observation system. The system could be used to give undergraduate students the chance to participate clinically in nursing research activities. Students involved in research projects, theses, or dissertations might gather or analyze data for the observational system.

The observational methods used and the extent of observations vary with the financial and personnel resources available. The development of the observation system should be based on knowledge acquired through the information-gathering process. The observation system must include measures of variables in the setting that might affect the problem, the intervention, or the outcomes. Possible elements of the observation system are listed in Table 13–11.

The observation system must be designed carefully and must include methods for measuring the elements of interest. The procedures should be specified in enough detail that they can be replicated. Observers must be carefully trained. Observations must be made before initiation of the intervention, during the intervention, and after the intervention. The observation system must be developed to allow monitoring of the extent to which the intervention was implemented as planned during the period in which it was provided.

The types of measurement used depend on a number of factors, such as (1) the number of individuals and behaviors to be observed, (2) the length of observations, (3) the size of observation intervals during an observation session, and (4) the availability of observers. Measures that might be used include tape-recorded interviews, field notes of observers, coding forms, checklists, knowledge tests, scales to measure aspects such as attitudes or beliefs, measures of physiological dimensions of the patient state, videotapes of the intervention being provided, and event logs. In addition to measures for direct observation, measures for self-monitoring or self-reporting by patients or interveners may be

necessary for events that are difficult to observe directly (Barlow et al., 1989).

The validity and reliability of measurement methods used must be evaluated. Criteria for use by the observer to determine whether or not the event being studying has occurred must be developed. These criteria may be used to determine the start of an observation period (Fawcett et al., 1994). Steps of the observation process are listed in Table 13–12.

In Powe and Weinrich's (1990) study, an observation system, designed to gather data from a number of studies testing the intervention, might have observed and measured the following elements:

Before the Intervention. The proportion of the target population obtaining FOBT; sources of FOBT in the study region; costs of FOBT from various sources; reasons for not obtaining FOBT, including cost concerns, access to care, income, fatalism, hope, coping, health beliefs, health care behaviors, spirituality, knowledge about cancer, and experience with family members who have cancer.

During the Intervention. Intervener characteristics, such as age, ethnicity, gender, spirituality, and previous experience with target population; setting characteristics; subject characteristics gathered

---

TABLE 13–12
STEPS OF THE OBSERVATION PROCESS

1. Determine elements that must be observed on the basis of the intervention theory.
2. Develop methods of measuring essential elements.
3. Develop criteria for determining whether or not the event to be observed has occurred.
4. Select observers.
5. Train observers.
6. Develop scoring instructions to guide recording of desired behaviors or products.
7. Develop schedule of observations to include:
   a. What is happening before the intervention is implemented.
   b. What is happening during the intervention.
   c. What changes occur after the intervention.
8. Perform preliminary analysis of preintervention data.
9. Apply preliminary analysis results to further develop the intervention.
10. Analyze changes in environment and behaviors before, during, and after the intervention.
11. Refine intervention theory.

before the intervention, such as age, gender, and ethnicity; number and characteristics of individuals choosing not to participate in the study.

After the Intervention. Use of FOBT; longitudinal follow-up to determine changes in health beliefs, health care behaviors, hope, and coping over time.

Testing the Intervention

The intervention is tested in stages, revised, and retested until a satisfactorily designed intervention emerges. The stages of testing are (1) development of a prototype, (2) analogue testing, (3) pilot testing, (4) formal testing, (5) advanced testing, and (6) field testing.

DEVELOPING A PROTOTYPE

A *prototype* is a primitive design that has evolved to the point that it can be tested clinically. The prototype is defined by the intervention theory. Developing a prototype involves establishing and selecting a mode of delivery of the intervention. Ulbrich's (1999) intervention, described previously, is a prototype. Considerable refinement would be required before it could be used in an intervention study (Fawcett et al., 1994).

ANALOGUE TESTING

For some interventions, before the pilot test, it is useful to test prototypes in analogue situations, using actors to play roles in the intervention. Members of the project team, staff from the settings to be used for the project, or nursing students might play roles in provision of the prototype intervention. The actor interveners follow the intervention steps prescribed by the prototype. Videotapes of the proceedings allow careful analysis of the adequacy of the prototype. Observers also make notes during the prototype test of missing elements, insights gained, or questions that must be explored by the project team (Fawcett et al., 1994).

PILOT TESTING

Multiple pilot tests are needed for intervention research. These pilot studies are used for the following purposes:

1. To determine whether the prototype will work.
2. To guide refinement of the prototype. The intervention is first evaluated according to standards established in that particular care situation. The established design criteria are then used to evaluate the effectiveness of the prototype. This evaluation enables the researchers to optimize the intervention before further testing.
3. To test and refine instructions, manuals, or training programs.
4. To determine whether the description of the intervention is provided in sufficient detail to allow replication by clinicians and other researchers. Clinicians should also be queried about their reasoning and decisions during the implementation of the intervention.
5. To examine reliability, validity, and usability of measurement methods in the target population.
6. To test the design.
7. To determine unanticipated effects.

Pilot tests should be conducted in settings similar to those in which the intervention will be used and with subjects similar to those who will typically be receiving the intervention. Observation techniques are used to gather the information needed to revise the prototype. Pilot tests are ideal for graduate nursing student research projects, theses, or dissertations conducted in collaboration with the project team.

FORMALLY TESTING AN INTERVENTION

The most desirable formal test of the intervention is a conventional experimental design to determine whether the intervention causes the intended effects. The design should be as rigorous as possible. Power analyses should be used to determine a sample size sufficient to avoid a Type II error. Analyses should be performed to ensure that the treatment and control groups are comparable on important variables. Measurement instruments with documented reliability and validity should be used. The effect size should be reported for each outcome examined. The observation system established before the initiation of testing is continued, and patient characteristics, intervener characteristics, and setting characteristics are measured (Sidani & Braden, 1998). Two-way analysis of variance (ANOVA) or multivariate analysis of covariance (ANCOVA) is commonly used to test for effects of the intervention. These analyses are described in Chapter 22.

Identifying the Required Resources

The formal test of an intervention must occur in a setting that can provide the required resources to implement the intervention optimally. The resources needed are defined by the nature of the intervention and its level of complexity. The resources required include (1) institutional support for testing the intervention, (2) availability of equipment and materials needed to administer the intervention, (3) availability of target participants who would benefit most from the intervention, and (4) interveners with the full range of skills needed to implement the intervention. If any of these resources is at a level less than required, variability in delivery of the intervention may occur, affecting the intervention outcomes (Chen, 1990; Lipsey, 1993; Rosen & Proctor, 1978; Sidani & Braden, 1998).

Maintaining the Integrity of the Intervention

In a formal test of an intervention, it is critical that the integrity of the intervention be maintained. *Integrity* is the extent to which the intervention is implemented as it was designed. The design defines what activities are to be done and when, where, how, and by whom they are to be carried out.

Lack of integrity is a discrepancy between what was planned and what was actually delivered. It may occur if the intervention is not clearly described or if the interveners do not have a clear understanding of what activities to perform, when, or with whom. Lack of integrity can occur because of insufficient training or lack of guidance during the period of formal testing. In some cases, interveners may not interpret instructions as expected by the researchers. This is most likely to occur when

elements of the intervention are not well defined and clearly circumscribed, leading to different interpretations by the interveners (Kirchhoff & Dille, 1994; Rezmovic, 1984; Sechrest et al., 1983; Sidani & Braden, 1998; Yeaton & Sechrest, 1981).

Loss of integrity can also occur because participants are exposed to different elements of the intervention or given different levels of strengths of the intervention. Loss of integrity may occur because the intervention is not provided in a consistent manner, interveners tailor the intervention to the needs of individual patients, or the intervention requires active involvement of the participants in implementing the intervention in settings away from the intervener's immediate supervision. These differences lead to differences in levels of outcomes and can result in an inability to detect significant treatment effects; thus, they may lead to incorrect conclusions about the effectiveness of the intervention (Rezmovic, 1984; Rossi & Freemen, 1993; Sidani & Braden, 1998; Yeaton & Sechrest, 1981). Level of response and motivation of subjects is another variation on outcomes. Factors affecting intervention integrity are listed in Table 13–13.

Kirchhoff and Dille (1994) described problems they experienced in maintaining the integrity of

---

TABLE 13–13
FACTORS AFFECTING INTEGRITY OF INTERVENTION

Inadequate training of interveners
Poorly defined intervention
Variation in strength of intervention provided
Variation in elements of intervention provided
Ease in implementing intervention activities
Intervention's level of complexity
Inadequate planning
Inadequate guidance during study
Level of skill of interveners
Level of staff commitment to the intervention
Level of organizational commitment to the intervention
Number of interveners
Number of sites involved in implementing the intervention
Level of compliance of staff with treatment protocol
Interactional style of interveners
Changes in organization policies after initiation of study
Changes in brand of equipment used
Changes in composition of interveners

their study intervention; the following excerpt is taken from their study.

· ·

"In 1983 a study was conducted on the Rehabilitation Nursing Unit at University of Utah Hospital to test the effectiveness of a decontamination procedure on vinyl urinary leg and bed bags. Rehabilitation patients with bladder dysfunction use two urine bags, a daytime leg bag (for concealment under clothing) and a nighttime larger-volume bed bag. Because the usually closed urinary drainage system is disrupted at least twice daily, a procedure for decontamination was necessary if the bags were to be reused safely rather than discarded daily. . . .

"The solution instilled into bags daily was a 1:3 solution of bleach to water with a contact time of at least 30 minutes (Hashisaki et al., 1984). Based on that study's results of effective decontamination, the bag replacement schedule was changed from daily to weekly at a considerable savings. . . .

"Four years later cost-conscious nurses proposed a 4-week in-hospital reuse for the bags. Because the bags are marketed as single-use disposable items, this time frame needed to be carefully tested. . . .

"In the decontamination study, the frequency, regularity, and daily nature of the intervention called for several individuals participating solely from a scheduling perspective. Because of the long-term nature of this study (3-year funding period), vacation time and other leave time had to be considered. . . .

"In this study, communication occurred with the obvious: the Rehabilitation Unit nursing staff, the attending physicians, nursing and hospital administration, and the epidemiology nurses. Inadvertently, the not so obvious did not receive or recall study information: the per diem nurses who floated to the unit, the rehabilitation residents who rotated in and out of the unit every 3 months, and the housekeepers. These three groups of people had the potential to influence results, affect subject accrual, and contribute to missing or altered data if they were not informed about the study requirements. Per diem staff either had not been taught about the protocol

or performed the former standard for the procedure. Residents who were not informed believed that the study would limit a patient's progression in bladder management and were reluctant to have their patients entered into the study. At times the housekeepers inadvertently discarded the drainage equipment as it was air drying, which resulted in the loss of data and affected costs of the grant.

"Using the procedure as a performance checklist, observations of the staff's performance of the procedure were completed before and during the study at least every 6 months. At the same time, the study progress was reviewed and the staff was questioned about activities they were required to perform for the study. These included how to label and use the bags, what to do when problems arise, the criteria for inclusion in the study, and the differences between the experimental and control groups. On subsequent observations, this time period also was used to discuss reported or discovered concerns about the individual's performance. . . .

"Despite the intensive planning and compliance checks, problems arose. Housekeeping personnel discarded bags that were air-drying. Per diem staff discarded the bags, performed the procedure incorrectly, or neglected to do it at all. Discoveries were made by the nursing staff or study staff that bags had been mislabeled, applied to the wrong patient, or had incomplete information on the bag label. When a few staff devised a method of hanging the leg bag to dry by knotting its tubing, the effect of air-drying was reduced. In all these instances, individual staff members were contacted and the situation was corrected. . . .

"Although it appears that a number of problems were uncovered, close monitoring showed these problems before there was major impact on the integrity of the study. When close monitoring does not occur, a lack of problems may really be a lack of discovery. A false sense of security can result." (Kirchhoff & Dille, 1994, pp. 32–36) ■

On the basis of these experiences, which they were good enough to share with us, Kirchhoff and colleagues modified their intervention protocol for future studies (Dille & Kirchhoff, 1993; Dille et al., 1993).

ADVANCED TESTING OF THE INTERVENTION

Advanced testing of the intervention occurs after sufficient evidence is available that the intervention is effective in achieving desired outcomes. This stage of testing might begin after a single well-designed study indicates a satisfactory effect size but is more likely to be initiated after a series of studies in which the intervention is modified or the findings are replicated. Advanced testing focuses on identifying variations in effectiveness based on patient characteristics, intervener characteristics, and setting characteristics.

Testing Variations in Effectiveness Based on Variations in Patient Characteristics

Intervention effects that have been determined through the use of a sample of white, middle-class Americans may not have the same effect with other groups. The intervention should be tested in various ethnic groups. Pilot tests may indicate the necessity of refining the intervention to make it culturally appropriate. The poor and undereducated may respond differently to interventions, because (1) they have a different view of health and of preventive behaviors and (2) they may not understand educational components of interventions that were designed for people with a higher level of education. For the same reasons, scales designed for the white middle class may not be effective measures in different ethnic groups or in the undereducated. Thus, modifications in the intervention and in the design may be necessary.

Studies also must be conducted to examine the effect of the intervention on groups with comorbidities or differing levels of severity of illness. Other variations in patient characteristics, such as age, gender, and diagnosis, may be important to examine. Characteristics specific to the intervention may be identified as important to study in determining differential effects. If sufficiently large samples were obtained in the initial study, these patient characteristics may be available from the observa-tion system and may involve secondary analyses of available data.

Testing Variations in Effectiveness Based on Setting

If the setting is held constant, so that all interventions are provided in the same place, under the same conditions, and among all subjects, then the setting effects will be potentially confounded with the treatment effects. Therefore, one component of testing the intervention is to set up multisite projects, in which the settings are varied and the effects of the settings on outcomes are examined (Sidani & Braden, 1998).

Testing Variations in Effectiveness Based on Variations in Intervener Characteristics

The initial study examining the effectiveness of the intervention is usually conducted under ideal conditions. Ideal conditions involve the selection of highly educated interveners judged to be experts in the field of practice related to the intervention. However, after the intervention is found to be effective, questions arise regarding the use of less well-prepared interveners to provide the intervention. Studies should be conducted to determine variations in the effectiveness of the intervention based on competencies of interveners.

Testing Variations in Effectiveness Based on Strength of an Intervention

The strategy of testing the variations of an intervention's strength is used to determine the amount of treatment that provides optimal strength in achieving the desired outcome. To test this issue, the researcher must be able to provide varying doses of the intervention. The researcher might vary the intensity of the intervention, the length of time of a single treatment, or the span of time over which the intervention is continued or repeatedly given.

Path Analyses

Path analyses are used to examine the causal processes through which each component of an intervention has its effect, including moderator and mediator variables. The design tests the validity of the intervention theory. Reliable measures of each of the processes and each of the outcome variables are included in the design. Structural equation analysis is used to examine the contribution of each component to the outcome (Sidani & Braden, 1998). Path analysis is described in Chapter 21.

Preference Clinical Trials

In the typical clinical trial, subjects are randomized into groups. However, in some cases, patient preference is an important variable. The effect of active choice on outcomes is important to understand. Wennberg and colleagues (1993, p. 56) indicate that "when symptom reduction and improvement in the quality of life are the main effects of treatment and the proper decision involves the evaluation of risk aversion and degree of botheredness, then these topics cannot be ignored; they must be made the object of investigation." Thus, in *preference clinical trials,* rather than being randomized to subject groups, patients choose among all treatments available. The Standard Gamble Method (explain) is used to measure an individual's preferences in situations of uncertainty (Gafni, 1994).

Treatment Matching

Treatment matching is performed to compare the relative effectiveness of various treatments. Treatment matching designs are used when the following conditions are met: (1) there is no clearly superior treatment for all individuals with a given problem, (2) a number of treatments with some proven efficacy are relatively comparable in their effectiveness for undifferentiated groups of subjects, and (3) there is evidence of differential outcomes, either within or among treatments, for defined subtypes of patients (Donovan et al, 1994). No control group is used. Sampling criteria are selected to promote heterogeneity rather than homogeneity. Randomization is used, but stratification, matching, and other strategies can be used to obtain balanced distribution. Creative sampling methods may be required to fulfill sampling requirements (Carroll et al., 1994; Connors et al., 1994; DiClemente et al., 1994; Miller & Cooney, 1994; Zweben et al., 1994).

Testing the Effectiveness of Individual Components of Complex Interventions

In complex interventions, whether all elements of the intervention or only some of them are causing the expected outcomes is not always clear. It is important in such cases to conduct studies to examine the differential effects of intervention elements.

For example, in Powe and Weinrich's (1999) study, the cause of a higher rate of FOBT might be the provision of free testing rather than the video intervention. To examine this issue, the following groups would have to be studied: (1) subjects who received no intervention and no offer of free FOBT, (2) subjects who received an offer of free FOBT but no intervention, (3) subjects who received the intervention but no offer of free FOBT, and (4) subjects who received both the intervention and free FOBT.

West and associates (1993) have described a series of designs that can be used to test the effectiveness of various components of such a treatment; these strategies are summarized on the following pages. Used as components of an intervention effectiveness research program, these strategies must be conducted with the guidance of the intervention theory and implementation of the observation system.

Dismantling Strategy (Subtraction Design). The full version of the program is compared with a reduced version in which one or more components have been removed. Criteria for selecting components to delete vary but are often based on theory or on information from review of the literature. Components that are expensive or difficult to provide may also be selected for deletion. Components are removed one at a time, and the reduced set is tested against the full version until a single base component remains. When programs are complex and include many components, various mixes of components may be tested.

Constructive Strategy. A base intervention is identified. A component that is expected to increase the effectiveness of the base intervention is added, and the two interventions are tested. There must be a theoretical rationale for the selection of components to add to the base intervention. The components are added one at a time, and each set of components is tested for effectiveness until the full set of possible combinations has been studied. As with the dismantling strategy, with the use of dismantling strategy in large programs, various mixes of components may be tested.

Factorial ANOVA Designs. Commonly used in psychology, factorial ANOVA designs are potentially the most powerful way to examine all possible combinations of an intervention. Factorial designs used in intervention trials are usually limited to a 2 × 2 design, examining the presence or absence of two intervention components. Factorial ANOVA designs usually involve a multisite project with a very large sample size to achieve adequate statistical power. Complexity of the design increases with the number of components in the intervention. Factorial ANOVA is described in Chapter 22.

Fractional Factorial Designs. Fractional factorial designs are simplifications of the factorial designs. The researcher systematically selects a portion of all possible intervention component combinations to implement. Such a design requires the researcher to be willing to assume that the effects of higher-order interactions (multiple combination effects) are negligible.

Response Surface Methodology. With response surface methodology, the dose response can be applied to more than one dimension of a treatment. If several interventions are constructed that represent a number of combinations of differing levels of strength of each component and the outcome is plotted for each combination, the plotted figure is referred to as a *response surface*. This methodology can be used to determine which combination of components produces the optimum outcome.

Results of previous response surface analyses have shown that increasing the strength of a component does not always lead to increases in effectiveness. When two individually effective components are combined, the resulting program may be more or less effective than each component alone or may not change the effect. A researcher can improve a program sequentially by refining each component and then studying the combined effects. Developing an optimal program is often an evolutionary process.

FIELD TESTS

Field tests are conducted in clinical settings in which the intervention will typically be implemented. Field tests are ideal for graduate nursing student projects. The purpose of these studies is to evaluate the effectiveness of the intervention when implemented in uncontrolled situations. Rather than being controlled, patient characteristics are allowed to vary and are measured. Sampling criteria are limited to selection of only those patients experiencing the problem. No other constraints are imposed.

The observation system is in operation, and patient characteristics, intervener characteristics, and setting characteristics are measured. Outcome variables are measured at least once before the treatment and once afterward. Repeated measures of outcome variables are often performed during the posttest period (Fawcett et al., 1994; Sidani & Braden, 1998). Design criteria against which the intervention is judged are listed in Table 13–14.

Collecting and Analyzing Data

Data from the observation system, pilot tests, the formal study, and field tests are collected and analyzed continuously. Data analysis goes beyond testing for statistical significance. Two-way analysis of variance, regression analyses, path analyses, and residual analyses are commonly used; these statistical procedures are described in Chapters 20 to 22.

Exploratory analysis techniques provide impor-

TABLE 13–14
CRITERIA FOR INTERVENTION DESIGN

1. The intervention is effective.
2. The intervention is replicable by typical interveners.
3. The intervention is simple to use.
4. The intervention is practical.
5. The intervention is adaptable to various contexts.
6. The intervention is compatible with local customs and values.

Adapted from Fawcett S. B., Suarez-Belcazar, Y., Belcazar F. E., White, G. W., Paine, A. L., Blanchard, K. A., & Embree, M. G. (1994). Conducting intervention research—the design and development process. In J. Rothman & E. J. Thomas (Eds.), *Intervention research: Design and development for human service* (pp. 25–54). New York: Haworth Press.

tant information for determining, for instance, when initial interventions should be implemented and whether supplemental procedures are necessary. Residual analyses may identify subjects who respond differently to the intervention. Qualitative analyses are used when appropriate. Ongoing graphing of phases of the intervention and outcomes over time provide critical information. Data from the project constitute an excellent source for secondary analyses by nursing students.

Dissemination

Once field testing and evaluation are completed, the intervention is ready for dissemination. In nursing, dissemination has traditionally involved presenting the findings at professional meetings, describing the intervention in professional journals, and reporting studies documenting its effect on outcomes. Results may be reported by traditional means throughout the process of intervention development and evaluation. These contributions are vital to the development of science in nursing.

A higher level of dissemination must also be considered. Nurse researchers might consider viewing the intervention as a product and its dissemination in terms of marketing and selling a product (Fawcett et al., 1994). This would be an important consideration if initial implementation of the intervention by a user required considerable investment of time in consultation or assistance from members of the project team. In this case, the process of dissemination would involve choosing a brand name, establishing a price, and setting standards for the intervention's use.

CHOOSING A BRAND NAME

The name given to the intervention should be intuitively appealing. It may address the purpose, patients, or setting of the intervention. The name may link the intervention to an established concept in a theory. Establishing a brand name allows adopters to recognize the intervention and differentiate it from other similar, but perhaps less effective, interventions. The name of the intervention will come to be associated with its effectiveness, dependability, or efficiency (Fawcett et al., 1994).

SETTING A PRICE

In setting a price for the intervention, the researchers must determine or define the market for the product and the discretionary budget of potential adopters. In this period of managed care, when health care corporations are competing for patients by demonstrating more effective outcomes than their competitors, the motivation to purchase well-designed interventions with demonstrated positive outcomes is high.

Other factors that must be considered by the research team in setting the price are (1) the cost of providing materials related to the intervention, (2) the costs of staff time for phone calls, mailing material, maintaining files, and so on, (3) organizational requirements, (4) the cost of training, and (5) the cost of technical support that may be required after the intervention is implemented. If the goal of the researchers is widespread adoption of the intervention with a simple training procedure and little need for ongoing technical support, the price might be set very low, only sufficient to recover costs. A comprehensive or complex treatment program requiring considerable involvement of the researchers or other technical personnel might appropriately be set higher (Fawcett et al., 1994).

SETTING STANDARDS FOR USE

The project team must establish guidelines for using the intervention correctly that adopters must agree to before they receive it. Specifications should be developed regarding conditions under which the intervention can be used. The project should be protected by a patent or copyright until costs are recovered. This arrangement helps ensure the integrity of the process and the quality of the product (Fawcett et al., 1994).

IDENTIFYING POTENTIAL MARKETS

Careful consideration must be given to determining all the potential markets for the intervention.

The following questions should be asked to identify the market for the intervention:

- Which people can benefit personally from the intervention?
- Who (with the use of the intervention) could contribute most to solving the problem?
- Is the goal of dissemination broad-based adoption (i.e., saturation of the market) or more restricted use by selected adopters?
- Which market segments—types of health or human service organizations—would most likely adopt and benefit from the intervention if they were aware of it?
- Which media approach—public service announcements, direct mail, or other strategies—would be most appropriate and feasible for informing the targeted market segment?

Identifying potential early adopters may encourage others in the identified market to adopt the intervention. Early adopters tend to have relatively greater resources, sophistication, education, and willingness to try innovative practices. These characteristics may put them in more frequent contact with their colleagues, increasing the chances that other adopters will become aware of the benefits of using the intervention (Fawcett et al., 1994). See Chapter 27 for a discussion of early adopters.

CREATING A DEMAND FOR THE INTERVENTION

Anyone marketing the intervention must persuade potential purchasers that they will actually benefit from the intervention. Strategies designed to market innovations include modeling the innovation, arranging sampling of the innovation and its benefits, and advertising. *Modeling* involves showing experts, celebrities, or others easily identifiable by the market segment using the intervention and benefitting from its use.

In *sampling*, potential purchasers are allowed to try out portions of the product. This process might consists of demonstrations of the intervention and opportunities to review materials at regional and national professional conferences.

Advertising campaigns can highlight desired features of the intervention, such as its relative effectiveness, low cost, and decreased time and effort for users. Incentives to encourage adoption, such as describing support services available, can positively influence purchasers. Ultimately, however, these strategies will work only if the product is more effective, lower in cost, or requires less user time than other similar interventions on the market (Fawcett et al., 1994).

ENCOURAGING APPROPRIATE ADAPTATION

Adaptation involves changing the intervention to fit local conditions and is sometimes referred to as *reinvention*. Elements of the intervention may be modified or deleted, or new elements may be added. There is a tension between maintaining the quality of the intervention and allowing adaptation. Allowing adaptation may increase the speed with which an intervention is adopted but result in a loss of effectiveness. The project team should permit (or even encourage) necessary adaptation, but only under the condition defined by the team. The team should be allowed to collect and analyze data related to the adaptation or see reports of ongoing analysis by the adapting facility. It is important for the team to determine whether the changed intervention continues to meet the established standards for the intervention (Fawcett et al., 1994).

PROVIDING TECHNICAL SUPPORT FOR ADOPTERS

The researchers and their staff are the primary experts on the intervention. Adopters may require assistance with troubleshooting or adapting the intervention to their specific needs (Fawcett et al., 1994).

■ SUMMARY

This chapter describes a revolutionary new approach to intervention research that holds great promise for designing and testing nursing interventions. The current approach to testing interventions, the "true experiment," is being seriously questioned by a growing number of scholars. Nursing interventions are defined as "deliberative cognitive, physical, or verbal activities performed with, or on behalf of, individuals and their families [that] are directed toward accomplishing particular therapeutic objectives relative to individuals' health and well-being" (Grobe, 1996, p. 50). The terminology and operationalization of a nursing intervention vary with the clinical setting and among individual nurses. Traditionally, adherence to rigid rules were required to define a study as a "true experiment." Many of the traditional rules have been abandoned. The validity of a true experiment as it is currently operationalized is a concern.

An intervention research project consists of multiple studies conducted over a period of years by a project team that may include nursing students. Some teams use a participatory research method that involves community groups. The initial focus of the team will be to clarify the problem. The process of intervention research begins with an extensive search for relevant information that is applied to the development of an intervention theory.

An intervention theory must include (1) a careful description of the problem to be addressed by the intervention, (2) the intervening actions that must be implemented to address the problem, (3) moderator variables that might change the impact of the intervention, (4) mediator variables that might alter the effect of the intervention, and (5) expected outcomes of the intervention. The intervention theory guides the design and development of an intervention, which is then extensively tested, refined, and retested.

Advanced testing of the intervention occurs after sufficient evidence is available to determine that the intervention is effective in achieving desired outcomes. This testing focuses on identifying variations in effectiveness based on patient characteristics, intervener characteristics, and setting characteristics. When the intervention is sufficiently refined and evidence of effectiveness has been obtained, field testing is implemented to ensure that the intervention can be effectively implemented in clinical settings. Results of field tests are used to further refine the intervention to improve clinical application.

An observation system is developed for use throughout the design and development process. This system allows the researchers to observe events related to the intervention naturalistically and to perform analyses of these observations. Dissemination efforts are more extensive than in traditional experimental studies and involve choosing a brand name, establishing a price, and setting standards for the intervention's use.

●●●●●●●●●●●●●●●●●●●●●●●●●●●●●●●●●●●●●●●

REFERENCES

Abraham, I. L., Chalifoux, Z. L., & Evers, G. C. M. (1992). Conditions, interventions, and outcomes: A qualitative analysis of nursing research (1981–1990). In U.S. Department of Health & Human Services, Public Health Service. *Patient outcomes research: Examining the effectiveness of nursing practice. Proceedings of the State of the Science Conference sponsored by the National Center for Nursing Research, September 11–13, 1991* (DHHS Publication #93–3411, pp. 70–87). Rockville, MD: U.S. Government Printing Office.

Adelman, H. S. (1986). Intervention theory and evaluating efficacy. *Evaluation Review, 10*(1), 65–83.

American Cancer Society. (1998). *Cancer facts and figures, 1998.* Atlanta: Author.

American College of Sports Medicine. (1995). *ACSM's Guidelines for exercise testing & prescription* (5th ed.). Baltimore: Williams & Wilkins.

American Heart Association. (1997). *Heart and stroke statistical update.* Dallas, TX: Author.

Barlow, D. H., Hayes, S. C., & Nelson, R. O. (1989). *The scientist practitioner: Research and accountability in clinical and educational settings.* New York: Pergamon Press.

Baron, R. M., & Kenny, D. A. (1986). The moderator-mediator variable distinction in social psychological research: Conceptual, strategic, and statistical considerations. *Journal of Personality and Social Psychology, 51*(6), 1173–1183.

Bergmark, A., & Oscarsson, L. (1991). Does anybody really know what they are doing? Some comments related to methodology of treatment service research. *British Journal of Addiction, 86*(2), 139–142.

Bulechek, G. M., & McCloskey, J. C. (1999). *Nursing interventions: Effective nursing treatments.* Philadelphia: W. B. Saunders.

Bulechek, G. M., McCloskey, J. C., & Donahue, W. J. (1995). Nursing Interventions Classifications (NIC): A language to describe nursing treatments. In N. M. Lang (Ed.), *Nursing Data Systems: An emerging framework: Data system advances for clinical nursing practice.* Washington, D.C.: American Nurses Publishing.

Carroll, K. M., Kadden, R. M., Donovan, D. M., Zweben, A., & Rounsaville, B. J. (1994). Implementing treatment and protecting the validity of the independent variable in treatment matching studies. *Journal on Studies of Alcohol, 12*(Suppl.), 149–155.

Chen, H. T. (1990). *Theory-driven evaluations*. Newbury Park, CA: Sage.

Chen, H. T., & Rossi, P. H. (1989). Issues in the theory-driven perspective. *Evaluation and Program Planning*, 12(4), 199–306.

Clark, A. M. (1998). The qualitative-quantitative debate: Moving from positivism and confrontation to post-positivism and reconciliation. *Journal of Advanced Nursing, 27*(6), 1242–1249.

Connors, G. J., Allen, J. P., Cooney, N. L., DiClemente, C. C., Tonigan, J. S., & Anton, R. F. (1994). Assessment issues and strategies in alcoholism treatment matching research. *Journal of Studies on Alcohol, 12*(Suppl.), 92–100.

Conrad, K. J., & Conrad, K. M. (1994). Reassessing validity threats in experiments: Focus on construct validity. *New Directions for Program Evaluation, 63*, 5–26.

DiClemente, C. C., Carroll, K. M., Connors, G. J., & Kadden, R. M. (1994). Process assessment in treatment matching research. *Journal of Studies on Alcohol, 12*(Suppl), 156–162.

Dille, C. A., Kirchhoff, K. T., Sullivan, J. J., & Larson, E. (1993). Increasing the wearing time of vinyl urinary drainage bags by decontamination with bleach. *Archives of Physical Medicine & Rehabilitation, 74*(4), 431–437.

Dille, C. M., & Kirchhoff (1993). Decontamination of vinyl urinary drainage bags with bleach. *Rehabilitation Nursing, 18*(5), 292–295, 355–356.

Dombeck, M., & Karl, J. (1987). Spiritual issues in mental health care. *Journal of Religion and Health, 26*(3), 183–197.

Donovan, D. M., Kadden, R. M., DiClemente, C. C., Carroll, K. M., Longabaugh, R., Zweben, A., & Rychtarik, R. (1994). Issues in the selection and development of therapies in alcoholism treatment matching research. *Journal of Studies on Alcohol, 12*(Suppl.), 138–148.

Dwyer, J., Clarke, L., & Miller, M. (1990). The effect of religious concentration and affiliation on county cancer mortality rates. *Journal of Health and Social Behavior, 31*(2), 185–202.

Egan, E. C., Snyder, M., & Burns, K. R. (1992). Intervention studies in nursing: Is the effect due to the independent variable? *Nursing Outlook, 40*(4), 187–190.

Emblem, J. (1992). Religion and spirituality defined according to current use in nursing literature. *Journal of Professional Nursing, 8(1)*, 41–47.

Fawcett, S. B., Suarez-Belcazar, Y., Balcazar, F. E., White, G. W., Paine, A. L., Blanchard, K. A., & Embree, M. G. (1994). Conducting intervention research—the design and development process. In J. Rothman & E. J. Thomas (Eds.), *Intervention research: Design and development for human service* (pp. 25–54). New York: Haworth Press.

Finney, J. W., & Moos, R. H. (1989). Theory and method in treatment evaluation. *Evaluation and Program Planning, 12*(4), 307–316.

Fisher, R. A. (1935). *The design of experiments*. New York: Hafner.

Frank-Stromborg, M., Pender, N. J., Walker, S. N., & Sechrist, K. R. (1990). Determinants of health-promoting lifestyle in ambulatory cancer patients. *Social Science and Medicine, 31*(10), 1159–1168.

Freeman, H. (1989). *Cancer and the socioeconomic disadvantaged*. Atlanta: American Cancer Society.

Gafni, A. (1994). The standard gamble method: What is being measured and how it is interpreted. *Health Services Research, 29*(2), 207–224.

Griffith, C. J. (1993). Colorectal cancer: Reducing mortality through early detection and treatment. *Physician Assistant, 17*(1), 25–42.

Grobe, S. J. (1996). The Nursing Intervention Lexicon and Taxonomy: Implications for representing nursing care data in automated patient records. *Holistic Nursing Practice, 11*(1), 48–63.

Hansen, C. (1995). Colorectal cancer: A preventable disease. *Physician Assistant, 19*(1), 15–16, 21–22, 25–26.

Hashisaki, P., Swenson, J., Mooney, B., Epstein, B., & Bowcutt, C. (1984). Decontamination of urinary bags for rehabilitation patients. *Archives of Physical Medicine & Rehabilitation, 65*(8), 474–476.

Hegyvary, S. T. (1992). Outcomes research: Integrating nursing practice into the world view. In U.S. Department of Health & Human Services, Public Health Service. *Patient outcomes research: Examining the effectiveness of nursing practice. Proceedings of the State of the Science Conference sponsored by the National Center for Nursing Research, September 11–13, 1991* (DHHS Publication #93–3411). Rockville, MD: U.S. Government Printing Office.

Hoskins, D., & Rose, M. (1989). *Cancer and the poor: A report to the nation*. Atlanta: American Cancer Society.

Johnson, J. L., Ratner, P. A., Bottroff, J. L., & Hayduk, L. A. (1993). An exploration of Pender's health promotion model using LISREL. *Nursing Research, 42*(3), 132–138.

Kirchhoff, K. T., & Dille, C. A. (1994). Issues in intervention research: Maintaining integrity. *Applied Nursing Research, 7*(1), 32–46.

Landrine, H., & Klonoff, E. (1994). Cultural diversity in causal attributions for illness: The role of the supernatural. *Journal of Behavioral Medicine, 17* (2), 181–193.

Lincoln, C. E., & Mamiya, L. (1990). *The black church in the African American experience*. Durham, NC: Duke University Press.

Lindley, P., & Walker, S. N. (1993). Theoretical and methodological differentiation of moderation and mediation. *Nursing Research, 42*(5), 276–279.

Lipsey, M. W. (1993). Theory as method: Small theories of treatments. *New Directions for Program Evaluation, 57*, 5–38

Lloyd, J., McConnell, P., & Zahorik, P. (1994). Collaborative health education training for African American health ministers and providers of community services. *Educational Gerontology, 20*(3), 265–276.

Marcus, B. H., Rossi, J. S., Selby, V. C., Niaura, R. S., & Abrams, D. B. (1992). The stages and processes of exercise adoption and maintenance in a worksite sample. *Health Psychology, 11*(6), 386–395.

Marcus, B. H., Selby, V. C., Niaura, R. S., & Rossi, J. S. (1992). Self-efficacy and the stages of exercise behavior change. *Research Quarterly for Exercise and Sport, 63*(1), 60–66.

Martin, K. S. & Scheet, N. J. (1995). The Omaha System: Nursing diagnoses, interventions, and client outcomes. In N. M. Lang (Ed.), *Nursing data systems: An emerging framework: Data system advances for clinical nursing practice.* Washington, D.C.: American Nurses Publishing.

Martin, M., & Henry, M. (1989). Cultural relativity and poverty. *Public Health Nursing, 6*(1), 28–34.

McCloskey, J. C., & Bulechek, G. M. (Eds.). (1992*). Nursing interventions classification (NIC).* St. Louis: Mosby–Year Book.

Meade, C. (1996). Producing videotapes for cancer education: Methods and examples. *Oncology Nursing Forum, 23*(5), 837–846.

Miller, W. R., & Cooney, N. L. (1994). Designing studies to investigate client-treatment matching. *Journal of Studies on Alcohol, 12*(Suppl.), 38–45.

Nolan, M., & Grant, G. (1993). Service evaluation: Time to open both eyes. *Journal of Advanced Nursing, 18*(9), 1434–1496.

Olsen, S., & Frank-Stromborg, M. (1993). Cancer prevention and early detection in ethnically diverse populations. *Seminars in Oncology Nursing, 9*(3), 198–209.

Orchid, C. (1994). Comparing healthcare outcomes. *British Medical Journal, 308*(6942), 1493–1496.

Orem, D. E. (1995). *Nursing: Concepts of practice.* St. Louis: Mosby.

Ottenbacher, K. (1992). Impact of random assignment on study outcome: An empirical examination. *Controlled Clinical Trials, 13*(1), 50–61.

Powe, B. D. (1995a). Cancer fatalism among elderly Caucasians and African Americans. *Oncology Nursing Forum, 22*(9), 1355–1359.

Powe, B. D. (1995b). Fatalism among elderly African Americans: Effects on colorectal cancer screening. *Cancer Nursing, 18*(5), 385–392.

Powe, B. D. (1995c). Perceptions of fatalism among African Americans: The influence of education, income, and knowledge. *Journal of the National Black Nurses Association, 7*(2), 41–48.

Powe, B. D. (1997). Cancer fatalism . . . spiritual perspectives. *Journal of Religion and Health, 36*(2), 135–144.

Powe, B. D., & Johnson, A. (1995). Fatalism as a barrier to cancer screening among African Americans: Philosophical perspectives. *Journal of Religion and Health, 34*(2), 119–125.

Powe, B. D., & Weinrich, S. (1999). An intervention to decrease cancer fatalism among rural elders. *Oncology Nursing Forum, 26*(3), 583–588.

Prochaska, J. O., & Marcus, B. H. (1994). The transtheoretical model: Applications to exercise. In R. K. Dishman (Ed.), *Advances in exercise adherence* (p. 161–180). Champaign, IL: Human Kinetics.

Reed, P. G. (1992). An emerging paradigm for the investigation of spirituality in nursing. *Research in Nursing & Health, 15*(5), 349–357.

Rezmovic, E. L. (1984). Assessing treatment implementation amid the slings and arrows of reality. *Evaluation Review, 8*(2), 187–204.

Rosella, J.D., Regan-Kubinski, M.J., & Albrecht, S.A. (1994). The need for multi-cultural diversity among health professionals. *Nursing and Health Care, 15*(5), 242–246.

Rosen, A., & Proctor, E. K. (1978). Specifying the treatment process: The basis for effectiveness research. *Journal of Social Service Research, 2*(1), 25–43.

Rossi, P. H., & Freeman, H. E. (1993). *Evaluation: A systematic approach* (5th ed.). Newbury Park, CA: Sage.

Rothman, J., & Thomas, E. J. (Eds.). (1994). *Intervention research: Design and development for human service.* New York: Haworth Press.

Saba, V. K. (1995). Home Health Care Classifications (HHCCs): Nursing diagnoses and nursing interventions. In N. M. Lang (Ed.), *Nursing data systems: An emerging framework: Data system advances for clinical nursing practice.* Washington, D.C.: American Nurses Publishing.

Scandrett, A. (1994). Religion as a support component in the health behavior of black Americans. *Journal of Religion and Health, 33*(2), 123–129.

Schmelzer, M. (1999–2001). Safety and effectiveness of large volume enema solutions. National Institutes of Health Research Enhancement Award (AREA).

Schmelzer, M., Case, P., Chappell, S., & Wright, K. (2000). Colonic cleansing, fluid absorption, and discomfort following tap water and soapsuds enemas. *Applied Nursing Research, 13*(2), 83–91.

Schmelzer, M., & Wright, K. (1993a). Risky enemas: What's the ideal solution? *American Journal of Nursing, 93*(2), 21.

Schmelzer, M., & Wright, K. (1993b). Say nope to soap. *American Journal of Nursing, 93*(3), 21.

Schmelzer, M., & Wright, K. (1996). Enema administration techniques used by experienced registered nurses. *Gastroenterology Nursing, 19*(5), 171–175.

Scott, A. G., & Sechrest, L. (1989). Strength of theory and theory of strength. *Evaluation and Program Planning, 12*(4), 329–336.

Sechrest, L., Ametrano, D., & Ametrano, I. M. (1983). Evaluations of social programs. In C. E. Walker (Ed.), *The handbook of clinical psychology* (pp. 129–166). Homewood, IL: Dow Jones–Irwin.

Sidani, S. & Braden, C. J. (1998). *Evaluating nursing interventions: A theory-driven approach.* Thousand Oaks, CA: Sage.

Thomas, S. B. (1994). The characteristics of northern black churches with community health outreach programs. *American Journal of Public Health, 84*(4), 575–579.

Ulbrich, S. L. (1999). Nursing practice theory of exercise as self-care. *Image—The Journal of Nursing Scholarship, 31*(1), 65–70.

Underwood, S., & Hoskins, D. (1994). Increasing nursing involvement in cancer prevention and control among the economically disadvantaged: The nursing challenge. *Seminars in Oncology Nursing, 10*(2), 89–95.

Underwood, S., Hoskins, D., Cummins, T., Morris, K., & Williams, A. (1994). Obstacles to cancer care: Focus on the socioeconomically disadvantaged. *Oncology Nursing Forum, 21*(1), 47–52.

U.S. Department of Health and Human Services, Centers for Disease Control and Prevention. (1996). *A report of the surgeon general: Physical activity and health.* Washington, D.C.: U.S. Government Printing Office.

U.S. Department of Health and Human Services, Public Health Service. (1990). *Healthy people 2000: National health promotion and disease prevention objectives* (DHHS Publication No. PHS 91–50213). Washington, D.C.: U.S. Government Printing Office.

U.S. Preventive Services Task Force. (1996). *Guide to clinical preventive services* (2nd ed.). Baltimore: Williams & Wilkins.

Warren, J. J., & Hoskins, L. M. (1995). NANDA's nursing diagnosis taxonomy: A nursing database. In N. M. Lang (Ed.), *Nursing data systems: An emerging framework: Data system advances for clinical nursing practice.* Washington, D.C.: American Nurses Publishing.

Weinrich, S., Weinrich, M., Boyd, M., Atwood, J., & Cervanka, B. (1992). Effective approaches for increasing compliance with ACS's screening recommendations in socioeconomically disadvantaged populations. *Presented at the Second National Conference on Cancer Nursing Research.* Atlanta: American Cancer Society.

Wennberg, J. E., Barry, M. J., Fowler, F. J., & Mulley, K. A. (1993). Outcomes research, PORTs, and health care reform. *Annals of the New York Academy of Sciences, 703,* 52–62.

West, S. G., Aiken, L. S., & Todd, M. (1993). Probing the effects of individual components in multiple component prevention programs. *American Journal of Community Psychology, 21*(5), 571–605.

Yeaton, W. H., & Sechrest, L. (1981). Critical dimensions in the choice and maintenance of successful treatments: Strength, integrity, and effectiveness. *Journal of Consulting and Clinical Psychology, 49*(2), 156–167.

Zweben, A., Donovan, D. M., Randall, C. L., Barrett, D., Dermen, K., Kabela, E., McRee, B., Meyers, R., Rice, C., Rosengren, D., Schmidt, P., Show, M., Thevos, A. K., & Velasquez, M. (1994). Issues in the development of subject recruitment strategies and eligibility criteria in multisite trials of matching. *Journal of Studies on Alcohol, 12* (Suppl.), 62–69.

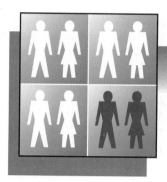

CHAPTER 14

SAMPLING

One tends to enter the field of research with preconceived notions about samples and sampling, many of which are acquired through exposure to television advertisements, polls of public opinion, market researchers in shopping centers, and newspaper reports of research findings. The commercial boasts that four of five doctors recommend their product; the newscaster announces that John Jones is predicted to win the senate election by a margin of 3 to 1; the newspaper reports that scientists have now shown that treatment of early breast cancer with lumpectomy and radiation is as effective as mastectomy.

All of the aforementioned examples use sampling techniques. Some of the outcomes, however, are more valid than others. The differences in validity are due, in part, to the sampling techniques used. In most instances, television, newspapers, and advertisements do not explain their sampling techniques. You may hold certain opinions about the adequacy of these techniques, but there is inadequate information from which to make a judgment.

In research, it is critical that the sampling component of the research process be carefully thought out and clearly described. Achieving these goals requires knowledge of the techniques of sampling and the reasoning behind them. With this knowledge, you can make intelligent judgments about sampling when critiquing studies or developing a sampling plan for your own study. This chapter examines sampling theory and concepts, sampling plans, probability and nonprobability sampling plans, sample size, and the process of acquiring a sample.

SAMPLING THEORY

Sampling involves selecting a group of people, events, behaviors, or other elements with which to conduct a study. A *sampling plan* defines the process of making the selections; *sample* denotes the selected group of people or elements. Sampling decisions have a major impact on the meaning and generalizability of the findings.

Sampling theory was developed to determine mathematically the most effective way to acquire a sample that would accurately reflect the population under study. The theoretical, mathematical rationale for decisions related to sampling emerged from survey research, although the techniques were first applied to experimental research by agricultural scientists. One of the most important surveys that stimulated improvements in survey techniques was the U.S. census. The assumptions of sampling theory have been adopted by researchers and incorporated within the research process.

Key concepts of sampling theory are (1) elements, (2) populations, (3) sampling criteria, (4) representativeness, (5) sampling errors, (6) randomization, (7) sampling frames, and (8) sampling plans. The following sections explain the meanings of these concepts. Later in the chapter, these concepts are used to explain a variety of sampling techniques.

Elements and Populations

The individual units of a population are called *elements*. An element can be a person, event, behavior, or any other single unit of a study. When

365

elements are persons, they are referred to as *subjects.* The *population,* sometimes referred to as the *target population,* is the entire set of individuals or elements who meet the sampling criteria. An *accessible population* is the portion of the target population to which the researcher has reasonable access. The accessible population might be elements within a state, city, hospital, or nursing unit. The sample is obtained from the accessible population, and findings are generalized first to the accessible population and then, more abstractly, to the target population.

Generalizing means that the findings can be applied to more than just to the sample under study. Because of the importance of generalizing, there are risks to defining the accessible population too narrowly. For example, a narrow definition of the accessible population reduces the ability to generalize from the study and, thus, diminishes the meaningfulness of the findings. Biases may be introduced that make generalization to the broader target population difficult to defend. If the accessible population is defined as individuals in a white, upper-middle-class setting, one cannot generalize to nonwhite or lower-income populations. These biases are similar to those that may be encountered in a nonrandom sample.

In some studies, the entire population is the target of the study. These studies are referred to as *population studies* (Barhyte et al., 1990). Many of these studies use data available in large databases, such as the census data or other government-maintained databases. Epidemiologists often use entire populations for their large database studies. In other studies, the entire population of interest in the study is very small and well defined. For example, one could conduct a study in which the defined population was all living recipients of heart transplants.

In some cases, a *hypothetical population* is defined. A hypothetical population assumes the presence of a population that cannot be defined according to sampling theory rules, which require a list of all members of the population. For example, individuals who successfully lose weight would be a hypothetical population. The number of individuals in the population, who they are, how much weight they have lost, how long they have kept it off, or

how they achieved the weight loss is unknown. Some populations are elusive and constantly changing. For example, listing all women in active labor in the United States, all people grieving the loss of a loved one, or all people coming into an emergency room would be impossible.

Sampling Criteria

Sampling criteria list the characteristics essential for membership in the target population. The criteria are developed from the research problem, the purpose, the conceptual and operational definitions of the study variables, and the design. The sample is selected from the population that meets the sampling criteria. When the study is completed, the findings are generalized to this population.

The sampling criteria may be designed to make the population as homogeneous as possible or to control for extraneous variables. In descriptive or correlational studies, the sampling criteria may be defined to ensure a heterogeneous population with a broad range of values for the variables being studied. In quasi-experimental or experimental studies, the primary purpose of sampling criteria is to limit the effect of extraneous variables on the particular interaction between the dependent and independent variables. Subjects are selected to maximize the effects of the independent variable and minimize the effects of variation in other variables. The number of restrictions that can be imposed by the sampling criteria depends on the typical patient load in the selected setting.

Sampling criteria may include characteristics such as the ability to read, to write responses on the data collection instruments or forms, and to comprehend and communicate using the English language. Age limitations are often specified, such as adults 18 years and older. Subjects may be limited to those who are not participating in any other study. Persons who are able to participate fully in the procedure for obtaining informed consent are often selected as subjects. If potential subjects have diminished autonomy or are unable to give informed consent, consent must be obtained from their legal representative. Thus, persons who are legally or mentally incompetent, terminally ill, or confined to an institution are more difficult to access as subjects. Sampling criteria can become so restrictive that an adequate number of subjects cannot be found. Narrow and restrictive sampling criteria reduce the sample size or make obtaining a sample difficult.

Inclusion criteria and exclusion criteria may be used to develop the desired sample. *Inclusion criteria* are characteristics that must be present for the element to be included in the sample. For example, for subjects to be included in the study, they must have been diagnosed with stage II breast cancer within the previous 3 months. *Exclusion criteria* are exceptions to the inclusion criteria. In the previous example with the inclusion criterion consisting of diagnosis with stage II breast cancer within the previous 3 months, subjects who meet that criterion might be excluded if they had a previous diagnosis of breast cancer.

The researcher must provide logical reasons for the inclusions and exclusions. Larson (1994) suggests that some groups, such as women, ethnic minorities, the elderly, and the poor, are unnecessarily excluded from many studies. A review of approved research protocols in one tertiary care center (1989–1990) revealed that 75% of studies listed exclusion criteria, many of which were not justified by the researchers (Larson, 1994). The most common exclusions for which no justification was provided were age, socioeconomic status, and race. Only 26.6% of nursing protocols included a justification for age. Exclusions limit generalizability and should be carefully considered.

Good (1995), in a study of the effects of jaw relaxation and music on postoperative pain, described the sampling criteria used in this study as shown in the following excerpt.

· ·

"The sampling frame included every eligible patient listed for elective abdominal surgery in two teaching and two community hospitals during a 7-month period. Patients were identified daily by the investigator from surgery lists, and eligibility was decided in consultation with office nurses. Inclusion criteria were: (a) aged 21 to 65 years, (b) scheduled for major abdominal surgery, (c) receiving intramuscular (IM) PRN analgesia, and (d) hospitalized 2 or

more days postoperatively. Patients who had laparoscopic surgeries or psychosis or retardation were excluded. All eligible patients ($N = 126$) were contacted in the nursing unit, holding area, clinic, or by telephone. Of the 102 patients who consented and were assigned, 2 patients later withdrew and 16 were excluded from the analysis because of canceled surgery ($n = 4$), inability to ambulate after surgery ($n = 2$), unforeseen patient-controlled analgesia ($n = 9$), or treatment error ($n = 1$). Thus, the sample consisted of 84 subjects, 25 men and 59 women aged 23 to 64 years." (Good, 1995, p. 53) ■

Note that this study excluded subjects older than 65 years and provided no justification for this exclusion. It is left to the imagination of the reader to guess the reasons for the exclusions. One might surmise that laparoscopic procedures would not generally be classified as major abdominal surgery and might have a different pain trajectory from that of procedures requiring an incision, or that providing instructions for relaxation and measuring differences in pain relief for patients with psychosis or retardation might require a different study design and different measurement methods.

Representativeness

For a sample to be *representative*, it must be like the population in as many ways as possible. It is especially important that the sample be representative in relation to the variables being studied and to other factors that may influence the study variables. For example, if a study examines attitudes toward acquired immunodeficiency syndrome (AIDS), the sample should be representative of the distribution of attitudes toward AIDS that exists in the specified population. In addition, a sample must be representative of characteristics such as age, gender, ethnicity, income, and education, which often influence study variables.

The accessible population must be representative of the target population. If the accessible population is limited to a particular setting or type of setting, the individuals seeking care at that setting may be different from those who would seek care for the same problem in other settings or from those who choose to use self-care to manage their problems. Studies conducted in private hospitals usually exclude the poor. Other settings could exclude the elderly or the undereducated, whereas people who do not have access to care are usually excluded from studies. Subjects in research centers and the care they receive are different from patients and the care they receive in community hospitals, public hospitals, veterans' hospitals, and rural hospitals. Obese individuals who chose to enter a program to lose weight may differ from those who did not enter a program. All of these factors limit representativeness, in turn limiting our understanding of phenomena important to the nursing body of knowledge.

Representativeness is usually evaluated through comparison of the numerical values of the sample (a *statistic* such as the mean) with the same values from the target population. A numerical value of a population is called a *parameter*. We can estimate the population parameter by identifying the values obtained in previous studies examining the same variables. The accuracy with which the population parameters have been estimated within a study is referred to as *precision*. These statistical concepts are discussed further in Chapter 18. Precision in estimating parameters requires well-developed methods of measurement that are used repeatedly among studies. The researcher can define parameters by conducting a series of descriptive and correlational studies, each of which examines a different segment of the target population. Meta-analysis can then be performed to estimate the population parameter.

Of major importance is whether the samples used to establish parameters were representative of the target population in terms of characteristics such as age, gender, ethnicity, educational level, and socioeconomic status. Assessment of this information may lead to redefining the target population for which we have a body of knowledge in a particular area of study.

Sampling Error

The difference between a sample statistic and a population parameter is called the *sampling error*

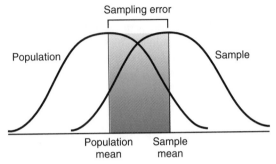

FIGURE 14–1 ■ Sampling error.

(see Figure 14–1). A large sampling error means that the sample is not providing a precise picture of the population; it is not representative. Sampling error is usually larger with small samples and decreases as the sample size increases. Sampling error, which reduces the *power* of a study (ability of the statistical analyses used to detect differences between groups or accurately to describe the relationships between or among variables), occurs as a result of random variation and systematic variation.

RANDOM VARIATION

Random variation is the expected difference in values that occurs when one examines different subjects from the same sample. If the mean is used to describe the sample, the values of individuals in that sample will not all be exactly the same as the sample mean. Individual subjects' values vary from the value of the sample mean. The difference is random because the value of each subject is likely to vary in a different direction. Some values are higher and others are lower than the sample mean. Thus, the values are randomly scattered around the mean. As the sample size becomes larger, overall variation in sample values decreases, with more values being close to the sample mean. As the sample size increases, the sample mean is also more likely to have a value similar to that of the population mean.

SYSTEMATIC VARIATION

Systematic variation, or *systematic bias,* is a consequence of selecting subjects whose measurement values are different, or vary, in some specific way from the population. Because the subjects have something in common, their values tend to be similar to those of others in the sample but different in some way from those of the population as a whole. These values do not vary randomly around the population mean. Most of the variation from the mean is in the same direction; it is systematic. All the values in the sample may tend to be higher or lower than the population mean.

For example, if all the subjects in a study examining some type of knowledge have an intelligence quotient (IQ) higher than 120, all their scores will likely be higher than the mean of a population that includes individuals with a wide variation in IQ. The IQs of the subjects have introduced a systematic bias. This situation could occur, for example, if all the subjects were college students, which has been the case in the development of many measurement methods in psychology.

Because of systematic variance, the sample mean is different from the population mean. The extent of the difference is the sampling error. Exclusion criteria tend to increase the systematic bias in the sample and thus, increase the sampling error. An extreme example of this problem is the highly restrictive sampling criteria used by clinical trials, which result in a large sampling error and greatly diminished representativeness.

If the method of selecting subjects produces a sample with a systematic bias, increasing the sample size will not decrease the sampling error. When a systematic bias occurs in an experimental study, it can lead the researcher to believe that a treatment has made a difference when, in actuality, the values would be different even without the treatment. This situation usually occurs because of an interaction of the systematic bias with the treatment. Systematic variation is most likely to occur when the sampling process is not random.

Random Sampling

From a sampling theory point of view, each individual in the population should have a greater than zero opportunity to be selected for the sample. The method of achieving this opportunity is referred to as *random sampling*. In experimental studies in which a control group is used, subjects are ran-

domly selected for placement in the control group and the experimental group as well as for participation in the study. The use of the term *control group* is limited to those studies using random sampling methods. If nonrandom methods are used for sample selection, the group not receiving a treatment is referred to as a *comparison group*, because there is a greater possibility of pre-existing differences between that group and the group receiving the treatment.

The purpose of random sampling is to increase the extent to which the sample is representative of the target population. However, the random sampling must take place in an accessible population that is representative of the target population. Exclusion criteria limit true randomness. Thus, a study that uses random sampling techniques may have such restrictive sampling criteria that the sample is not truly random. In any case, it is rarely possible to obtain a purely random sample for clinical nursing studies because of informed consent requirements. Persons who volunteer to participate in a study may differ in important ways from those who are not willing to participate. Methods of achieving random sampling are described later in the chapter.

Sampling Frames

In order for each person in the target or accessible population to have an opportunity to be selected for the sample, each person in the population must be identified. To accomplish this goal, a listing of every member of the population must be acquired, through the use of the sampling criteria to define membership. This listing is referred to as the *sampling frame*. The researcher then selects subjects from the sampling frame using a sampling plan.

Sampling Plans

A *sampling plan* describes the strategies that will be used to obtain a sample for a study. The plan is developed to enhance representativeness, reduce systematic bias, and decrease the sampling error (Brent et al., 1988). To accomplish this task, sampling theory has devised strategies for optimal sample selection. The sampling plan may use probability (random) sampling methods or nonprobability (nonrandom) sampling methods (see following discussion). A *sampling method* is similar to a design; it is not specific to a study. The sampling plan provides detail about the use of a sampling method in a specific study. The sampling plan must be described in detail for purposes of critique, replication, and future meta-analyses.

PROBABILITY (RANDOM) SAMPLING METHODS

Probability sampling methods have been developed to ensure some degree of precision in estimations of the population parameters. Thus, probability samples reduce sampling error. The term *probability sample* refers to the fact that *every* member (element) of the population has a probability higher than zero of being selected for the sample. Inferential statistical analyses are based on the assumption that the sample from which data were derived has been obtained randomly. Thus, probability samples are often referred to as *random samples*. Such a sample is more likely to be representative of the population than a nonprobability sample. All the subsets of the population, which may differ from one another but contribute to the parameters of the population, have a chance to be represented in the sample.

There is less opportunity for systematic bias if subjects are selected randomly, although it is possible for a systematic bias to occur by chance. Using random sampling, the researcher cannot decide that person X will be a better subject for the study than person Y. In addition, a researcher cannot exclude a subset of people from selection as subjects because he or she does not agree with them, does not like them, or finds them hard to deal with. Potential subjects cannot be excluded because they are too sick, not sick enough, coping too well, or not coping adequately. The researcher, who has a vested interest in the study, could tend (consciously or unconsciously) to select subjects whose conditions or behaviors are consistent with the hypothesis. It is tempting to exclude uncooperative or noncompliant individuals. Random sampling leaves the selection to chance and, thus, increases the validity of the study.

Theoretically, to obtain a probability sample, the researcher must identify every element in the population. A sampling frame must be developed, and the sample must be randomly selected from the sampling frame. Thus, according to sampling theory, it is not possible to select a sample randomly from a population that cannot be clearly defined. The following four sampling designs have been developed to achieve probability sampling: simple random sampling, stratified random sampling, cluster sampling, and systematic sampling.

Simple Random Sampling

Simple random sampling is the most basic of the probability sampling methods. To achieve simple random sampling, elements are selected at random from the sampling frame. This goal can be accomplished in a variety of ways, limited only by the imagination of the researcher. If the sampling frame is small, names can be written on slips of paper, placed in a container, mixed well, and then drawn out one at a time until the desired sample size has been reached. Another technique is assigning a number to each name in the sampling frame. In large population sets, elements may already have assigned numbers. For example, numbers are assigned to medical records, organizational memberships, and licenses. These numbers may then be selected randomly to obtain a sample.

There can be some differences in the probability for the selection of each element, depending on whether the selected element's name or number is replaced before the next name or number is selected. Selection with replacement, the most conservative random sampling approach, provides exactly equal opportunities for each element to be selected. For example, if the researcher draws names out of a hat to obtain a sample, each name must be replaced before the next name is drawn to ensure equal opportunity for each subject.

Selection without replacement gives each element different levels of probability of selection. For example, if the researcher is selecting 10 subjects from a population of 50, the first name has a 1 in 5 chance, or a .2 probability, of being selected. If the first name is not replaced, the second name has a 9 in 49 chance, or a .18 probability, of being selected.

As further names are drawn, the probability of being selected decreases.

There are many ways of achieving random selection. For example, a computer, bingo wheel, or roulette wheel could be used. The most common method of random selection is a table of random numbers. A section from a random numbers table is shown in Table 14–1. To use a table of random numbers, the researcher places a pencil or a finger on the random table with the eyes closed. The number touched is the starting place. Moving the pencil or finger up, down, right, or left, the researcher uses the numbers in order until the desired sample size is obtained. For example, the researcher places a pencil on 58 in Table 14–1, which is in the fourth column from the left and fourth row down. If five subjects are to be selected from a population of 100 and the researcher decides to go across the column to the right, the subject numbers chosen are 58, 25, 15, 55, and 38.

The table partially shown in Table 14–1 is useful only if the population number is less than 100. However, tables are available for larger populations. A larger random numbers table is available in Appendix A. With very large populations in which the sampling frame has been computerized, the simplest approach is to purchase a computer program to select subjects randomly.

Hart (1995) used random sampling in her study of pregnant women with Orem's self-care deficit theory as a framework. She describes her sample selection in the following excerpt from the study.

. . . .

"A random sample of women over 18 years of age who could read, write and speak English was chosen from a tertiary hospital obstetric clinic, a health department clinic, and a private federally-funded clinic in south Georgia. Women were in at least their 30th week of pregnancy. It was felt that by this time the subjects would have established a prenatal care routine and would have established the foundations for dependent-care agency. The researcher reviewed the daily appointment book to determine the list of eligible participants. Using a flip of the coin, a list of potential subjects was generated. Subjects were approached individually in the waiting room and asked to participate in the study. Data were collected over a period of 7 months. A total of 147 pregnant women were asked to participate; 127 completed the questionnaires. Most refusals were due to lack of interest or time and dealing with their children in the waiting room. An adequate number of participants was determined based on power analysis described by Cohen (1988). In this study, the number of independent variables is equal to eight. Because R^2 cannot be estimated, Cohen (1988) suggests a medium effect size of $R^2 = .13$ as adequate for correlational research. The power selected was .80." (Hart, 1995, pp. 121–122) ■

Stratified Random Sampling

Stratified random sampling is used in situations in which the researcher knows some of the variables in the population that are critical to achieving representativeness. Variables commonly used for stratification are age, gender, ethnicity, socioeconomic status, diagnosis, geographical region, type of institution, type of care, and site of care. The variable or variables chosen for stratification must be correlated with the dependent variables being examined in the study. Subjects within each stratum are expected to be more alike (homogeneous) in relation to the study variables than they are to be like subjects in other age strata or the total sample. In stratified random sampling, the subjects are randomly selected on the basis of their classification into the selected strata.

For example, if a sample of 100 subjects is planned, the researcher might plan to obtain 25 subjects younger than 20 years, 25 subjects in the age range 20 to 39 years, 25 subjects in the age range 40 to 59 years, and 25 subjects older than 60 years.

TABLE 14–1
SECTION FROM A RANDOM NUMBERS TABLE

06	84	10	22	56	72	25	70	69	43
07	63	10	34	66	39	54	02	33	85
03	19	63	93	72	52	13	30	44	40
77	32	69	58	25	15	55	38	19	62
20	01	94	54	66	88	43	91	34	28

Stratification ensures that all levels of the identified variables are adequately represented in the sample. Stratification allows the researcher to use a smaller sample size to achieve the same degree of representativeness as a large sample acquired through simple random sampling. Sampling error is decreased, power is increased, data collection time is reduced, and the cost of the study is lower if stratification is used.

One question that arises in relation to stratification is whether each stratum should have equivalent numbers of subjects in the sample (*disproportionate sampling*) or whether the numbers of subjects should be selected in proportion to their occurrence in the population (*proportionate sampling*). For example, if stratification is being achieved by ethnicity and the population is 60% white, 20% African American, 15% Mexican American, and 5% Asian, the researcher would have to decide whether to select equal numbers of each ethnic group or to calculate a proportion of the sample. Good arguments exist for both approaches. Stratification is not as useful if one stratum contains only a small number of subjects. In the aforementioned situation, if proportions are used and the sample size is 50, the study would include only two Asians, hardly enough to be representative. If equal numbers of each group are used, each group would contain at least 12 subjects; however, the white group would be underrepresented. In this case, mathematically weighting the findings from each stratum can equalize the representation to ensure proportional contributions of each stratum to the total score of the sample. This procedure is described in most textbooks on sampling (Cochran, 1977; Friday, 1967; Hansen et al., 1953; Levy & Lemsbow, 1980; Sudman, 1974; Williams, 1978; Yates, 1981).

Princeton and Gaspar (1991) used stratified random sampling in their study, "First-Line Nurse Administrators in Academe: How Are They Prepared, What Do They Do, and Will They Stay in Their Jobs?" The following excerpt is their description of the sampling procedure.

- -

"A random sample of 42 schools was drawn from the 114 nursing schools throughout the nation that were accredited by the National League for Nursing at the time, and that offered bachelor's degree and graduate nursing programs. The sample was stratified by geographic area and source of funding (public or private). The rationale for using these schools was that there was a high probability that they differentiated top-, mid-, and first-level administrative roles due to the size of the student population and the programs offered. This rationale was validated during the research project." (Princeton & Gaspar, 1991, p. 82) ▪

Cluster Sampling

Cluster sampling is used in two situations. The first situation is when a simple random sample would be prohibitive in terms of travel time and cost. Imagine trying to arrange personal meetings with 100 people, each in a different part of the United States. The second situation is in cases in which the individual elements making up the population are not known, thus preventing the development of a sampling frame. For example, there is no list of all the open-heart surgery patients in the United States. In these cases, it is often possible to obtain lists of institutions or organizations with which the elements of interest are associated.

In *cluster sampling,* a sampling frame is developed that includes a list of all the states, cities, institutions, or organizations with which elements of the identified population would be linked. States, cities, institutions, or organizations are selected randomly as units from which to obtain elements for the sample. In some cases, this random selection continues through several stages and is then referred to as multistage sampling. For example, the researcher might first randomly select states, then randomly select cities within the sampled states. Hospitals within the randomly selected cities might then be randomly selected. Within the hospitals, nursing units might be randomly selected. At this level, either all the patients on the nursing unit who fit the criteria for the study might be included or patients could be randomly selected.

Cluster sampling provides a means for obtaining a larger sample at a lower cost. However, it has some disadvantages. Data from subjects associated with the same institution are likely to be correlated and, thus, not completely independent. This correlation can lead to a decrease in precision and an increase in sampling error. However, such disadvantages can be offset to some extent by the use of a larger sample.

Mitchell and associates (1994) used multistage cluster sampling in their study differentiating women with three perimenstrual symptom patterns. They describe their sampling procedure as follows.

• •

"The community sample of healthy women participating in this study was obtained through a multistage sampling procedure commonly used in epidemiological studies. First, census block groups were selected using age, income, and ethnicity to facilitate the selection of a sample of menstruating women between the ages of 18 and 45 with a wide range of incomes. The ethnic mix was representative of the northwestern metropolitan area that was sampled. Second, street segments were identified and randomly ordered by computer from the selected census block groups. Third, residential telephone numbers for every household within the computer-generated street segments were obtained from a city directory. Finally, telephone contact was made with 5,755 households, and 1,135 women between the ages of 18 and 45 were identified.

"Criteria for inclusion were as follows: age between 18 and 45, not currently pregnant, not being treated for a gynecological problem, having menstrual periods, and the ability to write and understand English. Women taking birth control pills (BCPs) were included in the original data collection but were excluded from the analysis for this study to avoid confounding the sample selection and results with effects of exogenous hormones.

"Six hundred fifty-six eligible women who satisfied all the inclusion criteria completed an in-home interview and received instructions about keeping the Washington Women's Health Diary (WWHD). Three hundred forty-three women returned at least one complete cycle of daily data. Of these 343 women, 47 were taking BCPs, leaving 296 women who were not on any ovarian hormones. A total of 142 of these women fell into one of the three subgroups of interest for this study. The remaining 154

women fell into one of 25 other possible symptom severity subgroups that were not part of this study." (Mitchell et al., 1994, pp. 26–27) ▪

Systematic Sampling

Systematic sampling can be conducted when an ordered list of all members of the population is available. The process involves selecting every kth individual on the list, using a starting point selected randomly. If the initial starting point is not random, the sample is not a probability sample. To use this design, the researcher must know the number of elements in the population and the size of the sample desired. The population size is divided by the desired sample size, giving k, the size of the gap between elements selected from the list. For example, if the population size is $N = 1200$ and the desired sample size is $n = 50$, then $k = 24$. Every 24th person on the list would be included in the sample; this value is obtained by dividing 1200 by 50. There is argument that this procedure does not truly give each element an opportunity to be included in the sample; it provides a random but not equal chance for inclusion.

Care must be taken to determine that the original list has not been set up with any ordering that could be meaningful in relation to the study. The process is based on the assumption that the order of the list is random in relation to the variables being studied. If the order of the list is related to the study, systematic bias is introduced. In addition to this risk, computation of the sampling error with the use of this design is difficult. For additional information about systematic sampling, see Floyd (1993).

Youngblut and Brooten (1999) used systematic sampling in their study, "Alternate Child Care, History of Hospitalization, and Preschool Child Behavior." They described their sampling procedure as follows.

• •

"Families with preterm preschoolers were identified from the admission records of three level III neonatal intensive care units (NICUs); families with full-term preschoolers were identified from birth records of two normal newborn nurseries. A systematic random sample of families with full-terms and all families with preterms from four consecutive birth years were sent a letter that briefly described the study." (Youngblut & Brooten, 1999, p. 30) ■

NONPROBABILITY (NONRANDOM) SAMPLING METHODS

In *nonprobability sampling,* not every element of the population has an opportunity to be included in the sample. Although this approach to sampling raises the possibilities of samples that are not representative, it has been commonly used in nursing studies. An analysis of nursing studies published in six nursing journals from 1977 to 1986 revealed that only 9% used random sampling (Moody et al., 1988). The majority of the studies examined were descriptive or correlational in nature. Only 30% of the nursing studies reported during this period used quasi-experimental or experimental designs likely to require assignment of subjects to groups.

Kraemer and Thiemann (1987) classify studies as *exploratory* or *confirmatory.* According to their approach, confirmatory studies should be conducted only after a large body of knowledge has been gathered through exploratory studies. *Confirmatory* studies are expected to have large samples and to use random sampling techniques. These expectations are lessened for exploratory studies. *Exploratory* studies are not intended for generalization to large populations. They are designed to increase the knowledge of the field of study. For example, pilot or preliminary studies to test a methodology or provide estimates of an effect size are often conducted before a larger study. In other studies, the variables, not the subjects, are the primary area of concern. The same variables may be examined in several studies using different populations. In these types of studies, the specific population used may be somewhat incidental. Data from these studies may be used to define population parameters. This information can then be used to conduct confirmatory studies using large, randomly selected samples.

There are several types of nonprobability sampling designs. Each addresses a different research need. The four nonprobability sampling designs de-scribed here are convenience sampling, quota sampling, purposive sampling, and network sampling.

Convenience (Accidental) Sampling

Convenience sampling is considered a poor approach to sampling because it provides little opportunity to control for biases. In *convenience sampling,* subjects are included in the study because they happened to be in the right place at the right time. Available subjects are simply entered into the study until the desired sample size is reached. Multiple biases may exist in the sample, some of which may be subtle and unrecognized. However, serious biases are not always present in convenience samples.

The researcher needs to identify and describe known biases in the sample. Carefully thinking through the characteristics of the population, the researcher can identify the biases likely to occur. He or she can then take steps to improve the representativeness of the sample. For example, in a study of home care management of patients with complex health care needs, educational level would be an important extraneous variable. One solution for controlling this extraneous variable would be to redefine the sampling criteria to include only those individuals with a high school education. Doing so would limit the extent of generalization. Another option would be to select a population known to include individuals with a wide variety of educational levels. Data could be collected on educational level so that the description of the sample would include information on educational level. With this information, one could judge the extent to which the sample was representative in respect to educational level.

Decisions related to sample selection must be carefully described to enable others to evaluate the possibility of biases. In addition, data must be gathered to allow a thorough description of the sample. This information can be used to evaluate for possible biases. Data on the sample can be used to compare the sample with other samples and for estimating the parameters of populations through meta-analyses.

Many strategies are available for selecting a convenience sample. A classroom of students might be used. Patients who attend a clinic on a specific day, subjects who attend a support group, patients currently admitted to a hospital with a specific diagnosis or nursing problem, and every fifth person who enters the emergency room are examples of types of commonly selected convenience samples.

Convenience samples are inexpensive and accessible, and they usually require less time to acquire than other types of samples. Convenience samples provide means to conduct studies on topics that could not be examined through the use of probability sampling. They provide means of acquiring information in unexplored areas. As Kerlinger (1986, p. 120) states, "Used with reasonable knowledge and care, it [convenience sampling] is probably not as bad as it has been said to be." Kerlinger recommends using this type of sampling only if there is no possibility of obtaining a sample by other means. Convenience sampling is useful for exploratory studies but, in most cases, is unacceptable for confirmatory studies.

Tracy and colleagues (1999) used convenience sampling in their study, "Hope and Anxiety of Individual Family Members of Critically Ill Adults." The following excerpt describes their sample selection.

▪ ▪

"The study was conducted at a major hospital in central New Jersey using convenience sampling. Patients in any of five adult critical care units (medical, surgical/trauma, open heart, neurosurgical, and coronary care) were included in the study. With the approval from the Internal Review Board (IRB) and key administrative individuals in the critical care units, family members were identified by nursing staff and approached within 72 hours of patient admission." (Tracy et al., 1999, p. 123) ▪

Quota Sampling

Quota sampling uses a convenience sampling technique with an added feature, a strategy to ensure the inclusion of subject types that are likely to be underrepresented in the convenience sample, such as women, minority groups, the aged, the poor, the rich, and the undereducated. This method may also be used to mimic the known characteris-

tics of the target population or to ensure adequate numbers of subjects in each stratum for the planned statistical analyses. The technique is similar to that used in stratified random sampling. If necessary, mathematical weighting can be used to adjust sample values so that they are consistent with the proportion of subgroups found in the population. Quota sampling offers an improvement over convenience sampling and tends to decrease potential biases. In most studies in which convenience samples are used, quota sampling could be used and should be considered.

Gottlieb and Baillies (1995) used quota sampling in their study, "Firstborns' Behaviors During a Mother's Second Pregnancy." They described their sample selection as follows.

▪ ▪

"Eighty mothers and their only preschoolers agreed to participate. The study included four groups of 20 preschoolers: three groups of children of pregnant mothers (one each from the early, middle, and late phases of pregnancy); and a fourth group of children of non-pregnant mothers. Because the majority of pregnant do not see a physician until the end of the first trimester, the study was begun at 12 weeks and extended to the 38th week, close to the birth.

"The families were all intact families, and the preschoolers were their only children, 18 to 60 months of age. The mothers were employed less than 21 hours per week and had no intervening pregnancies between the first child and their participation in this study. To examine how behaviors differed as a function of a child's age and/or sex, each group was balanced for age (young: 18 to 36 months; old: 37 to 60 months) and sex. Thus, within each group, there were five young boys, five old boys, five young girls, and five old girls.

"Families were recruited from the practices of obstetricians and pediatricians. Of the 72 eligible families expecting a second child, five families refused, and seven mothers did not complete the data collection schedule. The design called for 26 children per group for each age and sex to attain a power of .8 with alpha equal to .05 to detect a large effect size, $d = .4$ (Cohen, 1988). Preliminary analyses indicated significant effects with 20 per group; therefore, the sample was considered adequate. Children of the comparison group were recruited from the practices of pediatricians and nursery schools. The groups were compared for equivalency on all major background characteristics and, with the exception of mothers' and fathers' ages, did not differ significantly. Parents in the three pregnancy groups were younger than parents in the comparison group, $p < .05$. Families were predominantly white, middle-class, and well educated. Parents had been together an average of 7 years." (Gottlieb & Baillies, 1995, p. 357) ■

Purposive Sampling

Purposive sampling is sometimes referred to as *judgmental sampling*. Purposive sampling involves the conscious selection by the researcher of certain subjects or elements to include in the study. Efforts might be made to include typical subjects or typical situations. Examples of good care and poor care or good patients and bad patients might be used. This approach is often used in qualitative studies. Using insights gained from initial data collection, the qualitative researcher may decide to seek subjects with particular characteristics to increase theoretical understanding of some facet of the phenomenon being studied. For example, the researcher might find, through subject interviews, that the views of a few subjects differed strikingly from the views of the group. The researcher might intentionally seek interviews with the individuals whose views differed.

The strategy has been criticized because there is no way to evaluate the precision of the researcher's judgment. How does one determine that the patient or element was typical, good, bad, effective, or ineffective? However, this sampling method may be a way to develop some initial ideas about an area not easily examined with the use of other sampling techniques. Sandelowski (1995) suggests that purposive samples can be too small to achieve informational redundancy or theoretical saturation or too large to perform the detailed analyses of data required in qualitative studies. Purposive sampling in qualitative research is discussed in more detail in Chapter 23.

Stewart and colleagues (1999) used purposive sampling in their study, "Development and Psycho-

metric Evaluation of the Environment-Behavior Interaction Code (EBIC)." The following excerpt describes the sample selection used in the study.

. . . .

"Three large (>100-bed) long-term care facilities provided the setting for the development and psychometric evaluation of the EBIC. These facilities had secure dementia care units for 34, 36, and 83 residents, respectively. . . . Residents were observed on two of the secure units during the development of the EBIC. Although time sampling was used, residents with dementia were not preselected. . . . A total of 158 participants were purposively selected for one of the components of the psychometric phase: (a) the initial psychometric study of the event formula (n = 82), (b) interrater reliability testing of the interval format (n = 23), and (c) replications on the event format for interrater reliability (n = 53) and stability (8 of the 53 replication subjects)." (Stewart et al., 1999, p. 262) ■

Network Sampling

Network sampling, sometimes referred to as *snowball sampling*, holds promise for locating samples that are difficult or impossible to obtain in other ways. Network sampling takes advantage of social networks and the fact that friends tend to have characteristics in common. When the researcher has found a few subjects with the needed criteria, the subjects are asked for their assistance in getting in touch with others who have similar characteristics. This strategy is particularly useful for finding subjects in socially devalued populations, such as alcoholics, prostitutes, child abusers, sex offenders, drug addicts, and criminals. These individuals are seldom willing to make themselves known to others. Other groups, such as widows, grieving siblings, and those successful at lifestyle changes, can be located with this strategy. These individuals are outside the existing health care system and are difficult to find. Obviously, biases are built into the sampling process, because the subjects are not independent of one another.

Stevens (1995) used network sampling to obtain subjects for her study, "Structural and Interpersonal Impact of Heterosexual Assumptions on Lesbian

Health Care Clients." She describes her sampling procedure as follows.

. . . .

"Through community-based snowball sampling (Watters & Biernacki, 1989) in San Francisco, 45 lesbians were recruited to participate in the study during 1990 and 1991; 32 were interviewed individually and 13 were involved in three focus groups. Participants met the inclusion criteria: self-identified as lesbian, at least 21 years old, and conversant in English." (Stevens, 1995, p. 26) ■

SAMPLE SIZE

One of the questions most commonly asked by beginning researchers is, "What size sample should I use?" Historically, the response to this question has been that a sample should contain at least 30 subjects. There is no logical reason for the selection of this number, and in most cases, 30 subjects is an inadequate sample size.

Currently, the deciding factor in determining an adequate sample size for correlational, quasi-experimental, and experimental studies is power. *Power* is the capacity of the study to detect differences or relationships that actually exist in the population. Expressed another way, power is the capacity to correctly reject a null hypothesis. The minimum acceptable power for a study is .80. If a researcher does not have sufficient power to detect differences or relationships that exist in the population, one might question the advisability of conducting the study. Determining the sample size needed to obtain sufficient power is made by performing a power analysis. The statistical procedures used to perform power analyses are described in Chapter 18.

Nurse researchers have only recently begun using power analysis to determine sample size, and they frequently fail to report the results of the power analyses in published results of their studies. This issue is a particular problem in studies that fail to detect significant differences or relationships, in which the results might be due to an inadequate sample size rather than to incorrect hypotheses.

Polit and Sherman (1990) evaluated the sample sizes in 62 studies published in 1989 in the journals *Nursing Research* and *Research in Nursing & Health.* The mean sample size for a group on which comparative data analysis was performed was 83. Two thirds of the studies had group samples of less than 100. Most of the studies had inadequate sample sizes to make comparisons between groups. The studies needed an average of 218 subjects per group to have a power level of .80. In only one of the studies did the researchers report having performed a power analysis to determine the adequacy of their sample size.

Beck (1994) reviewed the reporting of power analysis in three nursing research journals from 1988 through 1992. "During this 5-year period, in only 8 studies published in *Nursing Research,* 9 studies in *Research in Nursing & Health,* and 3 studies in *Western Journal of Nursing Research* had the researcher specified that power analysis had been done and supplied the readers with the particulars of their analysis." (Beck, 1994, p. 78)

The adequacy of sample sizes must be more carefully evaluated in future nursing studies *before data collection.* Studies with inadequate sample sizes should not be approved for data collection unless they are preliminary pilot studies conducted before a planned larger study. If it is not possible to obtain a larger sample because of time or numbers of available subjects, the study should be redesigned so that the available sample is adequate for the planned analyses. If one cannot obtain a sufficient sample size, one should not conduct the study.

Large sample sizes are difficult to obtain in nursing studies, require long data collection periods, and are costly. Therefore, in developing the methodology for a study, the researcher must evaluate the elements of the methodology that affect the required sample size. Kraemer and Thiemann (1987) identify the following factors that must be taken into consideration in determining sample size:

1. The more stringent the significance level (e.g., .001 versus .05), the greater the necessary sample size.
2. Two-tailed statistical tests require larger sample sizes than one-tailed tests. (Tailedness of statistical tests is explained in Chapter 18.)
3. The smaller the effect size, the larger the necessary sample size.
4. The larger the power required, the larger the necessary sample size.

5. The smaller the sample size, the smaller the power of the study.

Other factors that must be considered in decisions about sample size (because they affect power) are the effect size, the type of study, the number of variables, the sensitivity of the measurement tools, and the data analysis techniques.

Effect Size

Effect is the presence of a phenomenon. If a phenomenon exists, it is not absent, and thus, the null hypothesis is in error. However, effect is best understood when not considered in a dichotomous way, that is, as either present or absent. If a phenomenon exists, it exists to some degree. *Effect size* (ES) is the extent of the presence of a phenomenon. *Effect*, in this case, is used in a broader sense than that of "cause and effect."

For example, you might examine the impact of distraction on the experience of pain during an injection. To examine this question, you might obtain a sample of subjects receiving injections and measure differences in the experience of pain in a group who were distracted during injection and a group who were not distracted. The null hypothesis would be that there would be no difference in the amount of pain experienced by the two groups. If this were so, you would say that the effect of distraction on the experience of pain was zero. In another study, you might be interested in using the Pearson product moment correlation r to examine the relationship between coping and anxiety. Your null hypothesis would be that the population r would be zero. Coping would have no relationship to anxiety (Cohen, 1988).

In a study, it is easier to detect large differences between groups than to detect small differences. Thus, smaller samples can detect large ESs; smaller effect sizes require larger samples. Broadly speaking, a small ES would be about .2, a medium effect size .5, and a large ES .8. ES is smaller with a small sample and thus is more difficult to detect. Enlarging the sample size also increases the ES, making it more likely that the effect will be de-

tected. Extremely small ESs may not be clinically significant. Knowing the effect size that would be regarded as clinically important allows us to limit the sample to the size needed to detect that level of ES (Kraemer & Thiemann, 1987). A result is clinically significant if the effect is large enough to alter clinical decisions. For example, in a comparison of glass thermometers with electronic thermometers, an effect size of 0.1°F in oral temperature is probably not important enough to influence selection of a particular type of thermometer.

ESs vary according to the population being studied. Thus, we need to determine the ES for the particular effect being studied in a particular population. The most desirable source of this information is evidence from previous studies. Using such information as the mean and standard deviation, the researcher can calculate the ES. This calculation, however, can be used only as an estimate of ES for the study. If the researcher changes the measure used or the design or the population being studied, the ES will be altered. The best estimate of a population parameter of ES is obtained from a meta-analysis in which an estimated population effect size is calculated through the use of statistical values from all studies included in the analysis (Polit & Sherman, 1990).

If few relevant studies have been conducted in the area of interest, small pilot studies can be performed, and data analysis results used to calculate the effect size. If pilot studies are not feasible, dummy power table analysis can be used to calculate the smallest effect size with clinical or theoretical value. Yarandi (1991) describes the process of calculating a dummy power table. If all else fails, ES can be estimated as small, medium, or large. Numerical values would be assigned to these estimates, and the power analysis performed. Cohen (1988) has indicated the numerical values for small, medium, and large effects on the basis of specific statistical procedures. In new areas of research, effect sizes are usually small (Borenstein & Cohen, 1989).

In the nursing studies examined by Polit and Sherman (1990), 52.7% of the effect sizes computed were small. They found that in nursing studies, for small effects, average power was less than

.30. Thus, there was less than a 30% probability that acceptance of the null hypothesis was correct. This situation was, in most cases, due to an insufficient sample size. Even in the nursing studies in which the effect size was moderate, however, the average power was only .70. Only when the effect size was large did the nursing studies reach an acceptable level of power (0.8), and 11% of these studies were underpowered. Only 15% of the studies these researchers examined had sufficient power for all of their analyses.

Type of Study

Qualitative studies and case studies tend to use very small samples. Comparisons between groups are not being performed, and problems related to sampling error and generalization have little relevance for such studies. A small sample size may better serve the researcher who is interested in examining a situation in depth from various perspectives. The qualitative researcher stops seeking additional participants when theoretical saturation is achieved.

Descriptive studies, particularly those using survey questionnaires, and correlational studies often require very large samples. In these studies, multiple variables may be examined, and extraneous variables are likely to affect subject responses to the variables under study. Statistical comparisons are often made among multiple subgroups in the sample, requiring that an adequate sample be available for each subgroup being analyzed. In addition, subjects are likely to be heterogeneous in terms of demographic variables, and measurement tools are sometimes not adequately refined. Although target populations may have been identified, sampling frames may not be available, and parameters have not usually been well defined by previous studies. All of these factors lower the power of the study and require increases in sample size (Kraemer & Thiemann, 1987).

In the past, quasi-experimental and experimental studies often used smaller samples than descriptive and correlational studies. As control in the study increases, the sample size can decrease and still approximate the population. Instruments in these studies tend to be refined, thus improving precision. However, sample size must be sufficient to achieve an acceptable level of power (0.8) to reduce the risk of a Type II error (Kraemer & Thiemann, 1987).

The study design influences power, but the design with the greatest power may not always be the most valid design to use. The experimental design with the greatest power is the pretest-posttest design with a historical control group. However, this design may have questionable validity because of the historical control group. Can the researcher demonstrate that the historical control group is comparable to the experimental group? The repeated measures design will increase power if the trait being assessed is relatively stable over time. Designs that use blocking or stratification usually require an increase in the total sample size. The sample size increases in proportion to the number of cells included in the data analysis. Designs that use matched pairs of subjects have greater power and, thus, require a smaller sample. The higher the degree of correlation between subjects on the variable on which the subjects are matched, the greater the power (Kraemer & Thiemann, 1987).

Confirmatory studies, such as those testing the effects of nursing interventions on patient outcomes or those testing the fit of a theoretical model, require large sample sizes. Clinical trials are being conducted in nursing for these purposes. The power of these large, complex studies must be carefully analyzed (Leidy & Weissfeld, 1991). For the large sample sizes to be obtained, subjects are acquired in a number of clinical settings, sometimes in various parts of the country. Kraemer and Thiemann (1987) believe that these studies should not be performed until extensive information is available from exploratory studies. This information should include meta-analysis and the definition of a population effect size.

Number of Variables

As the number of variables under study grows, the needed sample size may also increase. Adding variables such as age, gender, ethnicity, and education to the analysis plan (just to be on the safe side) can increase the sample size by a factor of 5 to 10 if the selected variables are uncorrelated with the dependent variable. In this case, instead of a sample of 50, the researcher may need a sample of 500 if he or she plans to use the variables in the statistical analyses. (Using them only to describe the sample does not cause a problem in terms of power.) If the variables are highly correlated with the dependent variable, however, the effect size will increase, and the sample size can be reduced.

Therefore, variables included in the data analysis must be carefully selected. They should be essential to the research question or should have a documented strong relationship with the dependent variable (Kraemer & Thiemann, 1987). A number of the studies analyzed by Polit and Sherman (1990) had sufficient sample size for the primary analyses but failed to plan for analyses involving subgroups, such as analyzing the data by age categories or by ethnic groups. The inclusion of multiple dependent variables also increases the sample size needed.

Measurement Sensitivity

Well-developed instruments measure phenomena with precision. A thermometer, for example, measures body temperature precisely. Tools measuring psychosocial variables tend to be less precise. However, a tool with strong reliability and validity tends to measure more precisely than a tool that is less well developed. Variance tends to be higher in a less well-developed tool than in one that is well developed. An instrument with a smaller variance is preferred because the power of a test is always decreased by increased within-group variance (Kraemer & Thiemann, 1987). For example, if anxiety were being measured and the actual anxiety score for several subjects was 80, the subjects' scores on a less well developed tool might range from 70 to 90, whereas a well-developed tool would tend to show a score closer to the actual score of 80 for each subject. As variance in instrument scores increases, the sample size needed to gain an accurate understanding of the phenomenon under study increases.

The range of measured values influences power. For example, a variable might be measured in 10 equally spaced values, ranging from 0 to 9. Effect sizes vary according to how near the value is to the population mean. If the mean value is 5, effect sizes are much larger in the extreme values and lower for values near the mean. If the researcher decides to use only subjects with values of 0 and 9, the effect size will be large, and the sample could be small. The credibility of the study might be questionable, however, because the values of most individuals would not be 0 or 9 but rather would tend to be in the middle range of values. If the researcher decided to include subjects who have values in the range of 3 to 6, excluding the extreme scores, the effect size would be small, and a much larger sample would be required. The wider the range of values sampled, the larger the effect size (Kraemer & Thiemann, 1987).

Each measure of response should be used in as sensitive a form as can be reliably measured. If measurement on a continuum is reliable, the measure should not be reduced to a scale or dichotomized, because either maneuver would reduce the power. If an interval-level measure is reduced to an ordinal or nominal level, a much larger sample size is required to achieve adequate power (Kraemer & Thiemann, 1987).

Data Analysis Techniques

Data analysis techniques vary in their ability to detect differences in the data. Statisticians refer to this as the *power* of the statistical analysis. The most powerful statistical test appropriate to the data should be selected for data analysis. Overall, parametric statistical analyses are more powerful than nonparametric techniques in detecting differences and so should be used if the data meet criteria for parametric analysis. In many cases, however, nonparametric techniques are more powerful if the assumptions of parametric techniques are not met. Parametric techniques vary widely in their capacity to distinguish fine differences in the data. Parametric and nonparametric analyses are discussed in Chapter 18.

There is also an interaction between the measurement sensitivity and the power of the data analysis technique. The power of the analysis technique increases as precision in measurement increases.

Larger samples must be used when the power of the planned statistical analysis is low.

For some statistical procedures, such as the *t* test and analysis of variance (ANOVA), having equal group sizes increases power, because the effect size is maximized. The more unequal the group sizes are, the smaller the effect size. Therefore, in unequal groups, the total sample size must be larger (Kraemer & Thiemann, 1987).

The chi-squared (χ^2) test is the weakest of the statistical tests and requires very large sample sizes to achieve acceptable levels of power. As the number of categories grows, the sample size needed increases. Also, if there are small numbers in some of the categories, the sample size must be increased. Kraemer and Thiemann (1987) recommend that the chi-squared test be used only when no other options are available. In addition, the number of categories should be limited to those essential to the study.

RECRUITING AND RETAINING SUBJECTS

Once a decision has been made about the size of the sample, the next step is to develop a plan for recruiting subjects. Recruitment strategies differ, depending on the type of study and the setting. Special attention must focus on recruiting subjects who tend to be underrepresented in studies, such as minorities and women (Murdaugh, 1990). The sampling plan, initiated at the beginning of data collection, is almost always more difficult than is expected. Some researchers never obtain their planned sample size. Retaining acquired subjects is critical to the study and requires consideration of the effects of data collection strategies on subject mortality (loss of subjects from the study). Problems with retaining subjects increase as the data collection period lengthens.

Recruiting Subjects

Effective recruitment of subjects is crucial to the success of a study. Few studies have examined the effectiveness of various strategies of subject recruitment. Most information available to guide researchers comes from the personal experiences of skilled researchers. Schain (1994) suggests that the factors that influence subjects' decisions to participate are self-protectiveness, a high need for personal control, time and travel constraints, and the nature of the informed consent.

The initial approach to a potential subject usually strongly affects his or her decision about participating in the study. Therefore, the approach must be pleasant and positive. The importance of the study is explained, and the researcher makes clear exactly what the subject will be asked to do, how much of the subject's time will be involved, and what the duration of the study will be. Subjects are valuable resources. The recognition of this value must be communicated to the potential subject. High-pressure techniques, such as insisting that the subject make an instant decision to participate in a study, usually lead to resistance and a higher rate of refusals.

The researcher accepts refusals to participate gracefully—in terms of body language as well as words. The actions of the researcher can influence the decision of other potential subjects who observe or hear about the encounter. Studies in which a high proportion of individuals refuse to participate have a serious validity problem. The sample is likely to be biased, because usually, only a certain type of individual has agreed to participate. Therefore, records are kept of the numbers of persons who refuse and, if possible, their reasons for refusal.

Recruiting minority subjects for a study can be particularly problematic. Minority individuals may be difficult to locate and are often reluctant to participate in studies because of feelings of being "used" while receiving no personal benefit from their involvement. Pletsch and associates (1995, p. 211) recommend using "feasibility analysis, developing partnerships with target groups and community members, using active face-to-face recruitment, and using process evaluation techniques" to recruit members of minority groups as subjects of a study.

If data collectors are being used in the study, the researcher must verify that they are following the sampling plan, especially in random samples. When the data collectors encounter difficult subjects or are unable to make contact easily, they may simply shift to the next person without informing the principal investigator. This behavior could violate the rules of random sampling and bias the sample. If data collectors do not understand, or do not believe in, the importance of randomization, their decisions and actions can undermine the intent of the sampling plan. Thus, data collectors must be carefully selected and thoroughly trained. A plan must be developed for the supervision and follow-up of data collectors to increase their sense of accountability.

If you conduct a survey study, you may never have personal contact with the subjects. To recruit such subjects, you must rely on the use of attention-getting techniques, persuasively written material, and strategies for following up on individuals who do not respond to the initial written communication. Because of the serious problems of low response rates in survey studies, using strategies to raise the response rate is critical. For instance, we have received a teabag or packet of instant coffee with a questionnaire, accompanied by a recommendation in the letter to have a cup of tea or coffee "on" the researcher while we take a break from work to complete the questionnaire. Creativity is required in the use of such strategies, because they tend to lose their effect on groups who receive questionnaires frequently (such as faculty). In some cases, small amounts of money (fifty cents to a dollar) are enclosed with the letter, which may contain a suggestion that the recipient buy a soft drink or that the money is a small offering for completing the questionnaire. This strategy imposes some sense of obligation on the recipient to complete the questionnaire but is not thought to be coercive (Baker, 1985). Also, you should plan mailings to avoid holidays or times of the year when workloads are high for potential subjects, possibly reducing the return rate.

The letter to potential subjects must be carefully composed. It may be your only chance to persuade the subject to invest the time needed to complete the questionnaire. You need to "sell" the reader on the importance of both your study and his or her response. The tone of your letter will be the recipient's only image of you as a person; yet, for many subjects, their response to the perception of you as a person most influences their decision about completing the questionnaire. Seek examples of letters sent by researchers who had high response rates to questionnaires. Save letters you receive that you responded positively to. Pilot-test your letter on individuals who can give you feedback about their reactions to the tone of the letter.

The use of follow-up letters or cards has been repeatedly shown to raise response rates to surveys. The timing is important. If too long a period has lapsed, the questionnaire may have been discarded. Sending it too soon, however, could be offensive. Baker (1985) describes her strategy for following up on questionnaires.

• •

"Before the questionnaires were mailed, precise plans were made for monitoring the return of each questionnaire as a means of follow-up procedure. A bar graph was developed to record the return of each questionnaire as a means of suggesting when the follow-up mailing should occur (Babbie, 1973). Each square on the graph paper represented one questionnaire. Day 1 on the graph was the day on which the questionnaires were mailed. The cumulative number and percentage of responses were logged on the graph to reflect the overall data collection process. When the daily responses declined, a follow-up, first-class mailing was sent, containing another questionnaire, a modified cover letter, and a return envelope. Study participants and questionnaires were assigned the same code numbers, and nonrespondents were identified by checking the list of code numbers of unreturned questionnaires. A second follow-up questionnaire, with a further modified cover letter, and a return envelope were sent by certified mail. Should there still have been unreturned questionnaires, a dialogue was prepared for a final follow-up by telephone." (Baker, 1985, p. 119) ■

The factors involved in the decision whether to respond to a questionnaire are not well understood. One obvious factor is the time required to respond; this includes the time needed to orient to the directions and the emotional energy to deal with the threats and anxieties generated by the questions.

There is also a cognitive demand for thinking. Subjects seem to make a judgment about the relevance of the research topic and the potential for personal application of findings. Previous experience with mailed questionnaires is also a deciding factor (Baker, 1985).

To reduce costs, nurse researchers are now using the mail to collect far more extensive data than that of the simple questionnaire. In some cases, multiple scales are mailed to subjects, which are to be completed at home and returned. Recruitment strategies for these subjects may require some form of personal contact before the material is mailed as well as telephone contact during the data collection period.

Traditionally, subjects for nursing studies have been sought in the hospital setting. However, access to these subjects is becoming more difficult—in part because of the larger numbers of nurses now conducting research (Cronenwett, 1986). Nurse researchers are now recruiting subjects from a variety of sources. An initial phase of recruitment may involve obtaining community and institutional support for the study. Support from other health professionals, such as nurses and physicians, may be critical to the successful recruitment of subjects.

Studies may also benefit from endorsement by community leaders, such as city officials, key civic leaders, and leaders of social, educational, religious, or labor groups. In some cases, these groups may be involved in planning the study, leading to a sense of community ownership of the project. Community groups may also assist in recruitment of subjects for the study. Sometimes, subjects who meet the sampling criteria are found in the groups assisting with the study. Endorsement may involve letters of support and, in some cases, funding. These activities add legitimacy to the study and make involvement in the study more attractive to potential subjects (Diekmann & Smith, 1989).

Media support can be helpful in recruiting subjects. Advertisements can be placed in local newspapers and church and neighborhood bulletins. Radio stations can make public service announcements. Members of the research team can speak to groups relevant to the study population. Posters can be placed in public places, such as supermarkets, drugstores, and public laundries. With permission, tables can be placed in shopping malls with a member of the research team present to recruit subjects (Diekmann & Smith, 1989).

Lusk and associates (1994) used multiple recruitment strategies to obtain a sample of 645 workers for a study testing the effectiveness of the health promotion model to explain workers' use of hearing protection. The following excerpt from their study describes the strategies.

"A convenience sample of 645 workers (319 blue-collar, 209 skilled trades, and 117 white-collar) was recruited to complete written questionnaires. Supervisors were encouraged to give release time to workers who wished to participate. Posters, flyers, and the plant newsletter were used to publicize the study, and pairs of university football game tickets were offered as lottery prizes as an incentive for participation. To obtain sufficient power for analyses, data collection was designed to continue until at least 300 blue-collar, 200 skilled trades, and 100 white-collar subjects volunteered. The participants represented approximately 14.4% of the 4,473 workers employed at the plant (day and evening shifts only), in comparison to the 2 to 3% participation rate reported for other voluntary activities at the plant." (Lusk et al., 1994, p. 153) ▪

Recruitment of subjects for clinical studies requires a different set of strategies. For clinical trials, recruitment may be occurring simultaneously in several sites (perhaps in different cities). Many of these studies never achieve their planned sample size. The number of subjects meeting the sampling criteria who are available in the selected clinical sites may not be as large as anticipated. Researchers must often screen twice as many patients as are required for the study to obtain a sufficient sample size. Screening logs must be kept during the recruiting period to record data on patients who met the criteria but were not entered into the study. Researchers commonly underestimate the amount of time required to recruit subjects for a clinical study. In addition to defining the number of subjects and the time set aside for recruitment, it may be helpful to develop short-term or interim recruitment goals designed to maintain a constant rate of patient entry (Diekmann & Smith, 1989).

Retaining Subjects

One of the serious problems in many studies is subject retention. Often, subject mortality cannot be avoided. Subjects move, die, or withdraw from treatment. If data must be collected at several points over time, subject mortality can become a problem.

Subjects who move frequently and those without telephones pose a particular problem. A number of strategies have been found to be effective in maintaining the sample. For instance, names, addresses, and telephone numbers of at least two family members or friends are obtained when the subject is enrolled in the study. Consent may be sought from the subject to give the researcher access to unlisted telephone numbers in the event that the subject changes his or her phone number.

In some studies, the subject is reimbursed for participation. A bonus payment may be included for completing a certain phase of the study. Gifts can be used in place of money. Sending greeting cards for birthdays and holidays helps maintain contact. Rudy and associates (1994) compared the effect on recruitment and retention of money versus gifts. They found no differential effect on recruitment but found that money was more effective than gifts in retaining subjects in longitudinal studies. However, the researchers point out the moral issues related to providing monetary payment to subjects. This strategy can compromise the voluntariness of participation in a study and particularly has the potential of exploiting low-income persons.

Collecting data takes time. The researcher must always keep in mind that the subject's time is valuable and should be used frugally. During data collection, it is easy to begin taking the subject for granted. Taking time for social amenities with subjects may pay off. However, one needs to take care that these interactions do not influence the data being collected. Beyond that, nurturing subjects participating in the study is critical. In some situations, providing refreshments and pleasant surroundings is helpful. Often, during the data collection phase, others who interact with the subjects also

must be nurtured; these may be volunteers, family, staff, students, or other professionals. It is important to maintain a pleasant climate for the data collection process, which will "pay off" in the quality of data collected and the retention of subjects.

Some longitudinal studies require the completion of forms repeatedly at various intervals. Sometimes the forms are diaries requiring daily entries over a set period. These studies face the greatest risk of subject mortality.

Barnard and colleagues (1987) described the extensive sample maintenance procedures required for their longitudinal study in the following excerpt.

. . . .

"Sometimes the researcher needs to invest a great deal of time and money in sample maintenance. For example, for the 13-month assessment point in our current study of high-social-risk mothers and children, a research assistant picks up the mother and child at home (a 45-minute drive), brings them to the clinic for testing, and then drives them home again. In addition, the mother is given up to $10 to cover babysitting costs for her other children and is sent a free copy of the videotape we make of her and her child. Without these elaborate arrangements, we feel that our attrition rate would be very high." (Barnard et al., p. 47) ■

Subjects who have a personal investment in the study are more likely to continue in the study. This investment occurs through interactions with and nurturing by the researcher. A combination of the subject's personal belief in the significance of the study and the nurturing of the subject during data collection by the researcher may diminish subject mortality (Killien & Newton, 1990).

Gordon and Stokes (1989) describe strategies used in their longitudinal study of stressors and the onset of illness in individuals 65 years and older, which required subjects to keep a health diary and to complete a set of scales that were mailed to them every 3 months for 1 year. All materials were color-coded according to the quarter of the year. Oversized lettering was used on all forms. All forms were kept consistent throughout the year, so that subjects became increasingly familiar with them. Subjects remained anonymous throughout the study. Thus, telephone contact by the researcher was impossible. Materials were returned to the researchers by mail using preaddressed stamped envelopes of the same color as the data forms. Eighty-seven individuals participated in the study. The response rate the first quarter was 91%, the second quarter 86%, the third quarter 79%, and the fourth quarter 81%. The following excerpt describes further strategies these researchers used to achieve and maintain subject participation in the study.

. . . .

"Development of commitment began with the first letter sent to subjects. The letter emphasized the importance of the study to the health and well-being of people in the subject's age group. Subjects were told they would be providing an important service to their peers by participating in the study. All subsequent letters requesting data emphasized the importance of each individual's participation to successful completion of the study. Furthermore, as the study continued, subjects were told of the high response rate among their peers, in order to augment the feeling of being part of a larger group. They were encouraged to keep up the good work.

"Information regarding the use of data from the study was forwarded to the participants. For example, when the *New York Times* reported the study, a copy of the newspaper article was sent to each participant. They were informed of professional presentations, radio interviews, and grant proposals submitted for funding of related work.

"Personalized materials have been shown to raise response rates between 7 and 8% (Andreasen, 1970). Each letter was hand signed. The letters were phrased in an informal style using language of the cohort group. Pictures of the researchers and the school of nursing were included so the subjects could see those with whom they were communicating and the location to which they were sending their materials." (Gordon & Stokes, 1989, p. 375) ■

■ SUMMARY

. . . .

Sampling involves selecting a group of people, events, behaviors, or other elements with which to

conduct a study. *Sampling* denotes the process of making the selections; *sample* denotes the selected group of elements. *Sampling theory* was developed to determine mathematically the most effective way of acquiring a sample that would accurately reflect the population under study. Important concepts in sampling theory are target population, elements of the population, randomization, sampling frame, accessible population, representativeness, statistics, parameters, precision, sampling errors, and systematic bias.

A *sampling plan* is developed to increase representativeness, decrease systematic bias, and decrease the sampling error. The two main types of sampling plans are probability sampling and nonprobability sampling. Probability sampling plans have been developed to ensure some degree of precision in the accurate estimation of the population parameters. Thus, probability samples reduce sampling error. To obtain a probability (random) sample, the researcher must know every element in the population. A sampling frame must be developed, and the samples randomly selected from the sampling frame. Four sampling designs have been developed to achieve probability sampling: simple random sampling, stratified random sampling, cluster sampling, and systematic sampling.

In nonprobability (nonrandom) sampling, not every element of the population has an opportunity for selection in the sample. There is no sampling frame. Four nonprobability designs are described in this text: convenience sampling, quota sampling, purposive sampling, and network sampling.

A major concern in any study is determining the size of a sample. Sample size is determined by power analysis. Sampling error decreases as sample size increases. Many published nursing studies have an inadequate sample size and a high risk of a Type II error. One examination of published studies found that a nursing study needed an average of 218 subjects per group to have an acceptable power level. Factors that must be considered in making decisions about sample size are the type of study, the number of variables, the sensitivity of the measurement tools, the data analysis techniques, and the expected effect size. *Effect size* is the extent to which the null hypothesis is false. Calculating sample size requires that one know the level of significance, power, and effect size.

Another concern in conducting a study is acquiring and retaining subjects. This process is almost always more difficult than was expected. The problems encountered are usually associated with human interaction rather than with the sampling plan. Effective acquisition of subjects depends on the initial approach by the researcher. When surveys are used, the researcher may never have personal contact with the subjects. In this case, the researcher must rely on the use of attention-getting techniques, persuasively written material, and strategies for following up on individuals who do not respond to the initial written communication. Traditionally, subjects for nursing studies have been sought in the hospital setting. However, access to these subjects is becoming more difficult, and nurse researchers are now recruiting subjects from a variety of sources. An initial phase of recruitment may involve obtaining community or institutional support for the study. Endorsement may be obtained from individuals, such as city officials and key civic leaders, and social, educational, religious, or labor groups.

Retaining acquired subjects is critical to the study and requires consideration of the effects of data collection on subject mortality. A number of strategies have been found to be effective in maintaining the sample. Names, addresses, and telephone numbers of family members or friends of subjects may be obtained. A bonus payment may be given for completing a certain phase of the study. If subjects have a personal investment in the study, they are more likely to continue. This investment is developed through interactions with and nurturing by the researcher.

· ·

REFERENCES

Andreasen, A. R. (1970). Personalizing mail questionnaires. *Public Opinion Quarterly, 34*(2), 273–277.

Babbie, E. R. (1973). *Survey research methods.* Belmont, CA: Wadsworth.

Baker, C. M. (1985). Maximizing mailed questionnaire responses. *Image—The Journal of Nursing Scholarship, 17*(4), 118–121.

Barhyte, D. Y., Redman, B. K., & Neill, K. M. (1990). Popula-

tion or sample: Design decision. *Nursing Research, 39*(5), 309–310.

Barnard, K. E., Magyary, D. L., Booth, C. L., & Eyres, S. J. (1987). Longitudinal designs: Considerations and applications to nursing research. *Recent Advances in Nursing, 17,* 37–64.

Beck, C. T. (1994). Statistical power analysis in pediatric nursing research. *Issues in Comprehensive Pediatric Nursing, 17*(2), 73–80.

Borenstein, M., & Cohen, J. (1989). *Statistical power analysis* (Release: 1.00). Hillsdale, NJ: Lawrence Erlbaum Associates, Inc. (ISBN 0-8058-0222-3).

Brent, E. E., Jr., Scott, J. K., & Spencer, J. C. (1988). Ex-Sample™;: *An expert system to assist in designing sampling plans. User's guide and reference manual* (Version 2.0). Columbia, MO: The Idea Works, Inc. (100 West Briarwood, Columbia, MO 65203; phone [314] 445–4554).

Cochran, W. G. (1977). *Sampling techniques* (3rd ed.). New York: Wiley.

Cohen, J. (1988). *Statistical power analysis for the behavioral sciences* (2nd ed.). New York: Academic Press.

Cronenwett, L. R. (1986). Access to research subjects. *Journal of Nursing Administration, 16*(2), 8–9.

Diekmann, J. M., & Smith, J. M. (1989). Strategies for assessment and recruitment of subjects for nursing research. *Western Journal of Nursing Research, 11*(4), 418–430.

Floyd, J. A. (1993). Systematic sampling: Theory and clinical methods. *Nursing Research, 42*(5), 290–293.

Friday, F. A. (1967). *The elements of probability and sampling.* New York: Barnes & Noble.

Good, M. (1995). A comparison of the effects of jaw relaxation and music on postoperative pain. *Nursing Research, 44*(1), 52–57.

Gordon, S. E., & Stokes, S. A. (1989). Improving response rate to mailed questionnaires. *Nursing Research, 38*(6), 375–376.

Gottlieb, L. N., & Baillies, J. (1995). Firstborns' behaviors during a mother's second pregnancy. *Nursing Research, 44*(6), 356–362.

Hansen, M. H., Hurwitz, W. N., & Madow, W. G. (1953). *Sample survey methods and theory.* New York: Wiley.

Hart, M. A. (1995). Orem's self-care deficit theory: Research with pregnant women. *Nursing Science Quarterly, 8*(3), 120–126.

Kerlinger, F. N. (1986). *Foundations of behavioral research* (3rd ed.). New York: Holt, Rinehart & Winston.

Killien, M., & Newton, K. (1990). Longitudinal research—the challenge of maintaining continued involvement of participants. *Western Journal of Nursing Research, 12*(5), 689–692.

Kraemer, H. C., & Thiemann, S. (1987). *How many subjects? Statistical power analysis in research.* Newbury Park, CA: Sage.

Larson, E. (1994). Exclusion of certain groups from clinical research. *Image—The Journal of Nursing Scholarship, 26*(3), 185–190.

Leidy, N. K., & Weissfeld, L. A. (1991). Sample sizes and power computation for clinical intervention trials. *Western Journal of Nursing Research, 13*(1), 138–144.

Levy, P. S., & Lemsbow, S. (1980). *Sampling for health professionals.* Belmont, CA: Lifetime Learning.

Lusk, S. L., Ronis, D. L., Kerr, M. J., & Atwood, J. R. (1994). Test of the health promotion model as a causal model of workers' use of hearing protection. *Nursing Research, 43*(3), 151–157.

Mitchell, E. S., Woods, N. F., & Lentz, M. J. (1994). Differentiation of women with three perimenstrual symptom patterns. *Nursing Research, 43*(1), 25–30.

Moody, L. E., Wilson, M. E., Smyth, K., Schwartz, R., Tittle, M., & Van Cott, M. L. (1988). Analysis of a decade of nursing practice research: 1977–1986. *Nursing Research, 37*(6), 374–379.

Murdaugh, C. (1990). Recruitment issues in research with special populations. *Journal of Cardiovascular Nursing, 4*(4), 51–55.

Pletsch, P. K., Howe, C., & Tenney, M. (1995). Recruitment of minority subjects for intervention research. *Image—The Journal of Nursing Scholarship, 27*(3), 211–215.

Polit, D. F., & Sherman, R. E. (1990). Statistical power in nursing research. *Nursing Research, 39*(6), 365–369.

Princeton, T. C., & Gaspar, T. M. (1991). First-line nurse administrators in academics: How are they prepared, what do they do, and will they stay in their jobs? *Journal of Professional Nursing, 7*(2), 79–87.

Rudy, E. B., Estok, P. J., Kerr, M. E., & Menzel, L. (1994). Research incentives: Money versus gifts. *Nursing Research, 43*(4), 253–255.

Sandelowski, M. (1995). Sample size in qualitative research. *Research in Nursing & Health, 18*(2), 179–183.

Schain, W. S. (1994). Barriers to clinical trials. Part II: Knowledge and attitudes of potential participants. *Cancer, 74*(9) (Suppl.), 2666–2671.

Stevens, P. E. (1995). Structural and interpersonal impact of heterosexual assumptions on lesbian health care clients. *Nursing Research, 44*(1), 25–30.

Stewart, N. J., Hiscock, M., Morgan, D. G., Murphy, P.B., & Yamamoto, M. (1999). Development and psychometric evaluation of the environment-behavior interaction code (EBIC). *Nursing Research, 48*(5), 260–268.

Stuifbergen, A. K. (1995). Health-promoting behaviors and quality of life among individuals with multiple sclerosis. *Scholarly Inquiry for Nursing Practice: An International Journal, 9*(1), 31–55.

Sudman, S. (1974). *Applied sampling.* New York: Academic Press.

Tracy, J., Fowler, S., & Magarelli, K. (1999). Hope and anxiety of individual family members of critically ill adults. *Applied Nursing Research, 12*(3), 121–127.

Watters, J. K., & Biernacki, P. (1989). Targeted sampling: Options for the study of hidden populations. *Social Problems, 36*(4), 416–430.

Williams, B. (1978). *A sampler on sampling.* New York: Wiley.

Yarandi, H. N. (1991). Planning sample sizes: Comparison of factor level means. *Nursing Research, 40*(1), 57–58.

Yates, F. (1981). *Sampling methods for censuses and surveys.* New York: Macmillan.

Youngblut, J. M., & Brooten, D. (1999). Alternate child care, history of hospitalization, and preschool child behavior. *Nursing Research 48*(1), 29–34.

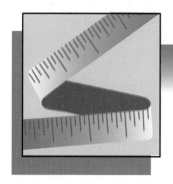

CHAPTER 15

THE CONCEPTS OF MEASUREMENT

Measurement is the process of assigning "numbers to objects (or events or situations) in accord with some rule" (Kaplan, 1963, p. 177). The numbers assigned can indicate numerical values or categories. *Instrumentation,* a component of measurement, is the application of specific rules to develop a measurement device (instrument). The purpose of instrumentation is to produce trustworthy evidence that can be used in evaluating the outcomes of research.

The rules of measurement ensure that the assignment of values or categories is performed consistently from one subject (or event) to another and, eventually, if the measurement strategy is found to be meaningful, from one study to another. The rules of measurement established for research are similar to those used in nursing practice. For example, when one is pouring a liquid medication, the rule is that the measuring container must be held at eye level. This practice ensures accuracy and consistency in the dose of medication. When one is measuring the abdominal girth to detect changes in ascites, the skin on the abdomen is marked to ensure that the measurement is always taken the same distance below the waist. With this method, any change in measurement can be attributed to a change in ascites rather than an inadvertent change in the measurement site. Developing consistent measures of concepts important to nursing practice is a major focus of nursing research.

An understanding of the logic within measurement theory is important to the selection, utilization, and development of measurement instruments. As with most theories, measurement theory uses terms with meanings that can be understood only within the context of the theory. The following explanation of the logic of measurement theory comprises definitions of directness of measurement, measurement error, levels of measurement, reference of measurement, reliability, and validity.

DIRECTNESS OF MEASUREMENT

Measurement begins by clarifying the object, characteristic, or element to be measured. Only then can strategies or techniques be developed to measure it. In some cases, identification of the measurement object and measurement strategies can be quite simple and straightforward, as when we are measuring concrete factors, such as a person's height or wrist circumference; this is referred to as *direct measurement.* The technology of health care has made direct measures of concrete elements, such as height, weight, temperature, time, space, movement, heart rate, and respiration, familiar to us. Technology is available to measure many bodily functions and biological and chemical characteristics. The focus of measurement theory in these instances is in the precision of measurement. Nurses are also experienced in gathering direct measures of attribute variables, such as age, gender, ethnic origin, diagnosis, marital status, income, and education.

Often in nursing, however, the characteristic to

be measured is an abstract idea, such as stress, caring, coping, anxiety, compliance, or pain. If the element to be measured is abstract, clarification is usually achieved through conceptual definition. The conceptual definition is then used to select or develop appropriate means of measuring the concept. The instrument used in the study must match the conceptual definition. When abstract concepts are measured, the concept is not directly measured; instead, indicators or attributes of the concept are used to represent the abstraction. This is referred to as *indirect measurement.* For example, indicators of coping might be the frequency or accuracy of problem identification, the speed or effectiveness of problem resolution, level of optimism, and self-actualization behaviors. Rarely, if ever, can a single measurement strategy completely measure all the aspects of an abstract concept.

MEASUREMENT ERROR

There is no perfect measure. Error is inherent in any measurement strategy. *Measurement error* is the difference between what exists in reality and what is measured by a research instrument. Measurement error exists in both direct and indirect measures and can be random or systematic. Direct measures, which are considered to be highly accurate, are subject to error. For example, the scale may not be accurate, the machine may be precisely calibrated but it may change with use, or the tape measure may not be held at exactly the same tightness.

There is also error in indirect measures. Efforts to measure concepts usually result in measuring only part of the concept or measures that identify an aspect of the concept but also contain other elements that are not part of the concept. Figure 15–1 shows a Venn diagram of the concept A measured by instrument A-1. As can be seen, A-1 does not measure all of A. In addition, some of what A-1 measures is outside the concept of A. Both of these situations are examples of errors in measurement.

Types of Measurement Errors

Two types of errors are of concern in measurement: random error and systematic error. To under-

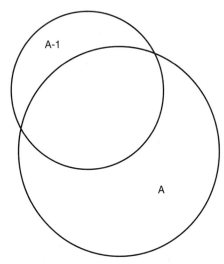

FIGURE 15–1 ■ Measurement error when measuring a concept.

stand these types of errors, we must first understand the elements of a score on an instrument or an observation. According to measurement theory, there are three components to a measurement score: the *true score* (T), the *observed score* (O), and the *error score* (E). The true score is what would be obtained if there were no error in measurement. Because there is always some measurement error, the true score is never known. The *observed score* is the measure obtained. The *error score* is the amount of random error in the measurement process. The theoretical equation of these three measures is as follows:

$$O = T + E$$

This equation is a means of conceptualizing random error, and not a basis for calculating it. Because the true score is never known, the random error is never known, only estimated. Theoretically, the smaller the error score, the more closely the observed score reflects the true score. Therefore, using measurement strategies that reduce the error score improves the accuracy of the measurement.

A number of factors can occur during the measurement process and can result in random error. They are (1) transient personal factors, such as fatigue, hunger, attention span, health, mood, mental set, and motivation, (2) situational factors, such as a hot stuffy room, distractions, the presence of significant others, rapport with the researcher, and the playfulness or seriousness of the situation, (3) variations in the administration of the measurement procedure, such as interviews in which wording or sequence of questions is varied, questions are added or deleted, or different coders code responses differently, and (4) processing of data, such as errors in coding, accidental marking of the wrong column, punching of the wrong key when the data are entered into the computer, or incorrect totaling of instrument scores.

Random error causes individuals' observed scores to vary haphazardly around their true score. For example, with random error, one subject's observed score may be higher than his or her true score, whereas another subject's observed score may be lower than his or her true score. According to measurement theory, the sum of random errors is expected to be zero, and the random error score (E) is not expected to be correlated with the true score (T). Thus, random error does not influence the direction of the mean but, rather, increases the amount of unexplained variance around the mean. When this occurs, estimation of the true score is less precise.

If a variable were measured for three subjects and the random error were diagrammed, it might appear as shown in Figure 15–2. The difference between the true score of subject 1 ($T1$) and the observed score ($O1$) is two positive measurement intervals. The difference between the true score ($T2$) and observed score ($O2$) for subject 2 is two negative measurement intervals. The difference between the true score ($T3$) and observed score ($O3$) for subject 3 is zero. The random error for these three subjects is zero ($+2 - 2 + 0 = 0$). In viewing this example, one must remember that this is only a means of conceptualizing random error.

Measurement error that is not random is referred to as *systematic error*. For example, use of a weight

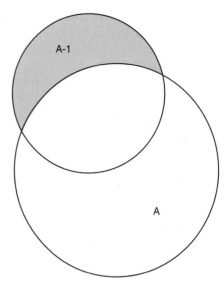

FIGURE 15–3 ■ Conceptualization of systematic error.

scale that weighed subjects 2 lb more than their true weights would result in systematic error. All of the body weights would be higher, and as a result, the mean would be higher than it should be. Systematic error occurs because something else is being measured in addition to the concept. A conceptualization of systematic error is presented in Figure 15–3. Systematic error (represented by shaded area in the figure) is due to the part of A-1 that is outside of A. This part of A-1 measures factors other than A and will bias scores in a particular direction.

Systematic error is considered part of T (true score) and reflects the true measure of A-1, not A. Adding the true score (with systematic error) to the random error (which is 0) yields the observed score, as shown by the following equations:

$$T + E = O$$

T (True Score with Systematic Error)
    + E (Random Error of 0) = O (Observed Score)

There will be some systematic error in almost any measure; however, a close link between the abstract theoretical concept and the development of the instrument can greatly decrease systematic error. Because of the importance of this factor in a study,

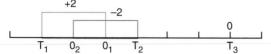

FIGURE 15–2 ■ Conceptualization of random error.

researchers spend considerable time and effort refining their measurement instruments to decrease systematic error.

Another effective means of diminishing systematic error is to use more than one measure of an attribute or a concept and to compare the measures. A variety of data collection methods, such as interview and observation, are used. This technique, which has been referred to as the *multimethod-multitrait technique*, was developed by Campbell and Fiske (1959). More recently, the technique is described as a version of methodological triangulation, as discussed in Chapter 10. Through the use of these techniques, more dimensions of the abstract concept can be measured, and the effect of the systematic error on the composite observed score decreases. Figure 15–4 illustrates how more dimensions of concept A are measured through the use of four instruments, designated A-1, A-2, A-3, and A-4.

For example, a researcher could decrease systematic error in measures of anxiety by (1) administering Taylor's Manifest Anxiety Scale, (2) recording blood pressure readings, (3) asking the subject about anxious feelings, and (4) observing the subject's behavior. The use of multimethod techniques

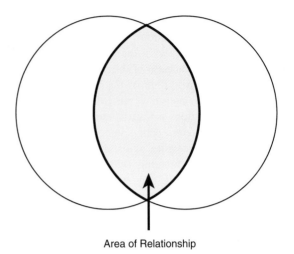

Area of Relationship

FIGURE 15–5 ■ True relationship of concepts A and B.

decreases systematic error by combining the values in some way to give a single observed score of anxiety for each subject. Sometimes, however, it may be difficult logically to justify combining scores from various measures, and triangulation may be the most appropriate approach. Using triangulation, the researcher decreases systematic error by performing a series of bivariate (two variable) correlations on the matrix of values.

In some studies, instruments are used to examine relationships. Consider a hypothesis in which the relationship between concept A and concept B is being tested. In Figure 15–5, the true relationship between concepts A and B is represented by the area enclosed in the dark lines. If two instruments (A-1 and B-1) are used to examine the relationship between concepts A and B, the part of the true relationship actually reflected by these measures is represented by shaded area in Figure 15–6. Because two instruments provide a more accurate measure of concepts A and B, more of the true relationship between concepts A and B can be measured.

If additional instruments (A-2 and B-2) are used to measure concepts A and B, more of the true relationship might be reflected. Figure 15–7 demonstrates the parts of the true relationship that might be reflected if two instruments are used to measure concept A (A-1 and A-2) and two instruments to measure concept B (B-1 and B-2).

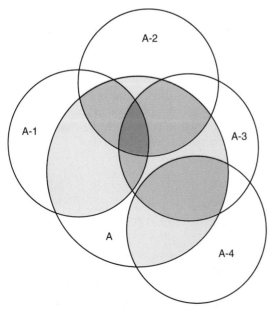

FIGURE 15–4 ■ Multiple measures of an abstract concept.

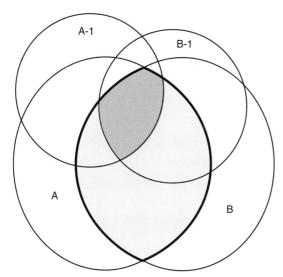

FIGURE 15–6 ■ Examining a relationship using one measure of each concept.

LEVELS OF MEASUREMENT

The traditional levels of measurement have been used for so long that the categorization system has been considered absolute and inviolate. The system was developed in 1946 by Stevens, who organized the rules for assigning numbers to objects so that a hierarchy in measurement was established. The levels of measurement, from lower to higher, are nominal, ordinal, interval, and ratio.

Nominal-Scale Measurement

Nominal-scale measurement is the lowest of the four measurement categories. It is used when data can be organized into categories of a defined property but the categories cannot be ordered. Thus, one cannot say that one category is higher than another or that category A is closer to category B than to category C. The categories differ in quality but not quantity. Therefore, one cannot say that subject A possesses more of the property being categorized than does subject B. (*Rule:* The categories must be unorderable.) Categories must be established in such a way that each datum will fit into only one of the categories. (*Rule:* The categories must be exclu-

sive.) All the data must fit into the established categories. (*Rule:* The categories must be exhaustive.)

Data such as gender, ethnicity, marital status, and diagnoses are examples of nominal data. When data are coded for entry into the computer, the categories are assigned numbers. For example, gender may be classified as 1 = male, 2 = female. The numbers assigned to categories in nominal measurement are used only as labels and cannot be used for mathematical calculations.

Ordinal-Scale Measurement

Data that can be measured at the *ordinal-scale level* can be assigned to categories of an attribute that can be ranked. There are rules for how one ranks data. As with nominal-scale data, the categories must be exclusive and exhaustive. With ordinal-scale data, the quantity of the attribute possessed can be identified. However, it cannot be demonstrated that the intervals between the ranked categories are equal. Therefore, ordinal data are considered to have unequal intervals. Scales with unequal

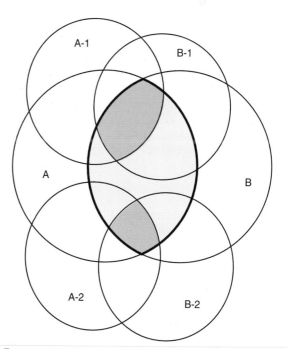

FIGURE 15–7 ■ Examining a relationship using two measures of each concept.

intervals are sometimes referred to as *ordered metric scales*.

Many scales used in nursing research are ordinal levels of measure. For example, one could rank intensity of pain, degrees of coping, levels of mobility, ability to provide self-care, or daily amount of exercise on an ordinal scale. For daily exercise, the scale could be 0 = no exercise; 1 = moderate exercise, no sweating; 2 = exercise to the point of sweating; 3 = strenuous exercise with sweating for at least 30 minutes per day; 4 = strenuous exercise with sweating for at least 1 hour per day. This type of scale may be referred to as a *metric ordinal scale*.

Interval-Scale Measurement

In *interval-scale measurements*, distances between intervals of the scale are numerically equal. Such measurements also follow the previously mentioned rules: mutually exclusive categories, exhaustive categories, and rank ordering. Interval scales are assumed to be a continuum of values. Thus, the magnitude of the attribute can be much more precisely identified. However, it is not possible to provide the absolute amount of the attribute because of the absence of a zero point on the interval scale.

Fahrenheit and centigrade temperatures are commonly used as examples of interval scales. A difference between a temperature of 70° and one of 80° is the same as the difference between a temperature of 30° and one of 40°. Changes in temperature can be precisely measured. However, it is not possible to say that a temperature of 0° means the absence of temperature.

Ratio-Level Measurement

Ratio-level measurements are the highest form of measure and meet all the rules of the lower forms of measures: mutually exclusive categories, exhaustive categories, rank ordering, equal spacing between intervals, and a continuum of values. In addition, ratio-level measures have absolute zero points. Weight, length, and volume are common examples of ratio scales. Each has an *absolute zero point*, at which a value of zero indicates the absence of the property being measured: Zero weight means the absence of weight. In addition, because of the absolute zero point, one can justifiably say that object A weighs twice as much as object B, or that container A holds three times as much as container B.

The Importance of Level of Measurement for Statistical Analyses

An important rule of measurement is that one should use the highest level of measurement possible. For example, data can be collected on age (measured) in a variety of ways: (1) the actual age of each subject can be obtained, (2) subjects can be asked to indicate their age by selecting from a group of categories, such as 20 to 29, 30 to 39, and so on, or (3) a bivariate measure such as under 65–over 65 can be used. The highest level of measurement in this case is the actual age of each subject. These data can be entered into the computer, and if categories are needed for specific analyses, the computer can be instructed to establish them from the initial age data.

The level of measurement is associated with the types of statistical analyses that can be performed on the data. Mathematical operations are limited in the lower levels of measurement. With nominal levels of measurement, only summary statistics, such as frequencies, percentages, and contingency correlation procedures, can be used. In the age example, however, more sophisticated analyses can be performed if the actual age of each subject has been obtained.

Controversy over Measurement Levels

In recent years, controversy has erupted over justification for the categorization of measurement levels, leading to two factions in regard to the system: the fundamentalists and the pragmatists. *Pragmatists* regard measurement as occurring on a continuum rather than by discrete categories, whereas *fundamentalists* adhere rigidly to the original system of categorization.

The primary focus of the controversy is related to classification of data into the categories ordinal and interval. The controversy developed because, according to the fundamentalists, many of the current statistical analysis techniques can be used only with interval data. Many pragmatists believe that if Stevens' rules were rigidly adhered to, few if any measures in the social sciences would meet the criteria to be considered interval-level data. They also believe that violating Stevens' criteria does not lead to serious consequences for the outcomes of data analysis. Thus pragmatists often treat ordinal data as interval data, using statistical methods to analyze them such as the *t* test and analysis of variance, which are traditionally reserved for interval data. Fundamentalists insist that analysis of ordinal data be limited to statistical procedures designed for ordinal data, such as nonparametric procedures.

There is also a controversy about the statistical operations that can justifiably be performed with scores from the various levels of measure (Armstrong, 1981, 1984; Knapp, 1984, 1990). For example, can one calculate a mean using ordinal data? Fundamentalists believe that appropriate statistical analysis is contingent on the level of measurement. They disagree with the contention that the scaling procedures used for most psychosocial instruments provide interval-level data. This is related to scale definition, which is discussed in Chapter 16.

For example, the Likert Scale uses the scale points "strongly disagree," "disagree," "uncertain," "agree," and "strongly agree." Numerical values (e.g., 1, 2, 3, 4, and 5, respectively) are assigned to these categories. Fundamentalists claim that equal intervals do not exist between these categories. It is not possible to prove that there is the same magnitude of feeling between "uncertain" and "agree" as there is between "agree" and "strongly agree." Therefore, they hold, parametric analyses cannot be used. Pragmatists believe that with many measures taken at the ordinal level, such as scaling procedures, an underlying interval continuum is present that justifies the use of parametric statistics.

Our position is more like that of the pragmatists than of the fundamentalists. However, many data in nursing research are obtained through the use of crude measurement methods that can be classified only into the lower levels of measurement. Therefore, we have included the nonparametric statistical procedures needed for their analysis in the statistical chapters.

REFERENCE OF MEASUREMENT

Referencing involves comparing a subject's score against a standard. Two types of testing involve referencing: norm-referenced testing and criterion-referenced testing. *Norm-referenced testing* addresses the question "How does the average person score on this test?" It involves the use of standardization that has been developed over several years, with extensive reliability and validity data available. Standardization involves collecting data from thousands of subjects expected to have a broad range of scores on the instrument. From these scores, population parameters such as the mean and standard deviation (described in Chapter 19) can be developed. Evidence of the reliability and validity of the instrument can also be evaluated through the use of the methods described later in this chapter. The best-known norm-referenced test is the Minnesota Multiphasic Personality Inventory (MMPI), which is used commonly in psychology and occasionally in nursing research.

Criterion-referenced testing asks the question "What is desirable in the perfect subject?" It involves the comparison of a subject's score with a criterion of achievement that includes the definition of target behaviors. When these behaviors are mastered, the subject is considered proficient in the behavior. The criterion might be a level of knowledge or desirable patient outcome measures. Criterion measures are not as useful in research as they might be in evaluation studies.

RELIABILITY

The *reliability* of a measure denotes the consistency of measures obtained in the use of a particular instrument and is an indication of the extent of random error in the measurement method. For example, if the same measurement scale is administered to the same individuals at two different times, the measurement is reliable if the individuals' responses to the items remain the same (assuming that nothing has occurred to change their responses). For example, if you measure oral temperatures of 10 individuals every 5 minutes 10 times using the same thermometer for all measures of all individuals, and at each measurement the individuals' temperatures change, being sometimes higher than before and sometimes lower, you begin to question the reliability of the thermometer. If two data collectors are observing the same event and recording their observations on a carefully designed data collection instrument, the measurement would be reliable if the recordings from the two data collectors are comparable. The equivalence of their results would indicate the reliability of the measurement technique. If responses vary each time a measure is performed, there is a chance that the instrument is not reliable—that is, that it yields data with a large random error.

Reliability plays an important role in the selection of scales for use in a study. Researchers need instruments that are reliable and provide values with only a small amount of random error. Reliable instruments enhance the power of a study to detect significant differences or relationships actually occurring in the population under study. Therefore, it is important to test the reliability of an instrument before using it in a study. Estimates of reliability are specific to the sample being tested. Thus, high-reported reliability values on an established instrument do not guarantee that its reliability will be satisfactory in another sample or with a different population. Therefore, reliability testing must be performed on each instrument used in a study before other statistical analyses are performed. The reliability values must be included in published reports of the study.

Reliability testing examines the amount of random error in the measurement technique. It is concerned with characteristics such as dependability, consistency, accuracy, and comparability. Because all measurement techniques contain some random error, reliability exists in degrees and is usually expressed as a form of correlation coefficient, with a 1.00 indicating perfect reliability and .00 indicating no reliability. A reliability coefficient of .80 is considered the lowest acceptable value for a well-

developed psychosocial measurement instrument. Higher levels are required for physiological measures that are "critical." For a newly developed psychosocial instrument, a reliability of .70 is considered acceptable. Reliability testing focuses on the following three aspects of reliability: stability, equivalence, and homogeneity.

Stability

Stability is concerned with the consistency of repeated measures of the same attribute with the use of the same scale or instrument. It is usually referred to as *test-retest reliability*. This measure of reliability is generally used with physical measures, technological measures, and paper and pencil scales. Use of the technique requires an assumption that the factor to be measured remains the same at the two testing times and that any change in the value or score is a consequence of random error.

Physical measures and equipment can be tested and then immediately retested, or the equipment can be used for a time and then retested to determine the necessary frequency of recalibration. With paper and pencil measures, a period of 2 weeks to a month is recommended between the two testing times. After retesting, correlational analysis is performed on the scores from the two measures. A high correlation coefficient indicates high stability of measurement by the instrument.

Test-retest reliability has not proved to be as effective with paper and pencil measures as was originally anticipated. There are a number of problems with the procedure. Subjects may remember their responses at the first testing time, leading to overestimation of the reliability. Subjects may actually be changed by the first testing and therefore may respond to the second test differently, leading to underestimation of the reliability.

Test-retest reliability requires the assumption that the factor being measured has not changed between the measurement points. Many of the phenomena studied in nursing, such as hope, coping, and anxiety, do change over short intervals. Thus, the assumption that if the instrument is reliable, values will not change between the two measurement periods may not be justifiable. If the factor being measured does change, the test is not a measure of reliability. In fact, if the measures stay the same even though the factor being measured actually has changed, the instrument may lack reliability.

Equivalence

The focus of *equivalence* is the comparison of two versions of the same paper and pencil instrument or of two observers measuring the same event. Comparison of two observers is referred to as *interrater reliability*. Comparison of two paper and pencil instruments is referred to as *alternate forms reliability* or *parallel forms reliability*. Alternative forms of instruments are of more concern in the development of normative knowledge testing. When repeated measures are part of the design, however, alternative forms of measurement, although not commonly used, would improve the design. Demonstrating that one is actually testing the same content in both tests is extremely complex, and thus, the procedure is rarely used in clinical research.

Determining interrater reliability is a more immediate concern in research and is used in many observational studies. Interrater reliability values must be reported in any study in which observational data are collected or judgments are made by two or more data gatherers. Two techniques determine interrater reliability. Both techniques require that two or more raters independently observe and record the same event using the protocol developed for the study or that the same rater observe and record an event on two occasions. For adequate judgment of interrater reliability, the raters need to observe at least 10 subjects or events (Washington & Moss, 1988). Recording the same event on two occasions can be accomplished by videotaping the event. Every data collector used in the study must be tested for interrater reliability.

The first procedure for calculating interrater reliability requires a simple computation involving a comparison of the agreements obtained between raters on the coding form with the number of possible agreements. This calculation is performed through the use of the following equation:

$$\frac{\text{Number of agreements}}{\text{Number of possible agreements}}$$

This formula tends to overestimate reliability, a particularly serious problem if the rating requires only a dichotomous judgment. In this case, there is a 50% probability that the raters will agree on a particular item through chance alone. Appropriate correlational techniques can be used to provide a more accurate estimate of reliability. If more than two raters are involved, a statistical procedure to calculate coefficient alpha (discussed later in this chapter) may be used. Analysis of variance may also be used to test for differences among raters. There is no absolute value below which interrater reliability is unacceptable. However, any value below .80 should generate serious concern about the reliability of the data. The interrater reliability value must be included in research reports.

When raters know they are being watched, their accuracy and consistency are considerably better than when they believe they are not being watched. Thus, interrater reliability declines (sometimes dramatically) when the raters are assessed covertly (Topf, 1988). Strategies can be used to monitor and reduce the decline in interrater reliability, but they may entail considerable time and expense.

The coding of data into categories has received little attention in regard to reliability. Two types of reliability are related to categorizing data, unitizing reliability and interpretive reliability. *Unitizing reliability* assesses the extent to which each judge (data collector, coder, researcher) consistently identifies the same units within the data as appropriate for coding. This is of concern in observational studies and studies using text transcribed from interviews. In observational studies, the data collector needs to select particular units of what is being observed as appropriate to record and code. Of concern is the extent to which two data collectors observing the same event would select the same units to record. In studies using transcribed text from interviews, the researcher must select particular units of the transcribed text to code into preselected categories. To what extent would two individuals reading the same text select the same passages to code into categories (Garvin et al., 1988)?

In some studies, selection of units for coding is simple and straightforward. For example, a unit may begin when a person starts talking. In other studies, however, the identification of an appropriate unit for coding may require some level of inference or judgment on the part of the rater. For example, if the unit began when the baby awakened, the rater would have to determine at what point the baby was indeed awake. Studies in which every event in the unit is coded require less inference than studies in which only select acts in the unit are to be coded. In all cases, reliability improves when the researcher clearly identifies the units to be coded rather than relying on the judgment of the coder (Washington & Moss, 1988). Unitizing reliability can be calculated with the use of Guetzkow's (1950) index (U) (Garvin et al., 1988).

Interpretive reliability assesses the extent to which each judge assigns the same category to a given unit of data. Most studies using categories report only a global level of reliability in which the overall rate of reliability is examined. The most commonly used measure of global reliability is Guetzkow's (1950) P, which reports the extent to which the judges agree in the selection of categories. A more desirable method of calculating the extent of agreement between judges is Cohen's (1960) Kappa statistic. However, global measures of interpretive reliability provide no information on the degree of consistency in assigning data to a particular category. Category-by-category measures of reliability include the assumption that some categories are more difficult to use than others, and thus, have a lower reliability. Using this method of evaluating reliability, the researcher must (1) statistically analyze the reliability category by category, (2) determine the equality of the frequency distribution among categories, and (3) examine the possibility that coders may be systematically confusing some categories (Garvin et al., 1988).

Homogeneity

Tests of instrument *homogeneity*, used primarily with paper and pencil tests, address the correlation of various items within the instrument. The original approach to determining homogeneity was *split-half reliability.* This strategy was a way of obtaining test-retest reliability without administering the test twice. Rather, the instrument items were split in odd-even or first-last halves, and a correlational procedure was performed between the two halves. The Spearman-Brown correlation formula has generally been used for this procedure. One of the problems with the procedure was that although items were usually split into odd-even items, it was possible to split them in a variety of ways. Each approach to splitting the items would yield a different reliability coefficient. Therefore, the researcher could continue to split the items in various ways until a satisfactorily high coefficient was obtained.

More recently, testing the homogeneity of all the items in the instrument has been seen as a better approach to determining reliability. Although the mathematics of the procedure are complex, the logic is simple. One way to view it is as though one conducted split-half reliabilities in all the ways possible and then averaged the scores to obtain one reliability score. Homogeneity testing examines the extent to which all the items in the instrument consistently measure construct. It is a test of internal consistency. The statistical procedures used for this process are Cronbach's alpha coefficient and, when the data are dichotomous, K-R 20 (Kuder-Richardson formula).

If the coefficient value were 1.00, each item in the instrument would be measuring exactly the same thing. When this occurs, one might question the need for more than one item. A slightly lower coefficient (.8 to .9) indicates an instrument that will reflect more richly the fine discriminations in levels of the construct. Magnitude can then be discerned more clearly.

Other approaches to testing internal consistency are (1) Cohen's Kappa statistic, which determines the percent of agreement with the probability of chance being taken out, (2) correlating each item with the total score for the instrument, and (3) correlating each item with each other item in the instrument. In this procedure, often used in instrument development, items that do not correlate highly may be deleted from the instrument. Factor analysis may also be used to develop reliability of instruments. Consistency of measure is influenced by the number of factors being measured. Total scores may be more reliable than subscores in determining reliability. After the factor analysis has been performed, instrument items with low factor weights can be deleted. After deletion of these items, reliability scores on the instrument will be higher. If there is more than one factor, correlations can be performed between items and factor scores.

An instrument that has low reliability values cannot be valid because it is inconsistent in its measurement. An instrument that is reliable cannot be assumed to be valid for a particular study or population.

VALIDITY

The *validity* of an instrument is a determination of the extent to which the instrument actually reflects the abstract construct being examined. Validity has been discussed in the literature in terms of three primary types: content validity, predictive validity, and construct validity. Within each of these types, subtypes have been identified. These multiple types of validity were very confusing, especially because the types were not discrete but interrelated.

Currently, validity is considered a single broad method of measurement evaluation referred to as *construct validity* (Berk, 1990; Rew et al., 1988). All of the previously identified types of validity are now considered evidence of construct validity. Standards used to judge the evidence of validity were published in the *Standards for Educational and Psychological Testing* in 1985 by the American Psychological Association (APA). This important work greatly extends our understanding of what validity is and how to achieve it. According to the APA, validity addresses the appropriateness, meaningfulness, and usefulness of the specific inferences made from instrument scores. It is important to note that it is the inferences made from the scores, not the scores themselves, that are important to validate (Goodwin & Goodwin, 1991).

Validity, like reliability, is not an all-or-nothing phenomenon but, rather, a matter of degree. No instrument is completely valid. Thus, one determines the degree of validity of a measure rather than whether or not it has validity. Defining the validity of an instrument requires years of work. Many equate the validity of the instrument with the rigorousness of the researcher. The assumption is that because the researcher develops the instrument, the researcher also must develop the validity. How-

ever, this assumption is to some extent an erroneous view, as pointed out by Brinberg and McGrath (1985):

• •

"Validity is not a commodity that can be purchased with techniques. Validity, as we will treat it, is a concept designating an ideal state—to be pursued, but not to be attained. As the roots of the word imply, validity has to do with truth, strength, and value. The discourse of our field has often been in tones that seem to imply that validity is a tangible "resource," and that if one can acquire a sufficient amount of it, by applying appropriate techniques, one has somehow "won" at the game called research. We reject this view. In our views, validity is not like money—to gain and lose, to count and display. Rather, validity is like integrity, character, or quality, to be assessed relative to purposes and circumstances." (Brinberg & McGrath, 1985, p. 13) ■

In Figure 15–8, validity (the shaded area) is illustrated by the extent to which the instrument A-1 reflects concept A. As measurement of the concept improves, validity improves. The extent to which the measurement instrument measures items other than the concept is referred to as systematic

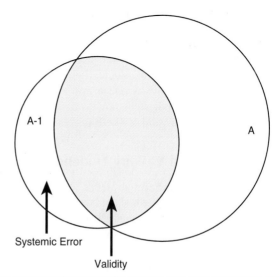

FIGURE 15–8 ■ Representation of instrument validity.

error (also identified as the unshaded area of Figure 15–8). As systematic error decreases, validity increases.

Validity varies from one sample to another and from one situation to another; therefore, validity testing actually validates the use of an instrument for a specific group or purpose rather than the instrument itself. An instrument may be very valid in one situation but not valid in another. Therefore, validity must be reexamined in each study situation.

Although many instruments used in nursing studies were developed for use in other disciplines, it is important that any measure chosen for a nursing study be valid in terms of nursing knowledge. Nagley and Byers (1987) give an example of a study in which a measure of cognitive function was used to measure confusion. However, the instrument did not capture the nursing meaning of *confusion*. Nurses consider persons confused who do not know their age or location. The aforementioned measure of cognitive function does not categorize such persons as confused.

Beck and associates (1974) developed an instrument to measure hopelessness with a sample of hospitalized suicidal patients. Later, one of us (Burns, 1981) used the instrument in a study examining family members of cancer patients. Burns had to question whether an instrument developed to measure hopelessness in the original population would be valid to measure hopelessness in family members of cancer patients. A computer search revealed that although the instrument had been used in 17 studies, none of the studies had reexamined the validity or reliability of the instrument. Further statistical analyses indicated, however, that the instrument was indeed valid for both purposes.

Content-Related Validity Evidence

Content-related validity evidence examines the extent to which the method of measurement includes all the major elements relevant to the construct being measured. This evidence is obtained from the following three sources: the literature, representatives of the relevant populations, and content experts.

Thirty years ago, the only type of validity addressed in most studies was referred to as *face validity,* which verified basically that the instrument looked like or gave the appearance of measuring the content. This approach is no longer considered acceptable evidence for validity. However, it is still an important aspect of the usefulness of the instrument, because the willingness of subjects to complete the instrument is related to their perception that the instrument measures the content they agreed to provide (Lynn, 1986; Thomas, 1992).

Documentation of content-related validity evidence begins with development of the instrument. The first step of instrument development is to identify *what* is to be measured; this is referred to as the *universe* or *domain* of the construct. The domain may be determined through a concept analysis or an extensive literature search. Qualitative methods can also be used for this purpose. Macnee and Talsma (1995), in developing the Barriers to Cessation scale, asked subjects to identify what made it most difficult for them to resist smoking. Their responses and the new scale were given to five individuals familiar with smoking cessation and with research. These individuals were asked to determine whether the subjective responses of the subjects could be considered examples of specific items in the scale. Of 38 responses, 29 were categorized as examples of an item in the scale. The remaining nine items could not be categorized and may have to be included in further development of the instrument.

The procedures used to develop or select items for the instrument that are representative of the domain of the construct must be described. One helpful strategy commonly used is to develop a blueprint or matrix, such as is used in developing test items for an examination. However, before development of such items, the blueprint specifications must be submitted to an expert panel to validate that they are appropriate, accurate, and representative. Selection of at least five experts is recommended, although a minimum of three experts is acceptable if it is not possible to locate additional individuals with expertise in the area (Lynn, 1986). Individuals with expertise in various fields might be sought, for example, one with knowledge of instrument development, a second with clinical expertise in an appropriate field of practice, and a third with expertise in another discipline relevant to the content area.

The experts must be given specific guidelines for judging the appropriateness, accuracy, and representativeness of the specifications. Berk (1990) recommends that the experts first make independent assessments and then meet for a group discussion of the specifications. The specifications are then revised and resubmitted to the experts for a final independent assessment. Davis (1992) recommends that expert reviewers be provided with theoretical definitions of concepts and a list of which instrument items are expected to measure each of the concepts. Reviewers are asked to judge how well each of the concepts has been represented in the instrument.

The researcher then needs to determine how the domain is to be measured. The item format, item content, and procedures for generating items must be carefully described. Items are then constructed for each cell in the matrix, or observational methods are designated to gather data related to a specific cell. The researcher is expected to describe the specifications used in constructing items or selecting observations. Sources of content for items must be documented. The items are then assembled, refined, arranged in a suitable order, and submitted to the content experts for evaluation. Specific instructions for evaluating each item and the total instrument must be given to the experts.

A numerical value reflecting the level of content-related validity evidence can be obtained by using the index of content validity (CVI) developed by Waltz and Bausell (1981). With this instrument, experts rate the content relevance of each item using a 4-point rating scale. Lynn (1986, p. 384) recommends standardizing the options on this scale to read as follows: "1 = not relevant; 2 = unable to assess relevance without item revision or item is in need of such revision that it would no longer be relevant; 3 = relevant but needs minor alteration; 4 = very relevant and succinct." In addition to evaluating existing items, the experts must be asked to identify important areas not included in the in-

strument. Berk (1990) suggests that judges also be asked to evaluate the items in terms of readability and possible offensiveness of the language to subjects or data gatherers.

Before sending the instrument to experts for evaluation, the researcher must decide how many experts must agree on each item and on the total instrument in order for the content to be considered valid. Items that do not achieve minimum agreement by the expert panel must be either eliminated from the instrument or revised.

With some modifications, this procedure can also be used with existing instruments, many of which have never been evaluated for content-related validity. With the permission of the author or researcher who developed the instrument, revision of the instrument could be implemented to improve the content-related validity (Lynn, 1986).

Berk (1990) describes the use of the foregoing procedure to obtain evidence of content-related validity for an instrument measuring the nursing care needs of patients with acquired immunodeficiency syndrome (AIDS). The matrix used to develop items related to respiratory and circulatory function is shown in Table 15–1. Berk used four AIDS nurses, one each from hospital, ambulatory care, home care, and nursing home settings, as experts. These nurses attended nine sessions of 2 to 3 hours each, for a total of 22.5 hours, to assist in the development of this complex instrument.

Readability is an essential element of the validity and reliability of an instrument. Assessing the level of readability of an instrument is relatively simple and takes about 20 minutes. There are more than 30 readability formulas. These formulas use counts of language elements to provide an index of the probable degree of difficulty of comprehending the text. Readability formulas are now a standard part of word-processing software. Evanoski (1990) used the Fog formula to calculate the level of readability of literature developed to provide health education for patients with ventricular tachycardia. Instructions for use of the Fog formula are presented in Table 15–2.

Although readability has never been formally identified as a component of content validity, it

TABLE 15–1
EXAMPLE OF A MATRIX DEVELOPED TO TEST CONTENT-RELATED VALIDITY

INDICATOR	LEVEL 1	LEVEL 2	LEVEL 3	LEVEL 4
A. Airway	Effective clearance	Congested, clears with coughing	Ineffective clearance requiring suction, chest PT	Obstruction threatening life
B. Breathing	Effective patterns with adequate gas exchange	SOB or DOE after moderate activity (e.g., climbing stairs); diminished or adventitious breath sounds (e.g., wheezing/rales/ronchi)	Dyspnea at rest or during ADL/minimal activity; impairment (e.g., retractions, nasal flaring)	Inadequate to meet survival needs (e.g., apnea periods)
C. Cardiovascular status	Unimpaired, normal pulse and BP	Fluctuates (e.g., decreased cardiac output and/or BP abnormality controlled by medication/diet); irregular heartbeat; abnormal heart sounds; chest pain	Decompensation as evidenced by poorly controlled arrhythmia, vertigo, syncope; poorly controlled BP or BP with orthostatic changes	Life-threatening abnormality in flow patterns or cardiac output (e.g., uncontrolled arrhythmia or BP)
D. Endurance	Sufficient	Fatigue; does not interfere with ADLs	Limited; affects ability to perform ADLs	Unable to perform ADLs

ADLs, activities of daily living; BP, blood pressure; DOE, dyspnea on exertion; PT, physiotherapy; SOB, shortness of breath.
Revised Domain Specifications: Sample of Respiratory and Circulatory Function Subdomain (Respiratory and circulatory function revised: The body functions concerned with (a) the transfer of gases to meet ventilatory needs, and (b) the supply of blood to body tissues via the cardiovascular system).
From Berk, R. A. (1990). Importance of expert judgement in content-related validity evidence. *Western Journal of Nursing Research, 12*(5), 663.

TABLE 15–2
HOW TO FIND THE FOG INDEX (FOG FORMULA)

1. Pick a sample of writing 100 to 125 words long. Count the average number of words per sentence. In counting, treat independent clauses as separate sentences. "In school we studied; we learned; we improved" is three sentences.
2. Count the words of three syllables or more. Do not count: (a) capitalized words; (b) combinations of short words like butterfly or manpower; or (c) verbs made into three syllables by adding "—es" or "—ed." such as trespasses or created. Divide the count of long words by the number of words in the passage to get the percentage.
3. Add the results from No. 1 (average sentence length) and No. 2 (percentage of long words). Multiply the sum by 0.4. Ignore the numbers after the decimal point.
4. The result is the years of schooling needed to understand the passage tested easily. Few readers have over 17 years' schooling, so give any passage higher than 17 a Fog Index of 17-plus.

Adapted from Gunning, R. (1968). *The technique of clear writing* (rev. ed.). New York: McGraw–Hill. "Fog Index" is a service mark of Gunning-Mueller Clear Writing Institute, Santa Barbara, California.

should be. How valid is content that is incomprehensible? Miller and Bodie (1994) suggest that the reading comprehension level of the population to be studied be assessed directly before the readability of the instrument is calculated with a formula. They indicate that the assumption that literacy is equivalent to the last grade level completed is likely to be erroneous. They recommend use of the Classroom Reading Inventory (CRI), which is based on the Flesch, Space, Dale, and Fry reading comprehension scales (Silvaroli, 1986). This instrument determines the level at which an individual can comprehend written material without assistance.

Ahijevych and Bernhard (1994), in discussing the use of the Health-Promoting Lifestyle Profile (HPLP), reported on a study of health-promoting behaviors of African American women. An excerpt from their study follows.

. . . .

"Readability of the HPLP instrument could have affected its reliability and validity. Anecdotal information with this sample is pertinent. Women asked the investigator the meaning of the HPLP items 'Enthusiastic and optimistic about life' and 'Like myself.' These were not among the terms clarified by Foster (1987) in her use of the HPLP with older African American adults, for whom she developed explanatory prompts. However, Kerr and Ritchey (1990) reported that Mexican American migrant farm workers frequently asked questions about several items, including 'Like myself.'

Analysis using RightWriter (RightSoft, Inc., Sarasota, FL) revealed the HPLP is written at a seventh-grade level, but there were 21 words readers may not understand, such as 'interpersonal.' Meade, Byrd, and Lee (1989) reported that educational grade level completion was a poor predictor of reading skill among subjects recruited at primary care clinics. They found that although subjects had a reported mean educational level of grade 11, their reading skills as estimated on the Wide Range Achievement Test were at grade 7. Since mean educational level in this study was 12.4 years and 28% of the women had completed 11 or fewer years of education, this may have influenced understanding of the HPLP.

The instrument may have a middle-class bias that is inappropriate for poor people who have, for example, little or no time, desire, or energy to 'Attend educational programs on improving the environment,' one item on the scale. The item, 'Find my living environment pleasant and satisfying,' yielded comments such as 'Yes, when the doors are locked, I feel safe.'" (Ahijevych & Bernhard, 1994, p. 89) ■

Evidence of Validity from Factor Analysis

Exploratory factor analysis can be performed to examine relationships among the various items of the instrument. Items that are closely related are clustered into a factor. The analysis may reveal the presence of several factors, which may indicate that the instrument reflects several constructs rather than a single construct. The number of constructs in the instrument and measurement equivalence among comparison groups can be validated through the use

of confirmatory factor analysis (Goodwin & Goodwin, 1991; Stommel et al., 1992; Teel & Verran, 1991). Items that do not fall into a factor (and thus do not correlate with other items) may be deleted. Factor analysis is further described in Chapter 20.

Evidence of Validity from Structural Analysis

Structural analysis is now being used to examine the structure of relationships among the various items of an instrument. This approach provides insights beyond that provided by factor analysis. Structural analysis is described in Chapter 20.

Evidence of Validity from Contrasting Groups

Validity of the instrument can be tested by identifying groups that are expected to have contrasting scores on the instrument. Hypotheses are generated about the expected response of various groups to the construct. Samples are selected from at least two groups that are expected to have opposing responses to the items in the instrument. Hagerty and Patusky (1995) developed a measure called the Sense of Belonging Instrument (SOBI). The instrument was tested on the following three groups: community college students, clients diagnosed with major depression, and retired Roman Catholic nuns, as described in the following excerpt.

"The community college sample was chosen for its heterogeneous mix of students and ease of access. Depressed clients were included based on the literature and the researcher's clinical experience that interpersonal relationships and feeling 'connected' are difficult when one is depressed. It was hypothesized that the depressed group would score significantly lower on the SOBI than the student group. The nuns were selected to examine the performance of the SOBI with a group that, in accordance with the theoretical basis of the instrument, should score significantly higher than the depressed and student groups." (Hagerty & Patusky, 1995, p. 10) ■

Analysis of variance (described in Chapter 22) can be used to determine whether the groups chosen are significantly different in the directions proposed.

Evidence of Validity from Examining Convergence

In many cases, other instruments are available to measure the same construct. For a number of possible reasons, the existing instruments may not be satisfactory for a particular purpose or a particular population. However, it is important to determine how closely these instruments measure the same construct as the newly developed instrument. Selecting instruments that used a variety of measurement strategies strengthens the test of validity. All of the selected instruments are administered to a sample concurrently. The results are examined with the use of correlational analyses. If the measures are highly positively correlated, the validity of each instrument is strengthened.

Evidence of Validity from Examining Divergence

Sometimes, instruments can be located that measure a construct opposite to the construct measured by the newly developed instrument. For example, if the newly developed instrument is a measure of hope, a search could be made for an instrument that measures hopelessness. If possible, this instrument is administered at the same time as the instruments used to test convergent validity. Correlational procedures are performed with all the measures of the construct. If the divergent measure is negatively correlated with other measures, validity for each of the instruments is strengthened.

Evidence of Validity from Discriminant Analysis

Sometimes, instruments have been developed to measure constructs closely related to the construct measured by the newly developed instrument. If such instruments can be located, the validity of the two instruments can be strengthened by testing the extent to which the two instruments can finely discriminate between these related concepts. Testing of

this discrimination involves administering the two instruments simultaneously to a sample and then performing a discriminant analysis. This procedure is described in Chapter 19.

Evidence of Validity from Prediction of Future Events

The ability to predict future performance or attitudes on the basis of instrument scores adds to the validity of an instrument. For example, nurse researchers might determine the ability of a scale that measures health-related behaviors to predict the future health status of individuals. The future level of health of individuals might be predicted by examining reported stress levels of these individuals for the past 3 years. Validity of the Holmes and Rahe Life Events Scale, for example, could be tested in this manner. Miller (1981) discussed the validity and reliability of the Holmes and Rahe Life Events Scale in measuring stress levels in a variety of populations. The accuracy of predictive validity is determined through correlational analysis.

Evidence of Validity from Prediction of Concurrent Events

Validity can be tested by examining the ability to predict the current value of one measure on the basis of the value obtained on the measure of another concept. For example, one might be able to predict the self-esteem score of an individual who had a high score on an instrument to measure coping.

Successive Verification of Validity

After the initial development of an instrument, other researchers begin using the instrument in unrelated studies. Each of these studies adds to the validity information on the instrument. Thus, there is a successive verification of the validity of the instrument over time.

RELIABILITY AND VALIDITY OF PHYSIOLOGICAL MEASURES

Reliability and validity of physiological and biochemical measures tend not to be reported in published studies. These routine physiological measures are assumed to be valid and reliable, an assumption that is not always correct. The most common physiological measures used in nursing studies are blood pressure, heart rate, weight, and temperature. These measures are often obtained from the patient's record with no consideration given to their accuracy. It is important to consider the possibility of differences between the obtained value and the true value of physiological measures. Thus, researchers using physiological measures need to provide evidence of the validity of their measures (Gift & Soeken, 1988).

Evaluation of physiological measures may require a slightly different perspective from that of behavioral measures, in that standards for physiological measures are defined by the National Bureau of Standards rather than the APA. The construct by which physiological validity is judged consists of human physiology and the mechanics of physiological equipment. However, the process is similar to that for behavioral measures and must be addressed (Gift & Soeken, 1988).

Gift and Soeken (1988) identify the following five terms as critical to the evaluation of physiological measures: accuracy, selectivity, precision, sensitivity, and error.

Accuracy

Accuracy is comparable to validity, in which evidence of content-related validity addresses the extent to which the instrument measured the domain defined in the study. For example, measures of pulse oximetry could be compared with arterial blood gas measures. The researcher needs to be able to document the extent to which the measure is an effective predictive clinical instrument. For example, peak expiratory flow rate can predict asthma episodes.

Selectivity

Selectivity, an element of accuracy, is "the ability to identify correctly the signal under study and to distinguish it from other signals" (Gift & Soeken, 1988, p. 129). Because body systems interact, instruments must be chosen that have selectivity for the dimension being studied. For example, electrocardiographic readings allow one to differentiate electrical signals coming from the myocardium from similar signals coming from skeletal muscles.

Content validity of biochemical measures can be determined by contacting experts in the laboratory procedure and asking them to evaluate the procedure used for collection, analysis, and scoring. They may also be asked to judge the appropriateness of the measure for the construct being measured. Contrasted groups' techniques can be used by selecting a group of subjects known to have high values on the biochemical measures and comparing them with a group of subjects known to have low values on the same measure. In addition, to obtain concurrent validity the results of the test can be compared with results from the use of a known, reliable method (DeKeyser & Pugh, 1990).

Precision

Precision is the degree of consistency or reproducibility of measurements made with physiological instruments. Precision is comparable to reliability. The reliability of most physiological instruments is determined by the manufacturer and is part of quality control testing. Because of fluctuations in most physiological measures, test-retest reliability is inappropriate. Engstrom (1988, p. 389) states that assessment of reliability for physiological variables that yield continuous data must include "mean, minimal, and maximal differences; standard deviation of the net differences; technical error of measurement; and indices of agreement." She suggests displaying these differences graphically and recommends exploratory data analysis (EDA) techniques for summarizing differences; EDA techniques are described in Chapter 19. Correlation coefficients are not adequate tests of reliability of physiological measures.

Two procedures are commonly used to determine precision of biochemical measures. One is the Levy-Jennings Chart. For each analysis method, a control sample is analyzed daily for 20 to 30 days. The control sample contains a known amount of the substance being tested. The mean, the standard deviation, and the known value of the sample are used to prepare a graph of the daily test results. Only 1 value of 22 is expected to be greater than or less than 2 standard deviations from the mean. If 2 or more values are more than 2 standard deviations from the mean, the method is unreliable in that laboratory. Another method of determining precision of biochemical measures is the duplicate measurements method. Duplicate measures are performed on randomly selected specimens for a specific number of days by the same technician. Results will be the same each day if there is perfect precision. Results are plotted on a graph, and the standard deviation is calculated on the basis of difference scores. The use of correlation coefficients is not recommended (DeKeyser & Pugh, 1990).

Sensitivity

Sensitivity of physiological measures is related to "the amount of change of a parameter that can be measured precisely" (Gift & Soeken, 1988, p. 130). If changes are expected to be very small, the instrument must be very sensitive to detect the changes. Thus, sensitivity is associated with effect size. With some instruments, sensitivity may vary at the ends of the spectrum. This is referred to as the frequency response. The stability of the instrument is also related to sensitivity. This feature may be judged in terms of the ability of the system to resume a steady state after a disturbance in input. For electrical systems, this feature is referred to as *freedom from drift* (Gift & Soeken, 1988).

Error

Sources of *error* in physiological measures can be grouped into the following five categories: environment, user, subject, machine, and interpretation. The environment affects both the machine and the subject. Environmental factors include temperature, barometric pressure, and static electricity. User errors are caused by the person using the instrument and may be associated with variations by the same user, different users, changes in supplies, or procedures used to operate the equipment. Subject errors occur when the subject alters the machine or the machine alters the subject. In some cases, the machine may not be used to its full capacity. Machine

error may be related to calibration or to the stability of the machine. Signals transmitted from the machine are also a source of error and can result in misinterpretation (Gift & Soeken, 1988).

Sources of error in biochemical measures are biological, preanalytical, analytical, and postanalytical. Biological variability in biochemical measures is due to factors such as age, gender, and body size. Variability in the same individual is due to factors such as diurnal rhythms, seasonal cycles, and aging. Preanalytical variability is due to errors in collecting and handling of specimens. These errors include sampling the wrong patients; using an incorrect container, preservative, or label; lysis of cells; and evaporation. Preanalytical variability may also be due to patient intake of food or drugs, exercise, or emotional stress. Analytical variability is associated with the method used for analysis and may be due to materials, equipment, procedures, and personnel used. The major source of postanalytical variability is transcription error. This source of error can be greatly reduced by direct entry of the data into the computer (DeKeyser & Pugh, 1990).

OBTAINING VALIDITY IN QUALITATIVE RESEARCH

One of the most serious concerns related to qualitative research has been the lack of strategies to determine the validity of the measurements that led to the development of theory. Qualitative researchers tend to work alone. Biases in their work, which threaten validity, can easily go undetected. Miles and Huberman (1994) caution the qualitative researcher to be alert to the occurrence of the *holistic fallacy*. This fallacy occurs as the researcher becomes more and more sure that his or her conclusions are correct and that the model does, in fact, explain the situation. This feeling should arouse suspicion and alert the researcher to take action to validate the findings. Miles and Huberman (1994) have described 12 strategies for examining the validity of qualitative measures, as follows.

Checking for Representativeness. Qualitative measurement can be biased by either the attention of the researcher or a bias in the people from whom they obtain their measures. To ensure that measures are representative of the entire population, the researcher looks for sources of data not easily accessible. The researcher assumes that observed actions are representative of actions that occur when the researcher is not present. However, efforts must be made to determine whether this is so.

Checking for Researcher Effects. In many cases, the researcher's presence can alter behavior, leading to invalid measures. To avoid this effect, the researcher must (1) remain on the site long enough to become familiar, (2) use unobtrusive measures, and (3) seek input from informants.

Triangulating. The qualitative researcher must compare all the measures from different sources to determine the validity of the findings.

Weighing the Evidence. Qualitative research involves reducing large amounts of data during the process of coming to conclusions. In this process, some evidence is captured from this mass of data and is used in reaching conclusions. The researcher needs to review the strength of the captured data to validate the conclusions. The researcher determines the strength of the evidence from the source, the circumstances of data collection, and the researcher's efforts to validate the evidence. The researcher must search actively for reasons why the evidence should not be trusted.

Making Contrasts and Comparisons. Contrasts between subjects or events in relation to the study conclusions must be examined. An example would be an action that nursing supervisors consider to be very important but that staff nurses regard as simply another administrative activity. The two extreme positions must be examined. A decision must then be made about whether the difference is a significant one.

Checking the Meaning of Outliers. Exceptions to findings must be identified and examined. These exceptions are referred to as *outliers*. The outliers provide a way to test the generality of the findings. Therefore, in the selection of subjects, it may be important to seek individuals who seem to be outliers.

Using Extreme Cases. Certain types of outliers, referred to as *extreme cases*, can be useful in confirming conclusions. The researcher can compare the extreme case with the theoretical model that was developed and determine the key factor that causes the model not to fit the case. Purposive sampling is often used to ensure that extreme cases are included.

Ruling Out Spurious Relations. The strategy of ruling out spurious relations requires the examination of relationships identified in the model to consider the possibility of a third variable influencing the situation.

Replicating a Finding. Documenting the findings from several independent sources increases the dependability of the findings and diminishes the risk of the holistic fallacy. The findings can be tested either with new data collected later in the study or with data from another site or data set. The second option is more rigorous.

Checking Out Rival Explanations. The qualitative researcher is taught to keep several hypotheses in mind and constantly to compare the plausibility of each with the possibility that one of the others is more accurate. Near the end of data analysis, however, when the researcher is more emotionally "wedded to" one idea, it is useful to have someone not involved in the research act as a devil's advocate. Questions such as "What could disprove the hypothesis?" or, conversely, "What does the present hypothesis disprove?" should be asked. Evidence that does not fit the hypothesis must be carefully examined.

Looking for Negative Evidence. A search for negative evidence naturally flows from the searches for outliers and rival explanations. In this step, there is an active search for disconfirmation of what is believed to be true. The researcher goes back through the data, seeking evidence to disconfirm the conclusions. However, the inability to find disconfirming evidence never decisively confirms the conclusions reached by the researcher. In some cases, independent verification, through examination of the data by a second qualitative researcher, is sought.

Obtaining Feedback from Informants. Conclusions must be given to the informants, and feedback is sought from them about the accuracy of the causal network developed. Although researchers have been getting feedback from informants throughout the analysis period, feedback after completion of the model provides a different type of verification of the information.

■ SUMMARY

Measurement is the process of assigning numbers to objects, events, or situations in accord with some rule. The numbers assigned can indicate numerical values or categories. A component of measurement is instrumentation. *Instrumentation* is the application of specific rules to develop a measurement device or instrument. A variety of measurement strategies are necessary to examine the concrete and abstract concepts relevant to nursing.

Measurement theory and the rules within this theory have been developed to direct the measurement of abstract and concrete concepts. Measurement theory addresses the directness of measurement, measurement error, levels of measurement, reference of measurement, reliability, and validity. There is direct measurement and indirect measurement. The technology of health care has made direct measures of concrete elements, such as height, weight, heart rate, temperature, and blood pressure, very familiar. Indirect measurement is used with abstract concepts, when the concepts are not measured directly, but when the indicators or attributes of the concepts are used to represent the abstraction. Measurement error is the difference between what exists in reality and what is measured by a research instrument. Measurement exists in both direct and indirect measures and can be random or systematic. The levels of measurement, from lower to higher, are nominal, ordinal, interval, and ratio. *Referencing* involves comparing a subject's score against a standard. There are two types of testing that involve referencing: norm-referenced testing and criterion-referenced testing.

Reliability in measurement is concerned with how consistently the measurement technique measures the concept of interest. Reliability testing is considered a measure of the amount of random error in the measurement technique. Reliability testing focuses on three aspects of reliability: stability, equivalence, and homogeneity. The validity of an instrument is a determination of the extent to which the instrument actually reflects the abstract construct being examined. Validity, as well as reliability, is not an all-or-nothing phenomenon but, rather, a matter of degree. No instrument is completely valid. Validity is considered a single, broad method of measurement evaluation referred to as *construct validity*. Validity testing validates the use of an instrument for a specific group or purpose, rather than being directed toward the instrument itself. An instrument may be very valid in one situation but not valid in another. Therefore, validity must be reexamined in each study situation.

There are a number of sources for obtaining evidence of the validity of an instrument. Content-related validity evidence examines the extent to which the method of measurement includes all the major elements relevant to the construct being measured. This evidence is obtained from three sources: the literature, representatives of the relevant populations, and content experts. Exploratory factor analysis can be performed to examine relationships among the various items of the instrument. The validity of the instrument can be tested through identification of groups that are expected to have contrasting scores on the instrument. Other instruments can be compared with the instrument to determine how closely correlated the scores are.

Sometimes, instruments can be located that measure a construct opposite to the construct measured by the instrument. If the divergent measure is negatively correlated with values from the instrument, validity of the instruments is strengthened. Sometimes, instruments have been developed to measure constructs closely related to the construct measured by the instrument. If such instruments can be located, the researcher can strengthen the validity of the two instruments by testing the extent to which they can finely discriminate between the related concepts. The ability to predict future performance or attitudes on the basis of instrument scores adds to the validity of an instrument. Validity can also be tested by examining the ability to predict the current value of one measure on the basis of the value obtained on the measure of another concept. After initial development of an instrument, other researchers begin using it in unrelated studies. Each of these studies adds to the validity information on the instrument. Thus, there is successive verification of the validity of the instrument over time.

Reliability and validity of physiological and biochemical measures tend not to be reported in published studies. The assumption is erroneously made that routine physiological measures are valid and reliable. Evaluation of physiological measures requires a different perspective from that of behavioral measures. Five terms are critical to evaluation of physiological measures: accuracy, selectivity, precision, sensitivity, and error.

One of the most serious concerns related to qualitative research has been the lack of strategies to determine the validity of the measurements that led to the development of theory. However, strategies are being identified to examine the validity of qualitative measures.

▪ ▪

REFERENCES

Ahijevych, K., & Bernhard, L. (1994). Health-promoting behaviors of African American women. *Nursing Research, 43*(2), 86–89.

American Psychological Association's Committee to Develop Standards. (1985). *Standards for educational and psychological testing.* Washington, DC: American Psychological Association.

Armstrong, G. D. (1981). Parametric statistics and ordinal data: A pervasive misconception. *Nursing Research, 30*(1), 60–62.

Armstrong, G. D. (1984). Parametric statistics [letter]. *Nursing Research, 33*(1), 54.

Beck, A., Weissman, A., Lester, D., & Trexler, L. (1974). The measurement of pessimism: The hopelessness scale. *Journal of Consulting and Clinical Psychology, 42*(6), 861–865.

Berk, R. A. (1990). Importance of expert judgment in content-related validity evidence. *Western Journal of Nursing Research, 12*(5), 659–671.

Brinberg, D., & McGrath, J. E. (1985). *Validity and the research process.* Beverly Hills, CA: Sage.

Burns, N. (1981). *Evaluation of a supportive-expressive group for families of cancer patients.* Unpublished doctoral dissertation, Texas Woman's University, Denton, TX.

Campbell, D. T., & Fiske, D. W. (1959). Convergent and discriminant validation by the multitrait-multimethod matrix. *Psychological Bulletin, 56*(2), 81–105.

Cohen, J. A. (1960). A coefficient of agreement for nominal scales. *Education and Psychological Measurement, 20*(1), 37–46.

Davis, L. L. (1992). Instrument review: Getting the most from a panel of experts. *Applied Nursing Research, 5*(4), 194–197.

DeKeyser, F. G., & Pugh, L. C. (1990). Assessment of the reliability and validity of biochemical measures. *Nursing Research, 39*(5), 314–317.

Engstrom, J. L. (1988). Assessment of the reliability of physical measures. *Research in Nursing & Health, 11*(6), 383–389.

Evanoski, C. A. M. (1990). Health education for patients with ventricular tachycardia: Assessment of readability. *Journal of Cardiovascular Nursing, 4*(2), 1–6.

Foster, M. (1987). A study of the relationships among perceived current health, health-promoting activities, and life satisfaction in older black adults. Unpublished doctoral dissertation, The University of Texas at Austin, TX.

Garvin, B. J., Kennedy, C. W., & Cissna, K. N. (1988). Reliability in category coding systems. *Nursing Research, 37*(1), 52–55.

Gift, A. G., & Soeken, K. L. (1988). Assessment of physiologic instruments. *Heart & Lung, 17*(2), 128–133.

Goodwin, L. D., & Goodwin, W. L. (1991). Estimating construct validity. *Research in Nursing & Health, 14*(3), 235–243.

Guetzkow, H. (1950). Unitizing and categorizing problems in coding qualitative data. *Journal of Clinical Psychology, 6*(1), 47–58.

Gunning, R. (1968). *The technique of clear writing* (Rev. ed.). New York: McGraw-Hill.

Hagerty, B. M. K., & Patusky, K. (1995). Developing a measure of sense of belonging. *Nursing Research, 44*(1), 9–13.

Kaplan, A. (1963). *The conduct of inquiry: Methodology for behavioral science.* New York: Harper & Row.

Kerr, M. J., & Ritchey, D. A. (1990). Health-promoting lifestyles of English-speaking and Spanish-speaking Mexican-American migrant farm workers. *Public Health Nursing, 7*(2), 80–87.

Knapp, T. R. (1984). Parametric statistics [letter]. *Nursing Research, 33*(1), 54.

Knapp, T. R. (1990). Treating ordinal scales as interval scales: An attempt to resolve the controversy. *Nursing Research, 39*(2), 121–123.

Lynn, M. R. (1986). Determination and quantification of content validity. *Nursing Research, 35*(6), 382–385.

Macnee, C. L., & Talsma, A. (1995). Development and testing of the Barriers to Cessation Scale. *Nursing Research, 44*(4), 214–219.

Meade, C., Byrd, J., & Lee, M. (1989). Improving patient comprehension of literature on smoking. *American Journal of Public Health, 79*(10), 1411–1412.

Miles, M. B., & Huberman, A. M. (1994). *Qualitative data analysis: A sourcebook of new methods* (2nd ed.). Beverly Hills, CA: Sage.

Miller, B., & Bodie, M. (1994). Determination of reading comprehension level for effective patient health-education materials. *Nursing Research, 43*(2), 118–119.

Miller, T. W. (1981). Life events scaling: Clinical methodological issues. *Nursing Research, 30*(5), 316–320A.

Nagley, S. J., & Byers, P. H. (1987). Clinical construct validity. *Journal of Advanced Nursing, 12*(5), 617–619.

Rew, L., Stuppy, D., & Becker, H. (1988). Construct validity in instrument development: A vital link between nursing practice, research, and theory. *Advances in Nursing Science, 10*(4), 10–22.

Silvaroli, N. J. (1986). *Classroom reading inventory* (5th ed.). Dubuque, IA: William C. Brown.

Stevens, S. S. (1946). On the theory of scales of measurement. *Science, 103*(2684), 677–680.

Stommel, M., Wang, S., Given, C. W., & Given, B. (1992). Confirmatory factor analysis (CFA) as a method to assess measurement equivalence. *Research in Nursing & Health, 15*(5), 399-405.

Teel, C., & Verran, J. A. (1991). Factor comparison across studies. *Research in Nursing & Health, 14*(1), 67–72.

Thomas, S. (1992). Face validity. *Western Journal of Nursing Research, 14*(1), 109–112.

Topf, M. (1988). Interrater reliability decline under covert assessment. *Nursing Research, 37*(1), 47–49.

Waltz, C. W. & Bausell, R. B. (1981). *Nursing Research: Design, statistics and computer analysis*. Philadelphia: F. A. Davis.

Washington, C. C. & Moss, M. (1988). Pragmatic aspects of establishing interrater reliability in research. *Nursing Research, 37*(3), 190–191.

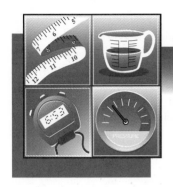

CHAPTER 16

MEASUREMENT STRATEGIES IN NURSING

Nursing studies examine a wide variety of phenomena and thus require the availability of an extensive array of measurement tools. However, nurse researchers have often found that there were no tools available to measure phenomena central to the development of nursing science. Tools used in older nursing studies tended to be developed for a specific study and had little if any documentation of validity and reliability. In the early 1980s, development of valid and reliable tools to measure phenomena of concern to nursing was identified as a priority. The number and quality of measurement methods developed have greatly increased since the first edition of this text.

Knowledge of measurement methods in nursing is important at all levels of nursing. An adequate critique of a study requires that you have some knowledge of not only measurement theory but also the state of the art in developing measures to examine the phenomena included in the study. You might want to know whether the researcher was using an older tool that had been surpassed by a number of more recently developed instruments. It might help you to know that measuring a particular phenomenon has been a problem with which nurse researchers have struggled for a number of years. Your understanding of the successes and struggles in measuring nursing phenomena may stimulate your creative thinking as a nursing research user and eventually lead to a contribution of your own to the development of measurement approaches. Many nursing phenomena have not been examined

because no one has thought of a way to measure them, which is a problem for clinical practice as well as for research.

This chapter describes the common measurement approaches used in nursing research, including physiological measures, observations, interviews, focus groups, questionnaires, and scales. Other methods of measurement discussed include Q methodology, visual analogue scales, the Delphi technique, projective techniques, and diaries. This presentation is followed by discussions concerned with selecting an existing instrument, locating existing instruments, examining existing instruments, assessing the readability of existing instruments, and describing an instrument in a written report. The chapter also includes a description of the process of scale construction and issues related to translating an instrument into another language.

PHYSIOLOGICAL MEASUREMENT

Much of nursing practice is oriented toward physiological dimensions of health. Therefore, many of our questions require the measurement of these dimensions. Of particular importance are studies linking physiological and psychosocial variables. In 1993, the National Institute of Nursing Research (NINR) expressed a need for increased numbers of physiologically based nursing studies inasmuch as 85% of NINR-funded studies involved nonphysiological variables. According to NINR staff, a review of physiological studies funded by the NINR found that "the biological measurements used in the funded grants often were not state-of-the-science, and the biological theory underlying the measurements often was underutilized" (Cowan et al., 1993, p. 4). This report would suggest that there needs to be an increase not only in the number of biologically based studies but also in the quality of measurements used in these studies. The Second Conference on Nursing Research Priorities identified biobehavioral studies as one of the five priority areas and proposed targeting the following biobehavioral foci: (1) assessment of the effectiveness of biobehavioral nursing interventions in HIV/AIDS, (2) development of biobehavioral and environmental approaches to remediating cognitive impairment, and (3) identification of biobehavioral factors related to immunocompetence (Pugh & DeKeyser, 1995).

Physiological measures can be obtained by using a variety of methods. The following sections describe how to obtain physiological measures by self-report, observation, direct or indirect measurement, laboratory tests, electronic monitoring, and creative development of new methods of measurement. Measurement of physiological variables across time is also addressed. The section concludes with a discussion of how to select physiological variables for a particular study.

Obtaining Physiological Measures by Self-Report

Self-report or paper-and-pencil scales can be used to obtain physiological information. These means may be particularly useful when the subjects are not in a closely monitored setting such as a hospital. For example, Heitkemper and colleagues (1991) used self-reporting to obtain information on stool frequency and stool consistency for their study. Other phenomena of possible nursing research interest that could be measured by self-report scales are sleep patterns, patterns of daily activities, eating patterns, patterns of joint stiffness, variations in degree of mobility, and exercise patterns. For some variables, self-reporting may be the only means of obtaining the information. Such may be the case, for example, when the physiological phe-

nomenon is experienced by the subjects but cannot be observed or measured by others. Nonobservable physiological phenomena include pain, nausea, dizziness, indigestion, patterns of hunger or thirst, variations in cognition, visual phenomena, tinnitus, itching, and fatigue. Pope (1995) points out that sound is an essential and constant component of the human condition, but its importance to health has been little recognized. Although one can measure sounds, one cannot measure sound perception and sensitivity. Pope recommends the development of instruments to measure these responses and specifically points out the potential impact of these variables in settings such as critical care units. Covey and associates (1999) used self-reporting to obtain information on symptoms of perceived breathlessness and leg fatigue in subjects during exercise.

· ·

"Subjects rated symptoms of perceived breathlessness (RPB) and leg fatigue (RPLF) during the last 10 seconds of each minute of exercise using the Borg Category-Ratio Scale (Borg, 1982). Subjects were introduced to the scale before the exercise test, and directions were given verbatim according to a script. The Borg scale is a vertical numeric scale with a range of 0 to 10 and is anchored with descriptors beside many of the numbers (range, *nothing at all* to *maximal*)." (Covey et al., 1999, p. 11) ■

Using self-report measures may enable nurses to ask research questions not previously considered, which could be an important means to build knowledge in areas not yet explored. The insight gained could alter the nursing management of patient situations now considered problematic and improve patient outcomes.

Obtaining Physiological Measures by Observation

Data on physiological parameters are sometimes obtained by using observational data collection measures and recording the results on a scale or index. The scale provides criteria for quantifying various levels or states of physiological functioning. In addition to collecting clinical data, this method provides a means to gather data from the observations of caregivers. This source of data has been particularly useful in studies involving persons with Alzheimer disease or advanced cancer and in the frail elderly living in the community. Studies involving home health agencies and hospices often use observation tools to record physiological dimensions of patient status. These data are sometimes stored electronically and are available for large database analysis by researchers.

Stevens and coworkers (1999) used the Premature Infant Pain Profile (PIPP; Stevens et al., 1996) in their study to assess developmentally sensitive interventions for relieving procedural pain in very low birth weight neonates. They describe the PIPP as follows.

• •

"The PIPP is a 7-indicator 4-point composite pain scale consisting of 3 behavioral (facial actions: brow bulge, eye squeeze, and nasolabial furrow), 2 physiologic (heart rate, oxygen saturation), and 2 contextual (gestational age, behavioral state) indicators of infant pain. The behavioral indicators were derived from the Neonatal Facial Coding System (NFCS)." (Grunau & Craig, 1987, p. 16) ▪

Obtaining Physiological Measures Directly or Indirectly

Measurement of physiological variables can be either direct or indirect. Direct measures are more valid. Norman and colleagues (1991) used both direct and indirect measures of blood pressure in their study. Measurement of arterial pressure waveforms through an arterial catheter provides a direct measure of blood pressure, whereas use of a stethoscope and sphygmomanometer provides an indirect measure. Keefe and associates (1996) used the Infant State Monitor to measure physiological parameters of the preverbal infant. They describe the measurement as follows.

• •

"The Infant State Monitor has been described by Keefe, Kotzer, Reuss, and Sander (1989). Sensors embedded within a mattress monitor the infant's respiratory pattern and body movement continuously for up to 24 hours. The Sleep State Evaluation

program (SSEP) reads the analog data stored on disk and uses a role-based algorithm to classify the activity pattern into the following primary infant states: quiet sleep, active sleep, awake, and indeterminate. In addition, the following additional sleep characteristics are summarized and reported: sleep transitions, sleep breaks, startles, sleep cycles, sleep periods, and noncyclic sleep sessions. In total, 62 variables reflecting the minimum, maximum, average, standard deviation, and totals of these sleep parameters are generated and reported by the SSEP software program. The concurrent validity of this system was assessed in a preliminary study (Keefe et al., 1988). In the current study, interrater reliability was assessed for a subset of 25 randomly selected records. Agreement between the computerized categorization of infant state and live reviewer scoring ranged from 67% to 94%. The overall average percentage of agreement was 78%." (Keefe et al., 1996, p. 6) ▪

Obtaining Physiological Measures from Laboratory Tests

Biochemical measures such as the activated partial thromboplastin time must be obtained through invasive procedures. Sometimes these invasive procedures are part of the routine care of the patient and can be gotten from the patient's record. Although nurses are now performing some biochemical measures on the nursing unit, these measures often require laboratory analysis. When invasive procedures are not part of routine care but are instead performed specifically for a study, great care needs to be taken to protect the subjects and to follow guidelines for informed consent and institutional approval.

Obtaining Physiological Measures Through Electronic Monitoring

The availability of electronic monitoring equipment has greatly increased the possibilities of physiological measurement in nursing studies, particularly in intensive care environments. Understanding the processes of electronic monitoring can make the procedure less formidable to those critiquing published studies and those considering using the method for measurement. The study of Keefe and colleagues (1996) described previously used electronic sensing.

To use electronic monitoring, sensors are usually placed on or within the subject. The sensors measure changes in body functions such as electrical energy. For many sensors, an external stimulus is needed to trigger measurement by the sensor. Transducers convert the electrical signal. Electrical signals often include interference signals as well as the desired signal, so an amplifier may be used to decrease interference and amplify the desired signal. The electrical signal is then digitized (converted to numerical digits or values) and stored on magnetic tape. In addition, it is immediately displayed on a monitor. The display equipment may be visual or auditory, or both. A writing recorder provides a printed version of the data. One type of display equipment is an oscilloscope that displays the data as a waveform, and it may provide information such as time, phase, voltage, or frequency of the data. Some electronic equipment provides simultaneous recording of multiple physiological measures that are displayed on a monitor. The equipment is often linked to a computer, which allows review of data, and the computer often contains complex software for detailed analysis of the data and will provide a printed report of the analysis (DeKeyser & Pugh, 1991). Figure 16–1 illustrates the process of electronic measurement.

One disadvantage of using sensors to measure physiological variables is that the presence of a transducer within the body can alter the reading. For example, the presence of a flow transducer in a blood vessel can partially block the vessel and thus alter flow. The reading, then, is not an accurate reflection of the flow.

Norman and colleagues (1991) used electronic sensing in their study evaluating three blood pressure methods in a stabilized acute trauma population and described their instrumentation.

· ·

"A Littmann Classic II Medallion Combination Stethoscope (model 2100), 3M Medical-Surgical Division (St. Paul, Minnesota), was used for all indirect blood pressure readings. Bell and diaphragm values for K1, K4, and K5 were measured with a Hawksley random-zero (R) sphygmomanometer (W. A. Baum Company Inc., Copiague, NY). The RZ is a conventional mercury sphygmomanometer with calibrations from 0 to 300 mm Hg. The singular feature of this instrument is a zero shifting device that allows the mercury column to be stopped randomly between 0 and 20 mm Hg. According to the manufacturers, the zero shifting device effectively eliminates observer bias because true blood pressure values remain unknown until after auscultation (personal communication, November 1987).

"Direct blood pressure was measured via radial arterial catheter. The catheters were connected to transducers which sent arterial pressure waveforms

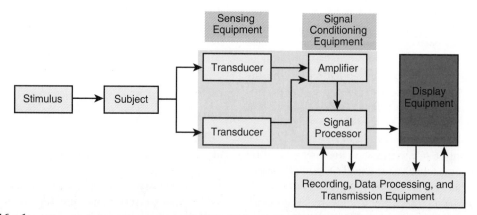

FIGURE 16–1 ■ Process of electronic measurement. (From Waltz, C. F., Strickland, O. L., & Lentz, E. R. [1991]. *Measurement in nursing research.* Philadelphia: F. A. Davis, p. 389.)

to Hewlett-Packard (H-P) four-channel monitors (#78534C). H-P monitors have strip chart recorders with frequency responses ranging from 0.05 to 100 Hz. Simultaneous EKG, pulmonary artery pressure, and arterial pressure waveforms were recorded from these monitors.

"Procedure: Demographic information was obtained from patient charts. The catheter-tubing-transducer system was visually assessed for bubbles, and monitor waveforms were checked for damping. Phlebostatic axis was noted before leveling, calibrating, and flushing the pulmonary artery and radial arterial lines. Core body temperature, right atrial pressure, cardiac output, and heart rate were recorded for each subject.

"The fidelity and accuracy of the radial catheter-tubing-transducer systems were assessed by calculating natural frequency (Fn) and damping coefficient (zeta) values using Gardner's formula (1981). Natural frequency (Fn) is the ability of a system to oscillate between fast and slow waves (Henneman & Henneman, 1989). Damping coefficient (zeta) refers to how quickly the system comes to rest. Specialists believe a lack of familiarity with natural frequency and damping coefficient calculations is a major reason for inconsistent blood pressure measurement (Gibbs & Gardner, 1988; Henneman & Henneman, 1989)." (Norman et al., 1991, p. 87) ■

Creative Development of Physiological Measures

Some studies require imaginative approaches to measuring phenomena that are traditionally observed in clinical practice but are not measured. The first step in this process is the recognition that the phenomenon being observed by the nurse could be measured. Once that idea has emerged, one can begin envisioning various means of measuring the phenomenon. The innovative approach of Fahs and Kinney (1991) to measuring the extent of bruising illustrates creativity. They traced the outline of the bruise onto polyethylene wrap with a ballpoint pen. This outline was then traced onto a graph with carbon paper. The surface area of the bruise was calculated in units of millimeters squared.

Ziemer and coworkers (1995) used photographic slides to measure the damage to nipple skin during the first week of breast-feeding. The following is their description of the measurement process.

. . . .

"To optimize visualization of the nipple skin, serial photographic slides were obtained for later assessment of skin characteristics. The slides provided a magnified image of the nipple skin and areola, which could not be readily observed with the naked eye. To generate reliable documentation of nipple skin condition, the serial photographs were taken with a 35 mm camera fitted with a macro lens and a ring light flash and loaded with Eastman Kodak ASA 25 Kodachrome film. All film was purchased at the same time to ensure similarity of the film emulsions. To obtain consistent exposure distance from the film plate (approximately 10 in.), the automatic focus was disabled and the lens length maximized. This approach resulted in a 1:1 exposure of the film. The same laboratory was used for photographic development in an effort to ensure consistency and reduce variation in color tones. Slide images of nipple skin were assessed to identify the amount of surface area covered by eschar and to rate the severity of erythema and fissures visible on the nipple skin. Eschar was measured by projecting the image downward onto a 20 × 20-in. digitizing tablet with a magnification ratio of 1:22. Visible eschar was then traced and its area calculated." (Ziemer et al., 1995, p. 348) ■

Some physiological phenomena are sufficiently complex that a combination of measures is necessary to obtain adequate data for evaluation. For example, measuring nutritional status requires combining a variety of strategies. Brown and Radke (1998) recommend that nutritional assessment include a nutritional history, physical examination, anthropometrical measures of weight and height, and biochemical indicators of protein stores and immune function.

Obtaining Physiological Measures Across Time

Most studies using physiological measures of interest in nursing are focused on a single point in time. However, there is insufficient information on normal variations in physiological measures across time, much less changes in physiological measures across time in individuals with abnormal physiological states. In some cases, physiological states demonstrate cyclic activity and are associated with circadian rhythms and day-night patterns. When a clinician observes variation in a physiological value, it is important to know whether the variation is within the normal range or is a signal of a change in the patient's condition. Studies need to be performed to describe patterns of physiological function. Thomas (1995) lists findings from studies examining infant biorhythms in Table 16–1. Dunbar and Farr (1996) studied heart rate, systolic blood pressure, and diastolic blood pressure in cardiac and noncardiac patients older than 65 years and described the measurement process.

• •

"Heart rate (HR), systolic blood pressure (SBP), and diastolic blood pressure (DBP) were measured by the indirect automatic oscillometrical technique with a Dinamap 8100T (Critikon). The validity of this noninvasive technique was established in several studies that compared BPs obtained with the Dinamap and intraarterial measures. Correlations ranged from $r = .97$ for SBP to $r = .90$ for DBP (Park & Menard, 1987; Ramsey, 1979). The Critikon Company reports the Dinamap 8100T to be accurate in measuring BP to a standard deviation range from 2.4 to 4.1 mm Hg, compared with the standard of direct aortic pressures. Appropriate cuff size was determined according to the circumference of the subject's upper arm.

"Rate-pressure product (RPP) was calculated by multiplying HR $\times$ SBP at each time of measurement. RPP is considered a noninvasive index of myocardial oxygen consumption (mVO_2) (Amsterdam, Hughes, DeMaria, Zellis, & Mason, 1974). Correlations between direct measures of mVO_2 and RPP of $r = .83$ have been reported (Gobel, Nordstrom, Nelson, Jorgenson, & Wang, 1978). . . .

"For 4 consecutive days, HR, SBP, and DBP were measured when subjects woke in the morning and then every 2 hours while they were awake. Subjects were asked to maintain their normal routines during this period. If they awoke during the night, they were instructed to turn on their call

light, and HR and BP measures were obtained. These procedures yielded approximately 36 to 48 measures per subject. HR and BP were taken after subjects assumed a sitting position for at least 5 minutes. Initial BP was measured in both arms, with all subsequent measures obtained from the arm with the highest BP." (Dunbar & Farr, 1996, p. 45) ■

Selecting a Physiological Measure

Researchers designing a physiological study have less assistance available in selecting methods of measurement than do those conducting studies using psychosocial variables. Multiple books discuss various means to measure psychosocial variables. In addition, numerous articles in nursing journals describe the development of psychosocial variables or discuss various means of measuring a particular psychosocial variable. However, literature guiding the selection of physiological variables is less available.

A number of factors need to be considered when selecting a physiological measure for a study. The first step is to identify the physiological variables relevant to the study. Do the variables need to be measured continuously or at a particular point in time? Are repeated measures needed? Do certain characteristics of the population under study place limits on the measurement approaches that can be used?

The next step is to determine how that variable has been measured in previous research. This process is more difficult for physiological measures than for psychosocial measures. Few books and articles address the options available for particular physiological measures, and the sources most commonly used are previous studies that have measured that variable. Literature reviews or meta-analyses can provide reference lists of relevant studies. Because the measure is likely to have been used in studies unrelated to the current research topic, it is usually necessary to examine the research literature broadly.

Physiological measures need to be carefully linked conceptually with the framework of the study. The logic of operationalizing the concept in a

TABLE 16–1
EXAMPLES OF INFANT BIORHYTHMS RESEARCH FINDINGS

AUTHOR	SUBJECTS	FINDINGS
Abe et al., 1978[25]	118 subjects, 5 days' PNA to adult	Adult-like temperature rhythm at 7 yr; diurnal at 1 mo; phase similar to that of adult at 10–11 mo
Anders, 1975[20]		Sleep-wake diurnal pattern at 16 wk PNA
Bamford et al., 1990[47]	174 term infants	Circadian pattern in sleep at 6 wk PNA
Brown et al., 1992[48]	30 infants, 2–26 wk PNA	1-hr periodic oscillations in temperature in 24 of 30; amplitude, 0.2–0.3°C
Cornelissen et al., 1990[49]	Neonates, 1–7 days' PNA	Circadian, circaseptan, and circannual heart rate and blood pressure rhythms present in first week of life
de Roquefeuil et al., 1993[50]	12 term infants	Sleep-wake circadian pattern at 4 mo PNA; sleep consolidation at 6–7 mo
Finley and Nugent, 1983[51]	11 term infants, 1 day–4 wk PNA	Periodicity of respiration and heart rate
Franks, 1967[52]	75 infants and children	Adult-like pattern of 17-hydroxycorticosteroid between 1 and 3 yr
Gupta, 1986[13]	Infants and children	Melatonin diurnal rhythm at 3–9 mo PNA
Hellbrugge et al., 1964[10]	Infants and children	Body temperature and sleep-wake pattern diurnal at 2–3 wk PNA; heart rate diurnal at 4–20 wk PNA; circadian rhythms synchronized to day/night after 23 wk PNA
Mirmiran and Kok, 1991[53]	12 preterm infants, 26–32 wk GA, 29–35 wk PCA	No circadian rhythm in any variable in 4 infants; many variables with ultradian rhythms; number of subjects demonstrating circadian rhythms: temperature, 7; heart rate, 5; motor pattern, 1
Mirmiran et al., 1990[54]	9 infants, 28–34 wk PCA	5 of 9 had circadian rhythm body temperature
Putet et al., 1990[37]	7 preterm infants, mean GA of 31 wk, mean PNA of 21.3 ± 11.7 days	5 of 7 had 3- to 4-hr cycle of oxygen consumption, meal frequency strong zeitgeber, handling with feeding a factor
Sankaran et al., 1989[55]	17 preterm infants, 26–41 wk GA, 3–4 days' PNA	Diurnal rhythm of β-endorphin evident at mean GA of 31.7 ± 4.8 wk and mean PNA of 3.3 ± 4.8 days
Sitka et al., 1994[56]	17 term infants at 2 days' PNA; 11 at 4 wk PNA	On day 2 of life, 12 of 17 had circadian rhythm of systolic blood pressure and heart rate; 16 of 17 had circadian skin temperature; 17 of 17 had circadian rectal temperature
Sostek et al., 1976[46]	12 infants, 37–43 wk GA	Diurnal sleep-wake pattern by 8 wk PNA
Thomas, 1991[57]	5 preterm infants, 30–34 wk GA, 5–10 days' PNA	Ultradian rhythm of temperature in 3 of 5; period length of 2–6 hours
Updike et al., 1985[58]	6 preterm infants, 34–37 wk GA, 10–20 days' PNA	Circadian cycles of body temperature; TcPO$_2$ and respiratory pauses showed diurnal pattern
Vermes et al., 1980[59]	45 neonate to 3-year-olds	Cortisol rhythm at 3 mo PNA
Wailoo et al., 1989[26]	Term infants, 3–4 mo PNA	Well-organized temperature endogenous rhythm at 4 mo PNA but not linked to time of day
Wu et al., 1990[60]	Term infants	Circaseptan and circannual rhythms present in first week of life; circannual acrophase in winter

Superscript reference numbers apply to original source.
GA = gestational age; PCA = postconceptional age; PNA = postnatal age.
From Thomas, K. A. (1995). Biorhythms in infants and role of the care environment. *Journal of Perinatal and Neonatal Nursing, 9*(2), 68–69.

particular way needs to be well thought out and expressed clearly. Triangulation of diverse physiological measures of a single concept is often advisable to reduce the impact of extraneous variables that might affect measurement. The operationalization and its link to concepts in the framework need to be made explicit in the published report of the study.

The validity and reliability of physiological measures need to be evaluated. Until recently, researchers commonly used information from the manufacturer of equipment to describe the accuracy of measurement. This information is useful but not sufficient to evaluate validity and reliability. The validity and reliability of physiological measures are discussed in Chapter 15.

One field of research in which considerable effort has been put forth to develop and evaluate measures is in wound healing. Identifying valid and reliable measurement methods is important for comparing the effectiveness of various methods of treating the wound. Measurement strategies that have been applied include tracing the outline of the wound, scanning the wound with a hand-held scanner, use of electronic cameras, use of a structured light-scanning device, and a computer vision method based on image processing. Other strategies involve measuring wound volume by filling it with various substances such as normal saline, plaster of Paris, or a high-viscosity vinyl polysiloxane (Gentzkow, 1995; Harding, 1995). Thomas (1997) developed a model for the perfect wound healing instrument and evaluated existing tools in terms of the model. A number of studies have been conducted to compare the validity and reliability of these measures (Etris et al., 1994; Hanson et al., 1997; Liskay et al., 1993; Melhuish et al., 1994; Plassman et al., 1994). Consensus on the most desirable method of measurement has not yet been reached, and methodological studies in this area continue.

Researchers need to consider problems that might be encountered when using various approaches to physiological measurement. One factor of concern is the sensitivity of the measure. Will the measure detect differences finely enough to avoid a Type II error? Physiological measures are usually norm referenced. Thus data obtained from a subject will be compared with a norm, as well as with other subjects. Researchers need to determine whether the norm used for comparison is relevant for the population under study. For example, if the norm is for healthy adults, is it relevant for chronically ill children? How labile is the measure? Some measures vary within the individual from time to time, even when conditions are similar. Circadian rhythms, activities, emotions, dietary intake, or posture can also affect physiological measures. To what extent will these factors affect the ability to interpret measurement outcomes?

Many measurement strategies require the use of specialized equipment. In many cases the equipment is available in the patient care area and is part of routine patient care in that unit. Otherwise, the equipment may need to be purchased, rented, or borrowed specifically for the study. Researchers need to be skilled in operating the equipment or obtain the assistance of someone who has these skills. Care should be taken that the equipment operate in an optimal fashion and be used in a consistent manner. In some cases, the equipment needs to be recalibrated regularly to ensure consistent readings. Recalibration means that the equipment is reset to ensure precise measurements. For example, weight scales are recalibrated periodically to ensure that the weight indicated is accurate.

According to federal guidelines, recalibration must be performed

- In accordance with the manufacturers' instructions
- In accordance with criteria set up by the laboratory
- At least every 6 months
- After major preventive maintenance or replacement of a critical part
- When quality control indicates a need for recalibration

When publishing the results of a physiological study, the measurement technique needs to be described in considerable detail to allow an adequate critique of the study, facilitate replication of the study by others, and promote clinical application of the results. At present, few replications of physiological studies have been reported in the literature. Detailed description of physiological measures in a research report includes the exact procedure followed and the specifics of the equipment used in the measurement. The examples in this section can be used as models for describing the method practiced to obtain a physiological measure.

OBSERVATIONAL MEASUREMENT

Although measurement by observation is most common in qualitative research, it is used to some extent in all types of studies. Observation is a particularly important measurement method in research involving children (Lobo, 1992). Measurement in qualitative research is not distinct from analysis; rather, the two occur simultaneously. For more detail on measurement and analysis in qualitative research, refer to Chapter 23. Measurement by observation is not as simple as it sounds. One first needs to decide what is to be observed and then determine how to ensure that every variable is observed in a similar manner in each instance. Observational measurement tends to be more subjective than other types of measurement and is thus often seen as less credible. However, in many cases, observation is the only possible approach to obtain important data for nursing's body of knowledge.

As with any means of measurement, consistency is important. Therefore, much attention must be given to training data collectors. If the measurement technique is complex, written instructions need to be provided. Opportunities for pilot testing of the technique are necessary, and data on interrater reliability need to be generated.

Unstructured Observations

Unstructured observation involves spontaneously observing and recording what is seen with a minimum of prior planning. Although unstructured observations give freedom to the observer, there is a risk of loss of objectivity and a possibility that the observer may not remember all the details of the observed event. If possible, notes are taken during observation periods. If this is not possible, the researcher needs to record the observations as soon afterward as possible. In some studies, the observation period is videotaped for extensive examination at a later time.

One type of unstructured observation is the chronolog. A *chronolog* provides a detailed description of an individual's behavior in a natural environment. Observational procedures used in a chronolog are designed to reduce the effect of the presence of an observer on the behavior being observed. The method of observation is intense. Therefore, the recommended maximal length of time for observation by one researcher is 30 minutes. If longer periods of observation are necessary, a team of observers may need to take turns observing. For details on the methodology of a chronolog, see Hodson (1986).

Structured Observations

The first step in *structured observational* measurement is to define carefully what is to be observed. From that point, concern is directed toward how the observations are to be made, recorded, and coded. In most cases, a category system is developed for organizing and sorting the behavior or events being observed. The extent to which these categories are exhaustive varies with the study.

CATEGORY SYSTEMS

The observational categories should be mutually exclusive. If the categories overlap, the observer will be faced with making judgments regarding what category should contain each observed behavior, and data collection may not be consistent. In some category systems, only the behavior that is of interest is recorded. Most category systems require some inference by the observer from the observed event to the category. The greater the degree of inference required, the more difficult the category system to use. Some systems are developed to be used in a wide variety of studies, whereas others are specific to the study for which they were designed. The number of categories used varies considerably with the study. An optimal number for ease of use and therefore effectiveness of observation is 15 to 20 categories.

CHECKLISTS

Checklists are techniques to indicate whether a behavior occurred. In this case, tally marks are generally placed on a data collection form each time the behavior is observed. Behavior other than that on the checklist is ignored. In some studies, multiple tally marks may be placed in various categories while one is observing a particular event. However, in other studies, the observer is required to select a single category at which to place the tally mark. Checklists can be used as self-report instruments. Sutherland and colleagues (1999) used a Behavioral

Documentation Instrument (BDI) in their study of foot acupressure and massage for patients with Alzheimer disease and related dementias. They describe the instrument as follows: "A Behavioral Documentation Instrument (BDI) was developed by the researchers with validation by an expert panel and used to obtain pre-test measures . . . on wandering, pulse, respirations, and quiet-time behaviors. Interrater reliability was established on the BDI by obtaining an index of equivalence" (Sutherland et al., 1999, p. 347). The authors provide a figure showing the checklist in the article.

RATING SCALES

Rating scales, which will be discussed in a later section of this chapter, can be used for observation as well as for self-reporting. A rating scale allows the observer to rate the behavior or event on a scale. This method provides more information for analysis than does the use of dichotomous data, which indicate only that the behavior either occurred or did not occur.

Keefe and coworkers (1996) used a rating scale in their study of irritable and nonirritable infants and described the instrument.

• •

"The Fussiness Rating Scale was originally adapted from the Intensity Rating Scale developed by Emde, Gauensbauer, and Harmon (1976). The scale defines fussiness as a state of irritability not easily explained, which may include crying, fussing, and restlessness. Parents are asked to rate their child's typical unexplained fussy behavior over the past week on the following three dimensions: amount of fussiness, intensity of fussiness, and hours of fussiness per day. For this study, parents were also asked the number of fussy episodes the infant had per week. Response options ranged from no episodes to every day of the week. Independent mother and father ratings of infant fussiness revealed interrater correlations ranging from $r = .91$ to $r = .72$." (Keefe et al., 1996, p. 6) ■

Interviews

Interviews involve verbal communication between the researcher and the subject, during which information is provided to the researcher. Although this measurement strategy is most common in qualitative and descriptive studies, it can be used in other types of studies. A variety of approaches can be used to conduct an interview, ranging from a totally unstructured interview in which the content is completely controlled by the subject to interviews in which the content is similar to a questionnaire with the possible responses to questions carefully designed by the researcher. Although most interviews are conducted face to face, interviewing by telephone is becoming more common (Burnard, 1994). Chapple (1997) points out that most interviews in nursing studies have concerned those in relatively powerless positions in society. Successfully interviewing persons in positions of power requires some variations in approach.

Planning measurement by interview requires careful, detailed work and has almost become a science in itself. Many excellent books are available on the techniques of developing interview questions (Bedarf, 1986; Briggs, 1986; Converse & Presser, 1986; Dillman, 1978; Dillon, 1990; Fowler, 1990; Gorden, 1987; McCracken, 1988; McLaughlin, 1990; Mishler, 1986; Schuman, 1981). Researchers planning to use this strategy need to consult a text on interview methodology before designing their instrument. Because nurses frequently use interview techniques in nursing assessment, the dynamics of interviewing are familiar; however, using this technique for measurement in research requires greater sophistication.

UNSTRUCTURED INTERVIEWS

Unstructured interviews are used primarily in descriptive and qualitative studies. The researcher may be seeking to understand how the subject organizes ideas on a particular topic or to identify attitudes. In some cases, this type of interview may be used as a step in developing a more precise measurement tool in a particular area of study.

The interview may be initiated by asking a broad question such as, "Describe for me your experience with. . . ." After the interview is begun, the role of the interviewer is to encourage the subject to continue talking by using techniques such as nodding the head or making sounds that indicate interest. In some cases, the subject may be encouraged to further elaborate on a particular dimension of the topic of discussion.

STRUCTURED INTERVIEWS

Structured interviews include strategies that provide increasing amounts of control by the researcher over the content of the interview. Questions asked by the interviewer are designed by the researcher before the initiation of data collection, and the order of the questions is specified. In some cases, the interviewer is allowed to further explain the meaning of the question or modify the way in which the question is asked so that the subject can better understand it. In more structured interviews, the interviewer is required to ask the question precisely as it has been designed. If the subject does not understand the question, the interviewer can only repeat it. The subject may be limited to a range of responses previously developed by the researcher, similar to those in a questionnaire. If the possible responses are lengthy or complex, they may be printed on a card that is handed to the subject for selection of a response.

Designing Interview Questions

The process of development and sequencing of interview questions is similar to that used in questionnaires and will be elaborated on in the section on questionnaires. Briefly, questions progress from broad and general to narrow and specific. Questions are grouped by topic, with fairly "safe" topics being addressed first and sensitive topics reserved until late in the interview process. Less interesting data such as age, educational level, income, and other demographic information are usually collected last. These data should not be collected in an interview if they can be obtained from another source such as a patient record. The wording of questions in an interview is dependent on the educational level of the subjects. The wording of certain questions may have a variety of interpretations by different subjects, and the researcher needs to anticipate this possibility. After the interview protocol has been developed, feedback needs to be sought from an expert in interview technique and also from a content expert. De Jong and Miller (1995) have developed interview questioning strategies for determining client strengths that could contribute to the nursing body of knowledge.

Pretesting the Interview Protocol

When the protocol has been developed satisfactorily, it needs to be pilot-tested on subjects similar to those who will be used in the study so that the researcher can identify problems in the design of questions, sequencing of questions, or procedure for recording responses. It also allows an assessment of the reliability and validity of the interview instrument.

Training Interviewers

Developing skills in interviewing requires practice. Interviewers need to be very familiar with the content of the interview. They must anticipate situations that might occur during the interview and develop strategies for dealing with them. One of the most effective methods of developing a polished approach is role-playing. Playing the role of the subject can give the interviewer insight into the experience of a subject and thus facilitate an effective response to particular situations.

The interviewer needs to learn how to establish a permissive atmosphere in which the subject will be encouraged to respond to sensitive topics. Methods of maintaining an unbiased verbal and nonverbal manner must also be developed. The wording of a question, the tone of voice, raising an eyebrow, or shifting body position can all communicate a positive or negative reaction of the interviewer to the subject's responses. Positive as well as negative verbal or nonverbal communications can alter the data.

Preparing for an Interview

If the interview is to be lengthy, an appointment needs to be made. The researcher needs to be nicely dressed but not overdressed and should be prompt for the appointment. The site selected for the interview must be quiet, allow privacy for the interaction, and provide a pleasant environment. Instructions given to the subject about the interview are carefully planned before the interview. For example, the interviewer might say, "I am going to ask you a series of questions about. . . . Before you answer each question you need to . . . select your answer from the following . . . and then you may elaborate on your response. I will record your answer and then, if it is not clear, I may ask you to explain some aspect further."

Probing

Probing is used by the interviewer to obtain more information in a specific area of the interview. In some cases the question may be repeated. If the subject has said "I don't know," the interviewer may press for a response. In other situations the interviewer may explain the question further or ask the subject to explain statements that have been made. At a deeper level, the interviewer may pick up on a comment made by the subject and begin asking questions to obtain further meaning from the subject. Probes should be neutral to avoid biasing the subject's responses. Probing needs to be done within reasonable guidelines to prevent the subject from feeling that he or she is being cross-examined or "grilled" on a topic.

Recording Interview Data

Data obtained from interviews are recorded either during the interview or immediately afterward. The recording may be in the form of handwritten notes or tape recordings. If notes are hand-recorded, the interviewer needs to have skills in identifying key ideas (or capturing essential data) in an interview and concisely recording this information. Recording data needs to be done without distracting the interviewee. In some situations, interviewees have difficulty responding if note taking or taping is obvious. Sometimes the interviewer may need to record data after completing the interview. Tape recording requires permission of the subject, and verbatim transcriptions of tapes are made before data analysis. Data from unstructured interviews are difficult to analyze. In some studies, content analysis is used to capture the meaning within the data.

ADVANTAGES AND DISADVANTAGES OF INTERVIEWS

Interviewing is a flexible technique that can allow the researcher to explore greater depth of meaning than can be obtained with other techniques. Interpersonal skills can be used to facilitate cooperation and elicit more information. The response rate to interviews is higher than that to questionnaires, and thus a more representative sample can be obtained with interviews. Interviews allow collection of data from subjects unable or unlikely to complete questionnaires, such as the very ill or those whose reading, writing, and ability to express themselves are marginal.

Interviews are a form of self-report, and the researcher must assume that the information provided is accurate. Interviewing requires much more time than needed for questionnaires and scales and is thus more costly. Because of time and cost, sample size is usually limited. Subject bias is always a threat to the validity of the findings, as is inconsistency in data collection from one subject to another.

Dzurec and Coleman (1995) used hermeneutics to study the experience of interviewing from the perspective of the interviewer. They found that an unspoken power gradient was present during an interview that made the process difficult for the interviewer. The insight from the interview process and from relating to the interviewee as a person made the process seem worthwhile. As respondents indicated, "You find out stuff you never even thought to ask" (Dzurec & Coleman, 1995, p. 245). Recommendations emerging from the study included "(a) identifying one's agenda for conducting an interview and sharing it with interviewees in a way comfortable for the interviewer; (b) staying in touch with personal discomforts of the interviewer-interviewee relationship, for example, their disparate roles, knowledge levels, and health and social status; (c) allowing the interview to follow its own course, even if structured by an interview format; and (d) conducting retrospective analyses of interview data to guide subsequent interviews" (Dzurec & Coleman, 1995, p. 245).

Interviewing children requires some special understanding of the art of asking children questions. The interviewer needs to use words that children tend to use to define situations and events, and understand the development of language at varying stages of development. Children view topics differently than adults do. Their perception of time, past and present, is also different. Holaday and Turner-

Henson (1989) provided detailed suggestions for developing an interview guide or questionnaire appropriate for children.

Knafl and associates (1988) used a structured telephone interview with subjects across the United States to study the role of the nurse researcher employed in a clinical setting. Interviews were recorded and transcribed verbatim. Development of the interview guide is described in the following excerpt.

. . . .

"Throughout the instrument development process, the research team was guided by the literature on nurse researchers in clinical settings, Lofland's (1971) discussion of interview guide development and Dillman's (1978) guidelines for questionnaire construction.

"The literature on nurse researchers, although limited and not research based, indicated that the following topics were salient for the study of clinical nurse researchers: their education, personality, and research experience; relationships of the clinical nurse researcher to others in the organization; ability of the clinical nurse researcher to meet the needs of the nursing department; and the range and nature of the clinical nurse researcher's activities. Once a list of topics consistent with the literature on clinical nurse researchers and with the proposed research questions had been generated, Lofland's general guidelines for interview guide construction were followed." (Knafl et al., 1988, p. 31) ■

The resulting instrument contained elements characteristic of the qualitative intensive interviewing technique combined with more structured quantitative elements. Thus, method triangulation was used. A sample of the questions is shown in Table 16–2. Data collection using the interview instrument was described in the following excerpt.

. . . .

"During the course of data collection, questions arose regarding the extent to which interviewers should be guided by the canons of flexibility associated with conducting intensive interviews or of standardization associated with much of survey research. Guidelines needed to be established regarding how much freedom individual interviewers had

TABLE 16–2
NUMBER AND EXAMPLES OF HIGHLY, MODERATELY, AND MINIMALLY STRUCTURED QUESTIONS USED IN CLINICAL NURSE RESEARCHER AND CHIEF NURSE EXECUTIVE INTERVIEW GUIDES

CLINICAL NURSE RESEARCHER GUIDE

Highly Structured Questions (n = 2)
Example: We have talked about the activities in which you are involved. Can you tell me approximately what percentage of your time is spent in each type of activity?

Type of Activity	% Time
Administrative	
Staff development	
Research	
Other	

Moderately Structured Questions (n = 5)
Example: Now I'd like to ask how you go about evaluating your performance. In general, what is your feeling about how well you are doing in your job?
  What criteria or cues do you use to decide how well you are doing?
  How do you think the clinical nurse researcher's contributions to an organization should be judged or evaluated?

Minimally Structured Questions (n = 11)
Example: What advice would you have for a new clinical nurse researcher or someone considering taking a job as a clinical nurse researcher?

CHIEF NURSE EXECUTIVE GUIDE

Highly Structured Questions (None)
Moderately Structured Questions (n = 6)
Example: In general, what is your overall feeling about how well the clinical nurse researcher is doing in her or his job?
  What do you see as his or her major accomplishments?
  Are there things you wanted the clinical nurse researcher to accomplish that he or she has not?
  How do you think a clinical nurse researcher's contribution to an organization should be judged or evaluated?

Minimally Structured Questions (n = 8)
Example: What do you see as the advantages of having a clinical nurse researcher?

From Knafl, K. A., Pettengill, M. M., Bevis, M. E., & Kirchhoff, K. T. (1988). Blending qualitative and quantitative approaches to instrument development and data collection. *Journal of Professional Nursing, 4*(1), 30–37.

to vary the wording and sequencing of questions on the interview guide.

"In the clinical nurse researcher study, interviews were conducted by five persons with variable experiences with conducting interviews. In order to fulfill the intent of the study, it was necessary to obtain comparable data across all subjects in general and clinical nurse researcher–chief nurse executive pairs in particular. This goal pulled the research team in the direction of standardization. At the same time, the investigators wanted to allow interviewers sufficient flexibility to follow up on interesting leads, probe for additional information as they judged appropriate, and interact naturally with subjects.

"Regarding standardization of the use of the interview guide, it was decided that all questions would be asked in the order specified. If a subject addressed a question on the guide before it was asked, the question was still asked in sequence. When this happened, the interviewer acknowledged that the topic already had been addressed and prefaced the asking of the question in sequence with a statement such as, 'I know you've already talked a bit about this, but perhaps there's more you'd like to say.' This approach both communicated that the interviewer had been paying attention, gave the subject an opportunity to expand on what had been said originally, and precluded omission or cursory investigation of a question by the interviewer. Furthermore, it was agreed that interviewers were not to engage in major rewordings of the questions; when revisions were suggested these were negotiated during the weekly staff meetings of the research team.

"In an effort to keep the use of the guide flexible, interviewers were encouraged to engage in 'minor' rewordings of the questions in order to make them more consistent with the interviewer's own style, thereby making the interview more conversational in nature. Interviewers also reworded questions when it was necessary to clarify their meaning to subjects. . . . In addition, interviewers were asked to follow up on any responses that they judged to be of interest but were not covered by a specific question in the guide and to probe for additional information and clarification as they thought appropriate. Probing was less frequent than minor rewordings and focused on asking for additional information (e.g., 'Are there other things you would like to mention?') or in clarifying data (e.g., 'Can you talk just a little more about that?')." (Knafl et al., 1988, pp. 32–33) ■

Focus Groups

Focus groups are a relatively recent strategy that began to be used in nursing studies in the late 1980s. However, they have been in use in other fields for a long time. The idea of focus groups emerged in the 1920s as a strategy for examining the effectiveness of marketing strategies. They re-emerged during World War II with efforts to determine ways to improve the morale of the troops. The technique serves a variety of purposes in nursing research. It is used in performing qualitative studies (Twinn, 1998), making policy analyses (Straw & Smith, 1995), assessing consumer satisfaction, evaluating the quality of care (Beaudin & Pelletier, 1996), examining the effectiveness of public health programs, assisting in professional decision making (Bulmer, 1998; Southern et al., 1999), developing instruments, exploring patient care problems and strategies for developing effective interventions, developing education programs (Halloran & Grimes, 1995), studying various patient populations (Disney & May, 1988; Goss, 1998; Quine & Cameron, 1995; Reed & Payton, 1997), and taking part in participatory research. A focus group study might include from 6 to 50 groups.

The following assumptions underlie focus groups:

1. A homogeneous group provides the participants with freedom to express thoughts, feelings, and behaviors candidly.
2. Individuals are important resources of information.
3. People are able to report and verbalize their thoughts and feelings.
4. A group's dynamics can generate authentic information.
5. Group interviews are superior to individual interviews.
6. The facilitator can help people recover forgotten information through focusing the interview. (Morrison & Peoples, 1999)

Effective use of focus groups requires careful planning. Questions that must be addressed include the following:

1. What are the aims of the focus groups?
2. How many focus groups should be assembled?

3. How many individuals should be in each focus group?
4. How will you recruit for the focus groups?
5. Can you locate sufficient people for the focus groups?
6. Are you selecting the right people for the focus groups?
7. Where should the focus groups meet?
8. What skills should the groups' moderators have?
9. How will moderators interact with participants?
10. What questions will the moderators ask?
11. How should the data be analyzed?

Focus groups were designed to obtain the participants' perceptions in a focused area in a setting that is permissive and nonthreatening. One of the assumptions underlying the use of focus groups is that group dynamics can assist people to express and clarify their views in ways that are less likely to occur in a one-to-one interview. The group may give a sense of "safety in numbers" to those wary of researchers or those who are anxious. Many different communication forms are used in focus groups, including teasing, arguing, joking, anecdotes, and nonverbal approaches such as gesturing, facial expressions, and other body language. Kitzinger (1995) suggests that "people's knowledge and attitudes are not entirely encapsulated in reasoned responses to direct questions. Everyday forms of communication may tell us as much, if not more, about what people know or experience. In this sense focus groups reach the parts that other methods cannot reach, revealing dimensions of understanding that often remain untapped by more conventional data collection techniques."

Recruiting appropriate participants for each of the focus groups is critical. Recruitment is the most common source of failure in focus group research. Each focus group should include 6 to 10 participants. Fewer participants tend to result in inadequate discussion. In most cases, participants are expected to be unknown to each other. However, when targeting professional groups such as clinical nurses or nurse educators, such anonymity usually is not possible. The researcher may use purposive sampling in which individuals known to have the desired expertise are sought. In other cases, partici-

pants may be sought through the media, posters, or advertisements. A single contact with an individual who agrees to attend a focus group is not sufficient to ensure that this person will attend the group. Success in prompting individuals to attend will require repeated phone calls and reminders by mail. Inform them at the initial time of consent that you will be calling them to remind them of the group and check to see whether the phone number they have given is the best number to call. Incentives may need to be provided. Cash payments are, of course, the most effective if such resources are available through funding. Other incentives include refreshments at the focus group meeting, T-shirts, coffee mugs, gift certificates, or coupons. Overrecruiting may be necessary, with a good rule being to invite two more potential participants than you need for the group (Morgan, 1995).

Segmentation is the process of sorting participants into focus groups with common characteristics. Selecting participants who are similar to each other in lifestyle or experiences, views, and characteristics facilitates more open discussion. Validity will be increased by conducting multiple focus groups and placing participants with differing characteristics in separate groups. These characteristics might be age, gender, social class, ethnicity, culture, lifestyle, or health status. Groups may include, for example, users of a program versus nonusers or satisfied customers versus dissatisfied customers. In some cases, groups may occur naturally such as those who work together. One must be cautious about bringing together participants with considerable variation in social standing, education, or authority because of the increased possibility of decreased input from some group members or discounting of the input of those with lower standing (Kitzinger, 1995; Morgan, 1995).

Selecting effective moderators is as critical as selecting appropriate participants. The moderator must be successful in encouraging participants to talk about the topic. In some cases, a moderator and assistant moderator should be included. Participants should be encouraged to talk to one another rather than addressing all comments to the moderator. A successful moderator will encourage participants to interact with one another and will formulate ideas and draw out cognitive structures not previously articulated. Moderators should remain neutral and nonjudgmental. If the topic is sensitive, moderators need to be able to put participants at ease. This goal may be accomplished by using a moderator with characteristics similar to those of the group participants. Extreme dominance or extreme passiveness on the part of the moderator will lead to problems (Kitzinger, 1995; Morgan, 1995; Morrison & Peoples, 1999).

The setting for the focus group should be relaxed, with space for participants to sit comfortably in a circle and maintain eye contact with all participants. The acoustics of the room should be sufficient to allow quality tape recording of the sessions. However, it may be necessary for the moderator or assistant moderator to take notes when the speaker's voice is soft or when several individuals are speaking at once. Sessions will usually last 1 to 2 hours, although some may extend to an entire afternoon or continue to a series of meetings.

It is important for the researcher to clarify the aims of the focus groups and communicate these aims to the moderators and the participants before the group session. Questions to be asked during the focus group should be carefully planned and, in some cases, pilot-tested. Limit the number of questions to those most essential so that sufficient time is left for discussion. Participants may be given some of the questions before the group meeting to enable them to give careful thought to their responses. A common problem in focus groups is to dive right into the topic of interest to the researcher with little emphasis on the interests of the participants. Early in the session, provide opportunities for participants to express their views on the topic of discussion. Next, proceed with the questions. Probes may be used if the discussion wanders too far. The discussion tends to express group norms, and individual voices of dissent may be stifled. However, when the discussion is on sensitive topics, the group may actively facilitate the discussion because less inhibited members break the ice for those who are more reticent. Participants may also provide group support for expressing feelings, opinions, or experiences. Late in the session, the moderator may encourage group members to go beyond the current discussion or debate and discuss inconsistencies

among participants and within their own thinking. Disagreements among group members can be used by the moderator to encourage participants to state their point of view more clearly and provide a rationale for their position (Kitzinger, 1995).

Analysis of data follows that of qualitative studies, as described in Chapter 23. However, data from focus groups are complex in that analysis requires that one analyze at the individual level and at the group level to consider interactions among individuals and the group and to make comparisons across groups. It is important to attend to the amount of consensus and interest in topics generated in the discussion. Analysis of deviance and minority opinions is important. Attending to the context within which statements were made is critical to the analysis (Morgan, 1995).

Carey (1995) makes the following suggestions regarding analyzing focus group data:

• •

"If the unit of analysis is limited to the group, then the evolving interaction of members and the impact on opinions will be unobserved. Because the interaction within the group will affect the data elicited, an appropriate description of the nature of the group dynamics is necessary to incorporate in analysis—for example, heated discussion, a dominant member, little agreement." (Carey, 1995, p. 488) ■

Questionnaires

A *questionnaire* is a printed self-report form designed to elicit information that can be obtained through the written responses of the subject. The information obtained through questionnaires is similar to that obtained by interview, but the questions tend to have less depth. The subject is unable to elaborate on responses or ask for clarification of questions, and the data collector cannot use probe strategies. However, questions are presented in a consistent manner, and there is less opportunity for bias than in an interview.

Questionnaires can be designed to determine facts about the subject or persons known by the subject, facts about events or situations known by the subject, or beliefs, attitudes, opinions, levels of knowledge, or intentions of the subject. They can be distributed to very large samples, either directly or through the mail. The development and administration of questionnaires have been the topic of many excellent books focusing on survey techniques that can be helpful in the process of designing a questionnaire (Berdie et al., 1986; Converse & Presser, 1986; Fox & Tracy, 1986; Kahn & Cannell, 1957; Sudman & Bradburn, 1982). Two nursing methodology texts (Shelley, 1984; Waltz et al., 1991) provide detailed explanations of the questionnaire development procedure. Although questions on a questionnaire appear easy to design, a well-designed item requires considerable effort.

Like interviews, questionnaires can have varying degrees of structure. Some questionnaires ask open-ended questions that require written responses from the subject. Others ask closed-ended questions that have options selected by the researcher.

Data from open-ended questions are often difficult to interpret, and content analysis may be used to extract meaning. Open-ended questionnaire items are not advised when data are being obtained from large samples. Computers are now being used to gather questionnaire data (Saris, 1991). Computers are provided at the data collection site, the questionnaire is shown on screen, and subjects respond by using the keyboard or mouse. Data are stored in a computer file and are immediately available for analysis. Data entry errors are greatly reduced.

DEVELOPMENT OF QUESTIONNAIRES

The first step in either selecting or developing a questionnaire is to identify the information desired. For this purpose, a blueprint or table of specifications is developed. The blueprint identifies the essential content to be covered by the questionnaire, and the content needs to be at the educational level of the potential subjects. It is difficult to stick to the blueprint when designing the questionnaire because it is tempting to add "just one more question" that seems a "neat idea" or a question that someone insists "really should be included." As the questionnaire becomes longer, fewer subjects are willing to respond and more questions are left blank.

The second step is to search the literature for questionnaires or items in questionnaires that match the blueprint criteria. Sometimes published studies include questionnaires, but frequently you must contact the authors of a study to receive a copy of their questionnaire. Unlike scaling instruments, questionnaires are seldom copyrighted. Researchers are encouraged to use questions in exactly the same form as those in previous studies to facilitate comparison of results between studies. However, questions that are poorly written need to be modified, even if rewriting interferes with comparison with previous results.

For some studies, the researcher can find a questionnaire in the literature that matches the questionnaire blueprint that has been developed for the study. However, the researcher must frequently add items to or delete items from an existing questionnaire to accommodate the blueprint developed. In some situations, items from two or three questionnaires are combined to develop an appropriate questionnaire.

An item on a questionnaire has two parts: a lead-in question (or stem) and a response set. Each lead-in question needs to be carefully designed and clearly expressed. Problems include ambiguous or vague meaning of language, leading questions that influence the response of the respondent, questions that assume a preexisting state of affairs, and double questions.

In some cases, respondents will interpret terms used in the lead-in question in one way, whereas the meaning to the researcher is different. For example, the researcher might ask how heavy the traffic is in the neighborhood in which the family lives. The researcher might be asking about automobile traffic but the respondent interprets the question in relation to drug traffic. The researcher might define *neighborhood* as a region composed of a three-block area, whereas the respondent considered a neighborhood to be a much larger area. Family could be defined as those living in one house or all close blood relations (Converse & Presser, 1986). If a question includes a term with which the respondent may not be familiar or for which several meanings are possible, the term needs to be defined.

Leading questions suggest the answer desired by the researcher. These types of questions often include value-laden words and indicate the bias of the researcher. For example, a questioner might ask, "Do you believe physicians should be coddled on the nursing unit?" or "All hospitals are bad places to work, aren't they?" These examples are extreme, and leading questions are usually constructed more subtly. The degree of formality with which the question is expressed and the permissive tone of the question are, in many cases, important for obtaining a true measure. A permissive tone suggests the acceptableness of any of the possible responses.

Questions implying a preexisting state of affairs lead the respondent to admit to a previous behavior regardless of how the question is answered. The favorite example of professors teaching questionnaire development is the question, "When did you stop beating your wife?" Similar questions more relevant to our times are, "How long has it been since you used drugs?" or, to an adolescent, "Do you use a condom when you have sex?"

Double questions ask for more than one bit of information. For example, a question might ask, "Do you like intensive care nursing and working closely with physicians?" It would be possible for the respondent to be affirmative about working in intensive care settings and negative about working closely with physicians. In this case, the question would be impossible to answer. A similar question is, "Was the in-service program educational and interesting?"

Questions with double negatives are also difficult to answer. For example, one might ask, "Do you believe nurses should not question doctors' orders?" Yes or No. In this case, it is difficult to determine the meaning of a yes or no. Thus the sample responses are uninterpretable.

Each item in a questionnaire has a *response set* that provides the parameters within which the question is to be answered. This response set can be open and flexible, as it is with open-ended questions, or it can be narrow and directive, as it is with closed-ended questions. For example, an open-ended question might have a response set of three blank lines. With closed-ended questions, the response set includes a specific list of alternatives from which to select.

Response sets can be constructed in a variety of ways. The cardinal rule is that every possible answer must have a response category. If the sample may include respondents who might not have an answer, include a response category of "don't know" or "uncertain." If the information sought is factual, this requirement can be accomplished by including "other" as one of the possible responses. However, it must be recognized that the item "other" is essentially lost data. Even if the response is followed by a statement such as "Please explain," it is rarely possible to analyze the data meaningfully. If a large number of subjects (greater than 10%) select the alternative "other," the alternatives included in the response set might not be appropriate for the population studied.

The simplest response set is the dichotomous yes/no option. Arranging responses vertically preceded by a blank will reduce errors. For example,

_____ Yes
_____ No

is better than

_____ Yes _____ No

because in the latter, the respondent might not be sure whether to indicate Yes by placing a response before or after the Yes.

Response sets need to be mutually exclusive, which might not be the case in the following response set:

working full-time
full-time graduate student
working part-time
part-time graduate student

Burns (1986) used a questionnaire to examine smoking patterns of nurses in the state of Texas. Items from that questionnaire, which demonstrates a variety of response sets, are given in Figure 16–2. Each question should clearly instruct the subject how to respond (i.e., choose one, mark all that apply), or instructions should be included at the beginning of the questionnaire. The subject needs to know whether to circle, underline, or fill in a circle as he or she responds to items. Clear instructions

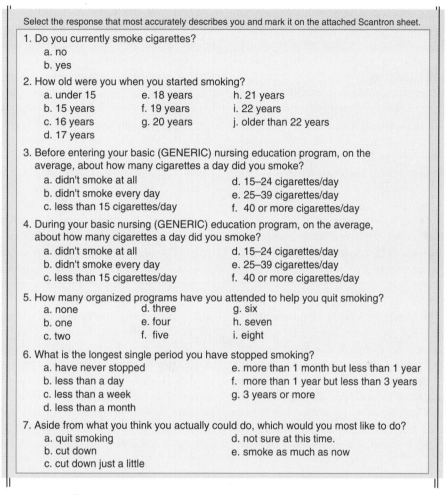

Select the response that most accurately describes you and mark it on the attached Scantron sheet.

1. Do you currently smoke cigarettes?
   a. no
   b. yes

2. How old were you when you started smoking?
   a. under 15   e. 18 years   h. 21 years
   b. 15 years   f. 19 years   i. 22 years
   c. 16 years   g. 20 years   j. older than 22 years
   d. 17 years

3. Before entering your basic (GENERIC) nursing education program, on the average, about how many cigarettes a day did you smoke?
   a. didn't smoke at all   d. 15–24 cigarettes/day
   b. didn't smoke every day   e. 25–39 cigarettes/day
   c. less than 15 cigarettes/day f. 40 or more cigarettes/day

4. During your basic nursing (GENERIC) education program, on the average, about how many cigarettes a day did you smoke?
   a. didn't smoke at all   d. 15–24 cigarettes/day
   b. didn't smoke every day   e. 25–39 cigarettes/day
   c. less than 15 cigarettes/day f. 40 or more cigarettes/day

5. How many organized programs have you attended to help you quit smoking?
   a. none   d. three   g. six
   b. one   e. four   h. seven
   c. two   f. five   i. eight

6. What is the longest single period you have stopped smoking?
   a. have never stopped   e. more than 1 month but less than 1 year
   b. less than a day   f. more than 1 year but less than 3 years
   c. less than a week   g. 3 years or more
   d. less than a month

7. Aside from what you think you actually could do, which would you most like to do?
   a. quit smoking   d. not sure at this time.
   b. cut down   e. smoke as much as now
   c. cut down just a little

FIGURE 16–2 ■ Example of items from a smoking questionnaire.

are difficult to construct and usually require several attempts, and each pilot should be tested on naive subjects who are willing and able to express their reactions to the instructions.

After the questionnaire items have been developed, the order of the items needs to be carefully planned. Questions related to a specific topic need to be grouped together. General items are included first, with progression to more specific items. More important items might be included first, with subsequent progression to items of lesser importance. Questions of a sensitive nature or those that might

be threatening should appear last on the questionnaire. In some cases, the response to one item may influence the response to another. If so, their order needs to be carefully considered. Any open-ended questions should be included last because their responses will require more time than needed for closed-ended questions. The general trend is to include demographic data about the subject at the end of the questionnaire.

In large studies, optical scanning sheets may be used to speed up data entry on computer and decrease errors. This decision needs to be carefully thought out, however, because subjects who are not familiar with these sheets may make errors when entering their responses (thus decreasing measurement validity), and fewer subjects may be willing to complete the questionnaire.

A cover letter explaining the purpose of the study, the name of the researcher, the approximate amount of time required to complete the form, and organizations or institutions supporting the study must accompany the questionnaire. Instructions include an address to which the questionnaire can be returned. This address needs to be at the end of the questionnaire as well as on the cover letter and envelope. Respondents will often discard both the envelope and the cover letter and, after completion of the questionnaire, will not know where to send it. It is also wise to provide a stamped, addressed envelope for the subject to return the questionnaire.

A pilot test of the questionnaire needs to be performed to determine the clarity of questions, effectiveness of instructions, completeness of response sets, time required to complete the questionnaire, and success of data collection techniques. As with any pilot test, the subjects and techniques need to be as similar to those planned for the main study as possible. In some cases, some open-ended questions are included in a pilot test to obtain information for the development of closed-ended response sets for the main study.

QUESTIONNAIRE VALIDITY

One of the greatest risks in developing response sets is leaving out an important alternative or response. For example, if the questionnaire item addressed the job position of nurses working in a hospital and the sample included nursing students, a category must be included that indicates the student role. When seeking opinions, there is a risk of obtaining a response from an individual who actually has no opinion on the subject. When an item requests knowledge that the respondent does not possess, the subject's guessing interferes with obtaining a true measure.

The response rate to questionnaires is generally lower than that with other forms of self-reporting, particularly if the questionnaires are mailed out. If the response rate is lower than 50%, the representativeness of the sample is seriously in question. The response rate for mailed questionnaires is usually small (25–30%), so the researcher is frequently unable to obtain a representative sample, even with randomization. Strategies that can increase the response rate include enclosing a stamped, addressed envelope and sending a postcard 2 weeks after the questionnaire was mailed to those who have not returned it. Sometimes a phone call follow-up is made to increase the return rate of questionnaires (Baker, 1985). Gordon and Stokes (1989) were successful in maintaining an 80% response rate in a study in which subjects were monitored quarterly for 1 year and asked to keep a diary. The impressive strategies that they used to achieve this high response rate are described in detail in their paper.

Commonly, respondents fail to mark responses to all the questions, which is a problem especially with long questionnaires and can threaten the validity of the instrument. In some cases, responses will be written in if the respondent does not agree with the available choices, or comments may be written in the margin. Generally, these responses cannot be included in the analysis; however, a record needs to be kept of such responses. It is advisable to decide before distributing the questionnaires those questions that are critical to the research topic. If any of these questions is omitted in a questionnaire, the results of that questionnaire are not included in the analysis.

Consistency in the way the questionnaire is administered is important to validity. For example, administering some questionnaires in a group setting and mailing out others is not wise. There should not be a mix of mailing to business addresses and to home addresses. If questionnaires are administered in person, the administration needs to be consistent. Several problems in consistency can occur: (1) Some subjects may ask to take the form home to complete it and return it later, whereas others will complete it in the presence of the data collector; (2) some subjects may complete the form themselves, whereas others may ask a family member to write the responses that the respondent dictates; and (3) in some cases, the form may be completed by a secretary or colleague rather than by the individual. These situations lead to biases in responses that are unknown to the researcher and alter the true measure of the variables.

ANALYSIS OF QUESTIONNAIRE DATA

Data from questionnaires are usually ordinal in nature, which limits analysis for the most part to summary statistics and nonparametrical statistics. However, in some cases, ordinal data from questionnaires are treated as interval data, and *t*-tests or analyses of variance (ANOVA) are used to test for differences between responses of various subsets of the sample. Discriminant analysis may be used to determine the ability to predict membership in various groups from responses to particular questions.

Scales

Scales, a form of self-report, are a more precise means of measuring phenomena than are questionnaires. The majority of scales have been developed to measure psychosocial variables. However, self-reports can be obtained on physiological variables such as pain, nausea, or functional capacity by using scaling techniques. Scaling is based on mathematical theory, and there is a branch of science whose primary concern is the development of measurement scales. From the point of view of scaling theory, considerable measurement error (random error) and systematic error are expected in a single item. Therefore, in most scales, the various items on the scale are summed to obtain a single score, and these scales are referred to as summated scales. Less random error and systematic error exist when using the total score of a scale. Using several items in a scale to measure a concept is comparable to using several instruments to measure a concept (see Figure 15–7). The various items in a scale increase the dimensions of the concept that are reflected in the instrument. The types of scales described include rating scales, the Likert scale, and semantic differentials.

RATING SCALES

Rating scales are the crudest form of measure involving scaling techniques. A rating scale lists an ordered series of categories of a variable that are assumed to be based on an underlying continuum. A numerical value is assigned to each category, and the fineness of the distinctions between categories varies with the scale. Rating scales are commonly used by the general public. In conversations one can hear statements such as "On a scale of 1 to 10, I would rank that. . . ." Rating scales are easy to develop; however, one needs to be careful to avoid end statements that are so extreme that no subject will select them. A rating scale could be used to rate the degree of cooperativeness of the patient or the value placed by the subject on nurse-patient interactions. This type of scale is often used in observational measurement to guide data collection. Burns (1974) used the rating scale in Figure 16–3 to examine differences in nurse-patient communication with cancer patients and other medical-surgical patients.

LIKERT SCALE

The *Likert scale* is designed to determine the opinion or attitude of a subject and contains a number of declarative statements with a scale after each statement. The Likert scale is the most commonly used of the scaling techniques. The original version of the scale included five response categories. Each response category was assigned a value, with a value of 1 given to the most negative response and a value of 5 to the most positive response (Nunnally, 1978).

Response choices in a Likert scale most commonly address agreement, evaluation, or frequency. Agreement options may include statements such as *strongly agree, agree, uncertain, disagree,* and *strongly disagree.* Evaluation responses ask the respondent for an evaluative rating along a good/bad dimension, such as positive to negative or excellent to terrible. Frequency responses may include statements such as *rarely, seldom, sometimes, occasionally,* and *usually.* The terms used are versatile and need to be selected for their appropriateness to the stem (Spector, 1992). Sometimes seven options are given, sometimes only four.

Use of the uncertain or neutral category is controversial because it allows the subject to avoid

1. Nurses come into my room
   a. rarely
   b. sometimes
   c. whenever I call them
   d. frequently just to speak or check me

2. I would <u>like</u> nurses to come into my room
   a. rarely
   b. sometimes
   c. whenever I call them
   d. frequently just to speak or check me

3. When a nurse enters my room, she usually
   a. talks very little
   b. tries to talk about things I do not wish to discuss
   c. talks only about casual things
   d. is willing to listen or discuss what concerns me

4. When a nurse enters my room, I would <u>prefer</u> that she
   a. talk very little
   b. talk only when necessary
   c. talk only about casual things
   d. be willing to listen or discuss what concerns me

5. When a nurse talks with me she usually seems
   a. not interested
   b. in a hurry
   c. polite but distant
   d. caring for me as a person

6. When a nurse talks with me, I would <u>prefer</u> that she be
   a. not interested
   b. in a hurry
   c. polite but distant
   d. caring for me as a person

7. When a nurse talks with me she usually
   a. stands in the doorway
   b. stands at the foot of the bed
   c. stands at the side of the bed
   d. sits beside the bed

8. When a nurse talks with me, I would <u>prefer</u> that she
   a. stand in the doorway
   b. stand at the foot of the bed
   c. stand at the side of the bed
   d. sit beside the bed

9. When a nurse talks with me, she is
   a. strictly business
   b. casual
   c. friendly but does not talk about feelings
   d. open to talking about things I worry or think about

10. When a nurse talks with me, I would <u>prefer</u> that she keep the conversation
    a. strictly business
    b. casual
    c. friendly but does not talk about feelings
    d. open to talk about things I worry or think about

FIGURE 16–3 ▪ A rating scale used to measure the nature of nurse-patient communications.

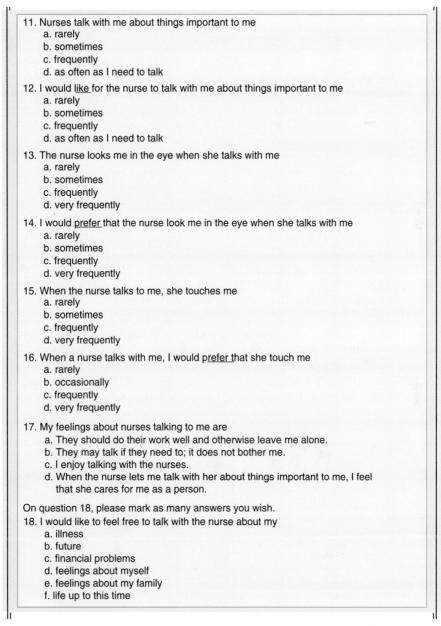

11. Nurses talk with me about things important to me
   a. rarely
   b. sometimes
   c. frequently
   d. as often as I need to talk

12. I would <u>like</u> for the nurse to talk with me about things important to me
   a. rarely
   b. sometimes
   c. frequently
   d. as often as I need to talk

13. The nurse looks me in the eye when she talks with me
   a. rarely
   b. sometimes
   c. frequently
   d. very frequently

14. I would <u>prefer</u> that the nurse look me in the eye when she talks with me
   a. rarely
   b. sometimes
   c. frequently
   d. very frequently

15. When the nurse talks to me, she touches me
   a. rarely
   b. sometimes
   c. frequently
   d. very frequently

16. When a nurse talks with me, I would <u>prefer</u> that she touch me
   a. rarely
   b. occasionally
   c. frequently
   d. very frequently

17. My feelings about nurses talking to me are
   a. They should do their work well and otherwise leave me alone.
   b. They may talk if they need to; it does not bother me.
   c. I enjoy talking with the nurses.
   d. When the nurse lets me talk with her about things important to me, I feel that she cares for me as a person.

On question 18, please mark as many answers you wish.
18. I would like to feel free to talk with the nurse about my
   a. illness
   b. future
   c. financial problems
   d. feelings about myself
   e. feelings about my family
   f. life up to this time

FIGURE 16–3 ■ *Continued*

making a clear choice of positive or negative statements. Thus sometimes only four or six options are offered, with the uncertain category omitted. This type of scale is referred to as a *forced choice* version. Sometimes respondents will become annoyed at forced choice items and refuse to complete them. Researchers who use the forced choice version consider an item that is left blank as a response of "uncertain." However, responses of "uncertain" are difficult to interpret, and if a large number of respondents select that option or leave the question blank, the data may be of little value.

The phrasing of item stems depends on the type of judgment that the respondent is being asked to make. Agreement items are declarative statements such as "Nurses should be held accountable for managing a patient's pain." Frequency items can be behavior, events, or circumstances to which the respondent can indicate how often they occur. A frequency stem might be "You read research articles in nursing journals." An evaluation stem could be "The effectiveness of 'X' drug for relief of nausea after chemotherapy." Items need to be clear, concise, and concrete (Spector, 1992).

An instrument using a Likert scale usually consists of 10 to 20 items, each addressing an element of the concept being measured. Half the statements should be expressed positively and half negatively to avoid inserting bias into the responses. Scale values of negatively expressed items must be reversed before analysis. Usually, the values obtained from each item in the instrument are summed to obtain a single score for each subject. Although the values of each item are technically ordinal-level data, the summed score is often treated as interval-level data, thus allowing more sophisticated statistical analyses. Some researchers now treat each item as interval-level data. The items (not actually part of a scale) in Figure 16–4 indicate the types of statements commonly used in Likert scales.

Flaskerud (1988) reports difficulty using the Likert scale with some cultural groups. Hispanic and Vietnamese subjects had difficulty understanding the request to select one of four or five possible responses and insisted on responding to each item with a simple yes or no. Additional explanation did not sway them from this position. The reason for this difficulty is not understood.

SEMANTIC DIFFERENTIALS

The *semantic differential* was developed by Osgood and colleagues (1957) to measure attitudes or beliefs. It is now used more broadly to measure variations in views of a concept. A semantic differential scale consists of two opposite adjectives with a seven-point scale between them. The subject is to select one point on the scale that best describes his or her view of the concept being examined. The scale is designed to measure the connotative mean-

	Strongly Disagree	Disagree	Uncertain	Agree	Strongly Agree
People with cancer almost always die					
Chemotherapy is very effective in treating cancer					
We are close to finding a cure for cancer					
I would work next to a person with cancer					
I could develop cancer					
Nurses take good care of patients with cancer					

FIGURE 16–4 ■ Example of items that could be included in a Likert Scale.

ing of the concept to the subject. Although the adjectives may not seem to be particularly related to the concept being examined, the technique can be used to distinguish varying degrees of positive and negative attitudes toward a concept. Figure 16–5 illustrates the form used for this type of scale.

Some semantic differentials use descriptive phrases rather than the original adjectives used by Osgood and colleagues (1957) to develop the semantic differential instrument. Burns (1981, 1983) developed a semantic differential to measure beliefs about cancer that uses descriptive phrases. Figure 16–6 includes some of the descriptive phrases from a 23-item scale.

In a semantic differential, values from 1 to 7 are assigned to each of the spaces, with 1 being the most negative response and 7 the most positive. Placement of negative responses to the left or right of the scale should be randomly varied to avoid global responses (in which the subject places checks in the same column of each scale). Each line is considered one scale. The values for the scales are summed to obtain one score for each subject. Factor analysis is used to determine the factor structure, which is expected to reflect three factors or dimensions: evaluation, potency, and activity. The researcher needs to explain theoretically why particular items on the scale cluster together in the factor analysis. Thus, development of the instrument contributes to theory development. Factor analysis is also used to evaluate the validity of the instrument. With some of these instruments, three factor scores, each representing one of the dimensions, are used

NURSING RESEARCH		
hot	__|__|__|__|__|__|__|	cold
sweet	__|__|__|__|__|__|__|	sour
pleasant	__|__|__|__|__|__|__|	unpleasant
worthless	__|__|__|__|__|__|__|	valuable
weak	__|__|__|__|__|__|__|	strong
beautiful	__|__|__|__|__|__|__|	ugly
passive	__|__|__|__|__|__|__|	active

FIGURE 16–5 ■ Example of items in the original semantic differential.

CANCER		
Certain Death	|__|__|__|__|__|__|__|	Being Cured
Punishment	|__|__|__|__|__|__|__|	No Punishment
Painless	|__|__|__|__|__|__|__|	Severe Constant Untreatable Pain
Abandoned	|__|__|__|__|__|__|__|	Cared For

FIGURE 16–6 ■ Example of items from the Burns Cancer Beliefs scales.

to describe the subject's responses and are a basis for further analysis (Nunnally, 1978).

Q METHODOLOGY

Q methodology is a technique of comparative rating that preserves the subjective point of view of the individual (McKeown & Thomas, 1988). Cards are used to categorize the importance placed on various words or phrases in relation to the other words or phrases in the list. Each phrase is placed on a separate card. The number of cards should range from 40 to 100 (Tetting, 1988). The subject is instructed to sort the cards into a designated number of piles, usually 7 to 10 piles ranging from the most to least important. However, the subject is limited in the number of cards that may be placed in each pile. If the subject must sort 59 cards, category 1 (of greatest importance) may allow only 2 cards; category 2, 5 cards; category 3, 10 cards; category 4, 25 cards; category 5, 10 cards; category 6, 5 cards; and category 7 (the least important), 2 cards. Thus placement of the cards fits the patterns of a normal curve. The subject is usually advised to select first the cards that he or she wishes to place in the two extreme categories and then work toward the middle category, which contains the largest number of cards, until they are satisfied with the results.

The Q-sort method can also be used to determine the priority of items or the most important items to include in the development of a scale. In the previously mentioned example, the behaviors sorted into categories 5, 6, and 7 might be organized into a 17-item scale. Correlational or factor analysis is used to analyze the data (Dennis, 1986; Tetting, 1988).

Simpson (1989) suggests using the Q-sort method for cross-cultural research, with pictures rather than words used for nonliterate groups.

The Q-sort technique is used in the Control Preferences Scale, a general measure of a unidimensional construct involving consumer preferences about participating in treatment decision making. The Control Preferences Scale is administered by having each subject sort a series of cards through successive paired comparisons (Degner, 1998). Luniewski and associates (1999) used a Q-sort technique in their study of effective education of patients with heart failure. Patients were asked to sort 12 cards with questions related to the content of discharge teaching for patients with heart failure.

VISUAL ANALOGUE SCALES

One of the problems of concern in scaling procedures is the difficulty of obtaining fine discrimination of values. A recent effort to resolve this problem is the *visual analogue scale,* sometimes referred to as magnitude scaling (Gift, 1989). This technique seems to provide interval-level data, and some researchers argue that it provides ratio-level data (Sennott-Miller et al., 1988). It is particularly useful in scaling stimuli (Lodge, 1981). This scaling technique has been used to measure mood, anxiety, alertness, craving for cigarettes, quality of sleep, attitudes toward environmental conditions, functional abilities, and severity of clinical symptoms (Wewers & Lowe, 1990, p. 229).

The stimuli must be defined in a way that is clearly understandable to the subject. Only one major cue should appear for each scale. The scale is a line 100 mm in length with right-angle stops at each end. The line may be horizontal or vertical. Bipolar anchors are placed beyond each end of the line. The anchors should *not* be placed underneath or above the line before the stop. These end an-chors should include the entire range of sensations possible in the phenomenon being measured. Examples include "all" and "none," "best" and "worst," and "no pain" and "pain as bad as it could possibly be." These scales can be developed for use with children by using pictorial anchors at each end of the line rather than words (Lee & Kieckhefer, 1989).

The subject is asked to place a mark through the line to indicate the intensity of the stimulus. A ruler is then used to measure the distance between the left end of the line and the mark placed by the subject. This measure is the value of the stimulus. The scale is designed to be used while the subject is seated. Whether use of the scale from the supine position influences the results by altering perception of the length of the line has yet to be determined (Gift, 1989).

Wewers and Lowe (1990) have published an extensive evaluation of the reliability and validity of visual analogue scales, although reliability is difficult to determine. Because most of the variables measured with the tool are labile, test-retest consistency is not applicable, and because a single measure is obtained, examination of internal consistency is not possible. The visual analogue scale is much more sensitive to small changes than numerical and rating scales are and can discriminate between two dimensions of pain. Comparisons of the scale with other instruments measuring the same construct have had varying results and are difficult to interpret. An example of a visual analogue scale is shown in Figure 16–7.

Delphi Technique

The *Delphi technique* is used to measure the judgments of a group of experts for the purpose of making decisions, assessing priorities, or making

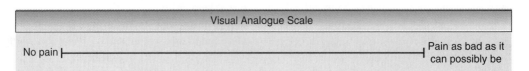

FIGURE 16–7 ▪ Example of a visual analogue scale.

forecasts. It provides a means to obtain the opinion of a wide variety of experts across the United States to provide feedback without the necessity of meeting together. When the Delphi technique is used, the opinions of individuals cannot be altered by the persuasive behavior of a few people at a meeting. Three types of Delphi techniques have been identified: classic Delphi, policy Delphi, and decision Delphi. In classic Delphi, the focus is on reaching consensus. In policy Delphi, the aim is not consensus but rather to identify and understand a variety of viewpoints. In decision Delphi, the panel consists of individuals in decision-making positions. The purpose is to come to a decision (Beretta, 1996; Crisp et al., 1997). A number of nursing specialty organizations have established their research priorities by using Delphi techniques (Rudy, 1996). Mitchell (1998) assessed the validity of the Delphi technique in nursing education planning and found that 98.1% of the predicted events had either occurred or were still expected to occur.

To implement the technique, a panel of experts is identified, but the criteria used to determine that a member of the panel is an expert are unclear. Members of the panel remain anonymous, even to each other. A questionnaire is developed that addresses the topics of concern. Although most questions call for closed-ended responses, the questionnaire usually contains opportunities for open-ended responses by the expert. The questionnaires are then returned to the researcher, and results are analyzed and summarized. Methods used for this analysis are undefined. The role of the researcher is to maintain objectivity. The outcome of the statistical analysis is returned to the panel of experts, along with a second questionnaire. Respondents with extreme responses to the first round of questions may be asked to justify their responses. The second round of questionnaires is returned to the researcher for analysis. This procedure is repeated until the data reflect a consensus among the panel. Limiting the process to two or three rounds is not a good idea if consensus is the goal. In some studies true consensus is reached, whereas in others it is a notion of "majority rules." Some question whether the agreement reached is genuine (Beretta, 1996; Crisp et al., 1997). A model of the Delphi technique was devel-

oped by Couper (1984) and is presented in Figure 16–8.

Goodman (1987) identified several potential problems that could be encountered during use of the Delphi technique. There has been no documentation that the responses of "experts" are different from those one would receive from a random sample of subjects. Because the panelists are anonymous, they have no accountability for their responses. Respondents could make hasty, ill-considered judgments because they know that no negative feedback will result. Feedback on the consensus of the group tends to centralize opinion, and traditional analysis with the use of means and medians may mask the responses of those who are resistant to the consensus. Thus conclusions could be misleading.

Lindeman (1975) conducted a Delphi survey to determine research priorities in clinical nursing research. She used a panel of 433 experts, both nurses and nonnurses, with a wide range of interests. Four rounds of a 150-item questionnaire were sent to the panel. The report, published in *Nursing Research,* had an important influence on the direction of research program development in nursing.

Projective Techniques

Projective techniques are based on the assumption that the responses of individuals to unstructured or ambiguous situations reflect the attitudes, desires, personality characteristics, and motives of the individual. The technique is most frequently used in psychology and includes techniques such as the Rorschach Inkblot Test, Machover's Draw-A-Person Test, word association, sentence completion, role-playing, and play techniques. The technique is an indirect measure of data that are unlikely to be obtained directly. Analysis of the data requires that inferences be made about the meaning and is therefore subjective. Many of the tests require extensive training for administration and interpretation and thus have not been frequently used in nursing research. However, with the increased frequency of interdisciplinary research, their use in nursing studies may increase. At present, the technique is used in nursing primarily in studying children (Waltz et al., 1991). Johnson (1990) provides an excellent

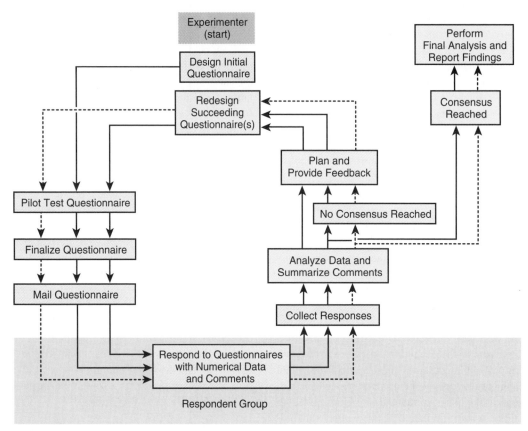

FIGURE 16–8 ■ Delphi technique sequence model. (From Couper, M. R. [1984]. The Delphi technique: characteristics and sequence model. *Advances in Nursing Science, 7*[1], 75.)

explanation of the techniques used to interpret children's drawings.

Diaries

A recent approach to obtaining information that must be collected over time is to ask the subjects to keep a record or *diary* of events. The data in this diary can then be collected and analyzed by researchers. A diary, which allows recording shortly after an event, is more accurate than obtaining the information through recall at an interview, the reporting level of incidents is higher, and one tends to capture the participant's perception of situations.

This technique provides a means to obtain data on topics of particular interest within nursing that have not been accessible by other means. Some potential topics for diary collection include expenses related to a health care event (particularly out-of-pocket expenses), self-care activities (frequency and time required), incidence of symptoms, eating behavior, exercise behavior, and care provided by family members in a home care situation. Although diaries have been used primarily with adults, they are also an effective means of data collection with school-aged children. Butz and Alexander (1991) reported an 88% completion rate in a study of children with asthma, with most children (72.3%) keeping the diary without assistance from their parents.

Health diaries have been used to document health problems, responses to symptoms, and efficacy of responses. Diaries may also be used to determine how people spend their days; this information could be particularly useful in managing the care needs of individuals with chronic illnesses. In experimental studies, diaries may be used to determine subjects' responses to experimental treatments. Two types of health diaries are used: a ledger in which different types of events are recorded, such as the occurrence of a symptom, and a journal in which entries related to specific topics are made daily. An example of a ledger is shown in Figure 16–9, and an example of a journal is shown in Figure 16–10. Figure 16–11 shows a sample patient diary. Validity and reliability have been examined by comparing the results with data obtained through interviews and have been found to be acceptable. Participation in studies using health diaries has been good, and attrition rates are reported as low. Adequate instructions related to completing the diary and arranging for pickup are critical (Burman, 1995).

Burman (1995) makes some recommendations regarding the general use of health diaries.

1. Critically analyze the phenomenon of interest to ensure that it can be adequately captured using a diary. Infrequent major events, very minor health events or behaviors, and vague symptoms are less likely to be reported than more frequent, definable acute problems. The use of a diary should be evaluated in light of other data collection approaches such as interviews and mail surveys, that may lead to higher data quality depending on the specific phenomenon of interest.
2. Determine which format—ledger or journal—should be used to decrease participant burden while minimizing missing data. The ledger format may be less burdensome but evaluation of missing data is more complicated.
3. Evaluate whether closed- or open-ended questions will result in clearer reporting. Closed-ended questions reduce respondent burden, but may result in overreporting of symptoms.
4. Pilot test any new or refined diary with the target population of interest to identify possible problems, to ensure that the phenomenon can be recorded with this approach, and to evaluate the ability of participants to complete diaries. Participation rates in diary studies vary, although those with high incomes and education levels, and better writing skills may be overrepresented. However, diaries have been used successfully with ill and general-community populations.
5. Determine the diary period that is necessary to adequately record changes and fluctuations in the phenomenon of interest, balancing this with respondent burden. Typical diary periods are 2 to 4 weeks.
6. Provide clear instructions to all participants on the use of a diary before participation begins to enhance data quality. Participants need to know how to use the diaries, what types of events are to be reported, and how to contact the investigator or clinician with questions.
7. Use follow-up procedures during data collection to enhance completion rates. Telephone contacts enhance completion rates. Diaries may be mailed; however, returning diaries through the mail may result in somewhat lower completion rates.
8. Plan analysis procedures during diary development or refinement to be sure the data are in the appropriate form for the analyses. Diary data are very dense and rich, carefully prepared plans can minimize problems. (Burman, 1995, p. 151)

Problems related to the diary method include costs, subject cooperation, quality of the data, conditioning effects on the subject of keeping a diary, and the complexity of data analysis. Costs include interview time, mail and telephone expenses, and remuneration to subjects. Costs are higher than single face-to-face interviews but lower than repeated interviews. Costs are lowest when diaries are used with telephone interviews and highest when diaries are used with repeated face-to-face interviews. Costs are lower when diaries are mailed rather than picked up. Most subject noncooperation occurs in the first month, with only 1% to 2% subject loss after that point. Diary completion rates are higher (80–88%) than the completion rates of other data collection methods such as surveys. Picking up the diary increases the completion rate (Butz & Alexander, 1991).

The use of diaries, however, has some disadvantages. Keeping the diary may, in some cases, alter the behavior or events under study. For example, if a person were keeping a diary of the nursing care that he or she was providing to patients, the insight that the person gained from recording the information in the diary might lead to changes in care. Subjects can become more sensitive to items (such as symptoms or problems) reported in the diary, which could result in overreporting. Subjects may also become bored with keeping the diary and become less thorough in recording items, which could result in underreporting (Butz & Alexander, 1991). Pfister (1999) used a diary to study urinary incontinence and daily voiding patterns of residents of retirement settings.

Date	What symptom did you have?	Did you talk wiih a family member or friend about the symptom?		Did you talk with a health professional about it?		Did you take any pills or treatments for the symptom?	
		No	Yes	No	Yes	No	Yes, Specify

FIGURE 16−9 ■ Sample ledger diary. (From Burman, M. E. [1995]. Health diaries in nursing research and practice. *Image: Journal of Nursing Scholarship, 27*[2], 148.)

---

1. Did you have any symptoms today?
   a. NO → Go to question 5

   b. YES, Please specify _____
   _____
   _____

2. Did you talk to a family member about the symptom(s)?
   a. NO

   b. YES

3. Did you talk to a health care professional about the symptom(s)?
   a. NO

   b. YES

4. Did you take any pills for the symptom(s)?
   a. NO → Go to question 5

   b. YES, Please specify _____
   _____
   _____

5. How would you rate your health today?

   _____
   Excellent   Poor

FIGURE 16−10 ■ Sample journal diary. (From Burman, M. E. [1995]. Health diaries in nursing research and practice. *Image: Journal of Nursing Scholarship, 27*[2], 148.)

The following samples are provided as a guide to keeping your diary. <u>Every day</u> when you write in the diary, please:

1. Record any <u>health problem</u> or problems you had (for example: constipation, skin rash on back, need bandages for surgery wound).

2. For each health problem, list the type of contact and person you contacted outside your home (such as nurse, doctor, social worked, pharmacist, or family member) and the place or agency (name of hospital, agency or facility, for example: Visiting Nurse Association).

3. Check (√) whether you made the contact by telephone or in person for each contact.

4. Record the date of each contact. If you visited or called the same place at different times list each contact separately.

5. Identify, "yes" or "no," if the visit or telephone call helped you with your health problem.

6. Record the <u>health problem</u> even if you did not contact someone outside your home for help with it.

Sample Patient Diary

What health problem did you have?	What person and place did you contact for this health problem?	What type of contact did you make? Check √ one		When did you call/visit? (Record date)	Did you receive the help you needed?	
		Telephone call	Visit		Yes	No
skin irritation on back	*Nurse, St. Jude Hospital*	√		*Dec. 6, 1980*	√	
needed cold pack for leg pain	*Pharmacist Mitchel's Pharmacy*		√	*Jan. 6, 1981*		√
difficulty in walking, needed a cane	*Counselor, American Cancer Society*	√		*Jan. 26, 1981*	√	
feeling depressed	*Minister, St. Paul's Church*		√	*Jan. 26, 1981*	√	

FIGURE 16–11 ■ Patient diary reports of home nursing. (From Oleske, D. M., Heinze, S., & Otte, D. M. [1990]. The diary as a means of understanding the quality of life of persons with cancer receiving home nursing care. *Cancer Nursing, 13*[3], 161.)

SELECTION OF AN EXISTING INSTRUMENT

Selecting an instrument for measurement of the variables in a study is a critical process in research. The method of measurement must closely fit the conceptual definition of the variable. An extensive search of the literature may be required to identify appropriate methods of measurement. In many cases, instruments will be found that measure some of the needed elements but not all, or the content may be related to but somehow different from that needed for the study being planned. Instruments found in the literature may have little or no documentation of their validity and reliability.

The initial reaction of a beginning researcher is that no methods of measurement exist and a tool must be developed by the researcher. At the time, this solution seems to be the most simple because the researcher has a clear idea of what needs to be measured. This solution, however, should not be used unless all else fails. The process of tool development is lengthy and requires considerable research sophistication. Using a new instrument in a study without first evaluating its validity and reliability is unacceptable; it is a waste of subject and investigator time.

Locating Existing Instruments

Locating existing measurement methods has become easier in recent years. A relatively new computer database, the Health and Psychological Instruments Online (HAPI), is available in many libraries and can search for instruments that measure a particular concept or for information on a particular instrument.

Many reference books have compiled published measurement tools, some that are specific to instruments used in nursing research. Dissertations often contain measurement tools that have never been published, so a review of *Dissertation Abstracts* might be helpful. *Dissertation Abstracts* is now on-line on the World Wide Web (WWW).

Another important source of recently developed measurement tools is word-of-mouth communication among researchers. Information on tools is often presented at research conferences years before publication. There are often networks of researchers conducting studies on similar nursing phenomena. These researchers are frequently associated with a nursing organization and keep in touch through newsletters, correspondence, telephone, electronic mail, computer bulletin boards, and WWW pages. Thus questioning available nurse researchers can lead to a previously unknown tool. These researchers are often easily contacted by telephone or letter and are usually willing to share their tools in return for access to the data to facilitate work on developing validity and reliability information. The Sigma Theta Tau *Directory of Nurse Researchers* provides address and phone information of nurse researchers. In addition, it lists nurse researchers by category according to their area of research.

Evaluating Existing Instruments

Several instruments must be examined to find the one most appropriate for your study. Selection of an instrument for research requires careful consideration of how the instrument was developed, what the instrument measures, and how to administer it. The following questions need to be addressed when examining an instrument:

1. Does this instrument measure what you want to measure?
2. Is the instrument reflective of your conceptual definition of the variable?
3. Is the instrument well constructed?

4. Does your population resemble populations previously studied with the instrument?
5. Is the readability level of the instrument appropriate for your population?
6. How sensitive is the instrument in detecting small differences in the phenomenon being measured (what is the effect size)?
7. What is the process for obtaining, administering, and scoring the instrument?
8. What skills are required to administer the instrument?
9. How are the scores interpreted?
10. What is the time commitment of the subjects and researcher for administration of the instrument?
11. What evidence is available related to reliability and validity of the instrument?

Particular populations may require further assessment to determine their instrumentation requirements. Burnside and coworkers (1998) provide an excellent discussion of research instrumentation for elderly subjects. They identify four factors that should be considered when selecting research instruments for use with older adults: fatigue, anxiety, ethnic background, and education.

Assessing Readability Levels of Instruments

The readability level of an instrument is a critical factor when selecting an instrument for a study. Regardless of how valid and reliable the instrument is, it cannot be used effectively in a study if the items are not understandable to the subjects. Calculating readability is relatively easy and can be performed in about 20 minutes. Many word processing programs and computerized grammar checkers will report the readability level of written material. The Fog formula described in Chapter 15 provides a quick and easy way to assess readability.

CONSTRUCTING SCALES

Scale construction is a complex procedure that should not be undertaken lightly. However, in many cases, measurement methods have not been developed for phenomena of concern to nurse researchers. Measurement tools that have been developed may be poorly constructed and have insufficient evidence of validity to be acceptable for use in studies. It is possible for the researcher to carry out instrument development procedures on an existing scale before using it in a study. Neophyte nurse researchers could assist researchers in carrying out some of the field studies required to complete the development of a scale. The procedures for developing a scale have been well defined. The following discussion describes this theory-based process and the mathematical logic underlying it.

The theories on which scale construction is most frequently based include classic test theory (Nunnally, 1978), item response theory (Hulin et al., 1983), multidimensional scaling (Davison, 1983; Kruskal & Wish, 1990), and unfolding theory (Coombs, 1950). Most existing instruments used in nursing research have been developed with classic test theory, which assumes a normal distribution of scores.

Constructing a Scale by Using Classic Test Theory

In classic test theory, the following process is used to construct a scale.

1. **Define the concept.** A scale cannot be constructed to measure a concept until the nature of the concept has been delineated. The more clearly the concept is defined, the easier it is to write items to measure it (Spector, 1992). Concept definition is achieved through concept analysis, a procedure discussed in Chapters 4 and 7.

2. **Design the scale.** Items should be constructed to reflect the concept as fully as possible. The process of construction will differ somewhat depending on whether the scale is a rating scale, Likert scale, or semantic differential scale. Items previously included in other scales can be used if they have been shown empirically to be good indicators of the concept (Hulin et al., 1983). A blueprint may be helpful in ensuring coverage of all elements of the concept. Each item needs to be stated clearly and concisely and express only one idea. The read-

ing level of items needs to be identified and considered in terms of potential respondents. The number of items constructed needs to be considerably larger than planned for the completed instrument because items will be discarded during the item analysis step of scale construction. Nunnally (1978) suggests developing an item pool at least twice the size of that desired for the final scale.

3. **Seek item review.** As items are constructed, it is advisable to ask qualified individuals to review them. Crocker and Algina (1986, p. 71) recommend asking for feedback in relation to accuracy, appropriateness, or relevance to test specifications; technical flaws in item construction; grammar; offensiveness or appearance of bias; and level of readability. Revise items according to the critique.

4. **Conduct preliminary item tryouts.** While items are still in draft form, it is helpful to test them on a limited number of subjects (15–30) representative of the target population. Observe the reactions of respondents during testing to note behavior such as long pauses, answer changing, or other indications of confusion about specific items. After testing, a debriefing session needs to be held during which respondents are invited to comment on items and offer suggestions for improvement. Descriptive and exploratory statistical analyses are performed on data from these tryouts while noting means, response distributions, items left blank, and outliers. Revise items on the basis of this analysis and comments from respondents.

5. **Perform a field test.** Administer all the items in their final draft form to a large sample of subjects representative of the target population. Spector (1992) recommends a sample size of 100 to 200 subjects. However, the sample size needed for the statistical analyses to follow is somewhat dependent on the number of items. Some recommend including 10 subjects for each item being tested. If the final instrument was expected to have 20 items and 40 items were constructed for the field test, as many as 400 subjects could be required.

6. **Conduct item analyses.** The purpose of item analysis is to identify items that form an inter-

nally consistent scale and eliminate items that do not meet this criterion. Internal consistency implies that all the items measure the same concept. Before these analyses, negatively worded items need to be reverse-scored. The analyses examine the extent of intercorrelation among the items. The statistical computer programs currently providing (as a package) the set of statistical procedures needed to perform item analyses are SPSS, SPSS/PC, and SYSTAT. This package performs item-item correlations and item-total correlations. In some cases, the value of the item being examined is subtracted from the total score and an item-remainder coefficient is calculated. This latter coefficient is most useful in evaluating items for retention in the scale.

7. **Select items to retain.** Depending on the number of items desired in the final scale, items with the highest coefficients are retained. Alternatively, a criterion value for the coefficient (e.g., .40) can be set and all items greater than this value retained. The greater the number of items retained, the smaller the item-remainder coefficients can be and still have an internally consistent scale. After this selection process, coefficient alpha is calculated for the scale. This value is a direct function of the number of items and the magnitude of intercorrelation. Thus one can increase the value of coefficient alpha by increasing the number of items or raise the intercorrelations through inclusion of more highly intercorrelated items. Values of coefficient alpha range from 0 to 1. The alpha value should be at least .70 to indicate sufficient internal consistency (Nunnally, 1978). An iterative process of removing or replacing items, or both, recalculating item-remainder coefficients, and then recalculating the alpha coefficient is repeated until a satisfactory alpha coefficient is obtained. Deleting poorly correlated items will raise the alpha coefficient, but decreasing the number of items will lower it (Spector, 1992).

The initial attempt at scale development may not achieve a sufficiently high coefficient alpha. In this case, additional items will need to be written, more data collected, and the item analysis redone. This scenario is most likely to occur when too few items were developed initially or when many of the initial items were poorly written. It may also be a consequence of attempts to operationalize an inadequately defined concept (Spector, 1992).

8. **Conduct validity studies.** When scale development is judged to be satisfactory, studies must be performed to evaluate the validity of the scale. (Refer to the discussion of validity in Chapter 15). These studies require the collection of additional data from large samples. As part of this process, scale scores need to be correlated with scores on other variables proposed to be related to the concept being put into operation. Hypotheses need to be generated regarding variations in mean values of the scale in different groups. Exploratory and then confirmatory factor analysis (discussed in Chapter 20) is usually performed as part of establishing the validity of the instrument. As many different types of evidence of validity should be collected as possible (Spector, 1992).

9. **Evaluate the reliability of the scale.** Various statistical procedures need to be performed to determine the reliability of the scale. These analyses can be performed on the data collected to evaluate validity. (See Chapter 15 for a discussion of the procedures performed to examine reliability.)

10. **Compile norms on the scale.** Determination of norms requires administration of the scale to a large sample representative of the groups to which the scale is likely to be given. Norms should be acquired for as many diverse groups as possible. Data acquired during validity and reliability studies can be included for this analysis. To obtain the large samples needed for this purpose, many researchers give permission to others to use their scale with the condition that data from these studies be provided for compiling norms.

11. **Publish the results of development of the scale.** Scales are often not published for a number of years after the initial development because of the length of time required to validate

the instrument. Some researchers never publish the results of this work. Studies using the scale are published, but the instrument development process may not be available except by writing to the author. This information needs to be added to the body of knowledge, and instrument developers need to be encouraged by their colleagues to complete the work and submit it for publication (Lynn, 1989; Norbeck, 1985).

Constructing a Scale by Using Item Response Theory

Using item response theory to construct a scale proceeds initially in a fashion similar to that of classic test theory. There is an expectation of a well-defined concept to operationalize. Initial item writing is similar to that previously described, as are item tryouts and field testing. However, with the initiation of item analysis, the process changes. The statistical procedures used are more sophisticated and complex than those used in classic test theory. Using data from field testing, item characteristic curves are calculated by using logistic regression models (Hulin et al., 1983). After selecting an appropriate model based on information obtained from the analysis, item parameters are estimated. These parameters are used to select items for the scale. This strategy is used to avoid problems encountered with classic test theory measures.

Scales developed by using classic test theory are effective in measuring the characteristics of subjects near the mean. The statistical procedures used assume a linear distribution of scale values. Items reflecting responses of subjects closer to the extremes tend to be discarded because of the assumption that scale values should approximate the normal curve. Therefore, scales developed in this manner often do not provide a clear understanding of subjects at the high or low end of values.

One of the purposes of item response theory is to choose items in such a way that estimates of characteristics at each level of the concept being measured are accurate. This goal is accomplished by using maximal likelihood estimates. A curvilinear distribution of scale values is assumed. Rather than choosing items on the basis of the item-remainder coefficient, the researcher specifies a test information curve. The scale can be tailored to have a desired measurement accuracy. By comparing a scale developed by classic test theory with one developed from the same items with item response theory, one would find differences in some of the items retained. Biserial correlations would be lower in the scale developed from item response theory than in the scale developed from classic test theory. Item bias is lower in scales developed by using item response theory and occurs when respondents from different subpopulations having the same amount of an underlying trait have different probabilities of responding to an item positively (Hulin et al., 1983, p. 152).

Constructing a Scale by Using Multidimensional Scaling

Multidimensional scaling is used when the concept being operationalized is actually an abstract construct believed to be represented most accurately by multiple dimensions. The scaling techniques used allow the researcher to uncover the hidden structure in the construct. The analysis techniques use proximities among the measures as input. The outcome of the analysis is a spatial representation, or a geometrical configuration of data points, that reveals the hidden structure. The procedure tends to be used for examining differences in stimuli rather than differences in people. Thus differences in perception of light or pain might be examined. Scales developed by using this procedure are effective in revealing patterns among items. The procedure is used in the development of rating scales and semantic differentials (Kruskal & Wish, 1990).

Constructing a Scale by Using Unfolding Theory

During construction of a scale with the use of unfolding theory, subjects are asked to respond to the items in the rating scale. Next, they are asked to rank the various response options in relation to the response option that they selected for that item. This procedure is followed for each item in the scale. By using this procedure, the underlying continuum for each scale item is "unfolded." As an example, suppose you developed the following item:

My favorite ice cream flavor is

1. chocolate
2. vanilla
3. strawberry
4. butter pecan

You would ask subjects to select their response to the item. They would then be asked to rank the other options according to the proximity to their choice. The subject might choose strawberry as No. 1, vanilla as No. 2, butter pecan as No. 3, and chocolate as No. 4. Although the preferences of other subjects would differ, the results can be plotted to reveal patterns of an underlying continuum. Items selected for the scale would be those with evidence of a pattern of responses. Degner (1998) used unfolding in analyzing the results of patient responses to the Control Preferences Scale, a measure of consumer preferences about participating in treatment decision making.

TRANSLATING A SCALE TO ANOTHER LANGUAGE

Contrary to expectations, translating an instrument from the original language to a target language is a complex process. The goal of translating a scale is to allow comparisons of concepts among respondents of different cultures. Such comparison requires that one first infer and then validate that the conceptual meaning in which the scale was developed is the same in both cultures. This process is highly speculative, and conclusions about the similarities of meanings in a measure must be considered tentative (Hulin et al., 1983).

Four types of translations can be performed: pragmatic translations, aesthetic-poetic translations, ethnographic translations, and linguistic translations. The purpose of pragmatic translations is to communicate the content from the source language accurately in the target language. The primary concern is the information conveyed. An example of this type of translation is the use of translated instructions for assembling a computer. The purpose of

aesthetic-poetic translations is to evoke moods, feelings, and affect in the target language that are identical to those evoked by the original material. In ethnographic translations, the purpose is to maintain meaning and cultural content. In this case, translators must be very familiar with both languages and cultures. Linguistic translations strive to present grammatical forms with equivalent meanings. Translating a scale is generally done in the ethnographic mode (Hulin et al., 1983).

One strategy for translating scales is to translate from the original language to the target language and then back-translate from the target language to the original language by using translators not involved in the original translation. Discrepancies are identified, and the procedure is repeated until troublesome problems are resolved. After this procedure, the two versions are administered to bilingual subjects and scored by standard procedures. The resulting sets of scores are examined to determine the extent to which the two versions yield similar information from the subjects. This procedure assumes that the subjects are equally skilled in both languages. One problem with this strategy is that bilingual subjects may interpret meanings of words differently from monolingual subjects. This difference in interpretation is a serious concern because the target subjects for most cross-cultural research are monolingual (Hulin et al., 1983). Phillips and colleagues (1994) provide an excellent description of this process in their cross-cultural study of family caregiving. Krozy and McCarthy (1999) describe the development of bilingual assessment tools designed to facilitate nursing assessment of the individual, family, and community in Ecuador.

Hulin and colleagues (1983) suggest the use of item response theory procedures to address some of the problems of translation. These procedures can provide direct evidence about the meanings of items in the two languages. Item characteristic curves for an item in the two languages can be compared, as can scale scores in the two languages. This procedure eliminates the need for bilingual samples. It also eliminates the need for the two populations to be equivalent in terms of the distributions of their scores on the trait being measured.

Rather than translating an instrument into each

language, Turner and associates (1996) tested the use of electronic technology involving multilingual audio computer-assisted self-interviewing (Audio-CASI) to enable researchers to include multiple linguistic minorities in nationally representative studies and clinical studies. This system uses electronic translation from one language to another. In the funded project to develop and test the system, a backup phone bank was available to provide multilingual assistance if needed. Whether this strategy will provide equivalent validity of a translated tool is unclear.

■ SUMMARY
. . . .

Common measurement approaches that are used in nursing research include physiological measures, observations, interviews, questionnaires, and scales. Specialized measurements include the Q-sort method, visual analogue scale, Delphi technique, projective techniques, and diaries. Much of nursing practice is oriented toward the physiological dimensions of health. Therefore, many of our questions require measurement of these dimensions. Measurements of physiological variables can be either direct or indirect. Many physiological measures require the use of specialized equipment, and some require laboratory analysis. In publishing the results of a physiological study, the measurement technique must be described in great detail.

Measurement of observations requires that one first decide what is to be observed and then determine how to ensure that every variable is observed in a similar manner in each instance. Careful attention is given to training data collectors. Observational measurement may be unstructured or structured. In structured observational studies, category systems must be developed. Checklists or rating scales are developed from the category systems and used to guide data collection.

Interviews involve verbal communication between the researcher and the subject, during which information is provided to the researcher. Approaches range from a totally unstructured interview in which the content is completely controlled by the subject to interviews in which the content is similar to a questionnaire, with the possible responses to questions carefully designed by the researcher. Interview questions are grouped by topic, with fairly safe topics being addressed first and sensitive topics reserved until late in the interview process. Interviewers need to be trained in the skills of interviewing, and the interview protocol needs to be pretested.

A questionnaire is a printed self-report form designed to elicit information through written responses of the subject. The information obtained through questionnaires is similar to that obtained by interview, but the questions tend to have less depth. The subject is unable to elaborate on responses or ask for clarification of questions, and the data collector cannot use probe strategies. Like interviews, questionnaires can have varying degrees of structure. An item on a questionnaire has two parts: a lead-in question and a response set. Each lead-in question needs to be carefully designed and clearly expressed to avoid influencing the response of the respondent.

Scales, another form of self-reporting, are a more precise means of measuring phenomena than are questionnaires. The majority of scales have been developed to measure psychosocial variables. However, self-reports can be obtained on physiological variables such as pain, nausea, or functional capacity by using scaling techniques. Rating scales are the crudest form of measure using scaling techniques. A rating scale lists an ordered series of categories of a variable, which are assumed to be based on an underlying continuum. A numerical value is assigned to each category. The Likert scale is designed to determine the opinion or attitude of a subject and contains a number of declarative statements with a scale after each statement. A semantic differential scale consists of two opposite adjectives with a seven-point scale between them. The subject is to select one point on the scale that best describes that subject's view of the concept being examined. The scale is designed to measure the connotative meaning of the concept to the subject.

One of the problems of concern in scaling procedures is the difficulty in obtaining fine discrimination of values. An effort to resolve this problem is the visual analogue scale, sometimes referred to as magnitude scaling. It is particularly useful in scaling stimuli. The scale is a line 100 mm in length with right-angle stops at each end. Bipolar anchors are placed beyond each end of the line. These end anchors should include the entire range of sensations possible in the phenomenon being measured.

The Delphi technique is used to measure the judgments of a group of experts, assess priorities, or make forecasts. It provides a means to obtain the opinion of a wide variety of experts across the United States without the necessity of meeting. Projective techniques are based on the assumption that the responses of individuals to unstructured or ambiguous situations reflect the attitudes, desires, personality characteristics, and motives of the individuals. The technique is most frequently used in psychology and includes techniques such as the Rorschach Inkblot Test, Machover's Draw-A-Person Test, word association, sentence completion, role-playing, and play techniques.

An approach to obtaining information that must be collected over time is to ask subjects to keep a record or diary of events. The data in this diary can then be collected and analyzed by researchers. A diary, which allows recording shortly after an event, is more accurate than obtaining the information through recall at an interview, the reporting level of incidents is higher, and one tends to capture the participant's perception of situations.

The choice of tools for use in a particular study is a critical decision that will have a major impact on the significance of the study. The researcher first needs to conduct an extensive search for existing tools. When tools are found, they need to be carefully evaluated. Tools that are selected for a study need to be described in great detail in the proposal or publication. Scale construction is a complex procedure that should not be undertaken lightly. Theories on which scale construction is most frequently based include classic test theory, item response theory, multidimensional scaling, and unfolding theory. Most existing instruments used in nursing research have been developed by using classic test theory.

Translating a scale to another language is a complex process. The goal of translating is to allow comparisons of concepts among respondents of different cultures. Item response theory can be useful in evaluating the effectiveness of translated scales.

REFERENCES

Amsterdam, E. A., Hughes, J. L., DeMaria, A. M., Zellis, R., & Mason, D. T. (1974). Indirect assessment of myocardial oxygen consumption in the evaluation of mechanisms and therapy of angina pectoris. *American Journal of Cardiology, 33*(6), 737–743.

Baker, C. M. (1985). Maximizing mailed questionnaire responses. *Image—Journal of Nursing Scholarship, 17*(4), 118–121.

Beaudin, C. L., & Pelletier, L. R. (1996). Consumer-based research: Using focus groups as a method for evaluating quality of care. *Journal of Nursing Care Quality, 10*(3), 28–33.

Bedarf, E. W. (1986). *Using structured interviewing techniques.* Washington, DC: Program Evaluation and Methodology Division, United States General Accounting Office.

Berdie, D. R., Anderson, J. F., & Niebuhr, M. A. (1986). *Questionnaires: Design and use.* Metuchen, NJ: Scarecrow Press.

Beretta, R. (1996). A critical review of the Delphi technique. *Nurse Researcher, 3*(4), 79–89.

Borg, G. A. (1982). Psychophysical bases of perceived exertion. *Medicine and Science in Sports and Exercise, 14,* 377–381.

Briggs, C. L. (1986). *Learning how to ask: A sociolinguistic appraisal of the role of the interview in social science research.* Cambridge, UK: Cambridge University Press.

Brown, J. K., & Radke, K. J. (1998). Nutritional assessment, intervention, and evaluation of weight loss in patients with non–small cell lung cancer. *Oncology Nursing Forum, 25*(3), 547–553.

Bulmer, C. (1998). Clinical decisions: Defining meaning through focus groups. *Nursing Standard, 12*(20), 34–36.

Burman, M. E. (1995). Health diaries in nursing research and practice. *Image—Journal of Nursing Scholarship, 27*(2), 147–152.

Burnard, P. (1994). The telephone interview as a data collection method. *Nurse Education Today, 14*(1), 67–72.

Burns, N. (1974). *Nurse-patient communication with the advanced cancer patient.* Unpublished master's thesis, Texas Woman's University, Denton, TX.

Burns, N. (1981). *Evaluation of a supportive-expressive group for families of cancer patients.* Unpublished doctoral dissertation, Texas Woman's University, Denton, TX.

Burns, N. (1983). Development of the Burns cancer beliefs scale. *Proceedings of the American Cancer Society Third West Coast Cancer Nursing Research Conference,* 308–329.

Burns, N. (1986). *Research in progress.* American Cancer Society, Texas Division.

Burnside, I., Preski, S., & Hertz, J. E. (1998). Research instrumentation and elderly subjects. *Image—Journal of Nursing Scholarship, 30*(2), 185–190.

Butz, A. M., & Alexander, C. (1991). Use of health diaries with children. *Nursing Research, 40*(1), 59–61.

Carey, M. A. (1995). Comment: Concerns in the analysis of focus group data. *Qualitative Health Research, 5*(4), 487–495.

Chapple, A. (1997). Personal recollections on interviewing GPs and consultants. *Nurse Researcher, 5*(2), 82–91.

Converse, J. M., & Presser, S. (1986). *Survey questions: Handcrafting the standardized questionnaire.* Newbury Park, CA: Sage.

Coombs, C. H. (1950). Psychological scaling without a unit of measurement. *Psychological Review, 57*(3), 145–158.

Couper, M. R. (1984). The Delphi technique: Characteristics and sequence model. *Advances in Nursing Science, 7*(1), 72–77.

Covey, M. K., Larson, J. L., Alex, C. G., Wirtz, S., & Langbein, W. E. (1999). Test-retest reliability of symptom-limited cycle ergometer tests in patients with chronic obstructive pulmonary disease. *Nursing Research, 48*(1), 9–19.

Cowan, M. J., Heinrich, J., Lucas, M., Sigmon, H., & Hinshaw, A. S. (1993). Integration of biological and nursing sciences: A 10-year plan to enhance research and training. *Research in Nursing & Health, 16*(1), 3–9.

Crisp, J., Pelletier, D., Duffield, C., Adams, A., & Nagy, S. (1997). The Delphi method? *Nursing Research, 46*(2), 116–118.

Crocker, L., & Algina, J. (1986). *Introduction to classical modern test theory.* New York: Holt, Rinehart and Winston.

Davison, M. L. (1983). *Multidimensional scaling.* New York: Wiley.

Degner, L. F. (1998). Preferences to participate in treatment decision making: The adult model. *Journal of Pediatric Oncology Nursing, 15*(3, Suppl 1), 3–9.

De Jong, P., & Miller, S. D. (1995). How to interview for client strengths. *Social Work, 40*(6), 729–736.

DeKeyser, F. G., & Pugh, L. C. (1991). Approaches to physiologic measurement. In C. F. Waltz, O. L. Strickland, & E. R. Lenz (Eds.), *Measurement in nursing research* (2nd ed., pp. 387–412). Philadelphia: Davis.

Dennis, K. E. (1986). Q methodology: Relevance and application to nursing research. *Advances in Nursing Science, 8*(3), 6–17.

Dillman, D. (1978). *Mail and telephone surveys: The total design method.* New York: Wiley.

Dillon, J. T. (1990). *The practice of questioning.* New York: Routledge.

Disney, J. A., & May, K. M. (1998, August). Focus group method for nursing research: Pleasures and pitfalls [7 pp]. Nursing Research Methods: An Electronic Journal for Nursing Researchers [Online serial], 3 (*http://www.nursing.uc.edu/nrm/disney81598.htm*).

Dunbar, S. B., & Farr, L. (1996). Temporal patterns of heart rate and blood pressure in elders. *Nursing Research, 45*(1), 43–49.

Dzurec, L. C., & Coleman, P. A. (1995). A Hermeneutic analysis of the process of conducting interviews. *Image—Journal of Nursing Scholarship, 27*(3), 245.

Emde, R. M., Gauensbauer, T. J., & Harmon, R. J. (1976). The early postnatal period: Unexplained fussiness. Emotional expression in infancy: A bio-behavioral study. *Psychological Issues, 10*(37), 80–85.

Etris, M. B., Pribble, J., & LaBrecque, J. (1994). Evaluation of two wound measurement methods in a multi-center, controlled study. *Ostomy/Wound Management, 40*(7), 44–48.

Fahs, P. S. S., & Kinney, M. R. (1991). The abdomen, thigh, and arm as sites for subcutaneous sodium heparin injections. *Nursing Research, 40*(4), 204–207.

Flaskerud, J. H. (1988). Is the Likert scale format culturally biased? *Nursing Research, 37*(3), 185–186.

Fowler, F. J. (1990). *Standardized survey interviewing: Minimizing interviewer-related error.* Newbury Park, CA: Sage.

Fox, J. A., & Tracy, P. E. (1986). *Randomized response: A method for sensitive surveys.* Beverly Hills, CA: Sage.

Gardner, R. M. (1981). Direct blood pressure measurement—dynamic response requirements. *Anesthesiology, 54*(3), 227–236.

Gentzkow, G. D. (1995). Methods for measuring size in pressure ulcers. *Advances in Wound Care, 8*(4), 43–45.

Gibbs, N. C., & Gardner, R. M. (1988). Dynamics of invasive monitoring systems: Clinical and laboratory evaluation. *Heart & Lung, 17*(1), 43–51.

Gift, A. G. (1989). Visual analogue scales: Measurement of subjective phenomena. *Nursing Research, 38*(5), 286–288.

Gobel, F. L., Nordstrom, L. A., Nelson, R. R., Jorgenson, C. R., & Wang, Y. (1978). The rate-pressure product as an index of myocardial oxygen consumption during exercise in patients with angina pectoris. *Circulation, 57*(3), 549–556.

Goodman, C. M. (1987). The Delphi technique: A critique. *Journal of Advanced Nursing, 12*(6), 729–734.

Gorden, R. L. (1987). *Interviewing: Strategy, techniques, and tactics.* Chicago: Dorsey Press.

Gordon, S. E., & Stokes, S. A. (1989). Improving response rate to mailed questionnaires. *Nursing Research, 38*(6), 375–376.

Goss, G. L. (1998). Focus group interviews: A methodology for socially sensitive research. *Clinical Excellence for Nurse Practitioners, 2*(1), 30–34.

Grunau, R. V. E., & Craig, K. D. (1987). Pain expression in neonates: Facial action and cry. *Pain, 28*(3), 395–410.

Halloran, J. P., & Grimes, D. E. (1995). Application of the focus group methodology to educational program development. *Qualitative Health Research, 5*(4), 444–453.

Hanson, G. L., Sparrow, E. M., Kokate, J. Y., Leland, K. J., & Iaizzo, P. A. (1997). *IEEE Transactions on Medical Imaging, 16*(1), 78–86.

Harding, K. G. (1995). Methods for assessing change in ulcer status. *Advances in Wound Care, 8*(4), 37–42.

Heitkemper, M., Jarrett, M., Bond, E. F., & Turner, P. (1991). GI symptoms, function, and psychophysiological arousal in dysmenorrheic women. *Nursing Research, 40*(1), 20–26.

Henneman, E. A., & Henneman, P. L. (1989). Intricacies of blood pressure measurement: Reexamining the ritual. *Heart & Lung, 18*(31), 263–271.

Hodson, K. E. (1986). Research in nursing education and practice: The ecological methods perspective. *Western Journal of Nursing Research, 8*(1), 33–48.

Holaday, B., & Turner-Henson, A. (1989). Response effects in surveys with school-age children. *Nursing Research, 38*(4), 248–250.

Hulin, C. L., Drasgow, F., & Parsons, C. K. (1983). *Item response theory: Application to psychological measurement.* Homewood, IL: Dow Jones–Irwin.

Johnson, B. H. (1990). Children's drawings as a projective technique. *Pediatric Nursing, 16*(1), 11–17.

Kahn, R., & Cannell, C. F. (1957). *The dynamics of interviewing.* New York: Wiley.

Keefe, M. R., Kotzer, A. M., Froeser-Fretz, A., & Curtin, M. (1996). A longitudinal comparison of irritable and nonirritable infants. *Nursing Research, 45*(1), 4–9.

Keefe, M. R., Kotzer, A. M., Reuss, J. L., & Sander, L. W. (1989). Development of a system for monitoring infant state behavior. *Nursing Research, 38*(6), 344–347.

Keefe, M. R., Pepper, G., & Stoner, M. (1988). Toward research-based nursing practice: The Denver Collaborative Research Network. *Applied Nursing Research, 1*(3), 109–115.

Kitzinger, J. (1995). Introducing focus groups. *British Medical Journal, 311*(7000), 299–302.

Knafl, K. A., Pettengill, M. M., Bevis, M. E., & Kirchhoff, K. T. (1988). Blending qualitative and quantitative approaches to instrument development and data collection. *Journal of Professional Nursing, 4*(1), 30–37.

Krozy, R. E., & McCarthy, N. C. (1999). Development of bilingual tools to assess functional health patterns; Ecuador. *Nursing Diagnosis, 10*(1), 21.

Kruskal, J. B., & Wish, M. (1990). *Multidimensional scaling.* Newbury Park, CA: Sage.

Lee, K. A., & Kieckhefer, G. M. (1989). Measuring human responses using visual analogue scales. *Western Journal of Nursing Research, 11*(1), 128–132.

Lindeman, C. A. (1975). Delphi survey of priorities in clinical nursing research. *Nursing Research, 24*(6), 434–441.

Liskay, A. M., Mion, L. C., & Davis, B. R. (1993). Comparison of two devices for wound measurement. *Dermatology Nursing, 5*(6), 437–441.

Lobo, M. L. (1992). Observation: A valuable data collection strategy for research with children. *Journal of Pediatric Nursing, 7*(5), 320–328.

Lodge, M. (1981). *Magnitude scaling: Quantitative measurement of opinions.* Beverly Hills, CA: Sage.

Lofland, H. (1971). *Analyzing social settings: A guide to qualitative observation and analysis.* Belmont, CA: Wadsworth.

Luniewski, M., Riegle, J. K., & White, B. (1999). Card sort: An assessment tool for the educational needs of patients with heart failure. *American Journal of Critical Care, 8*(5), 297–302.

Lynn, M. R. (1989). Instrument reliability: How much needs to be published? *Heart & Lung, 18*(4), 421–423.

McCracken, G. D. (1988). *The long interview.* Newbury Park, CA: Sage.

McKeown, B., & Thomas, D. (1988). *Q methodology.* Newbury Park, CA: Sage.

McLaughlin, P. (1990). *How to interview: The art of asking questions* (2nd ed.). North Vancouver, BC: International Self-Counsel Press.

Melhuish, J. M., Plassman, P., & Harding, K. G. (1994). Circumference, area and volume of the healing wound. *Journal of Wound Care, 3*(8), 380–384.

Mishler, E. G. (1986). *Research interviewing: Context and narrative.* Cambridge, MA: Harvard University Press.

Mitchell, M. P. (1998). Nursing education planning: A Delphi study. *Journal of Nursing Education, 37*(7), 305–307.

Morgan, D. L. (1995). Why things (sometimes) go wrong in focus groups. *Qualitative Health Research, 5*(4), 516–523.

Morrison, R. S., & Peoples, L. (1999). Using focus group methodology in nursing. *The Journal of Continuing Education in Nursing, 30*(2), 62–65.

Norbeck, J. S. (1985). What constitutes a publishable report of instrument development? *Nursing Research, 34*(6), 380–381.

Norman, E., Gadaleta, D., & Griffin, C. C. (1991). An evaluation of three blood pressure methods in a stabilized acute trauma population. *Nursing Research, 40*(2), 86–89.

Nunnally, J. C. (1978). *Psychometric theory* (2nd ed.). New York: McGraw-Hill.

Oleske, D. M., Heinze, S., & Otte, D. M. (1990). The diary as a means of understanding the quality of life of persons with cancer receiving home nursing care. *Cancer Nursing, 13*(3), 158–166.

Osgood, C. E., Suci, G. J., & Tannenbaum, P. H. (1957). *The measurement of meaning.* Urbana, IL: University of Illinois Press.

Park, M. K., & Menard, S. M. (1987). Accuracy of blood pressure measurement by the Dinamap monitor in infants and children. *Pediatrics, 79*(6), 907–914.

Pfister, S. M. (1999). Bladder diaries and voiding patterns in older adults. *Journal of Gerontological Nursing, 25*(3), 36–41.

Phillips, L. R., Hernandez, I. L., & Ardon, E. T. (1994). Strategies for achieving cultural equivalence. *Research in Nursing & Health, 17*(2), 149–154.

Plassmann, P., Melhuish, J. M., & Harding, K. G. (1994). Methods of measuring wound size: A comparative study. *Ostomy/Wound Management, 40*(7), 50–60.

Pope, D. S. (1995). Music, noise, and the human voice in the nurse-patient environment. *Image—Journal of Nursing Scholarship, 27*(4), 291–296.

Pugh, L. C., & DeKeyser, F. G. (1995). Use of physiologic variables in nursing research. *Image—Journal of Nursing Scholarship, 27*(4), 273–276.

Quine, S., & Cameron, I. (1995). The use of focus groups with the disabled elderly. *Qualitative Health Research, 5*(4), 454–462.

Ramsey, M. (1979). Noninvasive automatic determination of mean arterial pressure. *Medical and Biological Engineering and Computing, 17*(1), 11–18.

Reed, J., & Payton, V. R. (1997). Focus groups: Issues of analysis and interpretation. *Journal of Advanced Nursing, 26*(4), 765–771.

Rudy, S. F. (1996). Research forum. A review of Delphi surveys conducted to establish research priorities by specialty nursing organizations from 1985 to 1995. *ORL-Head & Neck Nursing, 14*(2), 16–24.

Saris, W. E. (1991). *Computer-assisted interviewing.* Newbury Park, CA: Sage.

Schuman, H. (1981). *Questions and answers in attitude surveys: Experiments on question form, wording, and context.* New York: Academic Press.

Sennott-Miller, L., Murdaugh, C., & Hinshaw, A. S. (1988). Magnitude estimation: Issues and practical applications. *Western Journal of Nursing Research, 10*(4), 414–424.

Shelley, S. I. (1984). *Research methods in nursing and health.* Boston: Little, Brown.

Simpson, S. H. (1989). Use of Q-sort methodology in cross-cultural nutrition and health research. *Nursing Research, 38*(5), 289–290.

Southern, D. M., Batterham, R. W., Appleby, N. J., Young, D., Dunt, D., & Guibert, R. (1999). The concept mapping method: An alternative to focus group inquiry in general practice. *Australian Family Physician, 28*(Suppl 1), 35–40.

Spector, P. E. (1992). *Summated rating scale construction: An introduction.* Newbury Park, CA: Sage.

Stevens, B., Johnston, C., Franck, L., Petryshen, P., Jack, A., & Foster, G. (1999). The efficacy of developmentally sensitive interventions and sucrose for relieving procedural pain in very low birth weight neonates. *Nursing Research, 48*(1), 35–43.

Stevens, B. J., Johnston, C., Petryshen, P., & Taddio, A. (1996). The Premature Infant Pain Profile: Development and initial validation. *Clinical Journal of Pain, 12*(1), 13–22.

Straw, R. B., & Smith, M. W. (1995). Potential uses of focus groups in Federal policy and program evaluation studies. *Qualitative Health Research, 5*(4), 421–427.

Sudman, S., & Bradburn, N. (1982). *Asking questions: A practical guide to questionnaire design.* San Francisco: Jossey-Bass.

Sutherland, J. A., Reakes, J., & Bridges, C. (1999). Foot acupressure and massage for patients with Alzheimer's disease and related dementias. *Image—Journal of Nursing Scholarship, 31*(4), 347–348.

Tetting, D. W. (1988). Q-sort update. *Western Journal of Nursing Research, 10*(6), 757–765.

Thomas, D. R. (1997). Existing tools: Are they meeting the challenges of pressure ulcer healing? *Advances in Wound Care, 10*(5), 86–90.

Thomas, K. A. (1995). Biorhythms in infants and role of the care environment. *Journal of Perinatal and Neonatal Nursing, 9*(2), 61–75.

Turner, C. F., Rogers, S. M., Hendershot, T. P., Miller, H. G., & Thornberry, J. P. (1996). Improving representation of linguistic minorities in health surveys. *Public Health Reports, 111*(3), 276–279.

Twinn, S. (1998). An analysis of the effectiveness of focus groups as a method of qualitative data collection with Chinese populations in nursing research. *Journal of Advanced Nursing, 28*(3), 654–661.

Waltz, C. F., Strickland, O. L., & Lenz, E. R. (1991). *Measurement in nursing research.* Philadelphia: Davis.

Wewers, M. E., & Lowe, N. K. (1990). A critical review of visual analogue scales in the measurement of clinical phenomena. *Research in Nursing & Health, 13*(4), 227–236.

Ziemer, M. M., Cooper, D. M., & Pigeon, J. G. (1995). Evaluation of a dressing to reduce nipple pain and improve nipple skin condition in breast-feeding women. *Nursing Research, 44*(6), 347–351.

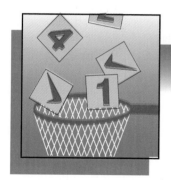

CHAPTER 17

COLLECTING AND MANAGING DATA

The initiation of data collection is one of the most exciting parts of research. After all the planning, writing, and negotiating, you are getting to the real part of research—the doing part. There is a sense of euphoria and excitement—an eagerness to get on with it. However, before you jump into data collection, spend some time carefully planning this adventure. It may save you some headaches later. Consider problems you might encounter during data collection and develop strategies for addressing them. You need to make careful plans for managing data as you collect it. This chapter is divided into three sections to assist you in planning data collection, collecting data, and managing data for quantitative studies. Data collection strategies for qualitative studies are described in Chapter 23.

PLANNING DATA COLLECTION

A *data collection plan* details how the study will be implemented. The data collection plan is specific to the study being conducted and requires consideration of some of the more prosaic elements of research. Elements that need to be planned include the procedures to be used to collect data, the time and cost of data collection, development of data collection forms that facilitate data entry, and development of a codebook.

Planning Data Collection Procedures

To plan the process of data collection, the researcher needs to determine step by step how and in what sequence data will be collected from a single subject. The timing of this process also needs to be determined. For example, how much time will be required to identify potential subjects, explain the study, and obtain consent? How much time is needed for activities such as completing questionnaires or obtaining physiological measures? Next, one needs to envision the overall activities that will be occurring during data collection. At what point are subjects assigned to groups? Will data be collected from more than one subject at a time, or is it necessary to focus attention on one subject at a time? How many subjects per day can be accessed for data given the study design and the setting? It might be helpful to conduct a trial run by collecting data from two or three subjects to get a better feel for the process. Developing a data collection tree to illustrate the process of collecting data can be helpful. An example of such a tree is shown in Figure 17–1.

Decision Points

Decision points that occur during data collection need to be identified and all options considered.

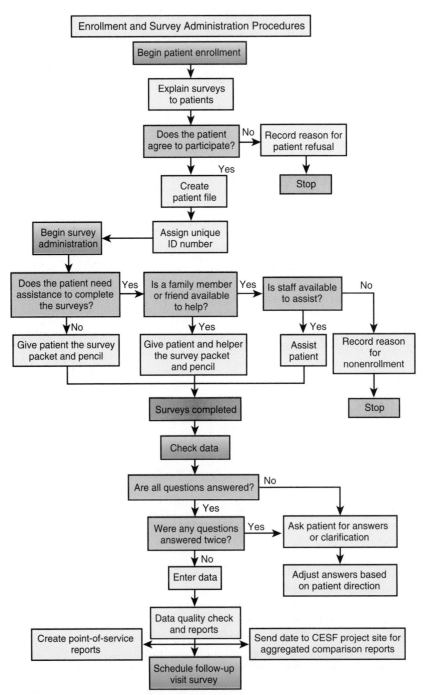

FIGURE 17–1 ▪ Data collection tree. (From Alles, P. [1995]. CESF medical outcomes research project: Implementing outcomes research in a clinical setting. *Wisconsin Medical Journal 94*[1], 27–31.)

Decisions might include things such as whether potential subjects meet the sampling criteria, whether a subject understands the information needed to give informed consent, what group the subject will be assigned to, whether the subject comprehends instructions related to providing data, and whether the subject has provided all the data needed. Each point at which a decision is made should be indicated in your data collection tree.

Consistency

Consistency in data collection across subjects is critical. If more than one data collector is used, consistency among data collectors (interrater reliability) is also necessary. Identify situations in your study that might interfere with consistency and develop a plan that will maximize consistency. The specific days and hours of data collection may influence the consistency of the data collected and thus need to be carefully considered. For example, the energy level and state of mind of subjects from whom data are gathered in the morning may differ from that of subjects from whom data are gathered in the evening. Visitors are more likely to be present at certain times of day and may interfere with data collection or influence subject responses. Patient care routines vary with the time of day. In some studies the care recently received or the care currently being provided may alter the data you gather. Subjects who are approached to participate in the study on Saturday may differ from subjects approached on weekday mornings. Subjects seeking care on Saturday may have a full-time job, whereas those seeking care on weekday mornings may be either unemployed or too ill to work.

Decisions regarding who collects the data also need to be made. Will the data all be collected by the researcher, or will data collectors be employed for this purpose? Can data collectors be nurses working in the area? Researchers have experienced difficulties in studies in which they expected nurses providing patient care to also be data collectors. Patient care will take priority over data collection, which may lead to missing data or missed subjects.

If data collectors are used, they need to be informed about the research project, familiarized with the instruments to be used, and provided equivalent training in the data collection process. In addition to training, data collectors need written guidelines that indicate which instruments to use, the order in which to introduce the instruments, how to administer the instruments, and a time frame for the data collection process (Gift et al., 1991).

After training, data collectors must be evaluated to determine their consistency in the data collection process. Washington and Moss (1988) suggest that a minimum of 10 subjects need to be rated with the complete instrument before interrater reliability can be adequately assessed. The data collectors' interrater reliability is usually assessed intermittently throughout data collection to ensure consistency. Data collectors also need to be encouraged to identify and record any problems or variations in the environment that affect the data collection process.

Time Factors

The time required for data collection is often inadequately estimated when planning a study. Data collection frequently requires two to three times longer than anticipated. It is helpful to write out a time plan for the data collection period. A pilot study can be conducted to refine the data collection process and determine the time required to collect data from a subject.

Events during the data collection period sometimes are not under the control of the researcher. Events such as a sudden heavy staff workload may make data collection temporarily difficult or impossible, or the number of potential subjects might be reduced for a period. In some situations, approval for data collection stipulates that the physician's permission be obtained for each subject before collecting data on that subject. Activities required to meet this stipulation, such as contacting physicians, explaining the study, and obtaining permission, require extensive time. In some cases, many potential subjects are lost before permission can be obtained, thus extending the time required to obtain the necessary number of subjects.

Cost Factors

Cost factors must also be examined when planning a study. Measurement tools—such as Holter monitors, spirometers, infrared thermometers, pulse oximeters, or glucometers—that are used in physiological studies may need to be rented or purchased. If questionnaires or scales must be ordered, a fee may be charged for the scale and for analyzing the data. Data collection forms must be typed and duplicated. In some cases, printing costs for materials that are to be distributed during data collection must be factored in, such as teaching materials, questionnaires, or scales. In some studies, postage is an additional expense. There may be costs involved in coding the data for entry into the computer and for conducting data analyses. Consultation with a statistician early in the development of a research project and during data analysis must also be budgeted. Sometimes it is necessary to hire a typist for the final report.

In addition to these direct costs, there are also indirect costs. The researcher's time is a cost, and costs for travel to and from the study site and for meals eaten out while working on the study must be taken into account. The expense of presenting the research project at conferences also needs to be estimated and included in a budget. To prevent unexpected expenses from delaying the study, costs need to be examined in an organized manner during the planning phase of the study. A budget is best developed early in the planning process and revised as plans are modified (see Chapter 28 for a sample budget). Seeking funding for at least part of the study costs can facilitate the conduct of a study. (See Conducting Research on a Shoestring in Chapter 29.)

Neophyte researchers have difficulty making reasonable estimates of time and costs related to a study. We advise validating the time and cost estimates with an experienced researcher. If the cost and time factors are prohibitive, the study can be simplified so that fewer variables are measured, fewer instruments are used, the design is made less complex, and fewer agencies are used for data collection. These modifications are serious changes in a study, and their impact must be thoroughly examined before revisions are made. If time or cost estimates go beyond expectations, the time schedules and budget can be revised with a new projection for completing the study.

Developing Data Collection Forms

Before data collection begins, the researcher may need to develop or modify forms on which to record data. These forms can be used to record demographic data, information from the patient record, observations, or values from physiological measures. The demographic variables commonly collected in nursing studies include age, gender, race, education, income or socioeconomic status, employment status, diagnosis, and marital status. Other data that may be either extraneous or confounding need to be collected and might include variables such as the subject's physician, stage of illness, length of illness or hospitalization, complications, date of data collection, time of day and day of week of data collection, and any untoward events that occur during the data collection period. In some cases, the length of time required of individual subjects for data collection may be a confounding variable and needs to be recorded. If it is necessary to contact the subject at a later time, the subject's address and telephone number must be obtained, but only with that person's awareness and permission. Names and phone numbers of family members may also be useful if subjects are likely to move or be difficult to contact. The importance of each piece of datum and the amount of the subject's time required to collect it need to be considered. If the data can be obtained from patient records or any other written sources, the subject should not be asked to provide this information.

Data collection forms need to be designed to allow ease in recording during data collection and for easy entry into the computer. A decision must be made about whether data are collected in raw form or coded at the time of collection. *Coding* is the process of transforming data into numerical symbols that can be entered easily into the computer. For example, the measurement of variables such as gender, ethnicity, and diagnoses produces data that can be categorized and given numerical labels. Gender has two categories, female and male, and the female category could be identified by a 1 and the male category by a 2. The variable of ethnicity might include four categories: white, African American, Hispanic, and other. The white category could be represented by the numerical label of 1, African American by a 2, Hispanic by a 3, and other by a 4.

The coding categories developed for a study must be mutually exclusive but exhaustive, which means that the value for a specific variable fits into only one category, and each observation must fit into a category. For example, the salary ranges would not be mutually exclusive if they were categorized as (1) $30,000 to 35,000; (2) $35,000 to 40,000; (3) $40,000 to 45,000; (4) $45,000 to 50,000; and (5) $50,000 and more. These categories overlap, so a subject with a $45,000 income could mark category 3 or 4, or both. For many items, a code for "other" should be included for unexpected classifications of variables such as marital status or ethnicity.

A number of response styles can be selected for use on the data collection form. The person completing the form (subject or data collector) might be asked to check a blank space before or after the words male or female, to circle the word male or female, or to write a 1 or a 2 in a blank space before or after the word selected. If codes are used, the codes should be indicated on the collection forms for easy access by the individual completing the form.

Placement of data on data collection forms is important for ease in completing the form and locating responses for computer entry. Placement of blanks on the left side of the page seems to be most efficient for data entry but may be problematic when subjects are completing the forms. The least effective is the placement of data irregularly on the form. In this case, the risk of data being missed during data entry is high. Subjects' names should not be on the data collection forms; only the subject's identification number should appear. A master list of subjects and associated coding numbers can be kept separately by the researcher.

DATA COLLECTION FORM

Demographics

____ Subject Indentification Number
____ Age
____ Gender
1. Male
2. Female
____ Weight (in pounds)
____ Height (in inches)
__________ Surgical Procedure Performed
__/__/__ Surgery Date (Month/Day/Year)
__/__/__ Surgery Time (Hour/Minute/AM or PM)
Narcotics Ordered After Surgery__________
____

Narcotic Administation

	Date	Time	Narcotic	Dose
1.				
2.				
3.				
4.				
5.				

Instruction on Use of Pain Scale

__/__/__ Date (Month/Day/Year)
__/__/__ Time (Hour/Minute/AM or PM)
Comments:

____Treatment Group
1. TENS
2. Placebo-TENS
3. No-Treatment Control

Treatment Implemented

__/__/__ Date (Month/Day/Year)
__/__/__ Time (Hour/Minute/AM or PM)
Comments:

FIGURE 17–2 ■ Example of a data collection form.

A sample data collection form is provided in Figure 17–2. This data collection form includes four items that could be problematic in terms of coding or data analysis, or both. The blank used to enter Surgical Procedure Performed will lead to problems devising effective ways to enter the data into a computerized data set. Because multiple surgical procedures could have been performed, developing codes for the various surgical procedures would be difficult and time-consuming. In addition, the same surgical procedure could be recorded with different wording. It may be necessary to tally the surgical procedures manually. Unless this degree of

Dressing Change
__/__/__ Date (Month/Day/Year)
__/__/__ Time (Hour/Minute/AM or PM)
_____ Hours since surgery
Comments:

Measurement of Pain
_____Score on Visual Analogue Pain Scale
__/__/__ Date Pain Measured
           (Month/Day/Year)
__/__/__ Time Pain Measured
           (Hour/Minute/AM or PM)
Comments:

_____ Data Collector Code
Comments:

FIGURE 17–2 ■ *Continued.*

specification of procedures is important to the study, an alternative would be to develop larger categories of procedures before data collection and place the categories on the data collection form. A category of "other" might be useful for less commonly performed procedures. This method would require the data collector to make a judgment regarding which category was appropriate for a particular surgical procedure. Another option would be to write in the category code number for a particular surgical procedure after the data collection form is completed but before data entry. Similar problems occur with the items Narcotics Ordered After Surgery and Narcotic Administration. Unless these data are to be used in statistical analyses, it might be advisable to manually categorize this information for descriptive purposes. If these items are needed for planned statistical procedures, careful thought is required to develop appropriate codes. In this study, the researcher might be interested in determining differences in the amount of narcotics administered in a given period in relation to weight and height. Recording the treatment groups on the data collection

form may be problematic because the information could influence the data recorded by the data collector.

Developing a Codebook for Data Definitions

A *codebook* identifies and defines each variable in your study and includes an abbreviated variable name (limited to six to eight characters), a descriptive variable label, and the range of possible numerical values of every variable entered in a computer file. Some codebooks also identify the source of each datum, thus linking your codebook with your data collection forms and scales. The codebook keeps you in control and provides a safety net for you when accessing the data later. Some computer programs, such as SPSS for Windows, will allow you to print out your data definitions after setting up a database. Figure 17–3 is an example of data definitions from SPSS for Windows. Another example of coding is presented in Figure 17–4.

Developing a logical method of abbreviating variable names can be challenging. For example, you might use a quality-of-life (QOL) questionnaire in your study. It will be necessary for you to develop an abbreviated variable name for each item in the questionnaire. For example, the fourth item on a QOL questionnaire might be given the abbreviated variable name QOL4. A question asking the last time you visited your mother might be abbreviated Lstvisit. Although abbreviated variable names usually seem logical at the time the name is created, it is easy to confuse or forget these names unless they are clearly documented.

It is advisable that your codebook be developed before initiating data collection. This practice provides a means for you to identify places in your forms that might prove to be a problem during data entry because of lack of clarity. Also, you may find that a single question contains not one but five variables. For example, an item might ask whether the subject received support from her or his mother, father, sister, brother, or other relatives and ask that those who provided support be circled. You might think that you could code mother as 1, father as 2, sister as 3, brother as 4, and other as 5. However,

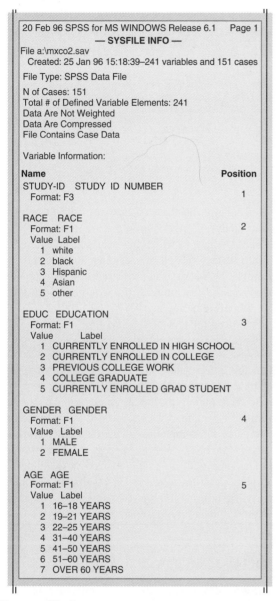

```
20 Feb 96 SPSS for MS WINDOWS Release 6.1    Page 1
             — SYSFILE INFO —
File a:\mxco2.sav
   Created: 25 Jan 96 15:18:39–241 variables and 151 cases

File Type: SPSS Data File

N of Cases: 151
Total # of Defined Variable Elements: 241
Data Are Not Weighted
Data Are Compressed
File Contains Case Data


Variable Information:

Name                                         Position
STUDY-ID   STUDY ID NUMBER
   Format: F3                                     1

RACE   RACE                                       2
   Format: F1
   Value  Label
      1  white
      2  black
      3  Hispanic
      4  Asian
      5  other

EDUC   EDUCATION
   Format: F1                                     3
   Value      Label
      1  CURRENTLY ENROLLED IN HIGH SCHOOL
      2  CURRENTLY ENROLLED IN COLLEGE
      3  PREVIOUS COLLEGE WORK
      4  COLLEGE GRADUATE
      5  CURRENTLY ENROLLED GRAD STUDENT

GENDER   GENDER
   Format: F1                                     4
   Value  Label
      1  MALE
      2  FEMALE

AGE   AGE
   Format: F1                                     5
   Value  Label
      1  16–18 YEARS
      2  19–21 YEARS
      3  22–25 YEARS
      4  31–40 YEARS
      5  41–50 YEARS
      6  51–60 YEARS
      7  OVER 60 YEARS
```

```
Name                                         Position
INCOME   ANNUAL INCOME                           6
   Format: F1
   Value  Label
      1  <$10,000
      2  $10,000–$19,999
      3  $20,000–$29,999
      4  $30,000–$39,999
      5  $40,000–$49,999
      6  >$50,000

AHEALTH   OVERALL HEALTH STATUS                  55
   Format: F1
   Value  Label
      1  EXCELLENT
      2  GOOD
      3  FAIR
      4  POOR

AEXP1   EXPECT PRE 1 EXPECT MEXICANS             56
TO BE FRIENDLY
FORMAT: F1
   Value  Label
      0  NO
      1  YES

AEXP2   EXPECT PRE 2 EXPECT TO USE PUBLIC        57
TRANSPORTATION
   Format: F1
   Value  Label
      0  NO
      1  YES

AEXP3   EXPECT PRE 3 EXPECT TO MAKE              58
FRIENDS WITH MEXICANS
   Format: F1
   Value  Label
      0  NO
      1  YES

AEXP4   EXPECT PRE 4 EXPECT TO UNDERSTAND  59
MEXICAN HUMOR
   Format: F1
   Value  Label
      0  NO
      1  YES

AEXP5   EXPECT PRE 5 EXPECT MEXICANS TO BE  60
POLITE/HELPFUL
   Format: F1
   Value  Label
      0  NO
      1  YES
```

FIGURE 17–3 ■ Example of data definitions from SPSS for Windows.

because the individual can circle more than one, each relative must be coded separately. Thus, mother is one variable and would be coded 1 if circled and 0 if not circled. The father would be coded similarly as a second variable, and so on.

Identifying these items before data collection may allow you to restructure the item on the questionnaire or data collection form to facilitate easier entry into the computer.

The codebook with its data definitions should be given to the individual or individuals who will enter

Name	Position
SOCMID1 SOC SIT MID 1 FRIENDS	78

Format: F1
Value Label
1 NEVER EXPERIENCED
2 NO DIFFICULTY
3 SLIGHT DIFFICULTY
4 MODERATE DIFFICULTY
5 GREAT DIFFICULTY
6 EXTREME DIFFICULTY

Name	Position
SOCMID2 SOC SIT MID 2 SHOPPING	79

Format: F1
Value Label
1 NEVER EXPERIENCED
2 NO DIFFICULTY
3 SLIGHT DIFFICULTY
4 MODERATE DIFFICULTY
5 GREAT DIFFICULTY
6 EXTREME DIFFICULTY

Name	Position
SOCMID3 SOC SIT MID 3 PUB TRANSPORTATION	80

Format: F1
Value Label
1 NEVER EXPERIENCED
2 NO DIFFICULTY
3 SLIGHT DIFFICULTY
4 MODERATE DIFFICULTY
5 GREAT DIFFICULTY
6 EXTREME DIFFICULTY

Name	Position
SOCMID5 SOC SIT MID 5 MAKING MEXICAN FRIENDS	82

Format: F1
Value Label
1 NEVER EXPERIENCED
2 NO DIFFICULTY
3 SLIGHT DIFFICULTY
4 MODERATE DIFFICULTY
5 GREAT DIFFICULTY
6 EXTREME DIFFICULTY

Name	Position
SOCMID12 SOC SIT MID 12 BEING WITH OLDER MEXICAN PEOLPLE	89

Format: F1
Value Label
1 NEVER EXPERIENCED
2 NO DIFFICULTY
3 SLIGHT DIFFICULTY
4 MODERATE DIFFICULTY
5 GREAT DIFFICULTY
6 EXTREME DIFFICULTY

FIGURE 17–3 ■ *See legend on preceding page.*

Name	Position
SOCMID13 SOC SIT MID 13 MEETING STRANGERS/NEW PEOPLE	90

Format: F1
Value Label
1 NEVER EXPERIENCED
2 NO DIFFICULTY
3 SLIGHT DIFFICULTY
4 MODERATE DIFFICULTY
5 GREAT DIFFICULTY
6 EXTREME DIFFICULTY

3. Information on the statistical package to be used for analysis of the data
4. The database in which the data will be entered
5. Information related to receiving the data, for example, whether you will deliver the data in batches or wait until all the data have been gathered before delivering it
6. Estimated number of subjects
7. Planned date for delivering the data

With this information, the assistant can develop the database in preparation for receiving the data for entry. Preparation of the database will require an average of 16 hours of concentrated work. Approximate dates for completion of the data entry work or analyses, or both, need to be negotiated before beginning data collection. If you have a deadline for completion or presentation of results at a conference, this information should be shared with those performing data entry/analysis.

COLLECTING DATA

Data collection is the process of selecting subjects and gathering data from these subjects. The actual steps of collecting the data are specific to each study and are dependent on the research design and measurement methods. Data may be collected on subjects by observing, testing, measuring, questioning, or recording, or any combination of these methods. The researcher is actively involved in this process either by collecting data or by supervising data collectors. Effective people management and problem-solving skills are used constantly as data collection tasks are implemented, kinks in the

your data into the computer *before initiating data collection,* in addition to the following information:

1. Copies of all scales, questionnaires, and data collection forms to be used in the study
2. Information on the location of every variable on scales, questionnaires, or data collection forms

Variable Name	Variable Label	Source	Value Levels	Valid Range	Missing Data	Comments
A1 to A5	Family Apgar	Q2Family Apgar	1=never 2=hardly ever 3=some of the time 4= almost always 5=always	1 – 5	9	Code as is (CAI)
MF3	Mother's feeling, Day 3	Tuesday diary, mother	1=poor 6=good	1 – 6	9	Code 1 to 6 left to right

FIGURE 17–4 ■ Example of coding. (From Lobo, M. L. [1993]. Code books—a critical link in the research process. *Western Journal of Nursing Research, 15*[3], 380.)

research plan are resolved, and support systems are used.

Data Collection Tasks

In both quantitative and qualitative research, the investigator performs four tasks during the process of data collection. These tasks are interrelated and occur concurrently rather than in sequence. The tasks include selecting subjects, collecting data in a consistent way, maintaining research controls as indicated in the study design, and solving problems that threaten to disrupt the study. Selecting subjects is discussed in Chapter 14. Data collection tasks for qualitative studies are discussed in more detail in Chapter 23.

COLLECTING DATA

Collecting data may involve administering written scales, asking subjects to complete data collection forms, or recording data from observations or from the patient record. Sometimes subjects are asked to enter data on Scantron sheets that can be entered directly into the computer by optic scanner (Dennis, 1994). This practice speeds up the process of entering data and reduces errors related to data entry. However, subjects may be reluctant to use scantron sheets, and some inaccuracies in data may occur because of subject error in completing these sheets.

With the advent of microcomputers, data collectors can code data directly into a microcomputer at the data collection site. If a computer is used for data collection, a program must be written for entering the data. If a computer programmer is hired for this purpose, there is, of course, a fee involved. A microcomputer enables collection of large amounts of data with few errors. Questionnaires might be placed within the microcomputer so that the subject could enter responses directly into the computer. Small data collection machines are also available to allow the researcher to code data into the machine from observations as they occur.

Advancements in technology have made it possible to interface bioinstruments with computers for data collection. The advantages of using computers for the acquisition and storage of physiological data from bioinstruments are listed by Harrison (1989).

1. Increased accuracy and reliability are achieved by reducing errors that may occur when manually recording or transcribing physiologic data from patient monitors or other clinical instruments.
2. Linking microcomputers with biomedical instruments (e.g., cardiac, respiratory, blood pressure, or oxygen saturation monitors) permits more frequent acquisition and storage of larger amounts of data (e.g., once or more per second) than is practical with manual recording procedures.
3. Once established, computerized data acquisition systems save researcher time during both the data collection and analysis phases of research.
4. Even though the initial cost of equipment may be high, over the long run computerized data collection systems are less expensive, more efficient, and more reliable than hiring and training multiple human data collectors. (Harrison, 1989, p. 131)

The use of computers for data collection also has disadvantages. The microcomputer and the equipment required to interface it with the bioinstruments take up space in an already crowded clinical setting. Purchasing the equipment, setting it up, and installing the software can be time-consuming and expensive at the start of the research project. Another concern is that the nurse researcher will focus mainly on the machine and neglect observing and interacting with the patient. The most serious disadvantage is the possibility of measurement error that can occur with equipment malfunctions and software errors, although these problems can be reduced with regular maintenance and reliability checks of the equipment and software.

Lookinland and Appel (1991) used a microcomputer interfaced with bioinstruments to collect data for their article "Hemodynamic and Oxygen Transport Changes Following Endotracheal Suctioning in Trauma Patients" (p. 133) .

. . . .

"Data from the transcutaneous oxygen sensor and the pulse oximeter were obtained via the analogue interfaces of the instruments. The voltage was converted by a specially designed 16-channel analogue to digital conversion board installed in a NEC PCII microcomputer. Custom database software was used for acquisition and storage of data at specified intervals. Data were then available for retrieval and display in numeric or graphic form by a variety of commercially available software packages. Use of analogue interfaces allowed continuous monitoring during the suction episodes." (Lookinland & Appel, 1991, p. 135) ■

MAINTAINING CONTROLS

Maintaining consistency and controls during subject selection and data collection protects the integrity or validity of the study. Research controls were built into the design to minimize the influence of intervening forces on the study findings. Maintenance of these controls is essential. These controls are not natural in a field setting, and letting them slip is easy. In some cases, these controls slip without the researcher realizing it. In addition to maintaining the controls identified in the plan, the re-

searcher needs to continually watch for previously unidentified extraneous variables that might have an impact on the data being collected. These variables are often specific to a study and tend to become apparent during the data collection period. The extraneous variables identified during data collection must be considered during data analysis and interpretation. These variables also need to be noted in the research report to allow future researchers to control them.

PROBLEM SOLVING

Problems can be perceived either as a frustration or as a challenge. The fact that the problem occurred is not as important as the success of problem resolution. Therefore, the final and perhaps most important task of the data collection period may be problem resolution. Little has been written about the problems encountered by nurse researchers. Research reports often read as though everything went smoothly. The implication is that if you are a good researcher, you will have no problems, which is not true. Research journals generally do not provide sufficient space to allow a description of the problems encountered, and inexperienced researchers may get a false impression. A more realistic picture can be obtained through personal discussions with researchers about the process of data collection. Some of the common problems experienced by researchers are discussed in the following section.

Data Collection Problems

Murphy's law (if anything can go wrong, it will, and at the worst possible time) seems to prevail at times in research, just as in other dimensions of life. For example, data collection frequently requires more time than was anticipated, and collecting the data is often more difficult than was expected. Sometimes changes must be made in the way the data are collected, in the specific data collected, or in the timing of data collection. People react to the study in unpredicted ways. Institutional changes may force modifications in the research plan, or unusual or unexpected events may occur. The researcher must be as consistent as possible in data collection but must also be flexible in dealing with unforeseen problems. Sometimes, sticking with the original plan at all costs is a mistake. Skills in finding ways to resolve problems that will protect the integrity of the study can be critical.

In preparation for data collection, possible problems need to be anticipated, and possible solutions for these problems need to be explored. In the following discussion, some of the common problems and concerns are described, and possible solutions are presented. Problems that tend to occur with some regularity in studies have been categorized as people problems, researcher problems, institutional problems, and event problems.

PEOPLE PROBLEMS

Nurses cannot place a subject in a test tube in a laboratory, instill one drop of the independent variable, and then measure the effect. Nursing studies are conducted by examining subjects in interaction with their environment. When research involves people, nothing is completely predictable. People, in their complexity and wholeness, have an impact on all aspects of nursing studies. Researchers, potential subjects, family members of subjects, health professionals, institutional staff, and others ("innocent bystanders") interact within the study situation. These interactions need to be closely observed and evaluated by the researcher for their impact on the study.

Problems Selecting a Sample

The first step in initiating data collection—selecting a sample—may be the beginning of people problems. The researcher may find that few available people fit the sample criteria or that many of those approached refuse to participate in the study even though the request seems reasonable. Appropriate subjects, who were numerous a month previously, seem to have disappeared. Institutional procedures may change, which might result in many potential subjects becoming ineligible for participation in the study. The sample criteria may have to be reevaluated or additional sources for potential subjects sought. In research institutions that provide care for the indigent, patients tend to be reluctant to participate in research. This lack of participation might be due to exposure to frequent studies, a

feeling of being manipulated, or a misunderstanding of the research. Patients may feel that they are being used or are afraid that they will be harmed.

Subject Mortality

After a sample has been selected, certain problems might cause subject mortality (a loss of subjects from the study). For example, some subjects may agree to participate but then fail to follow through. Some may not complete needed forms and questionnaires or may fill them out incorrectly. Researcher supervision while the subjects complete essential documents reduces these problems. Some subjects may not return for a second interview or may not be home for a scheduled visit. Although time has been invested in data collection with these subjects, their data may have to be excluded from analysis because of incompleteness.

Sometimes subjects must be dropped from the study because of changes in health status. For example, the patient may be transferred out of intensive care where the study is being conducted; the patient's condition may worsen, so he or she may no longer meet sample criteria; or the patient may die. Clinic patients may be transferred to another clinic or be discharged from the service. In the community, subjects may choose to discontinue services, or the limits of third-party reimbursement may force discontinuation of services that are being studied.

Subject mortality occurs, to some extent, in all studies. One way to deal with this problem is to anticipate the mortality rate and increase the planned number of subjects to ensure a minimally desired number of subjects who will complete the study. If subject mortality is higher than expected, the researcher may consider continuing data collection for a longer period to achieve an adequate sample size. Completing the study with a smaller than expected sample size may become necessary. If so, the effect of a smaller sample on the power of planned statistical analyses needs to be considered because the smaller sample may not be adequate to test the hypotheses.

Subject as an Object

The quality of interactions between the researcher and subjects during the study is a critical dimension for maintaining subject participation. When researchers are under pressure to complete a study, people can be treated as objects rather than as subjects. In addition to being unethical, such treatment also alters interactions, diminishes the subject's satisfaction in serving as a subject, and increases subject mortality. Subjects are scarce resources and must be treated with care. The researcher's treatment of the subject as an object can lead to similar treatment by other health care providers and result in poor quality of care. In this case, participation in the study becomes detrimental to the subject.

External Influences on Subject Responses

People interacting with the subject or researcher, or both, can have an important impact on the data collection process. Family members may not agree to the subject's participation in the study or may not understand the study process. These people will, in most cases, influence the subject's decisions related to the study. In many studies, time needs to be invested in explaining the study and seeking the cooperation of family members. Family cooperation is essential when the potential subject is critically ill and unable to give informed consent.

Family members or other patients may also influence the subject's responses to questionnaires or interview questions. In some cases, subjects may ask family members, friends, or other patients to complete study forms for them. Questions asked on the forms may be discussed with whomever happens to be in the room, and therefore the subjects' real feelings may not be those recorded on the questionnaire. If interviews are conducted while other persons are in the room, the subject's responses may be dependent on his or her need to respond in ways expected by the other persons. Sometimes, questions addressed verbally to the patient may be answered by a family member. Thus the setting in which a questionnaire is completed or an interview is conducted may determine the extent to which the answers are a true reflection of the subject's feelings. If the privacy afforded by the setting varies from one subject to another, the subjects' responses may also vary.

Usually, the most desirable setting is a private

area away from distractions. If such a setting is not possible, the presence of the researcher at the time that the questionnaire is completed may decrease the influence of others. If the questionnaire is to be completed later or taken home and returned at a later time, the probability of influence by others increases and the return of questionnaires greatly decreases. The impact of this problem on the integrity of the study depends on the nature of the questionnaire.

Passive Resistance

Health professionals and institutional staff working with the subject may affect the data collection process. Some professionals will verbalize strong support for the study and yet passively interfere with data collection. For example, nurses providing care may fail to follow the guidelines agreed on for providing the specific care activities being studied, or information needed for the study may be left off patient records. The researcher may not be informed of the admission of a potential subject, and a physician who has agreed that his or her patients can be study subjects may decide as each patient is admitted that this one is not quite right for the study. In addition, the physician might become unusually unavailable to the researcher.

Nonprofessional staff may not realize the impact of the data collection process on their work patterns until the process is initiated. Their beliefs about how care should be provided (and has been provided for the last 20 years) may be violated by the data collection process. If ignored, their resistance can lead to the complete undoing of a carefully designed study. For example, research on skin care may disrupt a nursing aide's bathing routine, so he or she continues the normal routine regardless of the study protocol and invalidates the study findings.

Because of the potential impact of these problems, the researcher needs to maintain open communication and nurture positive relationships with other professionals and staff during data collection. Problems that are recognized early and dealt with promptly have fewer serious consequences for the study than do those that are ignored. However, not all problems can be resolved. Sometimes it is necessary to find creative ways to work around an individual or to counter the harmful consequences of passive resistance.

RESEARCHER PROBLEMS

Some problems are a consequence of the interaction of the researcher with the study situation or lack of skill in data collection techniques. These problems are often difficult to identify because of the personal involvement of the researcher. However, their effect on the study can be serious.

Researcher Interactions

The researcher can become so involved in interactions with people involved in the study that data collection on the subject is not completed. Researcher interactions can also interfere with data collection in interview situations. If the researcher is collecting data while surrounded by familiar professionals with whom he or she typically interacts socially and professionally, it is sometimes difficult to focus completely on the study situation. This lack of attention usually leads to loss of data.

Lack of Skill in Data Collection Techniques

The researcher's skill in using a particular data collection technique can affect the quality of the data collected. A researcher who is unskilled at the beginning of data collection might practice the data collection techniques with the assistance of an experienced researcher. A pilot study to test data collection techniques can be helpful. If data collectors are being used, they also need opportunities to practice data collection techniques before the study is initiated. If skill is developed during the study itself, as skill increases the data being collected may change and thereby confound the study findings and threaten the validity of the study. If more than one data collector is used, changes in skill can occur more frequently than if the researcher is the data collector. The skills of data collectors need to be evaluated during the study to detect any changes in their data collection techniques.

Researcher Role Conflict

Professional nurses conducting clinical research often experience a conflict between the researcher role and the clinician role during data collection. As a researcher, one is observing and recording events. In some cases, involvement of the researcher in the event, such as providing physical or emotional care to a patient during an interview, could alter the event and thus bias the results. It would be difficult to generalize the findings to other situations in which the researcher was not present to intervene. In some situations, however, the needs of patients must take precedence over the needs of the study. The dilemma is to determine when the needs of patients are great enough to warrant researcher intervention.

Some patient situations are life threatening, such as respiratory distress and changes in cardiac function, and require immediate action by anyone present. Other patient needs are simple, are expected of any nurse available, and are not likely to alter the results of the study. Examples of these interventions include giving the patient a bedpan, informing the nurse of the patient's need for pain medication, or assisting the patient in opening food containers. These situations seldom cause a dilemma.

Solutions to other situations are not as easy. Suppose, for example, that the study involved examining emotional responses of patients' family members during and immediately after the patients' operations. The study included an experimental group that received one 30-minute family support session before and during the patients' operations and a control group that received no support session. Both sets of families are being monitored for 1 week after the surgeries to measure their levels of anxiety and coping strategies. The researcher is currently collecting data on the control group. The data consist of demographic information and scales measuring anxiety and coping. One of the family members is in great distress. After completing the demographic information, she verbally expresses her fears and the lack of support she has received from the nursing staff. Two other subjects from different families hear the expressed distress and concur; they move closer to the conversation and look to the researcher. In this situation, supportive responses from the researcher are likely to modify the results of the study because these responses are part of the treatment to be provided to the experimental group. This interaction is likely to narrow the difference between the two groups and thus decrease the possibility of showing a significant difference between the two groups. How should the researcher respond? Is there an obligation to provide support? To some extent, almost any response by the researcher will be supportive. One alternative is to provide the needed support and not include these family members in the control group. Another alternative is to recruit the help of a nonprofessional to collect the data from the control group. However, one must recognize that most people will provide some degree of support in the described situation, even though their skills in supportive techniques may vary.

Other dilemmas include witnessing unethical behavior that interferes with patient care or witnessing subjects' unethical or illegal behavior (Field & Morse, 1985). These dilemmas need to be anticipated before data collection whenever possible. Pilot studies can be helpful in identifying dilemmas likely to occur in a study, and strategies can be built into the design to minimize or avoid them. However, some dilemmas cannot be anticipated and must be responded to spontaneously. There is no prescribed way to handle difficult dilemmas; each case must be dealt with individually. We recommend discussing unethical and illegal behavior with colleagues, members of ethics committees, or legal advisors. After the dilemma is resolved, it is wise to reexamine the situation for its effect on study results and consider options in case the situation arises again.

Maintaining Perspective

Data collection includes both joys and frustrations. Researchers need to be able to maintain some degree of objectivity during the process and yet not take themselves too seriously. A sense of humor is invaluable. One must be able to feel the emotions experienced and then move to being the rational problem solver. Management skills and mental health are invaluable to a lifetime researcher.

INSTITUTIONAL PROBLEMS

Institutions are in a constant state of change. They will not stop changing for the period of a study, and these changes often affect data collec-

tion. A nurse who has been most helpful in the study may be promoted or transferred. The unit on which the study is conducted may be reorganized, moved, or closed during the study. An area used for subjects' interviews may be transformed into an office or a storeroom or may be torn down. Patient record forms may be revised, omitting data that were being collected. The record room personnel may be reorganizing their files and be temporarily unable to provide needed charts.

These problems are, for the most part, completely outside the control of the researcher. It is helpful to "keep an ear" to the internal communication network of the institution for advanced warning of impending changes. Contacts within the administrative decision-making system of the institution could facilitate communication about the impact of proposed changes on an ongoing study. However, in many cases, data collection strategies might have to be modified to meet the newly emerging situation. Again, flexibility while maintaining the integrity of the study may be the key to continuing successful data collection. Byers (1995) suggests that the home setting may be more desirable in the future as a data collection site than institutions and that the response rate in this setting is better than that in institutions. The disadvantage is that home visits are time intensive and the subject may not be home at the agreed appointment time.

EVENT PROBLEMS

Unpredictable events can be a source of frustration during a study. Research tools ordered from a testing company may be lost in the mail. The duplicating machine may break down just before 500 data collection forms are to be copied, or a machine to be used in data collection may break down and require 6 weeks for repair. A computer ordered for data collection may not arrive when promised, a tape recorder may become jammed in the middle of an interview, or after an interview the data collector may discover that the play button on the recorder had been pushed rather than the record button and there is no record of the interview. Data collection forms may be misplaced, misfiled, or lost.

Local, national, or world events and nature can also influence subjects' responses to a study. For example, one of our graduate students was examining patients' attitudes toward renal dialysis. She planned to collect data for 6 months. Three months into data collection, three patients died as a result of a dialysis machine malfunction in the city where the study was being conducted. The event made national headlines. Obviously, this event could be expected to modify subjects' responses. In attempting to deal with the impact of the event on the study, the graduate student could have modified the study and continued collecting data to examine the impact of news such as this on attitudes. However, the emotional climate of the clinics participating in the study was not conducive to this option. She chose to wait 3 months before collecting additional data and examined the data before and after the event for statistically significant differences in responses. Because no differences were found, she could justify using all the data for analysis.

Other less dramatic events can also have an impact on data collection. If data collection for the entire sample is planned for a single time, a snowstorm or a flood may require canceling the meeting or clinic. Weather may decrease attendance far below that expected at a support group or series of teaching sessions. A bus strike can disrupt transportation systems to such an extent that subjects can no longer get to the data collection site. A new health agency may open in the city, which may decrease demand for the care activities being studied. Conversely, an external event can also increase attendance at clinics to such an extent that existing resources are stretched and data collection is no longer possible. These events are also outside the control of the researcher and are impossible to anticipate. In most cases, however, restructuring the data collection period can salvage the study. To do so, it is necessary to examine all possible alternatives for collecting the study data. In some cases, data collection can simply be rescheduled; in other situations, the changes needed may be more complex.

SERENDIPITY

Serendipity is the accidental discovery of something useful or valuable. During the data collection phase of studies, researchers often become aware of elements or relationships not previously identified.

These aspects may be closely related to the study being conducted or have little connection with it. They come from increased awareness and close observation of the study situation. Because the researcher is focused on close observation, other elements in the situation can come into clearer focus and take on new meaning. This situation is similar to the open context discussed in Chapter 4. The researcher's perspective shifts, and new gestalts are formed.

Serendipitous findings are important to the development of new insights in nursing theory. They can be important in understanding the totality of the phenomenon being examined. Additionally, they lead to areas of research that generate new knowledge. Therefore, it is essential to capture these insights as they occur. These events need to be carefully recorded, even if their impact or meaning is not understood at the time. Sometimes, when these notes are reexamined at a later time, patterns begin to emerge.

Serendipitous findings can also lead the researcher astray. Sometimes researchers forget the original plan and move right into examining the newly discovered dimensions. Although modifying data collection to include data related to the new discovery may be valid, the researcher must remember that there has not been time to carefully plan a study related to the new findings. Examination of the new data should only be an offshoot of the initial study. Data collected as a result of serendipitous findings can guide future studies and need to be included in presentations and publications related to the study. Although the meaning of the discovery may not be understood, sharing the information may lead to insights by researchers studying related phenomena.

HAVING ACCESS TO SUPPORT SYSTEMS

The researcher must have access to individuals or groups who can provide support and consultation during the data collection period. Support systems themselves have been the subject of much study in recent years. In some cases, support systems can be the source of both stress and support. However, current theorists propose that to be classified as support, the individual or group must enhance the ego strength of the individual. Three dimensions of support have been identified: (1) physical assistance, (2) provision of money or other concrete needs such as equipment or information, and (3) emotional support. These types of support can usually be obtained from academic committees, from institutions serving as research settings, and from colleagues, friends, and family.

Support of Academic Committees

Although thesis and dissertation committees are basically seen as stern keepers of the sanctity of the research process, they also serve as support systems for neophyte researchers. In fact, committee members need to be selected from faculty who are willing and able to provide the needed support. Experienced researchers among faculty are usually more knowledgeable about the types of support needed. Because they are directly involved in research, they tend to be sensitive to the needs of neophyte researchers.

Institutional Support

A support system within the institution where the study is being conducted is also important. Support might be provided by people serving on the institutional research committee or by nurses working on the unit where the study is to be conducted. These people often have knowledge of how the institution functions, and their closeness to the study can increase their understanding of the problems experienced by the researcher and subjects. Their ability to provide useful suggestions and assistance must not be overlooked. Resolution of some of the problems encountered during data collection may be dependent on having someone within the power structure of the institution who can intervene.

Personal Support

In addition to professional support, it is helpful to have at least one significant other with whom one can share the joys, frustrations, and current problems of data collection. A significant other can often serve as a mirror to allow you to see the

situation clearly and perhaps more objectively. Through personal support, feelings can be shared and released so that the researcher can achieve distance from the data collection situation. Discussions of alternatives for problem resolution can then occur. Data collection is a demanding, but rewarding, time that increases the confidence and expertise of the neophyte researcher.

MANAGING DATA

When data collection begins, the researcher will have to handle large quantities of paper. The situation can quickly grow to a state of total confusion unless careful plans are made before data collection begins. Plans are needed to keep all data from a single subject together until analysis is begun. The subject code number is written on each form, and the forms for each subject are checked to ensure they are all present. Researchers have been known to sort their data by form, such as putting all the scales of one kind together, only to realize afterward that they had failed to code the forms with subject identification numbers first. They then had no idea which scale belonged to which subject, and valuable data were lost.

Space needs to be allotted for storing forms. File folders could be purchased, and a labeling method could be designed to allow easy access to data; color coding is often useful. For example, if multiple forms are being used, the subject's demographic sheet could be one color, with different colors for the visual analogue scale; the pain questionnaire; the physiological data sheet with blood pressure, pulse, and respiration readings; and the interview notes. Envelopes can be used to hold small pieces of paper or note cards that might fall out of a file folder. Plans need to be made to code data and enter them into the computer as soon as possible after data collection to help reduce the loss or disorganization of data.

Preparing Data for Computer Entry

Data need to be carefully checked and problems corrected before data entry is initiated. The data entry process should be essentially automatic and require no decisions regarding the data. Such simplicity in data entry will reduce the number of data entry errors and markedly decrease the time required for entry. It is not sufficient to establish general rules for those entering data such as "in this case always do X." This action still requires the data enterer to recognize a problem, refer to a general rule, and correct the data before entering them. Anything that alters the rhythm of data entry increases errors. The researcher needs to carefully examine each datum to search for the following problems and resolve them before data entry:

1. **Missing data.** Provide the data if possible or determine the impact of the missing data on your analysis. In some cases, the subject must be excluded from at least some of the analyses, so you must determine what data are essential.

2. **Items in which the subject provided two responses when only one was requested.** For example, if the item asked the subject to mark the most important in a list of 10 items and the subject selected 2, you must decide how to resolve this problem; do not leave the decision to an assistant who is entering the data. On the form indicate how the datum is to be coded.

3. **Items in which the subject has marked a response between two options.** This problem commonly occurs with Likert-type scales, particularly those using forced choice options. Given four options, the subject places a mark on the line between response 2 and response 3. On the form, indicate how the datum is to be coded.

4. **Items that ask the subject to write in some information such as occupation or diagnosis.** Such items are a data enterer's nightmare. A list of codes needs to be developed by the researcher for entering such data. Rather than leaving it up to the assistant to determine which code matches the subject's written response, this code should be indicated by the researcher before turning the data over for entry. After the data have been checked and needed codes written in, it is prudent to make a copy rather than turning over the only set of your data to an assistant.

The Data Entry Period

If you are entering your own data, develop a rhythm to your entry. Avoid distractions while entering data, and limit your data entry periods to 2 hours at a time to reduce errors. A backup of the database should be made after each data entry period and stored on a floppy disk or backup tape. It is possible for the computer to crash, with loss of your data. If an assistant is entering your data, make yourself as available as possible to respond to questions and address problems. After entry, the data should be checked for accuracy. Data checking is discussed in Chapter 18 in the section Preparation of the Data for Analysis.

STORAGE AND RETRIEVAL OF DATA

Storage of data from a study is relatively easy in this time of floppy disks and backup tapes. One decision that must be made is how long to store the data. The original data forms need to be stored as well as the database. Storage of data serves several purposes. The data can be used for secondary analyses of data. For example, individuals who are participating in a research program related to a particular research focus may pool data from various studies for access by all members of the group. The data are available to document the validity of your analyses and the published results of your study. Because of nationally publicized incidents of researchers inventing data from which multiple publications were developed, you are wise to preserve documentation that your data were obtained as you claim. Issues that have been raised include how long data should be stored, the need for institutional policy regarding storage of data, and whether graduate students who conduct a study should leave a copy of their data at the university. Thomas (1992) surveyed 153 researchers to determine their responses to these questions. She found that the length of data storage varied greatly, with 29% storing their data 5 years, 31% storing it 10 years, and 21% storing it forever. Most researchers stored their data in their office (84%), and a few used a central location (12%) or a laboratory (4%). The forms of data storage devices preferred were disk (54%), tape (47%), and paper/raw data (32%). Some researchers indicated a preference for more than one storage device for their data. The majority of the researchers (86%) indicated that their institutions did not have a policy for data storage, and most graduate students (74%) did not leave a copy of their data at the university.

■ SUMMARY

The initiation of data collection is one of the most exciting parts of research. However, some time needs to be carefully spent planning this adventure. A data collection plan details how the study will be implemented. To plan the process of data collection, the researcher needs to determine step by step how and in what sequence data will be collected and the timing of the process. Decision points that occur during data collection need to be identified and all options considered.

Consistency in data collection across subjects is critical, and so is consistency among data collectors if more than one data collector is used. Decisions regarding who collects the data also need to be made. If data collectors are used, they need to be informed about the research project, introduced to the instruments to be used, and provided equivalent training in the data collection process. After training, data collectors must be evaluated to determine their consistency.

The time required for data collection is often inadequately estimated when conducting a study. It is helpful to write out a time plan for the data collection period. Cost factors must also be examined when planning a study. Neophyte researchers have difficulty making reasonable estimates of the time and cost related to a study and might wish to validate estimates with an experienced researcher.

Before data collection begins, the researcher may need to develop forms on which to record data. Data collection forms need to be developed for easy recording during data collection and for easy entry into the computer. A decision must be made about whether data are collected in raw form or coded at the time of collection. Coding is the process of transforming qualitative data into numerical symbols that can be entered easily into the computer.

A codebook documents the variable name, abbreviated variable name, and possible values of every variable entered in a computer file. It is advisable to develop the codebook before initiating data collection to provide a means to identify places in data collection forms that might prove to be a problem during data entry. If the data are being given to an assistant for data entry, information on the data should be provided to the assistant before data entry. With this information, the assistant can develop the database in preparation for receiving the data for entry.

Data collection is the process of selecting subjects and gathering data from these subjects. Data collection involves four tasks: selecting subjects, collecting data in a consistent way, maintaining research controls, and solving problems that threaten to disrupt the study. Some of the common problems encountered by researchers during data collection include problems in selection of a sample, subject mortality, treatment of the subject as an object, external influences on subject responses, passive resistance, researcher interactions, lack of skill in data collection techniques, researcher role conflicts, and maintaining perspective.

Serendipity is the accidental discovery of something useful or valuable. During the data collection phase of studies, researchers often become aware of elements or relationships not previously identified. Serendipitous findings are important to the development of new insights in nursing and can lead to areas of research that generate new knowledge.

During data collection, the researcher needs access to individuals or groups who can provide support and consultation. Support needs to be available from academic committees, involved institutions, and significant others.

When data collection begins, the researcher will have to handle large quantities of paper. Plans need to be made for organizing and storing the data as they are gathered. Data need to be carefully checked and problems corrected before data entry is initiated. Storage of data after the study is completed must also be considered. The original data forms, as well as the database, need to be stored. Because of nationally publicized incidents of researchers inventing data from which multiple publications were developed, you are wise to preserve documentation that your data were obtained as you claim.

REFERENCES

Alles, P. (1995). CESF medical outcomes research project: Implementing outcomes assessment in a clinical setting. *Wisconsin Medical Journal, 94*(1), 27–31.

Byers, V. L. (1995). Overview of the data collection process. *Journal of Neuroscience Nursing, 27*(3), 188–193.

Dennis, K. E. (1994). Managing questionnaire data through optical scanning technology. *Nursing Research, 43*(6), 376–378.

Field, P. A., & Morse, J. M. (1985). *Nursing research: The application of qualitative approaches* (pp. 65–90). Rockville, MD: Aspen.

Gift, A. G., Creasia, J., & Parker, B. (1991). Utilizing research assistants and maintaining research integrity. *Research in Nursing & Health, 14*(3), 229–233.

Harrison, L. L. (1989). Interfacing bioinstruments with computers for data collection in nursing research. *Research in Nursing & Health, 12*(2), 129–133.

Lobo, M. L. (1993). Code books—a critical link in the research process. *Western Journal of Nursing Research, 15*(3), 377–385.

Lookinland, S., & Appel, P. L. (1991). Hemodynamic and oxygen transport changes following endotracheal suctioning in trauma patients. *Nursing Research, 40*(3), 133–138.

Thomas, S. P. (1992). Storage of research data: Why, how, where? *Nursing Research, 41*(5), 309–311.

Washington, C. C., & Moss, M. (1988). Methodology corner: Pragmatic aspects of establishing interrater reliability in research. *Nursing Research, 37*(3), 190–191.

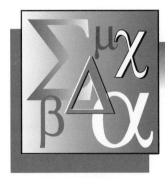

CHAPTER 18

INTRODUCTION TO
STATISTICAL ANALYSIS

The period of data analysis is probably the most exciting part of research. During this period, one finally obtains answers to the questions that initially generated the research activity. Nevertheless, nurses probably experience greater anxiety about knowledge of this phase of the research process than any other, whether the knowledge is needed to critique published studies or conduct research. To critique a quantitative study, the nurse needs to be able to (1) identify the statistical procedures used; (2) judge whether these statistical procedures were appropriate for the hypotheses, questions, or objectives of the study and for the data available for analysis; (3) comprehend the discussion of data analysis results; (4) judge whether the author's interpretation of the results is appropriate; and (5) evaluate the clinical significance of the findings. A neophyte researcher performing a quantitative study is confronted with many critical decisions related to data analysis that require statistical knowledge. To perform statistical analysis of data from a quantitative study, the nurse needs to be able to (1) prepare the data for analysis; (2) describe the sample; (3) test the reliability of measures used in the study; (4) perform exploratory analyses of the data; (5) perform analyses guided by the study objectives, questions, or hypotheses; and (6) interpret the results of statistical procedures. Both the critique of studies and performance of statistical analyses require an understanding of the statistical theory underlying the process of analysis.

This chapter and the following five will provide the information needed to critique the statistical sections of published studies or perform statistical procedures. The present chapter will introduce the concepts of statistical theory, followed by a discussion of some of the more pragmatic aspects of quantitative data analysis: the purposes of statistical analysis, the process of performing data analysis, choosing appropriate statistical procedures for a study, and resources for statistical analysis. Chapter 19 explains the use of statistics for descriptive purposes, Chapter 20 discusses the use of statistics to test proposed relationships, Chapter 21 explores the use of statistics for prediction, Chapter 22 will guide you in using statistics to examine causality, and Chapter 16 examines the use of statistics for developing methods of measurement.

THE CONCEPTS OF STATISTICAL THEORY

One reason that nurses tend to avoid statistics is that many were taught only the mathematical mechanics of calculating statistical formulas, with little or no explanation of the logic behind the analysis procedure or the meaning of the results. This mechanical process is usually performed by computer, and information about it is of little assistance in making statistical decisions or explaining results. We will approach data analysis from the perspective of enhancing the reader's understanding of the meaning underlying statistical analysis. This understanding can then be used either to critique or to perform data analyses.

As is common in many theories, theoretical ideas related to statistics are expressed by unique terminology and logic that is unfamiliar to many. Research ideas, particularly data analysis as expressed in the language of the clinician and the researcher, are perceived by statisticians to be relatively imprecise and vague because they are not expressed in the formal language of the professional statistician. To resolve this language barrier, developing a plan for data analysis requires translation from the common language (or even general research language) to the language of statisticians. When the analysis is complete, the results must be translated from the language of the statistician back to the language of the researcher and the clinician. Thus, explanation of the meaning of the results is a process of interpretation (Chervany, 1977). Figure 18–1 illustrates this process of translation and interpretation.

The ensuing discussion presents an explanation of some of the concepts commonly used in statistical theory. The logic of statistical theory is embedded within the explanations of these concepts. The concepts presented include probability theory, decision theory, inference, the theoretical normal curve, sampling distributions, sampling distribution of a statistic, shapes of distributions, standardized scores, confidence intervals, statistics and parameters, samples and populations, estimation of parameters, degrees of freedom, tailedness, Type I and Type II errors, level of significance, power, clinical signifi-cance, parametric and nonparametric statistical analyses, causality, and relationships.

Probability Theory

Probability theory addresses statistical analysis as the likelihood of accurately predicting an event or the extent of a relationship. Nurse researchers might be interested in the probability of a particular nursing outcome in a particular patient care situation. With probability theory, you could determine how much of the variation in your data could be explained by using a particular statistical analysis. In probability theory, the meaning of statistical results is interpreted by the researcher in light of his or her knowledge of the field of study. A finding that would have little meaning in one field of study might be an important finding in another (Good, 1983). Probability is expressed as a lowercase *p,* with values expressed as percentages or as a decimal value ranging from 0 to 1. If the exact probability is known to be .23, for example, it would be expressed as $p = .23$.

Decision Theory and Hypothesis Testing

Decision theory is inductive in nature and is based on assumptions associated with the theoretical normal curve. When using decision theory, one always begins with the assumption that all the groups are members of the same population. This assump-

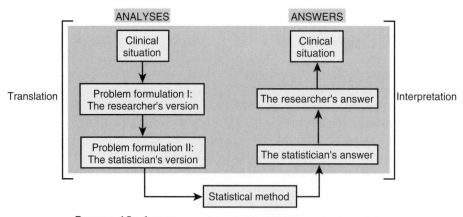

FIGURE 18–1 ■ Process of translation and interpretation in statistics.

tion is expressed as a null hypothesis. See Chapter 8 for an explanation of null hypothesis. To test the assumption, a cutoff point is selected before data collection. This cutoff point, referred to as alpha (α), or the level of significance, is the point on the normal curve at which the results of statistical analysis indicate a statistically significant difference between the groups. Decision theory requires that the cutoff point be absolute. Thus, the meaning applied to the statistical results is not based on interpretation by the researcher. Absolute means that even if the value obtained is only a fraction above the cutoff point, the samples are considered to be from the same population and no meaning can be attributed to the differences. Thus it is inappropriate when using this theory to make a statement that "the findings approached significance at the .051 level" if the alpha level was set at .05. By decision theory rules, this finding indicates that the groups tested are not significantly different and the null hypothesis is not rejected. On the other hand, if the analysis reveals a significant difference of .001, this result is not more significant than the .05 originally proposed (Slakter et al., 1991).

Inference

Statisticians use the term *inference* or *infer* in somewhat the same way that a researcher uses the term *generalize*. Inference requires the use of inductive reasoning. One infers from a specific case to a general truth, from a part to the whole, from the concrete to the abstract, from the known to the unknown. When using inferential reasoning, you can never prove things; you can never be certain. However, one of the reasons for the rules that have been established with regard to statistical procedures is to increase the probability that inferences are accurate. Inferences are made cautiously and with great care.

The Normal Curve

The theoretical *normal curve* is an expression of statistical theory. It is a theoretical frequency distribution of all *possible* scores. No real distribution exactly fits the normal curve. The idea of the normal curve was developed by an 18-year-old mathe-

matician, Johann Gauss, in 1795, who found that data measured repeatedly in many samples from the same population by using scales based on an underlying continuum can be combined into one large sample. From this very large sample, one can develop a more accurate representation of the pattern of the curve in that population than is possible with only one sample. Surprisingly, in most cases, the curve is similar, regardless of the specific data that have been examined or the population being studied.

This theoretical normal curve is symmetrical and unimodal and has continuous values. The mean, median, and mode (summary statistics) are equal (see Figure 18–2). The distribution is completely defined by the mean and standard deviation. The measures in the theoretical distribution have been standardized by using Z scores. These terms are explained further in Chapter 19. Note the Z scores and standard deviation values indicated in Figure 18–2. The proportion of scores that may be found in a particular area of the normal curve has been identified. In a normal curve, 68% of the scores will be within 1 SD or 1 Z score above or below the mean, 95% will be within 2 SD above or below the mean, and more than 99% will be within 3 SD above or below the mean. Even when statistics, such as means, come from a population with a skewed (asymmetrical) distribution, the sampling distribution developed from multiple means obtained from that skewed population will tend to fit the pattern of the normal curve. This phenomenon is referred to as the *central limit theorem*. One requirement for the use of parametric statistical analysis is that the data be normally distributed— *normal* meaning that the data approximately fit the normal curve. Many statistical measures from skewed samples also fit the normal curve because of the central limit theorem; thus, some statisticians believe that it is justifiable to use parametric statistical analysis even with data from skewed samples if the sample is large enough (Volicer, 1984).

Sampling Distributions

A *distribution* is the state or manner in which values are arranged within the data set. A *sampling distribution* is the manner in which statistical values

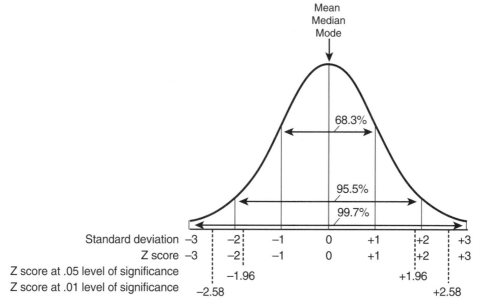

FIGURE 18–2 ■ The normal curve.

(such as means), obtained from multiple samples of the same population, are distributed within the set of values. The mean of this type of distribution is referred to as the *mean of means* (μ). Sampling distributions can also be developed from standard deviations. Other values, such as correlations between variables, scores obtained from specific measures, and scores reflecting differences between groups within the population, can yield values that can be used to develop sampling distributions.

The purpose of the sampling distribution is to allow us to estimate sampling error. *Sampling error* is the difference between the sample statistic used to estimate a parameter and the actual, but unknown value of the parameter. If we know the sampling distribution of a statistic, it allows us to measure the probability of making an incorrect inference. One should never make an inference without being able to calculate the probability of making an incorrect inference.

Sampling Distribution of a Statistic

Just as it is possible to develop distributions of summary statistics within a population, it is possible

to develop distributions of inferential statistical outcomes. For example, if one repeatedly obtained two samples of the same size from the same population and tested for differences in the means with a *t* test, a sampling distribution could be developed from the resulting *t* values by using probability theory. With this approach, a distribution could be developed for samples of many varying sizes. Such a distribution has, in fact, been generated by using *t* values. A table of *t* distribution values is available in Appendix C. Tables have been developed with this strategy to organize the statistical outcomes of many statistical procedures from various sample sizes. Because listing all possible outcomes would require many pages, most tables include only values that have a low probability of occurring in the present theoretical population. These probabilities are expressed as *alpha* (α), commonly referred to as the *level of significance,* and as beta (β), the probability of a Type II error.

By using the appropriate sampling distribution one could determine the probability of obtaining a specific statistical result if two samples being studied were really from the same population. Statistical analysis makes an inference that the samples being tested can be considered part of the population from which the sampling distribution was developed. This inference is expressed as a null hypothesis.

The Shapes of Distributions

The shape of the distribution provides important information about the data being studied. The outline of the distribution shape is obtained by using a histogram. Within this outline, the mean, median, mode, and standard deviation can then be graphically illustrated (see Figure 18–3). This visual presentation of combined summary statistics provides increased insight into the nature of the distribution. As the sample size becomes larger, the shape of the distribution will more accurately reflect the shape of the population from which the sample was taken.

SYMMETRY

Several terms are used to describe the shape of the curve (and thus the nature of a particular distribution). The shape of a curve is usually discussed in terms of symmetry, skewness, modality, and kurtosis. A symmetrical curve is one in which the left side of the curve is a mirror image of the right side (see Figure 18–2, the normal curve). In these curves, the mean, median, and mode are equal and are the dividing point between the left and right side of the curve.

SKEWNESS

Any curve that is not symmetrical is referred to as skewed or asymmetrical. Skewness may be exhibited in the curve in a variety of ways (see Figure 18–4). A curve may be positively skewed, which means that the largest portion of data is below the mean. For example, data on length of enrollment in hospice are positively skewed. Most of the people die within the first 3 weeks of enrollment, whereas increasingly smaller numbers survive as time increases. A curve can also be negatively skewed, which means that the largest portion of data is above the mean. For example, data on the occurrence of chronic illness by age in a population are negatively skewed, with most chronic illnesses occurring in older age groups.

In a skewed distribution, the mean, median, and mode are not equal. Skewness interferes with the validity of many statistical analyses; therefore, statistical procedures have been developed to measure the skewness of the distribution of the sample being studied. Very few samples will be perfectly symmetrical; however, as the deviation from symmetry increases, the seriousness of the impact on statistical analysis increases. A popular skewness measure is expressed in the following equation:

$$\text{skewness} = \frac{\Sigma (X - \bar{X})^3}{N(SD^3)}$$

In this equation, a result of zero indicates a completely symmetrical distribution, a positive number indicates a positively skewed distribution, and a negative number indicates a negatively skewed distribution. Statistical analyses conducted by computer will often automatically measure skewness, which is then indicated on the computer printout. Strongly skewed distributions must often be analyzed by nonparametric techniques, which make no assumptions of normally distributed samples. In a positively skewed distribution, the mean will be greater than the median, which will be greater than the mode. In a negatively skewed distribution, the mean

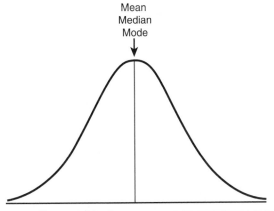

Mean
Median
Mode

FIGURE 18–3 ■ The symmetrical curve.

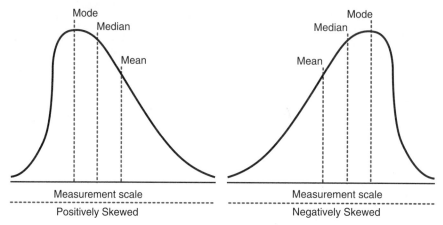

FIGURE 18–4 ■ Skewness.

will be less than the median, which will be less than the mode.

MODALITY

Another characteristic of distributions is their modality. Most curves found in practice are unimodal, which means that they have one mode and frequencies progressively decline as they move away from the mode. Symmetrical distributions are usually unimodal. However, curves can also be bimodal (see Figure 18-5) or multimodal. When you find a bimodal sample, it usually means that you have not adequately defined your population.

KURTOSIS

Another term used to describe the shape of the distribution curve is *kurtosis.* Kurtosis explains the degree of peakedness of the curve, which is related to the spread of variance of scores. An extremely peaked curve is referred to as *leptokurtic,* an intermediate degree of kurtosis as *mesokurtic,* and a

relatively flat curve as *platykurtic* (see Figure 18–6). Extreme kurtosis can affect the validity of statistical analysis because the scores have little variation. Many computer programs analyze kurtosis before conducting statistical analysis. A common equation used to measure kurtosis is

$$\text{kurtosis} = \frac{\sum (X - \bar{X})^4}{N(SD^4)} - 3$$

A kurtosis of zero indicates that the curve is mesokurtic. Values above zero indicate a platykurtic curve (Box et al., 1978).

Standardized Scores

Because of differences in the characteristics of various distributions, comparing a score in one distribution with a score in another distribution is difficult. For example, if you were comparing test scores from two classroom examinations and one test had a high score of 100 and the other had a high score of 70, the scores would be difficult to compare. To facilitate this comparison, a mechanism has been developed to transform raw scores into standard scores. Numbers that make sense only within the framework of the measurements used within a specific study are transformed to numbers

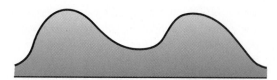

FIGURE 18–5 ■ Bimodal distribution.

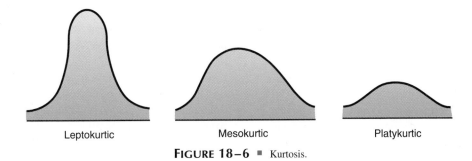

| Leptokurtic | Mesokurtic | Platykurtic |

FIGURE 18–6 ■ Kurtosis.

(standard scores) that have a more general meaning. Transformation to standard scores allows an easy conceptual grasp of the meaning of the score.

A common standardized score is called a *Z score*. It expresses deviations from the mean (difference scores) in terms of standard deviation units. The equation for a *Z* score is

$$Z = \frac{X - \bar{X}}{SD}$$

A score that falls above the mean will have a positive *Z* score, whereas a score that falls below the mean will have a negative *Z* score (see Figure 18-3). The mean expressed as a *Z* score is zero. The *SD* of *Z* scores is 1. Thus, a *Z* score of 2 indicates that the score from which it was obtained is 2 *SD* above the mean. A *Z* score of −.5 indicates that the score was .5 *SD* below the mean. The larger the absolute value of the *Z* score, the less likely the observation is to occur. For example, a *Z* score of 4 would be extremely unlikely. The cumulative normal distribution expressed in *Z* scores is given in Appendix B.

Confidence Intervals

When the probability of including the value of the parameter within the interval estimate is known (as described in Chapter 19), it is referred to as a *confidence interval.* Calculating the confidence interval involves the use of two formulas to identify the upper and lower ends of the interval. The formula for a 95% confidence interval when sampling from a population with a known standard deviation or from a normal population with a sample size greater than 30 is

$$\bar{X} - 1.96 \; SD/\sqrt{N} \qquad \bar{X} + 1.96 \; SD/\sqrt{N}$$

If one had a sample with a mean of 40, an *SD* of 5, and an *N* of 50, a confidence interval could be calculated.

$$40 - 1.96 \left(\frac{5}{\sqrt{50}}\right) = 40 - 1.386 = 38.6$$

$$40 + 1.96 \left(\frac{5}{\sqrt{50}}\right) = 40 + 1.386 = 41.4$$

Confidence intervals are usually expressed as "(38.6–41.4)," with 38.6 being the lower end and 41.4 being the upper end of the interval. Theoretically, we can produce a confidence interval for any parameter of a distribution. It is a generic statistical procedure. For example, confidence intervals can also be developed around correlation coefficients (Glass & Stanley, 1970, pp. 264–268). Estimation can be used for a single population or for multiple populations. In estimation, we are inferring the value of a parameter from sample data and have no preconceived notion of the value of the parameter. In contrast, in hypothesis testing we have an a priori theory about the value of the parameter or parameters or some combination of parameters.

Statistics and Parameters, Samples and Populations

Use of the terms *statistic* and *parameter* can be confusing because of the various populations referred to in statistical theory. A *statistic* ($\overline{X}$) is a numerical value obtained from a sample. A *parameter* is a true (but unknown) numerical characteristic of a population. For example, μ is the population mean or arithmetic average. The mean of the sampling distribution (mean of samples' means) can also be shown to be equal to μ. Thus, a numerical value that is the mean of the sample is a statistic; a numerical value that is the mean of the population is a parameter (Barnett, 1982).

Relating a statistic to a parameter requires an inference as one moves from the sample to the sampling distribution and then from the sampling distribution to the population. The population referred to is in one sense real (concrete) and in another sense abstract. These ideas are illustrated as follows:

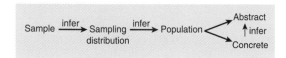

For example, perhaps you are interested in the cholesterol level of women in the United States. Your population is women in the United States. Obviously, you cannot measure the cholesterol level of every woman in the United States; therefore, you select a sample of women from this population. Because you wish your sample to be as representative of the population as possible, you obtain your sample by using random sampling techniques. To determine whether the cholesterol levels in your sample are like those in the population, you must compare the sample with the population. One strategy would be to compare the mean of your sample with the mean of the entire population. Unfortunately, it is highly unlikely that you *know* the mean

of the entire population. Therefore, you must make an estimate of the mean of that population. You need to know how good your sample statistics are as estimators of the parameters of the population.

First, you make some assumptions. You assume that the mean scores of cholesterol levels from multiple randomly selected samples of this population would be normally distributed. Implied by this assumption is another assumption: that the cholesterol levels of the population will be distributed according to the theoretical normal curve—that difference scores and standard deviations can be equated to those in the normal curve.

If you assume that the population in your study is normally distributed, you can also assume that this population can be represented by a normal sampling distribution. Thus, you infer from your sample to the sampling distribution, the mathematically developed theoretical population made up of parameters such as the mean of means and the standard error. The parameters of this theoretical population are those measures of the dimensions identified in the sampling distribution. You can then infer from the sampling distribution to the population. You have both a concrete population and an abstract population. The concrete population consists of all those individuals who meet your sampling criteria, whereas the abstract population consists of individuals who will meet your sampling criteria in the future or those groups addressed theoretically by your framework.

Estimation of Parameters

Two approaches may be used to estimate the parameters of a population: point estimation and interval estimation.

POINT ESTIMATION

A statistic that produces a value as a function of the scores in a sample is called an *estimator*. Much of inferential statistical analysis involves the use of *point estimation* to evaluate the fit between the estimator (a statistic) and the population parameter. A point estimate is a single figure that estimates a related figure in the population of interest. The best point estimator of the population mean is the mean of the sample being examined. However, the mean of the sample rarely equals the mean of the population. In addition to the mean, other commonly used estimators include the median, variance, standard deviation, and correlation coefficient.

INTERVAL ESTIMATION

When sampling from a continuous distribution, the probability of the sample mean being exactly equal to the population mean is zero. Therefore, we know that we are going to be in error if we use point estimators. The difference between the sample estimate and the true, but unknown parameter value is sampling error. The source of sampling error is the fact that we did not count every individual in the population. Sampling error is due to chance and chance alone. It is not due to some flaw in the researcher's methodology. Interval estimation is an attempt to overcome this problem by controlling the initial precision of an estimator. An interval procedure that gives a 95% level of confidence will produce a set of intervals, 95% of which will include the true value of the parameter. Unfortunately, after a sample is drawn and the estimate is calculated, it is not possible to tell whether the interval contains the true value of the parameter.

An *interval estimate* is a segment of a number line (or range of scores) where the value of the parameter is thought to be. For example, in a sample with a mean of 40 and an *SD* of 5, one might use the range of scores between 2 *SD* below the mean to 2 *SD* above the mean (30–50) as the interval estimation. This type of estimation provides a set of scores rather than a single score. However, it is not absolutely certain that the mean of the population lies within that range. Therefore, it is necessary to determine the probability that this interval estimate contains the population mean.

This need to determine probability brings us back to the sampling distribution. We know that 95% of the means in the sampling distribution lie within 2 *SD* of the mean of means (the population mean). If these scores are converted to *Z* scores, the unit normal distribution table can be used to determine how many standard deviations out from the

mean of means one must go to ensure a specified probability (e.g., 70%, 95%, or 99%) of obtaining an interval estimate that includes the population parameter that is being estimated.

By examining the normal distribution (see Figure 18–2), one finds that 2.5% of the area under the normal curve lies below a *Z* score of −1.96, or $\mu - (1.96\ SD/\sqrt{N})$, and 2.5% of the area lies above a *Z* score of 1.96, or $\mu + (1.96\ SD/\sqrt{N})$, where μ is the mean of means, *SD* is the standard deviation, and *N* is the sample size. The probability is .95 that a randomly selected sample would have a mean within this range. Calculation of confidence intervals is explained in Chapter 19.

Degrees of Freedom

The concept of *degrees of freedom* (*df*) is a product of statistical theory and is easier to calculate than it is to explain because of the complex mathematics involved in demonstrating justification for the concept. Degrees of freedom involve the freedom of a score's value to vary given the other existing scores' values and the established sum of these scores.

A simple example may provide beginning insight into the concept. Suppose difference scores are obtained from a sample of 4 and the mean is 4. The difference scores are −2, −1, +1, and +2. As with all difference scores, the sum of these scores is 0. As a result, if any three of the difference scores are calculated, the value of the fourth score is not free to vary. Its value will depend on the values of the other three to maintain a mean of 4 and a sum of 0. The degree of freedom in this example is 3 because only three scores are free to vary. In this case and in many other analyses, degree of freedom is the sample size (*N*) minus 1 (*N* − 1).

$$df = N - 1$$

In this example, $df = 4 - 1 = 3$ (Roscoe, 1969, p. 162). In some analyses, determination of levels of significance from tables of statistical sampling distributions requires knowledge of the degrees of freedom.

Tailedness

On a normal curve, extremes of statistical values can occur at either end of the curve. Therefore, the 5% of statistical values that are considered statistically significant according to decision theory must be distributed between the two extremes of the curve. The extremes of the curve are referred to as *tails.* If the hypothesis is nondirectional and assumes that an extreme score can occur in either tail, the analysis is referred to as a *two-tailed test of significance* (see Figure 18–7).

In a *one-tailed test of significance,* the hypothesis is directional, and extreme statistical values that occur on a single tail of the curve are of interest. Developing a one-tailed hypothesis requires sufficient knowledge of the variables and their interaction on which to base a one-tailed test. Otherwise, the one-tailed test is inappropriate. This knowledge may be theoretical or from previous research. (Refer to Chapter 8 for formulating hypotheses.) One-tailed tests are uniformly more powerful than two-tailed tests, which increases the possibility of rejecting the null hypothesis. In this case, extreme statistical values occurring on the other tail of the curve are not considered significantly different. In Figure 18–8,

which is a one-tailed figure, the portion of the curve where statistical values will be considered significant is in the right tail of the curve.

Type I and Type II Errors

According to decision theory, two types of error can occur when making decisions about the meaning of a value obtained from a statistical test: Type I errors and Type II errors. A *Type I error* occurs if the null hypothesis is rejected when, in fact, it is true. This error is possible because even though statistical values in the extreme ends of the tail of the curve are rare, they do occur within the population. In viewing Table 18–1, remember that the null hypothesis states that there is no difference or no association between groups.

The risk of making a Type I error is greater with a .05 level of significance than with a .01 level. As the level of significance becomes more extreme, the risk of a Type I error decreases, as illustrated in Figure 18–9. For example, suppose you studied the effect of a treatment in an experimental study consisting of two groups and found that the difference between the two groups was relatively equivalent in

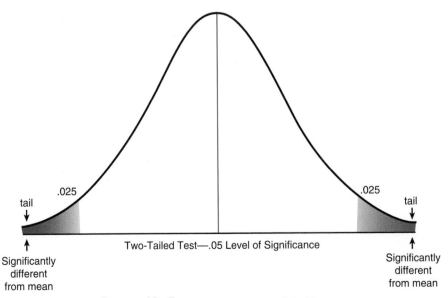

FIGURE 18–7 ■ The two-tailed test of significance.

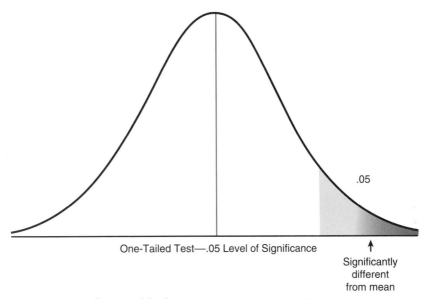

One-Tailed Test—.05 Level of Significance

.05

↑
Significantly
different
from mean

FIGURE 18–8 ■ The one-tailed test of significance.

magnitude to the standard error. The sampling distribution of the difference between the group means tells you that even if there is no real difference between the groups, a difference as large or larger than the one you detected would occur by chance about once in every three times. That is, the difference that you found is just what you could expect to occur if the true treatment effect were zero. This statement does not mean that the true difference is zero, but that on the basis of the results of the study you would not be justified in claiming a real difference between the groups. The data from your

samples do not establish a case for the position that a true treatment effect exists.

Suppose, on the other hand, that you find that the difference in your groups is over twice its standard error (Z score > 1.96). (Examine the Z scores in Figure 18–2.) A treatment difference of this magnitude would occur by chance less than 1 time in 20, and we say that these results are statistically significant at the .05 level. A difference of more than 2.6 times the standard error would occur by chance less than 1 time in 100, and we say that the difference is statistically significant at the .01 level. Cox (1958) states, "Significance tests, from this point of view, measure the adequacy of the data to support the qualitative conclusion that there is a true effect in the direction of the apparent difference" (p. 159). Thus, the decision is a judgment and can be in error. The level of statistical significance attained is an indication of the degree of uncertainty in taking the position that the difference between the two groups is real.

A *Type II error* occurs if the null hypothesis is regarded as true when, in fact, it is false. This type of error occurs as a result of some degree of overlap between the values of different populations in some cases, so a value with a greater than 5%

TABLE 18–1
OCCURRENCE OF TYPE I AND TYPE II ERRORS

DATA ANALYSIS INDICATES	IN REALITY THE NULL HYPOTHESIS IS	
	True	**False**
Results significant Null rejected	Type I error	Correct decision (power)
Results not significant Null not rejected	Correct decision	Type II error

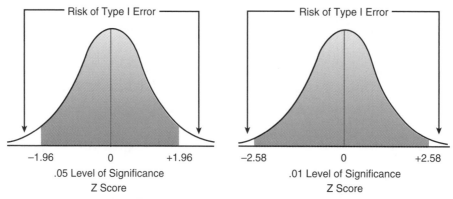

FIGURE 18–9 ■ Risk of Type I error.

probability of being within one population may in fact be within the dimensions of another population (see Figure 18–10).

As the risk of a Type I error decreases (by setting a more extreme level of significance), the risk of a Type II error increases. When the risk of a Type II error is decreased (by setting a less extreme level of significance), the risk of a Type I error increases. It is not possible to decrease both types of error simultaneously without a corresponding increase in sample size. Therefore, the researcher needs to decide which risk poses the greatest threat within a specific study. In nursing research, many studies are conducted with small samples and instruments that are not precise measures of the variables under study. In many nursing situations, multiple variables also interact to lead to differences within populations. However, when one is examining only a few of the interacting variables, small differences can be overlooked and could lead to a false conclusion of no differences between the samples. In this case, the risk of a Type II error is a greater concern, and a more lenient level of significance is in order.

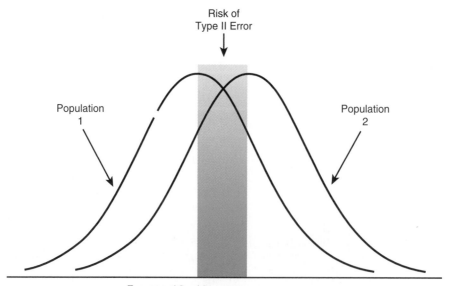

FIGURE 18–10 ■ Risk of Type II error.

As an example of the concerns related to error, consider the following problem. If you were to obtain three samples by using the same methodology, each sample would have a different mean. Yet you need to make a decision to accept or reject the null hypothesis. The null hypothesis states that the population mean is 50 and that the three samples below are all from the same population. Assume that you obtain the following results:

Sample Size	Sample Mean
$N = 50$ subjects	$\bar{X} = 52.0$
$N = 50$ subjects	$\bar{X} = 60.5$
$N = 50$ subjects	$\bar{X} = 52.2$

How much evidence would it take to convince you to switch from believing the null hypothesis to believing the alternative hypothesis? Will you choose correctly or will you make a Type I or a Type II error?

Level of Significance—Controlling the Risk of a Type I Error

The formal definition of the *level of significance* (α) is the probability of making a Type I error when the null hypothesis is true. The level of significance, developed from decision theory, is the cutoff point used to determine whether the samples being tested are members of the same population or from different populations. The decision criteria are based on the selected level of significance and the sampling distribution of the mean. For this example, the assumption is made that the sampling distribution of the mean is normally distributed. As mentioned previously, 68% of the means from samples in a population will fall within 1 SD of the mean of means (μ), 95% will fall within 2 SD, 99% within 3 SD, and 99.9% within 4 SD. This decision theory explanation of the expected distribution of means is equivalent to the confidence interval explanation described previously. It is simply expressed differently. In keeping with decision theory, the level of significance sought in a statistical test must be es-

tablished before conducting the test. In fact, the significance level needs to be established before collecting the data. In nursing studies, the level of significance is usually set at .05 or .01. However, in preliminary studies, it might be prudent to select a less stringent level of significance, such as .10.

If one wishes to predict with a 95% probability of accuracy, the level of significance would be $p \leq 1 - .95$, or $p \leq .05$. The mathematical symbol $\leq$ means "less than or equal to." Thus, $p \leq .05$ means that there is a probability of 5% or less of getting a test statistic at least as extreme as the calculated test statistic if the null hypothesis is true.

In computer analysis, the observed level of significance (p value) obtained from the data is frequently provided on the printout. For example, the actual level of significance might be $p \leq .03$ or $p \leq .07$. This level of significance should be provided in the research report, as well as the level of significance set before the analysis. This practice allows other researchers to make their own judgment of the significance of your findings.

Power—Controlling the Risk of a Type II Error

Power is the probability that a statistical test will detect a significant difference that exists. Often, reported studies failing to reject the null hypothesis (in which power is unlikely to have been examined) will have only a 10% power level to detect a difference if one exists. An 80% power level is desirable. Until recently, the researcher's primary interest was in preventing a Type I error. Therefore, great emphasis was placed on the selection of a level of significance but little on power. This point of view is changing as we recognize the seriousness of a Type II error in nursing studies.

A Type II error occurs when the null hypothesis is not rejected by the study even though a difference actually exists between groups. If the null hypothesis assumes no difference between the groups, the difference score in the measure of the dependent variable between groups would be zero. In a two-sample study, this relationship would be expressed mathematically as A − B = 0. The research hypothesis would be stated as A − B ≠ 0 where ≠

means "not equal to." A Type II error occurs when the difference score is not zero but is small enough that it is not detected by statistical analysis. In some cases, the difference is negligible and not of interest clinically. However, in other cases, the difference in reality is greater than indicated. This undetected difference is often due to research methodology problems.

Type II errors can occur for three reasons: (1) a stringent level of significance, (2) a small sample size, and (3) a small difference in measured effect between the groups. A difference in the measured effect can be due to a number of factors, including large variation in scores on the dependent variable within groups, crude instrumentation that does not measure with precision (e.g., does not detect small changes in the variable and thus leads to a small detectable effect size), confounding or extraneous variables that mask the effects of the variables under study, or any combination of these factors.

You can determine the risk of a Type II error through *power analysis* and modify the study to decrease the risk if necessary. Cohen (1988) has identified four parameters of power: (1) significance level, (2) sample size, (3) effect size, and (4) power. If three of the four are known, the fourth can be calculated by using power analysis formulas. Significance level and sample size are fairly straightforward. *Effect size* is "the degree to which the phenomenon is present in the population, or the degree to which the null hypothesis is false" (Cohen, 1988, pp. 9–10). For example, if one were measuring changes in anxiety levels, measured first when the patient is at home and then just before surgery, the effect size would be large if a great change in anxiety was expected. If only a small change in the level of anxiety was expected, the effect size would be small.

Small effect sizes require larger samples to detect these small differences. If the power is too low, it may not be worthwhile conducting the study unless a large sample can be obtained because statistical tests are unlikely to detect differences that exist. Deciding to conduct a study in these circumstances is costly in time and money, cannot add to the body of nursing knowledge, and can actually lead to false conclusions. Power analysis can be used to determine the sample size necessary for a particular

study. This use of power analysis is discussed in Chapter 14. Power analysis can be calculated by using a program in NCSS (Number Crunchers Statistical System) called PASS (Power Analysis and Sample Size). Sample size can also be calculated by a program called EX-SAMPLE produced by Idea Works, Inc. (Brent et al., 1988). SPSS (Statistical Packages for the Social Sciences) for Windows also now has the capacity to perform power analysis. Yarandi (1994) has provided the commands needed to perform power analysis for comparing two binomial proportions with SAS (Statistical Analysis System).

The power analysis should be reported in studies that fail to reject the null hypothesis. Results of power analysis should be presented in the results section of the study. If power is high, it strengthens the meaning of the findings. If power is low, the researcher needs to address this issue in the discussion of implications. Modifications in the research methodology that resulted from the use of power analysis also need to be reported.

Clinical Significance

The findings of a study can be statistically significant but may not be clinically significant. For example, one group of patients might have a body temperature .1°F higher than that of another group. Data analysis might indicate that the two groups are statistically significantly different. However, the findings have no clinical significance. In studies it is often important to know the magnitude of the difference between groups. However, a statistical test that indicates significant differences between groups (as in a *t* test) provides no information on the magnitude of the difference. The extent of the level of significance (.01 or .0001) tells you nothing about the magnitude of the difference between the groups. These differences can best be determined through descriptive or exploratory analysis of the data (see Chapter 19).

Parametric and Nonparametric Statistical Analysis

The most commonly used type of statistical analysis is *parametric statistics*. The analysis is referred to as parametric because the findings are inferred to the parameters of a normally distributed population. These approaches to analysis emerged from the work of Fisher and require meeting the following three assumptions before they can justifiably be used: (1) The sample was drawn from a population for which the variance can be calculated. The distribution is usually expected to be normal or approximately normal (Conover, 1971). (2) Because most parametric techniques deal with continuous variables rather than discrete variables, the level of measurement should be interval data or ordinal data with an approximately normal distribution. (3) The data can be treated as random samples (Box et al., 1978).

Nonparametric, or distribution-free, techniques can be used in studies that do not meet the first two assumptions just listed. However, the data still need to be treated as random samples. Most nonparametric techniques are not as powerful as their parametric counterparts. In other words, nonparametric techniques are less able to detect differences and have a greater risk of a Type II error if the data meet the assumptions of parametric procedures. However, if these assumptions are not met, nonparametric procedures are more powerful. The techniques can be used with cruder forms of measurement than required for parametric analysis. In recent years, there has been greater tolerance in using parametric techniques when some of the assumptions are not met if the analyses are robust to moderate violation of the assumptions. Robust means that the analysis will yield accurate results even if some of the assumptions are violated by the data used for the analysis. However, one needs to think carefully through the consequences of violating the assumptions of a statistical procedure. The validity of the results diminishes as the violation of assumptions becomes more extreme.

PRACTICAL ASPECTS OF DATA ANALYSIS

Purposes of Statistical Analysis

Statistics can be used for a variety of purposes, such as to (1) summarize, (2) explore the meaning of deviations in the data, (3) compare or contrast descriptively, (4) test the proposed relationships in a theoretical model, (5) infer that the findings from the sample are indicative of the entire population, (6) examine causality, (7) predict, or (8) infer from the sample to a theoretical model. Statisticians such as John Tukey (1977) divide the role of statistics into two parts: exploratory data analysis and confirmatory data analysis. *Exploratory data analysis* is performed to get a preliminary indication of the nature of the data and to search the data for hidden structure or models. *Confirmatory data analysis* involves traditional inferential statistics, which assists the researcher in making an inference about a population or a process based on evidence from the study sample.

The Process of Data Analysis

The process of quantitative data analysis consists of several stages: (1) preparation of the data for analysis; (2) description of the sample; (3) testing the reliability of measurement; (4) exploratory analysis of the data; (5) confirmatory analysis guided by the hypotheses, questions, or objectives; and (6) post hoc analysis. Although not all these stages are equally reflected in the final published report of the study, they all contribute to the insight that can be gained from analysis of the data. Many novice researchers do not plan the details of data analysis until the data are collected and they are confronted with the analysis task. This research technique is poor and often leads to collection of unusable data or failure to collect the data needed to answer the research questions. Plans for data analysis need to be made during development of the methodology.

Preparation of the Data for Analysis

Except in very small studies, computers are almost universally used for data analysis. This use of computers has increased as personal computers (PCs) have become more accessible and easy-to-use data analysis packages have become available. When computers are used for analysis, the first step of the process is entering the data into the computer.

Before entering data into the computer, the computer file that will hold the data needs to be carefully prepared with information from the codebook as described in Chapter 17. The location of each variable in the computer file needs to be identified. Each variable must be labeled in the computer so that the variables involved in a particular analysis will be clearly designated on the computer printouts. The researcher must develop a systematic plan for data entry that is designed to reduce errors during the entry phase, and data need to be entered during periods with few interruptions. However, entering data for long periods without respite results in fatigue and an increase in errors. If the data are being stored in a PC hard disk drive, a backup needs to be made on a floppy disk each time that more data are entered. It is wise to keep a second floppy disk of the data filed at a separate, carefully protected site. If the data are stored on a mainframe computer, request that a tape backup be made that you can keep in your possession, or download the data onto a floppy disk. After data entry, store the original data in locked files for safekeeping.

CLEANING THE DATA

Print the data file. When data size allows, crosscheck every piece of datum on the printout with the original datum for accuracy. Otherwise, randomly check the accuracy of data points. Correct all errors found in the computer file. Computer analysis of the frequencies of each value of every variable is performed as a second check of the accuracy of the data. Search for values outside the appropriate range of values for that variable. See Chapter 17 for more information on computerizing and cleaning data.

IDENTIFYING MISSING DATA

Identify all missing data points. Determine whether the information can be obtained and entered into the data file. If a large number of subjects have missing data on specific variables, a judgment needs to be made regarding the availability of sufficient data to perform analysis with those variables. In some cases, subjects must be excluded from the analysis because of missing essential data.

TRANSFORMING DATA

In some cases, data must be transformed before initiating data analysis. Items in scales are often arranged so that the location of the highest values for the item are varied. This arrangement prevents a global response by the subject to all items in the scale. To reduce errors, the values on these items need to be entered into the computer exactly as they appear on the data collection form. Values on the items are then reversed by computer commands.

Skewed, or nonlinear, *data* that do not meet the assumptions of parametric analysis can sometimes be transformed in such a way that the values are expressed in a linear fashion. Various mathematical operations are used for this purpose. Examples of these operations include squaring each value or calculating the square root of each value. These operations may allow the researcher insight into the data that is not evident from the raw data.

CALCULATING VARIABLES

Sometimes, a variable used in the analysis is not collected but calculated from other variables. For example, if data are collected on the number of patients on a nursing unit and on the number of nurses on a shift, one might calculate a ratio of nurse to patient for a particular shift. The data will be more accurate if this calculation is performed by the computer rather than manually. The results can then be stored in the data file as a variable rather than being recalculated each time that the variable is used in an analysis.

MAKING DATA BACKUPS

When the data-cleaning process is complete, backups need to be made again, labeled as the complete, cleaned data set, and carefully stored. Data cleaning is a time-consuming process one does not wish to repeat unnecessarily.

Description of the Sample

The next step is to obtain as complete a picture of the sample as possible. Begin with frequencies of descriptive variables related to the sample. Calculate measures of central tendency and measures of dispersion relevant to the sample. If the study is composed of more than one sample, comparisons of the various groups need to be performed. Relevant analyses might include examination of age, educational level, health status, gender, ethnicity, or other features for which data are available. If information is available on estimated parameters of the population from previous research or meta-analyses, measures in the present study need to be compared with these estimated parameters. If the samples are not representative of the population or if two groups being compared are not equivalent in ways important to the study, a decision will need to be made regarding the justification of continuing the analysis.

Testing the Reliability of Measurement

Examine the reliability of the methods of measurement used in the study. The reliability of observational measures or physiological measures may have been obtained during the data collection phase but needs to be noted at this point. Additional evaluation of the reliability of these measures may be possible at this point. If paper-and-pencil scales were used in data collection, alpha coefficients need to be calculated. The value of the coefficient needs to be compared with values obtained for the instrument in previous studies. If the coefficient is unacceptably low, a decision must be made regarding the justification of performing analysis on data from the instrument.

Exploratory Analysis of the Data

Examine all the data descriptively, with the intent of becoming as familiar as possible with the nature of the data. This step is often omitted by neophyte researchers, who tend to jump immediately into analysis designed to test their hypotheses, questions, or objectives. However, they omit this step at the risk of missing important information in the data and performing analyses on data inappropriate for the analysis. The researcher needs to examine data on each variable by using measures of central tendency and dispersion. Is the data skewed

or normally distributed? What is the nature of the variation in the data? Are there outliers with extreme values that seem unlike the rest of the sample? The most valuable insights from a study often come from careful examination of outliers (Tukey, 1977).

The methods of exploratory data analysis described in Chapter 19 provide simple, easy-to-use techniques for exploratory examination of your data. In many cases, as a part of exploratory analysis, inferential statistical procedures are used to examine differences and associations within the sample. From an exploratory perspective, these analyses are relevant only to the sample under study. There should be no intent to infer to a population. If group comparisons are made, effect sizes need to be determined for the variables involved in the analyses.

In many nursing studies, the purpose of the study is exploratory analysis. In such studies, it is often found that sample sizes are small, power is low, measurement is crude, and the field of study is relatively new. If treatments are tested, the procedure is approached as a pilot study. The most immediate need is tentative exploration of the phenomena under study. Confirming the findings of these studies will require more rigorously designed studies with much larger samples. Unfortunately, many of these exploratory studies are reported in the literature as confirmatory studies, and attempts are made to infer to larger populations. Because of the unacceptably high risk of a Type II error in these studies, negative findings should be viewed with caution.

USING TABLES AND GRAPHS FOR EXPLORATORY ANALYSIS

Although tables and graphs are commonly thought of as a way of presenting the findings of a study, these tools may be even more useful in providing a means for the researcher to become familiar with the data. Tables and graphs need to illustrate the descriptive analyses being performed, even though they will probably never be included in a research report. They are only for the benefit of the researcher; they assist in identifying patterns in the data and in interpreting exploratory findings. Visualizing the data in various ways can greatly increase insight regarding the nature of the data (see Chapter 19).

Confirmatory Analysis

As the name implies, confirmatory analysis is performed to confirm expectations regarding the data that are expressed as hypotheses, questions, or objectives. The findings are inferred from the sample to the population. Thus, inferential statistical procedures are used. The design of the study, the methods of measurement, and the sample size must be sufficient for this confirmatory process to be justified. A written analysis plan needs to describe clearly the confirmatory analyses that will be performed to examine each hypothesis, question, or objective. The following steps need to be followed for each analysis used when performing a systematic confirmatory analysis:

1. Identify the level of measurement of the data available for analysis with regard to the research objective, question, or hypothesis.
2. Select a statistical procedure or procedures appropriate for the level of measurement that will respond to the objective, answer the question, or test the hypothesis.
3. Select the level of significance that you will use to interpret the results.
4. Choose a one-tailed or two-tailed test if appropriate to your analysis.
5. Determine the sample size available for the analysis. If several groups will be used in the analysis, the size of each group needs to be identified.
6. Evaluate the representativeness of the sample.
7. Determine the risk of a Type II error in the analysis by performing a power analysis.
8. Develop dummy tables and graphics to illustrate the methods that you will use to display your results in relation to your hypotheses, questions, or objectives.
9. Determine the degrees of freedom for your analysis.
10. Perform the analysis manually or with a computer.

11. Compare the statistical value obtained with the table value by using the level of significance, tailedness of the test, and degrees of freedom previously identified. If you have performed your analysis on a computer, this information will be provided on the computer printout.
12. Reexamine the analysis to ensure that the procedure was performed with the appropriate variables and that the statistical procedure was correctly specified in the computer program.
13. Interpret the results of the analysis in terms of the hypothesis, question, or objective.
14. Interpret the results in terms of the framework.

Post Hoc Analysis

Post hoc analyses are commonly performed in studies with more than two groups when the analysis indicates that the groups are significantly different but does not identify which groups are different. This situation occurs, for example, in chi-squared analyses and in analysis of variance. In other studies, the insights obtained through the planned analyses generate further questions that can be examined with the available data. These analyses may be tangential to the initial purpose of the study but may be fruitful in providing important information and generating questions for further research.

Storing Computer Printouts from Data Analysis

Computer printouts tend to accumulate rapidly during data analysis. Results of data analysis can easily become lost in the mountain of computer paper. These printouts need to be systematically stored to allow easy access later when theses or dissertations are being written or research papers are being prepared for publication. We recommend storing the printouts by time sequence. Most printouts identify the date (and even the hour and minute) that the analysis was performed. Some mainframe computers also assign a job number to each printout, which can be recorded. This feature makes it easy to distinguish earlier analyses from those performed later. Sometimes, printouts can be sorted by variable or by hypothesis and then arranged within these categories by time.

When papers describing the study are being prepared, the results of each analysis reported in the paper need to be cross-indexed with the computer printout for reference as needed, with the job number, date, time, and page number of the printout listed. In addition, a printout of the program used for the analysis needs to be included. As interpretation of the results proceeds and you attempt to link various findings, you may question some of the results. They may not seem to fit with the rest of the results, or they may not seem logical. You may find that you have failed to include some statistical information that is needed. When rewriting the paper, you may decide to report results not originally included. The search for a particular data analysis printout can be time-consuming and frustrating if the printouts have not been carefully organized. It is easy to lose needed results and have to repeat the analysis.

After the paper has been submitted for publication (or to a thesis or dissertation committee), we recommend storing a copy of the page from the printout for each statistical value reported with the text. This copy needs to provide sufficient detail to allow you to gain access to the entire printout if needed. Thesis and dissertation committees and journal reviewers frequently recommend including additional information related to statistical procedures before acceptance. You often have only a short time frame within which to obtain the information and modify the paper to meet deadlines. Even after the paper is published, we have had requests from readers for validation of our results. If this request is made months (or years) after the study is complete, finding the information can be a nightmare if you have failed to store your printouts carefully.

RESOURCES FOR STATISTICAL ANALYSIS

Computer Programs

Packaged computer analysis programs such as SPSS, SAS, and BMDP (Biomedical Data Processing) are available on the mainframe computers of many universities. A variety of data analysis packages such as SAS, SPSS, ABSTAT, and NCSS are also available for the PC. Table 18–2 lists sources of data analysis packages for the PC. The emergence of more powerful, high-speed PCs has made it relatively easy to conduct most analyses on the PC. Although the mathematical formulas needed to conduct analysis with a packaged program have been written as part of the computer program, one needs to know how to instruct the computer program to perform the selected analysis. Manuals, available for each program, demonstrate how to perform the analyses and provide a detailed discussion of the mathematical logic behind each type of analysis. The researcher needs to understand this logic, even though the computer will perform the analysis. For each type of analysis, most manuals suggest up-to-date and comprehensive sources that may be helpful in further understanding the logic of the procedure.

Packaged computer programs can perform your data analysis and provide you with the results of the analysis on a computer printout. However, an enormous amount of information is provided on a computer printout, and its meaning can easily be misinterpreted. In addition, computers conduct anal-

---

TABLE 18–2
SOURCES OF DATA ANALYSIS PACKAGES FOR THE PC

NCSS (Number Cruncher Statistical System)
Dr. Jerry L. Hintze
329 North 1000 East
Kaysville, UT 84037
Phone: (801) 546-0445
Fax: (801) 546-3907

SPSS/PC (Statistical Packages for the Social Sciences)
SPSS, Inc.
444 N. Michigan Avenue
Chicago, IL 60611
Phone (312) 329-3500
Fax: (312) 329-3668

SAS (Statistical Analysis System)
SAS Institute, Inc.
SAS Circle, Box 8000
Cary, NC 27512-8000
Phone: (919) 467-8000

ABSTAT
Anderson-Bell
11479 S. Pine Drive
Suite 400-M
Parker, CO 80134
Phone: (303) 841-9755
Telex: 499-4230

ysis on whatever data are provided. If the data entered into the computer are garbage (e.g., numbers from the data are entered incorrectly or data are typed in the wrong columns), the computer output will be garbage. If the data are inappropriate for the particular type of analysis selected, the computer program is often unable to detect that error and will proceed to perform the analysis. The results will be meaningless, and the researcher's conclusions will be completely in error (Hinshaw & Schepp, 1984).

Statistical Assistance

Programmers assist in writing the programs that give commands to the computer to implement the mathematical processes selected. Programmers are skilled in the use of computer languages but are not statisticians; thus they do not interpret the outcomes of analysis. Computer languages are the messages used to give detailed commands to the computer. Even when packaged programs are being used, a programmer skilled in the use of common software packages can be of great help in selecting the appropriate programs, writing them according to guidelines, and speeding up the debugging process. In universities, computer science students are often available for programming services.

A statistician has an educational background that qualifies him or her as an expert in statistical analysis. Statisticians vary in their skill pertaining to specific statistical procedures and usually charge an hourly fee for services. However, some may contract to perform an agreed-upon analysis for a set fee. Although the extent of need for statistical consultation is dependent on the educational background of the researcher, most nurse researchers will benefit from statistical consultation. However, the researcher remains the content expert and must be the final authority in interpreting the meaning of the analyses in terms of the discipline's body of knowledge. Therefore, it is not acceptable to abdicate the total responsibility for data analysis to the statistician. The nurse researcher remains accountable for understanding the statistical procedures used and for interpreting these procedures to various audiences when the results of the study are communicated.

CHOOSING APPROPRIATE STATISTICAL PROCEDURES FOR A STUDY

Multiple factors are involved in determining the suitability of a statistical procedure for a particular study. Some of these factors are related to the nature of the study, some to the nature of the researcher, and others to the nature of statistical theory. Specific factors include (1) the purpose of the study; (2) hypotheses, questions, or objectives; (3) design; (4) level of measurement; (5) previous experience in statistical analysis; (6) statistical knowledge level; (7) availability of statistical consultation; (8) financial resources; and (9) access to computers. Statistical procedures that meet the requirements of the study are identified by using items 1 to 4. The options may then be further narrowed through the process of elimination based on items 5 through 9.

One approach to selecting an appropriate statistical procedure or judging the appropriateness of an analysis technique for a critique is to use a decision tree. A decision tree directs your choices by gradually narrowing your options through the decisions you make. Two decision trees that have been helpful in selecting statistical procedures are presented in Figures 18–11 and 18–12.

One disadvantage of decision trees is that if you make an incorrect or uninformed decision (guess), you can be led down a path in which you might select an inappropriate statistical procedure for your study. Decision trees are often constrained by space and therefore do not include all the information needed to make an appropriate selection. The most extensive decision tree that we have found is presented in *A Guide for Selecting Statistical Techniques for Analyzing Social Science Data* by Andrews and colleagues (1981). The following examples of questions designed to guide the selection or evaluation of statistical procedures were extracted from this book.

1. How many variables does the problem involve?
2. How do you want to treat the variables with respect to the scale of measurement?
3. What do you want to know about the distribution of the variable?
4. Do you want to treat outlying cases differently from others?

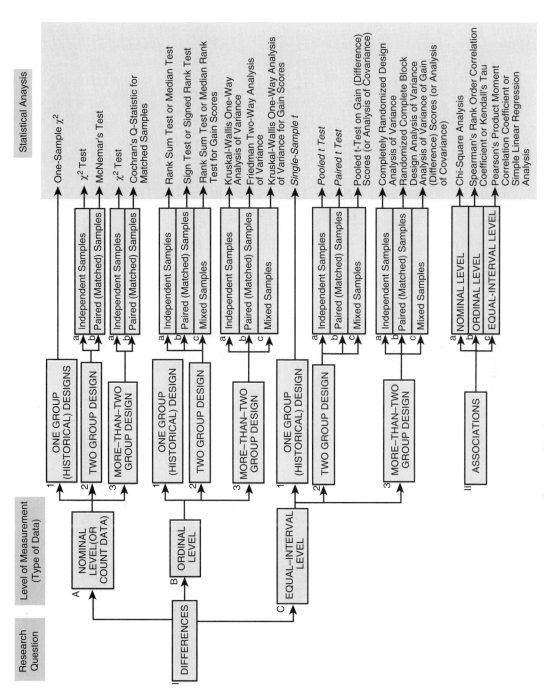

FIGURE 18–11 ■ Decision tree for choosing a statistical test.

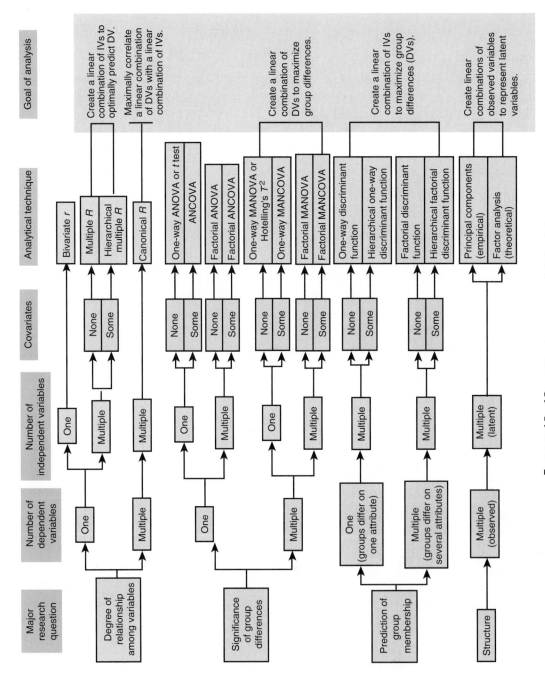

FIGURE 18–12 ■ Choosing among statistical techniques.

5. What is the form of the distribution?
6. Is a distinction made between a dependent and an independent variable?
7. Do you want to test whether the means of the two variables are equal?
8. Do you want to treat the relationship between variables as linear?
9. How many of the variables are dichotomous?
10. Is the dichotomous variable a collapsing of a continuous variable?
11. Do you want to treat the ranks of ordered categories as interval scales?
12. Do the variables have the same distribution?
13. Do you want to treat the ordinal variable as though it were based on an underlying normally distributed interval variable?
14. Is the interval variable dependent?
15. Do you want a measure of the strength of the relationship between the variables or a test of the statistical significance of differences between groups? (Kenny, 1979)
16. Are you willing to assume that an intervally scaled variable is normally distributed in the population?
17. Is there more than one dependent variable?
18. Do you want to statistically remove the linear effects of one or more covariates from the dependent variable?
19. Do you want to treat the relationships among the variables as additive?
20. Do you want to analyze patterns existing among variables or among individual cases?
21. Do you want to find clusters of variables that are more strongly related to one another than to the remaining variables?

Each question confronts you with a decision. The decision you make narrows the field of available statistical procedures. Decisions must be made regarding the following:

1. Number of variables (1, 2, more than 2)
2. Type of measurement (nominal, ordinal, interval)
3. Type of variable (independent, dependent, research)
4. Distribution of variable (normal, nonnormal)
5. Type of relationship (linear, nonlinear)
6. What you want to measure (strength of relationship, difference between groups)
7. Nature of the groups (equal or unequal in size, matched or unmatched, dependent or independent)
8. Type of analysis (descriptive, classification, methodological, relational, comparison, predicting outcomes, intervention testing, causal modeling, examining changes across time)

As you can see, selecting and evaluating statistical procedures requires that you make a number of judgments regarding the nature of the data and what you want to know. Knowledge of the statistical procedures and their assumptions is necessary for selection of the appropriate procedures. One must weigh the advantages and disadvantages of various statistical options. Access to a statistician can be invaluable in selecting the appropriate procedures.

▪ SUMMARY
. . . .

This chapter and the following five chapters provide the information that you need to critique the statistical sections of published studies or to perform statistical procedures. The present chapter introduces you to the concepts of statistical theory, followed by a discussion of some of the more pragmatic aspects of quantitative data analysis: the purposes of statistical analysis, the process of performing data analysis, choice of the appropriate statistical procedures for a study, and resources for statistical analysis. To critique a study, the nurse needs to be able to identify the statistical procedures used; judge whether these statistical procedures were appropriate for the hypotheses, questions, or objectives of the study and for the data available for the analysis; comprehend the discussion of data analysis results; judge whether the author's interpretation of the results is appropriate; and evaluate the clinical significance of the findings.

Statistical analysis procedures are based on statistical and mathematical theory. As is common in many theories, theoretical ideas related to statistics are expressed by unique terminology and logic that is unfamiliar to many. Evaluating the results of published research, developing a data analysis plan, and interpreting the results of a study require that you understand the language and logic of statistics. Inductive logic is used by statisticians to make inferences about the data. Probability theory addresses analyses from the perspective of explaining the likelihood of an event or the degree of a relationship. Decision theory is used when testing for differences between groups. A cutoff point is identified that will guide the decision of whether the groups are members of the same population. The cutoff point is the level of significance, or alpha (α).

The theoretical normal curve, a product of mathematical theory, is symmetrical and unimodal and has continuous values. The mean, median, and mode are equal. A sampling distribution is developed by using the statistical values of many samples obtained from the same population. The mean of a sampling distribution of means is referred to as the mean of means (μ). The purpose of the sampling distribution is to allow us to measure sampling error, which is the difference between the sample statistic used to estimate a parameter and the actual, but unknown value of the parameter. Just as it is possible to develop distributions of summary statistics within a population, it is also possible to develop distributions of inferential statistical outcomes. For example, a sampling distribution could be developed by testing for differences in the means with a t test.

Standardized scores have been developed to facilitate comparison of a score in one distribution with a score in another distribution. Raw scores are transformed into standard scores to allow easy conceptual grasp of the meaning of the score.

A statistic such as $\overline{X}$ is a numerical value obtained from a sample. The parameter μ refers to that same true (but unknown) value within a population. Relating a statistic to a parameter requires an inference as one moves from the sample to the sampling distribution and then from the sampling distribution to the population.

A statistic that produces a value as a function of the scores in a sample is called an estimator. Much of inferential statistical analysis involves the use of point estimation to evaluate the fit between the estimator (a statistic) and the population parameter. A point estimate is a single figure that estimates the related figure in the population of interest. Three characteristics of the estimator are considered important: (1) unbiasedness, (2) consistency, and (3) relative efficiency. The mean of the sample is the most unbiased estimator. When sampling from a continuous distribution, that is, one with either an interval or ratio scale, the probability of the sample mean being exactly equal to the population mean is zero. Therefore, we know that we are going to be in error if we use point estimators. Interval estimation is an attempt to overcome this problem by controlling the initial precision of an estimator. An interval estimate is a segment of a number line where the value of the parameter is thought to be.

The concept of degrees of freedom involves the freedom of a score's value to vary given the other existing scores' values and the established sum of these scores. On a normal curve, extremes of statistical values can occur at either end of the curve. Consequently, the 5% of statistical values that are considered statistically significant must be distributed between the two extremes of the curve. The extremes of the curve are referred to as tails. If the hypothesis is nondirectional and assumes that an extreme score can occur in either tail, the analysis is referred to as a two-tailed test of significance. In a one-tailed test of significance, the hypothesis is directional, and extreme statistical values that occur in a single tail of the curve are of interest.

Two types of error can occur when making decisions about the meaning of a value obtained from a statistical test: Type I errors and Type II errors. A Type I error occurs when the researcher concludes that the samples tested are from different populations (the difference between groups is significant) when, in fact, the samples are from the same population (no significant difference between groups). A Type II error occurs when the researcher concludes that the samples are from the same population when, in fact, they are from different populations. As the risk of a Type I error decreases (by setting a more extreme level of significance), the risk of a Type II error increases. When the risk of a Type II error is decreased (by setting a less extreme level of significance), the risk of a Type I error increases. It is not possible to decrease both types of error simultaneously without increasing the sample size. Therefore, the researcher needs to decide which risk poses the greatest threat within a specific study.

The formal definition of the level of significance, or alpha (α), is the probability of making a Type I error when the null hypothesis is true. The level of significance, developed from decision theory, is the cutoff point used to determine whether the samples being tested are members of the same population or from different populations. Power is the probability that a statistical test will detect a significant difference that exists. Many studies do not have the power to detect differences, and a Type II error results. The strategy used to determine the risk of a Type II error is power analysis.

When a statistical test determines that differences between groups are significant, the researcher has no information on the magnitude of the difference. Magnitude estimation is a strategy to estimate the degree of difference between groups.

Both parametric and nonparametric techniques are valuable methods to analyze data. The choice of technique is determined by the type of data available for analysis. The most commonly used procedures are parametric statistics, the use of which involves three assumptions: (1) the sample was drawn from a population for which the variance can be calculated, (2) the level of measurement should provide interval data or ordinal data with an approximately normal distribution, and (3) random sampling techniques were used to obtain the sample. Nonparametric techniques are not as powerful as parametric techniques but can be used with cruder forms of measurement that yield nominal or ordinal data. Correlational analysis provides important information about relationships within samples and populations. In addition to clarifying the relationship among theoretical concepts, correlational analysis can assist in identifying causal relationships, which can then be tested by inferential analysis.

A neophyte researcher performing a quantitative study is confronted with multiple critical decisions related to data analysis that require statistical knowledge. Statistics can be used for a variety of purposes, such as to (1) summarize, (2) explore the meaning of deviations in the data, (3) compare or contrast descriptively, (4) test the proposed relationships in a theoretical model, (5) infer that the findings from the sample are indicative of the entire population, (6) examine causality, (7) predict, or (8) infer from the sample to a theoretical model.

The role of statistics can be divided into two parts: exploratory data analysis and confirmatory data analysis. Exploratory data analysis is performed to get a preliminary vision of the nature of the data and to search the data for hidden structure or models. Confirmatory data analysis involves traditional inferential statistics that assist the researcher in making an inference about a population or a process based on evidence from the study sample. Quantitative data analysis consists of several stages: (1) preparation of the data for analysis; (2) description of the sample; (3) testing the reliability of measurement; (4) exploratory analysis of the data; (5) confirmatory analysis guided by the hypotheses, questions, or objectives; and (6) post hoc analysis.

Multiple factors are involved in determining the suitability of a statistical procedure for a particular study. One approach to selecting an appropriate statistical procedure or judging the appropriateness of an analysis technique for a critique is to use a decision tree. A decision tree directs your choices by gradually narrowing your options through the decisions you make. Statistical decision trees are provided in the chapter to guide your choice of statistical procedures.

REFERENCES

Andrews, F. M,. Klem, L., Davidson, T. N., O'Malley, P. M., & Rodgers, W. L. (1981). *A guide for selecting statistical techniques for analyzing social science data* (2nd ed). Ann Arbor, MI: Survey Research Center, Institute for Social Research, The University of Michigan.

Barnett, V. (1982). *Comparative statistical inference.* New York: Wiley.

Box, G. E. P., Hunter, W. G., & Hunter, J. S. (1978). *Statistics for experimenters.* New York: Wiley.

Brent, E. E., Jr., Scott, J. K., & Spencer, J. C. (1988). *Ex-Sample: An expert system to assist in designing sampling plans. User's guide and reference manual,* Version 2.0. The Idea Works, Inc., 100 West Briarwood, Columbia, MO 65203.

Chervany, N. L. (1977). *The logic and practice of statistics.* Written materials provided with a presentation at the Institute of Management Science. Bloomington, MN, Dec. 15, 1977.

Cohen, J. (1988). *Statistical power analysis for the behavioral sciences* (2nd ed.). New York: Academic Press.

Conover, W. J. (1971). *Practical nonparametric statistics.* New York: Wiley.

Cox, D. R. (1958). *Planning of experiments.* New York: Wiley.

Glass, G. V., & Stanley, J. C. (1970). *Statistical methods in education & psychology.* Englewood Cliffs, NJ: Prentice-Hall.

Good, I. J. (1983). *Good thinking: The foundations of probability and its applications.* Minneapolis: University of Minnesota Press.

Hinshaw, A. S., & Schepp, K. (1984). Problems in doing nursing research: How to recognize garbage when you see it! *Western Journal of Nursing Research, 6*(1), 126–130.

Kenny, D. A. (1979). *Correlation and causality.* New York: Wiley.

Knapp, R. G. (1985). *Basic strategies for nurses* (2nd ed.). New York: Wiley.

Roscoe, J. T. (1969). *Fundamental research statistics for the behavioral sciences.* New York: Holt, Rinehart & Winston.

Slakter, M. J., Wu, Y. B., & Suzuki-Slakter, N. S. (1991). *, **, and ***, statistical nonsense at the .00000 level. *Nursing Research, 40*(4), 248–249.

Tabachnick, B. G., & Fidell, L. S. (1983). *Using multi-variate statistics.* New York: Harper & Row.

Tukey, J. W. (1977). *Exploratory data analysis.* Reading, MA: Addison-Wesley.

Volicer, B. J. (1984). *Multivariate statistics for nursing research.* New York: Grune & Stratton.

Yarandi, H. N. (1994). Using the SAS system to estimate sample size and power for comparing two binomial proportions. *Nursing Research, 43*(2), 124–125.

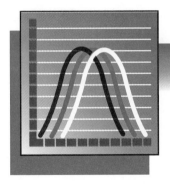

CHAPTER 19

USING STATISTICS TO DESCRIBE

Data analysis begins with description in any study in which the data are numerical, including some qualitative studies. *Descriptive statistics* allow the researcher to organize the data in ways that give meaning and facilitate insight and to examine a phenomenon from a variety of angles to understand more clearly what is being seen. Theory development and generation of hypotheses can emerge from descriptive analyses. For some descriptive studies, descriptive statistics will be the only approach to analysis of the data. This chapter will describe a number of uses of descriptive analysis: to summarize data, to explore deviations in the data, and to describe patterns across time.

USING STATISTICS TO SUMMARIZE DATA

Frequency Distributions

Frequency distributions are usually the first strategy used to organize data for examination. In addition, frequency distributions are used to check for errors in coding and computer programming. The two types of frequency distribution are ungrouped and grouped distribution. In addition to providing a means to display the data, these distributions may influence decisions concerning further analysis of the data.

UNGROUPED FREQUENCY DISTRIBUTION

Most studies have some categorical data that are presented in the form of ungrouped frequency distribution. To develop an ungrouped frequency distribution, list all categories of that variable on which you have data and tally each datum on the listing. For example, the categories of pets in the homes of elderly clients might include dogs, cats, birds, and rabbits. A tally of the ungrouped frequencies would have the following appearance:

Dogs 𝍷𝍷𝍷𝍷 𝍷𝍷𝍷𝍷 𝍷𝍷𝍷𝍷 𝍷𝍷𝍷

Cats 𝍷𝍷𝍷𝍷 𝍷𝍷𝍷𝍷 𝍷𝍷𝍷𝍷 𝍷𝍷𝍷𝍷 𝍷𝍷𝍷𝍷 𝍷𝍷𝍷

Birds 𝍷𝍷𝍷𝍷 𝍷𝍷𝍷𝍷 𝍷𝍷

Rabbits 𝍷𝍷

The tally marks are then counted, and a table is developed to display the results. This approach is generally used on discrete rather than continuous data. Examples of data commonly organized in this manner include gender, ethnicity, marital status, and diagnostic category. Continuous data, such as test grades or scores on a data collection instrument, could be organized in this manner; however, if the number of possible scores is large, it is difficult to extract meaning from examination of the distribution.

GROUPED FREQUENCY DISTRIBUTION

Some method of grouping is generally necessary when continuous variables are being examined. Age, for example, is a continuous variable. Many measures taken during data collection are continuous, including income, temperature, vital lung capacity, weight, scale scores, and time. Grouping requires that the researcher make a number of decisions that will be important to the meaning derived from the data.

Any method of grouping results in loss of information. For example, if age is being grouped, a breakdown of under 65–over 65 will provide considerably less information than will grouping by 10-year spans. The grouping should be made in such a manner to provide the greatest possible meaning in terms of the purpose of the study. If the data are to be compared with data in other studies, groupings should be similar to those of other studies in that field of research.

The first step in developing a grouped frequency distribution is to establish a method of classifying the data. The classes that are developed must be exhaustive; each datum must fit into one of the identified classes. The classes must be mutually exclusive; each datum can fit into only one of the established classes. A common mistake is to list ranges that contain overlaps. The range of each category must be equivalent. In the case of age, for example, if 10 years is the range, each category must include 10 years of ages. The first and last categories may be open-ended and worded to include all scores above or below a specified point. The precision with which the data will be reported is an important consideration. For example, data might be listed only in whole numbers, or decimals may be used. If decimals are used, you will need to decide at how many decimal places rounding off will be performed.

PERCENT DISTRIBUTION

Percent distribution indicates the percentage of the sample with scores falling in a specific group, as well as the number of scores in that group. Percent distributions are particularly useful in comparing the present data with findings from other studies that have varying sample sizes. A cumulative distribution is a type of percent distribution in which the percentages and frequencies of scores are summed as one moves from the top of the table to the bottom (or the reverse). Thus, the bottom category would have a cumulative frequency equivalent to the sample size and a cumulative percentage of 100 (Table 19–1). Frequency distributions can be displayed as tables, diagrams, or graphs. Four types of illustrations are commonly used: pie diagrams, bar graphs, histograms, and frequency polygons. Some examples of diagrams and graphs are presented in Chapter 25. Frequency analysis and graphic presentation of the results can be performed on the computer.

TABLE 19–1
EXAMPLE OF A CUMULATIVE FREQUENCY TABLE

SCORE	FREQUENCY	PERCENTAGE	CUMULATIVE FREQUENCY (f)	CUMULATIVE PERCENTAGE
1	4	8	4	8
3	6	12	10	20
4	8	16	18	36
5	14	28	32	64
7	8	16	40	80
8	6	12	46	92
9	4	8	$N = 50$	100

Measures of Central Tendency

A *measure of central tendency* is frequently referred to as an average. The term *average* is a lay term not commonly used in statistics because of its vagueness. Measures of central tendency are the most concise statement of the location of the data. The three measures of central tendency commonly used in statistical analyses are the mode, median (MD), and mean.

MODE

The *mode* is the numerical value or score that occurs with the greatest frequency; it does not necessarily indicate the center of the data set. The mode can be determined by examination of an ungrouped frequency distribution of the data. In Table 19–1, the mode is the score of 5, which occurred 14 times in the data set. The mode can be used to describe the typical subject or to identify the most frequently occurring value on a scale item. The mode is the appropriate measure of central tendency for nominal data and is used in the calculation of some nonparametric statistics. Otherwise, it is seldom used in statistical analysis. A data set can have more than one mode. If two modes exist, the data set is referred to as bimodal. More than two would be multimodal.

MEDIAN

The median (*MD*) is the score at the exact center of the ungrouped frequency distribution. It is the 50th percentile. The MD is obtained by rank-ordering the scores. If the number of scores is an uneven number, exactly 50% of the scores are above the MD and 50% are below it. If the number of scores is an even number, the MD is the average of the two middle scores. Thus, the MD may not be an actual score in the data set. It is not considered to be as precise an estimator of the population mean when sampling from normal populations as the sample mean is. In most other cases, it is actually the preferred choice because in these cases it is a more precise measure of central tendency. The MD is not affected by extreme scores in the data (outli-

ers), as is the mean. The MD is the most appropriate measure of central tendency for ordinal data and is frequently used in nonparametric analysis.

MEAN

The most commonly used measure of central tendency is the mean. The *mean* is the sum of the scores divided by the number of scores being summed. Thus, like the MD, the mean may not be a member of the data set. The formula for calculating the mean is as follows:

$$\bar{X} = \frac{\Sigma X}{N}$$

where

$\bar{X}$ = the mean
Σ = sigma (the statistical symbol for the process of summation)
X = a single raw score
N = number of scores being entered in the calculation

The mean was calculated for the data provided in Table 19–1.

$$\bar{X} = \frac{4 + 18 + 32 + 70 + 56 + 48 + 36}{50} = \frac{264}{50} = 5.28$$

The mean is an appropriate measure of central tendency for approximately normally distributed populations. This formula will be found repeatedly within more complex formulas of statistical analysis.

USING STATISTICS TO EXPLORE DEVIATIONS IN THE DATA

Although the use of summary statistics has been the traditional approach to describing data or describing the characteristics of the sample before inferential statistical analysis, it is limited as a means of understanding the nature of data. For example, using measures of central tendency, particularly the mean, to describe the nature of the data obscures the impact of extreme values or deviations in the data. Thus, significant features in the data may be concealed or misrepresented. Often, anomalous, unexpected, problematic data and discrepant patterns are seen but regarded as not meaningful (Ferketich & Verran, 1986; Fox, 1990). Measures of dispersion, such as the modal percentage, range, difference scores, sum of squares (*SS*), variance, and standard deviation (*SD*), provide important insight into the nature of the data.

Ferketich and Verran (1986) contend that there has been a tremendous push in nursing toward the use of inferential statistics. However, they consider the confirmatory approach to data analysis to be inefficient.

"When one basic hypothesis, the null, is tested we know only what is not supported in a study. The rejection or failure to reject a null hypothesis, which is all the statistical test can provide, is insufficient use of often rich data bases. For example, a null hypothesis that states there is no difference between groups on a particular parameter is the usual approach. However, through good exploratory techniques, it might be discovered that part of each group is similar to the corresponding part of the other group; but for the extremes of the group, differences are profoundly manifested. These extremes might have been missed if only summary statistics were used but could be discovered by various resistant statistics of exploratory data analysis (EDA). The most efficient use of the data base is to discover alternate hypotheses and to explore many instead of one single path. EDA provides such exploration without concern for restrictive model assumptions" (pp. 465–466). Chow (1996) defends the use of inferential analysis and suggests that the problems addressed are primarily due to inappropriate uses by researchers.

Measures of Dispersion

Measures of dispersion, or variability, are measures of individual differences of the members of the population and sample. They give some indication of how scores in a sample are dispersed around the mean. These measures provide information about the data that is not available from measures of central tendency. They indicate how different the scores are—the extent to which individual scores deviate from one another. If the individual scores are similar, measures of variability are small and the sample is relatively *homogeneous* in terms of those scores. *Heterogeneity* (wide variation in scores) is important in some statistical procedures, such as correlation. Heterogeneity is determined by measures of variability. The measures most commonly used are modal percentage, range, difference scores, *SS*, variance, and *SD*.

MODAL PERCENTAGE

The *modal percentage* is the only measure of variability appropriate for use with nominal data. It indicates the relationship of the number of data scores represented by the mode to the total number of data scores. To determine the modal percentage, the frequency of the modal scores is divided by the total number of scores. For example, in Table 19–2, the mode is 5 because 14 of the subjects scored 5, and the sample size is 50; thus, $14/50 = .28$. The result of that operation is then multiplied by 100 to convert it to a percentage. In the example given, the modal percentage would be 28%, which means that 28% of the sample is represented by the mode. The complete calculation would be $14/50(100) = 28\%$. This strategy allows comparison of the present data with other data sets.

RANGE

The simplest measure of dispersion is the *range*. The range is obtained by subtracting the lowest score from the highest score. The range for the scores in Table 19–2 is calculated as follows: $9 - 1 = 8$. The range is a difference score that uses only the two extreme scores for the comparison. It is a very crude measure and is sensitive to outliers.

TABLE 19–2
DATA FOR CALCULATION OF MEAN AND STANDARD DEVIATION

SCORE X	FREQUENCY (f)	fX	fX^2
1	4	4	$4(1) = 4$
3	6	18	$6(9) = 54$
4	8	32	$8(16) = 128$
5	14	70	$14(25) = 350$
7	8	56	$8(49) = 392$
8	6	48	$6(64) = 384$
9	4	36	$4(81) = 324$
	$N = 50$	$\Sigma X = 264$	$\Sigma X^2 = 1636$

Outliers are subjects with extreme scores that are widely separated from scores of the rest of the subjects. The range is generally reported but is not used in further analyses. It is not a very useful method of comparing the present data with data from other studies.

DIFFERENCE SCORES

Difference scores are obtained by subtracting the mean from each score. Sometimes a difference score is referred to as a deviation score because it indicates the extent to which a score deviates from the mean. The difference score will be positive when the score is above the mean and negative when the score is below the mean. Difference scores are the basis for many statistical analyses and can be found within many statistical equations. The sum of difference scores is zero, which makes the sum a useless measure. The formula for difference scores is

$$X - \bar{X}$$

THE SUM OF SQUARES

A common strategy used to allow meaningful mathematical manipulation of difference scores is to square them. These squared scores are then summed. The mathematical symbol for the operation of summing is Σ. When negative scores are squared, they become positive, and therefore the sum will no longer equal zero. This mathematical

maneuver is referred to as the *sum of squares (SS)*. In this case, the SS is actually the sum of squared deviations. The equation for SS is

$$SS = \Sigma (X - \bar{X})^2$$

The larger the value of SS, the greater the variance. Because the value of SS is dependent on the measurement scale used to obtain the original scores, comparison of SS with that obtained in other studies is limited to studies using similar data. SS is a valuable measure of variance and is used in many complex statistical equations. The importance of SS is due to the fact that when deviations from the mean are squared, the sum is smaller than the sum of squared deviations from any other value in a sample distribution. This relationship is referred to as the *least-squares principle* and is important in mathematical manipulations.

VARIANCE

Variance is another measure commonly used in statistical analysis. The equation for variance (V) is

$$V = \frac{\Sigma (X - \bar{X})^2}{N - 1}$$

As can be seen, variance is the mean or average of SS. Again, because the result is dependent on the measurement scale used, it has no absolute value and can be compared only with data obtained by using similar measures. However, in general, the larger the variance, the larger the dispersion of scores (Shelley, 1984).

STANDARD DEVIATION

Standard deviation (SD) is simply the square root of the variance. This step is important mathematically because squaring mathematical terms changes them in some important ways. Obtaining the square root reverses this change. The equation for obtaining *SD* is

$$SD = \sqrt{\frac{\Sigma (X - \bar{X})^2}{N - 1}}$$

Although this equation clarifies the relationships among difference scores, *SS*, and variance, using it requires that all these measures in turn be calculated. If *SD* is being calculated directly by hand (or with the use of a calculator), the following computational equation is easier to use. Data from Table 19–2 were used to calculate the *SD*:

$$SD = \sqrt{\frac{\Sigma X^2 - (1/N)(\Sigma X)^2}{N - 1}}$$

$$SD = \sqrt{\frac{1636 - (1/50)(264)^2}{50 - 1}}$$

$$SD = \sqrt{\frac{1636 - 1393.92}{49}}$$

$$SD = \sqrt{4.94}$$

$$SD = 2.22$$

Just as the mean is the "average" score, the *SD* is the "average" difference (deviation) score. *SD* provides a measure of the average deviation of a score from the mean in that particular sample. It indicates the degree of error that would be made if the mean alone were used to interpret the data. *SD* is an important measure, both in understanding dispersion within a distribution and in interpreting the relationship of a particular score to the distribution. Descriptive statistics (mean, MD, mode, and *SD*) are usually calculated by computer.

Exploratory data analysis, developed by Tukey (1977) and more recently expanded by Fox and Long (1990), is designed to detect the unexpected in the data and to avoid overlooking crucial patterns that may exist. In nursing, identification and expla-

nation of patterns are considered critical to both theory and practice. The procedures also facilitate comparison of groups. The outcome of EDA may be theory generation or the development of hypotheses for confirmatory data analysis. Graphic analysis of data, central to EDA, requires an element of subjective interpretation. However, when a series of visual displays continue to show evidence of the same pattern, subjectivity is minimized. Evidence is building to support the discovery of a basic pattern in the data (Ferketich & Verran, 1986). Using graphics as an element of data analysis is a relatively new strategy. More commonly, graphics has been used to present the results of data analysis. With EDA, the purpose of graphic displays is discovery. Even numeric summaries are presented in such a way that the researcher can visualize patterns in the data. Although EDA is a relative newcomer, most mainframe and personal computer (PC) data analysis programs perform the statistical procedures and graphic techniques of EDA.

The techniques of EDA use new terms and require different logical processes and a different mindset in the researcher than do those of summary statistics. The researcher must be flexible, open to the unanticipated, and sensitive to patterns that are revealed as the analysis proceeds. Tukey (1977) suggests that "exploratory data analysis is detective work" (p. 1); it is a search for clues and evidence. When using EDA, it is important for the researcher to get a feel for what the data are like. During analysis, the researcher will move back and forth among the techniques of numeric summaries, graphic displays of the data, pattern identification, and theoretical exploration of the meaning of discoveries (Ferketich & Verran, 1986).

Tukey's (1977) procedures make analysis fun rather than mysterious. EDA is somewhat akin to playing with numbers. It captures the right brain's playful, creative portion of the intellect, as well as the logical, deductive practical left brain portion. Tukey (1977) has even given the procedures playful, imaginative names. Moreover, EDA provides a depth of understanding not possible with previous approaches to data analysis. The following section describes some of the initial approaches to EDA. If you are interested in exploring some of the more advanced procedures of EDA, we refer you to Tukey (1977) and Fox and Long (1990). EDA procedures described in this chapter include stem-and-leaf displays, residual analysis, relationship plots, Q plots, box-and-whisker plots, symmetry plots, and Bland and Altman plots.

Stem-and-Leaf Displays

The *stem-and-leaf display* is a visual presentation of numbers that may provide important insight. It is useful for batches of data values from approximately 20 to 200 (Fox, 1990). To develop the display, the numbers are organized by lines. Each line of the display is a stem; each piece of information on the stem is a leaf. To develop a stem-and-leaf display, the last digit (or in some cases, the last two digits) of the number is used as the leaf; the rest of the number is the stem. An example is provided in the following sections.

DISTRIBUTION

Assume that we have a batch of numbers with the values shown in Table 19–3. There are 43 values with a mean of 57 and an *SD* of 6. However, these summary statistics would not be the primary interest of Tukey. He would want to see what the data looked like.

STEM AND LEAF

In a stem-and-leaf display, the stem is the first digit of each number and is placed to the left of the bar as in Table 19–4. When adding the leaves to the display, the last digit of each number is placed on the appropriate line of the stem. The first row includes the values of 12, 14, 16, and 18. The stem for the first row is 1 and the leaves are 2, 4, 6, and 8.

TABLE 19–3
SAMPLE DATA SET

12, 83, 59, 43, 26, 61, 66, 55, 84, 39, 75, 16, 125, 22, 65, 89, 28, 66, 40, 163, 73, 38, 21, 78, 35, 50, 42, 96, 32, 33, 59, 54, 47, 172, 18, 14, 68, 73, 52, 43, 49, 76, 25.

TABLE 19–4
STEM-AND-LEAF DISPLAY

1	2468
2	12568
3	23589
4	023379
5	024599
6	15668
7	33568
8	349
9	6
11	
12	5
13	
14	
15	
16	3
17	2

MEDIAN

The distribution in Table 19–4 appears positively skewed. This observation is validated by the difference in the mean (57) and the MD (52). Determining the MD from a stem-and-leaf display is relatively easy. The MD is either the single middle value or the mean of the two middle values (Tukey, 1977, p. 29). The equation for the position of the MD from the ends of the distribution is 1/2 (1 + N). In this set of 43 numbers, 1/2 (1 + 43) = 1/2 (44) = 22. The MD is the 22nd number to the right of the bar, or 52.

RANKING

Values in the distribution may be ranked from the lowest value to the highest value or from the highest value to the lowest value. Depth can also be ranked, with the MD being the greatest rank and the extremes being 1. Depth is the number of values between the MD and one of the extremes. These three rankings are illustrated in Table 19–5.

EXTREME VALUES

Extreme values are also of interest. In the distribution shown in Table 19–5, the upper extreme value (UE) is 172. The lower extreme value (LE) is 12.

TABLE 19-5
RANKED VALUES

UPWARD RANK	VALUE	DOWNWARD RANK	DEPTH
1	12 (LE)	43	1
2	14	42	2
3	16	41	3
4	18	40	4
5	21	39	5
6	22	38	6
7	25	37	7
8	26	36	8
9	28	35	9
10	32	34	10
11	33	33	11
12	35	32	12
13	38	31	13
14	39	30	14
15	40	29	15
16	42	28	16
17	43	27	17
18	43	26	18
19	47	25	19
20	49	24	20
21	50	23	21
22	52 (MD)	22	22
23	54	21	21
24	55	20	20
25	59	19	19
26	59	18	18
27	61	17	17
28	65	16	16
29	66	15	15
30	66	14	14
31	68	13	13
32	73	12	12
33	73	11	11
34	75	10	10
35	76	9	9
36	78	8	8
37	83	7	7
38	84	6	6
39	89	5	5
40	96	4	4
41	125	3	3
42	163	2	2
43	172 (UE)	1	1

LE = lower extreme value; MD = median; UE = upper extreme value.

HINGES

Hinges (H) are determined by calculating the value halfway from each extreme to the MD. A hinge is calculated in the same manner as the MD. Thus, 1/2 (1 + 22) = 11.5. However, Tukey (1977) drops the .5, instead preferring the simplicity of whole numbers, and the hinges will be the 11th

value from each extreme. In our distribution, the lower hinge (LH) is 33 and the upper hinge (UH) is 73. To allow you to see the positioning of the values more clearly, they are presented in folded form in Figure 19–1, in which the angle of the values changes at the hinge. These values may also be expressed as a five-number summary, as shown in Table 19–6.

Values that describe the spread of the distribution can also be expressed. The LH-LE spread in our distribution of 21 is obtained by subtracting 12 (LE) from 33 (LH). The LH-MD spread is 19. The UH-MD spread is 21 and the UE-UH spread is 99. The low spread (LS) is the spread between LE and MD, midspread (MS) is the spread between LH and UH (sometimes referred to as the hinge spread or H-spread), and high spread (HS) is the spread between MD and UH. These values can all be placed in a table that is referred to as the MD hinge number summary (Table 19–7). The values can be used in other displays to illustrate the shape of the distribution (Verran & Ferketich, 1987a).

If the distribution is symmetrical, the distance between LE and LH should be equal to the distance between UH and UE. Distances between the MD and the two hinges should also be equal, as should the distances between the hinges and the extremes. The distance between the MD and the two hinges should be smaller than the distance between the extremes and the hinges. The LS should be equal to the HS (Verran & Ferketich, 1987a). Clearly, the sample presented in Table 19–7 is not symmetrical.

FENCES

Two sets of fences, upper (Uf) and lower (Lf) and inner and outer, are used to identify outliers. These fences are defined by *steps,* a step being $1.5 \times MS$. The inner fences (f) are one step beyond the hinges. The fences can be calculated by using the following equation:

$$Uf = UH + 1.5 \times MS$$

$$Lf = LH - 1.5 \times MS$$

In our sample, the upper inner fence (Uf) is 133. The lower inner fence (Lf) is −27.

```
                          52 (MD)
   12 (LE)               50  54                    172(UE)
     14                 49    55                    163
      16               47      59                  125
       18             43        59                96
        21           43          61              89
         22         42            65            84
          25       40              66          83
           26     39                66        78
            28   38                  68      76
             32 35                    73  75
               33 (LH)                  73 (UH)
```

FIGURE 19–1 ■ Data distribution in folded form.

Outer fences (F) are two steps beyond the hinges and can be calculated by using the following equation:

$$UF = UH + 3 \times MS$$

$$LF = LH - 3 \times MS$$

In our sample, the upper outer fence (UF) is 193 and the lower outer fence (LF) is −87. Values beyond the inner fence are referred to as *outside,* whereas values beyond the outer fence are referred to as *far out.* However, Fox (1990) points out that "outside—and even far-outside—values are not necessarily 'outliers,' in the sense of not belonging with the rest of the data" (p. 75). They are displayed individually because they are unusual and should be looked at closely.

The decision regarding what to do about outliers is specific to the particular study. The researcher needs to be aware of their presence and their possible effect on outcomes of planned statistical analysis. In some cases, outliers are judged not to be representative of the population under study and are removed from the analyses. In others, specific analyses are planned to examine outliers. Information on outliers needs to be included in the research report because they can provide valuable insight into the phenomenon under study.

Residual Analysis

Most statistical procedures focus on measures of central tendency, which Tukey (1977) refers to as the *fit.* For any expression of fit that summarizes the data as a whole, there is a residual. For example, the result of regression analysis is a "line of best fit," which is drawn on a graph showing a plot of the individual values (see Chapter 21). For each point on that line (the fit), there are also individual values that vary from the fit. If the fit is the mean, the difference (or deviation) values would be the residuals. Combined, these variations are the residuals for that data set. This relationship can be expressed as

$$RESIDUALS = DATA - FIT$$

These residuals are the main tool of EDA. "They are to the data analyst what powerful magnifying glasses, sensitive chemical tests for bloodstains, and delicate listening devices are to a story-book detective" (Tukey, 1977, p. 125). Displays illustrating residuals are as important as displays of raw data or displays of the fit. Tukey (1977, p. 136) provides mathematical calculations for plotting residual values. These plots can provide evidence of hidden

TABLE 19–6
FIVE-NUMBER SUMMARY TABLE OF DATA DISTRIBUTION

12 (LE)	33 (LH)	52 (MD)	73 (UH)	172 (UE)

LE = lower extreme value; LH = lower hinge; MD = median; UH = upper hinge; UE = upper extreme value.

		TABLE 19–7		
		MEDIAN HINGE NUMBER SUMMARY		
12 (LE)	33 (LH)	52 (MD)	73 (UH)	172 (UE)
	21 (LH-LE)	19 (MD-LH)	21 (UH-MD)	99 (UE-UH)
	40 (LS)	40 (MS)	120 (HS)	

HS = high spread; LE = lower extreme value; LH = lower hinge; MD = median; UE = upper extreme value; UH = upper hinge.

structure or unusual values (Verran & Ferketich, 1987c). Figure 19–2 is an example of such a plot.

An important component of residual analysis is the identification of outliers. *Outliers* are extreme values in the data set. They occur for four main reasons (Slinkman, 1984). The first three reasons were identified by Barnett and Lewis (1978) and include inherent variability, measurement error, and execution error. *Inherent variability* means that in data you can naturally expect a few random observations to be in the extreme ends of the tail. For example, if you had 1000 observations from a normally distributed population, you could expect to find 2.6 observations to be more than 3 *SD* from the mean. Outliers also occur because of *measurement error*. This point was discussed in Chapter 15. If you can determine that the outlier is, in fact, caused by measurement error, the observation should be removed from the data set because it will have a negative influence on statistical analyses. *Execution errors* occur because of a defect in the data collection procedure. These erroneous observations, when detected, should also be removed from the data set.

However, the most important cause of outliers from the point of view of data analysis is *error in identifying the variables,* which is important in explaining the nature of the phenomenon under study (Weisberg, 1977). In this case, the summary statistics, the regression line, or the path analysis does not turn out as expected and the outlier provides new and unexpected information. This unexpected information is central to the discovery of new knowledge.

RELATIONSHIP PLOTS

In EDA, displays of the data such as plots are an important part of the process of analysis. They help the researcher get a feel for the data. A plot of relationship is a common way to illustrate the relationship of two variables graphically (Verran & Ferketich, 1987b). To develop a plot of relationship, you must first determine the units that you will use for the horizontal and vertical scales. For example, if you are using time for one scale, your units on the horizontal (or x) axis might be 1 day, 5 days, or 10 days. The vertical (or y) axis might be the occurrence and stage of a decubitus ulcer. The units are selected to provide the best image of the data. Scale units are indicated on the graph by marks or ticks along the axes. Units must be equal across the axes to avoid distorting the data. The marks (or ticks) along the axes are used to plot the points on the graph and to provide perspective to the information within the graph. Ticks should be sufficient to orient the viewer without distracting attention from the data presentation within the graph (see Figure 19–3).

The variables are usually expressed as *x* and *y*. The plot is constructed by using a scale for the values of each variable, with the scale for *y* placed vertically and the scale for *x* placed horizontally. For each unit or subject, there is a value for *x* and a value for *y*. The plot illustrates the relationship be-

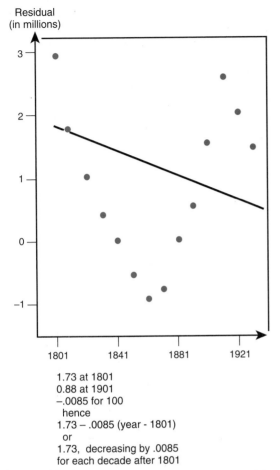

FIGURE 19–2 ▪ Example of a residual plot. (From Tukey, J. W. [1977]. *Exploratory data analysis.* Reading, MA. Addison-Wesley, 1977).

Text below figure 19-2:

1.73 at 1801
0.88 at 1901
−.0085 for 100
   hence
1.73 − .0085 (year - 1801)
   or
1.73, decreasing by .0085
for each decade after 1801

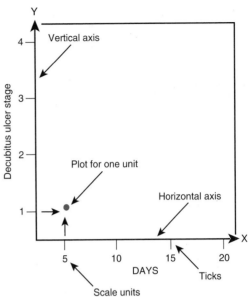

FIGURE 19–3 ▪ Structure of a plot.

viewer's eyes on the points. Symbols should be large enough to stand out; if more than one kind is used, each should be clearly different and equally noticeable. The graph should be constructed to facilitate the viewer's ability to see the behavior of the data. When exploring the data, plots of y against x may help even "when we know nothing about the logical connection from x to y—even when we do not know whether or not there is one—even when we know that such a connection is impossible" (Tukey, 1977, p. 131).

tween these two values. In one type of plot, a scatter plot, the point at which each value of x and y intersect is plotted on the graph (Figure 19–4). In other cases, a single line on the graph expresses the results of a statistical analysis summarizing the best fit for the overall data (Figure 19–5). Usually, the scatter plot and the line of best fit are overlaid (Figure 19–6).

The structure of the graph should be carefully planned to facilitate the visual impact of the presentation of the data. Graphs are for looking at the data; they are not stores of quantitative information. The graph should be constructed to keep the

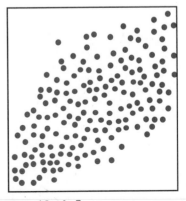

FIGURE 19–4 ▪ Example of a scatter plot.

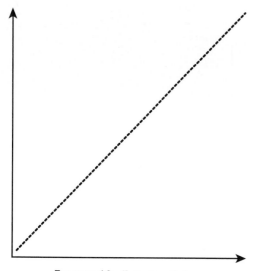

FIGURE 19–5 ▪ Best fit line.

Q PLOTS

Q plots display values in the distribution by quantile. A quantile shows the location of the score within the distribution, similar to that obtained by ranking the scores. However, it goes a step beyond ranking the scores. If i symbolizes the rank of a particular score, the quantile may be calculated by using the following formula:

$$(i - .5)/n$$

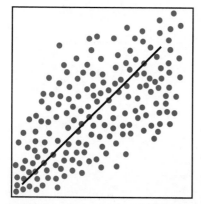

FIGURE 19–6 ▪ Overlay of scatter plot and best fit line.

For example, in our sample of 43, rank 1 is calculated as $(1 - .5)/43 = .0116$. Use of this calculation yielded the values for our distribution shown in Table 19–8. By using the actual value as y and the quantile value as x, a bivariate plot can

TABLE 19–8
ACTUAL VALUES AND QUANTILE VALUES

UPWARD RANK	VALUE	QUANTILE
1	12	.0116 (LE)
2	14	.0349
3	16	.0581
4	18	.0814
5	21	.1047
6	22	.1279
7	25	.1512
8	26	.1744
9	28	.1977
10	32	.2209
11	33	.2442 (LH)
12	35	.2674
13	38	.2907
14	39	.3140
15	40	.3372
16	42	.3605
17	43	.3837
18	43	.4070
19	47	.4302
20	49	.4535
21	50	.4767
22	52	.5 (MD)
23	54	.5233
24	55	.5465
25	59	.5698
26	59	.5930
27	61	.6163
28	65	.6395
29	66	.6628
30	66	.6860
31	68	.7093
32	73	.7326
33	73	.7558 (UH)
34	75	.7791
35	76	.8023
36	78	.8256
37	83	.8488
38	84	.8721
39	89	.8953
40	96	.9186
41	125	.9419
42	163	.9651
43	172	.9884 (UE)

LE = lower extreme value; LH = lower hinge; MD = median; UE = upper extreme value; UH = upper hinge.

be created (Figure 19–7). These plots reveal a pattern in the data (Verran & Ferketich, 1987a).

BOX-AND-WHISKER PLOTS

Box-and-whisker plots give fast visualization of some of the major characteristics of the data, such as the spread, symmetry, and outliers. The MD and upper and lower hinges are illustrated by the box in Figure 19–8. The whiskers (lines extending from the box) extend to the most extreme value within 1 MS of the hinge. Open circles represent values from 1 to 1.5 MS beyond the whisker. This display has two open circles. Extreme values or outliers (beyond 1.5 MS) are often represented by closed circles or asterisks. Our data set has no extreme values.

SYMMETRY PLOTS

Symmetry plots are designed to determine the presence of skewness in the data. Because symmet-

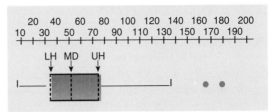

FIGURE 19–8 ■ A box-and-whisker plot.

rical distributions are equally balanced for each value above and below the MD, if values in the same position above and below the MD are plotted against each other, a straight line will result. This plot, then, can be a measure of symmetry. To develop the plot, one must first compute the distance from the MD to the next lower and next higher values. These distances are then plotted against each other (Verran & Ferketich, 1987a). In our sample, the MD is 52. The next lower value is 50; therefore, the distance between them is 2. The distance between the MD and the next higher value is 2. Thus 2 on the horizontal axis and 2 on the vertical axis will be plotted against each other. This procedure continues until all the values have been plotted. The results are illustrated in Figure 19–9. Although a line can be seen, some skewness is evident in the graph.

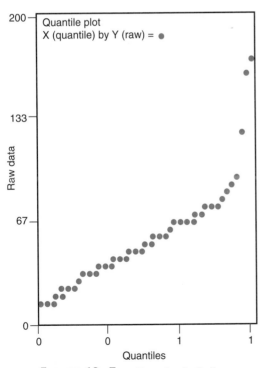

FIGURE 19–7 ■ Example of a Q plot.

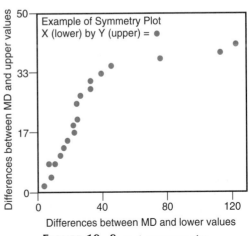

FIGURE 19–9 ■ A symmetry plot.

BLAND AND ALTMAN PLOTS

Bland and Altman plots are used to examine the extent of agreement between two measurement techniques. Generally, they are used to compare a new technique with an established one and have been used primarily with physiological measures. For example, one might wish to compare pulse oximeter values with arterial blood gas values (Figure 19–10). The method was developed by Bland and Altman (1986), and statistical programs to perform the plots are not yet available in the commonly used statistical packages but may be ordered from MedCalc Software (Schoonjans, 1993–1995). A World Wide Web page discussing the procedure is available at *http://allserv.rug.ac.be/~fschoonj/*.

In the plot, the difference between the measures of the two methods can be plotted against the average of the two methods. Thus, for each pair the difference between the two values would be calculated, as well as the average of the two values.

These values are then plotted on a graph displaying a scatter diagram of the differences plotted against the averages. Three horizontal lines are displayed on the graph to show the mean difference, the mean difference plus 1.96 times the *SD* of the differences, and the mean difference minus 1.96 times the *SD* of the differences. The purpose of the plot is to reveal the relationship between the differences and the averages, to look for any systematic bias, and to identify outliers. In some cases, two measures may be closely related near the mean but become more divergent as they move away from the mean. This pattern has been the case with measures of pulse oximetry and arterial blood gases (see Figure 19–10). Traditional methods of comparing measures such as correlation procedures will not identify such problems. Interpretation of the results is based on whether the differences are clinically important (Bland & Altman, 1986).

The repeatability of a single method of measurement may also be examined with this analysis tech-

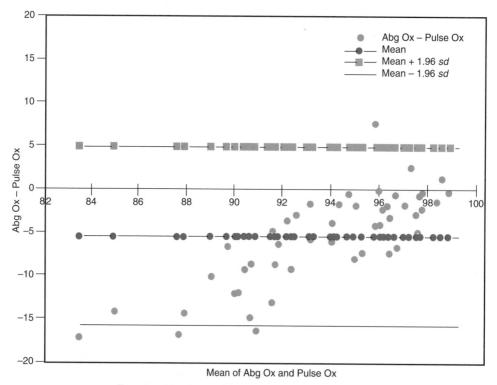

FIGURE 19–10 ■ Example of a Bland and Altman plot.

nique. By using the graph one can examine whether the variability or precision of a method is related to the size of the characteristic being measured. Because the same method is being repeatedly measured, the mean difference should be zero. A coefficient of repeatability (CR) can be calculated by using the following formula. MedCalc can perform this computation of CR (Schoonjans, 1993–1995).

$$CR = 1.96 \times \sqrt{\frac{\Sigma (d_2 - d_1)^2}{n - 1}}$$

where

d = the value of a measure

USING STATISTICS TO DESCRIBE PATTERNS ACROSS TIME

One of the critical needs in nursing research is to conduct studies examining patterns across time. Most nursing studies have examined events at a discrete point in time, and yet the practice of nursing requires an understanding of events as they unfold. This knowledge is essential for developing interventions that can have a positive effect on the health and illness trajectories of the patients in our care. Data analysis procedures that hold promise of providing this critical information include plots displaying variations in variables across time, survival analysis, and time-series analysis.

Analysis of Case Study Data

In case studies, large volumes of both qualitative and quantitative data are often gathered over a certain period. A clearly identified focus for the analysis is critical in a case study. Yin (1994) identified purposes for a case study:

1. To explore situations, such as those in which an intervention is being evaluated, that have no clear set of outcomes
2. To describe the context within which an event or intervention occurred

3. To describe an event or intervention
4. To explain complex causal links
5. To confirm or challenge a theory
6. To represent a unique or extreme case

Data analysis strategies will vary depending on the research questions posed. Because multiple sources of data (some qualitative and some quantitative) are usually available for each variable, triangulation strategies are commonly used in case study analyses. The qualitative data will be analyzed by methods described in Chapter 23. A number of analysis approaches may be used to examine the quantitative data. Some analytical techniques that might be used are pattern matching, explanation building, and time-series analysis (Yin, 1994). Pattern matching compares the pattern found in the case study with one that is predicted to occur. Explanation building is an iterative process that builds an explanation of the case. Time-series analysis may involve visual displays of variations in variables across time or may be the more complex analysis described later in this chapter. Plots are often used to display variables gathered across time. If more than one subject was included in the study, plots may be used to compare variables across subjects. Judgments or conclusions made during the analyses must be carefully considered. The researcher should clearly link information from the case to each conclusion.

Survival Analysis

Survival analysis is a set of techniques designed to analyze repeated measures from a given time (e.g., beginning of the study, onset of a disease, beginning of a treatment, initiation of a stimulus) until a certain attribute (e.g., death, treatment failure, recurrence of a phenomenon) occurs. The determinants of various lengths of survival can be identified. The risk (hazard or probability) of an event occurring at a given point in time for an individual can be analyzed.

A common feature in survival analysis data is the presence of censored observations. These data come from subjects who have not experienced the outcome attribute being measured. They did not die, the treatment continued to work, the phenomenon did not recur, or they were withdrawn from the study for some reason. Because of censored observations and the frequency of skewed data in studies examining such outcomes, common statistical tests may not be appropriate.

The distribution of survival times is explained by three functions: (1) the survivorship function, $S(t)$; (2) the density function, $f(t)$; and the hazard function, $h(t)$. The survivorship function is the probability that a specific individual's time (T) is greater than a specified time (t). The density function is the probability that the individual fails in a specific small interval of time. Thus, the density function reflects the failure rate. The hazard function is the conditional failure rate. It is the probability of failure within a specific small interval of time given that the individual has survived until that point. The results of survival analysis are often plotted on graphs. For example, one might plot the period between the initiation of cigarette smoking and the occurrence of smoking-related diseases such as cancer (Allison, 1984; Gross & Clark, 1975; Hintze, 1990; Lee, 1984; Nelson, 1982).

Survival analysis has been used most frequently in medical research. When a cancer patient asks what his or her chances of cure are from a specific treatment, the information that the physician provides was probably obtained by using survival analysis. The procedure has been used less commonly in nursing research. However, because of further development of statistical procedures and their availability in statistical packages such as NCSS (Number Cruncher Statistical System) for the PC, one can expect to see this analysis procedure more commonly in the nursing literature in the upcoming years.

With use of the procedure, it is possible to study many previously unexamined facets of nursing practice. Possibilities include the effectiveness of various pain relief measures, length of breast-feeding, maintenance of weight loss, abstinence from smoking, recurrence of decubitus ulcers, urinary tract infection after catheterization, and rehospitalization for the same diagnosis within the 60-day period in which Medicare will not provide reimbursement.

The researcher could examine variables that are effective in explaining recurrence within various time intervals or the characteristics of various groups who have received different treatments.

Time-Series Analysis

Time-series analysis is a technique designed to analyze changes in a variable across time and thus to uncover a pattern in the data. Multiple measures of the variable collected at equal intervals are required. Interest in these procedures in nursing is growing because of the interest in understanding patterns. For example, the wave-and-field pattern is one of the themes of Martha Rogers' (1986) theory. Pattern is also an important component of Margaret Newman's (1979) nursing theory. Pattern has been conceptually defined by Crawford (1982) as "the configuration of relationships among elements of a phenomenon" (quoted in Taylor, 1990, p. 256). Taylor has expanded this definition to incorporate time into the study of patterns and defines pattern as "repetitive, regular, or continuous occurrences of a particular phenomenon. Patterns may increase, decrease, or maintain a stable state by oscillating up and down in degree of frequency. In this way, the structure of a pattern incorporates both change and stability, concepts which are important to the study of human responses over time" (Taylor, 1990, p. 256).

Although certainly the easiest strategy for analyzing time-series data is to graph the raw data, this approach to analysis misses some important information. Important patterns in the data are often missed because of residual effects in the data. Therefore, various statistical procedures have been developed to analyze the data.

In the past, analysis of time-series data has been problematic because computer programs designed for this purpose were not easily accessible. The most common approach to analysis was ordinary least-squares multiple regression. However, this approach has been unsatisfactory for the most part. Better approaches to analyzing this type of data are now available (Box & Jenkins, 1976; Glass et al., 1975; Gottman, 1981). With easier access to computer programs designed to conduct time-series analysis, information in the nursing literature on these approaches has been increasing (Jirovec, 1986; Lentz, 1990a, 1990b; Metzger & Schultz, 1982; Taylor, 1990; Thomas, 1987, 1990).

One approach to the analysis of time-series data was developed and described by McCain and Mc-Cleary (1979), McCleary and Hay (1980), and McDowall and colleagues (1980). The most commonly used time-series analysis model is the *autoregressive integrated moving average (ARIMA) model,* which is based on work by Box and Jenkins (1976). A model is an equation or series of equations that explain a naturally occurring process (McCain & McCleary, 1979).

ARIMA modeling is based on the following four-step procedure: (1) identification, (2) estimation, (3) diagnostic checking, and (4) forecasting, with a feedback loop built into the process as shown in Figure 19–11.

The terminology and the problems that must be dealt with in time-series analysis are different from those that we are more familiar with when analyzing conventional data. A time series has two components: a deterministic component and a stochastic component. The *deterministic component* represents all the parameters of a time series that are not dependent on error (or random variation in the data). However, this parameter cannot perfectly predict the values in a time series because even though the underlying process may be systematic, a single observation will deviate from the expected value. The *stochastic component* describes what is referred to as *noise* (or random variance) in the data. The stochastic component has two parts, a systematic part and an unsystematic part. The systematic part is related to the autocorrelation inherent in time-series data. Autocorrelations, as the term implies, are repeated occurrences in the data that are systematic and to some extent patterned. Each of these events is correlated with both past and future occurrences of the same event. The unsystematic part is the typical error variance that leads to differences from measures of central tendency found in all data. The unsystematic part is the element in time series from which such measures as *SD* are calculated.

ARIMA models describe time series as stochastic or noise processes. The null hypothesis is that only the noise component is present and that no change has occurred. An ARIMA model has three parameters: *p, d,* and *q.* The integer values of these parameters are identified through a simple statistical analysis called *identification.* However, first it is important to understand the parameters.

STATIONARITY

To use an ARIMA (*p, d, q*) model, the data must be either stationary or nonstationary in a homogeneous sense. The noise in a time series drifts up and down across time. If the data are stationary, no decrease or increase has occurred in the level of the series as it drifts. However, most data in the social sciences are nonstationary. Nonstationary in the homogeneous sense means that differencing can be used to make the data stationary. To accomplish this task, difference scores are calculated between the sequences in the time series. The value of the first observation is subtracted from the second, the value of the second is subtracted from the third, and so on. For example, consider the following series of numbers as a time series:

2, 4, 6, 8, 10, 12. . .

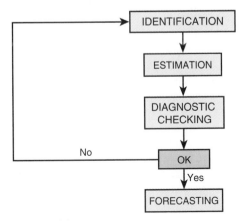

FIGURE 19–11 ■ Steps of autoregressive integrated moving average (ARIMA) modeling.

This series is nonstationary, but note the effect of differencing the series:

$$4 - 2 = 2$$
$$6 - 4 = 2$$
$$8 - 6 = 2$$
$$10 - 8 = 2$$

Now the series is stationary:

$$2, 2, 2, 2, 2, 2, \ldots 2$$

Fortunately, most social science data can be differenced to achieve stationarity. Differencing has no effect on the deterministic parameters of the model, which will be used in the analysis to detect changes. The model parameter d indicates the number of times that a series must be differenced before it becomes stationary. A zero in the model (ARIMA $[p, 0, q]$) indicates that the time series is stationary and does not require differencing.

AUTOREGRESSIVE MODELS

The parameter p indicates the autoregressive order of the model and has two elements: 0_1 and a_t. 0_1 is a correlation coefficient that describes the degree of dependency between observations. If a direct relationship exists between adjacent observations, the value of p exceeds zero. This direct relationship between observations means that the observations are dependent. If they are dependent, the current value can be predicted from the previous value in the series, and the present value can be used to predict future values. The p parameter of the model indicates the number of autoregressive terms included in the model. The a_t parameter is the error term and describes what is referred to as white noise or random shock. This term is the unsystematic element in the stochastic component of the model. In equations calculating this parameter, 0_1 and a_t are summed.

MOVING-AVERAGE MODELS

The q parameter in the ARIMA (p, d, q) model is an indication of the moving-average order. In some time series, a random shock may persist beyond a single observation. This persistence is similar to the effect of dropping a pebble in water. If this effect occurs, q exceeds zero. The statistic ϕ (phi) is a correlation coefficient that expresses the extent to which the current time-series observation can be predicted from preceding random shocks. Phi is used as the weight in a weighted term in a prediction equation. In some models, more than one weighted term may be used.

NOISE MODEL IDENTIFICATION

The systematic part of the stochastic component in an ARIMA (p, d, q) model is identified by using two functions: the autocorrelation function (ACF) and the partial autocorrelation function (PACF). When a likely model has been identified, the parameters are estimated by using special nonlinear computer software. The ACF and PACF are then used to diagnose the adequacy of the model. If the model is inadequate, a new ARIMA (p, d, q) model is identified, the parameters are estimated, and the residuals are diagnosed. This procedure continues until an adequate model is generated.

FORECASTING

When the first three steps of the modeling strategy—identification, estimation, and diagnosis—have been satisfactorily completed, the model can be used for forecasting. An ARIMA model could forecast variables such as infant mortality as a function of past infant mortality. The model cannot be used to explain causality. Three types of change can be detected by the model: abrupt, constant change; gradual, constant change; and abrupt, temporary change. In an adequate model, the residuals act like white noise, and the model can detect differences between the white noise and the effects of change.

Although the analysis process itself does not require extreme degrees of statistical sophistication, it will require some changes in the way that studies are designed in nursing. If a care process is being examined, each element of that care is an observation. Each behavioral response of the patient is an observation. Thus the process of observation may require that the situation be broken down into very discrete elements (McCain & McCleary, 1979; McCleary & Hay, 1980; McDowall et al., 1980; Metzger & Schultz, 1982).

Nursing studies using time-series analysis techniques have only recently begun appearing in the nursing literature. Taylor (1994) describes a study evaluating therapeutic change in symptom severity at the level of the individual woman experiencing severe premenstrual syndrome (PMS).

. . . .

"The purpose of this interrupted time-series study was to determine the effectiveness of a multi-model nursing intervention aimed at relieving the symptom severity and distress associated with PNA [perimenstrual negative affect], and to describe the occurrence of individual patterns of PNA symptoms and symptom pattern change. The use of a time-series design and methodology as an alternative to a cross-sectional group design allowed examination of individual responses over time, as well as an examination of the change in symptom patterns after treatment.

. . . .

"In this interrupted time-series design, each woman is considered as one experiment and serves as her own control. Internal validity is achieved in this design by accounting for the extraneous variables by multiple measures and planning for a stable baseline of data collection before introducing the independent variable (Gottman, 1984; Kazdin, 1982; Mitchell, 1988). Daily and weekly measures were collected across seven complete menstrual cycles in five women meeting restrictive sampling criteria. The baseline phase included three complete menstrual cycles followed by a seven-week intervention phase and a post-intervention phase of three menstrual cycles. Previous research had indicated that two complete menstrual cycles provide an adequate baseline (Mitchell, Woods, & Lentz, 1985, 1991, 1994; Taylor, 1986). Generalizability

is achieved through systematic replication of the design in additional women.

. . . .

"The experimental treatment is a system of non-pharmacologic strategies involving self-monitoring, personal choice, self-regulation and self/environmental modification, administered within a group format of peer support and professional guidance. The purpose of the multi-modal approach is to provide a therapeutic environment for women to incorporate non-pharmacologic treatments, adhere to difficult treatment plans and to provide a milieu to model behavioral, cognitive and environmental change strategies.

. . . .

"A group format (two hours weekly for seven weeks) included formal presentations by a nurse-facilitator. The formal presentations provided the knowledge base for the individual treatments which have been suggested as non-pharmacologic remedies for PMS: (a) specific dietary changes (decreased caffeine and sugar, increased complex carbohydrates, small frequent meals); (b) PMS-formula vitamin supplementation perimenstrually; (c) aerobic and relaxation/stretching exercises; (d) behavioral stress reduction techniques (stress identification, thought stopping, affirmations, self-esteem enhancement); and (e) lifestyle alterations and environmental control (time and role management, communication and social competency training). Demonstration and practice sessions allowed the women to try out the therapies and discussion sessions provided a means for the women to express their unique treatment concerns. A personalized treatment plan was developed for each woman at the end of the seven weeks. . . .

. . . .

"The analysis proceeded in two phases: within-individual, time-series analysis of pre-treatment baseline behavior and response; and an interrupted time-series analysis of treatment effect. For the baseline or pretreatment analysis, 90 data points were available for each woman for PNA symptom severity data. Examination of the shape and significance of the baseline PNA pattern permitted the analysis of symptom fluctuation within the menstrual cycle as well as confirmation of the initial classification of severe PNA. In the application of the interrupted time-series analysis to examine treatment effects, 120 daily data points were available for the post-treatment time-series. Simply, the time-series was 'interrupted' by the intervention. The pretreatment (or baseline) time-series data were analyzed for shape, structure and statistical significance, and compared with the shape, structure and statistical significance of the post-treatment time-series data (Abraham & Neundorfer, 1990; Gottman, 1984; Woods & Catanzaro, 1988).

● ●

"The auto-correlation function (ACF) was used to identify significant patterns within each woman's daily symptom data. The ACF measures the correlation between observations and can be defined as the shared variance of one observation and each successive observation taken from the same individual. In this case, each woman had approximately 200 daily symptom severity data points. . . . Since it was predicted that symptom severity would follow a menstrual cycle pattern, a 'lag' of 28 to 30 days was used for the ACF (depending on each individual menstrual cycle). For example, using a lag of 30 days, each daily symptom value was correlated, or 'lagged,' with the symptom severity value 30 days later (day one correlated with day 30). The ACF assumes serial dependency of the data points, since each data point is drawn from the same person.

● ●

"Each woman's symptom time-series was divided into a baseline time-series (90 days of symptom data) and a post-treatment time-series (120 days of symptom data) and analyzed as an interrupted time-series using the ACF. The auto-correlations were examined for their structure, pattern and significance. Analysis of the 'shape' of the correlogram (plot of the auto-correlations), along with examination of significant auto-correlations, can reveal deterministic patterns which recur within the whole time-series and between the baseline and post-treatment time-series (Gottman, 1984; Taylor, 1990). Auto-correlations greater than two times the standard deviation of the auto-correlation, called the Bartlett Band of significance, were considered statistically significant at the $p = .05$ level (Gottman, 1984).

● ●

"As expected by the use of careful sampling, a menstrual cycle pattern of PNA symptom severity was found in the baseline correlograms, but only in four of the five women. Due to space limitations, [Figure 19–12] represents the baseline pattern found in participant No. 1, No. 2, and No. 4 (e.g., similar patterns were found in each of the three women). [Figure 19–13] represents the menstrual cycle pattern found in participant No. 3. One woman (No. 5) did not demonstrate a menstrual cycle pattern in the baseline correlogram [Figure 19–14]. The ACF was applied to all five baseline time-series, allowing the determination of both pattern structure and statistical significance for each individual baseline time-series. The shape of the correlogram for the first four women revealed a menstrual cycle pattern [see Figures 19–12 and 19–13] with positive auto-correlations at lag 1 to 5 days and lag 27 to 32 days representing the menstrual and premenstrual phases. Negative auto-correlations occur at lag 10 to 21 representing the mid-cycle of the menstrual cycle. In both baseline patterns in [Figure 19–12] and [Figure 19–13], the auto-correlations fall outside the Bartlett Band of statistical significance indicating that these menstrual cycle patterns would not be found by chance at $p = .05$. Thus, four of the five women had confirmed PNA that followed a menstrual cycle pattern in the baseline phase. . . .

● ●

"In participant No. 1 and No. 2, the cyclic pattern of PNA changed significantly ($p = .05$) after treatment as represented by the interrupted time-series analyses [see Figure 19–12]. Perimenstrual negative affect was reduced in level and duration and postmenstrual negative affect was almost nonexistent after the treatment. Average PNA severity levels dropped sharply during the treatment period (cycle three to four) and remained low during the post-treatment phase (cycle five to seven). The average PNA severity score ranged from 0.0 to 4.6 postmenstrually (mean severity = 1.9), and from 4.7 to 8.1 perimenstrually (mean severity = 5.9). The menstrual cycle patterning the baseline correlo-

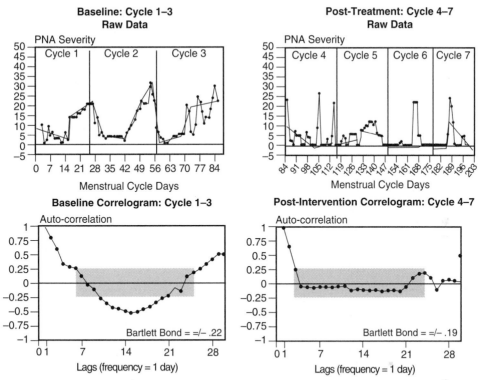

FIGURE 19–12 ■ "Normalizing" treatment effect pattern: PNA severity (participants No. 1, No. 2, and No. 4). (From Taylor, D. L. [1994]. Evaluating therapeutic change in symptom severity at the level of the individual woman experiencing severe PMS. *Image: Journal of Nursing Scholarship 26*[1], 28.)

gram was dampened after the intervention, and significant auto-correlations ($r = \pm.19$) were not apparent. There was a suggestion of a weak periodic process in the post-intervention series (day 23) which reflects the recurrence of low-intensity PNA in the premenstruum. For participants No. 1 and No. 2, the intervention clearly reduced the severity of cyclic PNA. The PNA symptom pattern became predictable and regular, with dramatic modification of symptom intensity, frequency, and duration. This pattern of therapeutic response was labeled a 'normalized' response pattern, whereby a high severity PNA pattern subsides to become a 'normal' menstrual cycle symptom pattern.

· ·

"In participant No. 4, PNA severity decreased during the third baseline cycle and there were many zero scores which mediated the cycle phase differences in symptom scores as well as the treat-

ment effect. Mean PNA severity levels in the premenstruum were low after treatment (1.7–3.5), as were the postmenstrual PNA severity levels (mean severity = .75–4.2). A weak, non-significant pattern emerged at day 31 to 33 ($r = \pm.19$) in the post-treatment correlogram. It is notable that the improvement in PNA severity was very rapid, indicating that treatment effects occurred prior to treatment onset. Because of the rapid response soon after the first baseline cycle, this therapeutic response pattern was also considered as a 'normalized' pattern. PNA symptom severity declined during the second and third baseline period and remained low during the post-intervention period, indicating a 'normal' menstrual symptom pattern.

· ·

"The intervention had little effect on PNA severity for participant No. 3, and the PNA pattern remained disorganized and unpredictable across the

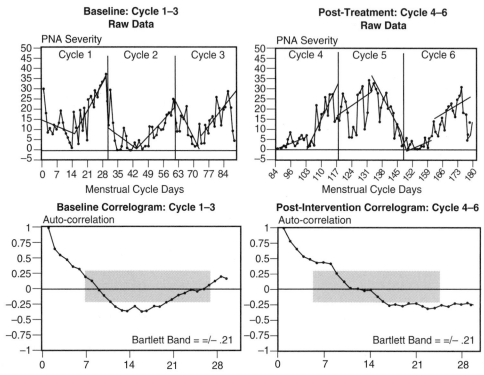

FIGURE 19–13 ▪ "Unstable" treatment effect pattern: PNA severity (participant No. 3). (From Taylor, D. L. [1994]. Evaluating therapeutic change in symptom severity at the level of the individual woman experiencing severe PMS. *Image: Journal of Nursing Scholarship 26*[1], 29.)

post-treatment cycles [see Figure 19–13]. While peri- and postmenstrual negative affect symptom severity was moderate to high in the three cycles comprising the baseline period (mean severity = 16.8 to 40 for three phases), only post-menstrual negative affect declined after treatment (mean severity = 4.4 to 20 for three phases). Perimenstrual negative affect severity remained high (16.8 to 18.0) with little respite from symptom frequency or intensity due to the intervention. The auto-correlations suggested little change in PNA severity after the intervention. Unlike the baseline correlogram, the shape of the auto-correlations did not reflect a menstrual cycle pattern after the intervention, and there were no significant auto-correlations after lag 8. This response pattern was labeled an 'unstable' therapeutic response, whereby PNA severity did not

decline to regular, low severity in the post-intervention period.

••••••••••••••••••••••••••••••••••••

"In participant No. 5, no menstrual cyclicity of PNA severity emerged before or after the treatment [see Figure 19–14]. PNA severity did not conform to a predictable pattern within cycles or across menstrual cycle phase (premenstrual PNA severity = 2.1 to 9.3; postmenstrual PNA severity = 4.3 to 9.7). After the intervention, the seven-day cyclic pattern in PNA severity became nonexistent and the shape of the correlogram revealed a non-cyclic PNA symptom pattern without statistical significance. This symptom pattern was labeled as a 'non–menstrual cycle' response pattern, whereby the shape of the auto-correlations did not resemble any cyclic pattern after the intervention.

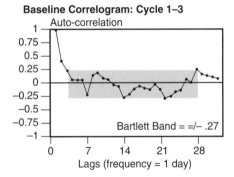

FIGURE 19–14 ■ "Nonmenstrual cycle" treatment effect pattern: PNA severity (participant No. 5). (From Taylor, D. L. [1994]. Evaluating therapeutic change in symptom severity at the level of the individual woman experiencing severe PMS. *Image: Journal of Nursing Scholarship 26*[1], 30.)

· ·

"Clear delineation of PMS and perimenstrual symptom clusters has plagued investigators attempting to understand the phenomena of symptoms that appear to follow a menstrual cycle pattern (Abplanalp, 1988). Certainly part of the problem has been the reliance on aggregate data that obscures individual differences. Furthermore, when individual differences are wildly diverse, conventional analytic strategies are not able to find significant differences without large sample sizes." (pp. 26–30) (Taylor, D. L., 1994)

─────────────────────────────

■ SUMMARY
· ·

Data analysis begins with descriptive statistics in any study in which the data are numerical, including some qualitative studies. Descriptive statistics

allow the researcher to organize the data in ways that give meaning and facilitate insight. Descriptive statistics include summary and exploratory procedures. Summary statistics include measures of central tendency and measures of dispersion. Frequency distributions are usually the first strategy used to organize the data for examination and consist of two types: ungrouped and grouped. Frequency distributions are often displayed in tables or graphs.

The measures of central tendency are the most concise statement of the nature of the data. The three measures of central tendency commonly used in statistical analysis are the mode, the median (MD), and the mean. The mode is the numerical value or score that occurs with greatest frequency, the MD is the score at the exact center of the ungrouped frequency distribution, and the mean is the sum of the scores divided by the number of scores being summed.

Although the use of summary statistics has been the traditional approach to describing data or describing the characteristics of the sample before inferential statistical analysis, it is limited as a means of understanding the nature of the data. For example, using measures of central tendency, particularly the mean, to describe the nature of the data obscures the impact of extreme values or deviations in the data. Thus, significant features in the data may be concealed or misrepresented. Measures of dispersion, such as the modal percentage, range, difference scores, sum of squares, variance, and standard deviation, provide important insight into the nature of the data. The modal percentage indicates the relationship of the number of data scores represented by the mode to the total number of data scores. The range is obtained by subtracting the lowest score from the highest score. Difference scores are obtained by subtracting the mean from each score. The sum of squares is the sum of squared difference scores. Variance is the mean or average of the sum of squares. The standard deviation is the square root of the variance.

Exploratory data analysis (EDA) is designed to detect the unexpected in the data and to avoid overlooking crucial patterns that may exist. EDA procedures described in this chapter include stem-and-leaf displays, residual analysis, relationship plots, Q plots, box-and-whisker plots, symmetry plots, and Bland and Altman plots. Probably the most important strategy in EDA for identifying patterns is visual or graphic examination of the data. EDA should begin by getting a general feel for what the numbers are like. The MD of the distribution is calculated. Values in the distribution may be ranked. Extreme values are also of interest. Hinges are determined by calculating the value halfway from each extreme to the MD. Values that describe the spread of the distribution can also be expressed. These values can all be placed in a table referred to as the MD hinge number summary. Two sets of fences are used to identify outliers: inner fences and outer fences.

One way of looking at data more closely is to examine residuals in the data. Residuals are essentially difference (or deviation) values. Displays illustrating residuals are as important as displays of raw data or displays of the fit.

The stem-and-leaf display is a visual presentation of numbers that may provide insight into the data. Scatter plots are also used. Box-and-whisker plots give a fast visualization of some of the major characteristics of the data, such as the spread, symmetry, and outliers. The MD and the upper and lower hinges are illustrated on the figure, and the whiskers extend to the most extreme value within one midspread of the hinge. A symmetry plot is designed to determine the presence of skewness in the data. Because symmetrical distributions are equally balanced for each value above and below the MD, if values in the same position above and below the MD are plotted against each other, a straight line will result. This display, then, can be a test of symmetry.

One of the critical needs in nursing research is to conduct studies examining patterns across time. Most nursing studies have examined events at a discrete point in time, and yet the practice of nursing requires an understanding of events as they unfold. This knowledge is essential for developing interventions that can have a positive effect on the health and illness trajectories of the patients in our care. Data analysis procedures that hold promise of providing this critical information include plots displaying variations in variables across time, survival analysis, and time-series analysis.

REFERENCES

Abplanalp, J. (1988). Psychosocial theories. In W. R. Keye (Ed.), *The premenstrual syndrome* (pp. 94–112). Philadelphia: Saunders.

Abraham, I. L., & Neudorfer, M. M. (1990). The design and analysis of time-series studies. In L. E. Moody (Ed.), *Advancing nursing science research* (Vol. 2, pp. 145–175). Newbury Park, CA: Sage.

Allison, P. D. (1984). *Event history analysis: Regression for longitudinal event data.* Beverly Hills, CA: Sage.

Box, G. E. P., & Jenkins, G. M. (1976). *Time-series analysis: Forecasting and control* (rev. ed.). San Francisco: Holden-Day.

Crawford, G. (1982). The concept of pattern in nursing: Conceptual development and measurement. *Advances in Nursing Science, 5*(1), 1–6.

Glass, G. V., Willson, V. L., & Gottman, J. M. (1975). *Design and analysis of time-series experiments.* Boulder, CO: Colorado University Associated Press.

Gottman, J. M. (1981). *Time-series analysis: A comprehensive introduction for social scientists.* Cambridge, MA: Cambridge University Press.

Gottman, J. M. (1984). *Time-series analysis.* Cambridge, MA: Cambridge University Press.

Gross, A. J., & Clark, V. (1975). *Survival distributions: Reliability applications in the biomedical sciences.* New York: Wiley.

Hintze, J. L. (1990). *Survival analysis. Number cruncher statistical system version 5.5.* Kaysville, UT: Hintze.

Jirovec, M. M. (1986). Time-series analysis in nursing research: ARIMA modeling. *Nursing Research, 35*(5), 315–319.

Kazdin, A. (1982). *Single-case research designs.* New York: Oxford University Press.

Lee, E. T. (1984). *Statistical methods for survival data analysis.* Belmont, CA: Wadsworth.

Lentz, M. J. (1990a). Time series—issues in sampling. *Western Journal of Nursing Research, 12*(1), 123–127.

Lentz, M. J. (1990b). Time-series analysis-Cosinor analysis: A special case. *Western Journal of Nursing Research, 12*(3), 408–412.

McCain, L. J., McCleary, R. (1979). The statistical analysis of the simple interrupted time-series quasi-experiment. In T. D. Cook & D. T. Campbell (Eds.), *Quasi-experimentation: Design and analysis issues for field settings* (pp. 233–293). Chicago: Rand McNally.

McCleary, R., & Hay, R. A., Jr. (1980). *Applied time-series analysis for the social sciences.* Beverly Hills, CA: Sage.

McDowall, D., McCleary, R., Meidinger, E. E., & Hay, R. A., Jr. (1980). *Interrupted time-series analysis.* Beverly Hills, CA: Sage.

Metzger, B. L., & Schultz, S., II. (1982). Time-series analysis:

An alternative for nursing. *Nursing Research, 31*(6), 375–378.

Mitchell, P. H. (1988). Designing small sample studies. In N. F. Woods & M. Catanzaro (Eds.), *Nursing research: theory and practice.* St. Louis, MO: Mosby.

Mitchell, E., Woods, N., & Lentz, M. (1985). Methodologic issues in the definition of perimenstrual symptoms. *Proceedings of the Society for Menstrual Cycle Research.* Chicago: Chicago University Press.

Mitchell, E., Woods, N., & Lentz, M. (1991). Distinguishing among menstrual cycle symptom severity patterns. In D. Taylor & N. Woods (Eds.), *Menstruation, health and illness* (pp. 89–101). Washington, D.C.: Hemisphere.

Mitchell, E. S., Woods, N. F., & Lentz, M. J. (1994). Differentiation of women with three perimenstrual symptom patterns. *Nursing Research, 43*(1), 25–30.

Nelson, W. B. (1982). *Applied life data analysis.* New York: Wiley.

Newman, M. A. (1979). *Theory development in nursing.* Philadelphia: Davis.

Rogers, M. (1986). Science of unitary human beings. In V. M. Malinski (Ed.), *Exploration on Martha Rogers' science of unitary human beings* (pp. 3–8). Norwalk, CT: Appleton-Century-Crofts.

Shelley, S. I. (1984). *Research methods in nursing and health.* Boston: Little, Brown.

Slinkman, C. W. (1984). *An empirical comparison of data analytic regression model building procedures.* Unpublished dissertation, University of Minnesota.

Taylor, D. (1986). Perimenstrual symptoms: Typology development. *Communicating Nursing Research, 19,* 168.

Taylor, D. (1990). Use of autocorrelation as an analytic strategy for describing pattern and change. *Western Journal of Nursing Research, 12*(2), 254–261.

Taylor, D. L. (1994). Evaluating therapeutic change in symptom severity at the level of the individual women experiencing severe PMS. *Image: Journal of Nursing Scholarship, 26*(1), 25–33.

Thomas, K. A. (1987). Exploration in time: Issues in studying response patterns. In *Western Institute of Nursing: Communicating nursing research, Vol. 20,* (p. 137). Boulder, CO: Western Commission on Higher Education.

Thomas, K. A. (1990). Time-series analysis—spectral analysis and the search for cycles. *Western Journal of Nursing Research, 12*(4), 558–562.

Tukey, J. W. (1977). *Exploratory data analysis.* Reading, MA: Addison-Wesley.

Verran, J. A., & Ferketich, S. L. (1987a). Exploratory data analysis—examining single distributions. *Western Journal of Nursing Research, 9*(1), 142–149.

Verran, J. A., & Ferketich, S. L. (1987b). Exploratory data analysis—Comparisons of groups and variables. *Western Journal of Nursing Research, 9*(4), 617–625.

Verran, J. A., & Ferketich, S. L. (1987c). Testing linear model assumptions: Residual analysis. *Nursing Research, 36*(2), 127–130.

Weisberg, S. (1977). *MULTREG user's manual* (Technical Report No. 298). St. Paul, MN: School of Statistics, University of Minnesota.

Woods, N. F., & Catanzaro, M. (1988). *Nursing research: Theory and practice.* St. Louis, MO: Mosby.

Yin, R. K. (1994). *Case study research: Design and methods.* Thousand Oaks: Sage.

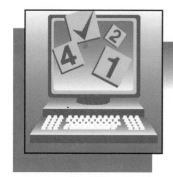

CHAPTER 20

USING STATISTICS TO EXAMINE RELATIONSHIPS

*C*orrelational analyses* are performed to identify relationships between or among variables. The purpose of the analysis may be to describe relationships between variables, clarify the relationships among theoretical concepts, or assist in identifying causal relationships, which can then be tested by inferential analysis. All the data for the analysis should have been obtained from a single population from which values are available on all variables to be examined in the correlational analyses. Data measured at the interval level will provide the best information on the nature of the relationship. However, analysis procedures are available for most levels of measurement. In preparation for correlational analysis, data collection strategies should be planned to maximize the possibility of obtaining the full range of possible values on each variable to be used in the analysis.

This chapter will discuss the use of scatter diagrams before correlational analysis, bipolar correlational analysis, testing the significance of a correlational coefficient, the correlational matrix, spurious correlations, the role of correlation in understanding causality, and multivariate correlational procedures, including factor analysis, canonical correlation, and structural equation modeling.

SCATTER DIAGRAMS

Scatter diagrams, which provide useful preliminary information about the nature of the relationship between variables, should be developed and examined before performing correlational analysis (methods of developing scatter diagrams are described in Chapter 19). Scatter diagrams may be useful for selecting appropriate correlational procedures, but most correlational procedures are useful for examining linear relationships only. Nonlinear relationships can be easily identified by a scatter plot; if the data are nonlinear, other approaches to analysis should be selected (see Figure 20–1). In addition, in some cases, data for correlational analysis have been obtained from two distinct populations. If the populations have different values for the variables of interest, inaccurate information will be obtained on relationships among the variables. Differences in values from distinctly different populations are clearly visible on a scatter plot, thus preventing inaccurate interpretation of correlational results (see Figure 20–2).

BIVARIATE CORRELATIONAL ANALYSIS

Bivariate correlation measures the extent of linear relationship between two variables and is performed on data collected from a single sample. Measures of the two variables to be examined must be available for each subject in the data set. Less commonly, data are obtained from two related subjects, such as blood lipid levels in father and son. The statistical analysis techniques used will depend on the type of data available. Correlational techniques are available for nominal, ordinal, or interval

Scatter Plot of Curvilinear Data

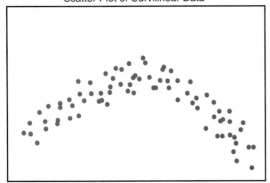

FIGURE 20–1 ■ Scatter plot of curvilinear data.

types of data. Many of the correlational techniques (gamma, Somers' *D*, Kendall's tau, contingency coefficient, phi, and Cramer's *V*) are used in conjunction with contingency tables. The Pearson product-moment correlation coefficient is the correlational technique used for interval data.

Correlational analysis provides two pieces of information about the data: the nature of the linear relationship (positive or negative) between the two variables and the magnitude (or strength) of the linear relationship. The outcomes of correlational analysis are symmetrical rather than asymmetrical. Symmetrical means that the direction of the linear relationship cannot be determined from the analysis.

Scatter Plot of Two Populations

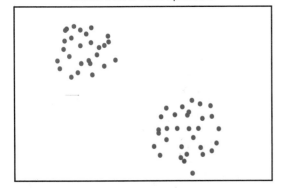

FIGURE 20–2 ■ Scatter plot showing data from two different populations.

One cannot say from the analysis that variable *A* leads to or causes variable *B*.

In a *positive linear relationship,* the scores being correlated vary together (in the same direction). When one score is high, the other score tends to be high; when one score is low, the other score tends to be low. In a *negative linear relationship,* when one score is high, the other score tends to be low. A negative linear relationship is sometimes referred to as an *inverse linear relationship.* These linear relationships can be plotted as a straight line on a graph. Sometimes, the outcome is not linear, but *curvilinear,* in which case a linear relationship plot will appear as a curved line rather than a straight one. Analyses designed to test for linear relationships, such as Pearson's correlation, cannot detect a curvilinear relationship.

The Spearman Rank-Order Correlation Coefficient

The *Spearman rho,* a nonparametric test, is an adaptation of the Pearson product-moment correlation, discussed later in this chapter. This test is used when the assumptions of Pearson's analysis cannot be met. For example, the data may be ordinal, or the scores may be skewed.

CALCULATION

The data must be ranked to conduct the analysis. Therefore, if scores from measurement scales are used to perform the analysis, the scores must be converted to ranks. As with all correlational analyses, each subject in the analysis must have a score (or value) on each of two variables (variable *x* and variable *y*). The scores on each variable are ranked separately. Calculation of rho is based on difference scores between a subject's ranking on the first and second set of scores. The formula for this calculation is

$$D = x - y$$

As in most statistical analyses, difference scores are difficult to use directly in equations because negative scores tend to cancel out positive scores; therefore, the scores are squared for use in the analysis. The formula is as follows:

$$rho = 1 - \frac{6 \Sigma D^2}{N^3 - N}$$

where

rho = Spearman correlation coefficient (derived from Pearson's r)

D = difference score between the ranking of a score on variable x and the ranking of a score on variable y

N = number of paired ranked scores

INTERPRETATION OF RESULTS

When the equation is used on data that meet the assumptions of Pearson's correlational analysis, the results are equivalent or slightly lower than Pearson's r, discussed later in this chapter. If the data are skewed, rho has an efficiency of 91% in detecting an existing relationship. The significance of rho must be tested as with any correlation; the formula used is presented in the following equation. The t distribution is presented in Appendix C, and $df = N - 2$.

$$t = rho \sqrt{\frac{N-2}{1 - rho^2}}$$

Kendall's Tau

Kendall's tau is a nonparametric measure of correlation used when both variables have been measured at the ordinal level. It can be used with very small samples. The statistic tau reflects a ratio of the actual concordance obtained between rankings with the maximal concordance possible. Marascuilo and McSweeney's (1977) explanation of this analysis technique is used in this text.

CALCULATION

To calculate tau, rank the scores on each of the two variables independently. Arrange the paired scores by subject, with the lowest ranking score on variable x at the top of the list and the ranking score on variable y for the same subject in the same row. An example of the ranking of scores for five subjects on variables x and y is presented in Table 20–1.

Comparisons are then made of the relative ranking position between each pair of subjects on variable y, shown in the last column in the table. (It is not necessary to compare rankings on variable x because the data have been arranged in order by rank.) If the comparison is concordant, the ranking of the score below will be higher than the ranking of the score above and is assigned a value of +1. If the comparison is discordant, the ranking of the score below will be lower than the ranking of the score above and is assigned a value of −1. In Table 20–2, the comparisons are identified as concordant (+1) or discordant (−1) for the ranked scores identified in Table 20–1. In this example, the number

SUBJECT	SCORE ON VARIABLE x	RANKING ON VARIABLE x	SCORE ON VARIABLE y	RANKING ON VARIABLE y
A	3	1	4	2
B	5	2	2	1
C	6	3	6	3
D	9	4	8	5
E	12	5	7	4

TABLE 20–1
RANKING OF SCORES FOR CALCULATION OF KENDALL'S TAU

TABLE 20–2
CALCULATION OF CONCORDANT-DISCORDANT STATES IN KENDALL'S TAU

COMPARISON OF SUBJECTS	VALUE FOR x	VALUE FOR y	STATE
AB	+1	−1	Discordant
AC	+1	+1	Concordant
AD	+1	+1	Concordant
AE	+1	+1	Concordant
BC	+1	+1	Concordant
BD	+1	+1	Concordant
BE	+1	+1	Concordant
CD	+1	+1	Concordant
CE	+1	+1	Concordant
DE	+1	−1	Discordant

of discordant pairs is two; the number of concordant pairs is eight. The statistic S is then calculated with the following equation:

$$S = N_c - N_d$$

Example:

$$S = 8 - 2 = 6$$

where

N_c = number of concordant pairs
N_d = number of discordant pairs

At this point, tau is calculated by using the following equation:

$$Tau = \frac{2S}{n(n-1)}$$

$$\text{Example: Tau} = \frac{(2)(6)}{5(5-1)} = .6$$

where

n = number of paired scores

INTERPRETATION OF RESULTS

If the ranking of values of x is not related to the ranking of values of y, any particular rank ordering of y is just as likely to occur as any other. The sample tau can be used to test the hypothesis that the population tau is 0. The significance of tau can be tested by using the following equation for the Z statistic. The Z statistic was calculated for the previous example.

$$Z = \frac{tau - mean}{SD_{tau}}$$

$$Z = \frac{.6 - 0}{\sqrt{\frac{2(10+5)}{(9)(5)(5-1)}}} = \frac{.6}{.408} = 1.47$$

where:

$$mean = \mu_{tau} = 0$$

$$SD_{tau} = \sqrt{\frac{2(2n+5)}{9n(n-1)}}$$

The Z values are approximately normally distributed, and therefore the table of Z scores available in Appendix B can be used. The Z score for the example was 1.47, which is nonsignificant at the .05 level.

Pearson's Product-Moment Correlation Coefficient

Pearson's correlation was the first of the correlation measures developed and is the most commonly used. All other correlation measures have been developed from Pearson's equation and are adaptations designed to control for violation of the assumptions that must be met to use Pearson's equation. These assumptions are

1. Interval measurement of both variables
2. Normal distribution of at least one variable
3. Independence of observational pairs
4. Homoscedasticity

Data that are *homoscedastic* are evenly dispersed both above and below the regression line, which indicates a linear relationship on a scatter diagram (plot). Homoscedasticity is a reflection of equal variance of both variables. A *regression line* is the line that best represents the values of the raw scores plotted on a scatter diagram.

CALCULATION

Numerous formulas can be used to compute Pearson's *r*. With small samples, Pearson's *r* can be generated fairly easily with a calculator by using the following formula:

$$r = \frac{n(\Sigma\, XY) - (\Sigma\, X)\,(\Sigma\, Y)}{\sqrt{[n(\Sigma\, X^2) - (\Sigma\, X)^2]\,[n(\Sigma\, Y^2) - (\Sigma\, Y)^2]}}$$

where

r = Pearson's correlation coefficient
n = number of paired scores
X = score of the first variable
Y = score of the second variable
XY = product of the two paired scores

An example is presented that demonstrates calculation of Pearson's *r*. Correlation between the two variables of functioning and coping was calculated. The functional variable (variable *X*) was operationalized by using Karnofsky's scale, and coping was operationalized by using a family coping tool. Karnofsky's scale ranges from 1 to 10; 1 is normal function, and 10 is moribund (fatal processes progressing rapidly). Nursing diagnosis terminology was used to develop the family coping tool (variable *Y*); scores ranged from 1 to 4, with 1 being effective family coping; 2, ineffective family coping, potential for growth; 3, ineffective family coping, compromised; and 4, ineffective family coping, disabling. The data for these two variables in 10 subjects are presented in Table 20–3. Usually, correlations are conducted on larger samples; this example serves only to demonstrate the process of calculating Pearson's *r*.

TABLE 20–3
DATA AND COMPUTATIONS FOR PEARSON'S R

SUBJECTS	X	Y	XY	X²	Y²
1	10	4	40	100	16
2	7	3	21	49	9
3	3	2	6	9	4
4	6	3	18	36	9
5	1	1	1	1	1
6	5	2	10	25	4
7	2	2	4	4	4
8	9	4	36	81	16
9	4	1	4	16	1
10	8	4	32	64	16
Sums	55	26	172	385	80

$$r = \frac{(10)(172) - (55)(26)}{\sqrt{[10(385) - (55)^2][10(80) - (26)^2]}}$$

$$= \frac{1720 - 1430}{\sqrt{(3850 - 3025)(800 - 676)}}$$

$$= \frac{290}{\sqrt{102{,}300}} = \frac{290}{319.844} = .907$$

INTERPRETATION OF RESULTS

The outcome of the Pearson product-moment correlation analysis is an *r* value of between −1 and +1. This *r* value indicates the degree of linear relationship between the two variables. A score of zero indicates no linear relationship.

−1 ———————— 0 ———————— +1

A value of −1 indicates a perfect negative (inverse) correlation. In a negative linear relationship, a high score on one variable is related to a low score on the other variable. A value of +1 indicates a perfect positive linear relationship. In a positive linear relationship, a high score on one variable is associated with a high score on the other variable. A positive correlation also exists when a low score on one variable is related to a low score on the other variable. As the negative or positive values of r approach zero, the strength of the linear relationship decreases. Traditionally, an r value of .1 to .3 is considered a weak linear relationship, .3 to .5 is a moderate linear relationship, and above .5 is a strong linear relationship. However, this interpretation depends to a great extent on the variables being examined and the situation within which they were observed. Therefore, interpretation requires some judgment on the part of the researcher. In the example provided, the r value was .907, which indicates a strong positive linear relationship between the Karnofsky scale and the family coping tool in this sample.

When Pearson's correlation coefficient is squared (r^2), the resulting number is the *percentage of variance* explained by the linear relationship. In the preceding computation based on data in Table 20–3, $r = .907$ and $r^2 = .822$. In this case, the linear relationship explains 82% of the variability in the two scores. Except for perfect correlations, r^2 will always be lower than r. This r value is very high. Results in most nursing studies will be much lower.

In nursing research, weak correlations have tended to be disregarded. However, such tendencies create a serious possibility of ignoring a linear relationship that may have some meaning within nursing knowledge when examined in the context of other variables. This situation is similar to a Type II error and commonly occurs for three reasons. First, many nursing measurements are not powerful enough to detect fine discriminations, and some instruments may not detect extreme scores. In this case, the linear relationship may be stronger than indicated by the crude measures available. Second, correlational studies must have a wide range of variance for linear relationships to be detected. If the study scores are homogeneous or if the sample is small, linear relationships that exist in the population will not show up as clearly in the sample. Third, in many cases, bivariate analysis does not provide a clear picture of the dynamics in the situa-

tion. A number of variables can be linked through weak correlations, but together they provide increased insight into situations of interest. Therefore, although one should not overreact to small Pearson coefficients, the information must be recorded for future reference. If the linear relationship is intuitively important, one may have to plan better-designed studies and reexamine the linear relationship.

Testing the Significance of a Correlational Coefficient

To infer that the sample correlation coefficient applies to the population from which the sample was taken, statistical analysis must be performed to determine whether the coefficient is significantly different from zero (no correlation). In other words, we can test the hypothesis that the population Pearson correlation coefficient is 0. The test statistic used is the t, distributed according to the t distribution, with $n - 2$ degrees of freedom. The formula for calculating the t statistic follows. This formula was used to calculate the t value for the example where $r = .907$.

$$t = \frac{r\sqrt{n-2}}{\sqrt{1-r^2}} \qquad t = \frac{.907\sqrt{10-2}}{\sqrt{1-(.907)^2}}$$

$$= \frac{2.565}{\sqrt{.177}} = \frac{2.565}{.421} = 6.09$$

where

r = Pearson's product-moment correlation coefficient
n = sample size of paired scores
$df = n - 2$

The significance of the t obtained from the formula is determined by using the t distribution table in Appendix C. With a small sample, a very high correlation coefficient (r) can be nonsignificant. With a very large sample, the correlation coefficient can be statistically significant when the degree of association is too small to be clinically significant.

Therefore, when judging the significance of the coefficient, one must consider both the size of the coefficient and the significance of the t test. The t value calculated in the example was 6.09, and the df for the sample was 8. This t value was significant at the .001 level. When reporting the results of a correlation coefficient, both the r value and the p value should be reported.

THE CORRELATIONAL MATRIX

A correlational matrix is obtained by performing bivariate correlational analysis on every pair of variables in the data set. The appearance of the matrix is shown in Figure 20–3. On the matrix the r value and the p value are given for each pair of variables. At a diagonal through the matrix are variables correlated with themselves. The r value for these correlations is 1.00 and the p value is 0.000 because when a variable is related to itself, the correlation is perfect. Note that to the left and the right of this diagonal, correlations for each pair of variables are repeated. Therefore, one needs to examine only half the matrix to obtain a full picture of the relationships.

When examining the matrix values, the researcher must place weight only on those r values with a p value of 0.05 or smaller. Once these pairs of variables are singled out, the researcher notes variable pairs with an r value sufficiently large to be of interest in terms of the study problem. Examination of these pairs of variables can provide theoretical insight into the dynamics of the variables within the problem of concern in the study. Of particular interest are pairs of variables that are unexpectedly significantly related. These results can sometimes provide new insight into the research problem.

Spurious Correlations

Spurious correlations are relationships between variables that are not logical. In some cases, these significant relationships are a consequence of chance and have no meaning. When you choose a level of significance of 0.05, 1 in 20 correlations that you perform in a matrix will be significant by chance. Other pairs of variables may be correlated because of the influence of other variables. For example, you might find a positive correlation between the number of deaths on a nursing unit and the number of nurses working on the unit. Clearly,

Correlations		AGE	educ12	HIGHER EDUCATION (fill one)	KNIDTOT
AGE	Pearson Correlation	1.000	.090	.175*	−.119†
	Sig. (2-tailed)		.118	.004	.038
	N	304	304	266	304
educ12	Pearson Correlation	.090	1.000	.390*	−.100
	Sig. (2-tailed)	.118		.000	.080
	N	304	305	267	305
HIGHER EDUCATION (fill one)	Pearson Correlation	−.119†	.390*	1.000	−.096
	Sig. (2-tailed)	.038	.000		.118
	N	304	267	267	267
KNIDTOT	Pearson Correlation	−.119†	−.100	−.096	1.000
	Sig. (2-tailed)	.038	.080	.118	
	N	304	305	267	305

* Correlation is significant at the 0.01 level (2-tailed).
† Correlation is significant at the 0.05 level (2-tailed).

FIGURE 20–3 ■ Correlational matrix using SPSS Version 9. KNIDTOT = knowledge of infant development by English-speaking Hispanic mothers.

the number of deaths cannot be explained as occurring because of increases in the number of nurses. It is more likely that a third variable (units having patients with more critical conditions) explains the increased number of nurses. In most cases, the "other" variable will remain unknown. Most of these correlations can be identified and excluded through reasoning.

The Role of Correlation in Understanding Causality

In any situation involving causality, a relationship will exist between the factors involved in the causal process. Therefore, the first clue to the possibility of a causal link is the existence of a relationship. However, a relationship does not mean causality. Two variables can be highly correlated but have no causal relationship whatsoever. However, as the strength of a relationship increases, the possibility of a causal link increases. The absence of a relationship precludes the possibility of a causal connection between the two variables being examined, given adequate measurement of the variables and absence of other variables that might mask the relationship. Thus a correlational study can be the first step in determining the dynamics important to nursing practice within a particular population. The best-known example of this type of relationship is the multitude of studies relating smoking to cancer. Determining these dynamics can allow us to increase our ability to predict and control the situation studied, regardless of whether we can ever clearly prove definite causal links (Kenny, 1979). However, correlation cannot be used alone to demonstrate causality.

MULTIVARIATE CORRELATIONAL PROCEDURES

Multivariate correlational procedures are more complex analysis techniques that examine linear relationships among three or more variables. The multivariate correlational procedures described here are factor analysis, canonical correlation, and structural equation modeling.

Factor Analysis

Factor analysis examines interrelationships among large numbers of variables and disentangles those relationships to identify clusters of variables that are most closely linked together. These closely related variables are grouped together into a *factor*, and several factors may be identified within a data set. Sample sizes must be large for factor analysis. Nunnally (1978) recommends 10 observations for each variable. Arrindell and van der Ende (1985) suggest that a more reliable determination is a sample size of 20 times the number of factors.

Once the factors have been identified mathematically, the researcher explains why the variables are grouped as they are. Thus, factor analysis aids in the identification of theoretical constructs. Factor analysis is also used to confirm the accuracy of a theoretically developed construct. For example, a theorist might state that the concept "hope" consists of the elements (1) anticipation of the future, (2) belief that things will work out for the best, and (3) optimism. Ways could be developed to measure these three elements, and factor analysis could be conducted on the data to determine whether subject responses clustered into these three groupings.

Factor analysis is frequently used in the process of developing measurement instruments, particularly those related to psychological variables such as attitudes, beliefs, values, or opinions. The instrument operationalizes a theoretical construct. The method can also be used with physiological data. For example, Woods and colleagues (1993) identified a large pool of symptoms commonly experienced during the perimenstruum, and daily rating of the severity of these symptoms by subjects was used to identify premenstrual symptom patterns. Testing of the validity of these patterns by factor analysis resulted in the selection of 33 symptoms for classification of women as having a low-severity symptom pattern, a premenstrual syndrome pattern, or a premenstrual magnification pattern. The analysis revealed that these patterns (factors) were consistent across menstrual cycle phases and had internal consistency reliability estimates above .70 (Woods et al., 1995). Factor analysis can be used as a data reduction strategy in studies examining large numbers of variables. It can also be used to attempt to sort out meaning from large numbers of items on survey instruments.

The two types of factor analysis are exploratory and confirmatory. *Exploratory factor analysis* is similar to stepwise regression, in which the variance of the first factor is partialed out before analysis is begun on the second factor. It is performed when the researcher has few prior expectations about the factor structure. *Confirmatory factor analysis* is more closely related to ordinary least-squares regression analysis or path analysis. It is based on theory and tests a hypothesis about the existing factor structure. In confirmatory factor analysis, statistical significance of the analysis outcomes is determined, and the parameters of the population are estimated. Confirmatory factor analysis is usually conducted after examination of the correlation matrix or after initial development of the factor structure through exploratory factor analysis.

EXPLORATORY FACTOR ANALYSIS

The first step in exploratory factor analysis is the development of a correlation matrix of the scores for all variables to be included in the factor analysis. This matrix is usually developed automatically by the computer program conducting the analysis. Although multiple procedures can be used for the actual factor analysis, the procedure described here is the one most commonly reported in the nursing literature.

The second step is a *principal components analysis*, which provides preliminary information needed by the researcher for making decisions before the final factoring. The computer printout of the principal components analysis will give (1) the eigenvalues, (2) the amount of variance explained by each factor, and (3) the weight for each variable on each factor. Weights (loadings) express the extent to which the variable is correlated with the factor. Weightings on the variables from a principal components factor analysis are essentially uninterpretable and are generally disregarded (Nunnally, 1978).

Eigenvalues are the sum of the squared weights for each factor. The researcher examines the eigenvalues to decide how many factors will be included

in the factor analysis. To decide the number of factors to include, the researcher determines the minimal amount of variance that must be explained by the factor to add significant meaning. This decision is not straightforward and has resulted in some criticism of the analysis as being subjective. Several strategies have been proposed for determining the number of factors to be included in a construct. One approach is to select factors that have an eigenvalue of 1.00 or above. Another strategy used is the scree test. Scree is a geological term that refers to the debris that collects at the bottom of a rocky slope. This test, which is considered by some to be the most reliable, requires that the eigenvalues be graphed (see Figure 20–4).

From this graph, one can see a change in the angle of the slope. A steep drop in value from one factor to the next indicates a large difference score between the two factors and an increase in the amount of variance explained. When the slope begins to become flat, which is an indication of small difference scores between factors, little additional information will be obtained by including more factors. In Figure 20–4, the slope begins to flatten at factor 6; therefore, six factors would be extracted to explain the construct.

The third step in exploratory factor analysis is *factor rotation*. The purpose of factor rotation is to simplify the factor structure, and the procedure most commonly used is referred to as varimax rotation.

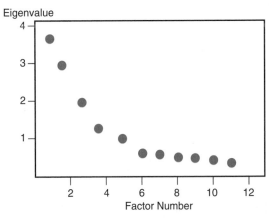

FIGURE 20–4 ■ Graphed eigenvalues from a factor analysis.

In varimax rotation, the factors are rotated for the best fit (best factor solution), and the factors are uncorrelated. An *oblique rotation* results in correlated factors.

The process of factor analysis is actually a series of multiple regression analyses (Kim & Mueller, 1978a, 1978b). The equation for a factor could be expressed as

$$F = b_1 X_1 + b_2 X_2 + b_3 X_3 + \cdots b_k X_k$$

where

F = factor score
X_k = original variables from the matrix
b_K = weights of the individual variables in the factor (if the scores used are standardized, b is a beta weight)

In exploratory factor analysis, regression analysis is performed for the first factor. The variance of each variable explained by the first factor is then partialed out. Next, a second regression analysis is performed for the second factor on the residual variance. The variance from that analysis is then partialed out, and a regression is performed for the third factor. This process is continued until all the factors have been developed. The computer printout will include a rotated factor matrix that contains information similar to that in Table 20–4.

Factor Loadings

A factor loading is actually the regression coefficient of the variable on the factor. In Table 20–4, the factor loading indicates the extent to which a single variable is related to the cluster of variables. In variable 1, the factor loading is .76 for factor I and .27 for factor II. Squaring the factor loadings ($[0.76]^2 = .578$, and $[.27]^2 = .073$) will give the amount of variance in variable 1, which explains factors I and II.

Communality

Communality (h^2) is the squared multiple regression coefficient for each variable and is closely related to the R^2 coefficient in regression. Thus the communality coefficient describes the amount of variance in a single variable that is explained across all the factors in the analysis. The communality for a variable can be obtained by summing the squared factor loadings on the variable for each factor. In Table 20–4, the communality coefficient for variable 1 is $(.76)^2 + (.27)^2 = .65$.

Identifying the Relevant Variables in a Factor

Only variables with factor loadings that indicate that a meaningful portion of the variable's variance is explained within the factor are included as elements of the factor. A cutoff point is selected for the purpose of identifying these variables, with the minimal acceptable cutoff point being .30. In Table 20–4, the factor loadings with asterisks indicate the variables that will be included in each factor. In this example, which uses a .50 cutoff, variables 1, 2, and 3 would be included in factor I, and variables 4, 5, and 6 would be included in factor II. Ideally, a variable will *load* (have a factor loading above

TABLE 20–4

FACTOR LOADINGS AND VARIANCE FOR TWO FACTORS

VARIABLE	FACTORS		
	I	*II*	*h²*
1	.76*	.27	.65
2	91*	.03	.83
3	.64*	.29	.49
4	.14	.67*	.47
5	.22	.59*	.40
6	.07	.77*	.60
Sum of squared loadings	1.89	1.55	
Variance	.22	.13	Total = .35

*Indicates the variables to be included in each factor.

the selected cutoff point) on only one factor. If the variable does have high loadings on two factors, the lowest loading is referred to as a *secondary loading*. When many secondary loadings occur, it is not considered a clean factoring, and the researcher re-examines the variables included in the analysis. Sometimes, researchers will attempt to set the cutoff point high enough to avoid secondary loadings of a variable.

"Naming" the Factor

At this point, the mathematics of the procedure takes a back seat, and the theoretical reasoning of the researcher takes over. The researcher examines the variables that have clustered together in a factor and explains that clustering. Variables with high loadings on the factor must be included, even if they do not fit the preconceived theoretical notions of the researcher. The purpose is to identify the broad construct of meaning that has caused these particular variables to be so strongly intercorrelated. Naming this construct is a very important part of the procedure because naming of the factor provides theoretical meaning.

Factor Scores

After the initial factor analysis, additional studies are conducted to examine changes in the phenomenon in various situations and to determine the relationships of the factors with other concepts. Factor scores are used during data analysis in these additional studies. To obtain factor scores, the variables included in the factor are identified, and the scores on these variables are summed for each subject. Thus each subject will have a score for each factor in the instrument. Because some variables explain a larger portion of the variance of the factor than others do, additional meaning can be added by multiplying the variable score by the weight (factor loading) of that variable in the factor. In the example in Table 20–4, variable 1 had a factor loading of .76 on factor I. If the subject score on variable 1 were 7, the score would be weighted by multiplying the variable score by the factor loading as follows:

$$7 \times .76 = 5.32$$

These weighted scores can be generated by com-puter. If comparisons between studies are to be made, standardized (Z) scores (for variable scores) and beta weights (for factor loadings) are used. Once analysis is complete, factor scores can be used as independent variables in multiple regression equations.

Woods and colleagues (1995) used factor analysis in a study examining social pathways to premenstrual symptoms. Women were recruited for the study through advertisements in local newspapers. They describe their study as follows:

• •

"Multiple indicators of the major constructs, feminine socialization, menstrual socialization, expectation of symptoms, stress, and support need, were included in the study. For purposes of data reduction, prior to comparing women with the LS [low symptom], PMS [premenstrual syndrome], and PMM [premenstrual magnification syndrome] symptom patterns, data from these indicators, obtained from all women who participated in the initial interview (N = 488), were included in a principal components factor analysis with a varimax rotation. This procedure yielded five factors with eigenvalues exceeding 1.0. . . . Socialization as a woman reflects the ways in which women were socialized about the roles of women in society, including in the workplace and their families. . . . Socialization for menstruation reflected what women had learned about menstruation through exposure to their mothers and sisters and through teaching about the effects of menstruation. Menstrual socialization was indicated by the respondent's rating of her mother's perimenstrual symptoms, a sister's symptoms, and the respondent's recollection of her menarcheal preparation. Expectations about menstrual symptoms reflected how women expected to experience menstruation and symptoms. . . . Respondents also were asked two single items, one from the Menstrual Attitudes Scale tapping whether women could anticipate menses by their symptoms, the other whether they perceived they had PMS. Stress was measured using indicators of major life events and daily stressors. Life events were assessed with Norbeck's (1984) woman-oriented revision of the Sarason Life Events Scale (LES). . . .

"Factor analysis results are presented in [Table 20–5]. Factor 1 (stress) included four variables:

TABLE 20–5

FACTOR LOADINGS FOR INDICATORS OF STRESS, FEMININE SOCIALIZATION, SUPPORT NEED, SYMPTOM EXPECTATION, AND MENSTRUAL SOCIALIZATION (N = 488)

VARIABLES	FACTORS				
	1	2	3	4	5
Stress					
Negative life events	.70	−.01	.09	.07	.09
Stress, family	.70	−.03	.10	−.19	.04
Stress, amount	.67	−.02	.21	−.09	−.08
Stress, personal	.64	.04	.23	−.01	.06
Feminine socialization					
Attitudes, women	.01	.90	.04	.03	−.07
Familism	−.01	.89	.04	.12	−.07
Support need					
Advice	.20	−.10	.63	.09	.15
Affirmation	.17	−.04	.62	−.09	−.04
Relaxation	−.04	.16	.57	.14	.14
Confidant	.38	.17	.54	−.10	.09
Help	−.06	−.03	.52	−.34	−.18
Expectation of symptoms[a]					
Have PMS	.23	.04	−.09	−.73	.19
Anticipate symptoms	.03	.04	−.06	.67	.04
Not debilitating	−.06	.34	−.06	.60	−.29
Menstrual socialization					
Menstrual effects	.01	.02	−.02	−.04	.65
Mother's symptoms	.04	−.15	−.15	−.00	.64
Sister's symptoms	−.01	−.02	−.02	−.13	.62
Eigenvalues	2.85	2.18	1.35	1.26	1.16
% Variance	16.8	12.8	7.9	7.4	6.8

[a]High scores equate with low symptom expectation.

From Woods, N. F., Mitchell, E. S., & Lentz, M. J. (1995). Social pathways to premenstrual symptoms. *Research in Nursing & Health, 18*(3), 230.

family-related stress, negative life events (LES scores), how stressed each woman felt over the past 3 months, and her rating of personal stress. Factor 2 (feminine socialization) included ratings of familism and attitudes toward women. High scores on this factor reflected more contemporary attitudes toward women and their roles vis-à-vis their families. Factor 3 (support needed) included women's ratings of need for more affirmation, advice, access to a confidant, someone to share fun and relax with them, and someone to help them. Factor 4 (symptom expectation) included three variables: anticipating symptoms, self-perceived PMS, and attitudes toward menstruation as debilitating. Low scores indicated high expectation of symptoms. Factor 5 (menstrual socialization) included exposure to a mother and/or sister with perimenstrual symptoms and having

been taught negative effects of menstruation. Of all the indicators analyzed, none had factor loadings of .40 or greater on any other factor. Each factor had an eigenvalue exceeding 1.0." (Woods et al., 1995, pp. 229–231) ■

CONFIRMATORY FACTOR ANALYSIS

Confirmatory factor analysis is a fairly recent development that is extremely complex mathematically. The procedure is usually performed by using the programs LISREL or EQS. Interpretation of results requires a high level of sophistication in statistical analysis. In confirmatory factor analysis, the researcher develops hypotheses about the factor structure. Because the elements of each factor are set in the analysis, factor rotation and partialing out of variance are not performed. Cutoff points for representation within the factor may also be preset and included in the analysis. As an outcome of the analyses, an estimate is made of the population parameters for the factor structure. The statistical significance of the results of the analyses is tested.

Wineman and associates (1994) used confirmatory factory analysis to examine the factor structure of the Ways of Coping Questionnaire in clinical populations. The original instrument was based on the responses of undergraduate psychology students. The researchers describe their work as follows:

· ·

"The original Ways of Coping Checklist (WCCL) (Folkman & Lazarus, 1985) contained 68 items rated with a simple 'yes or no' format. Scale items were categorized as emotion-focused or problem-focused coping based on expert judgment. This rating scale did not measure the frequency with which coping behaviors were used and was thus revised (Folkman & Lazarus, 1988). The newer version, now called the Ways of Coping Questionnaire (Folkman & Lazarus, 1988), includes 66 items measured in a 4-point Likert-type format. Potential responses include 0 (does not apply and/or not used), 1 (used somewhat), 2 (used quite a bit), and 3 (used a great deal). The factor structure of this revised scale was analyzed using data from two separate community samples (Folkman & Lazarus, 1985; Folkman et al., 1986). The 1986 study formed the basis for the information reported in the 1988 *Ways of Coping Manual* because it used a community sample experiencing diverse stressful encounters. Eight coping scales were identified using alpha and principal factoring with oblique rotation (Folkman et al., 1986). Reliability estimates for the eight scales ranged from alpha coefficients of .61 to .79 (*M* = .70). Folkman and Lazarus (1988) contended that construct validity was supported because results were consistent with theoretical predictions about the coping process. That is, both problem-focused and emotion-focused strategies were used to cope with almost all stressful situations, and coping strategies changed in relation to situational demands (Folkman & Lazarus, 1988). . . .

"The eight-factor structure guided initial scale construction (Wineman et al., 1994). Cronbach's al-

pha coefficients were less than .74 for all eight scales, with four of these less than .60. . . . These findings, consistent with the evidence of reliability insufficiency in the literature, led to the decision to compute an exploratory factor analysis (EFA).

"An EFA with orthogonal rotation (quartimax) was done to obtain the simplest factor structure possible (Nunnally, 1978). . . . Examination of the scree plot and eigenvalues suggested that two factors accounted for the covariation among the measured variables (Kim & Mueller, 1978a). The selection of items with factor loadings of .30 or greater on one factor (Nunnally, 1978) resulted in retention of 46 of the original 65 items (71%). Thirty-three items loaded on a problem-focused coping (PFC) scale and 13 items on an emotion-focused coping (EFC) scale. These scales supported coping theory that defines PFC as behaviors used to change a stressful situation and EFC as behaviors used to manage distressing feelings (Folkman et al., 1986). Acceptable reliability estimates were obtained: .90 for PFC and .76 for EFC. . . .

"Recent reports note that traditional factor analysis (EFC) does not allow for the specification of an exact factor structure, and that confirmatory factor analysis (CFA) with linear structural equation modeling provides the necessary control for testing theoretical expectations of the underlying relations among the variables (Long, 1983a; Youngblut, 1993). In other words, with CFA one can specify a priori which items (or measured indicators) are related to specific latent concepts (or factors). . . .

"In evaluating the goodness-of-fit of a model to observed data, no single statistic is sufficient for determining the adequacy of the fit (Raykov, Tomer, & Nesselroade, 1991). Four measures of overall fit were used to judge models in the present study: the chi-square statistic (χ^2), the goodness-of-fit index (GFI), the adjusted goodness-of-fit index (AGFI), and the root mean-squared residual (RMSR) (Joreskog & Sorbom, 1989). An acceptably small χ^2 value was determined by obtaining the ratio of the χ^2 value to its degrees of freedom (*df*). Ratios of 3:1 or less supported a good fit (Carmines & McIver, 1981). The GFI and the AGFI, which assess the relative amount of variance and covariance jointly explained by the model, were considered acceptable if values were .90 or greater (Boyd et al., 1988). The RMSR, a measure of the average of the fitted residuals, was acceptable if close to zero (Joreskog & Sorbom, 1989). The aim of this study was to reach a consensus of acceptable fit across all indicators of fit.

"A CFA with LISREL version 7.20, a structural equation modeling program (Jöreskog & Sörbom, 1988–1992), was performed to test the fit of data to the original hypothesized eight-factor structure (Folkman et al., 1986). Results indicated that the hypothesized factor structure did not provide a good fit to the data. . . . These findings indicated that the eight-factor coping model developed in a well community-residing sample (Folkman et al., 1986) was inadequate for describing coping in a community sample of individuals with a non–life-threatening chronic illness or disability. Because it was reasonable to assume that coping behaviors required to manage life with a chronic illness or disability would be quite different from those needed in daily living situations of well individuals, alternative models of the coping factor structure based on a more conservative approach were examined, rather than pursuing modifications based only on empirical parameter estimates within the structural equation modeling framework.

"The investigation of an alternative coping factor structure was conducted by randomly dividing the total study population into two samples and following a two-step procedure. This procedure generally consists of an initial EFA performed on one portion of the sample ($\frac{1}{3}$ of 655, $n = 218$) to derive an initial structure, followed by a CFA with the remaining sample ($\frac{2}{3}$ of 655, $n = 437$) to validate this structure. . . .

"In the following factor analyses, the two-step procedure described above was used twice to derive the best-fitting alternative factor structure. Using all 65 items, an EFA with a varimax rotation was performed on the smaller sample ($n = 218$). Selecting, as a more conservative estimate, a factor loading of .40 or greater (Nunnally, 1978), five factors were identified, with at least three items loading on each factor. If an item loaded on more than one factor it was not included. Twenty-five of the original 65 items were retained. To validate this 25-

item, five-factor solution, a CFA with the remaining sample ($n = 437$) was used. The fit was not acceptable ($\chi^2 = 680.42$, $p < .01$, $df = 265$; $\chi^2/df = 2.57$; GFI = .89; AGFI = .86; RMSR = .06). Next, the model was modified slightly by omitting items with lambda y loadings of $<.40$, resulting in a 21-item, five-factor model. A CFA was then used to confirm this modified five-factor model. The fit improved, but was still slightly less than desirable ($\chi^2 = 429.54$, $p < .01$, $df = 179$; $\chi^2/df = 2.40$; GFI = .91; AGFI = .89; RMSR = .05). Because the modification indices indicated that one item loaded on four of the five factors, the next CFA was performed with this item omitted. An acceptable fit was obtained with this 20-item, five-factor solution ($\chi^2 = 325.94$, $p < .01$, $df = 160$; $\chi^2/df = 2.04$; GFI = .93; AGFI = .91; RMSR = .04).

"Cronbach's alpha coefficients were acceptable for three of the five factors (.76, .709, and .69), but unacceptable for the other two (.55 and .61). Therefore, a final 14-item, three-factor model was tested using CFA, resulting in an acceptable fit ($\chi^2 = 149.16$, $p < .01$, $df = 74$; $\chi^2/df = 2.02$; GFI = .95; AGFI = .94; RMSR = .04). All standardized lambda y values were $>.40$ with the exception of one item that was .38. All but one of the goodness-of-fit indicators for this final three-factor model of coping were improved over earlier models." (Wineman et al., 1994, pp. 269–271) ■

Figure 20–5 shows the final results of the confirmatory factor analysis.

Canonical Correlation

Canonical correlation is an extension of multiple regression in which more than one dependent variable is involved. Researchers using the technique need to be very familiar with both regression analysis and factor analysis. The purpose of the test is to analyze the relationships between two or more dependent variables and two or more independent variables. The least-squares principle is used to partition and analyze variance. Two linear composites are developed: one associated with the dependent variables and the other associated with the independent variables. The relationship between the two

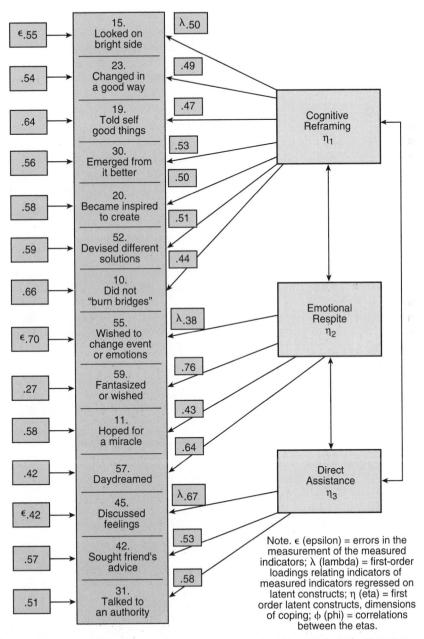

FIGURE 20–5 ■ Results of the confirmatory factor analysis for the three-factor model of coping. (From Wineman, N. M., Durand, E. J., & McCulloch, B. J. [1994]. Examination of the factor structure of the Ways of Coping Questionnaire with clinical populations. *Nursing Research 43*[5], 270.)

linear composites is then examined and expressed by the value R_c. The square of this canonical correlation coefficient indicates the proportion of variance explained by the analysis. When more than one source of covariation is involved, more than one canonical correlation can be identified. A more detailed explanation of canonical analysis can be found in Wikoff and Miller (1991).

Olson (1995) used canonical correlation in a study examining the relationships between nurse-expressed empathy, patient-perceived empathy, and patient distress. Olson described the study as follows:

· ·

"A correlational study examined relationships between nurse-expressed empathy and two patient outcomes: patient-perceived empathy and patient distress. Subjects ($N = 140$) were randomly selected from RNs and patients on medical and surgical units in two urban, acute care hospitals. Nurse-subjects ($N = 70$) completed two measures of nurse-expressed empathy: the Behavioral Test of Interpersonal Skills and the Staff-Patient Interaction Response Scale. Patient-subjects ($N = 70$) completed the profile of Mood States, the Multiple Affect Adjective Checklist, and the Barrett-Lennard Relationship Inventory.

"Nurse-expressed empathy is understanding what a patient is saying and feeling then communicating this understanding verbally to the patient. Patient-perceived empathy is the patient's feeling of being understood and accepted by the nurse. Patient distress is a negative emotional state. Three hypotheses were developed: (a) There will be negative relationships between measures of nurse-expressed empathy and measures of patient distress, (b) there will be negative relationships between patient-perceived empathy and measures of patient distress, and (c) there will be positive relationships between measures of nurse-expressed empathy and patient-perceived empathy.

"Hypotheses one and two were tested together using one canonical correlation. The canonical correlation was generated to analyze the relationships between a set of empathy variables and a set of patient-distress variables. The empathy set included the measures of nurse-expressed empathy and the

patient-perceived empathy score. The patient distress set included measures of patient distress. The overall relationship between the two sets of variables was significant beyond the .001 alpha level ($\chi^2(30) = 65.54$, $p = .001$) using Bartlett's test of Wilk's lambda. Canonical correlations are reported in [Table 20–6]. The first canonical correlation is .71 ($p = .0002$), representing 50% of the variance for the first pair of canonical variates. This means that 50% of the variation in patient distress scores can be accounted for by a combination of the factors that make up nurse-expressed empathy on the BTIS and patient-perceived empathy. The first pair of canonical variates, therefore, accounted for significant relationships between the two sets of variables. The remaining three canonical correlations were effectively zero and are not included in the table. Correlations (factor loadings) above .40 are reported. . . . Overall, patients of nurses who had high scores on nurse-expressed empathy . . . and

TABLE 20–6
CANONICAL RELATIONSHIP BETWEEN A SET OF EMPATHY VARIABLES AND A SET OF PATIENT DISTRESS VARIABLES

VARIABLES	FACTOR LOADINGS
Empathy Variables	
Nurse-expressed empathy (BTIS Feeling)	.68
Nurse-expressed empathy (BTIS Content)	.62
Nurse-expressed empathy (BTIS Don't Feeling)	−.42
Patient-perceived empathy (BLRI)	.85
Patient Distress Variables	
POMS Anxiety	−.89
POMS Depression	−.90
POMS Anger	−.68
MAACL Anxiety	−.72
MAACL Depression	−.88
MAACL Anger	−.63
First Canonical Correlation	
$R_c = .71386$	
$p = .0002$	

R_c = the canonical correlation coefficient or the maximal correlation that can be developed between two linear functions of variables.

BLRI = Barrett-Lennard Relationship Inventory; BTIS = Behavioral Test of Interpersonal Skills; MAACL = Multiple Affect Adjective Checklist; POMS = Profile of Mood States.

From Olson, J. K. (1995). Relationships between nurse-expressed empathy, patient-perceived empathy and patient distress. *Image—The Journal of Nursing Scholarship, 27*(4), 319.

who were rated by their patients as highly empathic (patient-perceived empathy) were less likely to be distressed (low scores on anxiety, depression, and anger)." (Olson, 1995, pp. 319–320) ■

Olson points out that this study is one of the first to link behavioral measures of nurse empathy to patient outcomes.

Structural Equation Modeling

Structural equation modeling is designed to test theories. In a theory, all the concepts are expected to be interrelated, and the web of relationships is often expressed as a conceptual map, as discussed in Chapter 7. Testing the structure of relationships within the theory as a whole provides much more information about the validity of the theory than does testing only specific propositions and can be achieved by structural equation modeling. The researcher hopes that the model derived from the structural equations is consistent with the proposed theory. Of course, this consistency does not prove the accuracy of the theory, but it does support it.

In any theory, elements external to the theory are related to variables within the theory and explain some of the variance within the theory. These elements are referred to as residual or exogenous variables and are important to structural equation modeling. Residual variables are not explained by the theory, and yet they introduce a source of error into the analyses. Thus, understanding residual variance is important when interpreting the results of structural equation modeling and validating the theory.

In a sample map initially described in Chapter 11 (see Figure 20–6), variables 1, 2, and 3 are proposed to be causally related to variable 4. Variable 4 is proposed to be a cause of variable 5. The map demonstrates unidirectional causal flow; variable 5 would not be considered a cause of variable 4. Because the causal relationships will not explain all the variance in the model, residual variables (shown here as *a* and *b*) are introduced to indicate the effect of variables not included in the analysis. Noncausal relationships such as those between variables 1 and 2, 1 and 3, and 2 and 3 are not included in the causal model.

Structural equation modeling requires that the following assumptions be made:

1. The relationships examined in the model are causal, linear, and additive.
2. The residual variables are not correlated with other residual variables or with variables being examined in the model.
3. The causal pathways are unidirectional.
4. The variables can be treated as interval-level measures.

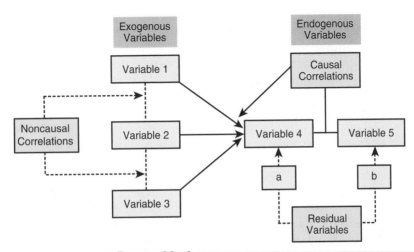

FIGURE 20–6 ■ Path analysis diagram.

Testing a theory by structural equation modeling occurs in stages and can be categorized into exploratory stages and the confirmatory stage. Initially, the researcher will seek information on beta weights concerning specific relationships between concepts from previous research. In the early exploratory period, correlational analyses are performed and a covariance matrix is obtained. A series of regression analyses may be performed as the researcher gets a feel for the data.

The reliability and validity of measures used in the analysis are critical to the validity of the model. When possible, it is desirable to use multiple indicators of parameters. As with regression analysis, a large sample is desirable, with at least 30 subjects for each variable being considered. Larger samples are more likely to yield the statistically significant path coefficients needed to validate the model, thus reducing the risk of a Type II error. Because of the importance of model building to theory development, a Type II error is a serious concern.

Data need to be carefully cleaned before analysis. Accuracy of the data is carefully checked. Subjects with missing data are removed, and outliers are identified and examined. Some statistical procedures will automatically exclude outliers from the analysis. However, the decision to retain or exclude outliers is a difficult one. The outliers may represent an important segment of the population under study, and yet the inclusion of a small amount of very divergent data can greatly alter the outcomes of the analysis.

In the exploratory stage, a path analysis is performed by using a series of regression analyses. In the analysis, a *path coefficient* indicates the effect of an independent variable on the dependent variable. The symbol for a path coefficient is P with two subscripts. The first subscript indicates the dependent variable; the second subscript indicates the independent variable. For example, the direct effect of variable 4 on variable 5 would be symbolized as P_{54}. Path coefficients are usually expressed in the form of beta weights. (Beta weights were discussed in the section on simple linear regression.)

The map in Figure 20–6 would require two regression analyses to identify the path coefficients. In the first analysis, path coefficients would be obtained by regressing variable 4 on variables 1, 2, and 3. Variable 5 would then be regressed on variable 4. In interpreting the results, the weight of the coefficient and its level of statistical significance are considered. A large coefficient that is highly significant validates the causal pathway.

Confirmatory structural equation modeling is performed with LISREL or EQS. When these procedures are used, the assumptions of regression are relaxed: all relevant variables are not assumed to be included in the model, and perfect measurement is not assumed. The analysis is concerned with the identification of latent variables—operationalizations of concepts that are not measurable by direct observation. Thus, one concept might be represented by a combination of several measures. In structural equation modeling, there are multiple dependent as well as independent variables. By using information obtained from previous studies and exploratory analyses, the researcher specifies the nature of the relationships and provides an initial estimation of the model as a starting point for the analysis. The analysis is an iterative procedure progressing in stages to a final estimation of the model (Mason-Hawkes & Holm, 1989).

Analysis involves three steps: specification, estimation, and assessing goodness of fit. In the specification step, the researcher specifies the parameters of the model, including variables and interrelationships (or paths)—similar to developing a conceptual map. The variance (or covariance) of some parameters of the model is specified (or held constant at a selected value). Selection of this value is based on previous studies and exploratory analyses. These parameters are referred to as *fixed*. All other variables are referred to as *free*. The analysis procedure has rules that govern the selection of parameters to be fixed or free.

In the estimation step, the free parameters are estimated by computer analysis. The results, including fixed parameters and estimated parameters, are then assessed for goodness of fit. Initially, the resulting model is examined in relation to the data. If the model is not a good fit, parameters can be added or dropped. The values of fixed parameters may be modified and the analysis rerun to achieve a better fit, a process referred to as *respecification*.

Some judgment is involved in determining what makes the model a fit. The initial evaluation is based on the statistical significance of each path proposed by the original model. Parameters that do not achieve significance in the analysis are carefully considered. Were the measures used to examine the parameter adequate? Was the sample size sufficient? Is it possible that the original theory is incorrect? Should the parameter be omitted from the map of the theory? How important is the parameter in explaining the phenomenon? In some cases, because of their theoretical importance, parameters may be retained in the model in spite of failing to achieve statistical significance. Validation of the final model is achieved by conducting further analyses on data from new samples.

Neuberger and colleagues (1994) used structural equation modeling to test their theoretical causal model of exercise and aerobic fitness in outpatients with arthritis.

. . . .

"Factors that influenced exercise behaviors and aerobic fitness were identified in 100 outpatients with rheumatoid arthritis or osteoarthritis. Data included perceived health status, benefits of and barriers to exercise, and impact of arthritis on health; demographic and biologic characteristics; and past exercise behavior. Exercise measures included range-of-motion [ROM] and strengthening exercises, 7-day activity recall, and the exercise subscale of the Health-Promoting Lifestyle Profile. An aerobic fitness level was obtained on each subject by bicycle ergometer testing. . . .

"To determine if rheumatoid arthritis ($n = 63$) subjects differed from osteoarthritis subjects ($n = 37$), the two groups were compared on the study variables using the t-statistic or chi-square. No statistically significant differences were found in the two groups on any of the study variables. Therefore, data on rheumatoid arthritis and osteoarthritis subjects were combined for analysis. . . .

"To simplify data analysis, a composite score of self-reported exercises was calculated by a principal component factor analysis of the four measures of exercise (ROM score, strengthening exercise score, MET [metabolic equivalents] score, and exercise subscale score) and calculating a factor score

by the regression technique. To determine if the theoretical model predicted the composite exercise scores and the resulting aerobic fitness levels of the subjects, path analysis was conducted based on the causal model. The analysis for the path model was done by a set of ordinary least squares regression equations. The first set of three equations had perceived health status, perceived benefits, and perceived barriers as predicted variables. The independent variables in the equations were the modifying factors in Stage I [Figure 20–7]. The three predicted variables were in turn used to predict participation in exercise. The last equation in the model was level of fitness predicted by participation in exercise. The standardized parameters from each equation were used as path coefficients to derive the indirect effects with the model.

"The theoretical model proposed that the eight modifying factors would produce direct effects on the cognitive-perceptual factors and that the modifying factors would affect exercise behaviors (composite exercise scores) and the resulting aerobic fitness levels indirectly through their effects on the cognitive perceptual factors of perceived health status, perceived benefits of exercise, and perceived barriers to exercise. As seen in [Figure 20–7], three modifying factors—impact of arthritis on health status, duration of arthritis, and age—had significant ($p = .05$) direct effects on perceived health status. Higher impact of arthritis scores and longer duration of arthritis were significantly ($p = .05$) associated with poorer perceived health status scores. Older age was associated ($p = .05$) with better perceived health status. When path coefficients of .10 and above are considered, education level, income level, and pain scores also affected perceived health status. Fewer years of education and high pain scores were related to poorer perceived health status, while higher income levels were associated with better perceived health status. The total variance in perceived health status scores accounted for by the eight modifying factors was 26% (adj. $R^2 = .26$).

"Subjects' scores on the eight modifying factors accounted for 18.4% of the variance in perceived benefits of exercise scores. Higher impact of arthritis scores were significantly ($p = .05$) associated

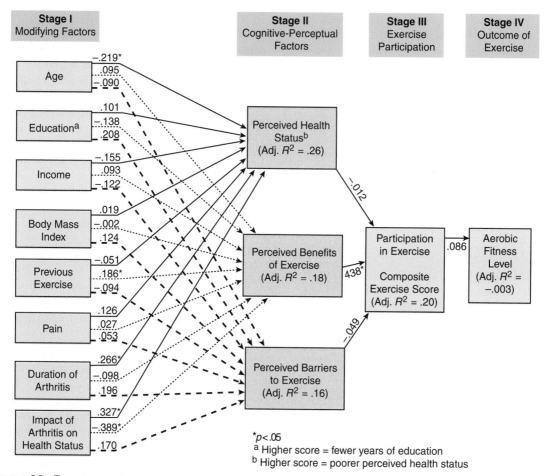

FIGURE 20–7 ■ Path coefficients of model testing determinants of exercise. (From Neuberger, G. B., Kasal, S., Smith, K. V., et al. [1994]. Determinants of exercise and aerobic fitness in outpatients with arthritis. *Nursing Research 43*[1], 12.)

with lower scores of perceived benefits of exercise. Previous exercise was significantly ($p = .05$) associated with higher perceived benefits of exercise scores. Longer duration of arthritis ($\beta = .098$), higher impact of arthritis scores ($\beta = .170$), higher body mass index scores ($\beta = .124$), and fewer years of education ($\beta = .122$) were related to lower perceived barriers to exercise. . . .

The total amount of variance in composite exercise scores accounted for by the model was 20%. Perception of more benefits of exercise was positively associated ($\beta = .438$, p = .05) with exercise participation. Poorer perceived health status ($\beta = -.012$) and higher perceived barriers to exercise

scores ($-.049$) were weakly ($\beta < .10$) associated with lower participation in exercise. As seen in Stage IV of the path model [Figure 20–7], regression of the aerobic fitness levels on composite exercise scores failed to predict any variance in aerobic fitness levels." (Neuberger et al., 1994, pp. 15–16) ■

■ SUMMARY

Correlational analyses are performed to identify relationships between or among variables. The purpose of the analysis may be to describe relationships between variables, clarify relationships among theoretical concepts, or assist in identifying causal relationships, which can then be tested by inferential analysis. All data for the analysis should have been obtained from a single population from which values are available on all variables to be examined in the correlational analysis. Data measured at the interval level will provide the best information on the nature of the relationship. However, analysis procedures are available for most levels of measurement. In preparation for correlational analysis, data collection strategies should be planned to maximize the possibility of obtaining the full range of possible values on each variable to be used in the analysis. Scatter diagrams, which provide useful preliminary information about the nature of the relationship between variables, should be developed and examined before performing correlational analysis.

Bivariate correlation measures the extent of the linear relationship between two variables and is performed on data collected from a single sample. Correlational analysis provides two pieces of information about the data: the nature of a linear relationship (positive or negative) between the two variables and the magnitude (or strength) of the linear relationship. The outcomes of correlational analysis are symmetrical rather than asymmetrical. Symmetrical means that the direction of the linear relationship cannot be determined from the analysis. One cannot say from the analysis that variable A leads to or causes variable B. In a positive linear relationship, the scores being correlated vary together (in the same direction). When one score is high, the other score tends to be high; when one score is low, the other score tends to be low. In a negative linear relationship, when one score is high, the other score tends to be low.

The Spearman rho, a nonparametric test, is used when the assumptions of Pearson's analysis cannot be met. The data must be ranked to conduct the analysis. Kendall's tau is a nonparametric measure of correlation used when both variables have been measured at the ordinal level. It can be used with very small samples. Pearson's correlation is used when both variables have been measured at the interval level. To infer that the sample Pearson correlation coefficient applies to the population from

which the sample was taken, statistical analysis must be performed to determine whether the coefficient is significantly different from zero (no correlation). With a small sample, a very high correlation coefficient (r) can be nonsignificant. With a very large sample, the correlation coefficient can be statistically significant when the degree of association is too small to be clinically significant. Therefore, when judging the significance of the coefficient, one must consider both the size of the coefficient and the significance of the t test.

A correlational matrix is obtained by performing bivariate correlational analysis on every pair of variables in the data set. During examination of the matrix values, the researcher must place weight only on r values with a p value of .05 or smaller. Once those pairs of variables are singled out, the researcher notes variable pairs with an r value sufficiently large to be of interest in terms of the study problem. Spurious correlations are relationships between variables that are not logical. In some cases, these significant relationships are a consequence of chance and have no meaning. When you choose a level of significance of .05, 1 in 20 correlations that you perform in a matrix will be significant by chance. Other pairs of variables may be correlated because of the influence of other variables.

In any situation involving causality, a relationship will exist between the factors involved in the causal process. Therefore, the first clue to the possibility of a causal link is the existence of a relationship, but a relationship does not necessarily mean causality. Two variables can be highly correlated but have no causal relationship whatsoever. However, as the strength of a relationship increases, the possibility of a causal link increases. The absence of a relationship precludes the possibility of a causal connection between the two variables being examined.

Multivariate correlational procedures are more complex analysis techniques that examine linear relationships among three or more variables. The multivariate correlational procedures described are factor analysis, canonical correlation, and structural equation modeling. Factor analysis examines interrelationships among large numbers of variables and disentangles those relationship to identify clusters of variables that are most closely linked together. Canonical correlation is an extension of multiple regression in which more than one dependent variable is present. The purpose of the test is to analyze the relationships between two or more dependent variables and two or more independent variables. Structural equation modeling is designed to test the interrelationships of all the concepts in a theory.

. . . .

REFERENCES

Arrindell, W. A., & van der Ende, J. (1985). An empirical test of the utility of the observations-to-variables ratio in factor and components analysis. *Applied Psychological Measurement, 9*(2), 165–178.

Boyd, C. J., Frey, M. A., & Aaronson, L. S. (1988). Structural equation models and nursing research. . . . LISREL: Part I. *Nursing Research, 37*(4), 249–252.

Carmines, E. G., & McIver, J. P. (1981). Analyzing models with unobserved variables: Analysis of covariance structures. In G. W. Bohrnstedt & E. F. Borgatta (Eds.), *Social measurement: Current issues* (pp. 65–115). Beverly Hills, CA: Sage.

Folkman, S., & Lazarus, R. S. (1985). If it changes it must be a process: Study of emotion and coping during three stages of a college examination. *Journal of Personality and Social Psychology, 48*(1), 150–170.

Folkman, S., & Lazarus, R. S. (1988). *Manual for the Ways of Coping Questionnaire*. Palo Alto, CA: Consulting Psychologists Press.

Folkman, S., Lazarus, R. S., Dunkel-Schetter, C., DeLongis, A., & Gruen, R. J. (1986). Dynamics of a stressful encounter: Cognitive appraisal, coping, and encounter outcomes. *Journal of Personality and Social Psychology, 50*(5), 992–1003.

Joreskog, K. G., & Sorböm, D. (1989). *LISREL 7: A guide to the program & applications* (2nd ed.). Chicago: SPSS.

Joreskog, K. G., & Sorböm, D. (1988–1992). *LISREL* [Computer Program]. Moorseville, IN: Scientific Software.

Kenny, D. A. (1979). *Correlation and causality*. New York: Wiley.

Kim, J., & Mueller, C. W. (1978a). *Introduction to factor analysis: What it is and how to do it*. Beverly Hills, CA: Sage.

Kim, J., & Mueller, C. W. (1978b). *Factor analysis: Statistical methods and practical issues*. Beverly Hills, CA: Sage.

Long, J. S. (1983a). *Confirmatory factor analysis*. Beverly Hills, CA: Sage.

Marascuilo, L. A., & McSweeney, M. (1977). *Nonparametric and distribution-free methods for the social sciences*. Monterey, CA: Brooks/Cole.

Mason-Hawkes, J., & Holm, K. (1989). Causal modeling: A comparison of path analysis and LISREL. *Nursing Research, 38*(5), 312–314.

Neuberger, G. B., Kasal, S., Smith, K. V., Hassanein, R., & DeViney, S. (1994). Determinants of exercise and aerobic fitness in outpatients with arthritis. *Nursing Research, 43*(1), 11–17.

Norbeck, J. S. (1984). Modification of life event questionnaire for use with female respondents. *Research in Nursing & Health, 7*(1), 61–71.

Nunnally, J. C. (1978). *Psychometric theory* (2nd ed.). New York: McGraw-Hill.

Olson, J. K. (1995). Relationships between nurse-expressed empathy, patient-perceived empathy and patient distress. *Image—The Journal of Nursing Scholarship, 27*(4), 317–322.

Raykov, T., Tomer, A., & Nesselroade, J. R. (1991). Reporting structural equation modeling results in *Psychology and Aging*: Some proposed guidelines. *Psychology and Aging, 6*(4), 499–503.

Wikoff, R. L., & Miller, P. (1991). Canonical analysis in nursing research. *Nursing Research, 40*(6), 367–370.

Wineman, N. M., Durand, E. J., & McCulloch, B. J. (1994). Examination of the factor structure of the Ways of Coping Questionnaire with clinical populations. *Nursing Research, 43*(5), 268–273.

Woods, N. F., Lentz, M. J., & Mitchell, E. S. (1993). Prevalence of perimenstrual symptoms. Unpublished report to National Center for Nursing Research.

Woods, N. F., Mitchell, E. S., & Lentz, M. J. (1995). Social pathways to premenstrual symptoms. *Research in Nursing & Health, 18*(3), 225–237.

Youngblut, J. M. (1993). Comparison of factor analysis options using the Home/Employment Orientation Scale. *Nursing Research, 42*(2), 122–124.

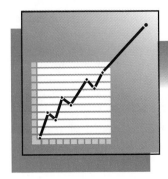

CHAPTER 21

USING STATISTICS TO PREDICT

The purpose of a regression analysis is to predict or explain as much of the variance in the value of a dependent variable as possible. In some cases, the analysis is exploratory and the focus is prediction. In others, selection of variables is based on a theoretical position, and the purpose is explanation, to confirm the theoretical position. The ability to predict future events is becoming increasingly important in our society. We are interested in predicting who will win the football game, what the weather will be like next week, or what stocks are likely to rise in the near future. In nursing practice, as in the rest of society, the capacity to predict is crucial. For example, we need to predict the length of stay of patients with varying severity of illness, as well as the response of patients with a variety of characteristics to nursing interventions. We need to know what factors play an important role in patients' responses to rehabilitation. One might be interested in knowing what variables were most effective in predicting a student's score on the State Board of Nurse Examiners' Licensure Examination.

Predictive analyses are based on probability theory rather than decision theory. Prediction is one approach to examining causal relationships between or among variables. The independent (predictor) variable or variables cause variation in the value of the dependent (outcome) variable. The goal is to determine how accurately one can predict the value of an outcome (or dependent) variable based on the value or values of one or more predictor (or independent) variables. This chapter will describe some of the more common statistical procedures used for prediction. These procedures include simple linear regression, multiple regression, and discriminant analysis.

SIMPLE LINEAR REGRESSION

Simple linear regression provides a means to estimate the value of a dependent variable based on the value of an independent variable. The regression equation is a mathematical expression of a causal proposition emerging from a theoretical framework. This linkage between the theoretical statement and the equation should be made clear before the analysis.

Simple linear regression is an effort to explain the dynamics within the scatter plot by drawing a straight line (the line of best fit) through the plotted scores. This line is drawn to provide the best explanation of the linear relationship between two variables. Knowing that linear relationship, we can, with some degree of accuracy, use regression analysis to predict the value of one variable if we know the value of the other variable. In addition, the following assumptions need to be met:

1. The presence of homoscedasticity equals scatter of values of y above and below the regression line at each value of x (constant variance).
2. The dependent variable is measured at the interval level.
3. The expected value of the residual error is zero.

Calculation

Simple linear regression is a method of determining parameters *a* and *b*. Mathematical development of the formula is based on the requirement that the squared deviation values (squared difference scores) be minimized. When squared deviation values are minimized, variance from the line of best fit is minimized. To understand the mathematical process, it is helpful to recall the algebraic equation for a straight line:

$$y = a + bx$$

In regression analysis, the straight line is usually plotted on a graph, with the horizontal axis representing x (the independent, or predictor, variable) and the vertical axis representing y (the dependent, or predicted, variable). The value represented by the letter a is referred to as the *y intercept,* or the point where the regression line crosses (or intercepts) the y-axis. At this point on the regression line, $x = 0$. The value represented by the letter b is referred to as the *slope,* or the coefficient of x. The slope determines the direction and angle of the regression line within the graph. The slope expresses the extent to which y changes for every 1-unit change in x. Figure 21–1 is a graph of these points.

In simple, or bivariate, regression, predictions are made in cases with two variables. The score on variable y (dependent variable) is predicted from the same subject's known score on variable x (independent variable). The predicted score (or estimate) is referred to as $\hat{y}$ (expressed y-hat) or occasionally as y' (expressed y-prime).

No single regression line can be used to predict with complete accuracy every y value from every x value. In fact, one could draw an infinite number of lines through the scattered paired values. However, the purpose of the regression equation is to develop the line to allow the highest degree of prediction possible—the line of best fit. The procedure for developing the line of best fit is the *method of least squares.*

To explain the method of least squares, we must return to difference scores. In a real sample in which values for both x and y are known, the regression line is plotted subject by subject, with both values used to determine the placement of each point. The multiple subjects with the same single value on x can have various values on y. Only the mean of these y values is located on the regression line. Therefore, at each point on the x-axis, one can determine difference scores from the mean on the y-axis. From these difference scores a sum of squares can be calculated. There can then be a sum of squares for each point on the x-axis. The sum of squares of all difference scores is an indicator of how good a fit the regression line is to the data.

The equations to estimate the regression line have been developed in such a way that the value of the sum of squares will be minimized, thus decreasing the variance and maximizing the predictive power of the resulting equation. The three equations for the method of least squares are

$$b = \frac{n(\Sigma\, xy) - (\Sigma\, x)(\Sigma\, y)}{n(\Sigma\, x^2) - (\Sigma\, x)^2}$$

$$a = \bar{y} - b\bar{x}$$

$$\hat{y} = a + bx$$

where

b = slope
n = number of paired values
x = known value of x
a = y intercept
$\hat{y}$ = predicted value of y

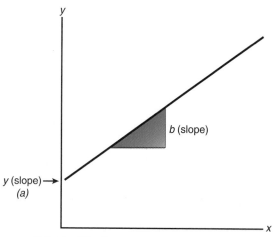

FIGURE 21–1 ■ Graph of a regression line.

The coefficient of x, which is b, can be determined from the analysis of raw data or from the analysis of Z scores. When the slope is determined from Z scores, it is no longer the coefficient of x but the coefficient of the Z score–transformed x. If b is determined from Z scores, it is referred to as *beta*. Beta is preferred when comparisons are made with the results of other analyses. Computer analyses usually provide both values.

Interpretation of Results

The outcome of analysis is the regression coefficient R. When R *is* squared, it indicates the amount of variance in the data that is explained by the equation. A null regression hypothesis states that the population regression slope is 0, which indicates that there is no useful linear relationship between x and y. (There are regression analyses that test for nonlinear relationships.) The test statistic used to determine the significance of a regression coefficient is t. However, the test uses a different equation than the t test used to determine significant differences between means. In determining the significance of a regression coefficient, t tends to become larger as b moves farther from zero. However, if the sum of squared deviations from regression is large, the t value will decrease. Small sample sizes also decrease the t value.

In reporting the results of a regression analysis, the equation is expressed with the calculated coefficient values. The R^2 value and the t values are also documented. The format for reporting the results of regression is as follows:

$$\underset{(2.79)\ \ \ (4.68)\ \leftarrow\ t\text{ value}}{\hat{y} = \overset{y\text{ intercept}}{3.45} + \overset{b\text{ (slope)}}{8.72x}\quad R^2 = .63}$$

The figures in parentheses are not always t values. They may be the standard error of the estimate. Therefore, the report must indicate which values are being reported. If t values are being used, the t value that indicates significance should also be re-

ported. A t value equal to or greater than the table value (Appendix C) indicates significance. From these results, a graph can be developed to illustrate the outcome. Additionally, a table can be developed to indicate the changes that are predicted to occur in the value of y with each increase in the value of x. Names are usually given to identify the variables of x and y. In the example in which the y intercept $= 3.45$ and $b = 8.72$, a table (see Table 21–1) of x and y values was developed. These values are graphed in Figure 21–2.

After a regression equation has been developed, the equation is tested against a new sample to determine its accuracy in prediction, a process called *cross-validation*. In some studies, data are collected from a holdout sample obtained at the initial data collection period but not included in the initial regression analysis. The regression equation is then tested against this sample. Some "shrinkage" of R^2 is expected because the equation was generated to best fit the sample from which it was developed. However, an equation is most useful if it maintains its ability to accurately predict across many and varied samples. The first test of an equation against a new sample should use a sample very similar to the initial sample.

MULTIPLE REGRESSION

Multiple regression analyses, which have become the most frequently used type of multivariate analysis in nursing studies, replaced the analysis of variance (ANOVA) models so popular a few years ago (ANOVA is described in Chapter 22). This change is a reflection of the move in nursing away from

TABLE 21–1

PREDICTED VALUES OF y FROM KNOWN VALUES OF x BY REGRESSION ANALYSIS

VALUE OF x	PREDICTED VALUE OF y
0	3.45 (y intercept)
1	12.17 (y intercept + b)
2	20.89 (+ b)
3	29.61 (+ b)
4	38.33 (+ b)

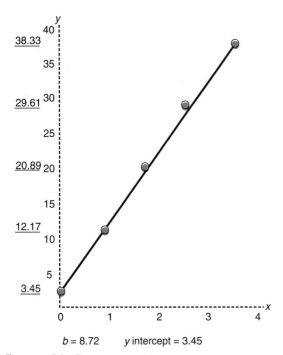

$b = 8.72$ y intercept $= 3.45$

FIGURE 21–2 ■ Regression line developed from values in Table 21–1.

decision theory reasoning to the logic of probability. Multiple regression is an extension of simple linear regression in which more than one independent variable is entered into the analysis.

Assumptions

The assumptions of multiple regression analysis are as follows:

1. The variables (dependent and independent) were measured without error.
2. Variables can be treated as interval-level measures.
3. The residuals are not correlated.
4. Dependent variable scores come from a normal distribution.
5. Scores are homoscedastic (equally dispersed about the line of best fit); thus there is a normal distribution of Y scores at each value of X.
6. Y scores have equal variance at each value of X; thus difference scores (residuals or error scores) are random and have homogeneous variance.

Determining whether these assumptions have been violated in a data set is difficult. Therefore, a set of statistical procedures, or residual analyses, have been developed to test for violation of the assumptions (Verran & Ferketich, 1987). The results of residual analysis need to be included in the research report.

Multicollinearity

Multicollinearity occurs when the independent variables in a multiple regression equation are strongly correlated. In nursing studies, some multicollinearity is inevitable; however, it can be minimized by careful selection of independent variables. Multicollinearity does not affect predictive power (the capacity of the independent variables to predict values of the dependent variable in that specific sample), but rather causes problems related to generalizability. If multicollinearity is present, the equation will not have predictive validity. The amount of variance explained by each variable in the equation will be inflated. The b values will not remain consistent across samples when cross-validation is performed because multicollinearity leads to the following problems:

1. It decreases the power of significance tests for the partial regression coefficients by increasing the sampling error of the coefficients. The values of b obtained in the analysis will not be found to be significant when, in reality, they are significant—a Type II error.
2. It sometimes causes the signs of the coefficients to be wrong.
3. It may adversely affect the accuracy of poorly written computer programs.
4. The removal of a single observation may cause a large change in the calculated coefficients.
5. The R^2 of the estimated regression will be large, but all the coefficients may be insignificant.

The first step in identification of multicollinearity is examination of correlations among the independent variables. Therefore, usually the researcher performs multiple correlation analyses before conducting the regression analyses. The correlation matrix is carefully examined for evidence of multicollinearity. Most researchers consider multicollinearity to exist if a bivariate correlation is greater than .65. However, some researchers use a stronger correlation of .80 or greater as an indication of multicollinearity (Schroeder, 1990).

The *coefficient of determination* (R^2), computed from a matrix of correlation coefficients, provides important information on multicollinearity. This value indicates the degree of linear dependencies among the variables. As the value of the determinant approaches zero, the degree of linear dependency increases. Thus it is preferable that this R^2 be large. Identifying the extent of multicollinearity is important when selecting regression procedures and interpreting results. Therefore, Schroeder (1990) describes additional procedures that researchers use to diagnose the extent of multicollinearity.

The extent of multicollinearity in the data needs to be examined by the researcher as part of the analysis procedure and reported in publication of the study. An example from Braden (1990) follows.

· ·

"A correlation matrix of model variables showed no evidence of multicollinearity in the multiple regression equations used to answer the research questions. Gordon's (1968) criteria of $r \leq .65$ for correlation of variables entered in the same equation was used." (Braden, 1990, p. 44) ■

Types of Independent Variables Used in Regression Analyses

Variables in a regression equation can take many forms. Traditionally, as with most multivariate analyses, variables are measured at the interval level. However, categorical or dichotomous measures (referred to as *dummy variables*), multiplicative terms, and transformed terms are also used. A mixture of types of variables may be used in a single regression equation. The following discussion describes the various terms used as variables in regression equations.

DUMMY VARIABLES

To use categorical variables in regression analysis, a coding system is developed to represent group membership. Categorical variables of interest in nursing that might be used in regression analysis

include gender, income, ethnicity, social status, level of education, and diagnosis. If the variable is dichotomous, such as gender, members of one category are assigned the number 1, and all others are assigned the number 0. In this case, for gender the coding could be

$$1 = \text{female}$$
$$0 = \text{male}$$

If the categorical variable has three values, two dummy variables are used; for example, social class could be classified as lower class, middle class, or upper class. The first dummy variable (X_1) would be classified as

$$1 = \text{lower class}$$
$$0 = \text{not lower class}$$

The second dummy variable (X_2) would be classified as

$$1 = \text{middle class}$$
$$0 = \text{not middle class}$$

The three social classes would then be specified in the equation in the following manner:

Lower class	$X_1 = 1, X_2 = 0$
Middle class	$X_1 = 0, X_2 = 1$
Upper class	$X_1 = 0, X_2 = 0$

When more than three categories define the values of the variable, increased numbers of dummy variables are used. The number of dummy variables is always one less than the number of categories.

TIME CODING

Time is commonly expressed in a regression equation as an interval measure. However, in some cases, codes may need to be developed for time periods. In this strategy, time is coded in a categorical form and used as an independent variable. For example, if 5 years' data were available, the following system could be used to provide dummy codes for the time variable:

$$-2 = \text{subjects cared for in the first year}$$
$$-1 = \text{subjects cared for in the second year}$$
$$0 = \text{subjects cared for in the third year}$$
$$+1 = \text{subjects cared for in the fourth year}$$
$$+2 = \text{subjects cared for in the fifth year}$$

EFFECT CODING

Effect coding is similar to dummy coding but is used when the effects of treatments are being examined by the analysis. Each group of subjects is assigned a code. The code numbers used are 1, 0, and −1. The codes are assigned in the same way as dummy codes. While using dummy codes, one category will be assigned 0; in effect coding, one group in each set will be assigned −1, one group will be assigned 1, and all others will be assigned 0 (Pedhazur, 1982).

MULTIPLICATIVE TERMS

The multiple regression model $Y = a + b_1X_1 + b_2X_2 + b_3X_3$ assumes that the independent variables have an additive effect on the dependent variable. In other words, each independent variable has the same relationship with the dependent variable at each value of the other independent variables. Thus, if variable X_1 increased as X_2 increased in lower values of X_2, X_1 would be expected to continue to increase at the same rate at higher values of X_2. However, in some analyses, such does not prove to be the case. For example, in a study of hospice care conducted by one of the authors (Burns & Carney, 1986), minutes of care (MC) was used as the dependent variable. Duration (DUR), or number of days of care, and age (AGE) were included as independent variables. When duration was short, minutes of care increased as age increased. However, when duration was long, minutes of care decreased as age increased.

In this situation, better prediction can occur if multiplicative terms are included in the equation. In this case, the regression model takes the following form:

$$Y = a + b_1X_1 + b_2X_2 + b_3X_1X_2$$

The last term ($b_3X_1X_2$) takes the form of a multiplicative term and is the product of the first two variables (X_1 multiplied by X_2). This term expresses the joint effect of the two variables. For example, duration (DUR) might be expected to interact with the subject's age (AGE). The third term would show the combined effect of the two variables

($DURAGE$). The example equation would then be expressed as

$$MC = a + b_1DUR + b_2AGE + b_3DURAGE$$

This procedure is similar to multivariate ANOVA, in which main effects and interaction effects are considered. Main effects are the effects of a single variable. Interaction effects are the multiplicative effects of two or more variables.

TRANSFORMED TERMS

The typical regression model assumes a linear regression in which the relationship between X and Y can be illustrated on a graph as a straight line. However, in some cases, the relationship is not linear but curvilinear. The fact that the scores are curvilinear can sometimes be demonstrated by graphing the values. In these cases, deviations from the regression line will be great and predictive power will be low; the F ratio will not be significant, R^2 will be low, and a Type II error will result. Adding another independent variable to the equation, a transformation of the original independent variable obtained by squaring the original variable, may accurately express the curvilinear relationship. This strategy will improve the predictive capacity of the analysis. An example of a mathematical model that includes a squared independent variable is

$$Y = a + b_1X + b_2X^2$$

This equation states that Y is related to both X and X^2 in such a way that changes in Y's values are a function of both X and X^2. The nonlinearity analysis can be extended beyond the squared term to add more transformed terms; thus, values such as X^3, X^4, and so on can be included in the equation. Each term adds another curve in the regression line. With this strategy, very complicated relationships can be modeled. However, small samples can incorrectly lead to a perfect fit. For these complex equations, the researcher needs a minimum of 30 observations per term (Cohen & Cohen, 1983). If the complex equation provides better prediction, R^2 will be increased and the F ratio will be significant.

Many versions of regression analyses are used in a variety of research situations. Some versions have been developed especially for situations in which some of the foregoing assumptions are violated.

The typical multiple regression equation is expressed as

$$Y = a + bX_1 + bX_2 + \cdots bX_i$$

The dependent variable (or predicted variable) is represented by Y in the regression equation. The independent variables (or indicators) are represented by X_i in the regression equation. The i indicates the number of independent variables in the equation. The coefficient of the independent variable, $b,$ is a numerical value that indicates the amount of change that occurs in Y for each change in the associated X and can be reported as a b weight (based on raw scores) or a beta weight (based on Z scores).

The outcome of a multiple regression is an R^2 value. For each independent variable, the significance of R^2 is reported, as well as the significance of b. Regression, unlike correlation, is one-way; the independent variables can predict the values of the dependent variable, but the dependent variable cannot be used to predict the values of the independent variables. If the b value of an independent variable is not significant, that independent variable is not an effective predictor of the dependent variable when that set of independent variables is used. In this case, the researcher may remove variables with non-significant coefficients from the equation and repeat the analysis. This action will often increase the amount of variance explained by the equation and thus raise the R^2 value. To be effective predictors, independent variables selected for the analysis should have strong correlations with the dependent variable but only weak correlations with other independent variables in the equation.

The significance of an R^2 value is tested with an F test. A significant F value indicates that the regression equation has been effective in predicting variation in the dependent variable and that the R^2 value is not a random variation from an R^2 value of zero.

Results

The outcome of regression analysis is referred to as a *prediction equation.* This equation is similar to that described for simple linear regression except that making a prediction is more complex. Consider the following sample equation:

DURATION =
  10.6 + .3 AGE + 2.4 INCOME + 3.5 COPING
  (4.56)   (2.78)   (4.43)   (7.52)

$R^2 = .51$ $n = 350$ $F = 1.832$ $p < .001$

If duration were measured as the number of days that the patient received care, the Y intercept would be 10.6 days. (This value is not meaningful apart from the equation.) For each increase of 1 year in age, the patient would receive .3 days more of care. For each increase in income level, the patient would receive an additional 2.4 days of care. For each increase in coping ability measured on a scale, the patient would receive an additional 3.5 days of care. In this example, $R^2 = .51$, which means that these variables explain 51% of the variance in the duration of care. The regression analysis of variance indicates that the equation is significant at a $p \leq .001$ level.

Relating these findings to real situations requires additional work. First, it is necessary to know how the variables were coded for the analysis; for example, one would need to know the range of scores on the coping scale, the income classifications, and the range of ages in the sample. Possible patient situations would then be proposed and the duration of care would be predicted for a patient with those particular dimensions of each independent variable. For example, suppose a patient is 64 years of age, in income level 3, and in coping level 5. In this case, the patient's predicted duration would be 10.6 + (64 × .3) + (3 × 2.4) + (5 × 3.5), or 54.5 days of care.

The results of a regression analysis are not expected to be sample specific. The final outcome of a regression analysis is a model from which values of the independent variables can be used to predict and perhaps explain values of the dependent variable in the population. If so, the analysis can be repeated in other samples with similar results. The equation is expected to have predictive validity. Knapp (1994) has listed the essential elements of a regression analysis that need to be included in a publication.

Cross-Validation

To determine the accuracy of the prediction, the predicted values are compared with actual values obtained from a new sample of subjects or values from a sample obtained at the time of the original data collection but held out from the initial analysis. This analysis is conducted on the difference scores between predicted values and the means of actual values. Thus in the new sample, the number of days of care for all patients 64 years of age, in income level 3, and in coping level 5 would be averaged, and the mean would be compared with 54.5 days of care. Each possible case within the new sample would be compared in this manner. An R^2 is obtained on the new sample and compared with the R^2 of the original sample. In most cases, R^2 will be lower in the new sample because the original equation was developed to most precisely predict scores in the original sample. This phenomenon is referred to as *shrinkage of R^2*. Shrinkage of R^2 is greater in small samples and when multicollinearity is great.

Mischel and colleagues (1991) performed a cross-validation procedure to test the uncertainty in illness theory by replicating a study examining the mediating effects of mastery and coping. They describe their methodology as follows.

• •

"To compare the results of this study with those of the prior research, regression equations were compared for consistency in variables entering the equations and for percent of variance explained. Additionally, the unstandardized regression coefficients were compared by using a 95% confidence interval to determine the comparability of the two models. For comparability to exist, the regression coefficients for this study should fall within the confidence interval calculated for those from previous research (Verran & Reid, 1987).

"Prescott (1987) notes that with highly homogeneous samples, the cross-validation procedure is likely to result in substantially similar findings.

Thus, if the goal of the replication is to determine the limits of the supported relationships and the population and contextual variability under which the relationships hold, then some heterogeneity in the sample and setting are desirable. To determine the heterogeneity of the samples, a series of chi-square and *t* test analyses were run on the demographic variables. The first sample had a significantly larger number of elderly subjects (above 70 years of age), more subjects with ovarian cancer, a greater number of ovarian cancer patients in Stages III and IV, and a greater number of subjects receiving chemotherapy as compared with the sample for the replication testing.

"Differences between the samples on the major predictor and dependent variables were explored through two MANOVA analyses. . . . Significant differences were found on all variables in this analysis. . . . The difference between the samples on the measures was not in a consistent direction, but supported that the two samples were not homogeneous. (p. 237)

"Regression analysis was used to test the mediating effects of mastery and coping following the procedure described by Baron and Kenny (1986) and applied in the initial test of the model (Mischel & Sorenson, 1991). To test for mediating effect of each mediator, three regression equations were run. The mediator was regressed on the independent variable, the dependent variable was regressed on the independent variable, and the dependent variable was regressed on both the independent variable and the mediator. In order to have the appropriate conditions to test the mediation effect of a variable, the independent variable must have a significant relationship with the mediating variable and with the dependent variable, plus the mediator must significantly account for variation in the dependent variable. When both the independent variable and mediating variable are entered on the dependent variable, the strength of the relationship between the independent and dependent variables should decrease. The ideal case is a reduction in the magnitude of the beta so that the path is insignificant. . . .

"Results of the model tests demonstrated significant relationships to be the same and in the same direction for uncertainty to mastery, mastery to danger, danger to an emotion-focused coping strategy, danger to emotional distress, the emotion-focused coping strategy to emotional distress, opportunity appraisal to a problem-focused coping strategy, and the problem-focused coping strategy to emotional distress. In considering the mediating function of mastery, mastery consistently reduced the strength of the impact of uncertainty on danger and opportunity but was inconsistent in its strength as a mediator in the relationship between uncertainty and opportunity. Both mastery and the emotion-focused coping strategy of wishful thinking were significant mediators in both tests of the model, although the mediation effect of wishful thinking was very small and not substantively meaningful. (p. 239)

"Although there were selected paths that replicated across testing with different samples, there was sufficient lack of fit between the two models to lead to speculation about moderating variables to explain the divergence. The finding that subjects differed in appraisal due to their location at data collection has some possible clinical implications. If the appraisal of uncertainty is held in abeyance during hospitalization or clinic visits, then it is an ideal time for the nurse to work with the patient to influence the course of uncertainty appraisal." (p. 240) (Mishel et al., 1991, pp. 236–240) ■

Exploratory Regression Analysis

A wide variety of regression analysis procedures are available. Selection of a particular procedure is based on the purpose of the study, the type of data available, and the experience of the researcher in performing regression procedures. Regression analyses can be broadly categorized into exploratory and confirmatory procedures. *Exploratory regression analysis* is the most commonly used strategy in nursing studies. In an exploratory mode, the researcher may not have sufficient information to determine which independent variables are effective predictors of the dependent variable. There may be no theoretical justification for the selection of variables or for considering one variable a more important predictor than another. In this case, many variables may be entered into the analysis simultaneously. During the analysis, the program enters variables into the equation or removes them,

or both, according to the amount of variance that the variable explains relative to other variables in the equation. An example of an exploratory procedure is stepwise regression.

STEPWISE REGRESSION

In *stepwise regression,* the independent variables are entered into or removed from the analysis one at a time. Although the researcher can control the sequence of movement of variables, most commonly, the computer program performs this task and bases the sequence on the amount of additional variance of the dependent variable explained by that particular independent variable. In *forward stepwise regression,* independent variables are entered into the analysis one at a time, and an analysis is made of the effect of including that variable on R^2. Thus, the computer printout indicates the increase in R^2 after addition of the new variable and the statistical significance (F value) of the change. In *backward stepwise regression,* all the independent variables are initially included in the analysis. One variable at a time is then removed from the equation and the effect of that removal on R^2 is evaluated.

During the process of stepwise regression analysis, the amount of variance of Y explained by X_1 is removed from the analysis before the variance explained by X_2 is analyzed. This procedure, referred to as *partialing out* the variance, continues throughout the analysis. Each additional variable included in the analysis will tend to explain a smaller additional amount of the variance in Y. As more variables are included, the increase in R^2 is less and the degrees of freedom decrease, and therefore it is more difficult to obtain a significant F statistic for the increase in R^2.

Kammer (1994) used stepwise regression in her study of stress and coping of family members responsible for nursing home placement of an older adult. She described her data analysis as follows:

. . . .

"Multiple regression analysis, using a backward elimination procedure (Pedhazur, 1982), was done to examine the relationship between 16 person-environment characteristics as independent variables and stress appraisal as the dependent variable. A second regression analysis using the same procedure with person-environment characteristics and stress appraisal as independent variables and coping as the dependent factor also was conducted. Stress appraisal, coping, and eight of the person-environment characteristics were entered as interval data. The remaining person-environment characteristics were coded as: (a) gender—male = 1, female = 2; (b) religions—Jewish = 1, other = 2; (c) employment—yes = 1, no = 2; (d) resident good health, considering age—yes = 1, no = 2; (e) resident physical impairment—yes = 1, no = 2; (f) resident mental impairment—yes = 1, no = 2; and (g) mutual admission decision—yes = 1, no = 2. The backward elimination procedure was chosen to determine the maximum R^2 that could be achieved when all variables were entered. The adjusted R^2 value is reported because of the exploratory nature of this study and the number of predictor variables. The maximum number of predictor variables remaining in any regression was seven; guidelines ($n \geq 10 \; v$) given by Marascuilo and Levin (1983). A probability level of .10 was set as the significance level for retaining a variable in the equations in order to see trends." (Kammer, 1994, p. 92) ■

The results of the first regression are presented below. The results of the second regression can be found in Kammer's paper.

● ●

"Person-environment characteristics significantly contributed to variance in stress appraisals as shown in [Table 21–2]. Higher *harm* appraisals were associated with more frequent visiting, higher satisfaction with nursing home resident relationship prior to admission, lack of mutual admission decision, lower present satisfaction with nursing home resident relationship, younger respondent age, and fewer number of respondent children at home. These six variables accounted for 23% of the variance in harm appraisals. Higher *benefit* appraisals were associated with younger respondent age, well older adult health status, less frequent visiting, and no respondent employment (16% variance). Higher *threat* appraisals were associated with more frequent visiting, respondents being employed, fewer children at home, and nursing home resident men-

tal impairment (20% variance). Higher *challenge* appraisals were associated with not being employed, higher present satisfaction with nursing home resident relationship, well resident health status, no resident physical impairments and younger respondent age (24% variance).

"Comparing the effect of person-environment variables across all stress appraisal categories showed *visit frequency* was the only variable significantly related to all appraisal. *Younger age* was associated with higher harm, benefit and challenge appraisals. *Fewer children at home* was associated with both harm and threat appraisals. Well nursing home resident *health* was associated with higher challenge and benefit appraisals. Being *employed* was associated with higher threat, while not being employed was associated with higher benefit and challenge appraisals." (Kammer, 1994, pp. 93–94) ■

The discussion related to these findings can be found in Kammer's paper.

Several problems should be considered when using stepwise regression. First, the strategy is somewhat akin to fishing in the data to find whatever significance is there. This approach is similar to conducting t tests between each two variables in a data set that includes many variables. With both strategies, researchers run a great risk of detecting significant differences in the data that are the result of random error, which greatly increases the risk of a Type I error. The shrinkage of R^2 when cross-validation is conducted is likely to be great; thus the value of R^2 in stepwise regression is likely to be inflated. Also, stepwise regression is very sample specific. If the data are collinear, small changes in data values will cause changes in the independent variables selected by the analysis. A good description of some of the difficulties with stepwise regression can be found in Aaronson (1989).

Second, in forward stepwise regression, the first variable to be included in the equation is the one that explains the greatest amount of variance in the dependent variable. This first step limits the possibility of inclusion of other variables that initially explain a lesser portion of the variance but, if joined with a different combination of variables, would explain a greater portion of the variance.

TABLE 21–2
FINAL STEP REGRESSION FOR PERSON-ENVIRONMENT CHARACTERISTICS WITH STRESS APPRAISALS AS DEPENDENT VARIABLES (N = 89)

VARIABLE	BETA	SE BETA	r	PARTIAL r	t VALUE
Harm Appraisal					
Visits	.23	.10	.27	.25	2.32*
Mutual decision†	.17	.09	.22	.19	1.79‡
Prior relationship	.27	.11	.10	.26	2.45*
Now relationship	−.31	.10	−.25	−.32	−3.02§
Age	−.33	.11	−.17	−.30	−2.88§
Child at home	−.20	.11	−.08	−.20	−1.89*
	Multiple R = .53	Adj. R^2 = .23	$F(6, 82) = 5.25^{\|\|}$		
Benefit Appraisal					
Visits	−.33	.10	−.34	−.34	−3.32‖
Employed†	.21	.11	.12	.21	1.92‡
Resident health well†	−.17	.10	−.20	−.18	−1.70‡
Age	−.19	.11	−.11	−.19	−1.73‡
	Multiple R = .44	Adj. R^2 = .16	$F(4, 84) = 5.08^{\|\|}$		
Threat Appraisal					
Visits	.28	.10	.28	.30	2.89§
Mental impairment†	−.17	.10	−.16	−.19	−1.74‡
Employed†	−.28	.10	−.17	−.30	−2.84§
Child at home	−.30	.10	−.28	−.32	−3.07§
	Multiple R = .49	Adj. R^2 = .20	$F(4, 84) = 6.53^{\|\|}$		
Challenge Appraisal					
Visits	−.20	.10	−.15	−.22	−2.03*
Employed†	.34	.11	.19	.33	3.19§
Resident health well†	−.41	.11	−.34	−.39	−3.82‖
Now relationship	.18	.10	.13	.20	1.87‡
Age	−.32	.11	−.13	−.31	−2.97§
Physical impairment†	−.22	.11	.04	−.21	−1.90‡
	Multiple R = .54	Adj. R^2 = .24	$F(6, 82) = 5.59^{\|\|}$		

*$p < .05$.
†Dummy coding: yes = 1, no = 2.
‡$p < .10$.
§$p < .01$.
‖$p < .001$.
From Kammer, C. H. (1994). Stress and coping of family members responsible for nursing home placement. *Research in Nursing & Health, 17*(2), 94.

Third, the variables selected in the procedure may be effective in *predicting* values of the dependent variable but not very effective in *explaining* the variance in the dependent variable. From a theoretical point of view, this lack of explanation is not satisfactory. Knowing why part of the variance of the dependent variable is explained by a particular independent variable is important because your ability to explain changes in values of the dependent variable is a prerequisite to controlling those values.

Confirmatory Regression Analysis

Regression analysis procedures designed to achieve confirmatory purposes assume a theoretically proposed set of variables. The purpose of *confirmatory regression analysis* is to test the validity of a theoretically proposed statement expressed as a regression equation. This equation is the hypothesis of the study. A number of regression procedures are used for this purpose. Procedures presented below include simultaneous regression, hierarchical regression, and logistic regression.

SIMULTANEOUS REGRESSION

In simultaneous regression, all independent variables are entered at the same time into a single analysis. A theoretical justification for the independent variables selected is presented by the author and expressed as a hypothesis before describing the analysis. Several simultaneous equations may be used as hypotheses for a study.

HIERARCHICAL REGRESSION

Sometimes, fully testing the theoretically proposed ideas requires a series of linked regression equations, which is referred to as hierarchical regression. Suppose the researcher had a set of four independent variables (age, education, attitudes about cancer, and social support) thought to explain variation in the dependent variable (coping). Nursing actions can have little effect on age and education, but perhaps the literature review indicates that these two variables are important predictors of coping. The researcher is interested in knowing whether, given the effects of age and education, attitudes and support also influence coping. One strategy for examining this question is to determine first the amount of variance explained by age and education by using regression analysis and then determine whether adding attitudes and support will increase the amount of variance in coping that can be explained. The series of equations would be expressed as follows:

$$Y = X_1$$

$$Y = X_1 + X_2$$

$$Y = X_1 + X_2 + X_3$$

$$Y = X_1 + X_2 + X_3 + X_4$$

The second equation controls for the variance explained by X_1 before testing the effect of X_2. If the addition of X_2 to the equation explains an increased amount of variance, it will be reflected by an increase in R^2. Additional variables are added, either one at a time or as a set, to test for their effect on R^2.

This technique can be extended to test the effect of the same set of independent variables on several dependent variables of interest in a particular area of study. An analysis might include three linked dependent variables designated Y_1, Y_2, and Y_3. The set of independent variables would be designated X_1, X_2, X_3, X_4. The independent variables may be entered into analysis one at a time, or some may be entered as a set. The entire set of hierarchical equations might have the following appearance:

$$Y_1 = X_1$$

$$Y_1 = X_1 + X_2$$

$$Y_1 = X_1 + X_2 + X_3$$

$$Y_1 = X_1 + X_2 + X_3 + X_4$$

$$Y_2 = X_1$$

$$Y_2 = X_1 + X_2$$

$$Y_2 = X_1 + X_2 + X_3$$

$$Y_2 = X_1 + X_2 + X_3 + X_4$$

$$Y_3 = X_1$$

$$Y_3 = X_1 + X_2$$

$$Y_3 = X_1 + X_2 + X_3$$

$$Y_3 = X_1 + X_2 + X_3 + X_4$$

Wu (1995) suggests the use of hierarchical regression to conduct multilevel data analysis. In *multilevel analysis,* the researcher is examining two or more units simultaneously. For example, the study might include a number of nursing homes, as well as the nurses employed within the nursing homes. Each nursing home would be one unit of measure and each nurse another unit of measure. By using hierarchical regression, the researcher can examine the random variation at both the individual and organizational level.

Johnson (1995) provided an excellent presentation of hierarchical regression in her study of healing determinants in older people with leg ulcers. This study was also used as an example of a predictive correlational design in Chapter 11. A summary of the descriptive statistics of all independent and dependent variables in Johnson's study is presented in Table 21–3. She describes her use of hierarchical analysis as follows:

· ·

"Each predictor variable was assessed to determine the best parameterization possible; nonmetric data (diuretic usage, clot history, and liposclerosis) were converted to dummy codings (absence, mild

TABLE 21–3
SUMMARY DESCRIPTIVE STATISTICS OF HEALING DETERMINANTS

CATEGORY OF VARIABLE	N	M (MODE)	SD
Independent Variables			
Physiological			
Edema	155	1.2 (1)	.94
Hyperpigmentation	155	1.1 (0)	1.30
Liposclerosis	155	.61 (0)	.89
Wound status	155	2.5 (2)	.65
Initial ulcer area	156	637	868
Clot history	153	0.2 (0)	.42
Pain on mobility	152	1.4 (1)	.78
Therapeutic			
Diuretics	150	0.5 (1)	.50
Ankle compression	152	29.2	19.0
Limb positioning			
Elevated	145	.87	2.7
Horizontal	145	13.01	4.44
Dependent	145	6.2	4.2
Dressing	145	32.07	8.77
Psychosocial			
Social support	134	22.25	10.09
Self-efficacy	145	5.7	3.08
Dependent Variable			
Healing rate	140	−.12	.94

From Johnson, M. (1995). Healing determinants in older people with leg ulcers. *Research in Nursing & Health, 18*(5), 399.

= 0; moderate, severe = 1) (Hair et al., 1992). Violations to statistical assumptions of multiple regression were examined using normal probability plots of the residuals (the difference between the observed and the predicted values for the dependent variable) versus the predictor variables for all models (Hair et al., 1992). The dependent variable, healing rate, was normally distributed. No evidence of curvilinear relationships were demonstrated in partial plots of the dependent and independent variables. Examination of standardized residuals identified one outlier, which was removed. Multicollinearity was also assessed with correlations between independent variables ranging from $r = .006$ to $r = .57$. Similarly, variance inflation factors (1.0–1.02), and tolerances (.97–.99) were within acceptable limits (Hair et al., 1992). In the initial analysis, the level of significance for entry into the model was ≤.10; this value was raised to .05 in the final reduced models.

"Hierarchical multiple regression procedures were applied to examine how much variance in healing rate was explained for each set of variables—physiologic, therapeutic, and psychosocial—and allowed for comparison with other studies that examined physiologic factors in venous subjects only. It was also important to identify variables significant (.05) in the venous-only sample and apply these to other disease groups not studied thus far. Data losses in individual variables have resulted in subject losses in these groups throughout the regression procedures. . . .

"Physiologic factors were the first set of variables entered into the venous disease model at step 1. . . . Hyperpigmentation was positively correlated with liposclerosis ($r = .51$) and was not included. Pain on mobility and moderate and severe liposclerosis were related to poorer healing, while improved wound status scores were associated with increased healing rates; these variables explained 41% of the variance in the healing rate, adj. $R^2 = .36$, $F = 7.04$, $p \geq .001$. A history of leg clots, initial ulcer areas, and edema were not significant. Therapeutic variables were included in the second step and did not significantly contribute to healing, although increased limb hours in horizontal positions were related to poorer healing rates (adj. $R^2 =$

.39). Hours with limbs elevated was negatively correlated with horizontal position hours ($r = -.57$), and was not included in the model. . . . Psychosocial factors were entered on the third step, and did not significantly contribute to the model (adj. $R^2 = .37$). Social support and self-efficacy beliefs were not significant.

"All variables involved in this model explained 49% of the variance in the healing rate, $F = 4.31$, $p < .0001$. In order to produce a simpler model, significant variables, $p \leq .05-.10$, were combined in one step and resulted in only four variables remaining significant at the .05 level: increased pain on mobility, $\beta = .46$, $p < .0001$, higher wound status scores, $\beta = -.33$, $p = .0007$, moderate or severe liposclerosis, $p = .003$, and increased hours in a horizontal position, $\beta = .24$, $p = .02$. These four variables explained 40% of the variance in the healing rate, $F = 11.74$, $p < .001$." (Johnson, 1995, pp. 398–399) ■

LOGISTIC REGRESSION

Logistic regression (sometimes called logit analysis) is used in studies in which the dependent variable is categorical. Although most regression analysis procedures are based on a least-squares approach to estimating parameters, logistic regression uses maximal likelihood estimation. The procedure estimates the likelihood of the fit of a theoretical model proposing the probability of various outcomes. It calculates the odds of one outcome occurring rather than other possible outcomes (Yarandi & Simpson, 1991). Because of the current clinical interest in predicting outcomes of nursing practice, this procedure is expected to become increasingly important to nursing research. A less theoretical alternative to logistic regression is discriminant analysis (described later), which is used to predict group membership.

Albers and colleagues (1995) used logistic regression in their study of maternal age and labor complications in healthy primigravidas at term. They describe their analysis as follows:

. . . .

"Multivariate analysis using logistic regression was used to assess predictors of labor complications for the study sample. This technique tests the effect of each variable in the model on the risk of labor complications, with simultaneous control of all other variables. A forward selection strategy was used to sequentially add one control variable at a time to a model containing only maternal age. Variables were added to the model based on statistical significance ($p < .05$) until no further variables were contributory.

"[Table 21–4] shows the results of logistic regression for predictors of cesarean section with simultaneous control of the other potential confounding factors. The odds ratios for the age/cesarean relationship are inflated compared with the risk ratios in stratified analysis. In most cases the odds ratio for maternal age in the final model are decreased slightly from the results of stratified analysis. This suggests minimal confounding in the simultaneous adjustment for epidural anesthesia and receipt of adequate prenatal care. Highly significant

---

TABLE 21–4
LOGISTIC REGRESSION ANALYSIS OF RISK FOR PRIMARY CESAREAN SECTION—ODDS RATIO (95% CONFIDENCE INTERVAL)

MODEL	AGE 20–29	AGE 30+	EPIDURAL	ADEQUATE PNC
C/S = age	1.4 (1.1–2.0)	3.0 (2.1–4.4)	—	—
C/S = age + epidural	1.3 (0.9–1.8)	2.5 (1.7–3.7)	3.5 (2.6–4.5)	—
C/S = age + epidural + adequate PNC	1.2 (0.9–1.7)	2.3 (1.4–3.4)	3.4 (2.6–4.5)	1.3 (1.0–1.8)

Reference group = age younger than 20 years.
C/S = cesarean section; PNC = prenatal care.
Reprinted by permission of Elsevier Science, Inc., from Albers, L. L., Lydon-Rochelle, M. T., & Krulewitch, C. J. (1995). Maternal age and labor complications in healthy primigravidas at term. *Journal of Nurse-Midwifery, 40*(1), 10.

predictors of cesarean delivery in this sample of healthy primigravidas were maternal age ≥ 30 and epidural anesthesia." (Albers et al., 1995, pp. 7–8) ■

DISCRIMINANT ANALYSIS

Discriminant analysis is designed to allow the researcher to identify characteristics associated with group membership and to predict group membership. The dependent variable is membership in a particular group. The independent variables (discriminating variables) measure characteristics on which the groups are expected to differ. Discriminant analysis is closely related to both factor analysis and regression analysis. However, in discriminant analysis, the dependent variable values are categorical in form. Each value of the dependent variable is considered a group. When the dependent variable is dichotomous, multiple regression is performed. However, when more than two groups are involved, analysis becomes much more complex. The dependent variable in discriminant analysis is referred to as the *discriminant function*. It is equivalent in many ways to a factor (Edens, 1987).

Two similar data sets are required for complete analysis. The first data set must contain measures on all the variables to be included in the analysis and the group membership of each subject. The purpose of analysis of the first data set is to identify variables that most effectively discriminate between groups. Selection of variables for the analysis is based on the researcher's expectation that they will be effective in this regard. The variables selected for the discriminant function are then tested on a second set of data to determine their effectiveness in predicting group membership (Edens, 1987).

The following are the assumptions of discriminant analysis:

1. The research problem must define at least two cases per group. The total sample size should be at least two or (preferably) three times the number of discriminating variables used.
2. The number of discriminating variables to be included in the analysis cannot exceed the total number of cases minus two ($n - 2$), nor should they be fewer than the number of groups being compared.

3. Variables can be treated as interval-level measures.
4. No discriminating variable can be a linear combination of other discriminating variables.
5. The covariance matrices for the groups must be equal.
6. Each group must be drawn from a population with a multivariate normal distribution on the discriminating variables. (Edens, 1987, p. 257)

The first step in the analysis is to determine whether the discriminating variables can be used to differentiate the groups. If significant group differences exist, further analyses are performed to determine the number of dimensions in which the groups differ and which variables are effective in defining group membership. An effort is made in the analysis to maximize between-group variance while minimizing within-group variance. Variables that are expected to achieve this maximization and minimization of variance are selected for the discriminant function (Edens, 1987).

Discriminant function analysis is then performed. The variables can be entered in a stepwise manner if desired. During the procedure, variables are added or eliminated, or both, and the procedure repeated until the best subset of discriminating variables is obtained. The outcomes of this procedure are linear discriminant functions (LDFs). Several variables may be associated with one LDF, or there may be as many LDFs as there are variables. Similar to the selection of factors in factor analysis, LDFs are arranged according to the amount of between-group variance that they explain. This property is determined by examination of eigenvalues, that is, the canonical correlation associated with each LDF or by examination of tests of significance, or both. The goal is to select LDFs that can achieve maximal group separation. The researcher eliminates LDFs that contribute little to group separation (Edens, 1987).

The results of the analysis must then be interpreted. This process is similar to that of explaining the variables that load on a factor in factor analysis. The researcher needs to determine the relative contribution of variables within the LDFs to effective discrimination among groups. Illustrating the LDFs graphically can provide useful insight. The coefficients associated with each LDF are also examined. The two types of coefficients are standardized coefficients and structured coefficients. Standardized coefficients are similar to the beta weights in regression analysis and allow the researcher to examine the relative contribution of each variable to an LDF. This examination is more difficult if multicollinearity exists. In this case, structured coefficients become important in the interpretation. Structured coefficients are correlations between each variable and each LDF (Edens, 1987).

To predict group membership by using the LDFs developed in this analysis, one must move from the exploratory mode to the confirmatory mode. First, the researcher needs to determine the power of the LDFs to predict group membership. This task is accomplished through cross-validation. Statistical procedures are then used to determine classifications. This step involves examining the distance between each individual case and each group. From this examination, the probability of each case being identified as a member of each group is calculated, and this probability is used to classify each case. Classification can be based on each group having an equal chance of having a case classified, or it may be based on the knowledge that a certain percentage of a population are members of a particular group. In some cases, discrimination is low or groups overlap. The researcher may need to determine whether each case must be assigned to one of the identified groups even when discrimination is low (Edens, 1987).

Woods and colleagues (1995) performed discriminant analysis as a component of their study of premenstrual symptoms, which was described in the section on factor analysis. The purpose of the discriminant analysis was to "differentiate women with an LS [low-symptom], PMS [premenstrual syndrome], or PMM [premenstrual magnification] symptom pattern with respect to their feminine and menstrual socialization, expectations about menstrual symptoms, stressful life context, and resources for responding to stressors" (p. 228). Factor scores from the factor analysis described in the section on factor analysis in this chapter were entered as follows.

• •

"[Factor scores were entered] along with indicators of health perception, health practices, depressed mood, pregnancies, income, education,

and age into three 2-group discriminant function analyses to differentiate women with LS versus PMS, LS versus PMM, and PMS versus PMM patterns. Structure coefficients (discriminant loadings) represent the simple correlation of a variable with the discriminant function and are not affected by multicollinearity. The square of the structure coefficient indicates the proportion of the variance in the function attributable to that variable. Canonical correlations [described below], which indicate the amount of variance accounted for by the function, are provided as a basis for judging the substantive value of the function (Dillon & Goldstein, 1984).

"The function differentiating women with LS and PMS patterns included six variables with a structure coefficient near or exceeding .3 (Dillon & Goldstein, 1984) [Table 21–5]. Expectation of symptoms, depressed mood, stress, confirmed pregnancies, health perception, and education differentiated the two groups. Women with PMS had greater expectation of having perimenstrual symptoms, higher depression scores, more stress in their lives, and more pregnancies, rated themselves as less healthy, and had less formal education than women with the LS pattern. Although the structure coefficient was less than .3, menstrual socialization also contributed significantly to this function, such that women with a PMS pattern had more negative menstrual socialization. This function explained 73% of the variance. Eighty-five percent of the women were correctly classified with similar prediction for the LS and PMS groups (LS = 85%; PMS = 86%).

"Expectation of symptoms, depressed moods, stress, health perception, and menstrual socialization differentiated the women with LS and PMM patterns. Those with PMM demonstrated greater expectation of perimenstrual symptoms, higher depression scores, more negative health ratings, and higher stress levels, and were exposed to more negative socialization about menstruation [Table 21–6] than the women with an LS pattern. This function explained 72% of the variance and correctly classified 85% of the women (PMS = 73%; PMM = 74%).

"Depressed mood, expectation of symptoms, stress, and menstrual socialization differentiated the women with a PMS and a PMM pattern. Women with a PMS pattern had lower scores on the depres-

TABLE 21–5
DISCRIMINANT ANALYSES DIFFERENTIATING WOMEN WITH LS, PMS, AND PMM SYMPTOM PATTERNS

LS VS. PMS (*n* = 109)		LS VS. PMM (*n* = 133)		PMS VS. PMM (*n* = 168)	
Factor/Variable	Structure Coefficient	Factor/Variable	Structure Coefficient	Factor/Variable	Structure Coefficient
Symptom expectation (4)*	.68†	Symptom expectation (4)	.70†	Depression	.76*
Depression	−.36	Depression	−.63†	Symptom expectation (4)	−.62†
Stress (1)	−.33†	Stress (1)	−.36†	Stress (1)	.40†
Confirmed pregnancy	−.32†	Health perception	−.31†	Menstrual socialization (5)	.31†
Health perception	.29	Menstrual socialization	−.27†	Income	−.29†
Education	.28†	Age	.19†	Health perception	−.27
Menstrual socialization (5)	−.24†	Income	.16†	Health practices	−.24
Health practices	.17	Education	.13	Feminine socialization (2)	.18†
Support need (3)	−.09†	Confirmed pregnancy	−.11†	Age	−.18
Income	.07	Health practices	.10	Support need (3)	.11
Feminine socialization (2)	.06†	Support need (3)	−.05†	Education	−.11
Age	−.01	Feminine socialization (2)	.01	Confirmed pregnancy	.00
Canonical correlation	.73	Canonical correlation	.72	Canonical correlation	.53
Centroids		. . .		Centroids	
LS	.74	LS	.96	PMS	−.47
PMS	−1.49	PMM	−1.10	PMM	.81

*Numbers in parentheses refer to factor numbers.
†$p < .05$.
LS = low symptom; PMM = premenstrual magnification; PMS = premenstrual syndrome.
From Woods, N. F., Mitchell, E. S., & Lentz, M. J. (1995). Social pathways to premenstrual symptoms. *Research in Nursing & Health, 18*(3), 233.

sion scale, fewer expectations of symptoms, less stress, less negative menstrual socialization, and higher incomes than women with the PMM pattern. The function explained only 53% of the variance and correctly classified 73% of the women, with a similar classification of the women with a PMS pattern (73% vs. 74%).

"These analyses provide support for inclusion of social as well as behavioral and biologic factors in a model distinguishing women who experience premenstrual symptoms (those with a PMS or PMM pattern) from those who do not (LS pattern). The ability to distinguish women with PMS and PMM patterns using the proposed model is limited. This may be a function of limited power, given the relatively modest sample sizes in these two groups, or it may reflect common social pathways for both symptom patterns." (Woods et al., 1995, pp. 232–234) ■

The results of this discriminant analysis have also been reported by Mitchell and associates (1994).

Discriminant analysis is also a useful strategy in clinical physiological studies, where understanding the variables important in explaining patient outcomes has become increasingly more critical. Hanneman (1994) used discriminant analysis in a study of multidimensional predictors of success or failure of early weaning from mechanical ventilation after cardiac surgery:

• •

"Empirically, postoperative cardiac surgery patients either fail early weaning attempts or have such attempts delayed for one or more of the following reasons: (a) hemodynamic instability, (b) poor gas exchange, and (c) poor pulmonary mechanics. The inadequate performance of weaning predictors may be explained by the inability of the dimensions to predict weaning outcome independently. Thus, the purpose of this study was to determine the interdependent contributions of hemodynamics, gas exchange, and pulmonary mechanics to the prediction of weaning outcome in cardiac surgery patients. Furthermore, given the desirability

TABLE 21–6
CARDIOPULMONARY STUDY VARIABLES ON MECHANICAL VENTILATION AND DURING A SPONTANEOUS VENTILATION TRIAL

On Mechanical Ventilation (MV)

Frequency of breaths (MVF)	Level of consciousness (LOC)
Tidal volume (MVVt)	Mixed venous oxygen saturation (Svo$_2$)
Peak inspiratory pressure (MVPIP)	Cardiac index (CI)
Dynamic compliance (CMPDYN)	Capillary wedge pressure (PCW)
Airway resistance (RAW)	Mean pulmonary artery pressure (PAM)
Static compliance (CMPST)	Central venous pressure (CVP)
Positive end-expiratory pressure (PEEP)	Heart rate (MVHR)
Fraction of inspired oxygen (FIO$_2$)	Systolic arterial blood pressure (MVSBP)
Pressure support (PS)	Diastolic arterial blood pressure (MVDBP)
pH of the arterial blood (MVpH)	Mean arterial blood pressure (MVMAP)
Arterial carbon dioxide tension (MVPaCO$_2$)	Oximeter oxygen saturation (MVPOX)
Arterial oxygen tension (MVPaO$_2$)	Cardiac rhythm (CR)
Arterial oxygen saturation (MVSaO$_2$)	Ratio of frequency to tidal volume (f/Vt)
Ratio of arterial oxygen tension to fraction of inspired oxygen (PaO$_2$/FIO$_2$)	

During Spontaneous Ventilation Trial (SVT)

Vital capacity (VC)	Diastolic arterial pressure (SVTDBP)
Negative inspiratory force (NIF)	Carbon dioxide tension (SVTPaCO$_2$)
Frequency of breaths (SVTF)	Arterial oxygen tension (SVTPaO$_2$)
Tidal volume (SVTVt)	Arterial oxygen saturation (SVTSaO$_2$)
Spontaneous minute volume (VES)	Cough effort (CE)
Total minute volume (VET)	Extubation date and time (EXT-TIME)
Fraction of inspired oxygen (SVTFIO$_2$)	Mechanical ventilation time (MVTIME)
Heart rate (SVTHR)	Number of SVT trials (TRIAL)
Pulse oximeter oxygen saturation (SVTPOX)	Reason for SVT trial failure (FAIL)
Systolic arterial blood pressure (SVTSBP)	Arterial pH (SVTpH)
Mean arterial blood pressure (SVTMAP)	Ratio of frequency to tidal volume (f/Vt)
Ratio of arterial oxygen tension to fraction of inspired oxygen (PaO$_2$/FIO$_2$)	

From Hanneman, S. K. G. (1994). Multidimensional predictors of success or failure with early weaning from mechanical ventilation after cardiac surgery. *Nursing Research, 43*(1), 6.

of predictors that can be used widely, a secondary purpose was to test common variables that are readily available to clinicians in all settings.

"One hundred sixty-five adult patients admitted to the cardiovascular critical care unit of a 950-bed tertiary private nonprofit teaching hospital in Houston were selected for study. . . . Three cases were discarded because the patients expired before a spontaneous ventilation trial. . . . One hundred thirty-four (83%) patients were weaned and extubated within 24 hours of unit admission and constituted the success group. Twenty-eight (17%) patients were not weaned from mechanical ventilation within 24 hours of unit admission; they constituted the failure group. Chi-square demonstrated no significant differences between success and failure groups in gender, admitting diagnosis, type of surgery, cardiac rhythm, and weaning technique." (Hanneman, 1994, p. 5) ■

Variables used in the study are shown in Table 21–7. Variables were measured at two points postoperatively: 2 hours after admission to the unit while the patient was on mechanical ventilation (MV) and during a spontaneous ventilation trial (SVT).

• •

"Given the consequences of erroneous prediction, the alpha was set at .01. Standard formulas (Griner, Mayewski, Mushlin, & Greenland, 1981; Yang & Tobin, 1991) were used to calculate the sensitivity [true positives/(true positives + false negatives)], specificity [true negatives/(true negatives + false positives)], positive predictive value [true positives/(true positives + false positives)], and negative predictive value [true negatives/(true negatives + false negatives)]. Diagnostic accuracy (Krieger et al., 1989) was calculated by the following formula: (true positives + true negatives)/(true positives + true negatives + false positives + false negatives).

"A greater percentage of the failure group (82%) had a depressed level of consciousness postoperatively than the success group (42%; $\chi^2 = 15.3$, $df = 2$, $p = .0005$). Strength of cough was different between groups ($\chi^2 = 17$, $df = 2$, $p = .0002$), with the failure group demonstrating a weaker voluntary cough effort. The number of weaning attempts in the early postoperative period was greater in failure patients ($M = 4.4$) than in successful patients ($M = 1.4$; $t = -10.11$, $df = 159$, $p < .001$). Reasons for failing SVT attempts also were different between success and failure groups ($\chi^2 = 34$, $df = 8$, $p = .00005$). Hemodynamic instability was prevalent in the failure group and prevented weaning within 24 hours, whereas depressed level of consciousness, carbon dioxide retention, and bleeding were dominant reasons in the success group but did not prevent weaning within 24 hours. Only 21 (13%) of the patients had left-atrial or pulmonary artery catheters. Therefore, the variables of venous oxygen saturation, cardiac index, pulmonary capillary wedge pressure, and pulmonary artery mean pressure were eliminated from the analysis. . . .

"The ratios during mechanical ventilation and spontaneous ventilation trials were included in the discriminant analysis. Half of the data cases ($n = 82$) were randomly selected for the analysis phase to examine the multivariate differences between success and failure groups, and half of the cases ($n = 80$) were left to test the predictive accuracy of the discriminant function variables. The proportion of variation in the discriminant function explained by the groups was 53% (canonical correlation = 0.733).

"Examination of the magnitude of the standardized coefficients showed that the greatest contributions were made by arterial pH during SVT, vital capacity standardized by weight (VCKG), and arterial pH during MV. Using a correlation coefficient of $> .30$ to denote strength of relationship, the structure coefficients having the most in common with the discriminant function were: pH during SVT and mean arterial pressure and pH during mechanical ventilation. VCKG and Pao_2/Fio_2 had less in common with the discriminant function. The classification results, adjusted for prior probabilities, are shown in [Table 21–7]. Sensitivity was .98, specificity .71, positive predictive value .94, and negative predictive value .87, yielding a diagnostic accuracy of .93 for the predictor set of variables. Eleven (7%) of the 162 cases were misclassified using the discriminant score to predict group membership." (Hanneman, 1994, pp. 6–7) ■

■ SUMMARY

The ability to predict future events is becoming increasingly important in our society. In nursing practice, as in the rest of society, the capacity to predict is crucial. For example, we need to predict the length of stay of patients with varying severity of illness, as well as the response of patients with a variety of characteristics to nursing interventions.

Predictive analyses are based on probability theory rather than decision theory. Prediction is one approach to examining causal relationships between or among variables. The independent (predictor) variable or variables cause variation in the value of

TABLE 21–7
ADJUSTED CLASSIFICATION RESULTS FOR ANALYSIS AND VALIDATION SAMPLES

SAMPLE	ACTUAL GROUP	NUMBER OF CASES	PREDICTED GROUP 1	PREDICTED GROUP 2
*Analysis Sample**
Success	1	67	66 (99%)	1 (1%)
Failure	2	15	3 (20%)	12 (80%)
Validation Sample†				
Success	1	67	65 (97%)	2 (3%)
Failure	2	13	5 (38%)	8 (62%)

*Ninety-five percent correctly classified ($n = 82$).
†Ninety-two percent correctly classified ($n = 80$).
From Hanneman, S. K. G. (1994). Multidimensional predictors of success or failure with early weaning from mechanical ventilation after cardiac surgery. *Nursing Research, 43*(1), 8.

the dependent (outcome) variable. The purpose of a regression analysis is to predict or explain as much of the variance in the value of the dependent variable as possible. In some cases, the analysis is exploratory and the focus is prediction. In others, selection of variables is based on a theoretical position, and the purpose is explanation, to confirm the theoretical position.

Simple linear regression provides a means to estimate the value of a dependent variable based on the value of an independent variable. Predictions are made by using two variables. The score on variable y (dependent variable) is predicted from the same subject's known score on variable x (independent variable). The outcome of analysis is the regression coefficient R. When R is squared, it indicates the amount of variance in the data that is explained by the equation. After a regression equation has been developed, the equation is tested against a new sample to determine its accuracy in prediction, a process called cross-validation.

Multiple regression analysis is an extension of simple linear regression in which more than one independent variable is entered into the analysis. Multicollinearity can be a problem in multiple regression analysis. Multicollinearity occurs when the independent variables in a multiple regression equation are strongly correlated. In nursing studies, some multicollinearity is inevitable; however, it can be minimized by careful selection of independent variables. Multicollinearity does not affect predictive power (the capacity of the independent variables to predict values of the dependent variable in that specific sample), but rather causes problems related to generalizability. If multicollinearity is present, the equation will not have predictive validity.

The variables in a regression equation can take many forms. Traditionally, as with most multivariate analyses, variables are measured at the interval level. However, categorical or dichotomous measures (referred to as dummy variables), multiplicative terms, and transformed terms are also used. A mixture of types of variables may be used in a single regression equation.

The outcome of regression analysis is referred to as a prediction equation. The final outcome of a regression analysis is a model from which values of the independent variables can be used to predict and perhaps explain values of the dependent variable in the population. If so, the analysis can be repeated in other samples with similar results, and the equation is expected to have predictive validity. To determine the accuracy of the prediction, the predicted values are compared with actual values obtained from a new sample of subjects or values from a sample obtained at the time of the original data collection but held out from the initial analysis. This analysis is conducted on the difference scores between predicted values and the means of actual values. An R^2 value is obtained on the new sample and compared with that of the original sample. In most cases, R^2 will be lower in the new sample because the original equation was developed to predict most precisely scores in the original sample, a phenomenon referred to as the shrinkage of R^2. Shrinkage of R^2 is greater in small samples and when multicollinearity is great.

A wide variety of regression analysis procedures are available. Selection of a particular procedure is based on the purpose of the study, the type of data available, and the experience of the researcher in performing regression procedures. Regression analyses can be broadly categorized into exploratory and confirmatory procedures. In the exploratory mode, the researcher may not have sufficient information to determine which independent variables are effective predictors of the dependent variable. There may be no theoretical justification for the selection of variables or for considering one variable a more important predictor than another. An example of an exploratory procedure is stepwise regression.

Regression analysis procedures designed to achieve confirmatory purposes assume a theoretically proposed set of variables. The purpose of confirmatory regression analysis is to test the validity of a theoretically proposed statement expressed as a regression equation. This equation is the hypothesis of the study. A number of regression procedures are used for this purpose, including simultaneous regression, hierarchical regression, and logistic regression.

Discriminant analysis is designed to allow the researcher to identify characteristics associated with group membership and to predict group membership. The dependent variable is membership in a particular group. The independent variables (discriminating variables) measure characteristics on which the groups are expected to differ. The dependent variable values are categorical in form. Each value of the dependent variable is considered a group.

• •

REFERENCES

Aaronson, L. S. (1989). A cautionary note on the use of stepwise regression. *Nursing Research, 38*(5), 309–311.

Albers, L. L., Lydon-Rochelle, M. T., & Krulewitch, C. J. (1995). Maternal age and labor complications in healthy primigravidas at term. *Journal of Nurse-Midwifery, 40*(1), 4–12.

Baron, R. M., & Kenny, D. A. (1986). The moderator-mediator variable distinction in social psychological research: Conceptual, strategic and statistical considerations. *Journal of Personality & Social Psychology, 51*(6), 1173–1182.

Braden, C. J. (1990). A test of the self-help model: Learned response to chronic illness experience. *Nursing Research, 39*(1), 42–47.

Burns, N., & Carney, N. (1986). Patterns of hospice care—the RN role. *The Hospice Journal, 2*(1), 37–62.

Cohen, J., & Cohen, P. (1983). *Applied multiple regression/ correlation analysis for the behavioral sciences.* Hillsdale, NJ: Lawrence Erlbaum.

Dillon, W., & Goldstein, M. (1984). *Multivariate analysis: Methods and applications.* New York: Wiley.

Edens, G. E. (1987). Discriminant analysis. *Nursing Research, 36*(4), 257–262.

Griner, P. F., Mayewski, R. J., Mushlin, A., & Greenland, P. (1981). Selection and interpretation of diagnostic tests and procedures: Principles and applications. *Annals of Internal Medicine, 94,* 553–600.

Hair, J. F., Anderson, R. E., Tatham, R. L., & Black, W. C. (1992). *Multivariate data analysis with readings.* New York: Macmillan.

Hanneman, S. K. G. (1994). Multidimensional predictors of success or failure with early weaning from mechanical ventilation after cardiac surgery. *Nursing Research, 43*(1), 4–10.

Johnson, M. (1995). Healing determinants in older people with leg ulcers. *Research in Nursing & Health, 18*(5), 395–403.

Kammer, C. H. (1994). Stress and coping of family members responsible for nursing home placement. *Research in Nursing & Health, 17*(2), 89–98.

Knapp, T. R. (1994). Regression analyses: What to report. *Nursing Research, 43*(3), 187–189.

Krieger, B. P., Ershowsky, P. F., Becker, D. A., & Gazeroglu, H. B. (1989). Evaluation of conventional criteria for predicting successful weaning from mechanical ventilatory support in elderly patients. *Critical Care Medicine, 17*(9), 858–861.

Marascuilo, L. A., & Levin, J. R. (1983). *Multivariate statistics in the social sciences.* Monterey, CA: Brooks/Cole.

Mischel, M. H., Padilla, G., Grant, M., & Sorenson, D. S. (1991). Uncertainty in illness theory: A replication of the mediating effects of mastery and coping. *Nursing Research, 40*(4), 236–240.

Mischel, M. H., & Sorenson, D. S. (1991). Coping with uncertainty in gynecological cancer: A test of the mediating functions of mastery and coping. *Nursing Research, 40*(3), 167–170.

Mitchell, E. S., Woods, N. F., & Lentz, M. J. (1994). Differentiation of women with three perimenstrual symptom patterns. *Nursing Research, 43*(1), 25–30.

Pedhazur, E. J. (1982). *Multiple regression in behavioral research: Explanation and prediction* (2nd ed.). New York: Holt, Rinehart & Winston.

Prescott, P. A. (1987). Multiple regression analysis with small samples: Cautions and suggestions. *Nursing Research, 36*(2), 130–133.

Schroeder, M. A. (1990). Diagnosing and dealing with multicollinearity. *Western Journal of Nursing Research, 12*(2), 175–187.

Verran, J. A., & Ferketich, S. L. (1987). Testing linear model assumptions: Residual analysis. *Nursing Research, 36*(2), 127–130.

Verran, J. A., & Reid, P. J. (1987). Replicated testing of the nursing technology model. *Nursing Research, 36*(3), 190–194.

Woods, N. F., Mitchell, E. S., & Lentz, M. J. (1995). Social pathways to premenstrual symptoms. *Research in Nursing & Health, 18*(3), 225–237.

Wu, Y. B. (1995). Hierarchical linear models: A multilevel data analysis technique. *Nursing Research, 44*(2), 123–126.

Yang, K. L., & Tobin, M. J. (1991). A prospective study of indexes predicting the outcome of trials of weaning from mechanical ventilation. *New England Journal of Medicine, 324*(21), 1445–1450.

Yarandi, H. N., & Simpson, S. H. (1991). The logistic regression model and the odds of testing HIV positive. *Nursing Research, 40*(6), 372–373.

CHAPTER 22

USING STATISTICS TO EXAMINE CAUSALITY

Causality is a way of knowing that one thing causes another. Statistical procedures that examine causality are critical to the development of nursing science because of their importance in examining the effects of interventions. The statistical procedures in this chapter examine causality by testing for significant differences between or among groups. Statistical procedures are available for nominal, ordinal, and interval data. The procedures vary considerably in their power to detect differences and in their complexity. The procedures presented are categorized as contingency tables, nonparametric procedures, t tests, and analysis of variance (ANOVA) procedures.

CONTINGENCY TABLES

Contingency tables, or cross-tabulation, allow visual comparison of summary data output related to two variables within the sample. Contingency tables are a useful preliminary strategy for examining large amounts of data. In most cases, the data are in the form of frequencies or percentages. With this strategy one can compare two or more categories of one variable with two or more categories of a second variable. The simplest version is referred to as a 2 × 2 table (two categories of two variables). Table 22–1 shows an example of a 2 × 2 contingency table from Knafl's (1985) study of how families manage a pediatric hospitalization.

The data are generally referenced in rows and columns. The intersection between the row and column in which a specific numerical value is inserted is referred to as a *cell.* The upper left cell would be row 1, column 1. In the example in Table 22–1, the cell of row 1, column 1 has the value of 18, the cell of row 1, column 2 has the value of 7, and so on. The output from each row and each column is summed, and the sum is placed at the end of the row or column. In the example, the sum of row 1 is 25, the sum of row 2 is 37, the sum of column 1 is 34, and the sum of column 2 is 28. The percentage of the sample represented by that sum can also be placed at the end of the row or column. The row sums and the column sums total to the same value, which is 62 in the example.

Although contingency tables are most commonly used to examine nominal or ordinal data, they can be used with grouped frequencies of interval data. However, one must recognize that information about the data will be lost when contingency tables are used to examine interval data. Loss of data usually causes loss of statistical power; that is, the probability of failing to reject a false null hypothesis is greater than if an appropriate parametric procedure could be used. Therefore, it is not generally the technique of choice. A contingency table is sometimes useful when an interval-level measure is being compared with a nominal- or ordinal-level measure.

In some cases, the contingency table is presented and no further analysis is conducted. The table is presented as a form of summary statistics. However, in many cases, statistical analysis of the relation-

TABLE 22–1
RELATIONSHIP BETWEEN PARENTS'
REPORTS OF IMPACT ON FAMILY LIFE AND
OUTSIDE HELP

PARENTS' REPORTS

OUTSIDE HELP	Neutral	Negative	Total
No*	18	7	25
Yes†	16	21	37
Total	34	28	62

$p < 0.05$; $\chi^2 = 4.98$; $df = 1$.
*Includes cases from "Alone" category.
†Combines cases from "Some Help" and "Delegation" categories.
Modified from Knafl, K. A. (1985). How families manage a pediatric hospitalization. *Western Journal of Nursing Research, 7*(2), 163.

ships or differences between the cell values is performed. The most familiar analysis of cross-tabulated data is use of the chi-squared (X^2) statistic. Chi-squared is designed to test for significant differences between cells. Some statisticians prefer to examine chi-squared from a probability framework and use it to detect possible relationships (Goodman & Kruskal, 1954, 1959, 1963, 1972).

Computer programs are also available to analyze data from cross-tabulation tables (contingency tables). These programs can generate output from chi-squared and many correlational techniques and indicate the level of significance for each technique. One should know which statistics are appropriate for one's data and how to interpret the outcomes from these multiple analyses. The information presented on each of these tests provides guidance in the selection of a test and interpretation of the findings.

Chi-Squared Test of Independence

The *chi-squared test of independence* tests whether the two variables being examined are independent or related. Chi-squared is designed to test for differences in frequencies of observed data and compare them with the frequencies that could be expected to occur if the data categories were actually independent of each other. If differences are

indicated, the analysis will not identify where these differences exist within the data.

ASSUMPTIONS

One assumption of the test is that only one datum entry is made for each subject in the sample. Therefore, if repeated measures from the same subject are being used for analysis, such as pretests and posttests, chi-squared is not an appropriate test. Another assumption is that for each variable, the categories are mutually exclusive and exhaustive. No cells may have an expected frequency of zero. However, in the actual data, the observed cell frequency may be zero. Until recently, each cell was expected to have a frequency of at least five, but this requirement has been mathematically demonstrated not to be necessary. However, no more than 20% of the cells should have less than five (Conover, 1971). The test is distribution-free, or nonparametric, which means that no assumption has been made of a normal distribution of values in the population from which the sample was taken.

CALCULATION

The formula is relatively easy to calculate manually and can be used with small samples, which makes it a popular approach to data analysis. The first step in the calculation of chi-squared is to categorize the data, record the observed values in a contingency table, and sum the rows and columns. Next, the expected frequencies are calculated for each cell. The expected frequencies are those frequencies that would occur if there were no group differences; these frequencies are calculated from the row and column sums by using the following formula:

$$E = \frac{(Tr)(Tc)}{N}$$

where

E = expected cell frequency
Tr = row total for that cell
Tc = column total for that cell
N = total number of subjects in the sample

Thus, the expected frequency for a particular cell is obtained by multiplying the row total by the column total and dividing by the sample size. When the expected frequencies have been calculated for all the cells, the sum should be equivalent to the total sample size. Calculations of the expected frequencies for the four cells in Table 22–1 follow; they total 62 (sample size).

Cell 1,1	**Cell 1,2**
$E = \dfrac{(25)(34)}{62} = 13.71$	$E = \dfrac{(25)(28)}{62} = 11.29$
Cell 2,1	**Cell 2,2**
$E = \dfrac{(37)(34)}{62} = 20.29$	$E = \dfrac{(37)(28)}{62} = 16.71$

By using this same example, a contingency table could be constructed of the observed and expected frequencies (see Table 22–2). The following formula is then used to calculate the chi-squared statistic:

$$\chi^2 = \Sigma \frac{(O - E)^2}{E}$$

where

O = observed frequency

E = expected frequency

TABLE 22–2
CONTINGENCY TABLE OF OBSERVED AND EXPECTED FREQUENCIES

PARENTS' REPORTS

OUTSIDE HELP	Neutral	Negative
No	O = 18	O = 7
	E = 13.71	E = 11.29
Yes	O = 16	O = 21
	E = 20.29	E = 16.71

E = expected frequencies; O = observed frequencies.

Note that the formula includes difference scores between the observed frequency for each cell and the expected frequency for that cell. These difference scores are squared, divided by the expected frequency, and summed for each cell. The chi-squared value was calculated by using the observed and expected frequencies in Table 22–2.

$$\chi^2 = \frac{(18 - 13.71)^2}{13.71} + \frac{(7 - 11.29)^2}{11.29}$$
$$+ \frac{(16 - 20.29)^2}{20.29} + \frac{(21 - 16.71)^2}{16.71} = 4.98$$
$$df = 1; p < .05$$

With any chi-squared analysis, the degrees of freedom (df) must be calculated to determine the significance of the value of the statistic. The following formula is used for this calculation:

$$df = (R - 1)(C - 1)$$

where

R = number of rows

C = number of columns

In the example presented previously, the chi-squared value was 4.98, and df was 1, which was calculated as follows:

$$df = (2 - 1)(2 - 1) = 1$$

INTERPRETATION Of RESULTS

The chi-squared statistic is compared with the chi-squared values in the table in Appendix E. The table includes the critical values of chi-squared for specific degrees of freedom at selected levels of significance (usually .05 or .01). A critical value is the value of the statistic that must be obtained to indicate that a difference exists in the two populations represented by the groups under study. If the value of the statistic is equal to or greater than the value identified in the chi-squared table, the difference between the two variables is significant. If the statistic remains significant at more extreme probability levels, the largest p value at which significance is achieved is reported. The analysis indicates that there are group differences in the categories of the variable and that those differences are related to changes in the other variable. Although a significant chi-squared value indicates difference, the magnitude of the difference is not revealed by the analysis. If the statistic is not significant, we cannot conclude that there is a difference in the distribution of the two variables, and they are considered independent (Siegel, 1956).

Interpretation of the results is dependent on the design of the study. If the design is experimental, causality can be considered and the results can be inferred to the associated population. If the design is descriptive, differences identified are associated only with the sample under study. In either case, the differences found are related to differences among all the categories of the first variable and all the categories of the second variable. The specific differences among variables and categories of variables cannot be identified with this analysis. Often, in reported research, the researcher will visually examine the data and discuss differences in the categories of data as though they had been demonstrated to be statistically significantly different. These reports must be viewed with caution by the reader. Partitioning, the contingency coefficient C, the phi coefficient, or Cramer's V can be used to examine the data statistically to determine in exactly which categories the differences lie. The last three strategies can also shed some light on the magnitude of the relationship between the variables. These strategies are discussed later in this chapter.

In reporting the results, contingency tables are generally presented only for significant chi-squared analyses. The value of the statistic is given, including the df and p values. Data in the contingency table are sufficient to allow other researchers to repeat the chi-squared analyses and thus check the accuracy of the analyses.

The chi-squared test of independence can be used with two or more groups. In this case, group membership is used as the independent variable. The chi-squared statistic is calculated with the same formula as above. If more than two categories of the dependent variable are present, differences in both central tendency and dispersion are tested by the analysis.

PARTITIONING Of CHI-SQUARE

Partitioning involves breaking up the contingency table into several 2×2 tables and conducting chi-squared analyses on each table separately. Partitioning can be performed on any contingency table greater than 2×2 with more than one degree of freedom. The number of partitions that can be conducted is equivalent to the degrees of freedom. The sum of the chi-squared values obtained by partitioning is equal to the original chi-squared value. Certain rules must be followed during partitioning to prevent inflating the value of chi-squared. The initial partition can include any four cells as long as two values from each variable are used. The next 2×2 must compress the first four cells into two cells and include two new cells. This process can continue until no new cells are available. By using this process it is possible to determine which cells have contributed to the significant differences found.

Phi

The *phi coefficient* (ϕ) is used to describe relationships in dichotomous, nominal data. It is also used with the chi-squared test to determine the location of a difference or differences among cells. Phi is used only with 2×2 tables (see Table 22–3).

CALCULATION

If chi-squared has been calculated, the following formula can be used to calculate phi. The data presented in Table 22–1 were used to calculate this phi coefficient. The chi-squared analysis indicated a significant difference, and the phi coefficient indicated the magnitude of effect.

$$\text{phi} = \sqrt{\frac{\chi^2}{N}} \quad \text{phi } (\phi) = \sqrt{\frac{4.98}{62}} = \sqrt{.0803} = .238$$

TABLE 22–3
FRAMEWORK FOR DEVELOPING A 2 × 2 CONTINGENCY TABLE

VARIABLE X

VARIABLE Y	0	1	Totals
0	A	B	A + B
1	C	D	C + D
Totals	A + C	B + D	N

where

N = the total frequency of all cells

Alternatively, phi can be calculated directly from the 2 × 2 table by using the following formula (Siegel, 1956). Again, the data from Table 22–1 are used to calculate the phi coefficient.

$$\text{phi} = \frac{AD - BC}{\sqrt{(A + C)(B + D)(A + B)(C + D)}}$$

$$= \frac{(18)(21) - (7)(16)}{\sqrt{(34)(28)(25)(37)}} = .283$$

INTERPRETATION OF RESULTS

The phi coefficient is similar to Pearson's product-moment correlation coefficient (r), except that two dichotomous variables are involved. Phi values range from -1 to $+1$, with the magnitude of the relationship decreasing as the coefficient nears zero. The results show the strength of the relationship between the two variables.

Cramer's V

Cramer's V is a modification of phi used for contingency tables larger than 2 × 2. It is designed for use with nominal data. The value of the statistic ranges from zero to 1.

CALCULATION

The formula can be calculated from the chi-squared statistic, and the data presented in Table 22–1 were used to calculate Cramer's V.

$$V = \sqrt{\frac{\chi^2}{N(L - 1)}} \quad V = \sqrt{\frac{4.98}{62(7 - 1)}}$$

$$= \sqrt{.01334} = .115$$

where

L = the smaller of the number of either columns or rows
N = total frequency of all cells

The Contingency Coefficient

The *contingency coefficient* (C) is used with two nominal variables and is the most commonly used of the three chi-squared–based measures of association.

CALCULATION

The contingency coefficient can be calculated with the following formula, which uses the data presented in Table 22–1:

$$C = \sqrt{\frac{\chi^2}{\chi^2 + N}} \quad C = \sqrt{\frac{4.98}{4.98 + 62}}$$

$$= \sqrt{.07435} = .273$$

The relationship demonstrated by C cannot be interpreted on the same scale as Pearson's r, phi, or Cramer's V because it does not reach an upper limit of 1. The formula does not consider the number of cells, and the upper limit varies with the size of the contingency table. With a 2 × 2 table, the upper limit is .71; with a 3 × 3 table, the upper limit is .82; and with a 4 × 4 table, the upper limit is .87.

Contingency coefficients from separate analyses can be compared only if the table sizes are the same.

Lambda

Lambda measures the degree of association (or relationship) between two nominal-level variables. The value of lambda can range from 0 to 1. Two approaches to analysis are possible: asymmetrical and symmetrical. The asymmetrical approach indicates the capacity to predict the value of the dependent variable given the value of the independent variable. Thus, when asymmetrical lambda is used, it is necessary to specify a dependent and an independent variable. Symmetrical lambda measures the degree of overlap (or association) between the two variables and makes no assumptions regarding which variable is dependent and which is independent (Waltz & Bausell, 1981).

NONPARAMETRIC TESTS

McNemar Test for Significance of Changes

The *McNemar test* analyzes changes that occur in dichotomous variables by using a 2 × 2 table. This nonparametric test is particularly appropriate for before-and-after or pretest-posttest designs in which the subjects serve as their own control and the data are nominal. For example, one might be interested in determining the number of nurses in a sample who changed from hospital nursing to home health care and vice versa. The two workplaces in the aforementioned example are nominal because it is not possible to rank one as being better than the other. Pluses and minuses are used to indicate the two conditions, and assignment of a plus or minus to a variable is at the discretion of the researcher. Data are placed in a 2 × 2 contingency table as exemplified in Table 22–4.

Subjects whose scores changed from positive to negative are tallied in cell A. In the example, nurses who changed from home health care to hospital nursing were tallied in cell A; five nurses were in this category. Those who changed from negative to positive are tallied in cell D. If the score remained negative, the subject is tallied in cell C, and if the

TABLE 22–4
2 × 2 CONTINGENCY TABLE FOR THE MCNEMAR TEST

		POSTTEST	
		−	+
Pretest	+	A	B
	−	C	D

score remained positive, the subject is tallied in cell B. Only subjects whose scores changed are included in the analysis; therefore, only the tally marks in cells A and D are considered. The null hypothesis is that the population probability of changing from negative to positive is the same as the population probability of changing from positive to negative.

If one were to study the nurses who changed from home health care to hospital nursing, the data might appear as presented in Table 22–5. Cell A contains the number of nurses who changed from home health nursing to hospital nursing; five nurses were included in this category. Fifteen (cell D) nurses changed from hospital nursing to home health care. Five nurses (cell B) stayed in home health nursing, and three nurses (cell C) remained in hospital nursing.

CALCULATION

If $\frac{1}{2}(A + D)$ is 5 or less, the binomial distribution is used to determine the level of probability. Otherwise, the chi-squared test with correction for continuity is used to test the hypothesis. The chi-

TABLE 22–5
EXAMPLE OF A 2 × 2 CONTINGENCY TABLE FOR THE MCNEMAR TEST

		POSTTEST	
		−	+
Pretest	+	A 5	B 5
	−	C 3	D 15

squared value is calculated for the data presented in Table 22–5.

$$\chi^2 = \frac{(|A - D| - 1)^2}{A + D}$$

$$\chi^2 = \frac{(|5 - 15| - 1)^2}{5 + 15} = \frac{(10 - 1)^2}{20}$$

$$= \frac{81}{20} = 4.05$$

INTERPRETATION OF RESULTS

The significance of the chi-squared value when $df = 1$ is determined from the chi-squared table in Appendix E. If the value is equal to or greater than the table value, the two groups are considered significantly different. In the example, $\chi^2 = 4.05$, and $df = 1$; the chi-squared value is significant at the .05 level.

Sign Test

The *sign test* is a nonparametric test that was developed for data for which it is difficult to assign numerical values. However, the data can be ranked on dimensions such as agree-disagree, easier-harder, earlier-later, more-less, and higher-lower.

The sign test acquired its name from use of the plus sign and the minus sign to rank or place value on the variables under study. The test makes no assumptions about the shape of the underlying distribution or that all subjects are from the same population. The null hypothesis states that the population probability of changing from negative to positive is the same as the population probability of changing from positive to negative.

CALCULATION

To conduct the sign test, the pretest-posttest or matched-pairs values are examined to determine whether the change from the first observation to the second observation was positive or negative. Subjects in whom no change was observed are dropped from the analysis, and N is reduced accordingly. N is the number of pairs of observations. The number of pluses and minuses for these paired observations is counted. If N is 25 or less, the binomial distribution is consulted for the level of probability. If N is greater than 25, the Z statistic is calculated by using the following equation:

$$Z = \frac{(x + 0.5) - \frac{1}{2} N}{\frac{1}{2} \sqrt{N}}$$

where

x = the smaller of either the sum of pluses or the sum of minuses

N = number of paired values retained for analysis

For a two-tailed test, a Z score of 1.96 indicates significance at the .05 level. For a one-tailed test, a Z score of 1.643 indicates significance at the .05 level. The table for the Z distribution (cumulative normal distribution) can be found in Appendix B.

Wilcoxon Matched-Pairs Signed-Ranks Test

The *Wilcoxon matched-pairs signed-ranks test,* like the sign test, is a nonparametric test that examines changes that occur in pretest-posttest measures or matched-pairs measures. It is more powerful than the sign test because it examines both the direction and the magnitude of change that occurs. A pair of scores in which a greater amount of change has occurred is given more weight than a pair in which very little change has occurred. This test requires that the researcher be able to assess the magnitude of a change between the first and second observation. When no change has occurred between the first and second observation, the subject or pair is dropped from the analysis and the sample size is decreased.

CALCULATION

Initially, a difference score (d) is calculated for each pair of scores. If the difference score is zero, the pair is omitted. The plus or minus sign associated with each difference score must be retained.

The plus and minus signs are ignored, and the difference scores are ranked, with the lowest difference score ranked 1. If some of the difference scores are tied, the ranks of the tied scores are averaged. For example, if ranks 3, 4, and 5 had the same difference score, the ranks would be summed and divided by the number of ranks [(3 + 4 + 5)/3 = 4], and the resulting rank would be assigned to each of the pairs. The next difference scores would then be assigned the rank of 6.

In the second step of analysis, the sign of the difference score is affixed to each rank to indicate which ranks resulted from a negative change and which ranks resulted from a positive change. If the two groups being examined are not different, the positive and negative ranks should be relatively interspersed, with the greatest difference scores occurring equally among positive and negative ranks. The third step in analysis is to sum the ranks having positive signs and sum the ranks having negative signs. If no difference is noted in the two groups, these two sums should be similar.

INTERPRETATION Of RESULTS

The smallest value of the two sums (T) and the number of pairs (N) are used to determine the significance of the difference in the two sums. If N is 25 or less, the Wilcoxon matched-pairs signed-ranks table in Appendix J is used to determine significance. If T is equal to or less than the table value, the null hypothesis that there is no difference in the values of the two sums is rejected. If N is greater than 25, the Z score is calculated by using the following equation:

$$Z = \frac{T - \frac{N(N+1)}{4}}{\sqrt{\frac{N(N+1)(2N+1)}{24}}}$$

where

 T = smallest value of the two sums
 N = number of matched pairs retained for analysis

In a two-tailed test, a Z score of 1.96 or less indicates a level of significance of .05. For a one-tailed test, a Z score of 1.68 or less indicates a level of significance of .05. The table for the Z distribution is in Appendix B.

Mann-Whitney U Test

The *Mann-Whitney* U *test* is the most powerful of the nonparametric tests, with 95% of the power of the t test to detect differences between groups of normally distributed populations. If the assumptions of the t test are violated, such as a nonnormal distribution or ordinal-level data, the Mann-Whitney U test is more powerful. Although ranks are used for the analysis, ties in ranks have little effect on the outcome of the analysis.

CALCULATION

Before calculation, the scores from the two samples must be combined and ranked, with the lowest score assigned the rank of 1. Each score should also be identified with regard to group membership. If one had two groups (males and females) and the males scored 50, 55, 62, and 70 on an anxiety tool and the females scored 45, 58, 75, 76, and 77 on the same tool, these scores could be combined and ranked. The groups, scores, and ranks of these scores are presented in Table 22–6. The formula for calculating the Mann-Whitney U test follows. The U statistic was calculated from the data presented in Table 22–6.

$$\hat{U} = n_1 n_2 + \frac{n_1(n_1 + 1)}{2} - R_1$$

$$U' = n_1 n_2 - \hat{U}$$

where

 n_1 = number of observations in the smallest group
 n_2 = number of observations in the largest group
 R_1 = sum of ranks assigned to n_1
 U = the smaller value of $\hat{U}$ or U'

TABLE 22–6
RANKED SCORES FROM TWO GROUPS

Group	F	M	M	F	M	M	F	F	F
Score	45	50	55	58	62	70	75	76	77
Rank	1	2	3	4	5	6	7	8	9

$$\hat{U} = (4)(5) + \frac{4(4+1)}{2} - (2 + 3 + 5 + 6)$$
$$= 20 + 10 - 16 = 14$$
$$U' = (4)(5) - 14 = 20 - 14 = 6$$

INTERPRETATION OF RESULTS

The equations for both $\hat{U}$ and U' must be calculated. Two tables are available to determine the significance of U. If n_2 is less than or equal to 8, the tables in Appendix F are used. If n_2 is between 9 and 20, the table in Appendix G is used. In the example, $U = 6$, $n_1 = 4$, and $n_2 = 5$. The probability (that the samples are from two different populations rather than one) listed in the table in Appendix F is .206, which is not significant. If n_2 is greater than 20, the Z statistic is calculated by using the following equation. The normal distribution (see Appendix B) is used to determine the level of significance.

$$Z = \frac{U - n_1 n_2 / 2}{\sqrt{\frac{(n_1 n_2)(n_1 + n_2 + 1)}{12}}}$$

Kolmogorov-Smirnov Two-Sample Test

The Kolmogorov-Smirnov two-sample test is a nonparametric test used to determine whether two independent samples have been drawn from the same population. This test uses the cumulative frequency from two samples for analysis. Either grouped or ungrouped frequencies can be used. If groupings are used, the same intervals must be used for developing the distribution of each sample.

Larger numbers of groups lead to a more meaningful analysis. For example, if age were being used, 5-year age spans would provide more meaningful analysis than 20-year spans. The test is sensitive to any differences in distribution of the two samples, including differences in measures of central tendency, dispersion, or skewness. The risk of a Type II error with this test is less than with chi-squared when small samples are being examined.

CALCULATION

The scores within two groups are ranked separately. The cumulative relative frequency is calculated for each rank by dividing the ranking by the number in the sample. In Table 22–7, a score of 2 is ranked 1 in a sample of 9; therefore, the relative frequency is $\frac{1}{9}$, or .11. A difference score is obtained for each point on the distribution by subtracting the smaller relative frequency from the larger relative frequency. For the score of 2, sample 1 had no scores that low, so the cumulative probability was .00 and the difference score was .11 − .00 = .11. The largest difference score in the example is indicated with an asterisk in Table 22–7.

INTERPRETATION OF RESULTS

One difficulty with the Kolmogorov-Smirnov two-sample test is that one cannot determine whether the difference is in central tendency, dispersion, or skewness; therefore, conclusions must be broad. The test compares the cumulative distributions of the two samples with the assumption that if they are from the same population, differences in distribution will be only random deviations. If the deviation is large enough, it is considered evidence for rejecting the null hypothesis.

The largest difference score is identified and used for comparison with the table values in Ap-

TABLE 22–7
RANKING OF SCORES FOR THE KOLMOGOROV-SMIRNOV TWO-SAMPLE TEST

SAMPLE 1 (*n* = 10)		SAMPLE 2 (*n* = 9)		ABSOLUTE VALUE OF THE DIFFERENCE
Scores	Cumulative Probability	Scores	Cumulative Probability	
	.00	2	1/9 = .11	.11
	.00	3	2/9 = .22	.22
	.00	5	3/9 = .33	.33
	.00	6	4/9 = .44	.44
	.00	9	5/9 = .56	.56
	.00	10	6/9 = .67	.67*
11	1/10 = .10		.67	.57
12	2/10 = .20	12	7/9 = .78	.58
13	3/10 = .30		.78	.48
14	4/10 = .40		.78	.38
15	5/10 = .50	15	8/9 = .89	.39
18	6/10 = .60	18	9/9 = 1.00	.40
19	7/10 = .70		1.00	.30
21	8/10 = .80		1.00	.20
23	9/10 = .90		1.00	.10
25	10/10 = 1.00		1.00	.00

*The largest difference score.

pendix H. If the difference score is equal to or greater than the table value, the test indicates a significant difference. In the example in Table 22-7, the largest difference score, .67, when compared with the table value of .578 at the .05 level for a two-tailed test, indicates that the samples are significantly different at the .05 level.

Wald-Wolfowitz Runs Test

The *Wald-Wolfowitz runs test,* a nonparametric test, is used to determine differences between two populations. The null hypothesis is false if the two populations differ in any way, including central tendency, variability, or skewness.

CALCULATION

The scores from the two samples are merged and ranked, and the group membership of each score is recorded with the rank. The number of runs in the ranked series of scores is then determined. A run is any sequence of scores from the same sample. In the following example given, sample 1 is coded as

A and sample 2 is coded as B. The merged scores from samples A and B are presented below. In this example, six runs were identified.

INTERPRETATION Of RESULTS

The runs test assumes that if the samples are from the same population, the scores will be well mixed. Therefore, *r*, the number of runs, will be large. When the null hypothesis is false, *r* is small. The table for the runs test is found in Appendix I. For the samples in the example, the table value of *r* is 5, which means that the number of runs must be equal to or less than 5 to be significant. Because the example has 6 runs, the null hypothesis is accepted.

The Kruskal-Wallis One-Way Analysis of Variance by Ranks

The *Kruskal-Wallis test* is the most powerful nonparametric test for examining three independent groups. It has 95% of the power of the *F* statistic to detect existing differences between groups. The technique tests the null hypothesis that all samples are from the same population. The main assumption with this test is an underlying continuous distribution.

CALCULATION

The initial step in analysis is to rank all scores from all samples together, with the smallest score being assigned a rank of 1. *N* is equal to the largest rank or the total number of observations from all samples. Next, the ranks from each sample are summed. The Kruskal-Wallis test determines whether the sum of ranks from each group is different enough that we can reject the hypothesis that the samples come from the same population. The statistic used in the Kruskal-Wallis test is *H*, and the following formula is used to calculate this statistic.

$$H = \frac{12}{N(N+1)} \sum \frac{R_j^2}{n_j} - 3(N+1)$$

where

j = number assigned to each sample
n_j = number of scores in sample j
N = total number of scores across all samples
R_j = sum of ranks from sample j

$\sum \dfrac{R_j^2}{n_j}$ indicates that $\dfrac{R_j^2}{n_j}$ is to be calculated separately for each sample and the results are to be summed

INTERPRETATION Of RESULTS

If each group has more than five subjects, the chi-squared table in Appendix E can be used to determine levels of significance. Degrees of freedom is calculated as the number of samples minus 1. If the value obtained for *H* is equal to or greater than the table value, the groups are considered statistically significantly different. If there are three samples and each sample contains fewer than five subjects, exact probabilities for these samples can be found in Appendix K.

The Cochran *Q* Test

The *Cochran* Q *test* is an extension of the McNemar test for two related samples. The Cochran *Q* test can be used in situations such as (1) when subjects have been matched and several levels of treatment have been administered, (2) when more than one matched control group has been used for comparison, or (3) for repeated measures of the dependent variable across time. Measures of the dependent variable must be coded dichotomously. For example, 1 could be coded if an event occurred, 0 if it did not occur; 1 could be coded for yes, 0 for no; or plus for a positive change, minus for a negative change.

CALCULATION

Data are arranged in a contingency table where *k* is equal to the number of columns and *N* is equal to the number of rows. The null hypothesis is that there is no difference in frequency or proportion of responses by category in each column except that of chance. The computational equation is as follows:

$$Q = \frac{(k-1)\,[k\sum G_j^2 - (\sum G_j)^2]}{k\sum L_i - \sum L_i^2}$$

where

i = number assigned to each row
j = number assigned to each column
k = number of columns
G_j = total number of positive responses (yes, 1 or +) in each column
L_i = total number of positive responses (yes, 1 or +) in each row

INTERPRETATION Of RESULTS

The value of Q is compared with the chi-squared table in Appendix E, using $df = k - 1$. If the value of Q is greater than or equal to the table value, the frequency or proportion of subjects coded as positive differs significantly among the samples. The power efficiency of Cochran's Q is not known because there are no parametric tests with which it can be compared.

The Friedman Two-Way Analysis of Variance by Ranks

The *Friedman two-way ANOVA* by ranks may be used with matched samples or in repeated measures. The null hypothesis is that the samples come from the same population. The Friedman test considers magnitude of differences and is therefore more powerful than the Cochran Q test in rejecting a false null hypothesis, given the same data.

CALCULATION

Data are placed in a contingency table with N rows and k columns. Rows represent groups of subjects, and columns represent conditions being studied. Scores within each cell are summed and ranked by row. In Figure 22–1, the scores and the row ranks for these scores are presented in contingency tables. The value of the Friedman test statistic χ_r^2 can be calculated by using the following equation:

$$\chi_r^2 = \frac{12}{Nk(k+1)} \Sigma(R_j)^2 - 3N(k+1)$$

where

N = number of rows
k = number of columns
j = column number
R_j = sum of ranks in column j
$\Sigma(R_j)^2$ = instruction to sum the squares of R_j over all columns

The χ_r^2 value was calculated for the data presented in Figure 22–1.

$$\chi_r^2 = \frac{12}{3(4)(4+1)}[(9)^2 + (8)^2 + (6)^2 + (7)^2]$$
$$- (3)(3)(4+1) = \frac{12}{60}(230) - 45$$
$$= (.2)(230) - 45 = 1.0$$

INTERPRETATION OF RESULTS

The value of the χ_r^2 statistic is compared with the values in Appendix L. If the value of the test statistic is equal to or greater than the table value for the selected level of significance (e.g., .05), the ranks in the various columns differ significantly; therefore, the value of a score depends on the condition. In the example, $\chi_r^2 = 1.0$, which is not significant, and the null hypothesis would be accepted. If k (number of columns) is greater than 4, the χ_r^2 statistic is compared with the chi-squared distribution in Appendix E. The power efficiency to reject the null hypothesis is equivalent to the F statistic when alpha is .05 and is 85% of the F statistic when alpha is .01.

SCORE TOTALS				
	Condition			
	I	II	III	IV
Group 1	22	16	8	2
Group 2	41	26	8	12
Group 3	2	8	36	44

ROW RANKS				
	Condition			
	I	II	III	IV
Group 1	4	3	2	1
Group 2	4	3	1	2
Group 3	1	2	3	4
R_j	9	8	6	7
R_j^2	81	64	36	49
$(R_j)^2 = 81 + 64 + 36 + 49 = 230$				

FIGURE 22–1 ■ Example of contingency tables for the Friedman test.

t TESTS

t Test for Independent Samples

One of the most common parametric analyses used to test for significant differences between statistical measures of two samples is the *t* test. The *t* test uses the standard deviation of the sample to estimate the standard error of the sampling distribution. The ease in calculating the formula is attractive to researchers who wish to conduct their analyses by hand. This test is particularly useful when only small samples are available for analysis. The *t* test being discussed here is for independent samples.

The *t* test is frequently misused by researchers who use multiple *t* tests to examine differences in various aspects of data collected in a study. Such practice leads to an escalation of significance that results in a greatly increased risk of a Type I error. The *t* test can be used only one time during analysis to examine data from the two samples in a study. The *Bonferroni procedure,* which controls for the escalation of significance, can be used if various *t* tests must be performed on different aspects of the same data. A Bonferroni adjustment is easily done by hand; you simply divide the overall significance level by the number of tests and use the resulting number as the significance level for each test. ANOVA is always a viable alternative to the pooled *t* test and is preferred by many researchers who have become wary of the *t* test because of its frequent misuse. Mathematically, the two approaches are the same when only two samples are being examined.

Use of the *t* test involves the following assumptions:

1. Sample means from the population are normally distributed.
2. The dependent variable is measured at the interval level.
3. The two samples have equal variance.
4. All observations within each sample are independent.

The *t* test is *robust* to moderate violation of its assumptions. Robustness means that the results of analysis can still be relied on to be accurate when one of the assumptions has been violated. The *t* test is not robust with respect to the between-samples or within-samples independence assumptions, nor is it robust with respect to extreme violation of the normality assumption unless the sample sizes are extremely large. Sample groups do not have to be equal for this analysis—the concern is, instead, for equal variance. A variety of *t* tests have been developed for various types of samples. Independent samples means that the two sets of data were not taken from the same subjects and that the scores in the two groups are *not* related.

CALCULATION

The *t* statistic is relatively easy to calculate. The numerator is the difference scores of the means of the two samples. The test uses the pooled standard deviation of the two samples as the denominator, which gives a rather forbidding appearance to the formula:

$$t = \frac{\bar{X}_a - \bar{X}_b}{\sqrt{\dfrac{\Sigma X_a^2 - \dfrac{(\Sigma X_a)^2}{n_a} + \Sigma X_b^2 - \dfrac{(\Sigma X_b)^2}{n_b}}{(n_a + n_b - 2)}\left(\dfrac{1}{n_a} + \dfrac{1}{n_b}\right)}}$$

$\bar{X}_a$ = mean of sample 1

$\bar{X}_b$ = mean of sample 2

n_a = number of subjects in sample 1

n_b = number of subjects in sample 2

ΣX_a^2 = Sum of Group a squared deviation scores

ΣX_b^2 = Sum of Group b squared deviation scores

$$df = n_a + n_b - 2$$

In the following example, the *t* test was used to examine the difference between a control group and an experimental group. The independent variable administered to the experimental group was a form of relaxation therapy. The dependent variable was pulse rate. Pulse rates for the experimental and control groups are presented in Table 22–8, along with calculations for the *t* test.

$$t = \frac{77 - 70}{\sqrt{\frac{71{,}376 - \frac{(924)^2}{12} + 58{,}944 - \frac{(840)^2}{12}}{(12 + 12 - 2)}\left(\frac{1}{12} + \frac{1}{12}\right)}}$$

$$= \frac{7}{\sqrt{\frac{(71{,}376 - 71{,}148 + 58{,}944 - 58{,}800)(.1667)}{22}}}$$

$$= \frac{7}{1.679} = 4.169$$

$$df = 12 + 12 - 2 = 22$$

INTERPRETATION OF RESULTS

To determine the significance of the t statistic, the degrees of freedom must be calculated. The value of the t statistic is then found in the table for the sampling distribution. If the sample size is 30 or less, the t distribution is used; a table of this distribution can be found in Appendix C. For larger sample sizes, the normal distribution may be used; a table of this distribution can be found in Appendix B. The level of significance and the degrees of freedom are used to identify the critical value of t.

This value is then used to obtain the most exact p value possible. The p value is then compared with the significance level. In the example presented in Table 22–8, the calculated $t = 4.169$ and $df = 22$. This t value was significant at the .001 level.

t Tests for Related Samples

When samples are related, the formula used to calculate the t statistic is different from the formula described above. Samples may be related because matching has been performed as part of the design or because the scores used in the analysis were obtained from the same subjects under different conditions (e.g., pretest and posttest). This test requires that differences between the paired scores be independent and normally or approximately normally distributed.

CALCULATION

The following formula assumes that scores in the two samples are in some way correlated (dependent).

TABLE 22–8
DATA AND COMPUTATIONS FOR THE T-TEST

PULSE RATE (CONTROL GROUP)

X_a	Frequency (f)	fX_a	X_a^2	fX_a^2
70	1	70	4900	4900
72	2	144	5184	10,368
76	5	380	5776	28,880
82	3	246	6724	20,172
84	1	84	7056	7056
$n_a = 12$	$\bar{X}_a = 77$	$\Sigma X_a = 924$		$\Sigma X_a^2 = 71376$

PULSE RATE (EXPERIMENTAL GROUP)

X_b	Frequency (f)	fX_b	X_b^2	fX_b^2
64	1	64	4096	4096
66	2	132	4356	8712
70	5	350	4900	24500
72	3	216	5184	15552
78	1	78	6084	6084
$n_b = 12$	$\bar{X}_b = 70$	$\Sigma X_b = 840$		$\Sigma X_b^2 = 58944$

$$t = \frac{\bar{d}}{\sqrt{\frac{\Sigma d^2}{n(n-1)}}}$$

where

$\bar{d}$ = mean difference between the paired scores

Σd^2 = sum of squared deviation difference scores

n = number of paired scores

$df = n - 1$

INTERPRETATION Of RESULTS

Results of the analysis are interpreted in the same way as those of the independent t test described above.

ANALYSIS OF VARIANCE PROCEDURES

ANOVA tests for differences between means. Expressed another way, it determines whether the samples under consideration were drawn from the same population and thus have the same population mean. As previously mentioned, the pooled variance t test is simply a specialized version of ANOVA in which only two means are examined. ANOVA has been considered a much more rigorous approach to statistical analysis than regression analysis is (which is often mistakenly equated with correlation analysis). However, statistically, ANOVA is simply a specialized version of regression analysis (Volicer, 1984). Regression analyses can be used for the same purpose of testing causality as ANOVA and are more flexible. According to Pedhazur and Schmelkin (1991), "the most compelling reason for a preference of the REGRESSION over the ANOVA approach is that it is more comprehensive from conceptual, design, and analytic perspectives. Conceptually, all variables, be they categorical or continuous, are viewed alike, in the sense of providing information to be used in attempts to explain or predict the dependent variable" (p. 541). Because both procedures can be used for the same purposes,

the choice is probably based on previous educational exposure, preference for particular computer programs, and taste.

One-Way Analysis of Variance

Although one-way ANOVA is a bivariate analysis, it is more flexible than other analyses in that it can examine data from two or more groups. This analysis is accomplished by using group membership as one of the two variables under examination and a dependent variable as the second variable.

ANOVA compares the variance within each group with the variance between groups. The outcome of the analysis is a numerical value for the F statistic, which will be used to determine whether the groups are significantly different. The variance within each group is a result of individual scores in the group varying from the group mean and is referred to as the *within-group variance*. This variance is calculated in the same way as that described in Chapter 19. The amount of variation about the mean in each group is assumed by ANOVA to be equal. The group means also vary around the grand mean (the mean of the total sample), which is referred to as the *between-groups variance*. One could assume that if all the samples were drawn from the same population, there would be little difference in these two sources of variance. The variance from within and between the groups explains the total variance in the data. When these two types of variance are combined, they are referred to as the total variance. Assumptions involved in ANOVA include

1. Homogeneity of variance
2. Independence of observations
3. Normal distribution of the populations from which the samples were drawn or random samples
4. Interval-level data

CALCULATION

Several calculation steps are required for ANOVA because the value of each source of variance must be determined and then compared with other sources of variance. ANOVA is usually calculated by computer. However, ANOVA is not difficult to calculate by hand with small groups. It is important to understand the process of calculation and the terms used for each step of the analysis. The mathematical logic follows easily from the formulas previously presented. To clarify this connection, conceptual formulas are used to explain the process.

To begin calculations, scores are separated by group and summed, and a mean is calculated for each group. Scores from all groups are then combined and summed, and a mean is obtained for all scores. This mean is referred to as the *grand mean*. Next, three different sums of squares are calculated: (1) the total sum of squares, (2) the sum of squares within, and (3) the sum of squares between. The sum of squares within and the sum of squares between will equal the total sum of squares. As with any sum of squares, difference scores are used for the calculation. The formula for the *total sum of squares* for three groups is

$$SS_T = \Sigma(X_1 - \bar{X})^2 + \Sigma(X_2 - \bar{X})^2 + \Sigma(X_3 - \bar{X})^2$$

where

SS_T = total sum of squares
X_1 = single score from group 1
X_2 = single score from group 2
X_3 = single score from group 3
$\bar{X}$ = grand mean

This formula indicates that the total sum of squares is obtained by summing the sum of squares from each group in the study. The formula for *sum of squares within* (or error) for three groups is

$$SS_W = \Sigma(X_1 - \bar{X}_1)^2 + \Sigma(X_2 - \bar{X}_2)^2 + \Sigma(X_3 - \bar{X}_3)^2$$

where

SS_W = sum of squares within
X_1 = single score from group 1
$\bar{X}_1$ = mean from group 1
X_2 = single score from group 2
$\bar{X}_2$ = mean from group 2
X_3 = single score from group 3
$\bar{X}_3$ = mean from group 3

The formula for *sum of squares between* for these groups is

$$SS_B = n_1(\bar{X}_1 - \bar{\bar{X}})^2 + n_2(\bar{X}_2 - \bar{\bar{X}})^2 + n_3(\bar{X}_3 - \bar{\bar{X}})^2$$

where

SS_B = sum of squares between
n_1 = number of scores in group 1
n_2 = number of scores in group 2
n_3 = number of scores in group 3

After these calculations, degrees of freedom are determined for the total sum of squares, sum of squares within, and sum of squares between by using the following formulas:

$$df_T = N - 1$$

$$df_W = N - k$$

$$df_B = k - 1$$

where

k = number of groups
N = total number of scores

By using the sum of squares and degrees of freedom, the mean square between (MS_B) and the mean square within (MS_W) are calculated from following formulas:

$$MS_B = \frac{SS_{between}}{k-1}$$

$$MS_W = \frac{SS_{within}}{N-k}$$

From these equations (MS_B and MS_W), the F statistic is calculated as follows:

$$F = \frac{MS_{between}}{MS_{within}}$$

Researchers who perform ANOVA on their data frequently record the results in an ANOVA summary table. Popkess (1981) examined self-image scores between two groups (obese and nonobese). The two variables studied were self-image and group membership. An ANOVA was performed on the data; a summary table of the results is presented in Table 22–9. In this example, the mean square between (MS_B), mean square within (MS_W), and F value were calculated as follows:

$$MS_B = \frac{776.69}{1} = 776.69$$

$$MS_W = \frac{11,228.74}{141} = 79.64$$

$$F = \frac{776.69}{79.64} = 9.75$$

INTERPRETATION OF RESULTS

The test for ANOVA is always one-tailed. The critical region is in the upper tail of the test. The F distribution for determining the level of significance of the F statistic can be found in Appendix D. Use of the table requires knowledge of the degrees of freedom of MS_B and MS_W, as well as the desired level of significance. If the F statistic (or ratio) is equal to or greater than the appropriate table value, the difference between the groups is significant. In the example, the df for MS_B was 1, the df for MS_W was 141, and the F value was 9.75, which is significant at the .002 level.

If only two groups are being examined, the location of a significant difference is clear. However, if more than two groups are being studied, it is not possible to determine from the ANOVA exactly where the significant differences lie. One cannot assume that all the groups examined are significantly different. Therefore, post hoc analyses are conducted to determine the location of the differences among groups. Several options are available for conducting post hoc analyses. When ANOVA has been conducted by computer, the computer usually automatically conducts several post hoc analyses and includes their levels of significance on the computer printout. The implications of each analysis must be understood to accurately interpret the meaning attached to the outcomes.

Post Hoc Analyses. One might wonder why a researcher would conduct a test that failed to provide the answer sought—namely, where the significant differences were in a data set. It would seem more logical to perform t tests or ANOVAs on the groups in the data set in pairs, thus clearly determining whether a significant difference exists between those two groups. However, when these tests are performed with three groups in the data set, the risk of a Type I error increases from 5% to 14%. As the number of groups increases (and with the increase in groups, an increase in the number of comparisons necessary), the risk of a Type I error increases strikingly.

Post hoc tests have been developed specifically to determine the location of differences after ANOVA. These tests were developed to reduce the incidence of a Type I error. Frequently used post hoc tests are the Bonferroni procedure, the Newman-Keuls test, the Tukey HSD test, the Scheffe test, and the Dunnett test. When these tests are

---

TABLE 22–9
ONE-WAY ANALYSIS OF VARIANCE OF WEIGHT GROUPS AND SELF-IMAGE

SOURCE	df	SS	MS	F	PROBABILITY
Between groups	1	776.69	776.69	9.75	.002
Within groups	141	11,228.74	79.64		
Total	142	12,005.43			

MS = mean square; SS = sum of squares.
From Popkess, S. A. (1981). Assessment scales for determining the cognitive-behavioral repertoire of the obese subject. *Western Journal of Nursing Research, 3*(2), 199–215. © 1981.

calculated, the alpha level is reduced in proportion to the number of additional tests required to locate statistically significant differences. As the alpha level is decreased, reaching the level of significance becomes increasingly more difficult.

The Newman-Keuls test compares all possible pairs of means and is the most liberal of the post hoc tests considered acceptable by publication editors. *Liberal* means that the alpha level is not as severely decreased. The Tukey HSD test computes one value with which all means within the data set are compared. It is considered more stringent than the Newman-Keuls test and requires approximately equal sample sizes in each group. The Scheffe test is the most conservative of the post hoc tests and has a good reputation among researchers. However, one must keep in mind that a test that is very conservative increases the risk of a Type II error. The Dunnett test requires a control group for its use. The mean for each experimental group is then compared with the mean for the control group. The test does not require a reduction of alpha and is thus advisable to use when the conditions for the test are met.

Factorial Analyses of Variance

A number of types of factorial ANOVAs have been developed to analyze data from specific experimental designs, including two-way ANOVA developed for studies with two independent variables, multifactorial ANOVA for studies with more than two independent variables, randomized block ANOVA, repeated measures ANOVA, and multivariate ANOVA for studies with more than one dependent variable (MANOVA). Mathematically, *factorial ANOVA* is a specialized version of multiple regression. In factorial ANOVA, the following assumptions can be made:

1. The dependent variable is treated as an interval-level measure.
2. At least one independent variable must have values that are categorical rather than continuous.
3. The variance of the dependent variable must be equal in the various groups included in the analysis.

4. Subjects should be randomly selected.
5. The sample size in each group should be equal or approximately equal.
6. No measurement error has been made.

ANOVA is generally robust to violation of its assumptions. However, it is relatively sensitive to variations in sample size between groups. This problem becomes increasingly important as the complexity of the design increases and, with it, the number of groups. Although computerized forms of ANOVA have included modifications of the analysis to control for different group sizes, there remains a problem of interpreting interaction effects when group sizes vary. In these cases, it may be advisable to use regression analysis with dummy variables.

In each type of ANOVA, the mathematical equations differ slightly. However, one element is characteristic of them all: partitioning of the sum of squares. The result of this partitioning is a lessening of the error term, or the amount of unexplained (within-group) variance. With a decrease in the unexplained (within-group) variance comes an increased probability of detecting existing differences between groups in the variables under study. Additionally, partitioning provides the opportunity to examine interactions between variables, which may illustrate effects not initially considered.

Two types of effects are considered when interpreting the results of a factorial ANOVA. Main effects are the effects of a single factor. Interaction effects are the multiplicative effects of two or more factors. In complex designs, interaction effects can be difficult to interpret, particularly when they are the combined effect of three or more variables.

A summary table is used to report both main effects and interaction effects, the *F* value of each, and the level of significance of the *F* value. Interaction effects are evaluated before consideration of main effects because interaction effects may render the main effects meaningless.

Jadack and colleagues (1995) conducted a MANOVA in their study of gender and knowledge about HIV, risky sexual behavior, and safer sex practices. The analysis procedure allowed them to incorporate a number of variables considered important in ex-

TABLE 22–10
MEAN RATINGS (*SD*) AND UNIVARIATE *F* TESTS OF THE PERCEIVED LIKELIHOOD OF BECOMING INFECTED WITH HIV FROM SELECTED BEHAVIOR

BEHAVIOR	WOMEN (*n* = 141)	MEN (*n* = 131)	*F* (1270)
Having vaginal intercourse with a person infected with HIV without using a condom	1.07 (.26)	1.28 (.62)	12.83*
Having anal intercourse with a person infected with HIV without using a condom	1.19 (.43)	1.15 (.40)	.42
Having multiple sexual partners	1.37 (.54)	1.83 (.75)	34.56*
Having sexual intercourse with prostitutes	1.39 (.57)	1.64 (.65)	11.60*
Having homosexual relationships	1.52 (.63)	1.58 (.65)	.65
Having bisexual relationships	1.54 (.61)	1.78 (.72)	9.33*
Having oral sex with a person infected with HIV	1.72 (.81)	2.04 (.85)	10.65*
Open mouth kissing with a person infected with HIV	3.20 (.88)	3.29 (.79)	.85
Donating blood	3.46 (.83)	3.68 (.67)	6.04†
Receiving a blood transfusion	2.75 (.96)	3.17 (.87)	14.01*
Using intravenous drugs	1.93 (.98)	2.20 (.99)	5.11†
Sharing needles with other intravenous drug users	1.19 (.43)	1.36 (.56)	7.81†

Ratings were made on 4-point scales (1 = very likely; 2 = somewhat likely; 3 = somewhat unlikely; 4 = very unlikely).
*$p < .001$.
†$p < .01$.
From Jadack, R. A., Hyde, J. S., & Keller, M. L. (1995). Gender and knowledge about HIV, risky sexual behavior, and safer sex practices. *Research in Nursing & Health, 18*(4), 318.

plaining sexual practices. They reported their results as follows:

· ·

"In general, respondents demonstrated accurate knowledge of the likelihood of transmission from various sexual behaviors. For example, persons reported that having vaginal intercourse without using a condom with a person infected with HIV, having multiple sexual partners, and having unprotected anal intercourse with a person infected with HIV carried risk of transmission.

"The hypothesis that predicted no gender differences in knowledge about HIV transmission was not supported for sexual and needle injection routes. Counter to theoretical predictions, a MANOVA testing for gender differences on multiple variables measuring knowledge about sexual routes of transmission indicated a significant overall effect for gender, $F(8,263) = 8.11$, $p < .001$. Univariate results are shown in [Table 22–10]. For most of the sexual behaviors listed, men reported less likelihood of transmission of HIV from risky sexual behaviors than women. That is, men were more likely

to downplay the likelihood of transmission in comparison to women." (Jadack et al., 1995, p. 317) ■

ANALYSIS OF COVARIANCE

Analysis of covariance (ANCOVA) is designed to reduce the error term (or the variance within groups) by using a somewhat different strategy than that used by factorial ANOVA. ANCOVA partials out the variance resulting from a confounding variable by performing regression analysis before performing ANOVA. This strategy removes the effect of differences between groups that are due to a confounding variable. The procedure is actually a general linear regression model with a mixture of dummy and nondummy independent variables.

This technique is sometimes used as a method of statistical control, which is an alternative to design control. ANCOVA allows the researcher to examine the effect of the treatment apart from the effect of the confounding variable; for example, variables such as age, education, social class, or anxiety level may appear to explain initial differences between groups in a study. The effects of these variables, which can have a bearing on subjects' responses to treatment, can be partialed out by using ANCOVA. However, whenever possible, it is better to use a randomized block design than ANCOVA.

ANCOVA is a useful approach to analysis in pretest-posttest designs in which differences occur in groups on the pretest. For example, individuals who achieve low scores on a pretest will tend to have lower scores on the posttest than will those whose pretest scores were higher, even if the treatment had a significant effect on posttest scores. Conversely, if an individual achieves a high pretest score, it is doubtful that the posttest will indicate a strong change as a result of the treatment. ANCOVA maximizes the capacity to detect differences in such cases.

By using multiple regression, it is also possible to partial out the effects of several covariates. For each covariate, a degree of freedom is lost, which somewhat decreases the possibilities of achieving significance, especially with small samples. Therefore, researchers need to be cautious in their use of multiple covariates. ANCOVA can be used with the more advanced types of ANOVA, including analyses of studies using complex designs such as factorial designs and repeated measures designs.

The assumptions on which ANCOVA is based are

1. randomization
2. homogeneity of within-group regression
3. statistical independence of covariate and treatment
4. fixed covariate values that are error-free
5. linearity of within-group regression
6. normality of conditional criterion scores
7. homogeneity of variance of conditional criterion scores
8. fixed treatment levels (Huitema, 1980, cited in Wu & Slakter, 1989).

Violating one or more of these assumptions will cause alpha (the level of significance) to deviate from the value that it would have if the assumptions had been met. The assumption of greatest concern is that the regression slopes for each treatment group are expected to be equal. The results, however, are relatively robust unless the deviation from equal slopes is extreme. In studies using ANCOVA,

design strategies should at least include random assignment and preferably total randomization. Subjects should be treated independently within groups. The covariate must be measured before the treatment is implemented because the treatment must not affect the covariate. In quasi-experimental studies in which randomization is not possible, ANCOVA needs to be interpreted with caution (Wu & Slakter, 1989).

Tollett and Thomas (1995) used ANCOVA in their examination of a theory-based nursing intervention to instill hope in homeless veterans. They described the analysis as follows.

· ·

"The hypothesis that there is greater hope, self-efficacy, and self-esteem and less depression in subjects receiving a specific nursing intervention to instill hope than in subjects who receive the usual and customary treatment was tested using an analysis of covariance (ANCOVA) procedure with pretest scores as the covariate. There was a significant difference in levels of hope between the control and treatment groups ($F = 8.93$, $p = .006$). There were no other significant differences between the groups on the dependent variables; however, the scores on each of the other variables changed in the hypothesized direction." (Tollett & Thomas, 1995, p. 87) ■

■ SUMMARY

Causality is a way of knowing that one thing causes another. Statistical procedures that examine causality are critical to the development of nursing science because of their importance in examining the effects of interventions. The statistical procedures described in this chapter examine causality by testing for significant differences between or among groups. Statistical procedures are available for nominal, ordinal, and interval data. The procedures vary considerably in their power to detect differences and in their complexity. The procedures presented are categorized as contingency tables, nonparametric procedures, t tests, and ANOVA procedures.

Contingency tables, or cross-tabulation, allow visual comparison of summary data output related to two variables within the sample. This preliminary strategy is useful for examining large amounts of data. In most cases, the data are in the form of frequencies or percentages. By using this strategy one can compare two or more categories of one variable with two or more categories of a second variable. The chi-squared test of independence uses a contingency table to examine whether the two variables being examined are independent or related. Chi-squared is designed to test for differences in frequencies of observed data and compare them with the frequencies that could be expected to occur if the data categories were actually independent of each other. If differences are indicated, the analysis will not identify where they exist within the data. These differences can be identified by using phi, Cramer's *V*, the contingency coefficient, or lambda as post hoc tests.

Nonparametric tests are used to examine nominal or ordinal data or data that do not meet the assumptions of the normal curve. The McNemar test uses a 2×2 table to analyze changes that occur in dichotomous variables. This nonparametric test is particularly appropriate for before-and-after or pretest-posttest designs in which the subjects serve as their own control and the data are nominal. The sign test was developed for data for which it is difficult to assign numerical values. However, the data can be ranked on such dimensions as agree-disagree, easier-harder, earlier-later, more-less, higher-lower. The Wilcoxon matched-pairs signed-ranks test, like the sign test, examines changes that occur in pretest-posttest measures or matched-pairs measures. It is more powerful than the sign test because it examines both the direction and the magnitude of change that occurs. The Mann-Whitney *U* test is the most powerful of the nonparametric tests, with 95% of the power of the *t* test to detect differences between groups of normally distributed populations. If the assumptions of the *t* test are violated, such as a nonnormal distribution or ordinal-level data, the Mann-Whitney *U* test is more powerful. The Kolmogorov-Smirnov two-sample test is a nonparametric test used to determine whether two independent samples have been drawn from the same population. The Wald-Wolfowitz runs test is used to determine differences between two populations. The test will determine whether the two populations differ in any way, including central tendency, variability, or skewness. The Kruskal-Wallis test is the most powerful nonparametric test for examining three independent groups. It has 95% of the power of the *F* statistic to detect existing differences between three or more groups. The Cochran *Q* test is an extension of the McNemar test for two related samples. The Cochran *Q* test can be used in situations such as (1) when subjects have been matched and several levels of treatment have been administered, (2) when more than one matched control group has been used for comparison, or (3) for repeated measures of the dependent variable across time. The Friedman two-way ANOVA by ranks may be used with matched samples or in repeated measures. The Friedman test considers the magnitude of differences and is therefore more powerful than the Cochran *Q* test in rejecting a false null hypothesis, given the same data.

The *t* test is one of the most commonly used parametric analyses to test for significant differences between statistical measures of two samples. The *t* test is frequently misused by researchers who use multiple *t* tests to examine differences in various aspects of data collected in a study. The use of multiple *t* tests causes an escalation of significance that results in a greatly increased risk of a Type I error. The *t* test can be used only one time during analysis to examine data from the two samples in a study. The Bonferroni procedure, which controls for the escalation of significance, can be used if various *t* tests must be performed on different aspects of the same data. When samples are related, the formula used to calculate the *t* statistic is different and the *t* test for related samples is used. Samples may be related because matching has been performed as part of the design or because the scores used in the analysis were obtained from the same subjects under different conditions (e.g., pretest and posttest).

ANOVA procedures test for differences between means. When two means are being examined, ANOVA is basically the same procedure as the *t* test. ANOVA can examine data from more than two groups and compares the variance within each group with the variance between groups. The outcome of the analysis is a numerical value for the *F* statistic, which is used to determine whether the groups are significantly different. The variance within each group is a result of individual scores in the group varying from the group mean and is referred to as the within-group variance. The amount of variation about the mean in each group is assumed by ANOVA to be equal. The group means also vary around the grand mean (the mean of the total sample), which is referred to as the between-groups variance. One could assume that if all the samples were drawn from the same population, there would be little difference in these two sources of variance. The variance from within and between the groups explains the total variance in the data. Researchers who perform ANOVA on their data frequently record the results in an ANOVA summary table. If only two groups are being examined, the location of a significant difference is clear. However, if more than two groups are being studied, it is not possible to determine from the ANOVA exactly where the significant differences lie. One cannot assume that all the groups examined are significantly different. Therefore, post hoc analyses are conducted to determine the location of the differences among groups. A number of types of factorial ANOVAs have been developed to analyze data from specific experimental designs, including two-way ANOVA for studies with two independent variables, multifactorial ANOVA for studies with more than two independent variables, randomized block ANOVA, repeated measures ANOVA, and MANOVA for studies with more than one dependent variable. ANCOVA is a useful approach to analysis in pretest-posttest designs in which differences occur in groups on the pretest. It is also used to remove the effect of a confounding variable, such as age, education, social class, or anxiety level. ANCOVA partials out the variance resulting from the confounding variable by performing regression analysis before performing ANOVA.

• •

REFERENCES

Conover, W. J. (1971). *Practical nonparametric statistics.* New York: Wiley.

Goodman, L. A., & Kruskal, W. H. (1954). Measures of association for cross classifications. *Journal of the American Statistical Association, 49,* 732–764.

Goodman, L. A., & Kruskal, W. H. (1959). Measures of association for cross classifications, II: Further discussion and references. *Journal of the American Statistical Association, 54(285),* 123–163.

Goodman, L. A., & Kruskal, W. H. (1963). Measures of association for cross classifications, III: Approximate sampling theory. *Journal of the American Statistical Association, 58(302),* 310–364.

Goodman, L. A., & Kruskal, W. H. (1972). Measures of association for cross classifications, IV: Simplification of asymptotic variances. *Journal of the American Statistical Association, 67(338),* 415–421.

Jadack, R. A., Hyde, J. S., & Keller, M. L. (1995). Gender and knowledge about HIV, risky sexual behavior, and safer sex practices. *Research in Nursing & Health, 18(4),* 313–324.

Knafl, K. A. (1985). How families manage a pediatric hospitalization. *Western Journal of Nursing Research, 7(2),* 151–176.

Pedhazur, E. J., & Schmelkin, L. P. (1991). *Measurement, design, and analysis: An integrated approach.* Hillsdale, NJ: Lawrence Erlbaum.

Popkess, S. A. (1981). Assessment scales for determining the cognitive-behavioral repertoire of the obese subject. *Western Journal of Nursing Research, 3(2),* 199–215.

Siegel, S. (1956). *Nonparametric statistics for the behavioral sciences.* New York: McGraw-Hill.

Tollett, J. H., & Thomas, S. P. (1995). A theory-based nursing intervention to instill hope in homeless veterans. *Advances in Nursing Science, 18(2),* 76–90.

Volicer, B. J. (1984). *Multivariate statistics for nursing research.* New York: Grune & Stratton.

Waltz, C., & Bausell, R. B. (1981). *Nursing research: Design, statistics and computer analysis.* Philadelphia: Davis.

Wu, Y. B., & Slakter, M. J. (1989). Analysis of covariance in nursing research. *Nursing Research, 38(5),* 306–308.

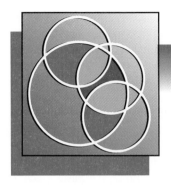

CHAPTER 23

QUALITATIVE RESEARCH METHODOLOGY

Researchers conducting a qualitative study will need to use methods of data collection and analysis that may be unique to qualitative research, although some of the techniques described in previous chapters may be useful, particularly methods of observation and interviewing as described in Chapter 16. Qualitative data analysis occurs concurrently with data collection rather than sequentially as is true in quantitative research. Therefore, the researcher is attempting to simultaneously gather the data, manage a growing bulk of collected data, and interpret the meaning of the data. Qualitative analysis techniques use words rather than numbers as the basis of analysis. However, the same careful skills in analytical reasoning are needed by qualitative researchers as in quantitative analysis. In qualitative analysis, the flow of reasoning moves from concreteness to increasing abstraction. This reasoning process guides the organization, reduction, and clustering of the findings and leads to the development of theoretical explanations.

This chapter describes some of the frequently used approaches to collection and analysis of qualitative data. Methods specific to the six qualitative approaches presented in Chapter 4 will be described, and detailed examples of published studies are provided to facilitate understanding of the techniques. The information in this chapter is sufficient to allow you to understand the process and to envision what the experience would be like if you choose to conduct this type of research. However, if you elect to conduct a qualitative study, we suggest that you seek additional sources of guidance for the process of collecting and analyzing qualitative data. Mentorship with someone experienced in the type of qualitative analysis you wish to perform is still the most useful approach to learning these skills (Morse, 1997; Sandelowski, 1997).

DATA ANALYSIS ISSUES

Researchers are confronted with several decisions regarding the approach to qualitative data analysis that will be used for a particular study. Will the analysis be performed manually or will computers be used? Will documentation of decisions related to the data analysis process be recorded? Will the researcher adhere to the methodology of a particular qualitative research approach or mix methodologies from several approaches? The following section will discuss these issues.

Using the Computer for Qualitative Analysis

Traditionally, qualitative data collection and analysis have been performed manually. The researcher recorded the data on small bits of paper or note cards, which were then carefully coded, organized, and filed at the end of a day of data gathering. Analysis requires cross-checking each bit of data with all the other bits of data on little pieces of paper. It is easy to lose data in the mass of paper.

Keeping track of connections between various bits of data requires meticulous record keeping. This method was developed because of the importance of the qualitative researcher maintaining a close link with—or being immersed in—the data being analyzed.

Some qualitative researchers believe that using the computer can make analysis of qualitative data quicker and easier without the researcher losing touch with the data (Anderson, 1987; Miles & Huberman, 1994; Pateman, 1998; Taft, 1993). Taft suggests that because of the ease of coding and recoding, the researcher feels more free to play with the data and experiment with alternative ways of coding. This freedom fosters analytical insight and thus facilitates data analysis. Researchers can also search for codes that tend to occur together. Because of easy access to the data, team research is facilitated. Pateman suggests that "some would argue that scientific, mathematically-minded people are more computer literate than those with more artistic, humanistic interests, in which case affinity with computing may have something to do with personal traits. . . . Some of the . . . arguments [by qualitative researchers against using computers] could simply be rationalisation by computer-phobic researchers." However, Taft expresses concern over the dark side of computer technology for qualitative researchers. The researcher may be tempted to study larger samples and sacrifice depth for breadth. Meaningful understanding of the data may also be sacrificed. Sandelowski (1995a) expresses concern that the use of computers will alter the aesthetics of qualitative research and suggests that the key motivation for using computer technology in qualitative research is to legitimate the claim that qualitative researchers are doing science. She states, "computer technology permits qualitative researchers to have computer printouts of data (with the veneer of objectivity they confer) comparable to their quantitative counterparts whose claims to doing science are often not questioned. Even so-called *soft* data can become *hard* when produced by *hard*ware. Qualitative work can now have the look and feel, or aesthetic features, of science" (p. 205).

The computer offers assistance in activities such as processing, storage, retrieval, cataloging, and sorting and leaves the analysis activities up to the researcher. Anderson (1987) points out that "the computer does not perform the thinking, reviewing, interpretative, and analytic functions that the researcher must do for himself or herself. Rather, the computer makes the researcher more efficient and effective in those high-level functions, and eases some of the tedious 'mindless' tasks that otherwise consume so much time and energy" (pp. 629–630). However, Sandelowski (1995a) argues that replacing and streamlining the cutting and pasting activities may be seen as desirable by some because they are uncomfortably reminiscent of childhood play. She argues against the claim that machine technology saves human labor and suggests that it may actually increase labor because of storage and retrieval of more data and that once the data are stored, one has more of a sense that it must all be accounted for in the report of results.

Computer use has several advantages over the more traditional methods of recording and storing data. Multiple copies can be made with ease, and files can be copied onto backup disks and stored at another site without the need for a large amount of storage space. Blocks of data can also be moved around in the file or copied to another file when data are being sorted by category. The same block of data could be inserted within several categories, if desired. At the same time, interviews or descriptions of observations can be kept intact for reference as needed. In addition, most word processing programs can perform sort operations and can search throughout a text file for a selected word or a string of words. Many of these activities can be performed with a traditional word processing program (Burnard, 1998). Files in a word processing program can be transferred to a database spreadsheet such as dBase or Lotus 1-2-3 to organize the data into matrices.

A number of computer programs have been developed specifically to perform qualitative analyses. One of the earliest attempts was described by Podolefsky and McCarty (1983). This program, Computer Assisted Topical Sorting (CATS), allowed the insertion of codes, designated as numbers, into a text file. A mainframe text editor provided the capacity to search for strings of characters such as words or phrases. Weitzman and Miles (1995) provide an evaluation of the currently available software used to assist in the analysis of qualitative data.

Auditability

The credibility of qualitative data analysis has been seriously questioned in some cases by the larger scientific community. The concerns expressed are related to the inability to replicate the outcomes of a study, even when using the same data set.

Miles and Huberman (1994) describe the problem as follows:

• •

"Most qualitative researchers work alone in the field. Each is a one-person research machine: defining the problem, doing the sampling, designing the instruments, collecting the information, reducing the information, analyzing it, interpreting it, writing it up. A vertical monopoly. And when we read the reports, they are most often heavy on the 'what' (the findings, the descriptions) rather than on the 'how' (how you got to the 'what'). We rarely see data displays—only the conclusions. In most cases, we don't see a procedural account of the analysis, explaining just how the researcher got from 500 pages of field notes to the main conclusions drawn. So we don't know how much confidence we can place in them. Researchers are not being cryptic or obtuse. It's just that they have a slim tradition to guide their analytic moves, and few guidelines for explaining to their colleagues what they did, and how." (Miles & Huberman, 1994, p. 262) ■

To respond to this concern, some qualitative researchers have attempted to develop strategies by which other researchers, using the same data, can follow the logic of the original researcher and arrive at the same conclusions. Guba and Lincoln (1982) refer to this strategy as auditability.

Auditability requires that the researcher establish decision rules for categorizing data, arriving at ratings, or making judgments. A decision rule might say, for example, that a datum would be placed in a specific category if it met specified criteria. Another decision rule might say that an observed interaction would be considered an instance of an emerging theoretical explanation if it met specific criteria. A record is kept of all decision rules used in the analysis of data. All raw data are stored so that they are available for review if requested. As the analysis progresses, the researcher documents the data and the decision rules on which each decision was based and the reasoning that entered into each decision. Thus, evidence is retained to support the study conclusions and the emerging theory and is made available on request (Burns, 1989). Marshall (1984, 1985), however, cautions against undermining the strengths of qualitative research by overly mechanistic data analysis. Marshall and Rossman (1989) express concern that efforts to increase validity will "filter out the unusual, the serendipitous—the puzzle that if tended to and pursued would provide a recasting of the entire research endeavor" (p. 113).

Method Mixing

Some studies are appearing in the literature in which the researchers have combined portions of various qualitative methodologies extracted from the philosophical bases for which the methodologies were developed. Morse (1989) expresses concern about the justification of this strategy and states, "Such mixing, while certainly 'do-able,' violates the assumptions of data collection techniques and methods of analysis of all the methods used. The product is not good science; the product is a sloppy mishmash" (p. 4).

It is likely that in this evolving research field, new qualitative methodologies will continue to emerge, some combining portions of previous methodologies. However, in qualitative research, the philosophy underlying the study is as important as the framework in a quantitative study and directs the interpretation of results. Therefore, it is essential that the researcher make the philosophical base of the study explicit and that the methodologies used be compatible with the philosophical base.

DATA COLLECTION METHODS

Because data collection is occurring simultaneously with data analysis, the process is complex.

The procedure of collecting data is not a mechanical process that can be carefully planned before initiation. The researcher as a whole person is totally involved—perceiving, reacting, interacting, reflecting, attaching meaning, recording. Such is the case whether the study involves observing and participating in social situations, as would occur in phenomenological, grounded theory, ethnographic, or critical social theory research, or whether the study deals with written communications of persons, as might occur in phenomenological, historical, philosophical, or critical social theory studies. For a particular study, the researcher may need to address data collection issues related to relationships between the researcher and the participants, reflections of the researcher on the meanings obtained from the data, and management and reduction of large volumes of data.

Researcher-Participant Relationships

One of the important differences between quantitative and qualitative research is the nature of relationships between the researcher and the individuals being studied. The nature of these relationships has an impact on the data collected and their interpretation. In many qualitative studies, the researcher observes social behavior and may participate in social interactions with those being studied. Field and Morse (1985) identify four types of participant observation: (1) *complete participation,* in which the observer becomes a member of the group and conceals the researcher role; (2) *participant as observer,* in which participants are aware of the dual roles of the researcher; (3) *observer as participant,* in which most of the researcher's time is spent observing and interviewing and less in the participation role; and (4) *complete observer,* in which the researcher is passive and has no direct social interaction in the setting.

In varying degrees, the researcher influences the individuals being studied and, in turn, is influenced by them. The mere presence of the researcher may alter behavior in the setting. This involvement, considered a source of bias in quantitative research, is thought by qualitative researchers to be a natural and necessary element of the research process. The researcher's personality is a key factor in qualitative research. Skills in empathy and intuition are cultivated. The researcher needs to become closely involved in the subject's experience to interpret it. It is necessary for the researcher to be open to the perceptions of the participants rather than attach his or her own meaning to the experience. Individuals being studied often participate in determining research questions, guiding data collection, and interpreting results.

The interface between the participant-observer role and the nurse role of the researcher is a concern. Because of the possible impact of the nursing role on the study, Robinson and Thorne (1988) claim that the nurse researcher has an obligation to explain in the study report the influence that his or her professional perspective had on the process and outcomes of the study. In some studies, the researcher is expected to interact with participants but to stay in the role of researcher and avoid relating to participants as a nurse. Some insist that the nurse researcher must always relate first as a nurse and second as a researcher (Cooper, 1988; Fowler, 1988). Connors (1988) suggests that qualitative researchers must be authentic and engaged as a whole person rather than just as a researcher or as a nurse.

In addition to the role one takes in the relationship, expectations of the study must be carefully considered. Munhall (1988) points out that ethically, it is essential that the qualitative researcher think through both the aims and the means of the study and determine whether these aims and means are consistent with those of the participants. For example, if the researcher's desire is to change the behavior of the participants, this goal also needs to be a desire of the participants. During the study, a level of trust develops between the researcher and the participant, who may provide information labeled as secret. Field and Morse (1985, pp. 72–73) describe situations with which the researcher may be confronted. "For example, [participants] may state that this is 'Just between you and me . . .' or 'Don't put this in your report, but. . . .' Alternatively, informants may provide information that is later regretted. They will state, 'I shouldn't have told you that yesterday. . . .' Because the researcher's first responsibility is to the informant, the informant has the right to retract information or to request that the information not be used in the report, and the researcher must respect the informant's wishes."

Establishing relationships with participants can cause harm that must be carefully considered. Participant observation requires a close relationship that invades the privacy of the individual. Although participants may experience confidence, commitment, and friendship from the encounter, they may also experience disappointment, perceived betrayal, and desertion as the researcher functions in the researcher role and then leaves (Munhall, 1988). The relationship can also cause harm to the researcher. Cowles (1988) described emotional pain and difficulty sleeping as she collected data from family members of murdered individuals. She frequently required support and opportunities to explore her feelings with colleagues during the process. Draucker (1999) cautions that little is known about the effects on participants in studies of sexual violence.

Reflexive Thought

Qualitative researchers need to critically think through the dynamic interaction between the self and the data occurring during analysis. This interaction occurs whether the data are communicated person to person or through the written word. The critical thinking used to examine this interaction is referred to as *reflexive thought* or *reflexivity* (Lamb & Huttlinger, 1989). During this process, the researcher explores personal feelings and experiences that may influence the study and integrates this understanding into the study. The process requires a conscious awareness of self.

Drew (1989), in a paper recounting her experience conducting a phenomenological study of caregiving behavior, described the impact of relationships on her study.

• •

"A session with a person who had been willing to talk about his or her experiences with caregivers, and who had invested energy into the interview session, often generated for me a sense of doing something worthwhile, as well as a feeling that I

would be competent to analyze the transcribed material in a meaningful way. This sense of competency dispelled any doubts about being an intruder. I became relaxed, unself-conscious, and more self-assured. However, an encounter with a person with blunt affect, abrupt answers, and a paucity of responses left me feeling awkward and self-conscious. A sense of doubt about the validity of my project encroached as I attempted to elicit that person's thoughts. At the time, my immediate reaction was to think that I had obtained nothing from these individuals, when in fact, as I was to discover later, the 'nothing' was something important that I was as yet unable to see.

"It was at the point of discouragement about my interviewing skills that I became aware that I was mentally classifying interviews as either 'good' or 'bad,' depending on my emotional response to the subjects. Good interviews were those in which I felt effective as an interviewer and was able to facilitate the person's recounting of experiences with caregivers. I enjoyed the interaction and felt that we connected on some level that produced meaningful discussion about the topic of relationships between patient and caregiver.

"Bad interviews, on the other hand, were those in which I could not seem to get subjects to talk about how they had experienced their caregivers. There seemed to be no questions that I could devise with which to explore feelings, either positive or negative, with them. They gave no indications of awareness of their feelings, or of feelings in others. Whereas the subjects of the good interviews were people I experienced as open, curious, and thoughtful, those of the bad interviews were experienced as distrustful and elicited in me a sense of anxiety and frustration; it seemed I could not get through to them. I felt inadequate as an interviewer and was ready to discard these interviews. Frustration and anxiety arose because I felt that I was not getting the information that I needed for the study.

"Subsequently, I discovered that my feelings of frustration and inadequacy were causing me to overlook data and that when I could put them aside, new data that were rich in meaning became apparent. . . . This discovery was a powerful experience for me, affecting my approach to subsequent interviews and influencing analysis of data thereafter." (Drew, 1989, pp. 433–434) ■

In some phenomenological research, especially for researchers using the Husserl interpretation of phenomenology, this critical thinking leads to bracketing, which is used to help the researcher avoid misinterpreting the phenomenon as it is being experienced by the individual. *Bracketing* is suspending or laying aside what is known about the experience being studied (Oiler, 1982). Other phenomenologists, especially those using Heideggerian phenomenology, do not bracket. However, they do identify beliefs, assumptions, and preconceptions about the research topic, which are put in writing at the beginning of the study for self-reflection and external review. These procedures are intended to facilitate openness and new insight.

Data Management and Reduction

Data collected during a qualitative study may be narrative descriptions of observations, transcripts from tape recordings of interviews, entries in the researcher's diary reflecting on the dynamics of the setting, or notes taken while reading written documents. In the initial phases of data analysis, you need to become very familiar with the data as you gather them. This process may involve reading and rereading notes and transcripts, recalling observations and experiences, listening to tapes, and viewing videotapes until you have become immersed in the data. Tapes contain more than words; they contain feeling, emphasis, and nonverbal communications. These aspects are at least as important to the communication as the words. In phenomenology, this immersion in the data is referred to as *dwelling with the data.*

Because of the volumes of data acquired in a qualitative study, initial efforts at analysis focus on reducing the volume of data to facilitate examination, a process referred to as *data reduction*. During data reduction, you begin attaching meaning to elements in your data. You will discover classes of things, persons, and events and detect properties that characterize things, persons, and events. You will also note regularities in the setting or the peo-

ple. These discoveries will lead to classifying elements in your data. In some cases, you may use the classification scheme used by participants or authors. In other cases, you may wish to construct your own classification scheme.

According to Sandelowski (1995b), "Although data preparation is a distinctive stage in qualitative work where data are put into a form that will permit analysis, a rudimentary kind of analysis often begins when the researcher proofs transcripts against the audiotaped interviews from which they were prepared. Indeed, the proofing process is often the first time a researcher gets a sense of the interview as a whole; it is, occasionally, the first time investigators will hear something said, even though they conducted the interview. During the proofing process, researchers will often underline key phrases, simply because they make some as yet inchoate impression on them. They may jot down ideas in the margins next to the text that triggered them, just because they do not want to lose some line of thinking" (p. 373).

TRANSCRIBING INTERVIEWS

Tape-recorded interviews are generally transcribed word for word. Field and Morse (1985) provide the following instructions for transcribing a tape-recorded interview.

• •

"Pauses are denoted in the transcript with dashes, while series of dots indicate gaps or prolonged pauses. All exclamations, including laughter and expletives, are included. Instruct the typist to type interviews single-spaced with a blank line between speakers. A generous margin on both sides of the page permits the left margin to be used for coding and the researcher's own critique of the interview style, and the right margin to be used for comments regarding the content. . . . Start a new paragraph each time a topic is changed. . . . Ensure that all pages are numbered sequentially and that each page is coded with the interview number and the informant's number." (Field & Morse, 1985, pp. 97–99) ■

Sandelowski (1994) indicates that the researcher must make choices of what features about the interview to preserve in print. These choices directly influence the nature and direction of the analysis. Once the interview is transcribed, the transcript takes on an independent reality and becomes the researcher's raw data. Sandelowski suggests that the process of transcription alters reality. The text is "many transformations removed from the so-called unadulterated reality it was intended to represent" (p. 312). She recommends asking the following questions regarding transcription:

1. Is a transcript necessary to achieve the research goals?
2. If a transcription is required, what features of the interview event should be preserved (if at all possible) and what features can be safely ignored?
3. What notation system should be used?
4. What purposes besides investigator analysis per se will the transcript serve? (Sandelowski, 1994, pp. 312–313)

Sandelowski points out that transcriptions require about 3½ hours for each 1 hour of interview time. The cost for this work may be as high as $20/hour for an experienced typist.

After transcriptions are completed, Field and Morse (1985) advise making at least three copies of transcripts and keeping the original separate from copies. One set of copies should be locked in a separate location to ensure against fire damage or loss. If the researcher is working in the field, one copy should be mailed home separately. Placing all data from your study in one suitcase when traveling is inviting disaster.

Listen to the tape recordings as soon after the interview as possible. Listen carefully to voice tone, inflection, and pauses of both the researcher and participant, as well as the content. These features may indicate that the topic is very emotional or very important. While you are listening, read the written transcript of the tape. Make notations of your observations on the transcript (Field & Morse, 1985).

Ayers and Poirier (1996) point out that "qualitative analysis results from the recontextualization of chunks of data, always with the caveat that the new context must in some way be faithful to its origins. Narrative data are meaningless without context" (p. 164). Using the reader response theory emerging from the work of Iser (1980) and Kermode (1983),

Ayers and Poirier indicate that "the meaning of a text arises from the interaction of the mind (including the personal history) of the reader with the content of the text (which in turn arose from the mind and personal history of the interview respondent)" (p. 164). Reading the text results in an interaction between the mind and personal history of the respondent and the mind and personal history of the researcher. This interaction results in the emergence of a "virtual text," which is the entity being interpreted. Thus, there is no real objective, authentic information from which only one correct interpretation can be made. The text does not explain everything. "Motives, histories, antecedents, and causal links, sometimes entire subplots are left to the reader, to the researcher, to infer" (Ayers & Poirier, 1996, p. 165). The process of interpretation occurs in the mind of the reader. The virtual text grows in size and complexity as the researcher reads and rereads. Throughout the process of analysis, the virtual text develops and evolves. Although multiple valid interpretations may occur if the text is examined by different researchers, all findings must remain trustworthy to the data. This trustworthiness applies to the unspoken meanings emerging from the totality of the data, not just the written words of the text.

The following is a description of some of the techniques used by qualitative researchers during the process of data analysis and interpretation. These techniques include coding, reflective remarks, marginal remarks, memoing, and developing propositions.

CODES AND CODING

Coding is a means of categorizing. A code is a symbol or abbreviation used to classify words or phrases in the data. Codes may be placed in the data at the time of data collection, when entering data into the computer, or during later examination of the data. Through the selection of categories, or codes, the researcher is defining the domain of the study. Therefore, it is important that the codes be consistent with the philosophical base of the study. Organization of data, selection of specific elements of the data for categories, and naming these categories will reflect the philosophical base used for the study. Later in the study, coding may progress to the development of a taxonomy. For example, you might develop a taxonomy of types of pain, types of patients, or types of patient education.

Field and Morse (1985) suggest that when selecting elements of the data to code, you note

1. the kinds of things that are going on in the context being studied;
2. the forms a phenomenon takes; and
3. any variations within a phenomenon. (Field & Morse, 1985, p. 104)

Characteristics such as "acts (one-shot events), activities (ongoing events), verbal productions that direct actions (meanings), participation of the actors, interrelationships among actions and the setting of the study [might be included]. . . . In the anthropological tradition, the history, social structure, recurring events, economy, authority, beliefs, and values of a community may constitute the initial list of universal categories used to organize data" (Field & Morse, 1985, p. 104). Although a classification system can identify the elements of interest and name them, it cannot identify processes.

Initial categories should be as broad as possible, but categories should not overlap. As more data are collected in relation to a particular category, the major category can be sectioned into smaller categories. Field and Morse (1985) find that "it is difficult during the initial data coding stage to work with more than ten major codes" (p. 101).

Field and Morse (1985) also suggest several innovative strategies for coding data. One approach is to use highlighter pens, with a different color for each major category. Another strategy, developed by Murdock (1971), is to assign each major category a number. The number is inserted in the computerized text. With this approach, a word or phrase in the text could easily have several codes indicated by numbers. Anthropologists have used McBee cards, which have holes punched in the top. The holes are used to sort data by category. Knafl and Webster (1988) suggest using colored markers, colored paper clips, colored index cards, or Post-it stickers to identify categories of data. Codes are often written in the margins. Data can then be sorted by cutting the pages into sections according to codes. Each section can be taped or pasted onto an index card for filing. This procedure can just as easily be performed by computer programs for qualitative analysis in which broad margins are available for coding. In this case, computerized data can be sorted by code into a separate file for each code while retaining identification by such identifiers as data and source.

Field and Morse (1985) color-code each page of a transcript in the left margin. One colored stripe is used for each participant and another for the interviewing sequence. When the pages are cut up according to topical codes, identification of the participant and the interviewing sequence is left intact.

Knafl and Webster (1988) described their coding process as follows:

• •

"In order to develop coding categories, the co-principal investigators (PIs) and research staff independently read through a sample of interview transcripts, taking notes on the major topics discussed in the interviews. The PIs and staff then met to compare and revise the categories individually arrived at and to determine 'semifinal' coding categories. Each category was assigned a number. Next, using the number system, the PIs and research staff independently applied the categories to a second sample of interview transcripts. The PIs and staff again met to compare their individual applications of the categories. The purpose of this second comparison was to identify ambiguities, overlap, and lack of clarity in the categories.

"During the entire process of developing coding categories, a record was maintained of criteria used in applying coding categories to the data. From this record, a codebook was developed in order to ensure consistent application of final coding categories. The codebook included the criteria for applying each category and a brief excerpt of data exemplifying each category.

"All data subsequently were coded by indicating the number of the appropriate category or categories in the margin of the interview transcript. Each of the PIs worked with one of the research assistants in coding the data. In order to enhance consistency in application of the coding categories, each member of a PI–research assistant pair coded data independently and then met to compare application of the categories and resolve any differences. In addition, the PIs and research assistants met as a group on a regularly scheduled basis to discuss issues and questions regarding coding.

"After completing the coding, the research assistant transferred the data to index cards. This was accomplished by photocopying the interview transcripts, cutting up the copies (with care taken to preserve wholeness and meaning of content) and taping the cut-up portions on 5 × 8 index cards. A color code system was devised, so that different categories of data were taped to different colored index cards." (Knafl & Webster, 1988, pp. 200–201) ■

The types of codes that can be used are descriptive, interpretative, and explanatory. *Descriptive codes* classify elements of the data by using terms that describe how the researcher is organizing the data. It is the simplest method of classification and is commonly used in the initial stages of data analysis. Descriptive codes remain close to the terms used by the participant being interviewed. For example, if you were reading a transcribed interview in which a participant was describing experiences in the first days after surgery, you might use descriptive codes such as PAIN, MOVING, FEAR, REST.

Interpretative codes are usually developed later in the data-collecting process as the researcher gains some insight into the processes occurring and begins to move beyond simply sorting statements. The participant's terms are used to attach meanings to these statements. For example, in a study of postoperative experiences, you might begin to recognize that the participant was investing much energy in seeking relief of symptoms and seeking information about how the health care providers believed that he or she is doing. These might be classified by using interpretative codes of RELIEF and INFO.

Explanatory codes are developed late in the data-collecting process after theoretical ideas from the study have begun to emerge. The explanatory codes are part of the researcher's attempt to unravel the meanings inherent in the situation. These codes connect the data to the emerging theory, and the

codes used may be specific to the theory or be more general, such as PATT (pattern), TH (theme), or CL (causal link). Typically, codes will not stay the same throughout the study. Some codes will have to be divided into subclassifications. Other codes may be discontinued because they do not work.

REFLECTIVE REMARKS

While the notes are being recorded, thoughts or insights often emerge into the consciousness of the researcher. These thoughts are generally included within the notes and are separated from the rest of the notes by double parentheses (( )). Later, they may need to be extracted and used for memoing (Miles & Huberman, 1994).

MARGINAL REMARKS

As the notes are being reviewed, observations about them need to be written immediately. These remarks are usually placed in the right-hand margin of the notes. The remarks often connect the notes with other parts of the data or suggest new interpretations. Reviewing notes can become boring, which is a signal that thinking has ceased. Making marginal notes assists the researcher in "retaining a thoughtful stance" (Miles & Huberman, 1994).

MEMOING

A *memo* is developed by the researcher to record insights or ideas related to notes, transcripts, or codes. Memos move the researcher toward theorizing and are conceptual rather than factual. They may link pieces of data together or use a specific piece of data as an example of a conceptual idea. The memo may be written to someone else in the study or may be just a note to oneself. The important thing is to value one's ideas and get them written down quickly. Whenever an idea emerges, even if it is vague and not well thought out, it needs to be written down immediately. One's initial feeling is that the idea is so clear in one's mind that it can be written later. However, the thought is soon forgotten and often cannot be retrieved again. As one becomes immersed in the data, these ideas will occur at odd times, such as 2 AM, when one is driving, or when one is preparing a meal. Therefore, it is advisable to keep paper and pencil handy. If one is awakened with an idea, it should be written down immediately; it may be gone by morning. Memos need to be dated, titled with the key concept discussed, and connected by codes with the field notes or forms that generated the thoughts (Miles & Huberman, 1994).

MULTIMEDIA ANALYSIS

The purpose of any sort of analysis of transcripts is to ascertain meaning. The type of meaning sought may vary. However, meaning in an interaction is not conveyed totally through the words that are used. The way in which the words were expressed may be critical to the meaning being conveyed. In addition, approximately 70% of communication is nonverbal. As Burnard (1995) wisely points out, "often the words used are not particularly relevant or are not 'registered' by the parties involved in a conversation. We do not, after all, usually pick our words very carefully when we speak, nor do we continually 'check each other' to ascertain that understanding has occurred. And yet we do understand one another, most of the time." In some cases, the words used have little or no meaning. They are used to convey unstated meanings. The meanings are "behind" the words. It may be impossible to capture this meaning through analyzing transcripts. The participant, asked for an exact interpretation of what was meant, may not be able to explain the meaning. Sometimes, "words do not convey any meaning at all but instead create a mood. . . . Sometimes words can be used as 'fillers' between pieces of information. . . . In summary, then, it seems possible that we communicate, using words, in many different ways. First, we may use words precisely and to convey very definite concepts. Second, we may use words to convey or to create moods. In this case, we are not conveying particular or precise meanings. Third, it may be that we communicate in chunks of words and phrases. Finally, in this summation, we may note that not everything we say is of equal importance—either to ourselves or to the listener. All of these factors make the likelihood of a researcher, using textual data and a method of textual analysis, uncovering the precise meaning of pieces of communication an unlikely scenario. . . . Transcripts are always post hoc—they always occur after and, sometimes, at some distance from the original interviews. This means that the reader of the transcripts—the researcher—always comes to the transcripts too late. What 'really happened' in the interview has been lost" (Burnard, 1995).

One way to address this problem is to use multiple data collection methods. Interviews might be videotaped as well as audiotaped. Analysis by the researcher might be strengthened by simultaneously reviewing video and audio transmissions while reviewing the transcript. Parse (1990) refers to this process as immersion in the data. Multimedia computers are now available in which text, video, graphical media, and sound can be used for such immersion. Burnard (1995) foresees a time when CD-ROM disks might be used to store these multimedia data sets. Use of this type of integrated and triangulated approach to analysis would provide a richer understanding of meaning.

DEVELOPING PROPOSITIONS

As the study progresses, relationships among categories, participants, actions, and events will begin to emerge. You will develop hunches about relationships that can be used to formulate tentative propositions. If the study is being conducted by a team of researchers, everyone involved in the study can participate in the development of propositions. Statements or propositions can be written on index cards and sorted into categories or entered into the computer. A working list can then be printed and shared among the researchers to generate further discussion (Miles & Huberman, 1994).

Displaying Data for Analysis and Presentation

Displays contain highly condensed versions of the outcomes of qualitative research. They are equivalent to the summary tables of statistical outcomes developed in quantitative research and allow the researcher to get the main ideas of the research across succinctly. Strategies for achieving displays are limited only by the imagination of the researcher. Some suggested ideas follow. Displays can be relatively easily developed by using computer spreadsheets, graphics programs, or desktop publishing programs. Miles and Huberman (1994) provide very helpful guidelines for the development of displays of qualitative data.

CRITICAL INCIDENT CHART

In some studies, the researcher, in an effort to gain increased insight into the dynamics of a process, identifies critical incidents occurring in the course of that process. The researcher can then compare these critical incidents in various subgroups of participants. The critical incidents and the subgroups can then be placed in a matrix listing the critical incidents in relation to time. Examination of the matrix can facilitate comparison of critical incidents in terms of timing and variation across participants or subgroups.

CAUSAL NETWORK

As the data are collected and analyzed, the researcher gains increasing understanding of the dynamics involved in the process under study. This understanding might be considered a tentative theory. The first tentative theories are vague and poorly pieced together. In some cases, they are altogether wrong. The best way to verify a tentative theory is to share it with others, particularly informants in the study situation. Informants have their own tentative theories, which have never been clearly expressed. The tentative theory needs to be expressed as a map. Developing a good map of the tentative theory is difficult and requires some hard work. The development of a tentative theory and an associated map is discussed in Chapter 7.

The validity of predictions developed in a tentative theory must be tested. However, finding effective ways to perform such testing is difficult. Predictions are usually developed near the end of the study. Because the findings are often context specific, the predictions must be tested on the same sample or on a sample that is very similar. One

strategy suggested is to predict outcomes expected to occur 6 months after completion of the study. Six months later, these predictions can be sent to informants who participated in the study. The informants can be asked to respond to the accuracy of (1) the predictions and (2) the explanation of why the prediction was expected to occur (Miles & Huberman, 1994).

COGNITIVE MAPPING

Cognitive mapping has been used for analysis and display as an alternative to transcribing taped interview data (Northcott, 1996). The technique might also be used as an adjunct to other approaches to analysis. A cognitive map is a visual representation of the information provided by a participant. It represents the conceptualizations and interpretations of the participant by the researcher. The ideas are mapped by the researcher onto a single page, including codes (concepts) and relationships among the codes (similar to the conceptual maps described in Chapter 7), as the researcher listens repeatedly to the taped interview. The interview is not transcribed. The procedure is designed to condense the process of coding, categorizing, and interpreting into one activity. Mapping is performed within 4 days of the interview. For a 45-minute interview, the researcher should allow 3 hours for cognitive mapping. Guidelines for performing cognitive mapping are as follows:

1. Generate field notes immediately after the interview and have them available for the cognitive mapping.
2. Use a large sheet of paper and a black pen (to facilitate photocopying) for the mapping.
3. Listen to the tape without stopping to write comments and rewind the tape.
4. Begin mapping. Start in the center of the paper with a pivotal word (code) and branch out as needed. Listen repeatedly to the tape as you develop the map to ensure that the map accurately reflects the participant's ideas.
5. Consider the data "cognitively." This process may require formulating codes, establishing relationships (or propositions), and recording non-

verbal data. You may need to take breaks to allow time for thought.

6. Keep verbatim quotes from the tape separately and indicate where they emerge on the map.

7. Annotate the map to indicate connections and respondent or researcher input.

8. As a second-level analysis, develop a "macro" map that combines content from all the individual cognitive maps. This map will initiate theory building from the analysis.

Drawing and Verifying Conclusions

Unlike the case in quantitative research, conclusions are formed throughout the data analysis process. Conclusions are similar to the findings in a quantitative study. Miles and Huberman (1994) identified 12 tactics used to draw and verify conclusions.

COUNTING

Qualitative researchers have tended to avoid any use of numbers. However, when judgments of qualities are made, counting is occurring. The researcher states that a pattern occurs "frequently" or "more often." Something is considered "important" or "significant." These judgments are made in part by counting. If the researcher is counting, it should be recognized and planned. Counting can help researchers see what they have, it can help verify a hypothesis, and it can help keep one intellectually honest. Qualitative researchers work by insight and intuition; however, their conclusions can be wrong. It is easier to see confirming evidence than to see disconfirming evidence. Comparing insights with numbers can be a good method of verification (Miles & Huberman, 1994).

NOTING PATTERNS, THEMES

People easily identify patterns, themes, and gestalts from their observations—almost too easily. The difficulty is in seeking real additional evidence of that pattern while remaining open to disconfirming evidence. Any pattern that is identified should be subjected to skepticism—that of the researcher and that of others (Miles & Huberman, 1994).

• •

"The researcher must distinguish between representative cases and anecdotal cases. Representative cases appear with regularity and encompass the range of behaviors described within a category. The anecdotal case appears infrequently and depicts a small range of events which are atypical of the larger group. . . . Negative cases are those episodes that clearly refute an emergent theory or proposition. Negative cases are important as they help to clarify additional causal properties which influence the phenomena under study." (Field & Morse, 1985, p. 106) ▪

SEEING PLAUSIBILITY

Often during analysis, a conclusion is seen as plausible. It seems to fit; it "makes good sense." When asked how one arrived at that point, the researcher may state that it "just feels right." These intuitive feelings are important in both qualitative and quantitative research. However, plausibility cannot stand alone. After plausibility must come systematic analysis. First, intuition occurs and, then, careful examination of the data to verify the validity of that intuition (Miles & Huberman, 1994).

CLUSTERING

Clustering is the process of sorting elements into categories or groups. It is the first step in inductive theorizing. To cluster objects, people, or behavior into a group, one must first conceptualize them as having similar patterns or characteristics. Clusters, however, like patterns, must be viewed with caution and verified. Alternative ways to cluster may be found that would be more meaningful (Miles & Huberman, 1994).

MAKING METAPHORS

Miles and Huberman (1994) suggest that qualitative researchers should think and write metaphorically. A metaphor uses figurative language to suggest a likeness or analogy of one kind of idea used in the place of another. Metaphors provide a strong image with a feeling tone that is powerful in communicating meaning. For example, stating rationally and logically that you are in a heavy work situation does not provide the emotional appeal and meaning that you could express by saying, "I am up to my ears in work!" Miles and Huberman also believe that metaphors add meaning to the findings and use the example of a mother's separation anxiety, a phrase "which is less appealing, less suggestive, and less theoretically powerful than the empty nest syndrome" (p. 221). The phrase "empty nest syndrome" communicates images loaded with meaning far beyond that conveyed by the words alone.

Metaphors are also *data-reducing devices* that involve generalizing from the particulars. They are *patternmaking devices* that place the pattern into a larger context. Metaphors are also effective *decentering devices*. They force the viewer to step back from the mass of particular observations to see the larger picture. Metaphors are also ways of *connecting findings* to theory. They are what initiates the researcher to think in more general terms. A few suggestions about developing metaphors may be of use: (1) It is unwise to look for metaphors early in the study. (2) To develop metaphors, one must be cognitively playful and move from the denotative to the connotative. Interacting with others in a cognitively playful environment can be useful. (3) Metaphors can be taken too far in terms of meaning; therefore, one must know when to stop.

SPLITTING VARIABLES

Qualitative research is strongly oriented toward integrating concepts. However, in some cases, researchers must recognize the need for differentiation. They must have the courage to question; Miles and Huberman refer to this early integration as *premature parsimony*. Splitting variables is particularly important during the initial stages of the analysis to allow more detailed examination of the processes that are occurring. It also often occurs with the development of matrices. During theorizing, if the variable does not seem to relate well with the rest of the framework, it may have to be split to allow a more coherent, integrated model to be developed (Miles & Huberman, 1994).

SUBSUMING PARTICULARS INTO THE GENERAL

This process is similar to clustering in that it involves the clumping of things together. Clustering tends to be intuitive and is similar to coding. Subsuming particulars into the general is a move from the specific and concrete to the abstract and theoretical.

FACTORING

The idea of factoring is taken from the quantitative procedure of factor analysis. If one has a list of characteristics, are there general themes within the list that allow one to explain more clearly what is going on? As with factor analysis, when clusters have been identified, they must be named. Factoring can occur at several levels of abstraction in the data. The important consideration is that they make a meaningful difference in clarity (Miles & Huberman, 1994).

NOTING RELATIONSHIPS BETWEEN VARIABLES

The development of relationships between variables was discussed previously. However, at this point, it is important to go beyond verifying that a relationship in fact exists to explain the relationship. The relationships described in Chapter 7 can be used to describe qualitative findings. Some relationships that might occur are as follows:

1. A+, B+ (both are high, or both low at the same time)
2. A+, B− (A is high, B is low, or vice versa)
3. A $\uparrow$, B $\uparrow$ (A has increased, and B has increased)
4. A $\uparrow$, B $\downarrow$ (A has increased, and B has decreased)
5. A $\uparrow$ then → B $\uparrow$ (A increased first, then B increased)
6. A $\uparrow$ then → B $\uparrow$ then A $\uparrow$ (A increased, then B increased, then A increased some more) (Miles & Huberman, 1994, p. 257)

FINDING INTERVENING VARIABLES

In some cases, the researcher believes that two variables should go together; however, the findings do not verify this thinking. In other cases, two variables are found during data analysis to go together, but their connection cannot be explained. In both these situations, a third variable may be responsible for the confusion. Therefore, the third variable must be identified. The matrices described earlier can be very useful in searching for this variable, and the search often requires some careful detective work. Finding an intervening variable is easiest when multiple cases of the two-variable relationship can be examined (Miles & Huberman, 1994).

BUILDING A LOGICAL CHAIN OF EVIDENCE

At first glance, this step would seem to be the same activity described earlier that resulted in the development of a tentative theory; however, this activity assumes the prior development of a tentative theory. Building a logical chain of evidence involves testing that theory. The researcher must go back and carefully trace evidence from the data through development of the tentative theory; the elements, relationships, and propositions of the theory are then tested against new data. The researcher looks for cases that closely fit the theory and for those that clearly do not fit the theory. The theory may then be modified.

This process is referred to as *analytical induction* and uses two interlocking cycles. The first cycle is *enumerative induction,* in which a number and variety of instances are collected that verify the model. The second cycle, *eliminative induction,* requires that the hypothesis be tested against alternatives. The researcher is required to check carefully for limits to generalizability of the theory. The process of constant comparisons used in grounded theory is related to eliminative induction (Miles & Huberman, 1994).

MAKING CONCEPTUAL/THEORETICAL COHERENCE

The previous steps have described a gradual move from empirical data to a conceptual overview of the findings. Inferences have been made as the analysis moved from the concrete to the more abstract. The steps then moved from metaphors to interrelationships, then to constructs, and from there to theories. The theory must now be connected with other existing theories in the body of knowledge.

To accomplish this step, one must develop familiarity with a wide variety of theories that could be used to explain the current phenomenon. If connections can be made with other theories, it further strengthens the present theoretical explanation (Miles & Huberman, 1994).

CONTENT ANALYSIS

Content analysis is designed to classify the words in a text into a few categories chosen because of their theoretical importance. Because content analysis uses counting, it is not considered a qualitative analysis technique by many qualitative researchers. Content analysis is frequently used in historical research. It is the primary approach to analysis used by Kalisch and colleagues (1977, 1982, 1983, 1985) in their series of studies examining the image of nursing as reflected in news media and prime-time television.

The technique provides a systematic means of measuring the frequency, order, or intensity of occurrence of words, phrases, or sentences. Initially, the specific characteristics of the content to be measured must be defined, and then rules are developed by the researcher for identifying and recording these characteristics. The researcher first selects a specific unit of analysis, which may be individual words, word combinations, or themes. This unit of analysis is considered a symbolic entity and is often an indicator of an abstract concept. Downe-Wamboldt (1992, p. 314) points out that "content analysis is more than a counting game; it is concerned with meanings, intentions, consequences, and context. To describe the occurrences of words, phrases, or sentences without consideration of the contextual environment of the data is inappropriate and inadequate."

To perform content analysis, text is divided into units of meaning (idea categories). These units are then quantified according to specific rules. Construction of idea categories along with selection of words considered representative of these idea categories is a crucial phase of content analysis. In more complex studies, more than one categorizing scheme may be used. One common approach to categorization is the use of a dictionary to identify terms and delineate their meaning (Kelly & Sime, 1990).

In some studies, the researcher is searching for latent meaning within the text. In these studies the text cannot be analyzed by direct observation or identification of specific terms. Meaning may have to be inferred by more indirect means. The researcher may be looking for relationships among ideas, reality, and language (Kelly & Sime, 1990).

Storytelling

During observation and interviewing, the researcher may record stories shared by participants. Banks-Wallace (1998) describes a story as "an event or series of events, encompassed by temporal or spatial boundaries, that are shared with others using an oral medium or sign language. Storytelling is the process or interaction used to share stories. People sharing a story (storytellers) and those listening to a story (storytakers) are the main elements of storytelling" (p. 17). Stories can be instructive in understanding a phenomenon of interest. In some qualitative studies, the focus of the research may be the gathering of stories. Gathering of stories can enable health care providers to develop storytelling as a powerful means to increase insight and facilitate health promotion behavior in clients. For example, Nwoga (1997, 2000) studied storytelling by African American mothers in guiding their adolescent daughters regarding sexuality. The stories used by these mothers, captured by Nwoga, could be useful in assisting other mothers struggling to help their daughters deal with sexuality issues.

Coffey and Atkinson (1996) discuss the importance of capturing stories in qualitative studies.

• •

"The story is an obvious way for social actors, in talking to strangers (e.g., the researcher), to retell key experiences and events. Stories serve a variety of functions. Social actors often remember and order their careers or memories as a series of narrative chronicles, that is, as series of stories marked by key happenings. Similarly, stories and legends are told and retold by members of particular social groups or organizations as a way of passing on a cultural heritage or an organizational culture. Tales of success or tales of key leaders/personalities are familiar genres with which to maintain a collective sense of the culture of an organization. The use of atrocity stories and morality fables is also well documented within organizational and occupational settings. Stories of medical settings are especially well documented (Atkinson, 1992; Dingwall, 1997). Here tales of professional incompetence are used to given warning of 'what not to do' and what will happen if you commit mistakes. . . . Narratives are also a common genre from which to retell or come to terms with particularly sensitive or traumatic times and events." (Coffey & Atkinson, 1996, p. 56) ■

Narrative analysis is a qualitative means of formally analyzing stories. In this method, the researcher "unpacks" the structure of the story. A story includes a sequence of events with a beginning, a middle, and an end. Stories have their own logic and are temporal (Coffey & Atkinson, 1996; Denzin, 1989). The structures can also be used to determine how people tell stories, how they give shape to the events that they describe, how they make a point, how they "package" events and react to them, and how they communicate their stories to audiences. The structure used for narrative analysis as identified by Coffey and Atkinson (1996, p. 58) is as follows:

Structure	Question
Abstract	What is this about?
Orientation	Who? What? When? Where?
Complication	Then what happened?
Evaluation	So what?
Result	What finally happened?
Coda	Finish narrative

The abstract initiates the narrative by summarizing the point of the story or by giving a statement of the proposition that the narrative will illustrate. Orientation provides an introduction to the major events central to the story. Complication continues the narrative by describing complications in the event that make it a story; it takes the form "and then what happened?" Evaluation is the point of the narrative, followed by the result, that gives the outcome or resolution of events. The coda ends the story and is a transition point at which talk may revert to other topics.

The narrative analysis can focus on social action embedded in the text or examine the effect of the story. Stories serve a purpose. They may make a point or be moralistic. They may be success stories or may be a reminder of what not to do or how not to be, with guidance on how to avoid the fate described in the story. The purpose of the story can be the starting point for a more extensive narrative analysis. Narrative analysis may examine multiple stories of key life events and gain greater understanding of the impact of these key events, it may assist in understanding the relationship between social processes and personal lives, and it may be used to understand cultural values, meanings, and personal experiences. Issues related to power, dominance, and opposition can be examined. Through stories, silenced groups can be given voice (Coffey & Atkinson, 1996).

Coding is not used in narrative analysis. Coding breaks data up into separate segments and is not useful in analyzing a story; the researcher can lose the sense that informants are providing an account or narrative of events.

Qualitative researchers may choose to communicate the findings of their study as a story. A story can be a powerful way to make a point. Stories can be presented to readers from a variety of perspectives: chronological order, the order in which the story was originally presented, progressive focusing, focusing only on a critical or key event in the story, describing the plot and characters as one would stage a play, following an analytical framework, providing versions of an event from the stories of several viewers, or presenting the story as one would write a mystery story and thus appealing to problem solvers.

Life Stories

A life story is a narrative analysis designed to reconstruct and interpret the life of an ordinary person. The methodology, which emerged from anthropology and more recently from phenomenology, has been described by a number of scholars (Bateson, 1989; Bertaux, 1981; Frank, 1979; Gergen & Gergen, 1983; Josselson & Leiblich, 1995; Linde, 1993; Mattingly & Garro, 1994; Polkinghorne, 1988; Sarbin, 1986; Tanner et al., 1993; Ventres, 1994). The life story can be used to understand the meanings of various states of health, chronic illness, and disability in the lives of patients, their families, and other caregivers. These stories can help us understand the meaning to patients of their health behavior, life styles, illnesses, or impairments; the meaning of symptoms; their experiences of treatment; how they adapt; and their hopes and the possibilities of reconstructing their lives. Interviews are tape-recorded and transcribed. Notes from observations may be important, and personal documents such as diaries or historical records may be used. Analysis involves more than just stringing events together; events should be linked in an interpretation that the researcher can make theoretical sense of. Materials are organized and analyzed according to theoretical interests. Constructing a life story often requires a long-term contact and extensive collaboration with the participant (Frank, 1996; Larson & Fanchiang, 1996; Mallinson et al., 1996).

RESEARCH METHODOLOGY OF SPECIFIC QUALITATIVE APPROACHES

Phenomenological Research Methods

In phenomenological studies, several strategies can be used for data collection, and it is possible to use combinations of strategies. To conduct these data collection strategies, the researcher involves his or her personality and uses intuiting. *Intuiting* is the process of actually looking at the phenomenon. During intuiting, the researcher focuses all awareness and energy on the subject of interest to allow an increase in insight. Thus, this process requires absolute concentration and complete absorption with the experience being studied (Oiler, 1982). Intuiting is a strange idea to those of us in the Western world. It is a more common practice in Eastern thought and is related to meditation practices and the directing of personal energy forces.

DATA COLLECTION STRATEGIES

In one data collection strategy, participants are asked to describe verbally their experiences of a phenomenon. These verbal data need to be collected in a relaxed atmosphere with sufficient time allowed to facilitate a complete description by the respondent. Alternatively, informants can be asked to provide a written description of their experiences. Ruffing-Rahal (1986) recommends the use of personal documents, particularly autobiographical accounts, as a source of data.

Another strategy requires that the researcher be more directly involved in the experience. During the participant's experience, the researcher simultaneously observes verbal and nonverbal behavior, the environment, and his or her own responses to the situation. Written notes may be used, or the experience may be tape-recorded or videotaped. When observed behavior is being recorded, the researcher describes rather than evaluates observations.

Several variations may be used to analyze phenomenological data. Porter (1998) clarifies the steps of the Husserlian method in Table 23–1. Beck (1994) compares the three methods of Van Kaam, Giorgi, and Colaizzi in Table 23–2. Within nursing, Parse (1990) has developed a methodology that is now being used in phenomenological nursing studies.

Van Kaam

Van Kaam (1966) suggests classifying data and ranking the classifications according to the frequency of occurrence. This ranking is verified by a panel of judges. The number of categories is then reduced to eliminate overlapping, vague, or intricate categories, and again, agreement of the panel of judges is sought. Hypotheses are developed to explain the categories theoretically, and these hypotheses are tested on a new sample. This process is continued until no new categories emerge.

Giorgi

Giorgi (1970) recommends a similar process but prefers to maintain more of the sense of wholeness. Although individual elements of the phenomenon are identified, their importance to the phenomenon is not established by the frequency of their occur-

rence but rather by the intuitive judgment of the researcher. Giorgi considers it important to identify the relationships of the units to each other and to the whole. In Table 23–3, Pallikkathayil and Morgan (1991) illustrate the steps of the Giorgi method of analysis by using examples from their study of suicide attempters.

Colaizzi

Colaizzi (1978) has developed a method that involves observing and analyzing human behavior within its environment to examine experiences that cannot be communicated. This strategy is useful in studying phenomena such as behavior of preverbal children, subjects with Alzheimer disease, combative behavior of an unconscious patient, and body motion of subjects with new amputations.

Parse

Parse (1990) describes a research methodology specific to the man-living-health theory. This methodology involves dialogical engagement, in which the researcher and respondent participate in an unstructured discussion about a lived experience. The experience is described as an I-Thou intersubjective *being with* the participant during the discussion. "The researcher, in true presence with the participant, engages in a dialogue surfacing the remembered, the now, and the not-yet all at once. Before the dialogue with the participant, the researcher 'dwells with' the meaning of the lived experience, centering self in a way to be open to a full discussion of the experience as shared by the participant. The discussion is audio and video tape-recorded (when possible), and the dialogue is transcribed to typed format for the extraction-synthesis process. Extraction-synthesis is a process of moving the descriptions from the language of the participants up the levels of abstraction to the language of science" (p. 11).

The researcher contemplates the phenomenon under study while listening to the tape, reading the transcribed dialogue, and viewing the videotape. Thus the researcher is multisensorily immersed in the data. According to Parse (1990), the details of this process include the following:

TABLE 23–1 HUSSERLIAN METHOD	
STEP	**PHILOSOPHIC REFERENT**
1. Explore the diversity of one's consciousness	"Each has his place whence he sees the things that are present, and each enjoys accordingly different appearances of the things" (p. 95)

2. Reflect on experiences
    Choose an experience to study
    Develop a phenomenological framework
    Specify a research question
	It is through reflection, one of the many spontaneities of consciousness that experiences are "brought under . . . [the] glance of the Ego [p. 197] [and become] objects *for* the Ego" (p. 196)

3. Bracket or perform the phenomenological reduction	"Not a single theorem [should] . . . be taken from any of the related sciences, nor allowed as premises for phenomenological purposes" (p. 165)
4. Explore the participants' life-world	Engage in a "thorough inspection, analysis, and description of the life-world as we encounter it" (p. 161)

5. Intuit the structures through descriptive analysis
    Perform the eidetic reduction (intuit the principle shared by the facts)
    Create a taxonomy for the experience: intention, component phenomenon
    Create a taxonomy for the context of experience: element, descriptor, and feature
	"We . . . must strive . . . to describe faithfully what we really see from our own point of view and after the most earnest consideration" (p. 259)
	"A living picture of the fruitfulness of phenomenology . . . can be won only when domain after domain has been actually tramped and the problem-vistas it possesses opened up for all to see" (p. 258)

6. Engage in intersubjective dialogue about the phenomena and contextual features	To develop a phenomenon fully, two "formations in the constituting of the Thing" (p. 387) are needed: the first formation (reflection, bracketing, and intuiting by the researcher) and the second formation ("the intersubjective identical thing" [p. 387]) to discuss phenomena and "counter-case" (p. 388)

7. Attempt to fill out the phenomena and features
    Cycle through reflection, bracketing, and intuiting
    Cycle between the first and second formations
    Integrate the bracketed material into the analysis
	"The possibility remains of changes in apprehension [but the goal is a] harmonious filling out" (pp. 131, 356) of phenomena

8. Determine uses for the phenomena and features	"In the end, the conjectures must be redeemed by the real vision of the essential connections" (p. 193)

From Husserl E., & Gibson, W. R. B. (Trans.) (1962). *Ideas: General introduction to pure phenomenology.* New York: Macmillan (original work published 1913).

1. Extracting essences from transcribed descriptions (participant's language). An extracted essence is a complete expression of a core idea described by the participant.
2. Synthesizing essences (researcher's language). A synthesized essence is an expression of the core idea of the extracted essence conceptualized by the researcher.
3. Formulating a proposition from each participant's description. A proposition is a non-directional statement conceptualized by the researcher joining the core idea of the synthesized essences from each participant.
4. Extracting core concepts from the formulated propositions of all participants. An extracted core concept is an idea (written in a phrase) that captures the central meaning of the propositions.
5. Synthesizing a structure of the lived experience from the extracted concepts. A synthesized structure is a statement conceptualized by the researcher joining the core concepts. The structure as evolved answers the research question, 'What is the structure of this lived experience?' (p. 11)

The results of this analysis are then moved up another level of abstraction to represent the meaning of the lived experience at the level of theory. The

TABLE 23–2
COMPARISON OF THREE PHENOMENOLOGICAL METHODS

COLAIZZI	GIORGI	VAN KAAM
1. Read all the subjects' descriptions to acquire a feeling for them	1. One reads the entire description to get a sense of the whole	1. Listing and preliminary grouping of descriptive expressions that must be agreed upon by expert judges. Final listing presents percentages of these categories in that particular sample
2. Return to each protocol and extract significant statements	2. Researcher discriminates units from the participants' description of the phenomenon being studied. Researcher does this from within a psychological perspective and with a focus on the phenomenon under study	2. In reduction the researcher reduces the concrete, vague, and overlapping expressions of the participants to more precisely descriptive terms. There again, intersubjective agreement among judges is necessary
3. Spell out the meaning of each significant statement, known as formulating meanings	3. Researcher expresses the psychological insight contained in each of the meaning units more directly	3. Elimination of elements that are not inherent in the phenomenon being studied or that represent a blending of this phenomenon with other phenomena that most frequently accompany it

4. Organize the formulated meanings into clusters of themes
  a. Refer these clusters of themes back to the original protocols to validate them
  b. At this point, discrepancies may be noted among and/or between the various clusters. Researchers must refuse temptation of ignoring data or themes that do not fit
	4. Researcher synthesizes all the transformed meaning units into a consistent statement regarding the participant's experiences. This is referred to as the structure of the experience and can be expressed on a specific or a general level	4. A hypothetical identification and description of the phenomenon being studied is written

5. Results so far are integrated into an exhaustive description of the phenomenon under study		5. The hypothetical description is applied to randomly selected cases of the sample. If necessary, the hypothesized description is revised. This revised description must be tested again on a new random sample of cases
6. Formulate the exhaustive description of the investigated phenomenon in as unequivocal a statement of identification as possible		6. When operations described in previous steps have been carried out successfully, the formerly hypothetical identification of the phenomenon under study may be considered to be a valid identification and description
7. A final validating step can be achieved by returning to each subject and asking about the findings so far		

From Beck, C. T. (1994). Reliability and validity issues in phenomenology. *Western Journal of Nursing Research, 16*(3), 254–267.

findings are interpreted in terms of the principles of the Parse theory.

OUTCOMES

Findings are often described from the orientation of the participants studied rather than being translated into scientific or theoretical language. For example, the actual words used by participants to describe an experience will often be used when reporting the findings. The researcher identifies themes found in the data. From these themes, a structural explanation of the findings is developed.

Descriptions of human experience need to produce a feeling of understanding in the reader. To do so, the author must focus not only on issues related to truth (validity) but also on issues related to beauty (aesthetics). Therefore, the author must com-

TABLE 23–3
APPLICATION OF GIORGI'S METHOD OF ANALYSIS OF PHENOMENOLOGICAL DATA

STEP NO.	THEORETICAL PROCESS	PRAGMATIC PROCESS USED IN EXAMPLE
One	Reading of the entire disclosure of the phenomenon straight through to obtain a sense of the whole	Reading and rereading the first three transcripts to look for emerging themes. Establishing the coding process and decision rules for coding
Two	Rereading the same disclosure again in a purposeful manner to delineate each time that a transition in meaning occurs. This is done with the intention of discovering the essence of the phenomenon under study. The end result is a series of meaning units or themes	Reading and coding each of the 20 transcripts for themes by each member of the research team. Weekly meetings of the coders to review the coding process and to reach consensus where questions or discrepancies had arisen. Intrarater and interrater reliability was established during this step
Three	Examining the previously determined meaning units for redundancies, clarification, or elaboration by relating meaning units to each other and to a sense of the whole	The meaning units or themes were examined and categories were developed that represented a higher level of abstraction. Themes not related to the research questions were categorized appropriately. The result was an extensive listing of data by categories
Four	Reflecting on the meaning units (still expressed essentially in the language of the subject) and extrapolating the essence of the experience for each subject. Systematic interrogation of each unit is undertaken for what it reveals about the phenomenon under study for each subject. During this process, each unit is transformed into the language of psychological science when relevant	After reflecting on the categories, such as thoughts, feelings, and responses of the subjects, a narrative capturing the essence of the phenomenon of an encounter with a suicide attempter was formulated for each subject. It was during this time that the true richness of the phenomenological method was realized
Five	Formalizing a consistent description of the structure of the phenomenon under study across subjects by synthesizing and integrating the insights achieved in the previous steps	Decisions were made regarding what to accept as the common experience for the phenomenon. Responses offered by 25% or more of the subjects were accepted as the structure of the phenomenon of an encounter with a suicide attempter

From Pallikkathayil, L., & Morgan, S. A. (1991). Phenomenology as a method for conducting clinical research. *Applied Nursing Research, 4*(4), 197.

municate in such a way that the reader is presented with both the structure and the texture of the experience (Todres, 1998).

PHENOMENOLOGICAL NURSING STUDY

One of the most significant nursing studies conducted with the phenomenological method was performed by Benner, from which emerged the critical description of nursing practice presented in her book *From Novice to Expert* (1984). This study was funded by a grant from the Department of Health and Human Services, Division of Nursing, at a time when external funding for qualitative research was almost unheard of. In Benner's study, the phenomenon explored was the experience of clinical practice. Benner's research question asked whether there were "distinguishable, characteristic differences in

the novice's and expert's descriptions of the same clinical incident. If so, how could these differences, if identifiable from the nurses' descriptions of the incidents, be accounted for or understood?" (p. 14).

Grounded Theory Methodology

Data collection for a grounded theory study is referred to as field work. Participant observation is a commonly used technique. The focus of observation is social interactions within the phenomenon of interest. Interviews may also be conducted to obtain the perceptions of participants. Data are coded in preparation for analysis, which begins with the initiation of data collection. Stern (1980) and Turner (1981) have described the methodology used for grounded theory analysis.

1. Category development. Categories derived

from the data are identified and named. These categories are then used as codes for data analysis. This process is the beginning stage of the development of a tentative theory.

2. **Category saturation.** Examples of the categories identified are collected until the characteristics of items that fit into the category become clear to the researcher. The researcher then examines all instances of the category in the data to determine whether they fit the emerging pattern of characteristics identified by the researcher.

3. **Concept development.** The researcher formulates a definition of the category (now properly referred to as a concept) by using the characteristics verified in step 2.

4. **Search for additional categories.** The researcher continues to examine the data and collect additional data to search for categories that were not immediately obvious but seem to be essential to understand the phenomenon under study.

5. **Category reduction.** Categories, which at this point in the research may have become numerous, are clustered by merging them into higher-order categories.

6. **Search for negative instances of categories.** The researcher continually seeks instances that contradict or otherwise do not fit the characteristics developed to define a category.

7. **Linking of categories.** The researcher seeks to understand relationships among categories. To accomplish this goal, data collection becomes more selective as the researcher seeks to determine conditions under which the concepts occur. Hypotheses are developed and tested with available data or by selecting additional interviews or observations specifically to examine proposed links among the categories. A narrative presentation of the emerging theory, including the concepts, conceptual definitions, and relationships, is developed. The narrative is rewritten repeatedly to achieve an explanation of an emerging theory that is clearly expressed, logically consistent, reflective of the data, and compatible with the knowledge base of nursing. A conceptual map may be provided to clarify the theory (Burns, 1989).

8. **Selective sampling of the literature.** Unlike the case in traditional research, the literature is not extensively searched at the beginning of the study to avoid development of a sedimented view. Background and significance of the research question are validated through the literature, and a brief review of previous research is conducted. A more extensive literature review is conducted during the interpretation phase of the study to determine the fit of findings from earlier studies with the present findings and the fit of existing theory with the emerging grounded theory.

9. **Emergence of the core variable.** Through the aforementioned activities, the concept most important to the theory emerges. This concept, or core variable, becomes the central theme or focus of the theory.

10. **Concept modification and integration.** This step is a wrapping-up process in which the theory is finalized and again compared with the data. "As categories and patterns emerge, the researcher must engage in the critical act of challenging the very pattern that seems so apparent. The researcher must search for other, plausible explanations for the data and the linkages among them" (Marshall & Rossman, 1989, p. 119). Sometimes, the fit between the data and the emerging theory is poor. A poor fit can occur when identification of patterns in the data takes place before the researcher can logically fit all the data within the emerging framework. In this case, the relationships proposed among the phenomena may be spurious. Miles and Huberman (1994) suggest that plausibility is the opiate of the intellectual. If the emerging schema makes good sense and fits with other theorists' explanations of the phenomena, the researcher may lock into it prematurely. Therefore, it is very critical to test the schema by rechecking the fit between the emerging theory and the original data.

GROUNDED THEORY STUDY

One significant study using a grounded theory approach that is relevant to clinical nursing practice is Fagerhaugh and Strauss's (1977) study of the politics of pain management. This study emerged from the previous work of Glaser and Strauss in care of the dying (Glaser & Strauss, 1965, 1968; Strauss & Glaser, 1970) and chronic illness care (Strauss, 1975; Strauss et al., 1984). The study of pain involved five researchers and 2 years of systematic observations in 20 wards, 2 clinics, and 9 hospitals. The purposes of the study were twofold: to develop an approach to pain management that was radically different from established approaches and to develop a substantive theory about "what happens in hospitals when people are confronted with pain and attempt to deal with it" (Fagerhaugh & Strauss, 1977, p. 13). The research questions were, "Under what conditions is pain encountered by staff?" and "How will it be handled?" In terms of accountability, the researchers found that pain work was not a major priority of staff. Staff tended to be more responsible for controlling the patient's expression of pain than controlling the experience of pain. Fagerhaugh and Strauss (1977) drew the following conclusions from their study.

• •

"Genuine accountability concerning pain work could only be instituted if the major authorities on given wards or clinics understood the importance of that accountability and its implications for patient care. They would then need to convert that understanding into a commitment that would bring about necessary changes in written and verbal communication systems. This kind of understanding and commitment can probably come about only after considerable nationwide discussion, such as now is taking place about terminal care, but that kind of discussion seems to lie far in the future." (Fagerhaugh & Strauss, 1977, p. 27) ■

Ethnographic Methodology

GAINING ENTRANCE

One of the critical steps in any study is gaining entry into the area being studied. This step can be particularly sensitive in ethnographic studies. The mechanics of this process may vary greatly, depending on whether one is attempting to gain entrance to another country or into a specific institution. The

researcher is responsible at this point for explaining the purposes and methods of the study to those with the power to grant entrance.

ACQUIRING INFORMANTS

To understand the culture, the researcher seeks out individuals who are willing to interpret the culture to them. These people (who are usually members of the culture) will not be research subjects in the usual sense of the word, but rather colleagues. The researcher must have the support and confidence of these individuals to complete the research. Therefore, maintaining these relationships is of utmost importance. Not only will the informants answer questions, but they may also have to help formulate the questions because they understand the culture better than the researcher does.

IMMERSION IN THE CULTURE

Ethnographic researchers must become very familiar with the culture being studied by living in it (active participation) and by extensive questioning. The process of becoming *immersed* in the culture involves gaining increasing familiarity with issues such as language, sociocultural norms, traditions, and other social dimensions, including family, communication patterns (verbal and nonverbal), religion, work patterns, and expression of emotion. Immersion also involves gradually increasing acceptance of the researcher into the culture.

GATHERING DATA (ELICITATION PROCEDURES)

The activity of collecting data is referred to as *field research* and requires taking extensive notes. The quality of these notes will depend on the expertise of the researcher. A skilled researcher experienced in qualitative research techniques will be able to discern more easily what observations need to be noted than will a less experienced researcher or assistant. During observations, the researcher will be bombarded with information. Intuition plays an important role in determining which data to collect. Although researchers must be actively involved in the culture that they are studying, they must avoid "going native," which will interfere with both data collection and analysis. In *going native,* the researcher becomes a part of the culture and loses all objectivity and, with it, the ability to observe clearly.

ANALYSIS OF DATA

Analysis of data is essentially analysis of the field notes and interviews. The notes themselves may be superficial. However, during the process of analysis, the notes are clarified, extended, and interpreted. Abstract thought processes (intuition, introspection, and reasoning discussed in Chapter 1) are involved in analysis. Interpretations are checked out with the informants. The data are then formed into categories and relationships developed between categories. Patterns of behavior are identified.

OUTCOMES

The analysis process in ethnography is used to provide detailed descriptions of cultures. These descriptions may be applied to existing theories of cultures. In some cases, the findings may lead to the development of hypotheses or theories, or both. The results are tested by whether another ethnographer, using the findings of the first ethnographic study, can accurately anticipate human behavior in the studied culture. Although the findings are not usually generalized from one culture or subculture to another, a case may be made for some degree of generalization to other similar cultures (Germain, 1986).

ETHNOGRAPHIC STUDY

Johnson (1993) used ethnographic analysis and discourse analysis in her study of nurse practitioner (NP)-patient discourse to "uncover the voice of nursing in primary care practice." Discourse analysis was used to "uncover the forms and functions guiding conversation." Ethnographic analysis was used "to discover the beliefs guiding conversation and to establish a context for the NP-patient dialogue" (p. 143). Although a number of studies have documented the effectiveness of NP outcomes versus those of the physician, the process of NP care

has not been examined. She sees the heart of the provider-patient relationship in primary care to be in the office visit. The focus of her study was "uncovering processes and skills used by NPs that could help expand understanding of their successful outcomes" (p. 143).

Historical Research Methodology

Historical researchers spend considerable time refining their research questions before the initiation of data collection. Sources of data relevant to the research question are then identified. Sources of data are often remote from the researcher, who will need to make travel plans to obtain access to the data. In many cases, the researcher must obtain special written permission of the relevant library to obtain access to needed data. The validity and reliability of the data are an important concern in historical research.

CLARIFYING VALIDITY AND RELIABILITY OF DATA

The validity and reliability concerns in historical research are related to the sources from which data are collected. The most valued source of data is the primary source. A primary source is material most likely to shed true light on the information being sought by the researcher. For example, material written by a person who experienced an event or letters and other mementos saved by the person being studied are primary source material. A secondary source is written by those who have previously read and summarized the primary source material. History books and textbooks are secondary source materials. Primary sources are considered more valid and reliable than secondary sources. "The presumption is that an eyewitness can give a more accurate account of an occurrence than a person not present. If the author was an eyewitness, he is considered a primary source. If the author has been told about the occurrence by someone else, the author is a secondary source. The further the author moves from an eyewitness account, the less reliable are his statements" (Christy, 1975, p. 191). Historiographers use primary sources whenever possible.

The historical researcher must consider the validity and reliability of primary sources used in the study. To do so, the researcher uses principles of historical criticism.

•••••••••••••••••••••••••••••• ▪ ••••••••

"One does not merely pick up a copy of Grandmother's diary and gleefully assume that all the things Grandma wrote were the unvarnished facts. Grandmother's glasses may at times have been clouded, at other times rose-colored. The well-prepared researcher will scrutinize, criticize, and analyze before even accepting its having been written by Grandma! And even after the validity of the document is established, every attempt is made to uncover bias, prejudice, or just plain exaggeration on Grandmother's part. Healthy skepticism becomes a way of life for the serious historiographer." (Christy, 1978, p. 6) ▪

Two strategies have been developed to determine the authenticity and accuracy of the source; these strategies are external and internal criticism.

External criticism determines the validity of source material. The researcher needs to know where, when, why, and by whom a document was written, which may involve verifying the handwriting or determining the age of the paper on which it was written. Christy (1975) describes some difficulties she experienced in establishing the validity of documents.

•••••••••••••••••••••••••••••• ▪ ••••••••

"An interesting problem presented by early nursing leaders was their frugality. Nutting occasionally saved stationery from hotels, resorts, or steamship lines during vacation trips and used it at a later date. This required double checking as to her exact location at the time the letter was written. When she first went to Teachers College in 1907, she still wrote a few letters on Johns Hopkins stationery. I found this practice rather confusing in early stages of research." (Christy, 1975, p. 190) ▪

Internal criticism involves examination of the reliability of the document. The researcher must determine possible biases of the author. To verify the accuracy of a statement, the researcher should have two independent sources that provide the same information. In addition, the researcher should ensure

that he or she understands the statements made by the writer because words and their meanings change across time and across cultures. It is also possible to read into a document meaning not originally intended by the author. This shortcoming is most likely to happen when one is seeking to find a particular meaning. Sometimes, words can be taken out of context (Christy, 1975).

DEVELOPING A RESEARCH OUTLINE

The research outline is a guide for the broad topics to be examined and also serves as a basis for a filing system for classifying the data collected. For example, data may be filed by time period. The materials may be cross-referenced for easy access. One piece of data may be filed under several classifications, and the researcher places a note in one file referring to data stored in another file. The research outline provides a checkpoint for the investigator during the process of data collection and can be used to easily identify gaps in the data collection process.

DATA COLLECTION

Data collection may require months or years of dedicated searching for pertinent material. Sometimes, one small source may open a door to an entire new field of facts. In addition, data collection has no clear, obvious end. By examining the research outline, the researcher must make the decision to discontinue collection of data. These facets of data collection are described by Newton (1965).

•••••••••••••••••••••••••••••• ▪ ••••••••

"The search for data takes the researcher into most unexpected nooks and corners and adds facet after facet to the original problem. It may last for months or years or a decade. Days and weeks may be fruitless and endless references may be devoid of pertinent material. Again, one minor reference will open the door to the gold mine of facts. The search becomes more exciting when others know of it and bring possible clues to the investigator. The researcher cultivates persistence, optimism, and patience in his long and sometimes discouraging quest. But one real 'find' spurs him on and he continues his search. Added to this skill is the training in the most meticulous recording of data with every detail complete, and the logical classification of the data." (Newton, 1965, p. 23) ■

Careful attention to note taking is critical. Lusk (1997) provides the following instructions related to note taking:

. . . .

"Note-taking begins as the first folder of documents is delivered. Each card or computer entry must clearly identify the archive, the collection, the folder, the file, and the document. References must be correct, for personal integrity, deference to the archivist and other researchers, and for being able to return to the source. In addition to careful note identification, a system of ordering the data by subject greatly facilitates the writing stage; Jensen (1992) suggests using colored pencils or stickers. Kruman (1985) recommends cross-referencing if information is applicable to two subjects.

"Whether to take notes on paper, cards, or laptop computers is a matter of personal preference. Paper may be cut into half-sheets and is lighter to carry than cards if notes become extensive. Some researchers use loose-leaf journals, leaving a wide margin for source identification. A computer, used at the discretion of the archivist, may be preferred and some consider it essential for voluminous notes. Hand-held scanners with parallel port interfaces have recently become available for use with laptop computers. Scanners have enormous potential to reduce time and expense, and are safer for fragile documents than photocopiers. Scanners typically come with text-recognition software to partially automate the note-taking process. Text-based management systems allow users to organize the data following entry." (Lusk, 1997, p. 358) ■

ANALYSIS OF DATA

Analysis of data involves synthesis of all the data collected. Data must be sifted and choices made about which to accept and which to reject. Sometimes, interesting data that do not contribute to the questions of the study are difficult to discard. Also, conflicting evidence must be reconciled. For example, if two primary sources give opposite information about an incident, the researcher will seek

to interpret the differences and determine, as nearly as possible, what actually occurred.

OUTCOMES

Interpreting the outcomes of a historical study is influenced by the perspective of the researcher inasmuch as competing explanations can be created from the same data set. Evidence for conclusions is always partial because of missing data. Historical interpretation is not about describing the progress of events but about ascribing meaning to them. Thus, the responsibilities of interpreting historical data are great. Lynaugh and Reverby (1987, p. 4) suggest that "historical scholarship is judged on its ability to assemble the best facts and generate the most cogent explanation of a given situation or period."

DEVELOPING A WRITING OUTLINE

Before proceeding to write the research report, the researcher must decide the most appropriate means of presenting the data. Some options include a biography, a chronology, and a paper organized to focus on issues. If the outline has been well organized and detailed, the writing that follows should flow easily and smoothly.

WRITING THE RESEARCH REPORT

Historical research reports do not follow the traditional formalized style of much research. The studies are designed to attract the interest of the reader and may appear deceptively simple. An untrained eye may not recognize the extensive work required to write the paper. As explained by Christy (1975, p. 192), "The reader is never aware of the painstaking work, the careful attention to detail, nor the arduous pursuit of clues endured by the writer of history. Perhaps that is why so many nurses have failed to recognize historiography as a legitimate research endeavor. It looks so easy."

Philosophical Studies

The purpose of philosophical research is to clarify meanings, make values manifest, identify ethics, and study the nature of knowledge (Ellis, 1983). A philosophical researcher is expected to consider a philosophical question from all perspectives by examining conceptual meaning, raising further questions, proposing answers, and suggesting the implications of those answers. The data source for most philosophical studies is written material and verbally expressed ideas relevant to the topic of interest. The researcher critically examines the text or the ideas for flaws in logic. A key element of the analysis is the posing of philosophical questions. The data are then searched for information relevant to the question. Ideas or values implied in the text are an important source of information because many philosophical analyses address very abstract topics. The researcher attempts to maintain an objective distance from perspectives in the data so that the logic of the idea can be abstractly examined. Ideas, questions, answers, and consequences are often explored or debated, or both, with colleagues during the analysis phase.

Three types of philosophical studies are foundational inquiry, philosophical analyses, and ethical analyses.

FOUNDATIONAL INQUIRIES METHODOLOGY

Foundational inquiries are critical and exploratory. The researcher asks questions that reveal flaws in the logic with which the ideas of the science were developed. These flaws may be an ambiguity, a discrepancy, or a puzzle in the way those within the science speak, think, and act. Generally, this knowledge is not seen as having logic problems by those within the science. The knowledge questioned could be in the form of ideas, concepts, facts, theories, or even various sorts of experiences and ways of doing things (Manchester, 1986). For example, one might question whether adaptation is a desired outcome of nursing action consistent with nursing's definition of health.

Outcomes

Foundational studies provide critical analyses of ideas and thought within a discipline and thereby facilitate further development of the body of knowledge. The critique of studies within the science is guided by the outcomes of foundational studies and entails use of the five traditional criteria for scientific thinking: accuracy, consistency, scope, simplicity, and fruitfulness (Manchester, 1986).

Example of a Foundational Study

By far, the best-known foundational inquiry in nursing is Carper's (1978) study of the ways of knowing in nursing. This study was her doctoral dissertation and only a portion of it has been published. In conducting the study, Carper examined nursing textbooks and journals from 1964 to 1974. She identified four ways of knowing in nursing: empirical, aesthetic, personal, and ethical.

PHILOSOPHICAL RESEARCH

The primary purpose of philosophical analysis is to examine meaning and to develop theories of meaning. This objective is usually accomplished through concept analysis or linguistic analysis (Rodgers, 1989). Concept analyses have become common exercises for graduate nursing students, although most have not been performed with philosophical research strategies. Many of them have been published and are providing an important addition to the body of knowledge in nursing. One of the best-known analyses, Smith's idea of health (1986), was performed by philosophical inquiry.

Example of Philosophical Inquiry

Smith searched the literature for fundamental concepts on the nature of health. Regardless of how health was defined, it was considered one extreme on a continuum of health and illness. Health was a relative term. A person was judged healthy when measured against some ideal of health. Who was considered healthy was based on the particular ideal of health being used. Smith identified four models (or ideals) of health: the eudaimonistic model, the adaptive model, the role performance model, and the clinical model. This analysis has proved useful in exploring many issues related to nursing, including differing expectations of clients in relation to their health. An instrument has been developed to put this concept into operation and will allow it to be examined in relation to a number of variables important to nursing (Smith, 1986).

ETHICAL ANALYSIS

In ethical inquiry, the researcher identifies principles to guide conduct that are based on ethical theories. Problems in ethics are related to obligation, rights, duty, right and wrong, conscience, justice, choice, intention, and responsibility. An analysis using a selected ethical theory is performed. The actions prescribed by the analysis may vary with the ethical theory used. The ideas are submitted to colleagues for critique and debate. Conclusions are associated with rights and duties rather than preferences.

Example of Ethical Analysis

An ethical analysis of an elder's treatment is an example of ethical research (Kayser-Jones et al., 1989). This case study was part of a 3-year project investigating the sociocultural factors likely to influence the evaluation and treatment of nursing home residents.

CRITICAL SOCIAL THEORY METHODOLOGY

Three means of collecting data for a critical social theory study may be used: verbal or written questions posed to individuals or groups, observation, or use of written documents. Data may be quantitative or qualitative and include numbers and stories. Methods are selected that are expected to yield the most compelling evidence, which is most likely to be a combination of stories and numbers. This strategy may use one of three basic approaches:

1. **Numbers foreground, stories background.** These studies are primarily quantitative with a lesser qualitative focus. This approach is used when the purpose of the study is to influence those in positions of power and the general public who are most likely to be influenced by "hard evidence" (numbers). In this case, stories are used to "put a face" on the numbers so that the intended audience can hear the voices of the participants and consider the meaning of the numbers.
2. **Stories foreground, numbers background.** These studies are primarily qualitative with a

lesser quantitative focus. The purpose of these studies is to provide opportunities for researchers and participants to engage in dialogue, reflection, and critique in relation to the phenomenon being studied. Telling a study enables the participants to "name their reality" and explore strategies for changing that reality. Emphasis is on personal change, growth, and empowerment. However, it must also be recognized that problems and concerns of individuals do not occur in isolation and are often beyond the control of the individual. Lasting changes must occur on many levels.
3. **Stories and numbers with equal emphasis.** A research program fostering individual empowerment and system change may use a full range of methods and types of data. This approach might include a combination of standardized instruments and various interview techniques. The data may be used to specify a theory, establish the prevalence of a phenomenon, explore the context of a phenomenon, test a nursing intervention, or any combination of these objectives (Berman et al., 1998).

The research process of critical social theory requires that researchers use oppositional thinking to perform a critique of the social situation under study by applying the following four steps: (1) critical examination of the implicit rules and assumptions of the situation under study in a historical, cultural, and political context; (2) use of reflection to identify the conditions that would make uncoerced knowledge and action possible; (3) analysis of the constraints on communication and human action to develop a theoretical framework that uses causal relationships to explain distortions in communications and repression; the theoretical framework is then tested against individual cases (Hedin, 1986); and finally, (4) participation in dialogue with those oppressed individuals within the social situation. Dialogue leads to raising of collective consciousness and identification of ways to take action against oppressive forces. The action for change must come from the groups and communities rather than the researcher. The groups and communities must consider "(a) their common interests; (b) the risks they are willing to undergo; (c) the consequences they can expect; and (d) their knowledge of the circumstances of their own lives" (Hedin, 1986, p. 146).

As with most qualitative research methodologies, it is difficult to separate the steps. Dialogue is used both to collect and to interpret the data, and researchers constantly move back and forth between collection and interpretation. Dialogue, which uses some of the techniques of phenomenology, includes conversations between the researcher and persons within the society and requires a relationship of equality and active reciprocity. In addition, by reflection and insight, the researcher dialogues with the data while collecting, analyzing, and interpreting it. "New meanings emerge, and phrases that have always been ignored suddenly come alive and demand explanation" (Thompson, 1987, p. 33). The process "exposes ways in which the self has been formed (or deformed) through the influence of coercive power relations. The work of critical scholarship is to make these power relations transparent, for these relations lose power when they become transparent" (Thompson, 1987, p. 33). Knowledge is created and this knowledge furthers autonomy and responsibility by enlightening individuals about how they may rationally act to realize their own best interests (Holter, 1988).

Feminist Research Methodology

Purpose. The purpose of feminist research is transformational and directed at social structures and social relationships, including logical arguments (Rafael, 1997).

Review of Literature. The review of literature focuses on a search for evidence of the relationship between power and knowledge. For example, who decides what counts as knowledge? How is power produced? What resistance to power exists? Whose interests are silenced, marginalized, or excluded? How open is power to change (Rafael, 1997)?

Participant-Research Relationships. The feminist method requires a leveling of the usual power imbalance between researcher and participant. The perspective of participants is considered primary, and yet they are assisted in gaining some distance from their views. A balance between objectivity and subjectivity is promoted (Rafael, 1997).

Methods of Inquiry. Feminist research methods include a broad range of quantitative and qualitative

methods. Qualitative methods commonly used in feminist research include narratives, advocacy oral history, and textual analyses.

Example of Critical Social Theory (Feminist) Study

Stevens (1995) has conducted a study to examine the structural and interpersonal impact of heterosexual assumptions on lesbian health care clients. "In this feminist narrative study using in-depth interviews and focus groups, a racially and economically diverse sample of 45 lesbians describe their access to and experience with health care" (p. 25). Stevens describes the problem as follows:

• •

"The existence of lesbians calls into question the universality of normative societal ideology about women. Many of society's institutions are based on heterosexual assumptions that reinforce the gender division of labor, sustain the secondary status of women wage earners, compel women's economic and emotional dependence on men, and confine women's identity to narrowly configured roles within traditional nuclear families (Allen, 1986; Jaggar, 1988; Rich, 1980). . . . Limited investigatory attention has been paid to the structural environments and interactional conditions in health that may act as barriers to help seeking by lesbian clients (Stevens, 1992b). Empirical efforts have generally focused on understanding the processes of how lesbians 'come out' (inform others that they are lesbian) in health care contexts (Hitchcock & Wilson, 1992; Smith et al., 1985; Stevens & Hall, 1988). These projects have also documented the risks entailed by such actions. Disclosure of lesbian identity is known to evoke a wide array of reactions from health care providers, ranging from embarrassment to overt hostility. Reported responses include fear, ostracism, refusal to treat, cool detachment, shock, pity, voyeuristic curiosity, demeaning jokes, avoidance of physical contact, insults, invasions of privacy, rough physical handling, and breaches of confidentiality." (Stevens, 1995, p. 25)

The feminist narrative study was designed to examine how lesbians experience clinical encounters. Stevens poses two research questions:

1. How do health care structures (i.e., economic,

political, and social environments) affect lesbians' access to health care?

2. How do interpersonal interactions with health care providers affect lesbians' access to health care?

Narrative analysis revealed that at the macrolevel, heterosexist structuring of health care delivery was obstructive to lesbians' seeking health care, their knowledge about health, and their behavior. At the micro, or individual, level, health care providers' heterosexual assumptions competed against potentially supportive interactions with lesbian clients.

■ SUMMARY

Qualitative data analysis occurs concurrently with data collection rather than sequentially as is true in quantitative research. Therefore, the researcher is simultaneously attempting to gather the data, manage a growing bulk of collected data, and interpret the meaning of the data. Qualitative analysis techniques use words rather than numbers as the basis of analysis. However, the same careful skills in analytical reasoning are needed by the qualitative researcher as those required by quantitative analysis.

The computer can make analysis of qualitative data much quicker and easier without the researcher losing touch with the data. The computer offers assistance in activities such as processing, storage, retrieval, cataloging, and sorting and leaves the analysis activities up to the researcher. A number of computer programs have been developed specifically to perform qualitative analyses.

The credibility of qualitative data analysis has been seriously questioned in some cases by the larger scientific community. The concerns expressed are related to an inability to replicate the outcomes of a study. To respond to this concern, some qualitative researchers have attempted to develop strategies by which other researchers, using the same data, can follow the logic of the original researcher and arrive at the same conclusions. This strategy is referred to as a decision trail.

Some studies are appearing in the literature in which researchers have combined portions of various qualitative methodologies extracted from the philosophical bases for which the methodologies were developed. This approach violates the assumptions of the methodologies. It is essential that the researcher make the philosophical base of the study explicit and that the methodologies used be compatible with the philosophical base.

Because data collection is occurring simultaneously with data analysis, the process is complex. The procedure of collecting data is not a mechanical process that can be carefully planned before initiation. The researcher as a whole person is totally involved. One of the important differences between quantitative and qualitative research is the nature of the relationships between the researcher and the individuals being studied. The nature of these relationships has an impact on the data collected and their interpretation. In varying degrees, the researcher influences the individuals being studied and, in turn, is influenced by them.

In the initial phases of data analysis, the researcher needs to become very familiar with the data that are gathered. This process may involve reading and rereading notes and transcripts, recalling observations and experiences, listening to tapes, and viewing videotapes until the researcher becomes immersed in the data. Initial efforts at analysis focus on reducing the volume of data to facilitate examination. During data reduction, you begin attaching meaning to elements in the data. Coding is a means of categorizing, and a code is a symbol or abbreviation used to classify words or phrases in the data. As the study progresses, relationships among categories, participants, actions, and events will begin to emerge.

Displays contain highly condensed versions of the outcomes of qualitative research. They are equivalent to the summary tables of statistical outcomes developed in quantitative research. The last stage of qualitative analysis is drawing and verifying conclusions. These steps result in a gradual move from empirical data to a conceptual overview of the findings.

The research methodologies of six approaches to qualitative research are discussed. A detailed presentation of a nursing study is used as an example of each approach. In addition, content analysis, an analysis strategy used by some of the qualitative methodologies, is described. Content analysis is designed to classify the words in a text into a few categories chosen because of their theoretical importance. The technique provides a systematic means of measuring the frequency, order, or intensity of occurrence of words, phrases, or sentences.

• •

REFERENCES

Allen, D. G. (1986). Professionalism, occupational segregation by gender and control of nursing. *Women and Politics, 6*(3), 1–24.

Anderson, N. L. R. (1987). Computer-assisted analysis of textual field note data. *Western Journal of Nursing Research, 9*(4), 626–630.

Atkinson, P. (1992). The ethnography of a medical setting: Reading, writing and rhetoric. *Qualitative Health Research, 2*(4), 451–474.

Ayers, L., & Poirier, S. (1996). Virtual text and the growth of meaning in qualitative analysis. *Research in Nursing & Health, 19*(2), 163–169.

Banks-Wallace, J. (1998). Emancipatory potential of storytelling in a group. *Image—The Journal of Nursing Scholarship, 30*(1), 17–21.

Bateson, M. C. (1989). *Composing a life*. New York: Penguin.

Beck, C. T. (1994). Phenomenology: Its use in nursing research. *International Journal of Nursing Studies, 31*(6), 499–510.

Benner, P. (1984). *From novice to expert: Excellence and power in clinical nursing practice*. Menlo Park, CA: Addison-Wesley.

Berman, H., Ford-Gilboe, M., & Campbell, J. C. (1998). Combining stories and numbers: A methodologic approach for a critical nursing science. *Advances in Nursing Science, 21*(1), 1–15.

Bertaux, D. (1981). *Biography and society: The life history approach in the social sciences*. Beverly Hills, CA: Sage.

Burnard, P. (1995). Unspoken meanings: Qualitative research and multi-media analysis. *Nurse Researcher, 3*(1), 55–64.

Burnard, P. (1998). Qualitative data analysis: Using a word processor to categorize qualitative data in social science research. *Social Sciences in Health, 4*(1), 55–61.

Burns, N. (1989). Standards for qualitative research. *Nursing Science Quarterly, 2*(1), 44–52.

Carper, B. (1978). Fundamental patterns of knowing in nursing. *Advances in Nursing Science, 1*(1), 13–24.

Christy, T. E. (1975). The methodology of historical research: A brief introduction. *Nursing Research, 24*(3), 189–192.

Christy, T. E. (1978). The hope of history. In M. L. Fitzpatrick (Ed.), *Historical studies in nursing* (pp. 3–11). New York: Teachers College, Columbia University.

Coffey, A., & Atkinson, P. (1996). *Making sense of qualitative data: Complementary research strategies*. Thousand Oaks, CA: Sage.

Colaizzi, P. (1978). Psychological research as the phenomenolo-gist views it. In R. S. Valle & M. King (Eds.), *Existential phenomenological alternatives for psychology* (pp. 48–71). New York: Oxford University Press.

Connors, D. D. (1988). A continuum of researcher-participant relationships: An analysis and critique. *Advances in Nursing Science, 10*(4), 32–42.

Cooper, M. C. (1988). Covenantal relationships: Grounding for the nursing ethic. *Advances in Nursing Science, 10*(4), 48–59.

Cowles, K. V. (1988). Issues in qualitative research on sensitive topics. *Western Journal of Nursing Research, 10*(2), 163–179.

Denzin, N. K. (1989). *Interpretive interactionism*. Newbury Park, CA: Sage.

Dingwall, R. (1977). Atrocity stories and professional relationships. *Sociology of Work and Occupations, 4,* 371–396.

Downe-Wamboldt, B. (1992). Content analysis: Method, applications, and issues. *Health Care for Women International, 13*(3), 313–321.

Draucker, C. B. (1999). The emotional impact of sexual violence research on participants. *Archives of Psychiatric Nursing, 13*(4), 161–169.

Drew, N. (1989). The interviewer's experience as data in phenomenological research. *Western Journal of Nursing Research, 11*(4), 431–439.

Ellis, R. (1983). Philosophic inquiry. In H. H. Werley & J. J. Fitzpatrick (Eds.), *Annual review of nursing research* (Vol. I, pp. 211–228). New York: Springer.

Fagerhaugh, S., & Strauss, A. (1977). *Politics of pain management: Staff-patient interaction*. Menlo Park, CA: Addison-Wesley.

Field, P. A., & Morse, J. M. (1985). *Nursing research: The application of qualitative approaches*. Rockville, MD: Aspen.

Fowler, M. D. M. (1988). Issues in qualitative research. *Western Journal of Nursing Research, 10*(1), 109–111.

Frank, G. (1979). Finding the common denominator: A phenomenological critique of life history method. *Ethos, 7,* 68–71.

Frank, G. (1996). Life histories in occupational therapy clinical practice. *American Journal of Occupational Therapy, 50*(4), 251–264.

Gergen, K. J., & Gergen, M. M. (1983). Narratives of the self. In T. R. Sarbin & K. E. Scheibe (Eds.), *Studies in social identity* (pp. 254–273). New York: Praeger.

Germain, C. P. H. (1986). Ethnography: The method. In P. L. Munhall & C. J. Oiler (Eds.), *Nursing research: A qualitative perspective* (pp. 147–162). E. Norwalk, CT: Appleton-Century-Crofts.

Giorgi, A. (1970). *Psychology as a human science: A phenomenologically based approach*. New York: Harper & Row.

Glaser, B. G., & Strauss, A. (1965). *Awareness of dying*. Chicago: Aldine.

Glaser, B. G., & Strauss, A. (1968). *Time for dying*. Chicago: Aldine.

Guba, E. G., & Lincoln, Y. S. (1982). *Effective evaluation*. Washington, DC: Jossey-Bass.

Hedin, B. A. (1986). Nursing, education, and emancipation: Applying the critical theoretical approach to nursing research. In P. L. Chinn (Ed.), *Nursing research methodology: Issues and implementation* (pp. 133–146). Rockville, MD: Aspen.

Hitchcock, J. M., & Wilson, H. S. (1992). Personal risking: Lesbian self-disclosure of sexual orientation to professional health care providers. *Nursing Research, 41*(3), 178–183.

Holter, I. M. (1988). Critical theory: A foundation for the development of nursing theories. *Scholarly Inquiry for Nursing Practice: An International Journal, 2*(3), 223–232.

Iser, W. (1980). The reading process: A phenomenological approach. In J. Tompkins (Ed.), *Reader-response criticism* (pp. 118–133). Baltimore: Johns Hopkins University Press.

Jaggar, A. M. (1988). *Feminist politics and human nature.* Sussex, England: Rowman & Littlefield.

Jensen, R. (1992). Text management—history and computing. III: Historians, computers and data, applications in research and teaching. *Journal of Interdisciplinary History, 22*(4), 711–722.

Johnson, R. (1993). Nurse practitioner–patient discourse: Uncovering the voice of nursing in primary care practice. *Scholarly Inquiry for Nursing Practice: An International Journal, 7*(3), 143–157.

Josselson, R., & Lieblich, A. (Eds.). (1995). *The narrative study of lives, Vol. 3: Interpreting experience.* Newbury Park, CA: Sage.

Kalisch, B. J., & Kalisch, P. A. (1977). An analysis of the sources of physician-nurse conflict. *Journal of Nursing Administration, 7*(1), 50–57.

Kalisch, B. J., Kalisch, P. A., & Belcher, B. (1985). Forecasting for nursing policy: A news-based image approach. *Nursing Research, 34*(1), 44–49.

Kalisch, P. A., Kalisch, B. J., & Clinton, J. (1982). The world of nursing on prime time television, 1950 to 1980. *Nursing Research, 31*(6), 358–363.

Kalisch, B. J., Kalisch, P. A., & Young, R. L. (1983). Television news coverage of nurse strikes: A resource management perspective. *Nursing Research, 32*(3), 175–180.

Kayser-Jones, J., Davis, A., Wiener, C. L., & Higgins, S. S. (1989). An ethical analysis of an elder's treatment. *Nursing Outlook, 37*(6), 267–270.

Kelly, A. W., & Sime, A. M. (1990). Language as research data: Application of computer content analysis in nursing research. *Advances in Nursing Science, 12*(3), 32–40.

Kermode, F. (1983). *The art of telling: Essays on fiction.* New York: Oxford University Press.

Knafl, K. A., & Webster, D. C. (1988). Managing and analyzing qualitative data: A description of tasks, techniques, and materials. *Western Journal of Nursing Research, 10*(2), 195–218.

Kruman, M. W. (1985). Historical method: Implications for nursing research. In M. M. Leininger (Ed.), *Qualitative research methods in nursing* (pp. 109–118). New York: Grune & Stratton.

Lamb, G. S., & Huttlinger, K. (1989). Reflexivity in nursing research. *Western Journal of Nursing Research, 11*(6), 765–772.

Larson, E. A., & Fanchiang, S. C. (1996). Life history and narrative research: Generating a humanistic knowledge base for occupational therapy. *The American Journal of Occupational Therapy, 50*(4), 247–250.

Linde, C. (1993). *Life stories: The creation of coherence.* New York: Oxford University Press.

Lusk, B. (1997). Historical methodology for nursing research. *Image—The Journal of Nursing Scholarship*, 29(4), 355–359.

Lynaugh, J., & Reverby, S. (1987). Thoughts on the nature of history. *Nursing Research, 36*(1), 4, 69.

Mallinson, T., Kielhofner, G., & Mattingly, C. (1996). Metaphor and meaning in a clinical interview. *American Journal of Occupational Therapy, 50*(5), 338–346.

Manchester, P. (1986). Analytic philosophy and foundational inquiry: The method. In P. L. Munhall & C. J. Oiler (Eds.), *Nursing research: A qualitative perspective* (pp. 229–249). E. Norwalk, CT: Appleton-Century-Crofts.

Marshall, C. (1984). Elites, bureaucrats, ostriches, and pussycats: Managing research in policy settings. *Anthropology and Education Quarterly, 15*(3), 235–251.

Marshall, C. (1985). Appropriate criteria of trustworthiness and goodness for qualitative research on education organizations. *Quality and Quantity, 19*(4), 353–373.

Marshall, C., & Rossman, G. B. (1989). *Designing qualitative research.* Newbury Park, CA: Sage.

Mattingly, C., & Garro, L. (1994). Introduction: Narratives of illness and healing. *Social Science and Medicine, 38,* 771–774.

Miles, M. B., & Huberman, A. M. (1994). *Qualitative data analysis: A sourcebook of new methods* (2nd ed.). Beverly Hills, CA: Sage.

Morse, J. M. (1989). Qualitative nursing research: A free-for-all? In J. M. Morse (Ed.), *Qualitative nursing research: A contemporary dialogue.* Rockville, MD: Aspen.

Morse, J. M. (1997). Learning to drive from a manual? *Qualitative Health Research, 7*(2), 181–183.

Morse, J. M., & Morse, R. M. (1989). QUAL: A mainframe program for qualitative data analysis. *Nursing Research, 38*(3), 188–189.

Munhall, P. L. (1988). Ethical considerations in qualitative research. *Western Journal of Nursing Research, 10*(2), 150–162.

Murdock, G. (1971). *Outline of cultural materials.* New Haven, CT: Human Relation Area Files Press.

Newton, M. E. (1965). The case for historical research. *Nursing Research, 14*(1), 20–26.

Northcott, N. (1996). Cognitive mapping: An approach to qualitative data analysis. *NTResearch, 1*(6), 456–464.

Nwoga, I. (1997). Mother-daughter conversation related to sex-role socialization and adolescent pregnancy. Unpublished dissertation, University of Flordia, Gainesville, Florida.

Nwoga, I. (2000). African American mothers use stories for family sexuality education. *MCN, American Journal of Maternal Child Nursing, 25*(1), 31–36.

Oiler, C. (1982). The phenomenological approach in nursing research. *Nursing Research, 31*(3), 178–181.

Pallikkathayil, L., & Morgan, S. A. (1991). Phenomenology as a method for conducting clinical research. *Nursing Research, 4*(4), 195–200.

Parse, R. R. (1990). Health: A personal commitment. *Nursing Science Quarterly, 3*(3), 136–140.

Pateman, B. (1998). Computer-aided qualitative data analysis: The value of NUD*IST and other programs. *Nurse Researcher, 5*(3), 77–89.

Podolefsky, A., & McCarty, C. (1983). Topical sorting: A technique for computer assisted qualitative data analysis. *American Anthropologist, 85*(4), 886–890.

Polkinghorne, D. E. (1988). *Narrative knowing and the human sciences.* Albany, NY: State University of New York Press.

Porter, E. J. (1998). On "being inspired" by Husserl's phenomenology: Reflections on Omery's exposition of phenomenology as a method of nursing research. *Advances in Nursing Science, 21*(1), 16–28.

Rafael, A. R. F. (1997). Advocacy oral history: A research methodology for social activism in nursing; Methods of Clinical Inquiry. *ANS, Advances in Nursing Science, 20*(2), 32–44.

Rich, A. (1980). Compulsory heterosexuality and lesbian existence. *Signs: Journal of Women in Culture and Society, 5*(4), 631–660.

Robinson, C. A., & Thorne, S. E. (1988). Dilemmas of ethics and validity in qualitative nursing research. *Canadian Journal of Nursing Research, 20*(1), 65–76.

Rodgers, B. L. (1989). Concepts, analysis and the development of nursing knowledge: The evolutionary cycle. *Journal of Advanced Nursing, 14*(4), 330–335.

Ruffing-Rahal, M. A. (1986). Personal documents and nursing theory development. *Advances in Nursing Science, 8*(3), 50–57.

Sandelowski, M. (1994). Notes on transcription. *Research in Nursing & Health, 17*(4), 311–314.

Sandelowski, M. (1995a). On the aesthetics of qualitative research. *Image—The Journal of Nursing Scholarship, 27*(3), 205–209.

Sandelowski, M. (1995b). Qualitative analysis: What it is and how to begin. *Research in Nursing & Health, 18*(4), 371–375.

Sandelowski, M. (1997). "To be of use": Enhancing the utility of qualitative research. *Nursing Outlook, 45*(3), 125–132.

Sarbin, T. R. (Ed.). (1986). *Narrative psychology: The storied nature of human conduct.* New York: Praeger.

Smith, E. M., Johnson, S. R., & Guenther, S. M. (1985). Health care attitudes and experiences during gynecological care among lesbians and bisexuals. *American Journal of Public Health, 75*(9), 1085–1087.

Smith, J. A. (1986). The idea of health: Doing foundational

inquiry. In P. L. Munhall & C. J. Oiler (Eds.), *Nursing research: A qualitative perspective* (pp. 251–262). E. Norwalk, CT: Appleton-Century-Crofts.

Stern, P. N. (1980). Grounded theory methodology: Its uses and processes. *Image—The Journal of Nursing Scholarship, 12*(1), 20–23.

Stevens, P. E. (1992a). Lesbian health care research: A review of the literature from 1970 to 1990. *Health Care for Women International, 13*(2), 91–120.

Stevens, P. E. (1992b). Who gets care? Access to health care as an arena for nursing action. *Scholarly Inquiry for Nursing Practice: An International Journal, 6*(3), 185–200.

Stevens, P. E. (1995). Structural and interpersonal impact of heterosexual assumptions on lesbian health care clients. *Nursing Research, 44*(1), 25–30.

Stevens, P. E., & Hall, J. M. (1988). Stigma, health beliefs, and experiences with health care in lesbian women. *Image—The Journal of Nursing Scholarship, 20*(2), 69–73.

Strauss, A. L. (1975). *Chronic illness and quality of life.* St. Louis: Mosby.

Strauss, A. L., Corbin, J., Fagerhaugh, S., Glaser, B. G., Maines, D., Suczek, B., & Wiener, C. L. (1984). *Chronic illness and the quality of life* (2nd ed.). St. Louis: Mosby.

Strauss, A. L., & Glaser, B. G. (1970). *Anguish.* Mill Valley, CA: Sociology Press.

Taft, L. B. (1993). Computer-assisted qualitative research. *Research in Nursing & Health, 16*(5), 379–383.

Tanner, C. A., Benner, P., Chesla, C., & Gordon, D. R. (1993). The phenomenology of knowing the patient. *Image—The Journal of Nursing Scholarship, 25*, 273–280.

Thompson, J. L. (1987). Critical scholarship: The critique of domination in nursing. *Advances in Nursing Science, 10*(1), 27–38.

Todres, L. (1998). The qualitative description of human experience: The aesthetic dimension. *Qualitative Health Research, 8*(1), 121–127.

Turner, B. (1981). Some practical aspects of qualitative data analysis: One way of organizing the cognitive processes associated with the generation of grounded theory. *Quality and Quantity, 15*(3), 225–247.

Van Kaam, A. L. (1966). *Existential foundations of psychology* (Vol. 3). Pittsburgh: Duquesne University Press.

Ventres, W. (1994). Hearing the patient's story: Exploring physician-patient communication using narrative case reports. *Family Practice Research Journal, 14*(2), 139–147.

Weitzman, E. A., & Miles, M. B. (1995). *A software sourcebook: Computer programs for qualitative data analysis.* Thousand Oaks, CA: Sage.

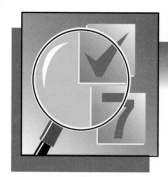

CHAPTER 24

INTERPRETING RESEARCH OUTCOMES

When data analysis is complete, there is a feeling that the answers are in and the study is finished. However, the results of statistical analysis, alone, are inadequate to complete the study. The researcher may know the results, but without careful intellectual examination, these results are of little use to others or to nursing's body of knowledge. To be useful, the evidence from data analysis needs to be carefully examined, organized, and given meaning, and both statistical and clinical significance needs to be assessed. This process is referred to as *interpretation*.

Data collection and analysis are action-oriented activities that require concrete thinking. However, when the results of the study are being interpreted, abstract thinking is used, including the creative use of introspection, reasoning, and intuition. In some ways, these last steps in the research process are the most difficult. They require a synthesis of the logic used to develop the research plan, strategies used in the data collection phase, and the mathematical logic or insight and gestalt formation used in data analysis. Evaluating the research process used in the study, producing meaning from the results, and forecasting the usefulness of the findings, all of which are involved in interpretation, require high-level intellectual processes.

Translation is frequently thought of as being synonymous with interpretation. Abstract theoretical statements are sometimes referred to as being translated into more concrete meaning, as, for example, in the operationalization of a variable. Although the two words *translate* and *interpret* are similar, their meanings have subtle differences. *Translation* means to transform from one language to another or to use terms that can be more easily understood. *Interpreting* involves explaining the meaning of information. Interpretation seems to include translation and to go beyond it to explore and impart meaning. Thus, in this step of the research process, the researcher translates the results of analysis into findings and then interprets by attaching meaning to the findings.

Within the process of interpretation are several intellectual activities that can be isolated and explored. These activities include examining evidence, forming conclusions, exploring the significance of the findings, generalizing the findings, considering implications, and suggesting further studies. Each of these activities is discussed in this chapter. The final chapter of theses and dissertations and the final sections of research articles and presentations include interpretation of research outcomes.

EXAMINING EVIDENCE

The first step in interpretation is a consideration of all the evidence available that supports or contradicts the validity of results related to the research objectives, questions, or hypotheses. To consider the evidence, one needs first to determine what the evidence is and then gather it together. The impact of each bit of evidence on the validity of results needs to be carefully considered; then the evidence as a whole needs to be synthesized for a final judgment. The process is somewhat like critiquing your own work. The temptation is to ignore flaws—certainly not to point them out. However, this process is essential to the building of a body of knowledge. It is a time not for confession, remorse, and apology, but rather for thoughtful reflection. Problems and strengths of the study need to be identified by the researcher and shared with colleagues at presentations and in publications. They affect the meaning of the results and can serve as guideposts for future researchers.

Evidence from the Research Plan

The initial evidence for the validity of the study results is derived from reexamination of the research plan. Reexamination requires reexploration of the logic of the methodology. This exploration will involve analyzing the logical links among the problem statement, purpose, research questions, variables, design, methods of observation, methods of measurement, and types of analyses. These elements of the study logically link together and are consistent with the research problem. Remember the old adage, a chain is only as strong as its weakest link? This saying is also true of research. Therefore, the study needs to be examined to identify its weakest links.

These weak links then need to be examined in terms of their impact on the results. Could the results, or some of the results, be a consequence of a weak link in the methodology rather than a true test of the hypotheses? Can the research objectives, questions, or hypotheses be answered from the methodology used in the study? Could the results be a consequence of an inappropriate conceptual or operational definition of the variable? Do the research questions clearly emerge from the framework? Can the results be related back to the framework? Are the analyses logically planned to test the questions?

If the types of analyses are inappropriate for examining the research questions, what do the results of analyses mean? For example, if the design failed to control extraneous variables, could some of these variables explain the results rather than the results being explained by the variables measured and examined through statistical analysis? Was the sample studied a logical group on which to test the hypotheses? Each link in the design needs to be carefully evaluated in this way to determine potential weaknesses. Every link is clearly related to the meaning given to the study results. If the researcher is reviewing a newly completed study and determines that the types of analyses were inappropriate, the analyses, of course, need to be redone. If the study is being critiqued, the findings may need to be seriously questioned.

Evidence from Measurement

One of the assumptions often made in interpreting study results is that the study variables were adequately measured. This adequacy is determined through examination of the fit of operational definitions with the framework and through validity and reliability information. Although reliability and validity of measurement strategies should be determined before their use in the study, the measures need to be reexamined at this point to determine the strength of evidence available from the results. For example, did the scale used to measure anxiety truly reflect the anxiety experienced in the study population? What was the effect size? Were the validity and reliability of instruments examined in the present study? Can this information be used to interpret the results? The validity and reliability of measurement are critical to the validity of results. If the instruments used do not measure the variables as defined conceptually and operationally in the study, the results of analyzed measurement scores mean little.

Scores from measurement instruments without validity and reliability can be used for statistical analyses just as easily as those with validity and reliability. The mathematical formula or the computer cannot detect the difference. Results of the analyses give the same information regardless of the validity and reliability. The difference is in the meaning attributed to the results. This difference is detectable only by scientists, not by computers.

Evidence from the Data Collection Process

Many activities that occur during data collection affect the meaning of results. Was the sample size sufficient? Did unforeseen events occur during the study that might have changed or had an impact on the data? Did strategies for acquiring a sample eliminate important groups whose data would have influenced the results? Were measurement techniques consistent? What impact do inconsistencies have on interpreting results? Sometimes data collection does not proceed as planned. Unforeseen situations alter the collection of data. What were these variations in the study? What impact do they have on interpreting the results? Sometimes data collection forms are completed by someone other than the subject. Variations may occur in events surrounding the administration of scales. For example, an anxiety scale may be given to one subject immediately before a painful procedure and to another subject on awakening in the morning. Values on these measures cannot be considered comparable. These types of differences are seldom reported and sometimes not even recorded. To some extent, only the researcher knows how consistently the measurements were taken. Reporting this information is dependent on the integrity of the researcher.

Evidence from the Data Analysis Process

The process of data analysis is an important factor in evaluating the meaning of results. One important part of this examination is to summarize the study weaknesses related to the data analysis process. A number of pertinent questions can be asked that are related to the meaning of results. How many errors were made in entering the data into the computer? How many subjects have missing data that could affect statistical analyses? Were the analyses accurately calculated? Were statistical assumptions violated? Were the statistics used appropriate

for the data? These issues need to be addressed initially before analyses are performed and again on completing the analyses before writing the final report. Before submitting a paper for publication, we recheck each analysis reported in the paper. We reexamine the analysis statements in the paper. Are we correctly interpreting the results of the analysis? Documentation on each statistical value or analysis statement reported in the paper is filed with a copy of the paper. The documentation includes the date of the analysis, page number of the computer printout showing the results (the printout is stored in a file by date of analysis), the sample size for the analysis, and the number of missing values.

Except in simple studies, data analysis in quantitative studies is usually performed by computer. With prepared statistical analysis programs, multiple analyses can be performed on the data that are not well understood by the researcher. To the neophyte researcher, the computer spits out reams of paper with incomprehensible printed information and, in the end, gives a level of significance. The appropriateness of the data and the logic behind the program may remain unknown, but the level of significance may be considered by a new researcher as absolute "proof" of an important finding.

The analysis process in qualitative studies is, to some degree, subjective. The process itself, however, requires great skill and can seldom be learned by reading a journal article. Sorting, organizing, and developing theoretical formulations from the data require great care and experience, yet the meaning derived from the analysis is dependent on the skill of conducting the analysis.

In gathering evidence for the implications of the study results, it is critical to reexamine the data analysis process. The researcher needs to examine the sufficiency of personal knowledge of the statistics and proficiency in the analyses used. Data need to be reexamined for accuracy and completeness. Mathematical operations performed manually need to be rechecked for accuracy. Computer printouts need to be reexamined for meaningful information that may have been overlooked. Tables of data need to be rechecked for accuracy and clarity. In qualitative studies, another qualitative researcher validates the analysis process by following the decision trail initially used to analyze the data. In all studies, researchers need to have a high level of confidence in the results they report.

Evidence from Data Analysis Results

The outcomes of data analysis are the most direct evidence available of the results. The researcher has intimate knowledge of the research and needs to evaluate its flaws and strengths carefully when judging the validity of the results. In descriptive and correlational studies, the validity of the results is dependent on how accurately the variables were measured in selected samples and settings. The value of evidence in any study is dependent on the amount of variance in the phenomenon explained within the study, a factor that is often not considered when interpreting the results (Tulman & Jacobsen, 1989). In quasi-experimental and experimental studies, in which hypothesized differences in groups are being examined, the differences or lack of differences do not indicate the amount of variance explained. This information needs to be reported in all studies and should serve as a basis for interpreting the results. (See Chapters 19–22 for discussions of methods of identifying the variance explained in an analysis.)

Interpretation of results from quasi-experimental and experimental studies is traditionally based on decision theory, with five possible results: (1) significant results that are in keeping with those predicted by the researcher, (2) nonsignificant results, (3) significant results that are opposite those predicted by the researcher, (4) mixed results, and (5) unexpected results.

SIGNIFICANT AND PREDICTED RESULTS

Results that are in keeping with those predicted by the researcher are the easiest to explain and, unless weak links are present, validate the proposed logical links among the elements of the study. These results support the logical links developed by the researcher among the framework, questions, variables, and measurement tools. This outcome is very satisfying to the researcher. However, in this situation, the researcher needs to consider alternative explanations for the positive findings. What other elements could possibly have led to the significant results?

NONSIGNIFICANT RESULTS

Unpredicted nonsignificant or inconclusive results are the most difficult to explain. These results are often referred to as negative results. The negative results could be a true reflection of reality. In this case, the reasoning of the researcher or the theory used by the researcher to develop the hypothesis is in error. If so, the negative findings are an important addition to the body of knowledge. Any report of nonsignificant results needs to indicate the results of power analysis to indicate the risk of a Type II error in relation to the nonsignificant results.

Negative results could also be due to inappropriate methodology, a deviant sample, a small sample, problems with internal validity, inadequate measurement, use of weak statistical techniques, or faulty analysis. This result may be a Type II error, which may mean that in reality the findings are significant but, because of weaknesses in the methodology, the significance was not detected. Unless these weak links are detected, the reported results could lead to faulty information in the body of knowledge (Angell, 1989). It is easier for the researcher to blame faulty methodology for nonsignificant findings than to find failures in theoretical or logical reasoning. If faulty methodology is blamed, the researcher needs to explain exactly how the breakdown in methodology led to the negative results. Negative results, in any case, do not mean that there are no relationships among the variables; they indicate that the study failed to find any.

SIGNIFICANT AND NOT PREDICTED RESULTS

Significant results opposite those predicted, if the results are valid, are an important addition to the body of knowledge. An example would be a study in which social support and ego strength were proposed to be positively related. If the study showed that high social support was related to low ego strength, the result would be opposite that predicted. Such results, when verified by other studies, indicate that we were headed in the wrong direction theoretically. Because these types of studies direct nursing practice, this information is important. In some of these cases, the researcher believes so strongly in the theory that the results are not believed. The researcher remains convinced that there was a problem in the methodology. Sometimes this belief remains entrenched in the minds of scientists for many years because of the bias that good research supports its hypotheses.

MIXED RESULTS

Mixed results are probably the most common outcome of studies. In this case, one variable may uphold the characteristics predicted whereas another does not, or two dependent measures of the same variable may show opposite results. These differences may be due to methodology problems, such as differing reliability or sensitivity of two methods of measuring variables. Mixed results may also indicate a need to modify existing theory.

UNEXPECTED RESULTS

Unexpected results are usually relationships found between variables that were not hypothesized and not predicted from the framework being used. These results are serendipitous. Most researchers examine as many elements of data as possible in addition to those directed by the questions. These findings can be useful in theory development or refinement and in the development of later studies. In addition, serendipitous results are important as evidence in developing the implications of the study. However, serendipitous results need to be dealt with carefully when considering meaning because the study was not designed to examine these results.

Evidence from Previous Studies

The results of the present study should always be examined in light of previous findings. It is impor-

tant to know whether the results are consistent with past research. Consistency in findings across studies is important in theory development and scientific progress. Therefore, any inconsistencies need to be explored to determine reasons for the differences. Replication of studies and synthesis of findings of existing studies are critical to the building of a body of knowledge and theory development.

FINDINGS

Results in a study are translated and interpreted; they then become findings. *Findings* are a consequence of evaluating evidence. Although much of the process of developing findings from results occurs in the mind of the researcher, evidence of such thinking can be found in published research reports. The 1994 study of McMillan and Mahon examining the quality of life of hospice patients on admission and at week 3 of hospice care presents the following research questions, results, and findings:

Research Question 1

"Is there a significant improvement in quality of life from admission to week 3 of hospice care as perceived by the patient?"

Results. "Only 31 of the original 67 patients who had a primary caregiver survived and were able to complete the SQLI (Sendra Quality of Life Index) a second time. The mean score for this group was 49.2 on admission and 49.7 at 3 weeks; there was no significant difference. Although grouped (mean) scores did not suggest a trend toward improvement, individual SQLI scores showed that approximately half of the subjects reported an improved quality of life with an increase of 10 points or more, whereas the other half reported a decrease in perceived quality of life. . . . Results of item analysis indicated that the greatest improvement in SQLI scores was in items related to support from nurses, worry about medical care, and sexual activity. The greatest decrease in SQLI scores was in items related to control over life and health, fun, being happy, and having a satisfying life. . . . Three items showed an improvement of more than six points. These items were subjected to paired *t* test comparisons to determine whether these improvements were statistically significant. The improvement in items related to sexual activity ($t = 6.18$, $p < 0.001$), worry over cost of medical care ($t = 6.6$, $p < 0.001$), and feeling support from the nurse ($t = 14.4$, $p < 0.0001$) were all found to be statistically significant with the greatest improvement being in feeling support from the nurse. Perceptions of physician support remained constant at about 62. The first item on the SQLI asks the patient, 'How much pain are you feeling?' The mean pain score from admission to week 3 shows a slight increase in mean scores on the pain item (from 56.9 to 59.3, $t = 1.86$, $p < 0.05$), indicating a slight but significant decrease in level of reported pain." (McMillan & Mahon , 1994, p. 56)

Findings. "Earlier research has found that for the vast majority of patients, quality of life declines rapidly near the end of life. However, the mean quality of life scores for patients remaining in this study remained at ~49. This result might suggest that hospice services in this case were unusually effective. However, individual scores showed that scores improved for some patients and decreased for others. Although the patient sample did not report a significant increase in their overall mean level of quality of life, when looked at individually it is encouraging to note that half of these patients did report summed scores that suggest such an improvement. Taken in the context of hospice where the average length of life after admission is 40 days, it is possible that the patients who did not report an overall increase in quality of life were those who were closer to death and thus were in a rapid decline." (McMillan & Mahon, 1994, p. 58) ■

● ●

Research Question 2

"Is there a significant improvement in quality of life from admission to week 3 of hospice care as perceived by the caregiver?" (McMillan & Mahon, 1994, p. 54)

Results. "The 31 caregivers who remained in the study until the third week reported a signifi-

cantly improved perception of the patient's quality of life from an admission mean of 48.2 to a week 3 mean of 53.3 ($t = 2.06$, $p < 0.05$)." (McMillan & Mahon, 1994, p. 56)

Findings. "It is also encouraging that caregivers reported a significant increase in their perceptions of the patient's quality of life. Although the increase was not large (5.3 points), it was statistically significant. There is more than one possible explanation for this finding. First, the patients' mean quality of life might really have improved. However, the patient data seem to refute this. Not only did patient scores not improve significantly, but the modest correlations between patient and caregiver scores suggest that patients' and caregivers' perceptions are not completely congruent. A second explanation for the overall increase in caregiver scores may be that the caregivers, after 3 weeks of involvement with the hospice team, want or need to believe that the patient quality of life has improved, regardless of the real situation. Or perhaps the support from the hospice team has improved the caregiver's quality of life in some way, causing a general improvement in caregiver attitude that was evident on the measure of the caregiver's perception of the patient's quality of life." (McMillan & Mahon, 1994, p. 58) ■

● ●

Research Question 3

"Is there a relationship between the patient's perceived quality of life and the demographic variables (age, gender, location of care)?" (McMillan & Mahon, 1994, p. 54)

Results. "At admission, there was a weak correlation between age and quality of life ($r = 0.30$). By week 3 there was no correlation. Using χ^2 analysis, there was no relationship found between gender and quality of life. Of the 80 subjects admitted to the study, data on location were available on 78. Sixty-five of these (83.3%) were being cared for in the home. The remaining subjects were receiving hospice care either in nursing homes ($n = 2$, 2.6%) or the hospital ($n = 11$, 14.1%)." (McMillan & Mahon, 1994, p. 57)

Findings. "No comparison was possible between location of care and perceived quality of life due to the small numbers of patients in nursing homes and hospitals." (McMillan & Mahon, 1994, p. 57) ■

. . . .

Research Question 4

"Is there a relationship between functional status as measured by the Karnofsky Performance Scale and quality of life as perceived by the patient?" (McMillan & Mahon, 1994, p. 54)

Results. "The mean Karnofsky Scale score at admission to hospice was 51.8. A weak relationship was found with SQLI scores at admission ($r = 0.25$). No Karnofsky scores were collected at week 3."

Findings. "The literature on quality of life included a number of studies that used the Karnofsky Performance Status Scale as a measure of quality of life. Although functional status is an important aspect of quality of life and may be correlated with it, functional status does not capture all of the aspects of quality of life that would be assessed by a multidimensional quality of life scale. The Karnofsky Performance Status Scale scores were available on these patients, so data were incorporated into the study. The correlations between the Karnofsky and SQLI scores were low ($r = 0.25$), as might be expected, providing evidence that the Karnofsky alone is not an adequate assessment of overall quality of life." (McMillan & Mahon, 1994, p. 58) ■

. . . .

Research Question 5

"Is there a correlation between quality of life as perceived by the patient and as perceived by the caregiver?" (McMillan & Mahon, 1994, p. 54)

Results. "Results showed a moderately weak to weak relationship, with the correlation decreasing slightly from admission ($r = 0.45$) to week 3 ($r = 0.39$)." (p. 57)

Findings. "Although it was expected, based on earlier research, that patient and caregiver scores would be correlated, it was expected that the corre-

lations would be weak to moderate, and they were weak. This seems to confirm that quality of life is a subjectively experienced phenomenon, and although caregivers are very 'tuned in' to the patients for whom they are providing care, the patients are the most reliable reporter of their own quality of life." (McMillan & Mahon, 1994, p. 58)

"It might be expected that although the correlation between patients and caregivers would be modest, the correlation would increase in magnitude from admission to week 3. That is, as the caregiver became increasingly involved in the patient's care, the ability to understand and report quality of life would increase. This was not the case. Although the correlations between patients and caregivers changed a little (from $r = 0.45$ to $r = 0.39$) from admission to week 3, it went in a downward direction. The reason for this slight decrease is unclear." (McMillan & Mahon, 1994, p. 58) ■

FORMING CONCLUSIONS

Conclusions are derived from the findings and are a synthesis of findings. Forming these conclusions requires a combination of logical reasoning, creative formation of a meaningful whole from pieces of information obtained through data analysis and findings from previous studies, receptivity to subtle clues in the data, and use of an open context in considering alternative explanations of the data.

When forming conclusions, it is important to remember that research never proves anything; rather, research offers support for a position. Proof is a logical part of deductive reasoning, but not of the research process. Therefore, formulation of causal statements is risky. For example, the causal statement that A *causes* B (absolutely, in all situations) cannot be scientifically proved. It is more credible to state conclusions in the form of conditional probabilities that are qualified. For example, it would be more appropriate to state in the study that if A occurred, then B occurred under conditions x, y, and z (Kerlinger, 1986), or that B had an 80% probability of occurring. Thus one could conclude that if preoperative teaching were given, postoperative anxiety was lowered as long as pain was controlled, complications did not occur, and family contacts were high.

McMillan and Mahon (1994) reached the following conclusions:

• •

"Results of this study suggest that hospice services are successful in improving the overall quality of life of some but not all patients who remain in care for 3 weeks. This is a very positive finding in light of previous research that suggests a rapid decline as death nears. Hospice services seemed to have a greater effect in some areas than in others. Patients felt increasingly supported by nurses from admission to week 3 and felt a constant level of support from their physicians. Patients seemed to worry less about the cost of medical care after 3 weeks in hospice care and reported an increase in sexual activity. Although some increase was seen in pain relief, pain management in hospice patients appears to need continued attention and monitoring." (McMillan & Mahon, 1994, p. 59) ■

The methodology of the study was examined when drawing conclusions from the findings. In spite of a researcher's higher motives to be objective, subjective judgments and biases will sometimes creep into the conclusions. A researcher needs to be alert and control subjectivity and biases. Students sometimes want positive findings so much that they will misinterpret statistical results on computer printouts as significant when they are clearly nonsignificant.

A researcher needs to identify the limitations of the study when forming conclusions about the findings. The limitations need to be included in the research report. McMillan and Mahon (1994) provided the following discussion of limitations:

• •

"A limitation of this study was the elimination of patients who were unable to self-report their quality of life. Thus, a large number of debilitated, comatose, or actively dying patients had to be eliminated. Although the quality of life of these patients could be reported by the caregivers, the data suggest that patient and caregiver reports are not com-

pletely congruent. Despite this lack of congruence, future studies should account for a wider sampling of all hospice patients even if the data source is less than ideal.

"A second limitation of this study was the inclusion of persons with diagnoses other than cancer. It is possible that persons with AIDS or cardiovascular disease may respond differently than would persons with cancer or that some cancers have a different course, affecting quality of life.

"A third limitation of the study was the lack of any quality of life tools designed especially for hospice patients. Because the SQLI is a fairly new instrument and has been validated for use with cancer patients rather than hospice patients per se, the appropriateness of the tool may be in question. However, the majority of patients in this study (80%) were cancer patients." (McMillan & Mahon, 1994, p. 59) ■

One of the risks in developing conclusions in research is going beyond the data, specifically, forming conclusions that are not warranted by the data. The most common example is a study that examines relationships between A and B by correlational analysis and then concludes that A causes B. Going beyond the data is due to faulty logic and occurs more frequently in published studies than one would like to believe. The researcher needs to check the validity of arguments related to conclusions before revealing findings.

EXPLORING THE SIGNIFICANCE OF FINDINGS

The word *significance* is used in two ways in research. Statistical significance is related to quantitative analysis of the results of the study. To be important, the results of quantitative studies that use statistical analysis must be statistically significant. *Statistical significance* means that the results are unlikely to be due to chance. However, statistically significant results are not necessarily important in clinical practice. The results can indicate a real difference that is not necessarily an important difference clinically. For example, Yonkman (1982, p. 356), in reporting results from her study of the effect of cool or heated aerosol on oral temperature, reported that "the statistical tests yielded small values which implied that differences were statistically significant. It is not clear that these differences in temperature are clinically significant."

The *practical significance of a study* is associated with its importance to nursing's body of knowledge. Significance is not a dichotomous characteristic because studies contribute in varying degrees to the body of knowledge. Statistically nonsignificant results can have practical significance. Significance may be associated with the amount of variance explained, control in the study design to eliminate unexplained variance, or detection of statistically significant differences. The researcher is expected to clarify the significance as much as possible. The areas of significance may be obvious to a researcher who has been immersed in the study but not to a reader or listener. Therefore, the researcher needs to delineate the areas of significance. Determining clinical significance is a judgment based on the researcher's clinical expertise. It is often based, in part, on whether treatment decisions or outcomes would be different in view of the study findings.

A few studies, referred to as landmark studies, become important referent points in the discipline, such as those by Johnson, 1972; Lindeman and Van Aernam, 1971; Passos and Brand, 1966; and Williams, 1972. The importance of a study may not become apparent for years after publication. However, some characteristics are associated with the significance of studies. Significant studies make an important difference in peoples' lives. The findings have external validity. Therefore, it is possible to generalize the findings far beyond the study sample so that the findings have the potential of affecting large numbers of people. The implications of significant studies go beyond concrete facts to abstractions and lead to the generation of theory or revisions in existing theory. A highly significant study has implications for one or more disciplines in addition to nursing. The study is accepted by others in the discipline and is frequently referenced in the literature. Over a period of time, the significance of a study is measured by the number of studies that it generates.

GENERALIZING THE FINDINGS

Generalization extends the implications of the findings from the sample studied to a larger population or from the situation studied to a larger situation. For example, if the study were conducted on diabetic patients, it may be possible to generalize the findings to persons with other illnesses or to well individuals. Highly controlled experimental studies, which are high in internal validity, tend to be low in generalizability because they tend to have low external validity.

How far can generalizations be made? The answer to this question is debatable. From a narrow perspective, one cannot really generalize from the sample on which the study was done. Any other sample is likely to be different in some way. The conservative position, represented by Kerlinger (1986), recommends caution in considering the extent of generalization. Generalization is considered particularly risky by conservatives if the sample was not randomly selected. According to Kerlinger (1986, p. 301), "Unless special precautions are taken and special efforts made, the results of research are frequently not representative, and hence not generalizable." This statement is representative of the classic sampling theory position. However, as discussed in Chapter 18, generalizations are often made to abstract or theoretical populations. Thus, conclusions need to address applications to theory. Judgments about the reasonableness of generalizing need to address issues related to external validity, as discussed in Chapter 10.

Generalizations based on accumulated evidence from many studies are called *empirical generalizations*. These generalizations are important for verification of theoretical statements or development of new theories. Empirical generalizations are the base of a science and contribute to scientific conceptualization. Nursing currently has few empirical generalizations.

CONSIDERING IMPLICATIONS

Implications are the meanings of conclusions for the body of knowledge, theory, and practice. Implications are based on the conclusions and are more specific than conclusions. They provide specific suggestions for implementing the findings. The researcher needs to consider the areas of nursing for which the study findings would be useful. For example, suggestions could be made about how nursing practice should be modified. If a study indicated that a specific solution was effective in decreasing stomatitis, the implications would state that the findings had implications for caring for patients with stomatitis. It would not be sufficient to state that the study had implications for nurses practicing in oncology.

McMillan and Mahon (1994) suggested the following implications:

"One important goal of hospice care is pain relief. Although pain is a symptom that can be brought under control in hours or days, there was only limited improvement in pain after 3 weeks of hospice care. Although a statistically significant decrease in pain intensity was reported, a decrease of only 2.4 points on a 100-point scale is not clinically significant. This finding of lack of improvement in pain is consistent with results of earlier studies. This finding would seem to suggest that greater attention needs to be paid to pain relief among these patients. . . . Even patients who are greatly debilitated and very near death should expect their level of pain to decrease." (McMillan & Mahon, 1994, p. 58) ■

SUGGESTING FURTHER STUDIES

Completing a study and examining its implications should culminate in recommendations for future studies that emerge from the present study and from previous studies in the same area of interest. Suggested studies or recommendations for further study may include replications or repeating the design with a different or larger sample. In every study, the researcher gains knowledge and experience that can be used to design "a better study next time." Formulating recommendations for future studies stimulates the researcher to define more clearly how to improve the study. From a logical or theoretical point of view, the findings should lead

directly to more hypotheses to further test the framework in use.

McMillan and Mahon (1994) provide the following suggestions for future research:

"Subsequent hospice quality of life studies should include number of days from death as part of the investigation. . . . Future studies might focus on what is actually done to assess and manage pain or might ask patients and caregivers whether they believe that everything possible was being done to relieve pain." (McMillan & Mahon, 1994, p. 58)

"The data suggest that patient and caregiver reports are not completely congruent. Despite this lack of congruence, future studies should account for a wider sampling of all hospice patients even if the data source is less than ideal." (McMillan & Mahon, 1994, p. 59)

"Future studies should control the diagnoses of hospice patients admitted to the study." (McMillan & Mahon, 1994, p. 59)

"Future studies should use an instrument that is specifically designed for hospice patients. In addition, a method should be formed to collect data from patients who are very debilitated when they are admitted to hospice so that the sample may be more representative of the population of interest." (McMillan & Mahon, 1994, p. 59) ■

■ SUMMARY

To be useful, evidence from data analysis needs to be carefully examined, organized, and given meaning. This process is referred to as interpretation. Data collection and analysis are action-oriented activities that are concrete. However, when the results of the study have been obtained, more abstract thinking is used to interpret the results. Within the process of interpretation, several intellectual activities can be isolated and explored, such as examining evidence, forming conclusions, exploring the significance of the findings, generalizing the findings, considering implications, and suggesting further studies.

The first step in interpretation is consideration of

all evidence available that supports or contradicts the validity of the results. Strengths and weaknesses of the study are explored. Evidence is obtained from a variety of sources, including the research plan, measurement validity and reliability, data collection process, data analysis process, data analysis results, and previous studies. Evidence of the validity of the results is derived from reexamination of the research plan. The reliability and validity of measurement strategies need to be determined before their use, and these measures need to be reexamined to determine the strength of evidence available from the results. Many factors can occur during the data collection process that affect the meaning of results, such as insufficient sample size, inappropriate sampling strategies, or unforeseen events. The evidence from data analysis is dependent on the researcher's knowledge of statistics and the proficiency of the analysis methods used.

The outcomes of data analysis are the most direct evidence available of the results related to the research objectives, questions, or hypotheses. Five possible results are (1) significant results that are in keeping with those predicted by the researcher, (2) nonsignificant results, (3) significant results that are opposite those predicted by the researcher, (4) mixed results, and (5) unexpected results. The results of a study should always be examined in light of previous findings.

The results of a study are translated and interpreted and then become findings. Findings are a consequence of evaluating evidence. Conclusions are derived from the findings and are a synthesis of the findings. Forming conclusions requires a combination of logical reasoning, creative formation of a meaningful whole from pieces of information obtained through data analysis and findings from previous studies, receptivity to subtle clues in the data, and use of an open context in considering alternative explanations of the data.

Implications are the meanings of study conclusions for the body of knowledge, theory, and practice. The significance of a study is associated with its importance to the body of knowledge. A study needs to be clinically significant as well as statistically significant. Significance is not a dichotomous characteristic because studies contribute in varying degrees to the body of knowledge. Generalization extends the implications of the findings from the sample studied to a larger population. Completion of a study and examination of implications should culminate in recommending future studies that emerge from the present study and previous studies. Suggested studies or recommendations for further study may include replications or repeating the design with a different or larger sample.

REFERENCES

Angell, M. (1989). Negative studies. *New England Journal of Medicine, 321*(7), 464–466.

Johnson, J. E. (1972). Effects of structuring patients' expectations on their reactions to threatening events. *Nursing Research, 21*(6), 499–503.

Kerlinger, F. N. (1986). *Foundations of behavioral research* (3rd ed.). New York: Holt, Rinehart & Winston.

Lindeman, C. A., & Van Aernam, B. (1971). Nursing intervention with the presurgical patient—the effects of structured and unstructured preoperative teaching. *Nursing Research, 20*(4), 319–332.

McMillan, S. C., & Mahon, M. (1994). A study of quality of life of hospice patients on admission and at week 3. *Cancer Nursing, 17*(1), 52–60.

Passos, J. Y., & Brand, L. M. (1966). Effects of agents used for oral hygiene. *Nursing Research, 15*(3), 196–202.

Tulman, L. R., & Jacobsen, B. S. (1989). Goldilocks and variability. *Nursing Research, 38*(6), 377–379.

Williams, A. (1972). A study of factors contributing to skin breakdown. *Nursing Research, 21*(3), 238–243.

Yonkman, C. A. (1982). Cool and heated aerosol and the measurement of oral temperature. *Nursing Research, 31*(6), 354–357.

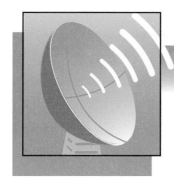

CHAPTER 25

COMMUNICATING RESEARCH FINDINGS

Imagine a nurse researcher conducting a study in which a unique phenomenon is described, a previously unrecognized relationship is detected, or the effectiveness of an intervention is determined. This information might make a difference in nursing practice; however, the nurse feels unskilled in presenting the information and overwhelmed by the idea of publishing. She places the study in a bottom drawer with an intent to communicate the findings "some day." This type of response results in many valuable nursing studies not being communicated and the information being lost. Winslow (1996) considers failure to publish a form of scientific misconduct.

Communicating research findings, the final step in the research process, involves developing a research report and disseminating it through presentations and publications to audiences of nurses, health care professionals, policymakers, and health care consumers. Disseminating research findings provides many advantages for the researcher, the nursing profession, and the consumer of nursing services. By presenting and publishing their findings, researchers are able to advance the knowledge of a discipline and receive personal recognition, professional advancement, and other psychological and financial compensation for their work. These rewards are essential for the continuation of research in a discipline. Communicating research findings also promotes the critique and replication of studies, identification of additional research problems, and the use of findings in practice. Using research find-

ings in practice promotes improved patient outcomes. To encourage and facilitate the communication of research findings in nursing, this chapter describes the content of a research report, the audiences for communication of findings, and the processes for presenting and publishing research findings.

CONTENT OF A RESEARCH REPORT

Both quantitative and qualitative research reports include similar sections. The report usually has four major sections: (1) introduction, (2) methods, (3) results, and (4) discussion of the findings (Field & Morse, 1985; Tornquist et al., 1989). The type and depth of information included in these sections depend on the type of study conducted, the intended audiences, and the mechanisms for disseminating the report. For example, theses and dissertations are research reports that are usually developed in-depth to demonstrate the student's understanding of the research problem and process to faculty members. Research articles for publication in journals are concisely written to communicate research findings efficiently and effectively to nurses and health professionals. The methods, results, and discussion sections of qualitative studies are usually more detailed than those of quantitative studies because of the complex data collection and analysis procedures and the comprehensive findings (Knafl & Howard, 1984).

Quantitative Research Report

An outline of the content covered in the four major sections of a quantitative research report is presented in Table 25–1.

INTRODUCTION

The introduction of a research report briefly identifies the problem that was studied, provides a rationale for studying that problem, and presents an empirical and theoretical basis for the study. An introduction includes the following content: a problem statement; significance of the problem; study purpose; a review of relevant literature; framework; and research objectives, questions, or hypotheses (if applicable). This content is developed for the research proposal and is then summarized in the final report. Depending on the type of research report, the review of literature and framework might be separate sections or even separate chapters.

Review of Literature

The review of literature documents the current knowledge of the problem investigated. The sources included in the literature review are those that were used to develop the study and interpret the findings. A review of literature can be two or three paragraphs or several pages in length. In journal articles, the review of literature is concise and usually includes 10 to 15 sources. Theses and dissertations frequently include an extensive literature review to document the student's knowledge of the research problem.

Framework

A research report needs to include an explicitly identified framework. The major concepts in the framework need to be defined and the relationships among the concepts described. A map or model can be developed to clarify the logic within the framework. If a particular proposition is being tested, that proposition should be clearly stated. Developing a framework map and identifying the proposition or propositions examined in a study provide a clear connection between the framework and the research objectives, questions, or hypotheses.

METHODS

The methods section of a research report describes how the study was conducted. This section needs to be concise, yet provide sufficient information for nurses to critique or replicate the study procedures. The study design, sample, setting, methods of measurement or instruments, and the data collection process are described in this section. If the research project included a pilot study, the planning, implementation, and results obtained from the pilot study are presented briefly. Any changes made in the research project based on the pilot study are described.

Design

The study design and level of significance (.05, .01, or .001) selected are identified in the research report. If the design included a treatment, the report needs to describe the treatment, including the protocol for implementing the treatment, training of people to implement the protocol, and a discussion of the consistency of administration of the treatment (Egan et al., 1992; Kirchhoff & Dille, 1994). A complex study design might be presented in a table

---

TABLE 25–1
OUTLINE FOR A QUANTITATIVE RESEARCH REPORT

INTRODUCTION
   Statement of the problem and significance
   Statement of the purpose
   Brief literature review
   Identification of the framework
   Identification of research objectives, questions, or hypotheses
     (if applicable)
METHODS
   Identification of the research design
   Description of the sample and setting
   Description of the methods of measurement
   Discussion of the data collection process
RESULTS
   Description of the data analysis procedures
   Presentation of results
DISCUSSION
   Discussion of major findings
   Identification of the limitations
   Presentation of conclusions
   Identification of the implications for nursing
   Recommendations for further research
REFERENCES

or figure, such as the examples provided in Chapter 11.

Sample and Setting

The research report usually includes the criteria for selecting the sample, the sample size, and sample characteristics. The use of power analysis to determine sample size needs to be discussed. Sample mortality is discussed, with reasons given for subject attrition. The number of subjects completing the study should be provided if it is different from the initial sample size. If the subjects were divided into groups (experimental and comparison groups), the method for assigning subjects to groups and the number of subjects in each group need to be identified. The protection of subjects' rights and the process of informed consent are also covered briefly. The setting of the study is often described in one or two sentences, and agencies are not identified by name unless permission has been obtained. The sample and setting for a study are often presented in narrative format; however, some researchers present the characteristics of their sample in a table.

Methods of Measurement

The variables of the study are operationalized by identifying the method of measurement for each. Details about the methods of measurement or instruments used in the data collection process are critical for nurses to critique and replicate a study. The report needs to describe what information is collected by each instrument, the frequency with which the instrument has been used in previous research, and any reliability and validity information previously published on the instrument. In addition, the report needs to include the reliability and any further validity development for the current study. If physiological measures are used, their accuracy, precision, selectivity, sensitivity, and sources of error need to be addressed.

Data Collection Process

The description of the data collection process in the research report details who collected the data, the procedure for collecting data, and the type and frequency of measurements obtained. In describing who collected the data, the report needs to indicate the experience of the data collector and any training provided. If more than one person collected data,

the precautions taken to ensure consistency in data collection need to be described.

RESULTS

The results section reveals what was found by conducting the study and includes the data analysis procedures, the results generated from these analyses, and sometimes the effect size achieved (Kraemer & Thiemann, 1987). For example, Lander and colleagues (1996) compared the effect of 5% lidocaine ointment with that of cream containing a eutectic mixture of local anesthetics (EMILA) on dermal anesthesia. The authors analyzed the data by a within-subject analysis of variance and found that "Significantly more pain was reported for 5% lidocaine ($M = 9.6$) than for EMILA ($M = 2.4$, $F = 11.5$, $p = .02$). The observed power was determined to be .77. The effect size for the study was .70" (p. 52).

The results section is best organized by the research objectives, questions, or hypotheses if stated in the study and, if not, by the study purpose. Research results can be presented in narrative format and organized into figures and tables. The methods used to present the results depend on the end product of data analysis and the researcher's preference. When reporting results in a narrative format, the value of the calculated statistic, the number of degrees of freedom, and probability or p value are identified. When insignificant results are reported, the power level for that analysis should also be reported to evaluate the risk of a Type II error. The *Publication Manual for the American Psychological Association* (APA) (1994) provides direction for citing a variety of statistical results in a research report. For example, the format for reporting chi-squared results is χ^2 (degrees of freedom, sample size) = statistical value, or p value. Wikblad and Anderson (1995) compared three wound dressings—conventional absorbent, semiocclusive hydroactive, and occlusive hydrocolloid—in patients undergoing heart surgery and expressed their results in narrative format according to the APA (1994) guidelines.

● ●

"Patients in the hydroactive dressing group had significantly poorer wound healing (27% of the wounds were well healed, and 25% were partially healed), compared with patients treated with the absorbent dressing (57% of the wounds were well healed, and 33% were partially healed); χ^2 (2, $n = 153$) $= 23.1$, $p < .0001$; and with patients in the hydrocolloid dressing group (50% of the wounds were well healed and 27% were partially healed); χ^2 (2, $n = 129$) $= 7.6$, $p < .02$. The differences in wound healing between the hydrocolloid and the absorbent dressing groups were not significant; χ^2 (2, $n = 150$) $= 5.3$, $p > .05$." (Wikblad & Anderson, 1995, p. 314) ■

Presentation of Results in Figures and Tables

Figures and tables are used to present a large amount of detailed information concisely and clearly. Researchers use figures and tables to demonstrate relationships, document change over time, and reduce the amount of discussion needed in the text of the report (Mirin, 1981). However, figures and tables are useful only if they are appropriate for the results generated and are well constructed (Wainer, 1984). Table 25–2 provides guidelines for the development of accurate and clear figures and tables for a research report.

Figures.   Figures or illustrations provide the reader with a picture of the results. Researchers often use computer programs to generate a variety of sophisticated black-and-white and color figures. Some common figures included in nursing research reports are bar graphs and line graphs. Bar graphs can have horizontal or vertical bars that represent the size or amount of the group or variable studied. The bar graph is also a means of comparing one item with another. McFarlane and colleagues (1996) studied abuse during pregnancy and the associations with maternal health and infant birth weight. The ethnic-specific birth weights by abuse status were presented in a figure (see Figure 25–1). The researchers' discussion of this figure was as follows: "Mean birth weights were lowest for women abused during pregnancy, followed by women abused within the last year but not during pregnancy. The highest mean birth weight infants were born to women reporting no abuse. Specific to ethnicity, abused African American women delivered infants weighing 127 g (grams) less, Hispanic 40 g less, and white 151 g less." (McFarlane et al., 1996, p. 39)

TABLE 25–2
GUIDELINES FOR DEVELOPING TABLES AND FIGURES IN RESEARCH REPORTS

1. Examine the results obtained from a study and determine what results are essential to include in the report. Determine which results are best conveyed in figure and table format.
2. Use figures and tables to explain or support only the major points of the report. Using too many figures and tables can overwhelm the rest of the report, but a few receive attention and are effective in conveying the main results. Statistically nonsignificant findings are not usually presented in tables.
3. Keep the figures and tables simple; do not try to convey too much information in a single table. Two simple tables are better than one complex one.
4. Tables and figures should be complete and clear to the reader without referring to the text.
5. Each table and figure needs a clear, brief title.
6. Tables and figures are numbered separately and sequentially in a report. Thus a report might have a Table 1 and Table 2 and a Figure 1 and Figure 2.
7. The headings, labels, symbols, and abbreviations used in figures and tables need to be appropriate, clear, and easy to read. Any symbols and abbreviations used need to be explained in a note included with the table or figure.
8. Probability values need to be identified with actual p values or with asterisks. If asterisks are used, a single asterisk is used for the least stringent significance level and two asterisks for more stringent significance, such as $*p < .05$ and $**p < .01$.
9. Figures and tables need to be referred to in the written text, such as "Table 3 presents . . . ." or "(see Figure 1)." Figures and tables also need to be placed as close as possible to the section of the text where they are discussed (APA, 1994; Shurter et al., 1965; Wainer, 1984).

A line graph is developed by joining a series of points with a line and shows how something varies over time. In this type of graph, the horizontal scale is used to measure time, and the vertical scale is used to measure number and quantity (Shurter et al., 1965). Figure 25–2 is a line graph developed by Swain and Steckel (1981, p. 219) to demonstrate the effects of three treatments (routine clinical care, health education, and contingency contracting) on patients' blood pressure over four visits. The discussion of this graph indicated that blood pressure for the three groups was significantly different ($F = 3.39$, $p < 0.05$), with the contingency contracting group demonstrating the greatest drop in diastolic blood pressure.

Tables.   Tables are used more frequently in research reports than figures are and can be developed to present results from numerous statistical analyses.

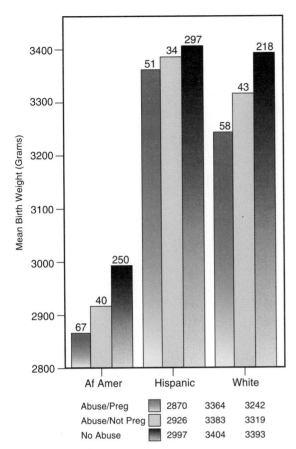

FIGURE 25–1 ■ Infant birth weight and abuse status. (From McFarlane, J., Parker, B., & Soeken, K. [1996]. Abuse during pregnancy: Associations with maternal health and infant birth weight. *Nursing Research, 45*[1], 39. Philadelphia: Lippincott-Raven.)

	Af Amer	Hispanic	White
Abuse/Preg	2870	3364	3242
Abuse/Not Preg	2926	3383	3319
No Abuse	2997	3404	3393

In tables, the results are presented in columns and rows for easy review by the reader. The sample tables included in this section present means, standard deviations, *t* values, chi-squared values, and correlations. The means and standard deviations for study variables should be included in the published study. These values provide a basis for comparison across studies and are important for future meta-analyses. During replication of a study, the means and standard deviations are used to calculate the effect size when performing a power analysis to determine sample size (Tulman & Jacobsen, 1989).

McKenna and associates (1995) examined coronary risk factors before and after percutaneous trans-luminal coronary angioplasty (PTCA). Table 25–3 presents the results of this study, including descriptive statistics (means, standard deviations, and frequencies) and inferential statistics (*t* test and chi-squared). The *t* test was used to analyze ratio-level data (serum cholesterol, body mass index, and number of cigarettes per day) and chi-squared to analyze nominal data (exercising and smoking habits). McKenna and colleagues (1995, p. 209) noted that "at post-PTCA follow-up, significant improvements had occurred in mean serum cholesterol levels, mean body mass index, and the number of subjects engaging in regular exercise ($p < .001$). . . . But the frequency of patients smoking after PTCA increased significantly ($p < .001$)."

Tables are used to identify correlations among variables, and often the table presents the correlation matrix generated from the data analysis. The significance of each correlation value needs to be indicated in the table. Reece (1995) studied the intercorrelations among dimensions of maternal adaptation and stress 1 year after delivery. The correlation matrix for the eight study variables is presented in Table 25–4, and the significance of each correlation is indicated by the use of asterisks. The discussion of this table was, "In addition to associations with stress, gratification with the labor and delivery experience were correlated additionally with spouse/partner relationship and satisfaction with the infant." (Reece, 1995, p. 65)

DISCUSSION

The discussion section ties the other sections of the research report together and gives them meaning. This section includes the major findings, limitations of the study, conclusions drawn from the findings, implications of the findings for nursing, and recommendations for further research. The major findings, which are generated through an interpretation of the results, should be discussed in relation to the research problem, purpose, and objectives, questions, or hypotheses (if applicable). Frequently, a study's findings are compared with the findings from previous research and are linked to the study's framework and the existing theoretical knowledge base. Discussion of the findings also includes the limitations that were identified in the proposal and

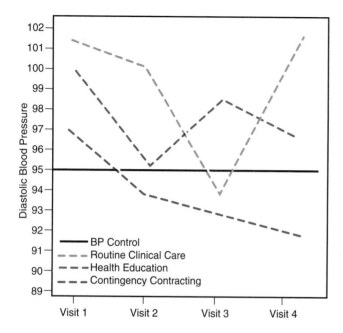

FIGURE 25–2 ■ Blood pressures by treatment group across four visits. (From Swain, M. A., & Steckel, S. B. [1981]. Influencing adherence among hypertensives. *Research in Nursing & Health, 4*[1], 219. Copyright © 1981, John Wiley & Sons. Reprinted by permission of John Wiley & Sons, Inc.)

during conduct of the study. For example, a study might have limitations related to sample size, design, or instruments. The generalizability of the findings is influenced by these limitations.

The research report includes the conclusions or the knowledge that was generated from the findings. Conclusions are frequently stated in tentative or speculative terms because one study does not produce conclusive findings (Tornquist et al., 1989). The researcher might provide a brief rationale for accepting certain conclusions and rejecting others. The conclusions need to be discussed in terms of their implications for nursing knowledge, theory, and practice. The researcher often describes how the

TABLE 25–3
CENTRAL TENDENCY, VARIABILITY, AND FREQUENCIES WITH CORRESPONDING STATISTICS FOR RISK FACTORS PRE-PTCA AND AT FOLLOW-UP

	DESCRIPTIVE STATISTICS			
RISK FACTOR	**Pre-PTCA**	**Follow-up**	**n**	**STATISTIC (TEST)**
Serum cholesterol	Mean = 240 SD = 47.5	Mean = 222 SD = 39.4	198	$t = 6.24*$
Body mass index	Mean = 26.58 SD = 3.65	Mean = 26.17 SD = 3.61	208	$t = 3.93*$
Currently exercising	f = 66 (31.7%)	f = 135 (64.9%)	208	$\chi^2 = 38.06*$
Currently smoking	f = 10 (4.8%)	f = 27 (13.0%)	208	$\chi^2 = 13.80*$
Cigarettes/day	Mean = 9.8 SD = 6.6	Mean = 20.4 SD = 11.9	208	$t = 2.38**$

$*p < .001.$
$**p < 0.05.$
PTCA = percutaneous transluminal coronary angioplasty; *SD* = standard deviation.
From McKenna, K. T., Maas, F., & McEniery, P. T. (1995). Coronary risk factor status after percutaneous transluminal coronary angioplasty. *Heart & Lung, 24*(3), 210.

TABLE 25-4
INTERCORRELATIONS AMONG DIMENSIONS OF MATERNAL ADAPTATION AND STRESS 1 YEAR AFTER DELIVERY ($N = 82$)

OUTCOME VARIABLES	1	2	3	4	5	6	7	8
Dimensions of maternal adaptation								
1. Quality of relationship with husband		.63*	.24**	.12	.09	.25**	.30**	.35*
2. Father's participation in infant care			.09	−.02	.11	.08	.07	.06
3. Gratification with delivery				.09	.24	.37*	.12	.32*
4. Satisfaction with life situation and life circumstance					.30*	.23	.22	.50*
5. Confidence in motherhood						.44*	.32*	.42*
6. Satisfaction with the infant and infant care tasks							.40*	.55*
7. Support for the parental role								.33*
Stress								
8. Global perceived stress								

Low scores on the Parent Symptom Questionnaire (PSQ) indicate maternal satisfaction and adaptation, and high scores indicate maladaptation, difficulty coping, and dissatisfaction.
*$p < .01$.
**$p < .05$.
From Reece, S. M. (1995). Stress and maternal adaptation in first-time mothers more than 35 years old. *Applied Nursing Research, 8*(2), 61–66.

findings and conclusions might be implemented in specific practice areas. The research report concludes with recommendations for further research. Specific problems that require investigation are identified, and procedures for replicating the study are described. The discussion section of the research report demonstrates the value of conducting the study and stimulates the reader to use the findings in practice or to conduct additional research.

Qualitative Research Report

Reports for qualitative research are as diverse as the different types of qualitative studies. (The different types of qualitative research are presented in Chapter 4, and results from specific qualitative studies are presented in Chapter 23.) The intent of a qualitative research report is to describe the flexible, dynamic implementation of the research project and the unique, creative findings obtained. Like the quantitative report, a qualitative research report usually includes the four sections of introduction, methods, results, and discussion (see Table 25–5).

INTRODUCTION

The introduction section of the report identifies the phenomenon under investigation and indicates the type of qualitative study that was conducted. The study purpose and specific research aims or questions flow from the phenomenon, clarify the study focus, and identify expected outcomes of the investigation. The significance of the study topic to nursing knowledge and practice is described, with documentation from the literature. Qualitative studies are based on a variety of assumptions and philosophies that are identified in the report to provide a basis for the methodology, results, and discussion sections. In a sense, the philosophy provides a theoretical perspective for the study (Burns, 1989). Some qualitative studies include a brief literature review in the introduction or as a separate section of the report. Other studies include a review of literature only in the discussion of findings.

METHODS

In the methods section, the researcher documents his or her credentials for conducting the study. This documentation is valuable in determining the worth of the study because the researcher serves as a primary data-gathering instrument and the data analyses occur within the reasoning processes of the researcher (Burns, 1989). The site and population selected for the study are described. The unique role of the researcher is also detailed, including training of project staff, entry into the setting, selection of subjects, and ethical considerations extended to the subjects during data collection and analysis.

The data collection process is time-consuming and complex. The research report includes a description of the variety of data collection tools used, such as observation guides, open-ended interviews, direct participation, documents, life histories, audiovisual media (photographs, videotapes), biographies, and diaries (Knafl & Howard, 1984; Leininger, 1985). The flexible, dynamic way in which the researcher collects data is described, including the time spent collecting data, how data were recorded, and the amount of data collected. For example, if data collection involved participant observation, the number, length, structure, and focus of the observation and participation periods need to be described. In addition, the tools (such as audiotapes or videotapes) for recording the information gained from these periods of observation and participation are identified.

Packard and coworkers (1991, p. 439) conducted a qualitative longitudinal investigation of "the stressful illness-related experiences reported by women living with one of three different diseases: nonmetastatic breast cancer, diabetes, and fibrocystic breast disease." The data were gathered through interviews conducted in the subjects' homes on "five occasions at 4-month intervals over a 17- to 18-month period." (p. 440) The subjects' responses to questions were recorded verbatim.

RESULTS

The results section of the research report includes data analysis procedures and presentation of the findings. The data, in the form of notes, tapes, and other materials from observations and interviews, must be synthesized into meaningful categories or organized into common themes by the researcher. The data analysis procedures (content, symbolic, structural, interactional, philosophical, ethnographic, phenomenological, semantic, historical, inferential, grounded theory, perceptual, and reflexive) are performed during and after the data collection process (Leininger, 1985). These analysis procedures and the process for implementing them are described in the report. Packard and colleagues (1991) used content analysis to analyze the verbatim reports from their subjects. They summarized their data analysis procedures in Table 25–6, which identifies the number of cycles of data analysis, the analysis procedures, and the number of categories identified.

The results are presented in a manner that clarifies the phenomenon under investigation for the reader. These results include gestalts, patterns, and theories that are developed to describe life experiences, cultures, and historical events, which are frequently expressed in narrative format. Sometimes, these theoretical ideas are organized into conceptual maps, models, or tables. Researchers often gather additional data or reexamine existing data to verify their theoretical conclusions, and this process is described in the report (Burns, 1989). Some of the results from the study of Packard and colleagues

		TABLE 25–6		
		DATA ANALYSIS PROCEDURE		
CYCLE	**SAMPLE SIZE**	**OCCASION**	**PROCEDURE**	**RESULTS**
1	66	1	Unitize data	41 categories
			Group data by category	
			Label categories	
2	49	1	Unitize data	35 categories
			Classify data	
			Revise schema	
			Revise labels	
3	115	2, 3	Repeat cycle 2 procedure	22 categories
			Reclassify data; cycles 1 and 2	
			Interrater reliability	85%
			Develop domains	7 domains
			Develop core constructs	3 constructs
4	115	1, 2, 3	Determine prevalence rates	See Figure 1

From Packard, N. J., Haberman, M. R., Woods, N. F., & Yates, B. C. (1991). Demands of illness among chronically ill women. *Western Journal of Nursing Research, 13*(4), 442.

(1991) are presented in Table 25–7. The discussion of Table 25–7 indicated that 22 categories were identified and organized into seven domains of illness demands, and these "domains were grouped into three overriding or core constructs of illness demands: (1) direct disease effects, (2) personal disruption, and (3) environmental transactions." (p. 442)

DISCUSSION

The discussion section includes conclusions, implications for nursing, and recommendations for further research. The conclusions are a summary of the findings and indicate what was and was not accomplished during the study. Each research question is answered, and the findings are linked to relevant theoretical and empirical literature. Implications of the findings for nursing practice and theory development are explored, and suggestions are provided for further research.

Theses and Dissertations

Theses and dissertations are research reports that are developed in depth by students as part of the requirements for a degree. The content included in a thesis or dissertation depends on the members of the student's research committee, but organization of the content usually follows the outline presented in Table 25–8. The introduction, review of relevant literature, framework, and the methods and procedures sections of this outline are described in Chapter 28. The content of the results and discussion sections is similar to that just described for a research report.

AUDIENCES FOR COMMUNICATION OF RESEARCH FINDINGS

Before developing a research report, the investigator needs to determine *who* will benefit from knowing the findings. The greatest impact on nursing practice can be achieved by communicating nursing research findings to a variety of audiences, including nurses, other health professionals, health care consumers, and policymakers. Nurses, including educators, practitioners, and researchers, must be aware of research findings for communication in academic programs, for use in practice, and as a basis for conducting additional studies. Other health professionals need to be aware of the knowledge generated by nurse researchers and facilitate the use of that knowledge in the health care industry. Con-

TABLE 25–7
CORE CONSTRUCTS, CONCEPTUAL DOMAINS, AND CATEGORIES

CORE CONSTRUCT	CONCEPTUAL DOMAIN	CATEGORY
Direct disease effects	Direct disease effects	1. Direct disease effects
Personal disruption	Disruption of continuity	2. Vulnerability
		3. Uncertainty
		4. Unmet expectations
		5. Future concerns
		6. Confrontation with time
		7. Reminders
	Disruption of integrity	8. Self-image
		9. Social comparisons
		10. Social-emotional disturbances
	Disruption of normality	11. Monitoring symptoms
		12. Monitoring coping (self and others)
Environmental trans- actions	Social response	13. Social network
		14. Role compensation
		15. Marital dynamics
	Treatment process	16. Financial costs
		17. Treatment effects
		18. Accommodation
		19. Waiting for results
		20. Additional treatment
	Patient provider interaction	21. Information exchange
		22. Negative relationships

From Packard, N. J., Haberman, M. R., Woods, N. F., & Yates, B. C. (1991). Demands of illness among chronically ill women. *Western Journal of Nursing Research, 13*(4), 443.

sumers are interested in the outcomes produced by nursing interventions that have been tested through research. Policymakers at the local, state, and federal level are using research findings to generate health policy that will have an impact on individual practitioners and the health care industry.

Strategies for Communicating Research to Different Audiences

Research findings can be communicated through written reports and oral and visual presentations. Various strategies for communicating findings to nurses, health care professionals, policymakers, and consumers are outlined in Table 25–9.

AUDIENCE OF NURSES

The most common mechanisms used by nurses to communicate research findings to their peers are presentations at conferences and meetings. An in-

creasing number of nursing organizations and institutions are sponsoring research conferences. The American Nurses' Association and many of its state associations sponsor annual nursing research conferences. The Western Council of Higher Education for Nursing has been sponsoring annual research conferences since 1968, and the proceedings from these conferences are published in a volume entitled *Communicating Nursing Research Findings.* The members of Sigma Theta Tau, the international honor society for nursing, sponsor international, national, regional, and local research conferences. Specialty organizations, such as the American Association of Critical Care Nurses, Oncology Nurses' Society, and Maternal-Child Health Nursing Association, sponsor research meetings and conferences. Many universities and some health care agencies sponsor or cosponsor research conferences. For a variety of reasons, many nurses are unable to attend research conferences. To increase the communication of research findings, conference sponsors provide audiotapes or videotapes of the research presentations. Some sponsors publish abstracts of studies with the conference proceedings or in a specialty journal or make them available electronically, such as on the World Wide Web (WWW).

The publishing opportunities in nursing continue to escalate—the number of nursing journals published in the United States has increased from 22 in 1977 (McCloskey, 1977) to 92 in 1991 (Swanson et al., 1991). Opportunities to publish research have expanded with the growth of research journals (*Advances in Nursing Science, Applied Nursing Research, Clinical Nursing Research, Nursing Research, Research in Nursing & Health, Scholarly Inquiry for Nursing Practice: An International Journal*, and *Western Journal of Nursing Research*) and with specialty journals publishing more studies.

TABLE 25–8
OUTLINE FOR THESES AND DISSERTATIONS

Chapter I	INTRODUCTION
	Statement of the problem
	Background and significance of the problem
	Statement of the purpose
Chapter II	REVIEW OF RELEVANT LITERATURE
	Review of relevant theoretical literature
	Review of relevant research
	Summary
Chapter III	FRAMEWORK
	Development of a framework
	Formulation of objectives, questions, or hypotheses
	Definition of research variables
	Definition of relevant terms
	Identification of assumptions
Chapter IV	METHODS AND PROCEDURES
	Identification of the research design
	Description of the population and sample
	Identification of the setting
	Presentation of ethical considerations
	Description of measurement methods
	Description of the data collection process
Chapter V	RESULTS
	Description of data analysis procedures
	Presentation of results
Chapter VI	DISCUSSION
	Presentation of major findings
	Identification of limitations
	Identification of conclusions
	Discussion of the implications for nursing
	Recommendations for further research
References	
Appendices	

TABLE 25–9
AUDIENCES AND STRATEGIES FOR COMMUNICATING RESEARCH

AUDIENCE	STRATEGIES FOR COMMUNICATING RESEARCH
Nurses—practitioners, researchers, and educators	Oral and visual presentations
	Nursing research conferences
	Professional nursing meetings and conferences
	Collaborative nursing groups
	Thesis and dissertation defenses
	Videotaped and audiotaped presentations
	Written reports
	Nursing-referred journals
	Nursing books
	Monographs
	Research newsletters
	Theses and dissertations
	Foundation reports
	Electronic databases
Other health care professionals	Oral and visual presentations
	Professional conferences and meetings
	Interdisciplinary collaboration
	Taped presentations
	Written reports
	Professional journals and books
	Newsletters
	Foundational reports
	Electronic databases
Policymakers	Oral and visual presentations
	Testifying on health problems to state and federal legislators
	Written reports
	Research reports to legislators
	Research reports to funding agencies
	Electronic databases
	AHRQ reports and presentations to policymakers, practitioners, and consumers
Health care consumers	Oral and visual presentations
	Television and radio
	Community meetings
	Patient and family teaching
	Written reports
	Newspaper
	News and popular magazines
	Electronic databases

AHRQ = Agency for Healthcare Research and Quality.

Heart & Lung is now 70% research publications, *Maternal-Child Nursing* is 75% research, and *Journal of Nursing Education* is 80% research (Swanson et al., 1991). The rapidly growing number of peer-reviewed electronic nursing journals also provides increased opportunity to publish research findings. An increasing number of researchers are also communicating their findings by publishing books or chapters in books.

Many universities and hospitals publish regular newsletters or monographs that include abstracts or articles about the research conducted by their members. The American Nurses' Association Council of Nurse Researchers publishes a newsletter that reports studies that have been presented at conferences and identifies ongoing studies of council members. Foundations and federal agencies publish reports of studies that have been conducted or are in progress. The American Nurses' Foundation publishes a newsletter, *Nursing Research Report,* that identifies the studies funded and includes abstracts of these studies. The National Institute for Nursing Research (NINR) publishes reports on its grants, including research project titles, names and addresses of researchers, period of support, a brief description of each project, and publication citations.

AUDIENCE OF HEALTH CARE PROFESSIONALS AND POLICYMAKERS

Nurse researchers communicate their research to other health professionals at meetings and conferences sponsored by such organizations as the American Heart Association, American Public Health Association, American Cancer Society, American Lung Association, National Hospice Organization, and National Rural Health Association. Nurses must believe in the value of their research and present their findings at conferences that attract a variety of health care professionals. Nurse researchers and other health professionals conducting research on the same or similar problems might publish a journal article, series of articles, book chapter, or even a book together. This type of interdisciplinary collaboration might increase the communication of research findings and the impact of the findings on health care.

In 1989, the Agency for Health Care Policy and Research (AHCPR) was established to enhance the quality, appropriateness, and effectiveness of health care services and access to these services. This agency has promoted the conduct of patient outcomes research and facilitated the dissemination and use of research findings in practice. To promote the communication of research findings, the AHCPR formed a work group for the dissemination of patient outcomes research. This work group included a variety of researchers and health practitioners, including nurses and physicians. The purpose of this group was to develop a plan for the dissemination of research findings that identified the audiences and strategies for communication of research. The audiences identified included consumers, health care practitioners, members of the health care industry, policymakers, researchers, and journalists. Strategies for the dissemination of research included printed materials provided through direct mail, technical journals, health journals, the popular press, and electronic media, with communication by radio, television, and the WWW. This group would review research and determine the knowledge that was ready for dissemination to practice. Other bodies within the AHCPR, such as the Forum for Effectiveness and Quality in Health Care and the Center for Research Dissemination, would then create and disseminate research-based clinical guidelines for use in practice (Goldberg et al., 1994). AHCPR is now the Agency for Healthcare Research and Quality (AHRQ).

Nurse researchers also need to communicate their findings to legislators through written reports and personal presentations so that their findings have an impact on health policies. Expert nurse researchers are being asked to testify in their areas of expertise, such as the prevention of pressure ulcers and the treatment of incontinence, to members of Congress as policies related to health care have been developed.

AUDIENCE OF HEALTH CARE CONSUMERS

An audience that is frequently neglected by nurse researchers is the health care consumer. The findings from nursing studies can be communicated to the public through news releases. A nursing research article published in a local paper has the potential of being picked up by the National Wire

Service and published in other papers across the United States. Thus the study findings can reach many potential health care consumers. Nurse researchers also need to make their findings available through electronic databases. An increasing amount of health care information is being made available electronically on the WWW, and consumers can access current research information from their home with their personal computer.

Nursing research findings could be communicated to consumers by being published in news magazines, such as *Time* and *Newsweek,* or popular women's and health magazines, such as *American Baby* and *Health.* Health articles published for consumer magazines can reach 20,000 to 24,000,000 readers at a time (Jimenez, 1991). Television and radio are other valuable sources for communicating research findings. Currently, the findings from many medical studies are covered through these media. Another important method of communicating research findings to consumers is through patient and family teaching. Nursing interventions and practice protocols based on research are more credible to consumers than unresearched actions are.

PRESENTING RESEARCH FINDINGS

Research findings are communicated at conferences and meetings through verbal and poster presentations. With presentations, researchers have an opportunity to share their findings, answer questions about their studies, interact with other interested researchers, and receive immediate feedback on their study. After completion of the research project, the findings are frequently presented at conferences with little delay, whereas when research findings are published, a 1- to 3-year delay in the communication process is typical.

Verbal Presentations

Researchers communicate their findings through verbal presentations at local, national, and international nursing and health care conferences. Presenting findings at a conference requires receiving acceptance as a presenter, developing a research report, delivering the report, and responding to questions.

RECEIVING ACCEPTANCE AS A PRESENTER

Most research conferences require submission of an abstract, and acceptance as a presenter is based on the quality of the abstract. An *abstract* is a clear, concise summary of a study that is usually limited to 100 to 250 words (Crosby, 1990; Juhl & Norman, 1989). Nine months to a year before a research conference, the sponsors circulate a call for abstracts. Many research journals and newsletters publish these calls for abstracts, and they are also available electronically. In addition, conference sponsors will mail the calls for abstracts to universities, major health care agencies, and known nursing researchers.

The call for abstracts will indicate the format for development of the abstract. Frequently, abstracts are limited to one page, single-spaced, and include the content outlined in Table 25–10. The title of an abstract must create interest while the body of the abstract "sells" the study to the reviewers. An example of an abstract is presented in Figure 25–3. Writing an abstract requires practice; frequently, a researcher will rewrite an abstract many times until it meets all the criteria outlined by the conference sponsors. Cason and associates (1988) identified six criteria that are often used in rating the quality of an abstract: (1) acceptability of a study for a spe-

---

TABLE 25–10

OUTLINE FOR AN ABSTRACT

I. TITLE OF THE STUDY
II. INTRODUCTION OF THE SCIENTIFIC PROBLEM
    Statement of the problem and purpose
    Identification of the framework
III. METHODOLOGY
    Design
    Sample size
    Identification of data analysis methods
IV. RESULTS
    Major findings
    Conclusions
    Implications for nursing
    Recommendations for further research

Title: Symptoms of Female Survivors of Child Sexual Abuse

Investigator: Polly A. Hulme

Research indicates that at least 20% of all women have been victims of serious sexual abuse involving unwanted or coerced sexual contact up to the age of 17 years. Women who suffered sexual abuse as children often experience a variety of physical and psychosocial symptoms as adults. Identifying this pattern of symptoms might assist health professionals in recognizing and treating nonreporting survivors of child sexual abuse. The framework for this study is Finkelhor and Browne's (1986) theory of traumagenic dynamics in the impact of child sexual abuse. This theory indicates that child sexual abuse is at the center of the adult survivor's existence and results in four trauma-causing dynamics: traumatic sexualization, betrayal, powerlessness, and stigmatization. These traumagenic dynamics lead to behavioral manifestations that collectively indicate a history of child sexual abuse. The severity of the behavioral manifestations is influenced by the contributing factors or characteristics of the abuse that affect the survivor's life.

The study design was descriptive correlation and the Adult Survivors of Incest (ASI) Questionnaire (Brown & Garrison, 1990) was used to determine the symptoms and contributing factors for 22 adult survivors of child sexual abuse. Six physical symptoms were experienced by 50% of the subjects, and over 75% of the subjects experienced 11 psychosocial symptoms. The number of physical symptoms correlated significantly with other victimizations ($r = .59$) and number of psychosocial symptoms ($r = .56$). The number of psychosocial symptoms also correlated significantly with other victimizations ($r = .40$) and duration of abuse ($r = .40$).

The findings suggest that the ASI Questionnaire was effective in identifying patterns of symptoms and contributing factors of adult survivors of child sexual abuse. Additional study is needed to determine the usefulness of this questionnaire in identifying nonreporting survivors in clinical situations (Hulme & Grove, 1994).

FIGURE 25–3 ■ Example of an abstract.

cific program; (2) overall quality of the work; (3) contribution to nursing scholarship; (4) contribution to nursing theory and practice; (5) originality of the work; and (6) clarity and completeness of the abstract, according to the content outlined in Table 25–10. These criteria might assist you in critiquing and refining your abstract.

DEVELOPING A RESEARCH REPORT

The report developed depends on the focus of the conference, the audience, and the time designated for each presentation. Some conferences focus on certain sections of the research report, such as tool development, data collection and analysis, findings, or implications of the findings for nursing practice. However, it is usually important to address the major sections of a research report (introduction, methods, results, and discussion) in a presentation. The content of a presentation varies with whether the audience consists of mainly researchers or clinical nurses (Jackle, 1989). If you do not know who your audience is, ask the sponsors of the conference.

Time is probably the most important factor in developing a presentation because many presenters are limited to 12 to 15 minutes, with 5 minutes for questions (Selby et al., 1989a). As a guideline, you might spend 10% of your time on the introduction, 20% on the methodology, 35% on the results, and 35% on the discussion. The introduction might in-

clude reasons for the study, a brief review of the literature, a simple discussion of the framework, and the research questions or hypotheses. The methodology content includes a brief identification of the design, sampling method, and measurement techniques. The content covered in the results section includes a simple rationale for the analysis methods used and the major statistical results. The presentation concludes with a brief discussion of findings, implications of the findings for nursing practice, and recommendations for future research (Miracle & King, 1994). Most researchers find that the shorter the presentation time, the greater the preparation time needed.

Many researchers develop a typed script of their study for presentation and include visuals such as slides or transparencies. The script for the presentation needs to indicate when a visual is to be shown. The information presented on each visual should be limited to eight lines or less, with six or fewer words per line. Thus, a single visual should contain information that can be easily read and examined in 30 seconds or a minute (Selby et al., 1989b). Only major points are presented on visuals, so single words or short phrases are used to convey ideas, not complete sentences. Figures such as bar graphs and line graphs usually convey ideas more clearly than tables do. Slides of the research setting, equipment, and researchers collecting data are effective in helping the audience visualize the research project. The use of color on a visual can increase the clarity of the information presented and can be appealing to the audience.

Preparing the script and visuals for a presentation is difficult, so the assistance of an experienced researcher and audiovisual expert can be valuable. Rehearse your presentation with an experienced researcher and use his or her comments to refine your script, visuals, and presentation style. If your presentation is too long, you need to synthesize your script and possibly provide handouts for important content. Audiovisual experts will ensure that your materials are clear and properly constructed, with the print large enough and dark enough to be easily read.

DELIVERING A RESEARCH REPORT AND RESPONDING TO QUESTIONS

A novice researcher might attend conferences and examine the presentation style of other researchers. Even though researchers need to develop their own presentation style, observing others can promote the development of an effective style. The research report can be read from a script, given from an outline, or delivered with slides or transparencies. An effective presentation requires practice. You need to rehearse your presentation several times, with the script, until you are comfortable with the timing, content, and your presentation style. When practicing a presentation, use the visuals so that you are comfortable with the audiovisual equipment. The presentation must be within the time frame designated by conference sponsors. Mathieson (1996) provides some practical advice for the novice presenter.

Some conferences include a presentation by the researcher, a critique of the study by another researcher, and a question period. When preparing for a presentation, you should try to anticipate the questions that might be asked and rehearse your answers. The presentation could be given to colleagues, who might be asked to raise questions. If you practice making clear, concise responses to specific questions, your anxiety will be decreased during the actual presentation. When giving a presentation, make notes of questions, suggestions, or comments made by the audience because they are

often useful when preparing a manuscript for publication or developing the next study.

Poster Sessions

Sometimes, your research will be accepted at a conference not as a presentation but as a poster session. A *poster session* is a visual presentation of your study. Before developing a poster, contact the conference sponsors regarding (1) size limitations or format restrictions for the poster, (2) the size of the poster display area, and (3) the background and potential number of conference participants (Lippman & Ponton, 1989). A poster usually includes the following content: the title of the study; investigator and institution names; brief abstract; purpose; research objectives, questions, or hypotheses (if applicable); framework; design; sample; instruments; essential data collection procedures; results; conclusions; implications for nursing; and recommendations for further research. For clarity and conciseness, a poster often includes pictures, tables, or figures to communicate the study. Often, one color is used for most of the poster and one or two additional colors for accents (McDaniel et al., 1993). The structure of a poster is provided in Figure 25–4.

A poster can be made from sturdy cardboard, or special display board can be purchased. Your budget will determine the type of poster you develop, but it should be easy to transport and assemble at the conference setting. A quality poster is complete in the presentation of a study, yet easily comprehended in 5 minutes or less (Ryan, 1989). Bold headings are used for the different parts of the research report, followed by clear, concise narratives. The size of the print on a poster needs to be large enough to be read easily at 4 to 6 feet (McDaniel et al., 1993). Poster sessions usually last from 1 to 2 hours; the researcher should remain with the poster during this time. Most researchers provide conference participants with copies of their abstract and other relevant handouts and offer to answer any questions.

Qualitative research posters are becoming more prevalent as the number of qualitative studies increases. Russell and coauthors (1996) reported the results of reviewing qualitative posters at research

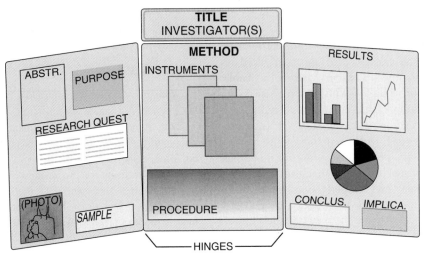

FIGURE 25–4 ■ Three-part hinged poster. (From Ryan, N. M. [1989]. Developing and presenting a research poster. *Applied Nursing Research, 2*[1], 53.)

conferences. One fourth of the posters had too little information; however, many of them had too much information. Narrative content does not lend itself to the concise presentation required on a poster.

The number of words should be kept to a minimum. As stated previously, the size of print should allow viewers to easily read it from 4 to 6 feet. They recommend having color-coordinated sections of the poster with written material provided in matted format. Summary and implications sections were frequently omitted in qualitative posters. This omission is a serious problem inasmuch as most viewers search for that content first. Because rich narrative text is so meaningful in qualitative studies, authors are advised to use a notebook with additional data examples and art work that viewers can examine.

An advantage of a poster session is the opportunity for one-to-one interaction between the researcher and those viewing the poster. At the end of the poster session, individuals interested in a study will frequently stay to speak to the researcher. A notepad is often needed to record comments and the names and addresses of those conducting similar research. This occasion is an excellent opportunity to begin networking with other researchers involved in the same area of research. Sometimes, conference participants will want study instruments or other items to be mailed, faxed, or e-mailed to them, so a record of their names, addresses, fax numbers, and requests must be kept.

PUBLISHING RESEARCH FINDINGS

Presentations are a valuable means of rapidly communicating findings, but their impact is limited. Published research findings are permanently recorded in a journal or book and usually reach a larger audience than presentations do (Diers, 1981). However, the research report developed for a presentation can provide a basis for writing an article for publication. Regrettably, many researchers present their findings at a conference and never submit the paper for publication. Hicks (1995) studied the publishing activities of 500 randomly selected nurses and found that only 10% submitted their studies for publication. Studies with negative findings, such as no significant differences or relationships, are frequently not submitted for presentation or publication. These negative findings can be as important to the development of knowledge as the positive findings (Angell, 1989).

Publishing research findings is a rewarding experience, but the process demands a great deal of time and energy. The manuscript rejections or requests for major revisions that most authors receive can be discouraging. However, one can take certain steps to increase the probability of having a manuscript accepted for publication. Plans for publishing a study should be outlined during proposal development. At this time, investigators should discuss and, if possible, determine authorship credit. This issue becomes complex when the research is a collaborative project among individuals from different disciplines. Some researchers develop the entire manuscript and are then faced with the decision of who will be first, second, or third author. There are many ways to determine authorship credit, but the decision should be one that is acceptable to all investigators involved (Hanson, 1988). Authorship credit should be given only to those who made substantial contributions to developing and implementing a study and in writing the final report (Shapiro et al., 1994).

Publishing Journal Articles

Developing a manuscript for publication includes the following steps: (1) selecting a journal, (2) developing a query letter, (3) preparing a manuscript, (4) submitting the manuscript for review, and (5) responding to requests for revision of the manuscript.

SELECTING A JOURNAL

Selecting a journal for publication of a study requires knowledge of the basic requirements of the journal, the journal's refereed status (see the next paragraph), and recent articles published in the journal. Swanson and colleagues (1991) studied publishing opportunities for nurses by surveying 92 U.S. nursing journals. The authors provided, in table format, the following basic information on each journal: circulation; number of issues published each year; article length; number of copies of the manuscript to be submitted; format for the manuscript; query letter; free reprints; and the percentage of staff-written, unsolicited, and research manuscripts published. Other information in the article that is of interest to potential authors is the number of unsolicited manuscripts received, number of un-

solicited manuscripts published, number of manuscripts rejected, percentage of manuscripts accepted, refereed status, review process, time for acceptance, and time until publication (Swanson et al., 1991, p. 35). Table 25–11 presents some essential publishing information for five research journals included in this survey.

A *refereed journal* uses referees or expert reviewers to determine whether a manuscript is accepted for publication. In nonrefereed journals, the editor makes the decisions for acceptance or rejection of manuscripts, but these decisions are usually made after consultation with a nursing expert (Carnegie, 1975). Most refereed journals require manuscripts to be reviewed anonymously by two or three reviewers. The reviewers are asked to determine the strengths and weaknesses of a manuscript, and their comments or a summary of the comments is sent to the author. Most academic institutions support the refereed system and will recognize only publications that appear in refereed journals. The five research journals presented in Table 25–11 are refereed and have the following review process: "Editor receives manuscripts, reviews, and distributes them to experts selected from an established group of reviewers. Decision on the manuscript is based on reviews and mediated by editor." (Swanson et al., 1991, p. 35)

Researchers often review articles recently published in the journal to which they plan to submit a manuscript. This review will indicate whether a research topic has recently been covered and whether the research findings would be of interest to the journal's readers. This selection process enables researchers to identify a few journals that would be appropriate for publishing their findings.

DEVELOPING A QUERY LETTER

A *query letter* is developed to determine an editor's interest in reviewing a manuscript. This letter should be no more than one or two pages and usually includes the research problem, a brief discussion of the major findings, the significance of the findings, and the researcher's qualifications for writing the article (Mirin, 1981). A query letter is addressed to the current editor of a journal; fre-

TABLE 25–11
PUBLISHING INFORMATION FOR SELECTED RESEARCH JOURNALS

JOURNAL	NUMBER OF ISSUES	QUERY LETTER	REFERRED	ARTICLE LENGTH (PAGES)	FORMAT	COPIES REQUIRED	ACCEPTANCE RATE (%)
Advances in Nursing Science	4	Optional	Yes	15–30	APA	3	13
Applied Nursing Research	4	Optional	Yes	8–12	APA	5	48
Nursing Research	6	Preferred	Yes	14–16	APA	3	15
Research in Nursing & Health	6	Optional	Yes	10–15	APA	4	22
Western Journal of Nursing Research	6	Optional	Yes	15	APA	4	20

APA = American Psychological Association.
Adapted from Swanson, E. A., McCloskey, J. C., & Bodensteiner, A. (1991). Publishing opportunities for nurses: A comparison of 92 U.S. journals. *Image—The Journal of Nursing Scholarship, 23*(1), 33–38.

quently, three or four letters are sent to different journals at the same time. Of the five journals presented in Table 25–11, only *Nursing Research* prefers a query letter; the other research journals indicated that these letters were optional. Some researchers send query letters because the response (positive or negative) enables them to make the final selection of a journal for submission of a manuscript. An example of a query letter is presented in Figure 25–5.

PREPARING A MANUSCRIPT

A manuscript is written according to the format outlined by the journal. Guidelines for developing a manuscript are usually published in an issue of the

January 31, 1997

Joyce J. Fitzpatrick, PhD, FAAN
Editor
Applied Nursing Research

Case Western Reserve University
Frances Payne Bolton School of Nursing
10900 Euclid Avenue
Cleveland, OH 44106

Dear Dr. Fitzpatrick:

An increasing number of nursing studies are focused on clinical problems and specifically on the outcomes of nursing interventions. Currently, many nursing interventions are implemented without adequate research, such as the treatments for pain. I have just completed a study to examine the effects of ice therapy versus heat therapy on patients who are experiencing chronic low back pain.

The framework for this study was the Melzack and Wall gate-control theory of pain. The independent variables, ice and heat therapies, were consistently implemented with structured protocols by nurses in a pain clinic. The dependent variable, perception of pain, was measured with a visual analogue scale. The sample included 90 clinic patients with low back pain. The subjects were randomly assigned to three groups: a comparison group that received no treatment, an experimental group that received ice therapy, and an experimental group that received heat therapy.

An analysis of variance (ANOVA) with post hoc analyses indicated that patients in the comparison group and heat therapy group perceived their pain to be significantly greater than the perception of pain by the patients receiving ice therapy. The findings suggest that ice therapy is more effective than heat in reducing chronic low back pain. Ice therapy is an intervention that can be prescribed and implemented by nurses to reduce patients' perception of pain.

I hope you will consider reviewing this manuscript for possible publication. I look forward to receiving a response from you.

Sincerely,

Susan K. Grove, PhD, R.N.
Professor, School of Nursing
The University of Texas at Arlington

FIGURE 25–5 ■ Example of a query letter.

journal; however, some journals require that you write and request the author guidelines. These guidelines should be followed explicitly to increase the probability of your manuscript being published. The information provided for authors includes (1) directions for manuscript preparation, (2) discussion of copyright, and (3) guidelines for submission of the manuscript.

Writing research reports for publication requires skills in technical writing that are not used in other types of publication. Technical writing condenses information and is stylistic. The *Publication Manual for the APA* (APA, 1994) and the *Chicago Manual of Style* (University of Chicago Press, 1993) are considered useful sources for quality technical writing. Some journals will stipulate the style manual required for their journal. A quality research report has no punctuation, spelling, or sentence structure errors; confusing words; clichés; jargon; or wordiness (Camilleri, 1987, 1988). Computer programs have been developed with the capacity to proof manuscripts for grammar, punctuation, spelling, and sentence structure errors. However, the writer still needs to respond and correct the sentences that are identified as problematic by the computer.

Knowledge about the author guidelines provided by the journal and a background in technical writing facilitate the process of developing an outline for a proposed manuscript. The initial brief outlines presented in Tables 25–1 and 25–5 must be expanded in detail to guide the writing of a manuscript. A rough draft of the article is developed from the outline and revised numerous times. The content of an article should be logically and concisely presented under clear headings, and the title selected for the manuscript needs to create interest and reflect the content.

Developing a clear, concise manuscript is difficult. Often, universities and other agencies offer writing seminars to assist students and other researchers in preparing a research report for publication. Some faculty members who chair thesis and dissertation committees will also assist their students in developing an article for publication. In this situation, the faculty member is almost always the second author for the article.

When researchers are satisfied with their manuscripts, they usually ask one or two colleagues to review it for organization, completeness of content, and writing style. Colleagues' comments can be used to make the final revisions in the manuscript (Hagemaster & Kerrins, 1984). The manuscript should be expertly typed according to the journal's specifications; most nursing research journals require the APA (1994) format. The reference list for the manuscript needs to be in a complete and correct format. Computer programs are available with bibliography systems that enable you to compile a complete, consistently formatted reference list in any style you desire. With these programs you can maintain a permanent collection of reference citations. When you need a reference list for a manuscript, you can select the appropriate references from the collection and use the program to print the list. Computer programs can also be used to scan your manuscript and create a reference list based on the citations in the manuscript.

SUBMITTING A MANUSCRIPT FOR REVIEW

Guidelines in each journal indicate the name of the editor and the address for manuscript submission. A manuscript must be submitted to only one journal at a time. The researcher should submit the number of copies of the manuscript requested and the original manuscript, if required. Research journal editors require from three to five copies of a manuscript (see Table 25–11), and some also request a disk of the manuscript. When submitting the manuscript, the researcher identifies his or her complete mailing address, phone number, fax number, and e-mail address. An author usually receives notification of receipt of the manuscript within 1 to 2 weeks.

PEER REVIEW

Most journals use some form of peer review process to evaluate the quality of manuscripts submitted for publication. The manuscript is usually sent to two or three reviewers with guidelines from the editor for performing the review. In most cases, the review is "blind," which means that the reviewers do not know who the author is and the author does not know who is reviewing the paper. For research papers, the reviewers are asked to evaluate the validity of the study. Broadly, of concern is whether the methodology was adequate to address the research objectives, questions, or hypotheses, whether the findings are trustworthy (for example, if the results were nonsignificant, was a power analysis performed), whether the discussion is appropriate given the findings, and whether the author discusses the clinical implications of the findings. A concern with some specialty journals is that reviewers, who may not be prepared at the Ph.D. level, may not have sufficient expertise in the research process to adequately evaluate the manuscript.

RESPONDING TO REQUESTS TO REVISE A MANUSCRIPT

Review of a manuscript results in one of four possible decisions: (1) acceptance of the manuscript as submitted, (2) acceptance of the manuscript pending minor revisions, (3) tentative acceptance of the manuscript pending major revisions, and (4) rejection of the manuscript. Accepting a manuscript as submitted is extremely rare. The editor will send the author a letter that indicates acceptance of the manuscript and a possible issue of publication.

Most manuscripts are returned for minor or major revisions before they are published. It is regrettable that many of these returned manuscripts are never revised. The author incorrectly interprets the request for revision as a rejection and assumes that the revised manuscript will also be rejected. This assumption is not usually true because revising a manuscript based on reviewers' comments improves the quality of the manuscript. When editors return a manuscript for revision, they include the reviewers' actual comments or a summary of the comments to direct the revision. The researcher must carefully review the comments and make those revisions that improve the quality of the research report without making inaccurate statements about the study. As you revise your manuscript, follow as carefully as possible the recommendations of the reviewers. When the revision is complete, return it with a cover letter explaining exactly how you responded

to each recommendation. List each recommendation and describe your modification. Indicate the page number of your manuscript for that revision. In some cases, you may disagree with the recommendation. If so, in the cover letter, provide rationale for your disagreement and indicate how you have chosen to respond to the comment. Do not ignore a recommendation. Sometimes a revised manuscript is returned to the reviewers, and yet further modifications are requested in the paper before it is published. Although these experiences are frustrating, they are also opportunities to improve your writing skills or your logic. Frequently, editors request that the final manuscript be submitted on disk.

An author who receives a rejection feels devastated, but he or she is not alone. All authors, even famous ones, have had their manuscripts rejected (Gay & Edgil, 1989). Manuscripts are rejected for a variety of reasons. Swanson and colleagues (1991, p. 38) asked journal editors to rate the frequency of 14 reasons for manuscript rejection. Table 25–12 identifies these reasons and their mean frequencies. "Poorly written" and "poorly developed idea" were the most frequent reasons for rejecting manuscripts. If you receive a rejection notice, give yourself a cooling-off period and then determine why the

TABLE 25–12
REASONS FOR MANUSCRIPT REJECTION

FACTOR	MEAN*
Poorly written	3.72
Poorly developed idea	3.62
Not consistent with purpose	3.37
Term paper style	3.28
Methodology problems	3.13
Content undocumented	2.98
Content inaccurate	2.94
Content not important	2.84
Clinically not applicable	2.83
Statistical problems	2.82
Data interpretation problems	2.80
Subject covered recently	2.39
Content scheduled for future	2.11
Too technical	1.66

*1 = rarely; 5 = very frequently.
From Swanson, E. A., McCloskey, J. C., & Bodensteiner, A. (1991). Publishing opportunities for nurses: A comparison of 92 U.S. journals. *Image—The Journal of Nursing Scholarship*, 23(1), 38.

manuscript was rejected. Most manuscripts, especially those that are poorly written, can be revised and submitted to another journal.

PUBLISHING RESEARCH FINDINGS IN ON-LINE JOURNALS

A number of print journals are moving to the Web. These journals continue to provide the traditional print version of their journal but also have a website with access to some or all the articles in the printed journal. The number of Web-only on-line nursing journals is also growing. These on-line–only journals have some distinct advantages for authors. E-mail links from author to editor to reviewer allow papers to be submitted and sent from editor to reviewer electronically and allow review comments to be sent back to the editor more quickly than usually occurs in print journals. Reviewer comments are sent back to the author by e-mail, after which the article is revised and resubmitted by e-mail, reviewed again, and if judged satisfactory, accepted for publication. This process is particularly important for international scientific communications. "Continuous publication" is used by on-line journals, which means that there is no wait for approved articles to be published because the editor does not have to wait until the next issue is scheduled to go to the printer. In fact, the notion of an "issue" is becoming antiquated as a result of electronic publishing. Approved articles are placed on-line almost immediately, which is important for research reports because it provides more rapid access to recent research findings for other researchers and clinicians interested in evidence-based practice. The possibilities of dialogue with readers, including other researchers in the same field of study, is great.

Not all on-line journals provide peer review. You may wish to check for information on the peer review process at the on-line journal website. Peer review is essential to scholars in the university tenure track system. Electronic publishing may result in a more open peer review process. Some journals are posting a submitted paper for peer review on a secure Internet site accessible only by the editor and reviewers. The review occurs by way of a discussion rather than individual comments. This arrangement provides a measure of quality control in the review process that is missing in the traditional process. Bingham describes the changes in peer review likely to occur because of on-line journals:

· ·

"By creating a more open peer review process, it is possible for reviewers, authors and editors to observe each other's behavior. . . . This may improve the trust in the system, and the quality of the outcomes. More open review systems widen the educational function of peer review for editors and authors, and extend it to readers for the first time. . . . Most articles will be reviewed online in a closed forum, then published for review in an open forum, then declared 'final.'" (Bingham, 1999) ■

Publishing in an on-line journal has other potential advantages. The constraints on length imposed because of the cost of print publishing do not exist. Multiple tables, figures, graphics, and even streaming audio and video are possibilities with on-line journals. Animations can be created to assist the reader in visualizing ideas. Links may be established with full text versions of citations from other on-line sources. It will be possible to track the number of times that the article has been accessed. This feature will provide the author with additional information, beyond citations of his or her paper, to assess its impact on the scientific community. Forward referencing will allow links to later works, which can be added to the article continuously. The reader will be able to see how the paper influenced later works. Electronic listservs and chat rooms may be available to discuss the paper. All these capabilities are not currently available with every on-line journal. The technology to provide them exists, but there is no free lunch. Most on-line journals in nursing are free. On-line journals with some of these advanced technologies may have to cover their costs by charging subscription fees or obtaining financing through advertisements (Holoviak & Seitter, 1997; Ludwick & Glazer, 2000; Sparks, 1999).

Because on-line journals are rapidly emerging,

providing a list of websites in this text is not feasible. However, a number of websites maintain a current list of on-line journals. Investigate the following websites:

http://www.nursefriendly.com/nursing/
linksections/nursingjournals.htm
http://www.lib.umich.edu/hw/nursing/
resources.html
http://www-sci.lib.uci.edu/HSG/
Nursing.html#NN3
http://www.nursing-portal.com/nursing—
journals.html

PUBLISHING RESEARCH FINDINGS IN BOOKS

Some qualitative studies and large, complex quantitative studies are published in books or chapters of books. Publishing a book requires extensive commitment on the part of the researcher. In addition, the researcher must select a publisher and convince the publisher to support the book project. A prospectus must be developed that identifies the proposed content of the book, describes the market for the book, and includes a rationale for publishing the book. The publisher and researcher must negotiate a contract that is mutually acceptable regarding (1) the content and length of the book, (2) the time required to complete the book, (3) the percentage of royalties to be received, and (4) the advances to be offered. The researcher must fulfill the obligations of the contract by producing the proposed book within the time frame agreed upon. Publishing a book is a significant accomplishment and an effective, but sometimes slow, means of communicating research findings.

DUPLICATE PUBLICATION IN THE NURSING LITERATURE

Duplicate publication is the practice of publishing the same article or major portions of the article in two or more print or electronic media without notifying the editors or referencing the other publication in the reference list (Blancett et al., 1995). Duplicate publication of studies is a poor practice because it limits the opportunities for publishing new knowledge, artificially inflates the importance of a study topic, clutters the literature with redundant information, rewards researchers for publishing the same content twice, and may violate the copyright law. Blancett and colleagues (1995) studied the incidence of duplicate publications in the nursing literature. In a sample of 642 articles published by 77 authors over 5 years, 181 of the articles were classified as duplicate publications. Forty-one of the 77 authors published at least one form of duplicate article, and 59 of the duplicate articles did not include a reference to the primary article. Thus, duplicate publications are a serious concern in the nursing literature.

Journals require the submission of an original manuscript or one that has not been previously published, so submitting a manuscript that has been previously published without referencing the duplicate work or notifying the editor of the previous publication is unethical and probably violates the copyright law. In 1994, the International Academy of Nursing Editors developed guidelines for nurse authors and editors regarding duplicate publications. Both authors and editors have the responsibility to inform readers and reviewers of duplicate publications. Authors must avoid unethical duplication by submitting original manuscripts or by providing full disclosure if portions or the entire manuscript has been previously published. Previous publications must be cited in the text of the manuscript and the reference list. Editors have the responsibility of developing a policy on duplicate publications and informing all authors, reviewers, and readers of this policy. In addition, editors must ensure that readers are informed of duplicate materials by adequate citation of the materials in the article's text and reference list (Yarbro, 1995).

■ SUMMARY

Communicating research findings, the final step in the research process, involves developing a research report and disseminating it through presentations and publications to audiences of nurses, health care professionals, policymakers, and health care consumers. Both quantitative and qualitative research reports include four basic sections: (1) introduction, (2) methods, (3) results, and (4) discussion. In a quantitative research report, the introduction briefly identifies the problem that was studied, provides a rationale for studying that problem, and presents an empirical and theoretical basis for the study. The methods section of the report describes how the study was conducted and includes the design, setting, sample, methods of measurement, and data collection process. The results section reveals what was found by conducting the study and includes the data analysis procedures, the results generated from these analyses, and the effect size determined for each analysis procedure. The discussion section ties the other sections of the research report together and gives them meaning. This section includes the major findings, limitations of the study, conclusions, implications of the findings for nursing, and recommendations for further research.

Research reports developed for qualitative research are as diverse as the different types of qualitative studies. However, qualitative research reports, like quantitative reports, usually include introduction, methods, results, and discussion sections. The introduction section identifies the phenomenon under investigation and indicates the type of qualitative study that was conducted. In the methods section, the researcher documents his or her credentials for conducting the study, identifies the site and sample, describes the researcher's role, and details the data collection process. The results section of the research report includes the data analysis procedures and presentation of the findings. The discussion section includes conclusions, limitations, implications for nursing, and recommendations for further research.

Before writing a research report, the investigator needs to determine who will benefit from knowing the findings. The greatest impact on nursing practice can be achieved by communicating nursing research findings to nurses, other health professionals, policymakers, and health care consumers. A variety of strategies for communicating to these audiences, such as oral and visual presentations and publications, are discussed in this chapter.

Research findings are presented at conferences and meetings through verbal and poster presentations. Presenting findings at a conference requires receiving acceptance as a presenter, developing a research report, delivering the report, and responding to questions. Most research conferences require the submission of an abstract, and acceptance as a presenter is based on the quality of the abstract. The report developed depends on the focus of the conference, the audience, and the time designated for each presentation. Delivering a research report and responding to questions involve practice to improve timing, content, and presentation style.

Sometimes a research project will be accepted at a conference not as a presentation but as a poster session. A poster session is a visual presentation of a study. The conference sponsors can guide the development of a poster by providing the following information: (1) size limitations or format restrictions for the poster, (2) the size of the poster display area, and (3) the background and potential number of conference participants.

Presentations are valuable means to rapidly communicate findings, but their impact is limited. Published research findings are permanently recorded in a journal or book and usually reach a larger audience than presentations do. Developing a manuscript for publication includes the following steps: (1) selecting a journal, (2) writing a query letter, (3) preparing a manuscript, (4) submitting the manuscript for review, and (5) responding to requests for revision of the manuscript. Selecting a journal for publication of a study requires knowledge of the basic requirements of the journal, the journal's refereed status, and recent articles published in the journal. A query letter is developed to determine an editor's interest in reviewing a manuscript. A manuscript is then written according to the format outlined by the journal and submitted to the journal editor. The manuscript is then reviewed and usually requires revisions before it is accepted for publication.

A concern that was recently identified in the nursing literature is the publication of duplicate articles. Duplicate publication is the practice of publishing the same article or major portions of the article in two or more print or electronic media without notifying the editors or referencing the other publication in the reference list. In 1994, the International Academy of Nursing Editors developed guidelines for nurse authors and editors regarding duplicate publications. Publishing research findings is a rewarding experience, but the process of publishing demands a great deal of time and energy. We hope that this information will stimulate researchers to present and publish their findings.

• •

REFERENCES

American Psychological Association. (1994). *Publication manual of the American Psychological Association* (4th ed.). Washington, DC: American Psychological Association.

Angell, M. (1989). Negative studies. *New England Journal of Medicine, 321*(7), 464–466.

Bingham, C. (1999). The future of medical publishing. *HMS Beagle* (*http://www.biomednet.com/hmsbeagle/46/cutedge/day1.htm*) [January 22, 1999].

Blancett, S. S., Flanagin, A., & Young, R. K. (1995). Duplicate publication in the nursing literature. *Image—The Journal of Nursing Scholarship, 27*(1), 51–56.

Brown, B. E., & Garrison, C. J. (1990). Patterns of symptomatology of adult women incest survivors. *Western Journal of Nursing Research, 12*(5), 587–600.

Burns, N. (1989). Standards for qualitative research. *Nursing Science Quarterly, 2*(1), 44–52.

Camilleri, R. (1987). Six ways to write right. *Image—The Journal of Nursing Scholarship, 19*(4), 210–212.

Camilleri, R. (1988). On elegant writing. *Image—The Journal of Nursing Scholarship, 20*(3), 169–171.

Carnegie, M. E. (1975). The referee system. *Nursing Research, 24*(4), 243.

Cason, C. L., Cason, G. J., & Redland, A. R. (1988). Peer review of research abstracts. *Image—The Journal of Nursing Scholarship, 20*(2), 102–105.

Crosby, L. J. (1990). The abstract: An important first impression. *Journal of Neuroscience Nursing, 22*(3), 192–194.

Diers, D. (1981). Why write? Why publish? *Image—The Journal of Nursing Scholarship, 13*(1), 3–8.

Egan, E. C., Snyder, M., & Burns, K. R. (1992). Intervention studies in nursing: Is the effect due to the independent variable? *Nursing Outlook, 40*(4), 187–190.

Field, P. A., & Morse, J. M. (1985). *Nursing research: The application of qualitative approaches.* Rockville, MD: Aspen.

Finkelhor, D., & Browne, A. (1986). Initial and long term effects: A conceptual framework. In D. Finkelhor (Ed.), *A source book on child sexual abuse* (pp. 180–198). Beverly Hills, CA: Sage.

Gay, J. T., & Edgil, A. E. (1989). When your manuscript is rejected. *Nursing & Health Care, 10*(8), 459–461.

Goldberg, H. I., Cummings, M. A., Steinberg, E. P., Ricci, E. M., Shannon, T., Soumerai, S. B., Mittman, B. S., Eisenberg, J., Heck, D. A., Kaplan, S., Kenzora, J. E., Vargus, A. M., Mulley, A. G., & Rimer, B. K. (1994). Deliberations on the dissemination of PORT products: Translating research findings into improved patient outcomes. *Medical Care, 32*(7), JS90–JS110.

Hagemaster, J. N., & Kerrins, K. M. (1984). Six easy steps to publishing. *Nurse Educator, 9*(4), 32–34.

Hanson, S. M. (1988). Collaborative research and authorship credit: Beginning guidelines. *Nursing Research, 37*(1), 49–52.

Hicks, C. (1995). The shortfall in published research: A study of nurses' research publication activities. *Journal of Advanced Nursing, 21*(3), 594–604.

Holoviak, J., & Seitter, K. L. (1997). Transcending the limitations of the printed page. *The Journal of Electronic Publishing, 3*(1) (*http://www.press.umich.edu/jep/033-01/EI.html*) [Accessed 3-12-00].

Hulme, P. A., & Grove, S. K. (1994). Symptoms of female survivors of child sexual abuse. *Issues in Mental Health Nursing, 15*(5), 519–532.

Jackle, M. (1989). Presenting research to nurses in clinical practice. *Applied Nursing Research, 2*(4), 191–193.

Jimenez, S. L. M. (1991). Consumer journalism: A unique nursing opportunity. *Image—The Journal of Nursing Scholarship, 23*(1), 47–49.

Juhl, N., & Norman, V. L. (1989). Writing an effective abstract. *Applied Nursing Research, 2*(4), 189–191.

Kirchhoff, K. T., & Dille, C. A. (1994). Issues in intervention research: Maintaining integrity. *Applied Nursing Research, 7*(1), 32–38.

Knafl, K. A., & Howard, M. J. (1984). Interpreting and reporting qualitative research. *Research in Nursing & Health, 7*(1), 17–24.

Kraemer, H. C., & Thiemann, S. (1987). *How many subjects? Statistical power analysis in research.* Newbury Park, CA: Sage.

Lander, J., Nazarali, S., Hodgins, M., Friesen, E., McTavish, J., Ouellette, J., & Abel, R. (1996). Evaluation of a new topical anesthetic agent: A pilot study. *Nursing Research, 45*(1), 50–53.

Leininger, M. M. (1985). *Qualitative research methods in nursing.* New York: Grune & Stratton.

Lippman, D. T., & Ponton, K. S. (1989). Designing a research poster with impact. *Western Journal of Nursing Research, 11*(4), 477–485.

Ludwick, R., & Glazer, G. (January 31, 2000). Electronic publishing. The movement from print to digital publication. *Online Journal of Issues in Nursing, 5*(5), Manuscript 2 (*http://www.nursingworld.org/ojin/topic11/tpe11 2.htm*) [Accessed: 3/12/00].

Mathieson, A. (1996). The principles and practice of oral presentation. *Nurse Researcher, 4*(2), 41–54.

McCloskey, J. C. (1977). Publishing opportunities for nurses: A comparison of 65 journals. *Nurse Educator, 11*(4), 4–13.

McDaniel, R. W., Bach, C. A., & Poole, M. J. (1993). Poster update: Getting their attention. *Nursing Research, 42*(5), 302–304.

McFarlane, J., Parker, B., & Soeken, K. (1996). Abuse during pregnancy: Associations with maternal health and infant birth weight. *Nursing Research, 45*(1), 37–42.

McKenna, K. T., Maas, F., & McEniery, P. T. (1995). Coronary risk factor status after percutaneous transluminal coronary angioplasty. *Heart & Lung, 24*(3), 207–212.

Miracle, V. A., & King, K. C. (1994). Presenting research: Effective paper presentations and impressive poster presentations. *Applied Nursing Research, 7*(3), 147–157.

Mirin, S. K. (1981). *The nurse's guide to writing for publication.* Wakefield, MA: Nursing Resources.

Packard, N. J., Haberman, M. R., Woods, N. F., & Yates, B. C. (1991). Demands of illness among chronically ill women. *Western Journal of Nursing Research, 13*(4), 434–457.

Reece, S. M. (1995). Stress and maternal adaptation in first-time mothers more than 35 years old. *Applied Nursing Research, 8*(2), 61–66.

Russell, C. K., Gregory, D. M., & Gates, M. F. (1996). Aesthetics and substance in qualitative research posters. *Qualitative Health Research, 6*(4), 542–552.

Ryan, N. M. (1989). Developing and presenting a research poster. *Applied Nursing Research, 2*(1), 52–54.

Selby, M. L., Tornquist, E. M., & Finerty, E. J. (1989a). How to present your research. Part I: What they didn't teach you in nursing school about planning and organizing the content of your speech. *Nursing Outlook, 37*(4), 172–175.

Selby, M. L., Tornquist, E. M., & Finerty, E. J. (1989b). How to present your research. Part II: The ABCs of creating and using visual aids to enhance your research presentation. *Nursing Outlook, 37*(5), 236–238.

Shapiro, D. W., Wenger, N. S., & Shapiro, M. F. (1994). The contributions of authors to multiauthored biomedical research papers. *JAMA, 271*(6), 438–442.

Shurter, R. L., Williamson, J. P., & Broehl, W. G. (1965). *Business research and report writing.* New York: McGraw-Hill.

Sparks, S. M. (1999). Electronic publishing and nursing research. *Nursing Research, 48*(1), 50–54.

Swain, M. A., & Steckel, S. B. (1981). Influencing adherence among hypertensives. *Research in Nursing & Health, 4*(1), 213–222.

Swanson, E. A., McCloskey, J. C., & Bodensteiner, A. (1991). Publishing opportunities for nurses: A comparison of 92 U.S. journals. *Image—The Journal of Nursing Scholarship, 23*(1), 33–38.

Tornquist, E. M., Funk, S. G., & Champagne, M. T. (1989). Writing research reports for clinical audiences. *Western Journal of Nursing Research, 11*(5), 576–582.

Tulman, L. R., & Jacobsen, B. S. (1989). Goldilocks and variability. *Nursing Research, 38*(6), 377–379.

University of Chicago Press. (1993). *The Chicago manual of style* (14th ed.). Chicago: University of Chicago Press.

Wainer, H. (1984). How to display data badly. *American Statistician, 38*(2), 137–147.

Wikblad, K., & Anderson, B. (1995). A comparison of three wound dressings in patients undergoing heart surgery. *Nursing Research, 44*(5), 312–316.

Winslow, E. H. (1996). Failure to publish research: A form of scientific misconduct? *Heart & Lung, 25*(3), 169–171.

Yarbro, C. H. (1995). Duplicate publication: Guidelines for nurse authors and editors. *Image—The Journal of Nursing Scholarship, 27*(1), 57.

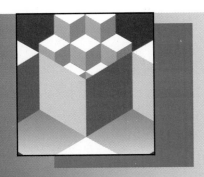

III

STRATEGIES FOR USING RESEARCH IN PRACTICE

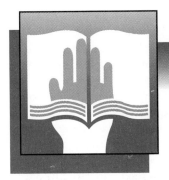

CHAPTER 26

CRITICAL ANALYSIS OF NURSING STUDIES

The critique of studies is an essential process in the synthesis of knowledge for use in practice or for the conduct of studies, yet this process is poorly understood by many nurses. The word *critique* is often linked with the word *criticize,* which has negative connotations and is often considered untherapeutic in nursing. However, in the arts and sciences, critique takes on another meaning. It is associated with critical thinking and appraisal and requires carefully developed intellectual skills. This type of critique is sometimes referred to as intellectual critique. An intellectual critique is directed not at the person who created but at the product of creation. For example, one might critique an art object, an architectural design, a ballet performance, a theory, or a study. One can even critique a critique, such as a faculty member critiquing a student's critique of a study.

An *intellectual critique of research* involves a systematic, unbiased, careful examination of all aspects of a study to judge the merits, limitations, meaning, and significance based on previous research experience and knowledge of the topic. Conducting a research critique requires a background in critical analysis and skills in logical reasoning to examine the credibility and integrity of a study. The intent of this chapter is to provide a background for critiquing studies. Evolution of the research critique in nursing and the different types of research critiques conducted by nurses are discussed. The critique processes for both quantitative and qualitative research are described, including the unique skills,

guidelines, and standards for critiquing different types of studies.

EVOLUTION OF THE RESEARCH CRITIQUE IN NURSING

The process for critiquing research has evolved gradually in nursing because until recently only a few nurses have been prepared to conduct comprehensive, scholarly critiques. During the 1940s and 1950s, presentations of nursing research were followed by critiques of the research. These critiques often focused on the faults or limitations of the studies and tended to be harsh and traumatic for the researcher (Meleis, 1991). As a consequence of these early unpleasant experiences, nurse researchers moved to a strategy of protecting and sheltering their nurse scientists from the threat of criticism. Public critiques, written or verbal, were rare in the 1960s and 1970s. Those responding to research presentations focused on the strengths of studies, and the limitations were either not mentioned or minimized. Thus the impact of the limitations on the meaning and significance of the study was often lost.

Incomplete critiques or the absence of critiques may have served a purpose as nurses gained basic skills in the conduct of research. However, the discipline of nursing has moved past this point, and intellectual critiques are essential to strengthen scientific investigation and use of research evidence in practice. Many nurses now have the preparation and

663

expertise for conducting intellectual critiques as a result of advances in the nursing profession during the 1980s and 1990s. Nursing research textbooks provide detailed information on the critique process. Nursing research skills, including critique, are introduced at the baccalaureate level of nursing education and are expanded at the master's and doctoral levels. Specialty organizations provide workshops on the critique process to promote the use of research findings in practice.

Intellectual critiques of studies are essential for the development and refinement of nursing knowledge. Nurses need the skills to examine the meaning of study findings and to ask searching questions. Are the findings an accurate reflection of reality? Do they lead to increased understanding of the nature of phenomena that are important in nursing? Are the findings from the present study consistent with those from previous studies? Can the study be replicated? Are the findings ready for use in nursing practice? The answers to these questions require careful examination of the research problem, the theoretical basis of the study, and the study's methodology. Not only must the mechanics of conducting the study be examined, but the abstract and logical reasoning used by the researcher in planning and implementing the study must also be evaluated. If the reasoning process used to develop the study has flaws, there are probably flaws in interpreting the meaning of the findings.

All studies have flaws, but if all flawed studies were discarded, there would be no scientific base for practice (Oberst, 1992). In fact, science itself is flawed. Science does not completely or perfectly describe, explain, predict, or control reality. However, improved understanding and increased ability to predict and control phenomena depend on recognizing the flaws in studies and in science. New studies can then be planned to minimize the flaws or limitations of earlier studies. Thus a researcher must critique previous studies to determine their limitations, and the study findings need to be interpreted in light of the limitations. These limitations can lead to inaccurate data, inaccurate outcomes of analysis, and decreased ability to generalize the findings. When using study findings in practice, one recognizes that knowledge is not absolute; however,

confidence in empirical knowledge grows as the number of quality studies conducted increases.

All studies have strengths as well as limitations. Recognition of these strengths is also critical to the generation of scientific knowledge and use of study findings in practice. If only weaknesses are identified, nurses might discount the value of the study and refuse to invest time in examining research (Oberst, 1992). The continued work of the researcher also depends on recognition of the study's strengths. If no study is good enough, why invest time conducting research? Points of strength in a study, added to points of strength from multiple other studies, slowly build a solid knowledge base.

Types of Research Critiques Conducted in Nursing

In general, research is critiqued to broaden understanding, summarize knowledge for use in practice, and provide a base for the conduct of a study. Formal research critiques are often conducted after verbal presentations of studies, after a published research report, for abstract or article selection, and for evaluation of research proposals. Thus, nursing students, practicing nurses, nurse educators, and nurse researchers are all involved in critiquing research.

STUDENT CRITIQUES

In nursing education, a critique is often seen as a first step in learning the research process. Moreover, it is true that part of learning the research process is being able to read and comprehend published research reports. However, comprehension of the research report is dependent on understanding the research process. Thus, conducting a critique is not a basic skill, and the content presented in previous chapters is essential for implementing the critique process. Basic knowledge of the research process and critique process is usually provided early in professional nursing education. More advanced critique skills are often taught at the master's and doctoral levels. Students' skills in the steps involved in performing a critique (comprehension, comparison, analysis, evaluation, and conceptual clustering) increase as their knowledge of the research process expands. By conducting research critiques, students strengthen their knowledge base and increase their use of research findings in practice.

CRITIQUES BY THE PRACTICING NURSE

Critiques of studies by practicing nurses are essential for the implementation of an evidence-based nursing practice (Brown, 1999; Omery & Williams, 1999). Nursing actions require updating in response to the current evidence that is generated through research and theory development. Practicing nurses need to design methods for remaining current in their practice areas. Reading research journals or posting current studies at work can make nurses aware of study findings but is not sufficient for critique to occur. Nurses need to question the quality of the studies and the credibility of the findings and share their concerns with other nurses. For example, a research journal club might be formed where studies are presented and critiqued by members of the group (Tibbles & Sanford, 1994). Skills in research critique enable the practicing nurse to synthesize the most credible, significant, and appropriate empirical evidence for use in practice (Brown, 1999).

CRITIQUES BY NURSE EDUCATORS

Educators conduct research critiques to expand their knowledge base and to develop and refine the educational process. Careful critique of current nursing studies provides a basis for updating the curricular content in clinical and classroom settings. Educators act as role models for their students by examining new studies, evaluating the information obtained from research, and using research knowledge as a basis for practice. In addition, educators collaborate in the conduct of studies, which requires a critique of previous relevant research.

CRITIQUES BY NURSE RESEARCHERS

Researchers conduct critiques to plan and implement a study. Many researchers focus their studies in one area, and they update their knowledge base

by critiquing new studies in this area. The outcome of the critique influences the selection of research problems, development of methodology, and interpretation of findings in future studies. Critique of previous studies to develop a review of literature section in a research proposal or report is described in Chapter 6.

VERBAL CRITIQUES AFTER PRESENTATIONS OF STUDIES

Verbal critiques need to be considered part of a research presentation. Through verbal critique, researchers can gain increased understanding of the strengths and weaknesses of their studies and generate ideas for further research. Participants listening to critiques might gain insight into the conduct of research. Experiencing the critique process can increase the participants' ability to critique studies and judge the usefulness of the findings for their practice.

CRITIQUES AFTER PUBLISHED RESEARCH REPORTS

Currently, at least two nursing research journals, *Scholarly Inquiry for Nursing Practice: An International Journal* and *Western Journal of Nursing Research,* include commentaries (partial critiques) after research articles. In these journals, authors receive critiques of their studies and have an opportunity to respond to the critiques. Published critiques increase readers' understanding of the study and their ability to critique research. Another more informal critique of a published study might appear in a letter to the editor. Readers have the opportunity to comment on the strengths and weaknesses of published studies by writing to the editor.

CRITIQUE FOR ABSTRACT SELECTION

One of the most difficult types of critique to perform is that of examining abstracts. The amount of information available is usually limited because many abstracts are restricted to 100 to 250 words (Crosby, 1990; Pyrczak, 1999). Nevertheless, reviewers must select the best-designed studies with the most significant outcomes for presentation at nursing conferences. This process requires an experienced researcher who needs few cues to determine the quality of a study. Critique of an abstract usually addresses the following criteria: (1) appropriateness of the study for the program; (2) completeness of the research project; (3) overall quality of the study problem, purpose, framework, methodology, and results; (4) contribution of the study to nursing's empirical knowledge base; (5) contribution of the study to nursing theory; (6) originality of the work (not previously published); (7) implication of the study findings for practice; and (8) clarity, conciseness, and completeness of the abstract (American Psychological Association [APA], 1994; Morse et al., 1993).

CRITIQUE OF AN ARTICLE FOR PUBLICATION

Nurse researchers serve as reviewers for professional journals to evaluate the quality of research papers submitted for publication. The role of these scientists is to examine the quality of the studies submitted to ensure that those accepted for publication are well designed and contribute to the body of knowledge. Most of these reviews are conducted anonymously so that friendships or reputations do not interfere with the selection process. In most refereed journals (82%), the research report is examined by experts selected from an established group of reviewers (Swanson et al., 1991). The reviewers' comments or a summary of these comments is sent to the researcher. These comments are also used by the editor in making selections for publication. The process for publishing research is described in Chapter 25.

CRITIQUE OF RESEARCH PROPOSALS

Critiques of research proposals are conducted to approve student research projects, to permit data collection in an institution, and to select the best studies for funding. Seeking approval to conduct a study is presented in Chapter 28. The peer review process in federal funding agencies involves an extremely complex critique. Nurses are involved in this level of research review through the National Institute of Nursing Research (NINR) and the Agency for Healthcare Research and Quality

(AHRQ). Kim and Felton (1993) identified some of the criteria used to evaluate the quality of a proposal for possible funding, such as the (1) appropriate use of measurement for the types of questions that the research is designed to answer, (2) appropriate use and interpretation of statistical procedures, (3) evaluation of clinical practice and forecasting of the need for nursing or other appropriate interventions, and (4) construction of models to direct the research and interpret the findings.

CRITIQUE PROCESS FOR QUANTITATIVE STUDIES

The critique process for quantitative research includes five steps: (1) comprehension, (2) comparison, (3) analysis, (4) evaluation, and (5) conceptual clustering. Conducting a critique is a complex mental process that is stimulated by raising questions. The level of critique conducted is influenced by the sophistication of the individual doing the critique (see Table 26–1). The initial critique of an undergraduate student often involves only the comprehension step of the critique process, which includes identification of the steps of the research process in a study. Some baccalaureate programs include more in-depth research courses that incorporate the comparison step of critique, wherein the quality of the research report is examined using expert sources. A research critique conducted by a master's level student usually involves the steps of comprehension, comparison, analysis, and evaluation. The analysis step involves examining the logical links among the steps of the research process, with evaluation focus-

TABLE 26–1
EDUCATIONAL LEVEL AND EXPECTED LEVEL OF EXPERTISE IN THE CRITIQUE

EDUCATIONAL LEVEL	EXPECTED LEVEL OF EXPERTISE IN THE CRITIQUE PROCESS
Baccalaureate	Step I—Comprehension
	Step II—Comparison
Master's	Step III—Analysis
	Step IV—Evaluation
Doctorate or experienced researcher, or both	Step V—Conceptual clustering

ing on the overall quality of the study and credibility of the findings. Conceptual clustering is a complex synthesis of critiqued study findings that provides a current, empirical knowledge base for a phenomenon. This critique step is usually perfected by doctoral students or experienced researchers as they develop integrated reviews of research for publication. These integrated research reviews provide a knowledge base for future research and current evidence for use in practice.

Conducting an intellectual critique of quantitative and qualitative research involves applying some basic guidelines such as outlined in Table 26–2. These guidelines stress the importance of examining the expertise of the authors; critiquing the entire study; addressing the study's strengths, weaknesses, and logical links; and evaluating the contribution of the study to nursing knowledge. These guidelines are linked to the first four steps of the critique process: comprehension, comparison, analysis, and evaluation. These steps occur in sequence, vary in depth, and presume accomplishment of the preceding steps. However, an individual with critique experience frequently performs several steps of this process simultaneously.

This section includes the steps of the critique process and provides relevant questions for each step. These questions are not comprehensive but have been selected as a means for stimulating the abstract reasoning necessary for conducting a critique. Persons experienced in the critique process formulate additional questions as part of their reasoning processes. The comprehension step is covered separately because those new to critique start with this step. The comparison and analysis steps are covered together because these steps often occur simultaneously in the mind of the person conducting the critique. Evaluation and conceptual clustering are covered separately because of the increased expertise needed to perform each step.

Step I—Comprehension

Initial attempts to comprehend research articles are often frustrating because the terminology and stylized manner of the report are unfamiliar. *Comprehension* is the first step in the critique process and involves understanding the terms and concepts

TABLE 26–2
GUIDELINES FOR CONDUCTING QUANTITATIVE AND QUALITATIVE RESEARCH CRITIQUES

1. **Read and critique the entire study.** A research critique requires identification and examination of all steps of the research process. (Comprehension)
2. **Examine the research and clinical expertise of the authors.** The authors need a clinical and scientific background that is appropriate for the study conducted. (Comprehension)
3. **Examine the organization and presentation of the research report.** The title of the research report needs to clearly indicate the focus of the study. The report usually includes an abstract, introduction, methods, results, discussion, and references. The abstract of the study needs to present the purpose of the study clearly and highlight the methodology and major results. The body of the report needs to be complete, concise, clearly presented, and logically organized. The references need to be complete and presented in a consistent format. (Comparison)
4. **Identify the strengths and weaknesses of a study.** All the studies have strengths and weaknesses, and you can use the questions in this chapter to facilitate identification of them. Address the quality of the steps of the research process and the logical links among the steps of the process. (Comparison and analysis)
5. **Provide specific examples of the strengths and weaknesses of a study.** These examples provide a rationale and documentation for your critique of the study. (Comparison and analysis)
6. **Be objective and realistic in identifying the study's strengths and weaknesses.** Try not to be overly critical when identifying a study's weaknesses or overly flattering when identifying the strengths.
7. **Suggest modifications for future studies.** Modifications should increase the strengths and decrease the weaknesses in the study.
8. **Evaluate the study.** Indicate the overall quality of the study and its contribution to nursing knowledge. Discuss the consistency of the findings of this study with those of previous research. Discuss the need for further research and the potential to use the findings in practice. (Evaluation)

in the report, as well as identifying study elements and grasping the nature, significance, and meaning of these elements. Comprehension is demonstrated as the reviewer identifies each element or step of the study.

GUIDELINES FOR COMPREHENSION

The first step involves reviewing the abstract and reading the study from beginning to end. As you read, address the following questions about the presentation of the study: Does the title of the research report clearly identify the focus of the study by including the primary variables and the population studied? Does the title indicate the type of study conducted—descriptive, correlational, quasi-experimental, or experimental? Was the abstract clear? Was the writing style of the report clear and concise? Were the different parts of the research report clearly identified? Were relevant terms clearly defined? (Brown, 1999; Crookes & Davies, 1998). You might underline the terms you do not understand and determine their meaning from the Glossary at the end of this book. Read the article a second time and highlight or underline each step of the quantitative research process. An overview of these steps is presented in Chapter 3. To write a research critique, you need to identify each step of the research process concisely and respond briefly to the following guidelines and questions:

I. Introduction
   A. Identify the reference style of the article (use APA format).
   B. Describe the qualifications of the authors (such as research expertise, clinical experience, educational preparation).
   C. Discuss the clarity of the article title (type of study, primary variables, and population identified).
   D. Discuss the quality of the abstract (includes purpose; highlights design, sample, intervention [if applicable], and key results).
II. State the problem.
   A. Significance of the problem
   B. Background of the problem
III. State the purpose.
IV. Examine the literature review.
   A. Are relevant previous studies and theories described?
   B. Are the references current? (Number of sources in the last five years?)
   C. Are the studies critiqued?
   D. Describe the current knowledge (what is known and not known) about the research problem.
V. Examine the study framework or theoretical perspective.
   A. Is the framework explicitly expressed or must the reviewer extract the framework from implicit statements in the literature review?
   B. Is the framework based on substantive theory or a tentative theory?
   C. Does the framework identify, define, and describe the relationships among the concepts of interest?
   D. Is a map of the framework provided for clarity? If a map is not presented, develop a map that represents the study's framework and describe the map.
   E. Link the study variables to the relevant concepts in the map.
   F. How is the framework related to nursing's body of knowledge?
VI. List any research objectives, questions, or hypotheses.
VII. Identify and define (conceptually and operationally) the study variables or concepts that were identified in the objectives, questions, or hypotheses. If objectives, questions, or hypotheses are not stated, identify and define the variables in the study purpose. If conceptual definitions are not found, identify possible definitions for each major study variable.
   A. Independent variables: Identify and define conceptually and operationally.
   B. Dependent variables: Identify and define conceptually and operationally.
   C. Research variables or concepts: Identify and define conceptually and operationally.
VIII. Identify attributes/demographic variables and other relevant terms.
IX. Identify the research design.
   A. Identify the specific design of the study and draw a model of the design by using the sample design models presented in Chapter 11.
   B. Identify the treatment or intervention if appropriate for the study conducted.
   C. Were pilot study findings used to design this study? If yes, briefly discuss the pilot and the changes made in this study based on the pilot.
X. Describe the sample and setting.
   A. Sampling criteria
   B. Method used to obtain the sample
   C. Sample size (indicate whether a power analysis was conducted)

D. Characteristics of the sample
E. Sample mortality
F. Type of consent obtained
G. How were subjects assigned to groups if groups were studied?
H. Identify the study setting and indicate if it is appropriate for the study purpose.
XI. Identify and describe each measurement strategy used in the study.
A. Identify the author of each instrument.
B. Identify the type of each measurement strategy (e.g., Likert scale, visual analogue scale, physiological measure) and the level of measurement (nominal, ordinal, interval, ratio) achieved.
C. Discuss how the instrument was developed.
D. Describe the validity and reliability of each instrument.
XII. Describe the procedures for data collection.
A. If appropriate, identify the intervention protocol.
B. How were the data collected?
XIII. Describe the statistical analyses used.
A. List the statistical procedures used to describe the sample.
B. Identify the statistical procedures used to establish the reliability and validity of the measurement methods in the study.
C. Was the level of significance or alpha identified? If so, indicate what it was (.05, .01, .001).
D. List each objective, question, or hypothesis and (1) identify the focus (description, relationships, or differences) of each objective, question, or hypothesis and (2) list the statistical procedures, statistics, specific results, and probability value (p value).
XIV. Describe the researcher's interpretation of findings.
A. Are the findings related back to the study framework?
B. Which findings are in keeping with those expected?
C. Which findings were not expected?
D. Are serendipitous findings described?
E. Are the findings consistent with previous research findings?
XV. What study limitations were identified by the researcher?

XVI. How did the researcher generalize the findings?
XVII. What were the implications of the findings for nursing?
XVIII. What suggestions for further study were identified?
XIX. Is the description of the study sufficiently clear for replication?

Step II—Comparison

The next step, *comparison,* requires knowledge of what each step of the research process should be like. The ideal is compared with the real. During the comparison step, you examine the extent to which the researcher followed the rules for an ideal study. You also need to gain a sense of how clearly the researcher grasped the study situation and expressed it. The clarity of researchers' explanation of the elements of the study demonstrates their skill in using and expressing ideas that require abstract reasoning.

Step III—Analysis

The *analysis step* involves a critique of the logical links connecting one study element with another. For example, the problem needs to provide background and direction for the statement of the purpose. In addition, the overall flow of logic in the study must be examined (Brown, 1999; Liehr & Houston, 1993). The variables identified in the study purpose need to be consistent with the variables identified in the research objectives, questions, or hypotheses. The variables identified in the research objectives, questions, or hypotheses need to be conceptually defined in light of the study framework. The conceptual definitions provide the basis for the development of operational definitions. The study design and analyses need to be appropriate for the investigation of the study purpose, as well as for the specific objectives, questions, or hypotheses (Ryan-Wenger, 1992).

Most of the limitations in a study result from breaks in logical reasoning. For example, biases caused by sampling and design impair the logical flow from design to interpretation of findings. The previous levels of critique have addressed concrete aspects of the study. During analysis, the process moves into examining abstract dimensions of the study, which requires greater familiarity with the logic behind the research process and increased skill in abstract reasoning.

GUIDELINES FOR COMPARISON AND ANALYSIS

To conduct the steps of comparison and analysis, you need to review Unit II of this text on the research process and other sources on the steps of the research process (Brown, 1999; Crookes & Davies, 1998; Gill, 1996; Liehr & Houston, 1993; LoBiondo-Wood & Haber, 1998; Mateo & Kirchhoff, 1999; Pyrczak, 1999; Polit & Hungler, 1999; Ryan-Wenger, 1992). After review, compare the elements in the study that you are critiquing with the criteria established for each element in this textbook or in other sources (Step II—Comparison), and then analyze the logical links among the steps of the study by examining how each step provides a basis for and links with the following steps of the research process (Step III—Analysis). The following guidelines will assist you in implementing the steps of comparison and analysis for each step of the research process. Questions relevant to analysis are identified; all other questions direct comparison of the steps of the study with the ideal. The written critique will be a summary of the *strengths* and *weaknesses* that you noted in the study.

I. Research problem and purpose
   A. Is the problem sufficiently delimited in scope without being trivial?
   B. Is the problem significant to nursing?
   C. Does the problem have a gender bias and address only the health needs of men to the exclusion of women's health needs? (Yam, 1994)
   D. Does the purpose narrow and clarify the aim of the study?
II. Review of literature
   A. Is the literature review organized to demonstrate the progressive development of ideas through previous research? (Analysis)
   B. Is a theoretical knowledge base developed for the problem and purpose? (Analysis)
   C. Does the literature review provide rationale and direction for the study? (Analysis)
   D. Is a clear, concise summary presented of the current empirical and theoretical knowledge in the area of the study?
III. Study framework
   A. Is the framework presented with clarity? If a model or conceptual map of the framework is present, is it adequate to explain the phenomenon of concern?
   B. Is the framework linked to the research purpose? Would another framework fit more logically with the study? (Analysis)
   C. Is the framework related to nursing's body of knowledge? (Analysis)
   D. If a proposition from a theory is to be tested, is the proposition clearly identified and linked to the study hypotheses? (Analysis and comparison)
IV. Research objectives, questions, or hypotheses
   A. Are the objectives, questions, or hypotheses expressed clearly?
   B. Are the objectives, questions, or hypotheses logically linked to the research purpose and framework? (Analysis)
V. Variables
   A. Are the variables reflective of the concepts identified in the framework? (Analysis)
   B. Are the variables clearly defined (conceptually and operationally) and based on previous research or theories?
   C. Is the conceptual definition of a variable consistent with the operational definition? (Analysis)
VI. Design
   A. Is the design used in the study the most appropriate design to obtain the needed data?
   B. Does the design provide a means to examine all the objectives, questions, or hypotheses? (Analysis)
   C. Is the treatment clearly described? Does the study framework explain the links between the treatment (independent variable) and the proposed outcomes (dependent variables) (Sidani & Braden, 1998)? Was a protocol developed to promote consistent implementation of the treatment? Did the researcher monitor implementation of

the treatment to ensure consistency (Egan et al., 1992)? If the treatment was not consistently implemented, what might be the impact on the findings? (Analysis and comparison)

D. Have the threats to design validity been minimized?

E. Is the design logically linked to the sampling method and statistical analyses? (Analysis)

VII. Sample, population, and setting

A. Is the sampling method adequate to produce a representative sample?

B. What are the potential biases in the sampling method? Are any subjects excluded from the study because of age, socioeconomic status, or race without a sound rationale? (Larson, 1994)

C. Were the sampling criteria appropriate for the type of study conducted?

D. Is the sample size sufficient to avoid a Type II error?

E. If more than one group is used, do the groups appear equivalent?

F. Are the rights of human subjects protected?

G. Is the setting used in the study typical of clinical settings?

H. Was sample mortality a problem? If so, how might this factor influence the findings?

VIII. Measurements

A. Do the instruments adequately measure the study variables? (Analysis)

B. Are the instruments sufficiently sensitive to detect small differences between subjects?

C. Does the instrument have adequate validity and reliability for use in a study?

D. Respond to the following questions, which are relevant to the measurement approaches used in the study:

1. Scales and questionnaires

(a) Are the instruments clearly described?

(b) Are techniques to complete and score the instruments provided?

(c) Are validity and reliability of the instruments described?

(d) Did the researcher reexamine the validity and reliability of instruments for the present sample?

(e) If the instrument was developed for the study, is the instrument development process described?

2. Observation

(a) Is what is to be observed clearly identified and defined?

(b) Is interrater reliability described?

(c) Are the techniques for recording observations described?

3. Interviews

(a) Do the interview questions address concerns expressed in the research problem? (Analysis)

(b) Are the interview questions relevant for the research purpose and objectives, questions, or hypotheses? (Analysis)

(c) Does the design of the questions tend to bias subjects' responses?

(d) Does the sequence of questions tend to bias subjects' responses?

4. Physiological measures

(a) Are the physiological measures or instruments clearly described? If appropriate, are the brand names, such as Space Labs or Hewlett-Packard, of the instruments identified?

(b) Are the accuracy, selectivity, precision, sensitivity, and error of the instruments discussed?

(c) Are the physiological measures appropriate for the research purpose and objectives, questions, or hypotheses? (Analysis)

(d) Are the methods for recording data from the physiological measures clearly described? Is the recording of data consistent?

IX. Data collection

A. Is the data collection process clearly described?

B. Are the forms used to collect data organized to facilitate computerizing the data?

C. Is the training of data collectors clearly described and adequate?

D. Is the data collection process conducted in a consistent manner?

E. Are the data collection methods ethical?

F. Do the data collected address the research objectives, questions, or hypotheses? (Analysis)

X. Data analysis
   A. Are data analysis procedures appropriate for the type of data collected?
   B. Are data analysis procedures clearly described?
   C. Are the results presented in an understandable way by narrative, tables, or figures, or a combination of methods?
   D. Are the statistical analyses logically linked to the design? (Analysis)
   E. Is the sample size sufficient to detect significant differences if they are present? Was power analysis used to determine sample size? (Analysis)
   F. Do data analyses address each research objective, question, or hypothesis? (Analysis)
   G. Are the analyses interpreted appropriately?

XI. Interpretation of findings
   A. Are findings discussed in relation to each objective, question, or hypothesis?
   B. Are various explanations for significant and nonsignificant findings examined?
   C. Are the findings clinically significant? (Brown, 1999; LeFort, 1993)
   D. Do the conclusions fit the findings from the analyses? Are the conclusions based on statistically significant and clinically significant results? (Analysis)
   E. Does the study have limitations not identified by the researcher? (Analysis)

Step IV—Evaluation

Evaluation involves determining the meaning and significance of the study by examining the links between the study process, study findings, and previous studies. The steps of the study are evaluated in light of previous studies, such as an evaluation of present hypotheses based on previous hypotheses, present design based on previous designs, and present methods of putting variables into operation based on previous approaches. The findings of the present study are also examined in light of the findings of previous studies. Evaluation builds on conclusions reached during the first three stages of the

critique and provides the basis for conceptual clustering.

GUIDELINES FOR EVALUATION

You need to reexamine the findings, conclusions, and implications sections of the study and the researcher's suggestions for further study. Using the following questions as a guide, summarize the *strengths* and *weaknesses* of the study.

1. What rival hypotheses can be suggested for the findings?
2. How much confidence can be placed in the study findings?
3. To what populations can the findings be generalized?
4. What questions emerge from the findings and are they identified by the researcher?
5. What future research can be envisioned?
6. Could the limitations of the study have been corrected?
7. When the findings are examined in light of previous studies, what is now known and not known about the phenomenon under study?

You need to read previous studies conducted in the area of the research being examined and summarize your responses to the following questions:

1. Are the findings of previous studies used to generate the research problem and purpose?
2. Is the design an advancement over previous designs?
3. Do sampling strategies show an improvement over previous studies? Does the sample selection have the potential for adding diversity to samples previously studied? (Larson, 1994)
4. Does the current research build on previous measurement strategies so that measurement is more precise or more reflective of the variables?
5. How do statistical analyses compare with those used in previous studies?
6. Do the findings build on the findings of previous studies?
7. Is current knowledge in this area identified?
8. Does the author indicate the implication of the findings for practice?

Step V—Conceptual Clustering

The last step of the critique process is *conceptual clustering,* which involves the synthesis of study findings to determine the current body of knowledge in an area (Pinch, 1995). Until the 1980s, conceptual clustering was seldom addressed in the nursing literature. However, in 1983, the initial volume of the *Annual Review of Nursing Research* was published to provide conceptual clustering of specific phenomena of interest to nursing in the areas of nursing practice, nursing care delivery, nursing education, and the profession of nursing (Werley & Fitzpatrick, 1983). These books continue to be published each year and provide integrated reviews of research on a variety of topics relevant to nursing. Conceptual clustering is also evident in the publication of several integrative reviews of research in clinical and research journals (Ganong, 1987; Massey & Loomis, 1988).

GUIDELINES FOR CONCEPTUAL CLUSTERING

Through conceptual clustering, current knowledge in an area of study is carefully analyzed, relationships are examined, and the knowledge is summarized and organized theoretically. Conceptual clustering maximizes the meaning attached to research findings, highlights gaps in knowledge, generates new research questions, and provides empirical evidence for use in practice.

I. Process for clustering findings and developing the current knowledge base
   A. Is the purpose for reviewing the literature clearly identified?
   B. Are the criteria for including studies in the review clearly identified and used appropriately?
   C. Is the process for clustering study findings clearly described?
   D. Is the current knowledge base clearly expressed? What is known and not known?
II. Theoretical organization of the knowledge base
   Draw a map showing the concepts and relationships found in the studies reviewed in the previous criteria (1) to detect gaps in understanding relationships. The map can also be compared with current theory in the area of study by asking the following questions:
   A. Is the map consistent with current theory?
   B. Are there differences in the map that are upheld by well-designed research? If so, modification of existing theory should be considered.
   C. Are there concepts and relationships in existing theory that have not been examined in the studies diagramed in the map? If so, studies should be developed to examine these gaps.
   D. Are there conflicting theories within the field of study? Do existing study findings tend to support one of the theories?
   E. Are there no existing theories to explain the phenomenon under consideration?
   F. Can current research findings be used to begin the development of nursing theory to explain the phenomenon more completely?
III. Use of research findings in practice
   A. Is there sufficient confidence in the findings to use them in nursing practice? If so, develop a protocol to promote the use of this empirical evidence in practice.
   B. If confidence in the findings is not sufficient, what further knowledge is needed before the findings can be used in practice?
   C. What are the benefits and risks of using the findings for patients, health care providers, and health care agencies?
   D. How will patient, care provider, and agency outcomes be affected by use of the findings?
   E. Would the changes in outcome make a significant difference in the health of the patient and family?
   F. Would the changes in outcome make a significant difference for health care providers or agencies, or both?

Meta-analysis is another form of conceptual clustering that goes beyond critique and integration of research findings to conducting statistical analysis on the outcomes of similar studies (Pillemer & Light, 1980). A meta-analysis statistically pools the results from previous studies into a single result or outcome that provides the strongest evidence about the efficacy of a treatment (LaValley, 1997). Conducting a quality meta-analysis requires a great deal of rigor in implementing the following steps: (1) development of a protocol to direct conduct of the meta-analysis, (2) location of relevant studies, (3) selection of studies for analysis that meet the criteria in the protocol, (4) conduct of statistical analyses, (5) assessment of the meta-analysis results, and (6) discussion of the relevance of the findings to nursing knowledge and practice. Chapter 27 discusses the use of meta-analysis to synthesize research for generating evidence to put into practice.

CRITIQUE PROCESS FOR QUALITATIVE STUDIES

Critique in qualitative research also requires comprehension, comparison, analysis, and evaluation; thus, the guidelines in Table 26–2 are helpful in conducting the critique. Critiquing a qualitative study involves examining the expertise of the researchers, noting the organization and presentation of the report, discussing the strengths and weaknesses of the study, suggesting modifications for future studies, and evaluating the overall quality of the study. However, other standards and skills are also useful for assessing the quality of a qualitative study and the credibility of the study findings (Burns, 1989; Cutcliffe & McKenna, 1999). The skills and standards for critiquing qualitative research are described in the following sections.

Skills Needed to Critique Qualitative Studies

The skills needed to critique qualitative studies include (1) context flexibility; (2) inductive reasoning; (3) conceptualization, theoretical modeling, and theory analysis; and (4) transformation of ideas across levels of abstraction (Burns, 1989).

CONTEXT FLEXIBILITY

Context flexibility is the capacity to switch from one context or world view to another, to shift perception to see things from a different perspective. Each world view is based on a set of assumptions through which reality is defined. Developing skills in the critique of qualitative studies requires that the

individual be willing to move from the assumptions of quantitative research to those of qualitative research. This skill is not new in nursing; beginning students are encouraged to see things from the patient's perspective. However, accomplishing this switch of context requires investing time and energy to learn more about the patient and setting aside personal, sometimes strongly held views. It is not necessary for one to become committed to a perspective to follow or apply its logical structure. In fact, all scholarly work requires a willingness and ability to examine and evaluate works from diverse perspectives. For example, analysis of the internal structure of a theory requires this same process.

INDUCTIVE REASONING SKILLS

Although all research requires skill in both deductive and inductive reasoning, the transformation process used during data analysis in qualitative research is based on inductive reasoning. Individuals conducting a critique of a qualitative study must be able to exercise skills in inductive reasoning to follow the logic of the researcher. This logic is revealed in the systematic move from the concrete descriptions in a particular study to the abstract level of science.

CONCEPTUALIZATION, THEORETICAL MODELING, AND THEORY ANALYSIS SKILLS

Qualitative research is oriented toward theory construction. Therefore, an effective reviewer of qualitative research needs to have skills in conceptualization, theoretical modeling, and theory analysis. The theoretical structure in a qualitative study is developed inductively and is expected to emerge from the data. The reviewer must be able to follow the logical flow of thought of the researcher and be able to analyze and evaluate the adequacy of the resulting theoretical schema, as well as its connection to theory development within the discipline.

TRANSFORMING IDEAS ACROSS LEVELS OF ABSTRACTION

Closely associated with the necessity of having skills in theory analysis is the ability to follow the transformation of ideas across several levels of abstraction and to judge the adequacy of the transformation. Whenever one reviews the literature, organizes ideas from the review, and then again modifies those ideas in the process of developing a summary of the existing body of knowledge, one is involved in the *transformation of ideas.* Developing a research proposal requires transforming ideas across levels of abstraction. Those critiquing the proposal evaluate the adequacy of this transformation process.

Standards for Critique of Qualitative Studies

Multiple problems can occur in qualitative studies, as in quantitative studies. However, the problems are likely to be different. Reviewers not only need to know the problems that are likely to occur but also must be able to determine the probability that the problem may have occurred in the study being critiqued. A scholarly critique includes a balanced evaluation of study strengths and limitations. Five standards have been proposed to evaluate qualitative studies: descriptive vividness, methodological congruence, analytical preciseness, theoretical connectedness, and heuristic relevance (Burns, 1989; Johnson, 1999). The following sections describe these standards and the threats to them.

STANDARD I: DESCRIPTIVE VIVIDNESS

Descriptive vividness or validity refers to the clarity and factual accuracy of the researcher's account of the study (Johnson, 1999). The description of the site, the subjects, the experience of collecting the data, and the thinking of the researcher during the process needs to be presented so clearly and accurately that the reader has the sense of personally experiencing the event. Glaser and Strauss (1965) say that the researcher should "describe the social world studied so vividly that the reader can almost literally see and hear its people" (p. 9). Because one of the assumptions of qualitative research is that all data are context-specific, the evaluator of a study must understand the context of that study. From this description, the reader gets a sense of the

data as a whole as they are collected and the reactions of the researcher during the data collection and analysis processes. A contextual understanding of the whole is essential and prerequisite to the capability of the reviewer to evaluate the study in light of the other four standards.

Threats to Descriptive Vividness

1. Failure to include essential descriptive information
2. Lack of clarity or depth, or both, of the description
3. Lack of factual accuracy in the description (Johnson, 1999)
4. Lack of credibility of the description (Beck, 1993)
5. Inadequate skills in writing descriptive narrative
6. Reluctance to reveal self in the written material (Burns, 1989; Kahn, 1993)

STANDARD II: METHODOLOGICAL CONGRUENCE

Evaluation of *methodological congruence* requires that the reviewer have knowledge of the philosophy and the methodological approach that was used by the researcher. The researcher needs to identify the philosophy and methodological approach and cite sources where the reviewer can obtain further information (Beck, 1994; Munhall & Boyd, 1999). Methodological excellence has four dimensions: rigor in documentation, procedural rigor, ethical rigor, and auditability.

Rigor in Documentation

Rigor in documentation requires a clear, concise presentation of the following study elements by the researcher: phenomenon, purpose, research question, justification of the significance of the phenomenon, identification of assumptions, identification of philosophy, researcher credentials, the context, the role of the researcher, ethical implications, sampling and subjects, data-gathering strategies, data analysis strategies, theoretical development, conclusions, implications and suggestions for further study and practice, and a literature review. The reviewer examines the study elements or steps for completeness and clarity and identifies any threats to rigor in documentation.

Threats to Rigor in Documentation

1. Failure to present all elements or steps of the study
2. Failure to present all elements or steps of the study accurately or clearly

Procedural Rigor

Another dimension of methodological congruence is the rigor of the researcher in applying selected procedures for the study. To the extent possible, the researcher needs to make clear the steps taken to ensure that data were accurately recorded and that the data obtained are representative of the data as a whole (Beck, 1993; Knafl & Howard, 1984). All researchers have bias, but reflexivity needs to be used in qualitative studies to reduce bias. Reflexivity is an analytical method in which the "researcher actively engages in critical self-reflection about his or her potential biases and predispositions" to reduce their impact on the conduct of the study (Johnson, 1999, p. 103). Methodological congruence can also be promoted by extended field work, where the researcher collects data in the study setting for an extended period to ensure accuracy of the data. When critiquing a qualitative study, the reviewer examines the description of the data collection process and the study findings for threats to procedural rigor.

Threats to Procedural Rigor

1. The researcher asked the wrong questions. The questions need to tap the subjects' experiences, not their theoretical knowledge of the phenomenon.
2. The questions included terminology from the theoretical orientation of the researcher (Kirk & Miller, 1986; Knaack, 1984).
3. The informant might have misinformed the researcher, for several reasons. The informant might have had an ulterior motive for deceiving the researcher. Some individuals might have been present who inhibit free expression by the informant. The informant might have wanted to impress the researcher by giving the response

that seemed the most desirable (Dean & Whyte, 1958).
4. The informant did not observe the details requested or was not able to recall the event and substituted instead what he or she supposed happened (Dean & Whyte, 1958).
5. The researcher placed more weight on data obtained from well-informed, articulate, high-status individuals (an elite bias) than on data from those who were less articulate, obstinate, or of low status (Miles & Huberman, 1994).
6. The presence of the researcher distorted the event being observed.
7. The researcher's involvement with the subject-participants distorted the data (LeCompte & Goetz, 1982).
8. Atypical events were interpreted as typical.
9. The informants lacked credibility (Beck, 1993; Becker, 1958).
10. An insufficient amount of data was gathered.
11. An insufficient length of time was spent in the setting gathering the data.
12. The approaches for gaining access to the site or the subjects, or both, were inappropriate.
13. The researcher failed to keep in-depth field notes.
14. The researcher failed to use reflexivity or critical self-reflection to assess his or her potential biases and predispositions.

Ethical Rigor

Ethical rigor requires recognition and discussion by the researcher of the ethical implications related to conduct of the study. Consent is obtained from subjects and documented. The report must indicate that the researcher took action to ensure that the rights of subjects were protected during the consent process, data collection and analysis, and communication of the findings (Munhall, 1999). The reviewer examines the consent process, data-gathering process, and the results for potential threats to ethical rigor.

Threats to Ethical Rigor

1. The researcher failed to inform the subjects of their rights.
2. The researcher failed to obtain consent from the subjects.

3. The researcher failed to ensure protection of the subjects' rights during conduct of the study.
4. The results of the study were presented in such a way to reveal the identity of individual subjects.

Auditability

A fourth dimension of methodological congruence is the rigorous development of a decision trail (Beck, 1993; Miles & Huberman, 1994). Guba and Lincoln (1982) refer to this dimension as *auditability*. To achieve this end, the researcher must report all decisions involved in the transformation of data to the theoretical schema. This reporting should be in sufficient detail to allow a second researcher, using the original data and the decision trail, to arrive at conclusions similar to those of the original researcher. When critiquing the study, the reviewer examines the decision trail for threats to auditability.

Threats to Auditability

1. The description of the data collection process was inadequate.
2. The researcher failed to develop or identify the decision rules for arriving at ratings or judgments.
3. The researcher failed to record the nature of the decisions, the data on which they were based, and the reasoning that entered into the decisions.
4. The evidence for conclusions was not presented (Becker, 1958).
5. Other researchers were unable to arrive at similar conclusions after applying the decision rules to the data (Beck, 1993).

STANDARD III: ANALYTICAL PRECISENESS

The analytical process in qualitative research involves a series of transformations during which concrete data are transformed across several levels of abstraction. The outcome of the analysis is a theoretical schema that imparts meaning to the phenomenon under study. The analytical process occurs primarily within the reasoning of the researcher and is frequently poorly described in published reports. Some transformations may occur intuitively. However, *analytical preciseness* requires that the researcher make intense efforts to identify and record the decision-making processes through which the transformations are made. The processes by which the theoretical schema are cross-checked with data also need to be reported in detail.

Premature patterning may occur before the researcher can logically fit all the data within the emerging schema. Nisbett and Ross (1980) have shown that patterning happens rapidly and is the way that individuals habitually process information. The consequence may be a poor fit between data and the theoretical schema (LeCompte & Goetz, 1982; Sandelowski, 1986). Miles and Huberman (1994) suggest that plausibility is the opiate of the intellectual. If the emerging schema makes sense and fits with other theorists' explanations of the phenomenon, the researcher locks into it. For that reason, it is critical to test the schema by rechecking the fit between the schema and the original data. The participants could be asked to provide feedback on the researcher's interpretations and conclusions to gain additional insight or verification of the theoretical scheme proposed (Johnson, 1999). Beck (1993) recommends that the researcher have the "data analysis procedures reviewed by a judge panel to prevent researcher bias and selective inattention" (p. 265). When critiquing a study, the reviewer examines the decision-making processes and the theoretical schema to detect threats to analytical preciseness.

Threats to Analytical Preciseness

1. The interpretive statements do not correspond with the findings (Parse et al., 1985).
2. The categories, themes, or common elements are not logical.
3. The samples are not representative of the class of joint acts referred to by the researcher (Denzin, 1989).
4. The set of categories, themes, or common elements fails to set forth a whole picture.
5. The set of categories, themes, or common elements is not inclusive of data that exist.
6. The data are inappropriately assigned to categories, themes, or common elements.
7. The inclusion and exclusion criteria for categories, themes, or common elements are not consistently followed.

8. The working hypotheses or propositions are not identified or cannot be verified by data.
9. Various sources of evidence fail to provide convergence.
10. The evidence is incongruent.
11. The subject-participants fail to validate findings when appropriate (Johnson, 1999).
12. The conclusions are not data based or do not encompass all the data.
13. The data are made to appear more patterned, regular, or congruent than they actually are (Beck, 1993; Sandelowski, 1986).

STANDARD IV: THEORETICAL CONNECTEDNESS

Theoretical connectedness requires that the theoretical schema developed from the study be clearly expressed, logically consistent, reflective of the data, and compatible with the knowledge base of nursing.

Threats to Theoretical Connectedness

1. The findings are trivialized (Goetz & LeCompte, 1981).
2. The concepts are inadequately refined.
3. The concepts are not validated by data.
4. The set of concepts lacks commonality.
5. The relationships between concepts are not clearly expressed.
6. The proposed relationships between concepts are not validated by data.
7. The working propositions are not validated by data.
8. Data are distorted during development of the theoretical schema (Bruyn, 1966).
9. The theoretical schema fails to yield a meaningful picture of the phenomenon studied.
10. A conceptual framework or map is not derived from the data.

STANDARD V: HEURISTIC RELEVANCE

To be of value, the results of a study need *heuristic relevance* for the reader. This value is reflected in the readers capacity to recognize the phenomenon described in the study, its theoretical significance, its applicability to nursing practice sit-

uations, and its influence on future research activities. The dimensions of heuristic relevance include intuitive recognition, relationship to the existing body of knowledge, and applicability.

Intuitive Recognition

Intuitive recognition means that when individuals are confronted with the theoretical schema derived from the data, it has meaning within their personal knowledge base. They immediately recognize the phenomenon being described by the researcher and its relationship to a theoretical perspective in nursing.

Threats to Intuitive Recognition

1. The reader is unable to recognize the phenomenon.
2. The description is not consistent with common meanings.
3. Theoretical connectedness is lacking.

Relationship to the Existing Body of Knowledge

The existing *body of knowledge,* particularly the nursing theoretical perspective from which the phenomenon was approached, must be reviewed by the researcher and compared with the findings of the study. The study should have intersubjectivity with existing theoretical knowledge in nursing and previous research. Reasons for differences with the existing body of knowledge should be explored by the researcher. When critiquing a study, the reviewer examines the strength of the link of study findings to the existing knowledge.

Threats to the Relationship to the Existing Body of Knowledge

1. The researcher failed to examine the existing body of knowledge.
2. The process studied was not related to nursing and health.
3. The results show a lack of correspondence with the existing knowledge base in nursing (Parse et al., 1985).

Applicability

Nurses need to be able to integrate the findings into their knowledge base and apply them to nursing practice situations. The findings also need to contribute to theory development. The reviewer examines the discussion section of the research report for threats to applicability.

Threats to Applicability

1. The findings are not significant for the discipline of nursing.
2. The report fails to achieve methodological congruence.
3. The report fails to achieve analytical preciseness.
4. The report fails to achieve theoretical connectedness.

Application of these five standards in critiquing qualitative studies determines the strengths and weaknesses of a study. A summary of the strengths will indicate adherence to the standards, and a summary of weaknesses will indicate potential threats to the integrity of the study. A final evaluation of the study involves application of the standard of heuristic relevance. This standard is used to critique the quality of the study and the usefulness of the study findings for the development and refinement of nursing knowledge and for the provision of evidence-based practice.

■ SUMMARY

An intellectual critique of research involves careful examination of all aspects of a study to judge its merits, limitations, meaning, and significance in light of previous research experience and knowledge of the topic. Intellectual critiques of studies are essential for the development and refinement of nursing knowledge and the use of research evidence in practice. In nursing, a critique is often seen as a first step in learning the research process. However, conducting a critique is not a basic skill, and the content presented in previous chapters is necessary for implementing the critique process.

Research is critiqued to improve practice, broaden understanding, and provide a base for conducting a study. Nursing students, practicing nurses, nurse educators, and nurse researchers perform research critiques. These critiques are often conducted after verbal presentations of studies, after a published research report, for abstract or article selection, and for evaluating research proposals. A critique process is described for both quantitative and qualitative research. Steps in the critique process include comprehension, comparison, analysis, evaluation, and conceptual clustering. These steps occur in sequence, vary in depth, and presume accomplishment of the preceding steps. However, a person with critique experience frequently performs several steps of this process simultaneously.

The first step, comprehension, involves understanding the terms and concepts in the report, as well as identifying study elements and grasping the nature, significance, and meaning of these elements. The next step, comparison, requires knowledge of what each step of the research process should be like. The ideal is compared with the real. The analysis step involves a critique of the logical links connecting one study element with another. The fourth step, evaluation, involves examining the meaning and significance of the study according to set criteria. During this step of the critique, the internal and external validity of the study are examined. The last step of the critique process is the clustering of present knowledge within a given area of study. Conceptual clustering is a means of generating new research questions, developing and refining theory, and synthesizing research for use in practice. Each step of the critique process is described and questions are provided to direct the critique of quantitative studies.

Critique in qualitative research requires the same steps as those of quantitative research. However, the skills and standards for critique of qualitative research are different. The skills needed to critique qualitative studies include (1) context flexibility; (2) inductive reasoning; (3) conceptualization, theoretical modeling, and theory analysis; and (4) transformation of ideas across levels of abstraction.

Standards proposed to evaluate qualitative studies include descriptive vividness, methodological congruence, analytical preciseness, theoretical connectedness, and heuristic relevance. Descriptive vividness means that the site, subjects, experience of collecting data, and the thinking of the researcher during the process are presented so clearly that the reader has the sense of personally experiencing the event. Methodological congruence has four dimensions: rigor in documentation, procedural rigor, ethical rigor, and auditability. Analytical preciseness is essential to perform a series of transformations in which concrete data are transformed across several levels of abstraction.

The outcome of the analysis is a theoretical schema that imparts meaning to the phenomenon under study. Theoretical connectedness requires that the theoretical schema developed from the study be clearly expressed, logically consistent, reflective of the data, and compatible with the knowledge base of nursing. Heuristic relevance includes intuitive recognition, a relationship to the existing body of knowledge, and applicability. These standards and the threats to these standards are presented to guide the process of critiquing qualitative studies.

REFERENCES

American Psychological Association (APA). (1994). *Publication manual of the American Psychological Association* (4th ed.). Washington, DC: Author.

Beck, C. T. (1993). Qualitative research: The evaluation of its credibility, fittingness, and auditability. *Western Journal of Nursing Research, 15*(2), 263–266.

Beck, C. T. (1994). Reliability and validity issues in phenomenological research. *Western Journal of Nursing Research, 16*(3), 254–267.

Becker, H. S. (1958). Problems of inference and proof in participant observation. *American Sociological Review, 23*(6), 652–660.

Brown, S. J. (1999). *Knowledge for health care practice: A guide to using research evidence.* Philadelphia: W.B. Saunders.

Bruyn, S. T. (1966). *The human perspective in sociology.* Englewood Cliffs, NJ: Prentice-Hall.

Burns, N. (1989). Standards for qualitative research. *Nursing Science Quarterly, 2*(1), 44–52.

Crookes, P., & Davies, S. (1998). *Essential skills for reading and applying research in nursing and health care.* Edinburgh: Baillière Tindall.

Crosby, L. J. (1990). The abstract: An important first impression. *Journal of Neuroscience Nursing, 22*(3), 192–194.

Cutcliffe, J. R., & McKenna, H. P. (1999). Establishing the credibility of qualitative research findings: The plot thickens. *Journal of Advanced Nursing, 30*(2), 374-380.

Dean, J. P., & Whyte, W. F. (1958). How do you know if the informant is telling the truth? *Human Organization, 17*(2), 34–38.

Denzin, N. K. (1989). *The research act* (3rd ed.). New York: McGraw-Hill.

Egan, E. C., Snyder, M., & Burns, K. R. (1992). Intervention studies in nursing: Is the effect due to the independent variable? *Nursing Outlook, 40*(4), 187–190.

Ganong, L. H. (1987). Integrative reviews of nursing research. *Research in Nursing & Health, 10*(1), 1–11.

Gill, H. (1996). Guidelines on conducting a critical research evaluation. *Nursing Standard, 11*(6), 40-43.

Glaser, B., & Strauss, A. L. (1965). Discovery of substantive theory: A basic strategy underlying qualitative research. *American Behavioral Scientist, 8*(1), 5–12.

Goetz, J. P., & LeCompte, M. D. (1981). Ethnographic research and the problem of data reduction. *Anthropology and Education Quarterly, 12*(1), 51–70.

Guba, E. G., & Lincoln, Y. S. (1982). *Effective evaluation.* Washington, DC: Jossey-Bass.

Johnson, R. B. (1999). Examining the validity structure of qualitative research. In F. Pyrczak (Ed.), *Evaluating research in academic journals: A practical guide to realistic evaluation* (pp 103-108). Los Angeles: Pyrczak Publishing.

Kahn, D. L. (1993). Ways of discussing validity in qualitative nursing research. *Western Journal of Nursing Research, 15*(1), 122–126.

Kim, M. J., & Felton, F. (1993). The current generation of research proposals: Reviewers' viewpoints. *Nursing Research, 42*(2), 118–119.

Kirk, J., & Miller, M. L. (1986). *Reliability and validity in qualitative research.* Beverly Hills, CA: Sage.

Knaack, P. (1984). Phenomenological research. *Western Journal of Nursing Research, 6*(1), 107–114.

Knafl, K. A., & Howard, M. J. (1984). Interpreting and reporting qualitative research. *Research in Nursing & Health, 7*(1), 17–24.

Larson, E. (1994). Exclusion of certain groups from clinical research. *Image—The Journal of Nursing Scholarship, 26*(3), 185–190.

LaValley, M. (1997). Methods article: A consumer's guide to meta-analysis. *Arthritis Care and Research, 10*(3), 208–213.

LeCompte, M. D., & Goetz, J. P. (1982). Problems of reliability and validity in ethnographic research. *Review of Educational Research, 52*(1), 31–60.

LeFort, S. M. (1993). The statistical versus clinical significance debate. *Image—The Journal of Nursing Scholarship, 25*(1), 57–62.

Liehr, P., & Houston, S. (1993). Critique and using nursing research: Guidelines for the critical care nurse. *American Journal of Critical Care, 2*(5), 407–412.

LoBiondo-Wood, G. L., & Haber, J. (1998). *Nursing research: Methods, critical appraisal, and utilization* (4th ed.). St. Louis: Mosby.

Massey, J., & Loomis, M. (1988). When should nurses use research findings? *Applied Nursing Research, 1*(1), 32–40.

Mateo, M. A., & Kirchhoff, K. T. (1999). *Using and conducting nursing research in the clinical setting* (2nd ed.). Philadelphia: W.B. Saunders.

Meleis, A. I. (1991). *Theoretical nursing: Development and progress* (2nd ed.). Philadelphia: J. B. Lippincott.

Miles, M. B., & Huberman, A. M. (1994). *Qualitative data*

analysis: A source book of new methods (2nd ed.). Beverly Hills, CA: Sage.

Morse, J. M., Dellasega, C., & Doberneck, B. (1993). Evaluating abstracts: Preparing a research conference. *Nursing Research, 42*(5), 308–310.

Munhall, P. L. (1999). Ethical considerations in qualitative research. In P. L. Munhall & C. O. Boyd (Eds.), *Nursing research: A qualitative perspective* (2nd ed.). New York: National League for Nursing.

Munhall, P. L., & Boyd, C. O. (1999). *Nursing research: A qualitative perspective* (2nd ed.). New York: National League for Nursing.

Nisbett, R., & Ross, L. (1980). *Human inference: Strategies and shortcomings of social judgment.* Englewood Cliffs, NJ: Prentice-Hall.

Oberst, M. T. (1992). Warning: Believing this report may be hazardous. . . . *Research in Nursing & Health, 15*(2), 91–92.

Omery, A., & Williams, R. P. (1999). An appraisal of research utilization across the United States. *Journal of Nursing Administration, 29*(12), 50-56.

Parse, R. R., Coyne, A. B., & Smith, M. J. (1985). *Nursing research: Qualitative methods.* Bowie, MD: Brady.

Pillemer, D. B., & Light, R. J. (1980). Synthesizing outcomes: How to use research evidence from many studies. *Harvard Educational Review, 50*(2), 176–195.

Pinch, W. J. (1995). Synthesis: Implementing a complex process. *Nurse Educator, 20*(1), 34–40.

Polit, D. F., & Hungler, B. P. (1999). *Nursing research: Principles and methods* (6th ed.). Philadelphia: J. B. Lippincott.

Pyrczak, F. (1999). *Evaluating research in academic journals: A practical guide to realistic evaluation.* Los Angeles: Pyrczak Publishing.

Ryan-Wenger, N. (1992). Guidelines for critique of a research report. *Heart & Lung, 21*(4), 394–401.

Sandelowski, M. (1986). The problem of rigor in qualitative research. *Advances in Nursing Science, 8*(3), 27–37.

Sidani, S., & Braden, C. J. (1998). *Evaluation of nursing interventions: A theory-driven approach.* Thousand Oaks, CA: Sage.

Swanson, E. A., McCloskey, J. C., & Bodensteiner, A. (1991). Publishing opportunities for nurses: A comparison of 92 U.S. journals. *Image—The Journal of Nursing Scholarship, 23*(1), 33–38.

Tibbles, L., & Sanford, R. (1994). The research journal club: A mechanism for research utilization. *Clinical Nurse Specialist, 8*(1), 23–26.

Werley, H. H., & Fitzpatrick, J. J. (1983). *Annual review of nursing research* (Vol. 1). New York: Springer.

Yam, M. (1994). Strategies for teaching nursing research: Teaching nursing students to critique research for gender bias. *Western Journal of Nursing Research, 16*(6), 724–727.

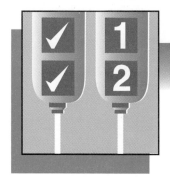

CHAPTER 27

UTILIZATION OF RESEARCH TO PROMOTE EVIDENCE-BASED NURSING PRACTICE

The generation of empirical knowledge to improve clinical practice was the major focus of researchers in the 1980s and 1990s. Since 1985, many quality clinical studies and an increasing number of replications have been conducted. In addition, dissemination of research findings has increased through presentations at conferences, communication through electronic media (radio, television, on-line journals, and a variety of websites), and publications in research and clinical journals. Thus the generation and diffusion of empirical knowledge are expanding, but greater emphasis needs to be placed on the use of research findings in practice, with the ultimate goal for nursing being evidence-based practice (EBP) (Brown, 1999; Mateo & Kirchoff, 1999; Omery & Williams, 1999).

With the current changes in the health care system, society is demanding more of nurses than ever before. Nurses now have the attention of health care policymakers and can influence the future delivery system. Meeting these policymakers' expectations will require increased scientific productivity for all nurses, including the conduct of high-quality research and the use of those findings in practice. In addition, EBP guidelines need to be developed and used by practicing nurses to produce measurable, quality patient outcomes in a variety of clinical settings (Brown, 1999; Davies et al., 1994). This chapter was developed to promote an understanding of the research utilization process and provide a back-

ground for implementing evidence-based nursing practice. Some of the problems or barriers related to knowledge utilization are identified, and theories relevant to research utilization are introduced. An example of a research utilization project is presented with Rogers' theory as the organizing framework. The chapter concludes with a presentation of strategies to facilitate the implementation of EBP in nursing.

PROBLEMS RELATED TO KNOWLEDGE UTILIZATION

Knowledge utilization is the process of disseminating and using research-generated information to make an impact on or change in the existing practices in society. The time lag between generating and using knowledge by society has been a concern for numerous years. For example, the time lag between the discovery of citrus juice as a preventive measure for scurvy and its use on British ships was 264 years. The span of time between the first conception of 10 important ideas and initial utilization of them are presented in Table 27–1 (Glaser et al., 1983). The table suggests that the average length of time between discovery and utilization is almost 20 years. Lynn (cited in Glaser et al., 1983) reports a decrease in time for utilization of discoveries made in the period between 1885 and 1965 from 30 years (1885–1919) to 9 years (1945–1965). Even today,

	TABLE 27–1		
	TIME SPAN BETWEEN IDEA AND UTILIZATION		
INNOVATION	**YEAR OF FIRST CONCEPTION**	**YEAR OF FIRST REALIZATION**	**DURATION IN YEARS**
Heart pacemaker	1928	1960	32
Input-output economic analysis	1936	1964	28
Hybrid corn	1908	1933	25
Electrophotography	1937	1959	22
Magnetic ferrites	1933	1955	22
Hybrid small grains	1937	1956	19
Green revolution: wheat	1950	1966	16
Organophosphorus insecticides	1934	1947	13
Oral contraceptive	1951	1960	9
Videotape record	1950	1956	6
Average duration			19.2

From Glaser, E. M., Abelson, H. H., & Garrison, K. N. (1983). *Putting knowledge to use* (p. 8). San Francisco: Jossey-Bass.

the gap between the discovery of research knowledge and use of that knowledge in practice can be extensive. For example, the research findings about the benefits of aspirin in protecting patients from myocardial infarction and stroke have been known since the mid-1980s, but only recently has the U. S. Food and Drug Administration approved the use of aspirin as a preventive measure in persons at risk for cardiovascular disease (Marwick, 1997). Why some findings require much longer to implement than others is not clearly understood. Historical events, attitudes toward researchers and research in general, and the necessity with some innovations to change attitudes before the findings can be accepted and used seem to influence the time required.

Problems Related to the Use of Research Findings in Nursing

Most people believe that a good idea will sell itself—the word will spread rapidly and the idea will quickly be used. Unfortunately, this is seldom true. Even today, research findings that clearly warrant utilization are not being used in nursing practice. Brett (1987) studied the extent to which 14 nursing research findings that met the Conduct and Utilization of Research in Nursing (CURN) Project's (1982) criteria for use in practice were being used by practicing nurses. A stratified sample of

216 nurses was obtained from small, medium, and large hospitals. One of the findings (innovations) examined was the following technique for giving intramuscular injections: "Internal rotation of the femur during injection into the dorsogluteal site, in either the prone or the side-lying position, results in reduced discomfort from the injection" (Brett, 1987, p. 346). Internal rotation of the femur is achieved by having patients point their toes inward. Forty-four percent of the nurses were aware of the finding, 34% were persuaded that the finding was useful for practice, 29% were implementing this finding in practice sometimes, but only 10% were implementing it always. Coyle and Sokop (1990) replicated Brett's (1987) study with a sample of 113 nurses in North Carolina. Thirty-four percent of these nurses were aware of this finding, 21% were persuaded that the finding was useful, but only 4% used the intervention sometimes and 22% used it always. These figures indicate a limited increase in the use of this innovation from 1987 to 1990.

The findings regarding positioning during an intramuscular injection would be comparatively simple to implement. The decision could be made by the nurse alone; no physician's order would be needed. Administrative personnel would not have to give approval, and no additional cost or nursing time would be involved. At the time of Brett's (1987) and Coyle and Sokop's (1990) studies, the findings on intramuscular injections (Kruszewski et al., 1979) had been available in the literature for more than 10 years. Why were more than 56% to 66% of the nurses unaware of the findings? Had the nurses not read the information in textbooks or journal articles? Was it not taught in nursing schools? Was the suggested change in nursing practice not considered important by those who did read the information? Did nurses who sometimes implemented the findings in practice not perceive a positive impact on patient care? What are the barriers that interfere with the use of research findings in practice? Nursing must address these questions to increase the utilization of research knowledge in practice.

BARRIERS TO KNOWLEDGE UTILIZATION IN NURSING

Several barriers to research utilization have been identified in the literature and seem to focus on the characteristics of nurse researchers and practicing nurses, organizations employing the practitioners, and quality of the research findings. A common barrier to research utilization is the communication gap between the university-based researcher and the institutional-based practitioner. This concern is not unique to nursing; it was a major topic of discussion at the think tanks convened by the federal government to promote utilization of research. Criticisms included the following: (1) Researcher-originated studies do not solve pressing clinical problems, (2) findings from researcher-originated studies often cannot be utilized in practice, (3) the studies conducted lack replication, (4) findings are communicated primarily to other researchers, (5) findings are not expressed in terms understood by practitioners, (6) practitioners do not value research, (7) practitioners are unaware of or unwilling to read research reports, (8) practitioners have inadequate education related to the research process, (9) practitioners do not have confidence in the research findings, and (10) practitioners do not know how to apply research findings or are not allowed to apply them (Bock, 1990; MacGuire, 1990; Omery & Williams, 1999). Every effort must be made to bridge the gap between researchers and practitioners by

enhancing the communication of research, synthesis of findings, and generation of protocols for use in practice.

Sometimes the organizations where nurses work do not support the use of research findings in practice. Organizational barriers might include lack of access to research journals and other sources of research findings, no time allocated for using research in practice, attitudes discouraging changes in practice, no funds to support research-based changes for practice, and no rewards for using research findings in practice. In addition to organizational barriers are barriers related to the research. For some areas of research, the quality of studies is inadequate to generate sound empirical evidence for practice. For example, the studies might lack replication, rigorous methodology, and clear interpretation of findings. Some studies do not provide clear recommendations for how the findings might be used in practice (Omery & Williams, 1999). More quality research is needed in nursing to generate sound empirical knowledge for practice, and organizations need to provide more resources for implementing evidence-based nursing care.

Several sources have identified the barriers to using research in practice, but the specific barriers need to be identified for different settings and situations. Funk and colleagues (1991) developed a scale to measure the barriers to research utilization. The BARRIERS Scale includes 29 items that were developed from the utilization literature, the CURN Project Research Utilization Questionnaire, and informal data gathered from nurses. The items were refined through input from research utilization consultants, nurse researchers, practicing nurses, and a psychometrician. The items on the scale cover four areas: (1) characteristics of the adopter, the nurse's research values, skills, and awareness; (2) characteristics of the organization, setting barriers and limitations; (3) characteristics of the innovation, qualities of the research; and (4) characteristics of the communication, presentation and accessibility of the research. The BARRIERS Scale provides a way to identify the research utilization problems in varied clinical settings and among groups of practicing nurses and administrators. Some of the most common barriers identified by practicing nurses included time, limited support of nursing administrators and others, and lack of knowledge of research findings (Pettengill et al., 1994). The greatest barriers to research utilization identified by administrators include nurses not aware of research findings, insufficient time, and research reports that are not understandable (Funk et al., 1995). Identifying barriers to research utilization can promote communication between researchers, practitioners, and administrators and can facilitate problem solving during the use of empirical evidence in practice.

THEORIES OF UTILIZATION

Problems related to knowledge utilization became a major concern in the 1970s when it was discovered that many of the findings from research funded by the federal government were not being used by society. A think tank of experts in the area of research utilization was convened by the government to examine reasons for the lack of utilization and to propose strategies to improve it. From the work done by this group, a field of study evolved that examines the process of utilization. With the increased focus on knowledge utilization, two prominent theories about diffusion and adoption of innovations were developed: Rogers' theory of diffusion of innovations and Havelock's theory of linker systems. These theories have provided frameworks for many of the studies in the area of utilization. In addition, Rogers' (1995) theory has provided theoretical guidance for the implementation of several funded nursing research utilization projects.

Rogers' Theory of Diffusion of Innovations

E. M. Rogers is an expert and noted theorist in the field of knowledge diffusion and utilization. For 25 years, Rogers has conducted research related to knowledge diffusion and utilization, and his theory is a synthesis of the findings from his and other scientists' research in this field. This text provides an introduction to Rogers' (1995) theory, including a definition of major concepts and description of the process for promoting diffusion of innovations or new knowledge into society.

KNOWLEDGE DIFFUSION

According to Rogers (1995), diffusion is the process by which an innovation or new idea is communicated through certain channels over time among the members of a social system. The word *dissemination* is considered synonymous with diffusion. The main elements of diffusion include (1) an innovation, (2) communication channels, (3) time, and (4) a social system. He defines an *innovation* as an idea, practice, or object that is perceived as new by an individual, group, or other unit of adoption. The idea might not necessarily be new, but it must be perceived as new by those considering adoption.

Communication channels may include one-to-one communication; one individual communicating to several others; or mass media such as books, journals, newspapers, television, and the Internet. Mass media are effective for achieving diffusion; however, interpersonal channels involving face-to-face exchange have been found to be more effective in facilitating adoption of an innovation. Communication is most effective when the two interacting individuals are similar in characteristics such as beliefs, values, education, social status, and profession. Rogers (1995) refers to these individuals as near-peers.

Time is another important element of the diffusion-adoption process. The three time-related elements of interest are (1) the time span from the point at which an individual first hears about an innovation to the point at which a decision is made to accept or reject the innovation, (2) the innovativeness of the individual or agency that determines the time needed to achieve adoption, and (3) the number of individuals within a social system who adopt an innovation within a given period.

Rogers (1995) defines a *social system* as a set of interrelated units that is engaged in problem solving to accomplish a common goal. Diffusion occurs within a social system, and the social structure of the system affects diffusion of the innovation. A social system has both formal and informal structure, with formal structure being related to authority and power. The informal structure is related to who interacts with whom under what circumstances. Every social system has *opinion leaders* who are in favor of innovations and those who oppose change. Opinion leaders are at the center of the system's interpersonal communication networks and tend to reflect the norms of the system. In seeking adoption of an innovation within a social system, one must identify the opinion leaders and seek their acceptance. Advanced practice nurses (nurse practitioners, clinical nurse specialists, nurse anesthetists, and nurse midwives) are often viewed as opinion leaders because of their clinical expertise, expanded education, and knowledge of research.

INNOVATION-DECISION PROCESS

Rogers (1995) conceptualizes that the diffusion of knowledge is best achieved by an *innovation-decision process* that consists of five stages: (1) knowledge, (2) persuasion, (3) decision, (4) implementation, and (5) confirmation (Fig. 27–1). The *knowledge stage* is the first awareness of the existence of the innovation, and the *persuasion stage* occurs when the individual forms an attitude toward

the innovation. A *decision stage* occurs when the individual chooses to adopt or reject the innovation. The *implementation stage* is when the individual uses the innovation, and the *confirmation stage* occurs when the individual evaluates the effectiveness of the innovation and decides to either continue or discontinue use of it.

Knowledge Stage

Knowledge of an innovation in nursing can be achieved by formal communication through media such as television, newspapers, computer networks, publications, or seminars. In addition, informal communication within an agency from one nurse to another can be effective in increasing awareness of an innovation. Certain prior conditions influence the knowledge stage, such as previous practice, perceived needs/problems, innovativeness, and norms of the social system. Dissatisfaction with previous practice can lead to recognizing the needs or problems that require change. A need might create a search for an innovation to improve practice, but knowledge of a new innovation might also create a need for change. For example, knowledge of a new

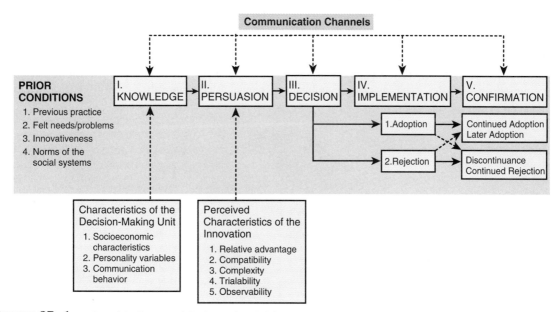

FIGURE 27–1 ■ A model of stages of the innovation-decision process. (From Rogers EM. [1983]. *Diffusion of innovations* [3rd ed.]. The Free Press.)

treatment for pressure sores might create a need to change the existing treatment policy.

Innovativeness is the degree and quickness with which an individual or other unit of adoption embraces new ideas (Rogers, 1995). Rogers uses five categories to describe adopters according to their degree of innovativeness: (1) innovators, (2) early adopters, (3) early majority, (4) late majority, and (5) laggards. *Innovators* are active information seekers of new ideas. They have a high level of mass media exposure and interpersonal networks that are widely extended and reach beyond their local social system. From these sources they receive early information about innovations. Innovators usually function outside the existing social structures and tend to have cosmopolitan relationships. They are the change agents that an agency might hire to implement an innovation. Their social support system is diverse and not tightly linked. Innovators can cope with higher levels of uncertainty related to an innovation than can other adopters and are the first to adopt a new idea. They do not rely on subjective evaluations of the innovation by other system members. Because innovators are less closely linked with the local social system, they have less influence on adoption of an innovation within the system than do early adopters.

Early adopters tend to be opinion leaders in existing social systems. They learn about new ideas rapidly, utilize them, and then serve as role models in their use. In the hospital, early adopters might be nurses in advanced roles such as administrators, acute care nurse practitioners, clinical nurse specialists, and in-service educators. The *early majority* are rarely leaders, but they are active followers and will readily follow in the use of a new idea. The *late majority* are skeptical about new ideas and will adopt them only if group pressure is great. *Laggards* are security oriented, tend to cling to the past, and are often isolates without a strong support system. By the time they adopt a new idea, it is considered by most to be an old idea.

Research has shown that the adopter distribution over time approaches a bell-shaped curve (Fig. 27–2). Innovators (2.5%) and early adopters (13.5%) are comparable in number to the laggards (16%). This distribution can assist agencies in realistically identifying the number of individuals who will and who will not support a change. The early adopters and early majority can form a powerful group to promote change of the late majority. All groups (innovators, early adopters, and early and late majority) can apply pressure to persuade the laggards to change, but many of the laggards will continue to resist change and some might leave the agency.

Norms, the expected behavior patterns within a social system, affect the diffusion of innovations. Norms can serve as barriers to change or can facilitate change. When the norms of the social system are oriented toward change, the opinion leaders tend to be innovative (early adopters), and change is facilitated. When the norms are opposed to change, so are the opinion leaders, thus creating barriers to change. When innovations are diffused and adopted

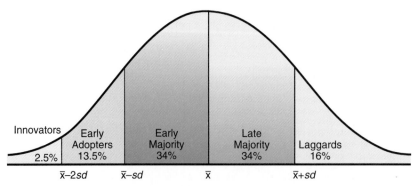

FIGURE 27–2 ▪ Adopter categorization on the basis of innovativeness. (From Rogers EM. [1983]. *Diffusion of innovations* [3rd ed.] The Free Press.)

or rejected within a social system, social change occurs and affects the norms of the system.

During the knowledge stage, the characteristics of the individual, administration, or institution that is considering the adoption of an innovation need to be examined (see Fig. 27–1). Characteristics requiring examination include socioeconomic elements, personality variables, and communication behavior of the decision-making unit. Socioeconomic characteristics include social status, interactional patterns, and economic level of those involved in adopting an innovation. Examination of personality variables will indicate individuals' innovativeness (early adopter or laggard) and whether they will facilitate or obstruct change. Communication behavior, whether it is open and honest or closed and subversive, has a strong impact on the diffusion process.

Persuasion Stage

During the persuasion stage, an individual or other decision-making unit develops a favorable or unfavorable attitude toward the change or innovation (Rogers, 1995). Characteristics of an innovation that determine the probability and speed of adoption include (1) relative advantage, (2) compatibility, (3) complexity, (4) trialability, and (5) observability (see Fig. 27–1). *Relative advantage* is the extent to which the innovation is perceived to be better than current practice. *Compatibility* is the degree to which the innovation is perceived to be consistent with current values, past experience, and priority of needs. *Complexity* is the degree to which the innovation is perceived to be difficult to understand or use. If the innovation requires the development of new skills, complexity increases. *Trialability* is the extent to which an individual or agency can try out the idea on a limited basis with the option of returning to previous practices. *Observability* is the extent to which the results of an innovation are visible to others. A highly visible innovation with beneficial results is usually rapidly diffused. In conclusion, innovations that have great relative advantage, are compatible, have trialability, are not complex, and are observable will be adopted more quickly than will innovations that do not meet these criteria.

Effective communication can occur through mass media at the knowledge stage because the individual seeks information to reduce uncertainty. However, at the persuasion stage and throughout the rest of the innovation-decision process, mass media are less effective than informal communication. Rather than information, the individual seeks evaluative statements related to the innovation. Have you used it? How do you feel about it? What are the consequences of using it? What are the advantages and disadvantages of using it in my situation? Would you advise me to use it? Will I still be approved of and accepted if I use it? Interpersonal networks with near-peers are much more likely to influence individuals during the persuasion and subsequent stages.

Decision Stage

At the decision stage, the individual either adopts or rejects the innovation (see Fig. 27–1). *Adoption* involves full acceptance of the innovation and implementation of the ideas in practice. Adoption can be continued infinitely or can be discontinued after evaluation of the innovation's effectiveness in the social system. *Rejection* is a decision not to use an innovation and can be active or passive. *Active rejection* indicates that the innovation was examined and a decision was made not to adopt it. With *passive rejection,* the innovation was never seriously considered. Over time, the social system might continue with the decision to reject or might initiate adoption later.

Implementation Stage

In the implementation stage, the innovation is put to use by an individual (or other decision-making unit). A detailed plan of implementation that addresses the risks and benefits of the innovation will facilitate diffusion. The three types of implementation are (1) direct application, (2) reinvention, and (3) indirect effects.

Direct application occurs when an innovation is used exactly as it was developed. In fact, some scientists would not consider the innovation to have been adopted unless its original form has been kept intact. For example, if a study demonstrated that a particular intervention, conducted in specifically defined steps, was effective in achieving an outcome, adoption would require that the nurse perform the steps of the intervention in exactly the same way in which they were described in the study. This expectation reflects the narrow, precise definition of an innovation that is necessary to the scientific endeavor. However, this preciseness is not compatible with typical practice behavior, and research has indicated that maintenance of the original innovation does not always occur.

With *reinvention,* adopters modify the innovation to meet their own needs. In this strategy, the steps of a procedure might be changed, or some of the steps might be combined with care activities emerging from previous experience. To some researchers, adding, deleting, altering, or rearranging steps in a procedure means that it is no longer the same innovation. Thus adoption has not occurred. However, from the practitioner's viewpoint, the innovation has been adopted.

The expectation is that the new knowledge will directly modify the actions of the individual, either in the original suggested way or as a reinvention. However, individuals usually incorporate the knowledge and use it in diffuse ways. Thus the implementation of knowledge can be indirect. For example, practitioners and researchers might discuss the findings, cite them in clinical papers and textbooks, and use them to provide strength to arguments. Thus the knowledge would be incorporated into the individual's thinking and combined with past experience, previous education, and current values. In this instance, determining that the innovation was being utilized would be more difficult, and therefore the use of certain nursing research findings may be underestimated.

Weiss (1980), another theorist in the field of knowledge utilization, suggests considering utilization as a continuum. One extreme of the continuum is that findings have a direct effect on decisions and activities, and the other extreme is that findings have a diffuse or indirect effect. This indirect effect involves awareness, insight, or cumulative understanding that may lead to subtle, gradual changes in behavior. The middle of the continuum reflects a modified impact in which the findings are combined with other types of information for problem solving and decision making.

Confirmation Stage

During the confirmation stage, the individual evaluates the effectiveness of the innovation and decides either to continue or to discontinue it. If an innovation is evaluated positively by those involved, the decision might be to continue the innovation and expand its use throughout an agency or a corporation. *Discontinuance* can consist of at least two types: (1) replacement and (2) disenchantment. With *replacement discontinuance,* the innovation is rejected to adopt a better idea. Thus innovations can occur in waves as new ideas replace outdated, impractical innovations. The computer is an excellent example in that users can constantly upgrade their systems with new, more powerful interactive innovations in hardware and software. *Disenchantment discontinuance* occurs when an idea is rejected because the user is dissatisfied with its outcome.

Rogers's (1995) theory has been used to facilitate the use of research findings in nursing practice. His innovation-decision process has provided the framework for implementation of some major research utilization projects discussed later in this chapter. The innovation-decision process could be very helpful in assisting individual nurses or groups of nurses within an agency to implement research findings to directly influence practice or to merge findings with other knowledge to affect nursing care indirectly.

Havelock's Linker Systems

Havelock (1970, 1974) added a new dimension to the current knowledge of utilization theory by proposing the development of a linker system. This linker system is used to transfer new knowledge, skills, or products (innovations) from resource systems (researchers and their publications) to user systems (practitioners) for utilization. Havelock's model (Fig. 27–3) illustrates the link of the user-client system to the resources and the interaction with a change agent (outside process consultant) (Havelock & Havelock, 1973). The change process is depicted as a six-step process in the linker system: (1) need felt, (2) problem diagnosis, (3) search for resources, (4) retrieval of ideas and information, (5) fabrication of a solution, and (6) application.

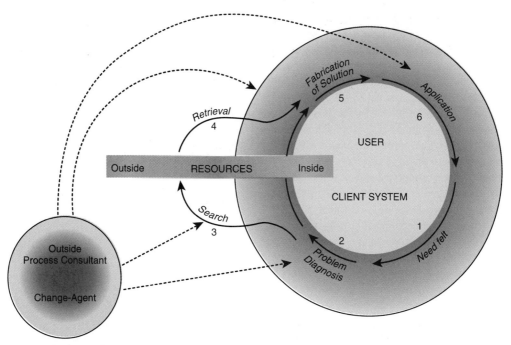

FIGURE 27–3 ■ The problem-solver view of the change process. (From Havelock, R. G., & Havelock, M. C. [1973]. *Training for change agents: A guide to the design of training programs in education and other fields.* Ann Arbor, MI: Litho Crafters, p 9.)

CHANGE PROCESS USING THE LINKER SYSTEM

Step 1 is the identification of a need by a client, who might be an individual, organization, or institution. The need is then translated into a diagnosis in step 2. The diagnosis represents a set of problems to be solved and should be based on values of the user-client system. At this point, the change agent shares diagnostic skills with the client system and facilitates the diagnostic process. Step 3 is the initiation of a link to resources outside the agency (including research publications and researchers' ideas) and inside the agency (administration, personnel, and financial support). Change is frequently more effective when initiated from inside rather than outside a client system. In step 4, which completes the link with the resource system, ideas and information are retrieved to solve the identified problem or problems. Step 5 is fabrication of a solution that involves selecting or formulating an innovation. The change agent assists in evaluation of the information and determination of the knowledge that is ready for use in practice. Step 6 is application of

the innovation, which includes adapting the innovation as needed, implementing it, and evaluating its effectiveness.

The change agent clearly identifies the desired outcome, and actions are selected to achieve this outcome. Persons or groups that will facilitate or resist change are identified. Careful plans are made to strengthen and promote factors facilitating the change. Strategies are designed to counter factors resisting the change. When the change has been adopted by most of the members, the agent leaves the system. Unfortunately, in some cases when the change agent is withdrawn, use of the innovation gradually declines. As indicated in Figure 27–3, the change process is continuous and consists of identification of additional problems, search and retrieval of information from resources, formulation of additional innovations, and application of innovations by the user.

LINKER

Havelock (1970, 1973) also suggests the establishment of a *linker,* an individual who could serve as a connection between the user system and the resource system. The linker would have extensive knowledge of research findings and strategies for implementing them and could serve as an advisor to the user system in implementing new ideas. The linker could package the innovation in a form that would increase its acceptability to the user system and thus increase utilization. The idea of packaging comes from the research and development programs of the technology in which researchers make a discovery; then another group (the linker system) takes the new idea and develops practical ways to use it (Havelock & Lingwood, 1973). The linker can also be involved in the transmission of user needs to the resource systems, thus increasing the probability of new studies addressing practitioner concerns.

The idea of using a linker and packaging innovations for practice is evident in the clinical practice guidelines that were developed by U.S. Department of Health and Human Services (DHHS). The Agency for Healthcare Research and Quality (AHRQ) within the DHHS has facilitated the organization of panels of expert clinicians (linkers) to summarize the research in selected areas and develop protocols for use in practice. These practice guidelines (packaged innovations) are available in formats that are suitable for health care practitioners, the scientific community, educators, and consumers. More details on these guidelines are presented later in this chapter.

RESEARCH UTILIZATION PROJECTS AND MODELS FOR NURSING

Since the 1970s, nursing has focused on defining and implementing the research utilization process to improve nursing care. *Research utilization in nursing* is a multiple-step process that involves (1) critique and synthesis of research findings in a selected area, (2) application of these findings to make a change in practice, and (3) measurement of the outcomes from the change in practice. Several research utilization projects based on the theories of Rogers and Havelock have been implemented in nursing. In 1976, Stetler and Marram developed a model to guide the utilization of research findings in nursing practice, and this model was later refined by Stetler.

Two major projects that were undertaken to promote the adoption of innovations in nursing included (1) the Western Interstate Commission for Higher Education (WICHE) Regional Nursing Research Development Project and (2) the CURN Project. In these projects, nurse researchers, with the assistance of federal funding, designed and implemented strategies for using research in practice. The works of Rogers (1995) and Havelock (1970) were used as the frameworks for these projects. Two models have also been developed by nurses to promote the utilization of research findings in practice, the WICHE project model and the Stetler (1994) Model for Research Utilization. These research utilization projects and models are presented in this section.

WICHE

The WICHE project, initiated in the mid-1970s, was the first major nursing project to address research utilization in nursing. The 6-year project was directed by Krueger and colleagues (Krueger, 1978; Krueger et al., 1978) and was funded by the Division of Nursing. The initial goal of the project was to increase nursing research activities within the western region of the United States.

The WICHE project involved development of the first model for the utilization of nursing research, the Five-Phase Resources Linkage Model (Fig. 27–4). This model was based on Havelock's linker system theory and focused on linking nursing resources with the users of research findings in practice. Phase 1 involved using resources, as outlined in Figure 27–4, to recruit members for the project and to prepare research-based materials. Phase 2 consisted of a workshop where participants were organized into dyads composed of a nurse educator and clinician. The objective of the workshop was to help participants develop skills in critiquing research and applying utilization theory. Each dyad selected a research-based intervention that they were willing to implement within an institution. The dyad was to function as a change agent in phase 3, when the utilization projects were implemented in the participants' agencies for 5 months. Phase 4 was a second workshop for reports, analysis, and evaluation of the project, and phase 5 was the follow-up

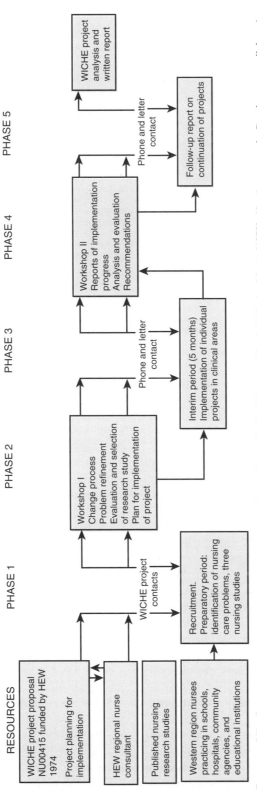

FIGURE 27–4 ■ The five-phase resources linkage model. (From Kruger, J. C., Nelson, A. H., & Wolanin, M. A. [1978]. *Nursing research: Development, collaboration, and utilization.* Aspen Pulishers.)

report on continuation of the utilization projects 3 and 6 months later.

The project staff and participants had difficulty identifying clinical studies with findings appropriate to implement in practice. Findings that were identified tended to be merged with other activities by the dyad and then implemented as a package. Because the project staff expected the findings to be implemented in pure form, this strategy was viewed with disfavor. Three reports from this project were published: (1) Axford and Cutchen (1977) developed a preoperative teaching program, (2) Dracup and Breu (1978) devised a care plan for grieving spouses and tested its effectiveness, and (3) Wichita (1977) developed a program to treat and prevent constipation in nursing home residents by increasing the fiber in their diets.

CURN

The CURN Project, directed by Horsley (Horsley et al., 1978, 1983), was awarded to the Michigan Nurses Association by the Division of Nursing. The 5-year (1975–1980) project was developed to increase the utilization of research findings by (1) disseminating findings, (2) facilitating organizational modifications necessary for implementation, and (3) encouraging collaborative research that was directly transferable to clinical practice. The theoretical base for this project included Rogers's theory of diffusion of innovations. Research utilization was seen as an organizational process rather than as a process to be implemented by an individual practitioner. Activities of the utilization process include (1) identification and synthesis of multiple research studies in a common conceptual area (research base), (2) transformation of the knowledge derived from a research base into a solution or clinical protocol, (3) transformation of the clinical protocol into specific nursing actions (innovations) that are administered to patients, and (4) clinical evaluation of the new practice to ascertain whether it produced the predicted result (Horsley et al., 1983, p. 2).

During this project, published clinical studies were critiqued for scientific merit, replication, and relevance to practice. The relevance of the research to practice involved examining (1) clinical merit or

significance in addressing patient problems, (2) the extent to which clinical control belonged to nursing, (3) the feasibility of implementing a change in an agency, and (4) an analysis of the cost-benefit ratio. The following 10 areas were considered to have research of sufficient quality to warrant implementation: (1) structured preoperative teaching, (2) reducing diarrhea in tube-fed patients, (3) preoperative sensory preparation to promote recovery, (4) prevention of decubitus ulcers, (5) intravenous cannula change, (6) closed urinary drainage systems, (7) distress reduction through sensory preparation, (8) mutual goal setting in patient care, (9) clean intermittent catheterization, and (10) pain: deliberative nursing interventions (CURN Project, 1981, 1982).

PROTOCOL DEVELOPMENT AND IMPLEMENTATION

The CURN Project involved the development of protocols from research findings to implement and evaluate a change in practice (Horsley et al., 1983). Each protocol contained the following content: (1) identification of the practice problem and the need for change; (2) summary of the research base, including limitations of the research; (3) design of the nursing practice innovation or intervention; (4) description of the research-based principle to guide the innovation; (5) description of the implementation of the innovation, or the clinical trial; (6) evaluation of the effects of the innovation, including evaluation procedures and recording forms; and (7) summary and references. The protocols were implemented in clinical trials and evaluated for effectiveness. Based on the evaluations, a decision was made to reject, modify, or adopt the intervention (innovation). Strategies could then be developed to extend the innovation to other appropriate nursing practice settings (Horsley et al., 1983).

The CURN Project was implemented on a test unit within a hospital, and baseline data and comparison groups were used to evaluate outcomes from the implementation. Follow-up questionnaires were sent to the 17 participating hospitals for a 4-year period to determine the long-term impact of the implementation on the organization. Pelz and Horsley (1981) reported that before the project, research utilization was low in both the comparison and experimental groups. One year after the intervention, significant differences were found, with experimental organizations having higher levels of utilization. The second year after the intervention, differences were still noted between the groups, but they were not significant for all 10 utilization activities. In the third year, experimental units continued to perform the protocols, but the rate of diffusion of the innovations to other units was not reported. The clinical protocols developed during the project were published to encourage nurses in other health care agencies to use these evidence-based interventions in their practice (CURN Project, 1981, 1982). Today, the CURN Project provides a valuable strategy for teaching baccalaureate students, master's students, and practicing nurses about using research findings in practice.

Stetler Model of Research Utilization

An initial model for research utilization in nursing was developed by Stetler and Marram in 1976 and expanded by Stetler in 1994. The Stetler Model for Research Utilization (Fig. 27–5) provides a comprehensive framework to enhance the use of research findings by nurses. The use of research findings can be at the institutional or individual level. At the institutional level, study findings are synthesized and the knowledge generated is used to develop or refine policy, procedures, protocols, or other formal programs implemented in the institution. Individual nurses, such as practitioners, educators, and policymakers, summarize research and use the knowledge to influence educational programs, make practice decisions, and have an impact on political decision making. The Stetler Model of Research Utilization is included in this text to promote the use of research findings by individuals and institutions. The phases of the Stetler model are presented in the following sections: (1) preparation, (2) validation, (3) comparative evaluation, (4) decision making, (5) translation/application, and (6) evaluation.

PHASE I: PREPARATION

The intent of Stetler's (1994) model is to make using research findings in practice a conscious, critical thinking process that is initiated by the user. Thus the first phase involves determination of the purpose and focus of the research review. The research literature might be reviewed to solve a difficult clinical, managerial, or educational problem; to provide the basis for a policy, standard, or protocol; or to prepare for an in-service program or other type of professional presentation. Sometimes the literature is reviewed just so that the nurse is kept current with the new content in a specialty area.

PHASE II: VALIDATION

In the validation phase, the research reports are critiqued to determine their scientific soundness. If the studies are limited in number or are weak, or both, the findings and conclusions are considered inadequate and the utilization process stops. If the research knowledge base is strong in the selected area, a decision must be made regarding whether the findings are applicable or useful for the institution or individual conducting the utilization project. Thus the purpose of the utilization project is examined in light of the research findings, and a decision is made either to proceed or not to proceed to phase III.

PHASE III: COMPARATIVE EVALUATION

Comparative evaluation includes four parts: substantiating evidence, fit of setting, feasibility, and current practice. Substantiating evidence is produced by replication, in which consistent, credible findings are obtained from studies in similar settings. In addition, substantial knowledge for change can be obtained from clinical articles, textbooks, theories, and standards and guidelines from professional organizations (Stetler, 1994). To determine the fit of the setting, the characteristics of the setting are examined to determine the forces that will facilitate or inhibit implementation of the research findings. The feasibility of using research findings in practice involves examining the three Rs related to making

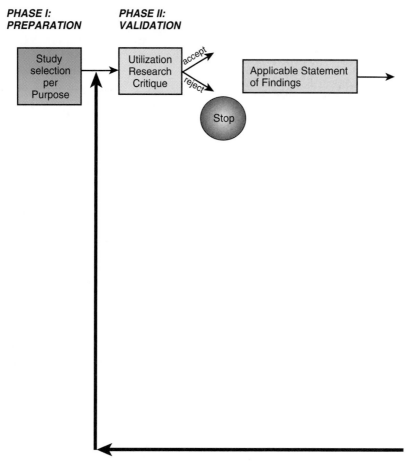

FIGURE 27–5 ▪ Stetler Model for Research Utilization. (From Stetler, C. B. [1994]. Refinement of the Stetler/Marram Model for application of research findings to practice. *Nursing Outlook 42*[1], 18–19.)

changes in practice: (1) potential risks, (2) resources needed, and (3) readiness of those involved. The final comparison involves determining whether the research information provides credible, empirical evidence for making changes in the current practice. Thus, research knowledge needs to promote increased quality in current practice by solving practice problems and improving patient outcomes. By conducting phase III, the overall benefits and risks of using the research base in a practice setting can be assessed. If the benefits are much greater than the risks for the organization or the individual nurse, or both, using the research findings to change practice is feasible.

PHASE IV: DECISION MAKING

Four types of decisions are possible during this phase: (1) to use the findings, (2) to consider using the findings, (3) to delay using the findings, and (4) to reject or not use the findings. Use of the research findings can be cognitive, instrumental, or symbolic (see Fig. 27–5). With cognitive application, the research base is a means of modifying a way of thinking or one's appreciation of an issue (Stetler, 1994). Thus, cognitive application may improve the nurse's understanding of a situation, allow analysis of practice dynamics, or improve problem-solving skills for clinical problems. Instrument

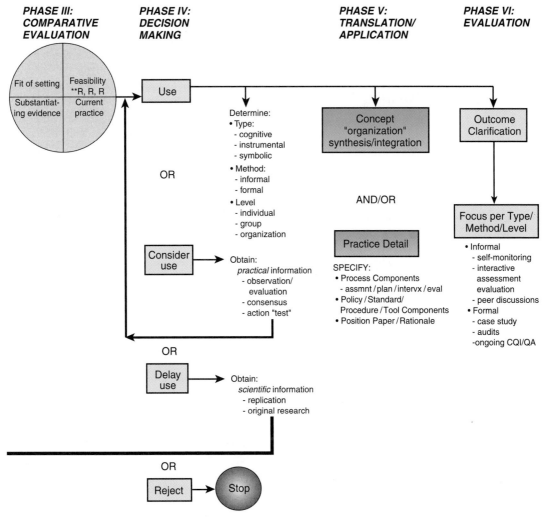

PHASE III:
COMPARATIVE
EVALUATION

PHASE IV:
DECISION
MAKING

PHASE V:
TRANSLATION/
APPLICATION

PHASE VI:
EVALUATION

Fit of setting | Feasibility **R, R, R

Substantiating evidence | Current practice

Use

OR

Determine:
• Type:
  - cognitive
  - instrumental
  - symbolic
• Method:
  - informal
  - formal
• Level
  - individual
  - group
  - organization

Concept
"organization"
synthesis/integration

AND/OR

Practice Detail

SPECIFY:
• Process Components
  - assmnt / plan / intervx / eval
• Policy / Standard/
  Procedure / Tool Components
• Position Paper / Rationale

Outcome
Clarification

Focus per Type/
Method/Level

• Informal
  - self-monitoring
  - interactive
    assessment
    evaluation
  - peer discussions
• Formal
  - case study
  - audits
  -ongoing CQI/QA

Consider use

Obtain:
practical information
  - observation/
    evaluation
  - consensus
  - action "test"

OR

Delay use

Obtain:
scientific information
  - replication
  - original research

OR

Reject   Stop

FIGURE 27–5 ▪ *Continued*

application involves using study findings to support the need for change in nursing interventions or practice protocols. For example, findings from research on the use of self-regulatory interventions to decrease blood pressure might be implemented to change the care provided to hypertensive patients (Massey & Loomis, 1988). Patients could be taught self-regulatory interventions such as progressive muscle relaxation, biofeedback, or transcendental meditation and then monitored for changes in their blood pressure. Symbolic or political utilization oc-

curs when information is used to support or change a current policy.

Another decision might be to consider use of the available findings in practice. When a change is complex and involves multiple disciplines, additional time is often needed to determine how the findings might be used and what measures will be taken to coordinate the involvement of different health professionals in the change. The use of findings can also be delayed until additional research is conducted or until agency personnel are ready to make changes in practice. A final option might be to reject or not use the findings in practice because the findings are not strong or the risks or costs of change in current practice are too high.

PHASE V: TRANSLATION/APPLICATION

The translation/application phase involves planning for and actual implementation of the findings in practice. The translation phase involves determining exactly what knowledge will be used and how that knowledge will be applied to practice. The application phase includes the following steps for planned change: (1) assess the situation to be changed, (2) develop a plan for change, and (3) implement the plan. During the application phase, the protocols, policies, or procedures developed with research knowledge are implemented in practice (Stetler, 1994).

PHASE VI: EVALUATION

The final stage in the research utilization process is to evaluate the impact of the research-based change on the health care agency, personnel, and patients. The evaluation process can include both formal and informal activities that are conducted by administrators, nurse clinicians, and other health professionals. Informal evaluations might include self-monitoring or discussions with patients, families, peers, and other professionals. Formal evaluations can include case studies, audits, or quality assurance projects (Stetler, 1994).

Because utilization is an essential component of professional nursing practice, nurses need to seek the outcomes of current research, evaluate the research for use in practice, and modify practice according to the results of this research. Utilization of research findings in practice needs to be continuous and considered the norm in an institution. Professional nurses could be viewed as knowledge oriented rather than rule oriented and could function as critical thinkers who use research to provide evidence-based care. The Stetler Model for Research Utilization can provide direction to practicing nurses and organizations to make the essential changes in practice based on research.

PROMOTING RESEARCH UTILIZATION IN NURSING

An examination of barriers to knowledge utilization and utilization theory provides a basis for encouraging you to summarize research and use the knowledge to change your practice. To assist you in conducting your first research utilization project, some strategies to facilitate research utilization are identified and an example research utilization project is presented that uses the steps in Rogers's (1995) Innovation-Decision Model.

Strategies to Facilitate Research Utilization

The lack of diffusion of research knowledge in nursing is a multifaceted problem that has many possible solutions. Educators, researchers, practitioners, and administrators need to collaborate in the application of a variety of strategies in order to increase the use of research knowledge to make essential changes in practice. Currently, many theses and dissertations are not being published, and educators could provide more assistance to new graduates in publishing their works. The graduate receives first-author credit, and the chair of the thesis or dissertation committee receives second-author credit. Educators might also encourage students to conduct a research utilization project that includes synthesis of research in an area of interest, development of a protocol for use of the findings in practice, measurement of the impact of the protocol on patient outcomes, and publication of the project. Doctorate students might be encouraged to conduct meta-analyses to synthesize research in selected areas to promote the development of evidence-based guidelines for practice.

Additional effort is needed to promote the dissemination of research findings to practicing nurses. Communication between researchers and practitioners has increased with the development of research journals for clinicians, such as *Applied Nursing Research* in 1988 and *Clinical Nursing Research* in 1992. The studies in these journals are presented in a format to promote the interest and understanding of practitioners. Some articles focus on summarizing research findings for use in practice. For example, Beyea and Nicoll (1995) conducted an integrative review of the literature and developed a research-based protocol for the administration of medications via the intramuscular route. This protocol is included in Appendix 27–A at the end of this chapter.

Many nurses lack the confidence to synthesize research findings for use in practice. They would benefit from interacting with nurses who have expert skills in conducting research critiques, integrative reviews, meta-analyses, and research utilization projects. These researchers might serve as role models in an agency to form networks of nurses to implement changes in practice based on research evidence (Omery & Williams, 1999). For example, practicing nurses might use research as a basis for evaluating products for purchase in an agency. Janken and associates (1992) used research in evaluating a new product, a closed-system catheter for endotracheal suctioning of mechanically ventilated patients, for possible purchase. Practicing nurses could also evaluate and revise agency procedure manuals, standards of care, and nursing care plans so that they are reflective of current research. In the future, accrediting agencies for health care institutions will require that nursing care measures be research or evidence based. Many progressive nursing executives realize the importance of research and are hiring nurse researchers to increase the use of research findings in practice and to promote the conduct of relevant studies. Another helpful strategy is the publication of papers by clinicians reporting effective clinical use of research findings.

Administrators can facilitate the use of research in agencies by showing support for and rewarding activities to base nursing care on research. Champion and Leach (1989) studied three variables related to research utilization in nursing: (1) availability of research findings, (2) attitude toward use of the findings in practice, and (3) perceived support for using the findings. Attitude ($r = .55$) and availability ($r = .52$) were strongly correlated with research utilization. In addition, key administrative persons such as the unit director ($r = .35$, $p = .004$), chairperson ($r = .32$, $p = .02$), and director of nursing ($r = .44$, $p = .001$) can significantly influence research utilization.

Agencies can also expand research utilization by incorporating it into their strategic plan. Mullem and coworkers (1999) conducted a study to assess nurses' knowledge, attitudes, and implementation of research activities in agencies providing strategic support for research utilization. The authors found that providing an environment that supports research utilization and educating nurses about research findings and the utilization process increase their accountability in using nursing research in their daily practice.

Example Research Utilization Project

Preparing to conduct a utilization project usually raises some important questions. Which research findings are ready for use in clinical practice? How can you use these findings to improve your practice? What are the most effective strategies for implementing findings in your practice? What are the outcomes from using the research findings in your practice? We suggest that effective strategies for using research findings will require a multifaceted approach that takes into consideration the research findings, practicing nurses, and the organizations where they practice. In this section, an example of research utilization is presented that uses Rogers's (1995) five-stage process: (1) knowledge, (2) persuasion, (3) decision, (4) implementation, and (5) confirmation (see Fig. 27–1). Research knowledge about the effects of heparin flush versus saline flush for irrigating peripheral heparin locks is evaluated for use in nursing practice. This knowledge is used to develop an evidence-based protocol example for making a change in practice, and outcome measures are identified for determining the impact of the practice change.

KNOWLEDGE

The body of nursing research must be evaluated for scientific merit and clinical relevance, and then the current findings need to be integrated in preparation for use in practice (Massey & Loomis, 1988; Mateo & Kirchhoff, 1999; Stetler et al., 1998b; Tanner & Lindeman, 1989). The integration of findings from scientifically sound research is referred to as *cognitive clustering.*

Evaluation for Scientific Merit

The scientific merit of nursing studies is determined by critiquing criteria such as (1) conceptualization and internal consistency, or the logical links of a study; (2) methodological rigor, or the strength of the design, sample, instruments, and data collection and analysis processes; (3) generalizability of the findings, or the representativeness of the sample and setting; and (4) the number of replications of the study (Tanner & Lindeman, 1989). The critique steps in Chapter 26 can be used to evaluate the scientific merit of quantitative and qualitative research.

Evaluation of Clinical Relevance

The nature and scope of research utilization are evaluated by determining clinical relevance. Research-based knowledge might be used to solve practice problems, enhance clinical judgment, or measure phenomena in clinical practice. The scope of utilization might be a single patient care unit, a hospital, or all hospitals in a corporation. A cost-benefit analysis is needed to determine the impact of the proposed change on the clinical setting. A practitioner desiring to implement an innovation must be able to assure the agency that the cost in time, energy, and money and any real or potential risks are outweighed by the benefits of the innovation (Tanner & Lindeman, 1989).

Cognitive Clustering

The research on a topic needs to be examined and clustered to determine what is currently known. These activities of cognitive clustering are accomplished through integrative reviews and meta-analyses of nursing research (Stetler, Morsi, et al., 1998b). The importance of cognitive clustering is evident by the increasing number of integrative reviews of nursing research that are being published. Ganong (1987) proposed that "integrative reviews should be held to the same standards of clarity, rigor, and replication as primary research" (p. 1). He compared 17 reviews from nursing journals and proposed the following steps for the review process: "(1) Formulate the purpose of the review and de-

velop related questions to be answered by the review or hypotheses to be tested, (2) establish tentative criteria for inclusion of studies in the review such that as data are gathered criteria may be changed on substantive or methodological grounds, (3) conduct a literature search making sampling decisions if the number of studies located is large, (4) develop a questionnaire with which to gather data from studies, (5) identify rules of inference to be used in data analyses and interpretation, (6) revise criteria for inclusion in the questionnaire as needed, (7) read the studies using the questionnaire to gather data, (8) analyze data in a systematic fashion, (9) discuss and interpret data, and (10) report the review as clearly and completely as possible" (pp. 10–11).

Pillemer and Light (1980) suggest that nursing must go beyond critique and integration of research findings to conducting meta-analyses on the outcomes of similar studies. *Meta-analysis* statistically pools the results from previous studies into a single quantitative analysis that provides the highest level of evidence for treatment efficacy (LaValley, 1997). This approach allows the application of scientific criteria to factors such as sample size, level of significance, and variables examined. Through the use of meta-analysis, the following can be generated:

1. the determination of the overall significance of probability of pooled data from confirmed studies;
2. the average of the effect size indicating the degree to which the null hypothesis is false, or the degree to which the phenomenon is present in the population; and
3. the relationship between variables (Hunt, 1987, pp. 104–105).

Meta-analyses make it possible to be objective rather than subjective in evaluating research findings for practice. Massey and Loomis (1988) developed a coding form to be used in gathering data for a meta-analysis (Table 27–2). This form could be used to conduct a meta-analysis on research findings to determine their usefulness for practice.

Goode and colleagues (1991) conducted a meta-analysis "to estimate the effects of heparin flush and saline flush solutions on maintaining patency, preventing phlebitis, and increasing duration of periph-

TABLE 27–2
CODING FORM FOR A META-ANALYSIS

I. Description

Topic area
Study ID number
Publication date _____
Source
  Journal, nursing
  Journal, nonnursing (area)
  Thesis, doctoral; master's nursing
  Thesis, doctoral; master's nonnursing (area)
  Other (specify)
Highest level of preparation of primary author
  Doctoral   Master's
  Baccalaureate   Other (specify)
Area of interest
  Nursing   Education
  Psychology   Social work
  Medicine   Psychiatry
  Health education   Religion
  Other (specify)

II. Study Characteristics

Design
  Descriptive   Correlational
  Experimental   Quasi-experimental
Appears representative of population?
  Yes   No
Medical diagnosis or treatment (ICDA)
Sample size (N)
Treatment group size (n)
Control group size (n)
Sex of subjects
  Male   Female
  Both
Age range of subjects
Mean age of subjects
Developmental level of subjects
  Infant   Child
  Adolescent   Young adult
  Middle-aged adult
  Geriatric   Mixed (specify)
  Other (specify)
Subject assignment to treatment
  Random   Matching
  Nonrandom

III. Intervention

Type of treatment (specify)
Special equipment with treatment condition (specify)
Treatment provider
  Nurse   Psychiatrist
  Educator   Health educator
  Psychologist   Religious
  Physician   Other (specify)
Treatment provider assignment
  Random   Single provider
  Matched   Other (specify)
  Nonrandom
Treatment duration
Number of treatments

Type of control
  Usual care   Other (specify)
  Placebo

IV. Validity

Internal
  High
  Medium
  Low
External
  High
  Medium
  Low
Number of threats
Percent subject mortality, treatment group
Percent subject mortality, control group

V. Reliability of Dependent Variables

Reliability (specify type)
  High
  Medium
  Low
Number of comparisons in study
Dependent variables (list)
Dependent variable of concern (name and code)
Type of measure
  Physiological   Psychological
Standardized
  Yes   No
Independent variables (other than treatment) of concern (name
  and code)
Reactivity of measure
  Very low   High
  Low   Very high
  Medium

VI. Overall Quality of Study

Significance of treatment effect
  $p < .01$ Nonsignificant
  $0.01 < p < .05$ $-0.01 < p < -0.5$
  $0.5 < p < .10$
Control group mean ($\overline{X}_c$)
Control group standard deviation (S_c)
Treatment group mean ($\overline{X}_e$)
Treatment group standard deviation (S_e)
Effect size calculation

$$ES = \frac{\overline{X}_e - \overline{X}_c}{S}$$

$$S = \sqrt{\frac{(n^e - 1)\,(S^e)^2 + (n^c - 1)\,(S^c)^2}{n^e + n^c - 2}}$$

ICDA = International Classification of Diseases, Adapted (for use in the United States).
From Massey, J., & Loomis, M. (1988). When should nurses use research findings? *Applied Nursing Research, 1*(1), 34–35.

eral heparin locks" (p. 324). The meta-analysis was conducted on 17 quality studies that are described in Table 27–3. The total sample size of the 17 studies was 4153, and the settings of these studies were a variety of medical-surgical and critical care units. The small effect size values (most are less than .20) for clotting, phlebitis, and duration indicate that saline flush is as effective as heparin flush in maintaining peripheral heparin locks. Goode and colleagues (1991) summarized current knowledge on the use of saline versus heparin.

• •

"It can be concluded that saline is as effective as heparin in maintaining patency, preventing phlebitis, and increasing duration in peripheral intravenous locks. Quality of care can be enhanced by using saline as the flush solution, thereby eliminating problems associated with anticoagulant effects and drug incompatibilities. In addition, an estimated yearly savings of $109,100,000 to $218,200,000 U.S. health care dollars could be attained." (Goode et al., 1991, p. 324) ■

The meta-analysis provides sound scientific evidence for making a change in practice from heparin flush to saline flush for irrigating heparin locks. Clinical relevance is evident in that the use of saline to flush heparin locks promotes quality outcomes for the patient (patent heparin lock and fewer problems with anticoagulant effects and drug incompatibilities), the nurse (decreased time to flush the lock and no drug incompatibilities with saline), and the agency (extensive cost savings and quality patient care).

If you plan on making this change in your practice setting, you need to examine the following prior conditions: (1) previous practice, (2) perceived needs or problems, (3) innovativeness, and (4) norms of the social system (Rogers, 1995). Does your institution currently use heparin, not saline, to irrigate heparin locks? Do the nurses believe that this is a problem? You need to highlight the problems with heparin that have been identified in the research literature. Are the nurses innovative and willing to change, or are they very resistant to change? Which nurses might be most helpful in assisting with the change? You also need to talk

with your administrator about the change. Is the administration in your agency open or resistant to change? Is the agency supportive of using research findings to make changes in practice?

PERSUASION

During the persuasion stage of the research utilization process, you want to encourage the administration and other nurses to change current practice. Persuasion might be accomplished by demonstrating the relative advantage, compatibility, complexity, trialability, and observability of changing from heparin to saline as a flush solution (see Fig. 27–1). The relative advantages of using saline are the improved quality of care and cost savings clearly documented in the research literature (Goode et al., 1991; Shoaf & Oliver, 1992). The cost savings for different sizes of hospitals is summarized in Table 27–4. The compatibility of the change can be determined by identifying the changes that will need to occur in your agency. What changes will the nurses have to make in irrigating heparin locks with saline? What changes will have to occur in the pharmacy to provide the saline flush? Are the physicians aware of the research in this area? Are the physicians willing to order the use of saline to flush heparin locks?

The change in peripheral heparin lock irrigant from heparin flush to saline flush has minimal complexity. The only thing changed is the flush, so no additional skills, expertise, or time is required by the nurse to make the change. Because saline flush, unlike heparin flush, is compatible with any drug that might be administered through the heparin lock, the number of potential complications is decreased. The change might be started on one unit as a clinical trial and then evaluated. Once the quality of care and cost savings become observable to nurses, physicians, and hospital administrators, the change will probably spread rapidly throughout the institution. Persuasion is strong to change irrigants from heparin flush to saline flush because the advantages are extensive and no disadvantages have been identified. This change is also compatible with existing nursing care and would be relatively simple to implement on a trial basis to demonstrate the

TABLE 27-3
STUDIES INCLUDED IN THE META-ANALYSIS

STUDY	N	SUBJECTS	ASSIGNMENT	HEPARIN DOSE (U/cc)	CLOTTING EFFECT SIZE (d_c)	PHLEBITIS EFFECT SIZE (d_p)	DURATION EFFECT SIZE (d_d)
Ashton et al., 1990	16 exp$_c$, 16 con$_c$; 13 exp$_p$, 14 con$_p$	Adult critical care	Random, double blind	10	.3590	−.1230	
Barrett & Lester, 1990	59 experimental, 50 control	Adult Med-Surg patients	Nonrandom double-blind crossover	10	−.1068	−.4718	
Craig & Anderson, 1991	129 exp, 145 con	Adult Med-Surg patients	Random double-blind crossover	10	.0095	−.0586	
Cyganski et al., 1987	225 exp, 196 con	Adult Med-Surg patients	Nonrandom	100	.2510		
Donhan & Denning, 1987	8 exp$_c$, 4 con$_c$; 7 exp$_p$, 5 con$_p$	Adult critical care	Random, double blind	10	.0000	.0548	
Dunn & Lenihan, 1987	61 experimental, 51 control	Adult patients	Nonrandom	50	−.2057	−.2258	
Epperson, 1984	138 exp, 120 con; 138 exp, 154 con	Adult Med-Surg patients	Random, double blind	10, 100			−.1176, −.1232
Garrelts et al., 1989	131 exp, 173 con	Adult Med-Surg patients	Random, double blind	10	−.1773	.1057	.2753
Hamilton et al., 1988	137 exp, 170 con	Adult patients	Random, double blind	100	.0850	−.1819	−.0604
Holford et al., 1977	39 experimental, 140 control	Young adult volunteers	Nonrandom, double blind	3.3, 10, 16.5, 100, 132	.6545		
Kasparek et al., 1988	49 exp, 50 con	Adult Med patients	Random, double blind	10	.3670	−.5430	
Lombardi et al., 1988	34 experimental, 40 control	Pediatric patients (4 wk to 18 yr)	Nonrandom, sequential, double blind	10		−.2324	.0000
Miracle et al., 1989	167 exp, 441 con	Adult Med-Surg patients	Nonrandom	100	−.0042		
Shearer, 1987	87 exp, 73 con	Med-Surg patients	Nonrandom	10	−.1170	−.0977	
Spann, 1988	15 experimental, 19 control	Adult telemetry step-down	Nonrandom, double blind	10	−.3163	−.3252	
Taylor et al., 1989	369 exp, 356 con	Adult Med-Surg patients	Nonrandom, time series	10	.0308	.0288	−.1472
Tuten & Gueldner, 1991	43 exp, 71 con	Adult Med-Surg patients	Nonrandom	100	.0000	.1662	

From Goode, C. J., Titler, M., Rakel, B., Ones, D. S., Kleiber, C., Small, S., & Triolo, P. K. (1991). A meta-analysis of effects of heparin flush and saline flush: Quality and cost implications. *Nursing Research, 40*(6), 325. Used with permission of Lippincott-Raven Publishers, Philadelphia, PA.

TABLE 27-4
ANNUAL COST SAVINGS FROM CHANGING TO SALINE

STUDY	COST SAVINGS	HOSPITAL
Craig & Anderson, 1991	$40,000/yr	525-bed tertiary care hospital
Dunn & Lenihan, 1987	$19,000/yr	530-bed private hospital
Goode et al., 1991 (this study)	$38,000/yr	879-bed tertiary care hospital
Kasparek et al., 1988	$19,000/yr	350-bed private hospital
Lombardi et al., 1988	$20,000–$25,000/yr	52-bed pediatric unit
Schustek, 1984	$20,000/yr	391-bed private hospital
Taylor et al., 1989	$30,000–$40,000/yr	216-bed private hospital

From Goode, C. J., Titler, M., Rakel, B., Ones, D. S., Kleiber, C., Small, S., & Triolo, P. K. (1991). A meta-analysis of effects of heparin flush and saline flush: Quality and cost implications. *Nursing Research, 40*(6), 328. Used with permission of Lippincott-Raven Publishers, Philadelphia, PA.

positive outcomes for patients, nurses, and the health care agency.

DECISION

The decision to use saline flush versus heparin flush as an irrigant requires institutional approval, physician approval, and approval of the nurses managing patients' heparin locks. When a change requires institutional approval, decision making may be distributed through several levels of the organization. Thus a decision at one level may lead to contact with another official who must approve the action. In keeping with the guidelines of planned change, institutional changes are more likely to be effective if all those affected by the change have a voice in the decision. In your institution, who needs to approve the change? What steps do you need to take to get the change approved within your institution? Do the physicians support the change? Do the nurses on the units support the change? Who are the leaders in the institution and can you get them to support the change? Try to get the nurses to make a commitment and take a public stand to make the change because their commitment increases the probability that the change will be made. Contact the appropriate administrative people and physicians and detail the pros and cons of making the change to saline flush for irrigating heparin locks. You need to clearly indicate to physicians and administrators that the change is based on extensive research evidence. Most physicians are positively influenced by research-based knowledge.

IMPLEMENTATION

Implementing a research-based change can be simple or complex, depending on the change. The change might be implemented as indicated in the research literature or may be modified to meet the agency's needs. In some cases, a long time might be spent in planning implementation of the change after the decision is made. In other cases, implementation can begin immediately. Usually, a great deal of support is needed during initial implementation of a change. As with any new activity, unexpected events often occur. The nurse adopter frequently does not know how to interpret these events. Contact with a person experienced in the change can make the difference between continuation and rejection of the innovation.

The change from heparin flush to saline flush will involve the physicians ordering saline for flushing heparin locks. You will need to speak with the physicians to gain their support for the change. You might convince some key physicians to support the change, and they will convince others to make the change. The pharmacy will have to package saline for use as an irrigant. The nurses will also be provided information about the change and the rationale for the change. It might be best to implement the change on one nursing unit and give the nurses on this unit an opportunity to design the protocol and plan for implementing the change. The nurses might develop a protocol similar to the one in Figure 27–6. This protocol directs you in preparing for irrigating a heparin lock, actually irrigating the heparin lock, and documenting your actions.

CONFIRMATION

After a change has been implemented in practice, the nurses who implemented the change need to confirm or document the effectiveness of the

1. Obtain the saline flush for irrigation from the pharmacy.
2. Wash hands, collect equipment for irrigating the heparin lock, and put on gloves.
3. Cleanse the heparin lock with alcohol before injection with saline solution.
4. Flush the peripheral heparin lock with 1 cc of normal saline every 8 hr (Goode et al., 1991; Shoaf & Oliver, 1992).
5. If a patient is receiving IV medication, administer 1 cc of saline, administer the medication, and follow with 1 cc of saline (Shoaf & Oliver, 1992).
6. Check the peripheral heparin lock site for complications of phlebitis or loss of patency. The symptoms of phlebitis include the presence of erythema, tenderness, warmth, and a tender or palpable cord. Loss of patency is indicated by resistance to flushing, "as evidenced by inability to administer 1 cc of flushing solution within 30 seconds" (Shoaf & Oliver, 1992).
7. Chart the time that the peripheral heparin lock was irrigated with saline and any complications of phlebitis or loss of patency.

FIGURE 27–6 ▪ Protocol for irrigating peripheral heparin locks. (Data from Goode, C. J., Titler, M., Rakel, B., et al. [1991]. A meta-analysis of effects of heparin flush and saline flush: Quality and cost implications. *Nursing Research, 40*[6], 324–330 and Shoaf, J., & Oliver, S. [1992]. Efficacy of normal saline injection with and without heparin for maintaining intermittent intravenous site. *Applied Nursing Research, 5*[1], 9–12.)

change. They need to document that the change improved quality of care, decreased the cost of care, or saved nursing time, or any combination of these benefits. If the outcomes from the change in practice are positive, nurses, administrators, and physicians will often want to continue the change. Nurses usually seek feedback from those around them. Their peers' reactions to the change in nursing practice will influence continuation of the change. If peers approve, the nurses will often adopt the change and even encourage others to do the same. If peers disapprove or provide negative feedback, nurses will often abandon the change.

You can confirm the effectiveness of the saline flush for peripheral heparin lock irrigation by examining patient care outcomes and cost-benefit ratios. Patient care outcomes can be examined by determining the number of clotting and phlebitis complications associated with peripheral heparin locks 1 month before the change and 1 month after the change. If no significant difference is seen, the use of saline flush is supported. The cost savings can be calculated for 1 month by determining the cost difference between heparin flush and saline flush. This cost difference can then be multiplied by the number of saline flushes conducted in 1 month. This cost savings can then be multiplied by 12 months and compared with the cost savings summarized in

Table 27–4. If positive patient outcomes and cost savings are demonstrated, the adoption of saline flush for irrigating peripheral heparin locks will probably continue and be used by all nurses in the agency.

In the future, accrediting agencies for health care organizations will require that protocols for nursing interventions be evidence based. Procedure manuals, standards of care, and nursing care plans will need to reflect current nursing research evidence. Many progressive nurse executives realize the importance of research and are encouraging their nursing staff to use research findings in their practice. However, to improve nursing practice with research knowledge effectively, research utilization must become a priority for all nurses.

Evidence-Based Practice for Nursing

A future goal for the United States is evidence-based health care systems. An evidence-based health care system incorporates research evidence, expertise of the practitioners, views of the patient, and the resources available in delivering care (Cullum, 1998). EBP for medicine and nursing is essential in providing evidence-based health care. EBP has been emphasized in medicine for years, and expert clinicians have developed numerous evidence-based guidelines for the prevention of illness and for diagnosis and management of disease conditions. Nurses are now faced with the challenge of developing EBP for nursing.

In some sources, the terms *research utilization* and *EBP* are used synonymously, but they are different phenomena. Research utilization is a more prescribed task of using research findings in a selected area in practice. In research utilization, the research literature is analyzed, findings are synthesized, a research-based protocol is developed for use in practice, and outcomes from the practice change are measured. Research utilization incorporates only empirical findings in making changes in practice. EBP is the "careful and practical use of current best evidence to guide health-care decisions" (Omery & Williams, 1999, p. 51). EBP is usually based on clinical practice guidelines that evolve from an integration of research findings and expert practitioners' opinions (Stetler, Brunell, et al., 1998a). The highest-quality guidelines are developed with sound empirical knowledge (quality studies, integrative reviews, and meta-analyses) and the consensus of expert clinicians and researchers. In EBP, implementation of quality guidelines by experienced practitioners is based on the patient's values and the resources available (Brown, 1999; Omery & Williams, 1999; Stetler, et al., 1998a).

MODEL FOR FACILITATING EVIDENCE-BASED PRACTICE

Nursing is in the initial stages of developing an EBP, and the discipline can learn a great deal from the practice guidelines that have been developed in medicine. In addition, advanced practice nurses (nurse practitioners, clinical nurse specialists, nurse midwives, and nurse anesthetists) will be responsible for both medical and nursing practice guidelines. A model is proposed in this textbook to promote an understanding of EBP and facilitate the use of EBP by nurses (Fig. 27–7).

As demonstrated in the model, a practice problem initiates a search for the best evidence that a practitioner might use in making health care decisions. The best evidence that nurses might use in providing care is a quality practice guideline. *Qual-*

ity practice guidelines are based on synthesized research findings from meta-analyses, supported by consensus from recognized national experts, and affirmed by outcomes obtained by clinicians (Stetler et al., 1998a). These guidelines are used in the delivery of EBP and might be obtained from the Internet, published sources (journal articles and textbooks), and clinical presentations. In 1989, the Agency for Health Care Policy and Research (AHCPR) within the U.S. DHHS began convening panels of expert health care providers and researchers to summarize research and develop clinical practice guidelines. These panels summarized research findings and developed guidelines for practice in areas such as (1) *Acute Pain Management in Infants, Children, and Adolescents: Operative and Medical Procedures*; (2) *Pressure Ulcers in Adults: Prediction and Prevention*; (3) *Urinary Incontinence in Adults*; (4) *Cataracts in Adults: Management of Functional Impairment*; (5) *Depression in Primary Care:* Volume I: *Detection and Diagnosis,* and Volume II: *Treatment of Major Depression*; (6) *Sickle Cell Disease: Screening, Diagnosis, Management, and Counseling in Newborns and Infants*; (7) *Evaluation and Management of Early HIV infection*; (8) *Benign Prostatic Hyperplasia: Diagnosis and Treatment*; (9) *Management of Cancer-Related Pain*; (10) *Diagnosis and Treatment of Heart Failure*; (11) *Low Back Problems*; (12) *Otitis Media in Children*; (13) *Post-stroke Rehabilitation;* (14) *Screening for Alzheimer's and Related Dementias*; (15) *Chest Pain Due to Unstable Angina*; (16) *Treatment of Pressure Ulcers in Adults*; (17) *Quality Determinants of Mammography;* and (18) *Cardiac Rehabilitation Services.* The AHCPR was renamed the AHRQ in 1999 and can be found on the Web at *http://www.ahcpr.gov/*. Within the AHRQ are EBP centers that synthesize scientific evidence to improve quality and effectiveness in clinical care (*http://www.ahcpr.gov/clinic/epc/*). Another source of practice guidelines is the National Guideline Clearinghouse (NGC) at *http://www. guideline.gov/*. The NGC provides nearly 700 practice guidelines within two categories: disease/condition and treatment/intervention.

The AHRQ and the NGC provide a variety of guidelines that were developed to promote evi-

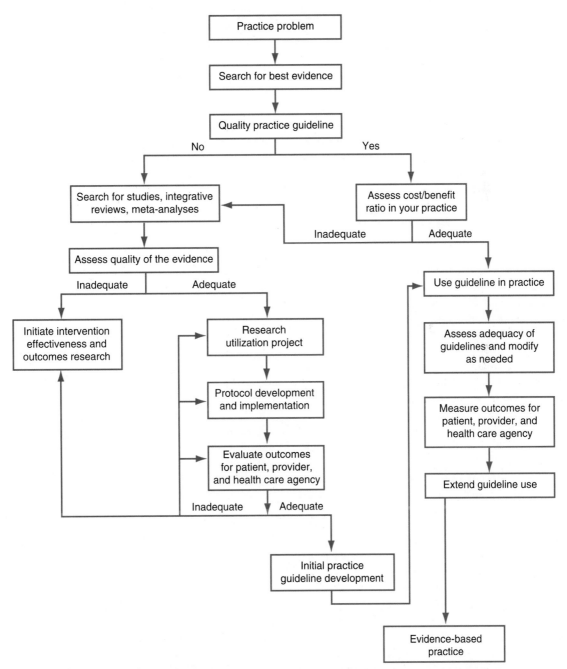

FIGURE 27–7 ■ Algorithm for facilitating evidence-based practice in nursing developed by Grove.

dence-based medical practice. Recently, nursing has implemented a best-practice network where professionals might collaborate in transforming health care. Best practice is defined as a service, function, or process that has been developed, refined, and implemented to produce high-quality outcomes for patients, families, and communities. The best-practice network was initiated to promote the development of protocols, guidelines, standards, and clinical pathways to ensure high-quality outcomes. Several best-practice projects are currently in progress, such as open visitation policy in intensive care units, justification of staffing, evidence-based hemodynamics, and smoke-free campuses. Nurses are encouraged to participate in best-practice projects by providing constructive feedback, networking with colleagues on a project, and mentoring less experienced colleagues. The website for the best-practice network provides extensive information about current guidelines, new projects, and future directions for developing EBP in health care and can be located at *http://www.best4health.org/*.

Progressing down the right side of the algorithm, you note that if a quality guideline exists, it must be assessed for cost and benefit in your practice (see Figure 27–7). If the cost-benefit ratio is not adequate, the practitioner needs to search for empirical evidence (quality studies, integrative review, and meta-analyses) to make a change in practice. If the ratio is adequate, the practitioner uses the guideline in his or her practice and measures the most appropriate outcomes to determine the impact on the patient, provider, and health care system. If the outcomes are adequate, use of the guidelines can be extended in a selected practice, a variety of practices, or several health care systems. At least for this practice problem, the practitioner is able to deliver EBP.

If a quality guideline does not exist for the practice problem, the practitioner needs to search for relevant evidence in studies, integrative reviews, and meta-analyses and to assess the quality of this evidence (see the left side of Figure 27–7). If the evidence is adequate, the practitioner can implement the research utilization process. The synthesized research knowledge can be used to develop a protocol for making a change in practice that can be imple-

mented and evaluated by the practitioner. If this protocol is effective, it might be tested in other clinical situations and evaluated by researchers and clinicians for its effectiveness and potential for development into a practice guideline. If the outcomes are not positive, the researcher needs to evaluate the research utilization process for problems and resolve them if possible (see the feedback loop in Figure 27–7).

If adequate evidence does not exist for a research utilization project, the practitioner might conduct or encourage others to conduct intervention effectiveness research (see Chapter 13) and outcome studies (see Chapter 12) to generate essential knowledge for relevant practice problems. The accumulation of essential research evidence leads to the implementation of a research utilization project, practice guideline development, and ultimately EBP. This model demonstrates the complexity of developing and implementing an EBP in nursing. Nurses are encouraged to continue the conduct of relevant clinical studies, to use research findings in practice, and to strive for an EBP.

■ SUMMARY

Most people believe that a good idea will sell itself. Unfortunately, this is seldom true. Even today, research findings that clearly warrant utilization are not being used. Nurses need to understand the process of research utilization and develop strategies to achieve this process. Two important theories in the area of research utilization are Rogers's theory of diffusion of innovations and Havelock's theory of linker systems. Rogers is an expert and noted theorist in the field of knowledge diffusion and utilization. He has conducted research related to diffusion for 25 years, and his theory is a synthesis of the findings from his research. The main elements of diffusion are innovation, communication channels, time, and social system. Rogers conceptualized the innovation-decision process as consisting of five stages: (1) knowledge, (2) persuasion, (3) decision, (4) implementation, and (5) confirmation. The types of utilization identified by Rogers include direct application, reinvention, and indirect effects.

Havelock added a new dimension to utilization theory by proposing the development of a linker system. This linker system is used to transfer new knowledge, skills, or products (innovations) from resource systems (researchers and their publications) to user systems (practitioners) for dissemination. Both theories focus on change and describe the use of a change agent external to the system to initiate and facilitate the change process.

Two federally funded projects that were developed to increase utilization of nursing research findings include the WICHE Regional Program for Nursing Research Development and the CURN Project. Rogers's and Havelock's theories were used as the theoretical frameworks for these projects. The WICHE project was the first major nursing project to address research utilization. This project focused on critiquing research, using change theory, and diffusing innovations. The CURN Project was developed to increase the utilization of research findings in the following ways: disseminating findings, facilitating organizational modifications necessary for implementation, and encouraging collaborative research that was directly transferable to clinical practice. Clinical studies were critiqued, protocols were developed from the findings, and implementation was initiated on test units within hospitals.

The Stetler/Marram model was developed in 1976 and refined by Stetler in 1994 to direct utilization of nursing research. In this model, utilization includes critical thinking and a series of judgmental activities that occur in phases. The phases of the revised Stetler Model for Research Utilization are (1) preparation, (2) validation, (3) comparative evaluation, (4) decision making, (5) translation/application, and (6) evaluation. The activities of each phase are identified in the model and can be used to critique and cluster findings for use in practice; direct the use of findings in practice; and evaluate the impact of the research knowledge on the practice setting, personnel, and patients.

Strategies are identified for educators, researchers, practitioners, and administrators to promote research utilization. Educators might encourage students to synthesize research in an area of interest and develop a protocol for implementation in practice. Researchers might publish findings in a way that facilitates the understanding of practitioners. Practicing nurses need to seek outcomes of current research, evaluate their potential for practice, and modify their practice with new knowledge. Administrators can facilitate the use of research in agencies by showing support for and rewarding activities to base nursing care on research. An example of a research utilization project is presented that incorporates some of the strategies identified and uses Rogers's five decision-making steps: knowledge, persuasion, decision, implementation, and confirmation.

A future goal for the United States is evidence-based health care systems that incorporate research evidence, expertise of the practitioner, views of the patient, and available resources. EBP for medicine and nursing is essential in providing evidence-based health care. EBP is the careful and practical use of current best evidence to guide health care decisions. In EBP, implementation of quality guidelines by experienced practitioners is based on the patient's values and the resources available. Nursing is in the initial stages of developing an EBP. An algorithm is proposed to promote an understanding of EBP and facilitate the use of EBP by nurses.

• •

TABLE 27–A
Procedure for Administration of Intramuscular Injections

PROCEDURE	RATIONALE	REFERENCES
1. For adults, select a 1.5-inch needle. For children, select a 1-inch needle. Use a needle of 21–23 gauge.	The needle must be long enough to reach the muscle. Injections into subcutaneous tissue cause the patient pain. The VG site provides the most consistent depth of subcutaneous tissue; in adults, the adipose tissue layer over the VG muscle is less than 3.75 cm (1.47 in chest) in depth. Using a smaller-gauge needle minimizes tissue injury and subcutaneous leakage.	Hick et al., 1989; Johnson & Raptou, 1965; Michaels & Poole, 1970; Shaffer, 1929; Talbert et al., 1967
2. The maximum volume to be administered in one injection should not exceed 4 mL in adults with well-developed muscles such as the VG. Children and individuals with less well developed muscles should receive no more than 1–2 mL. Children younger than 2 yr should not receive more than 1 mL. If using the deltoid, do not exceed a volume of 0.5–1 mL. The size of the syringe is determined by the volume to be administered and should correspond as closely as possible to the amount to be administered. Volumes less than 0.5 mL require a low-dose syringe such as a tuberculin syringe.	High-volume injections cause more pain. Finely graduated syringes such as tuberculin syringes ensure administration of the correct dose.	Farley et al., 1986; Losek & Gyuro, 1992; Zenk, 1982
3. Use a filter needle to draw up medication from a glass ampule or vial. Hold the vial or ampule down and do not draw up the last drop in the container. After drawing the medication into the syringe, change the needle before administration. If using a prefilled syringe such as Tubex or Carpuject and drawing from a vial or ampule, instill the medication into another syringe and ensure the use of a clean needle before injection. If using a prefilled unit-dose medication, take caution to avoid dripping medication on the needle before injection. If medication does drip, wipe it off the needle with sterile gauze.	Glass and rubber particulate matter has been found in medications withdrawn with a regular needle. Holding the vial or ampule down will allow particulate matter to precipitate out of solution, and leaving the last drops reduces the chance of withdrawing foreign particles. Changing the needle will prevent tracking the medication through subcutaneous tissue during insertion of the needle, which can cause pain. Similarly, medication should be wiped from the needle because it can cause pain when tracked through subcutaneous tissue.	Hahn, 1990; Keen, 1986; McConnell, 1982
4. Do not use an air bubble.	An air bubble affects the dose administered by causing an overdose of medication of at least 5% and as great as 100%, depending on the dose administered.	Chaplin et al., 1985; Zenk, 1982, 1993
5. Select the VG site as the injection site for children older than 7 mo and adults except for those with strict contraindication. Strict contraindications would include preexisting tissue injury and administration of hepatitis B vaccine, which should be administered only in the deltoid. In infants younger than 7 mo, the vastus lateralis should be used for administration of hepatitis B vaccine.	The VG site is free of nerves and blood vessels. No reports of complications from IM injections administered at this site have been documented. The VG muscle is a well-developed muscle in infants, children, and adults.	Beecroft & Redick, 1990; Brandt et al., 1972; Centers for Disease Control, 1985; Daly et al., 1992; Hochstetter, 1954, 1955, 1956

TABLE 27–A
PROCEDURE FOR ADMINISTRATION OF INTRAMUSCULAR INJECTIONS *Continued*

PROCEDURE	RATIONALE	REFERENCES
6. Before administration of any IM injection, carefully assess the site for evidence of induration, abscesses, or other contraindications to use of the site.	Injections are contraindicated in previously injured muscles or tissues.	Stokes et al., 1944
7. Position the patient to relax the muscle. Prone: Have the patient "toe in" to internally rotate the femur. Side-lying: Have the patient flex the upper part of the leg at 20 degrees. Supine: Have the patient flex both knees, if possible; if not possible, flex the knee on the side where the medication will be administered.	Pain is reduced with a relaxed muscle.	Keen, 1986; Kruszewski et al., 1979; Rettig & Southby, 1982
8. Identify the site by placing the palm of the hand on the greater trochanter, with the index finger toward the anterior superior iliac spine and the middle finger spread away to form a "V." Use the right hand on the left VG site and the left hand on the right VG site.	The landmarks are described by Hochstetter.	Hochstetter, 1954, 1955, 1956; Zelman, 1961
9. Pull the skin down to administer the injection in a Z-track manner at a 90-degree angle to the iliac crest in the middle of the "V."	The Z-track technique reduces discomfort and the incidence of lesions.	Keen, 1981, 1986, 1990
10. Cleanse the skin in a circular fashion in an area of approximately 5–8 cm (2–3 inches) and allow the alcohol to dry.	Deep tissues can be infected with skin contaminants injected via the needle; the skin is the first line of defense. Alcohol is irritating to subcutaneous tissue and causes pain.	Berger & Williams, 1992; Murphy, 1991
11. Insert the needle with steady pressure and then aspirate for at least 5–10 sec. Inject the medication slowly at a rate of approximately 10 sec/mL.	Aspirating for 5–10 sec is adequate to ensure that the needle is not in a small, low-flow blood vessel. A slow, steady injection rate promotes comfort and minimizes tissue damage.	Stokes et al., 1944; Zelman, 1961
12. Wait 10 sec after injecting the medication before withdrawing the needle.	Waiting 10 sec allows the medication to be deposited in the muscle and begin to diffuse through it.	Belanger-Annable, 1985; Hahn, 1990, 1991; Keen, 1990
13. Smoothly and steadily withdraw the needle and apply gentle pressure at the site with a dry sponge.	This technique minimizes tissue injury. Massaging the site can result in tissue irritation.	Newton et al., 1992
14. Encourage leg exercises.	Leg exercises will promote absorption of the medication.	Stokes et al., 1944
15. Whenever possible, assess the site 2–4 hr after injection and as needed to identify any side effects.	Given the number of complications reported in the literature, it is important to assess the site for any signs of redness, swelling, pain, or other iatrogenic effects from the injection.	Beecroft & Redick, 1989, 1990

IM = intramuscular; VG = ventrogluteal.

From Beyea, S. C., & Nicoll, L. H. (1995). Administration of medication via the intramuscular route: An integrative review of the literature and research-based protocol for the procedure. *Applied Nursing Research, 8*(1), 23–33.

REFERENCES

Ashton, J., Gibson, V., & Summers, S. (1990). Effects of heparin versus saline solution on intermittent infusion device irrigation. *Heart & Lung, 19*(6), 608–612.

Axford, R., & Cutchen, L. (1977). Using nursing research to improve preoperative care. *Journal of Nursing Administration, 7*(10), 16–20.

Barrett, P. J., & Lester, R. L. (1990). Heparin versus saline flush solutions in a small community hospital. *Hospital Pharmacy, 25*(2), 115–118.

Beecroft, P. C., & Redick, S. A. (1989). Possible complications of intramuscular injections on the pediatric unit. *Pediatric Nursing, 15*(4), 333–336, 376.

Beecroft, P. C., & Redick, S. A. (1990). Intramuscular injection practices of pediatric nurses: Site selection. *Nurse Educator, 15*(4), 23–28.

Belanger-Annable, M. C. (1985). Long acting neuroleptics: Technique for intramuscular injection. *The Canadian Nurse, 81*(8), 41–44.

Berger, K. J., & Williams, M. B. (1992). *Fundamentals of nursing: Collaborating for optimal health.* Norwalk, CT: Appleton & Lange.

Beyea, S. C., & Nicoll, L. H. (1995). Administration of medications via the intramuscular route: An integrative review of the literature and research-based protocol for the procedure. *Applied Nursing Research, 8*(1), 23–33.

Bock, L. R. (1990). From research to utilization: Bridging the gap. *Nursing Management, 21*(3), 50–51.

Brandt, P. A., Smith, M. E., Ashburn, S. S., & Graves, J. (1972). IM injections in children. *American Journal of Nursing, 72*(7), 1402–1406.

Brett, J. L. (1987). Use of nursing practice research findings. *Nursing Research, 36*(6), 344–349.

Brown, S. J. (1999). *Knowledge for health care practice: A guide to using research evidence.* Philadelphia: W.B. Saunders.

Centers for Disease Control. (1985). Diphtheria, tetanus and pertussis: Guidelines for vaccine prophylaxis and other preventive measures. Immunization Practices Advisory Committee. *MMWR. Morbidity and Mortality Weekly Report, 34*(27), 405–414.

Champion, V. L., & Leach, A. (1989). Variables related to research utilization in nursing: An empirical investigation. *Journal of Advanced Nursing, 14*(9), 705–710.

Chaplin, G., Shull, H., & Welk, P. C., III. (1985). How safe is the air-bubble technique for I.M. injections? Not very, say these experts. *Nursing85, 15*(9), 59.

Conduct and Utilization of Research in Nursing (CURN) Project. (1981–1982). *Using research to improve nursing practice.* New York: Grune & Stratton. (Series of clinical protocols: *Clean intermittent catheterization* [1982], *Closed urinary drainage systems* [1981], *Distress reduction through sensory preparation* [1981], *Intravenous cannula change* [1981], *Mutual goal setting in patient care* [1982], *Pain: Deliberative nursing interventions* [1982], *Preventing decubitus ulcers* [1981], *Reducing diarrhea in tube-fed patients* [1981], *Structured preoperative teaching* [1981].)

Coyle, L. A., & Sokop, A. G. (1990). Innovation adoption behavior among nurses. *Nursing Research, 39*(3), 176–180.

Craig, F. D., & Anderson, S. R. (1991). *A comparison of normal saline versus heparinized normal saline in the maintenance of intermittent infusion devices.* Manuscript submitted for publication.

Cullum, N. (1998). Evidence-based practice. *Nursing Management, 5*(3), 32–35.

Cyganski, J. M., Donahue, J. M., & Heaton, J. S. (1987). The case for the heparin flush. *American Journal of Nursing, 86*(6), 796–797.

Daly, J. M., Johnston, W., & Chung, Y. (1992). Injection sites utilized for DPT immunizations in infants. *Journal of Community Health Nursing, 9*(2), 87–94.

Davies, A. R., Doyle, M. A. T., Lansky, D., Rutt, W., Stevic, M. O., & Doyle, J. B. (1994). Outcome assessments in clinical settings: A consensus statement on principles and best practices in project management. *The Joint Commission Journal on Quality Improvement, 20*(1), 6–16.

Donham, J., & Denning, V. (1987). Heparin vs. saline in maintaining patency in intermittent infusion devices: Pilot study. *The Kansas Nurse, 62*(11), 6–7.

Dracup, K. A., & Breu, C. S. (1978). Using nursing research findings to meet the needs of grieving spouses. *Nursing Research, 27*(4), 212–216.

Dunn, D. L., & Lenihan, S. F. (1987). The case for the saline flush. *American Journal of Nursing, 87*(6), 798–799.

Epperson, E. L. (1984). Efficacy of 0.9% sodium chloride injection with and without heparin for maintaining indwelling intermittent injection sites. *Clinical Pharmacy, 3*(6), 626–629.

Farley, F., Joyce, N., Long, B., & Roberts, R. (1986). Will that IM needle reach the muscle? *American Journal of Nursing, 86*(12), 1327–1328.

Funk, S. G., Champagne, M. T., Tornquist, E. M., & Wiese, R. A. (1995). Administrators' views on barriers to research utilization. *Applied Nursing Research, 8*(1), 44–49.

Funk, S. G., Champagne, M. T., Wiese, R. A., & Tornquist, E. M. (1991). BARRIERS: The barriers research utilization scale. *Applied Nursing Research, 4*(1), 39–45.

Ganong, L. H. (1987). Integrative reviews of nursing research. *Research in Nursing & Health, 10*(1), 1–11.

Garrelts, J., LaRocca, J., Ast, D., Smith, D. F., & Sweet, D. E. (1989). Comparison of heparin and 0.9% sodium chloride injection in the maintenance of indwelling intermittent I.V. devices. *Clinical Pharmacy, 8*(1), 34–39.

Glaser, E. M., Abelson, H. H., & Garrison, K. N. (1983). *Putting knowledge to use.* San Francisco: Jossey-Bass.

Goode, C. J., Titler, M., Rakel, B., Ones, D. S., Kleiber, C., Small, S., & Triolo, P. K. (1991). A meta-analysis of effects of heparin flush and saline flush: Quality and cost implications. *Nursing Research, 40*(6), 324–330.

Hahn, K. (1990). Brush up on your injection technique. *Nursing90, 20*(9), 54–58.

Hahn, K. (1991). Extra points on injections (letter). *Nursing91, 21*(1), 6.

Hamilton, R. A., Plis, J. M., Clay, C., & Sylvan, L. (1988). Heparin sodium versus 0.9% sodium chloride injection for maintaining patency of indwelling intermittent infusion devices. *Clinical Pharmacy, 7*(6), 439–443.

Havelock, R. G. (1970). *A guide to innovation in education.* Ann Arbor, MI: Center for Research on Utilization of Scientific Knowledge, Institute for Social Research, University of Michigan.

Havelock, R. G. (1973). *The change agent's guide to innovation in education.* Englewood Cliffs, NJ: Educational Technology Publications.

Havelock, R. G. (1974). *Ideal systems for research utilization: Four alternatives.* Washington, DC: Social and Rehabilitation Service, U.S. Department of Health, Education & Welfare.

Havelock, R. G., & Havelock, M. C. (1973). *Training for change agents: A guide to the design of training programs in education and other fields.* Ann Arbor, MI: Center for Research on Utilization of Scientific Knowledge, Institute for Social Research, University of Michigan.

Havelock, R. G., & Lingwood, D. A. (1973). *R&D utilization strategies and functions: An analytical comparison of four systems.* Ann Arbor, MI: Center for Research on Utilization of Scientific Knowledge, Institute for Social Research, University of Michigan.

Hick, J. F., Charboneau, J. W., Brakke, D. M., & Goergen, B. (1989). Optimum needle length for DPT inoculation of infants. *Pediatrics, 84*(1), 136–137.

Hochstetter, V. A. V. (1954). Uber die intraglutaale Injektion, ihre Komplikationen und deren Verhutung. *Schweizerische Medizinische Wochenschrift, 84,* 1226–1227.

Hochstetter, V. A. V. (1955). Uber Probleme und Technik der intraglutaalen injektion, Teil I. Der Einfluß des Medikamentes und der Individualitat des Patienten auf die Entstehung von Spritzenschaden. *Schweizerische Medizinische Wochenschrift, 85,* 1138–1144.

Hochstetter, V. A. V. (1956). Uber Probleme und Technik der intraglutaalen Injektion, Teil II. Der Einfluβ der Injektionstechnick auf die Entstehung von Spritzenschaden. *Schweizerische Medizinische Wochenschrift, 86,* 69–76.

Holford, N. H., Vozeh, S., Coates, P., Porvell, J. R., Thiercelin, J. F., & Upton, R. (1977). More on heparin lock (letter). *The New England Journal of Medicine, 296*(22), 1300–1301.

Horsley, J. A., Crane, J., & Bingle, J. D. (1978). Research utilization as an organizational process. *Journal of Nursing Administration, 8*(7), 4–6.

Horsley, J. A., Crane, J., Crabtree, M. K., & Wood, D. J. (1983). *Using research to improve nursing practice: A guide* (CURN Project). New York: Grune & Stratton.

Hunt, M. (1987). The process of translating research findings into nursing practice. *Journal of Advanced Nursing, 12*(1), 101–110.

Janken, J. K., Rudisill, P., & Benfield, L. (1992). Product evaluation as a research utilization strategy. *Applied Nursing Research, 5*(4), 188–201.

Johnson, E. W., & Raptou, A. D. (1965). A study of intragluteal injections. *Archives of Physical Medicine and Rehabilitation, 46,* 167–177.

Kasparek, A., Wenger, J., & Feldt, R. (1988). *Comparison of normal versus heparinized saline for flushing or intermittent intravenous infusion devices* (pp. 1–18). Unpublished manuscript. Cedar Rapids, IA: Mercy Medical Center.

Keen, M. F. (1981). Comparison of two intramuscular injection techniques on the incidence and severity of discomfort and lesions at the injection site. *Dissertation Abstracts International, 42*(4), 1394B (University Microfilms No. 8120152).

Keen, M. F. (1986). Comparison of intramuscular injection techniques to reduce site discomfort and lesions. *Nursing Research, 35*(4), 207–210.

Keen, M. F. (1990). Get on the right track with Z-track injections. *Nursing90, 20*(8), 59.

Krueger, J. C. (1978). Utilization of nursing research: The planning process. *Journal of Nursing Administration, 8*(1), 6–9.

Krueger, J. C., Nelson, A. H., & Wolanin, M. A. (1978). *Nursing research: Development, collaboration, and utilization.* Germantown, MD: Aspen.

Kruszewski, A., Lang, S., & Johnson, J. (1979). Effect of positioning on discomfort from intramuscular injections in the dorsogluteal site. *Nursing Research, 28*(2), 103–105.

LaValley, M. (1997). Methods article: A consumer's guide to meta-analysis. *Arthritis Care and Research, 10*(3), 208–213.

Lombardi, T. P., Gunderson, B., Zammett, L. O., Walters, J. K., & Morris, B. A. (1988). Efficacy of 0.9% sodium chloride injection with or without heparin sodium for maintaining patency of intravenous catheters in children. *Clinical Pharmacy, 7*(11), 832–836.

Losek, J. D., & Gyuro, J. (1992). Pediatric intramuscular injections: Do you know the procedure and complications? *Pediatric Emergency Care, 8*(2), 79–81.

MacGuire, J. M. (1990). Putting nursing research findings into practice: Research utilization as an aspect of the management of change. *Journal of Advanced Nursing, 15*(5), 614–620.

Marwick, C. (1997). Aspirin's role in prevention now official. *Journal of the American Medical Association, 277*(9), 701–702.

Massey, J., & Loomis, M. (1988). When should nurses use research findings? *Applied Nursing Research, 1*(1), 32–40.

Mateo, M. A., & Kirchhoff, K. T. (1999). *Conducting and using nursing research in the clinical setting* (2nd ed.). Baltimore: Williams & Wilkins.

McConnell, E. A. (1982). The subtle art of really good injections. *RN, 45*(2), 25–35.

Michaels, L., & Poole, R. W. (1970). Injection granuloma of the buttock. *Canadian Medical Association Journal, 102*(6), 626–628.

Miracle, V., Fangman, B., Kayrouz, P., Kederis, K., & Pursell, L. (1989). Normal saline vs. heparin lock flush solution: One institution's findings. *The Kentucky Nurse, 37*(4), 1, 6–7.

Mullem, C. V., Burke, L. J., Dobmeyer, K., Farrell, M., Harvey, S., John, L., Kraly, C., Rowley, F., Sebern, M., Twite, K., &

Zapp, R. (1999). Strategic planning for research use in nursing practice. *Journal of Nursing Administration, 29*(12), 38–45.

Murphy, J. I. (1991). Reducing the pain of intramuscular (IM) injections. *Advancing Clinical Care, 6*(4), 35.

Newton, M., Newton, D., & Fudin, J. (1992). Reviewing the "big three" injection techniques. *Nursing92, 22*(2), 34–41.

Omery, A., & Williams, R. P. (1999). An appraisal of research utilization across the United States. *Journal of Nursing Administration, 29*(12), 50–56.

Pelz, D., & Horsley, J. (1981). Measuring utilization of nursing research. In J. Ciarlo (Ed.), *Utilizing evaluation.* Beverly Hills, CA: Sage.

Pettengill, M. M., Gillies, D. A., & Clark, C. C. (1994). Factors encouraging and discouraging the use of nursing research findings. *Image—The Journal of Nursing Scholarship, 26*(2), 143–147.

Pillemer, D. B., & Light, R. J. (1980). Synthesizing outcomes: How to use research evidence from many studies. *Harvard Educational Review, 50*(2), 176–195.

Rettig, F. M., & Southby, J. R. (1982). Using different body positions to reduce discomfort from dorsogluteal injection. *Nursing Research, 31*(4), 219–221.

Rogers, E. M. (1995). *Diffusion of innovations* (4th ed.). New York: Free Press.

Schustek, M. (1984). A cost-effective approach to PRN device maintenance . . . the change from heparin to saline. *Journal of the National Intravenous Therapy Association, 7*(6), 527.

Shaffer, L. W. (1929). The fate of intragluteal injections. *Archives of Dermatology and Syphilology, 19,* 347–363.

Shearer, J. (1987). Normal saline flush versus dilute heparin flush. *National Intravenous Therapy Association, 10*(6), 425–427.

Shoaf, J., & Oliver, S. (1992). Efficacy of normal saline injection with and without heparin for maintaining intermittent intravenous site. *Applied Nursing Research, 5*(1), 9–12.

Spann, J. M. (1988). Efficacy of two flush solutions to maintain catheter patency in heparin locks. *Dissertation Abstracts, 28*(1), 1337125, 1–58. *Dissertation Abstracts International, 42*(4), 1394B (University Microfilms No. 8120152).

Stetler, C. B. (1994). Refinement of the Stetler/Marram model for application of research findings to practice. *Nursing Outlook, 42*(1), 15–25.

Stetler, C. B., Brunell, M., Giuliano, K. K., Morsi, D., Prince, L., & Newell-Stokes, V. (1998a). Evidence-based practice and the role of nursing leadership. *Journal of Nursing Administration, 28*(7/8), 45–53.

Stetler, C. B., & Marram, G. (1976). Evaluating research findings for applicability in practice. *Nursing Outlook, 24*(9), 559–563.

Stetler, C. B., Morsi, D., Rucki, S., Broughton, S., Corrigan, B., Fitzgerald, J., Giuliano, K., Havener, P., & Scheridan, E. A. (1998b). Utilization-focused integrative reviews in a nursing service. *Applied Nursing Research, 11*(4), 195–206.

Stokes, J. H., Beerman, H., & Ingraham, N. R. (1944). *Modern clinical syphilology: Diagnosis, treatment, case study* (3rd ed.). Philadelphia: W.B. Saunders.

Talbert, J. L., Haslam, R. H. A., & Haller, J. A. (1967). Gangrene of the foot following intramuscular injection in the lateral thigh: A case report with recommendations for prevention. *Journal of Pediatrics, 70*(1), 110–117.

Tanner, C. A., & Lindeman, C. A. (1989). *Using nursing research.* New York: National League for Nursing.

Taylor, N., Hutchison, E., Milliken, W., & Larson, E. (1989). Comparison of normal versus heparinized saline for flushing infusion devices. *Journal of Nursing Quality Assurance, 3*(4), 49–55.

Tuten, S. H., & Gueldner, S. H. (1991). Efficacy of sodium chloride versus dilute heparin for maintenance of peripheral intermittent intravenous devices. *Applied Nursing Research, 4*(2), 63–71.

Weiss, C. J. (1980). Knowledge creep and decision accretion. *Knowledge: Creation, Diffusion, Utilization, 1*(3), 381–404.

Wichita, C. (1977). Treating and preventing constipation in nursing home residents. *Journal of Gerontological Nursing, 3*(6), 35–39.

Zelman, S. (1961). Notes on the techniques of intramuscular injection. *The American Journal of Medical Science, 241*(5), 47–58.

Zenk, K. E. (1982). Improving the accuracy of mini-volume injections. *Infusion, 6*(1), 7–12.

Zenk, K. E. (1993). Beware of overdose. *Nursing93, 23*(3), 28–29.

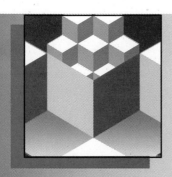

IV

SEEKING SUPPORT FOR RESEARCH ACTIVITIES

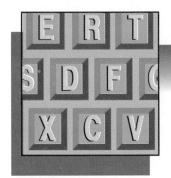

CHAPTER 28

PROPOSAL WRITING FOR RESEARCH APPROVAL

With a background in critique and utilization of research, you are ready to propose a study for implementation. A *research proposal* is a written plan that identifies the major elements of a study, such as the research problem, purpose, and framework, and outlines the methods and procedures to conduct the study. A proposal is a formal way to communicate ideas about a proposed study to receive approval for conducting the study and to seek funding. Seeking approval for the conduct or funding of a study involves submission of a research proposal to a selected group for review and, in many situations, verbally defending that proposal. Receiving approval to conduct research has become more complicated because of the increasing complexity of nursing studies, difficulty accessing subjects, and rising concern over legal and ethical issues. In many large hospitals, research proposals are reviewed by the lawyer in addition to the institutional research review committee. The expanded number of studies being conducted has led to conflict among investigators over who has the right to access potential research subjects. This chapter focuses on writing a research proposal and seeking approval to conduct a study. Chapter 29 presents the process of seeking funding for a study.

WRITING A RESEARCH PROPOSAL

A well-written proposal communicates a significant, carefully planned research project, demonstrates the qualifications of the researcher, and generates support for the project. Conducting research requires precision and rigorous attention to detail. Thus, reviewers often judge a researcher's ability to conduct a study by the quality of the proposal. A quality proposal is concise, clear, and complete (Dexter, 2000; Tornquist, 1986). Writing a quality proposal involves (1) developing ideas logically, (2) determining the depth or detail of the proposal's content, (3) identifying critical points in the proposal, and (4) developing an aesthetically appealing copy.

Developing Ideas Logically

The ideas in a research proposal must logically build on each other to justify or defend a study, just as a lawyer would logically organize information in the defense of a client. A case is built to justify why a problem should be studied, and appropriate methodology for conducting the study is proposed. Each step in the research proposal builds on the problem statement to give a clear picture of the study and its merit (Brink, 1993; Rogers, 1987). Websites have been developed to promote success in proposal writing, such as *http://www.research. umich.edu/research/proposals/proposals.html*. In addition, a variety of resources have been developed to assist individuals in improving their writing skills (American Psychological Association [APA], 1994; Dexter, 2000; Krathwohl, 1988; University of Chicago Press, 1993).

Determining the Depth of a Proposal

The depth of a proposal is determined by guidelines developed by schools of nursing, funding agencies, and institutions where research is conducted. Guidelines provide specific directions for the development of a proposal and should be followed explicitly. Omission or misinterpretation of a guideline is frequently the basis for rejection of a proposal. In addition to following the guidelines, you need to determine the amount of information necessary to describe each step of your study clearly. The content in a proposal needs to be detailed enough to inform the reader, yet concise enough to be interesting and easily reviewed. Often, the guidelines stipulate a page limit, which will determine the depth of the proposal. The relevant content of a research proposal is discussed later in this chapter.

Identifying Critical Points

The key or critical points in a proposal must be clear, even to a hasty reader. Critical points might be highlighted with bold type or underlined. Sometimes, headings are created to highlight critical content, or the content is organized into tables or graphs. Content considered to be critical in a proposal are the background and significance of the research problem; purpose; framework; research objectives, questions, or hypotheses; methodology/research design; and research production plans (data collection and analysis plan, personnel, schedule, and budget) (Brink, 1993).

Developing an Aesthetically Appealing Copy

An aesthetically appealing copy is typed without spelling, punctuation, or grammatical errors. Even a proposal with excellent content that is poorly typed or formatted will probably not receive the full attention or respect of the reviewer (Dexter, 2000). The format used in typing the proposal should follow the guidelines developed by the reviewer. If no particular format is requested, the APA (1994) format is commonly used. An appealing copy is legible (the print is dark enough to be read) and neatly organized in a folder for easy examination by the reviewer.

CONTENT OF A RESEARCH PROPOSAL

The content of a proposal is written with the interest and expertise of the reviewers in mind. Proposals are frequently reviewed by faculty, clinical agency members, and representatives of funding institutions. The content of a proposal varies with the reviewer, the guidelines developed for the review, and the type of study (quantitative or qualitative) proposed. This section addresses the content of (1) a student proposal for both quantitative and qualitative studies, (2) condensed research proposals, and (3) preproposals.

Content of a Student Proposal

Student researchers develop proposals to communicate their research projects to the faculty and members of university and agency research review committees. Student proposals are written to satisfy requirements for a degree and are usually developed according to guidelines outlined by the faculty. These guidelines are generally reviewed with the faculty member (the chair of the student's thesis or dissertation committee) who will be assisting with the research project. Each faculty member has a unique way of interpreting and emphasizing aspects of the guidelines. In addition, a student needs to evaluate the faculty member's background regarding a research topic of interest and determine whether a productive working relationship can be developed. Faculty members who are actively involved in their own research have extensive knowledge and expertise that can be helpful to a novice researcher. Both the student and the faculty member benefit when a student becomes involved in an aspect of the faculty's research. This collaborative relationship can lead to the development of essential knowledge for providing evidenced-based nursing practice.

The content of a student proposal usually requires greater detail than does a proposal developed for review by agency personnel or funding organizations. The proposal is often the first three or four chapters of the student's thesis or dissertation, and the proposed study is discussed in the future tense of what *will be* done in conducting the research. A title page, which includes the title of the proposal, name of the investigator, and the date that the proposal is submitted, and a table of contents often precede the proposal content.

CONTENT OF A QUANTITATIVE RESEARCH PROPOSAL

A quantitative research proposal usually includes the following chapters or sections: (1) introduction, (2) review of relevant literature, (3) framework, and (4) methods and procedures. Some graduate schools require an in-depth development of these sections, whereas others require a condensed version of the same content. Another approach is that proposals for theses and dissertations be written in a format that facilitates development into a publication. The content often covered in the chapters of a quantitative research proposal is outlined in Table 28–1.

Introduction

The introductory chapter identifies the research topic and problem and provides the background and significance of this problem. The background of a problem describes how the problem was identified and historically links the problem to nursing. The background information might also include one or two major studies conducted to resolve the problem, some key theoretical ideas related to the problem, and possible solutions to the problem. The significance of the problem addresses the importance of this problem in nursing practice and the expected generalizability of the findings. The interest of nurses, other health care professionals, policymakers, and health care consumers in the problem at the local, state, national, or international level is part of determining the significance of the problem. This interest can usually be documented with sources from the literature. The background and significance of the problem indicate the need for further research and are followed by a clear, concise statement of the research purpose.

Review of Relevant Literature

The review of relevant literature provides an overview of the essential information that will guide development of the study and includes relevant

---

TABLE 28–1

QUANTITATIVE RESEARCH PROPOSAL GUIDELINES FOR STUDENTS

CHAPTER I   Introduction
   A. Background and significance of the problem
   B. Statement of the problem
   C. Statement of the purpose

CHAPTER II   Review of Relevant Literature
   A. Review of relevant theoretical literature
   B. Review of relevant research
   C. Summary

CHAPTER III   Framework
   A. Development of a framework
      (Develop a map of the study framework, define concepts in the map, describe relationships in the map, indicate the focus of the study, and link concepts to study variables)
   B. Formulation of objectives, questions, or hypotheses
   C. Definitions (conceptual and operational) of research variables
   D. Definition of relevant terms
   E. Identification of assumptions

CHAPTER IV   Methods and Procedures
   A. Description of the research design
      (Model of the design, strengths and weaknesses of the design, and description of treatment if appropriate)
   B. Identification of the population and sample
      (Sample size; use of power analysis; sampling criteria; and sampling method, including strengths and weaknesses)
   C. Selection of a setting
      (Strengths and weaknesses of the setting)
   D. Presentation of ethical considerations
      (Protection of subjects' rights and review process)
   E. Selection of measurement methods
      (Reliability, validity, scoring, and level of measurement of the instruments, as well as plans for examining reliability and validity of the instruments, in the present study)
   F. Plan for data collection
      (Data collection process, data collector(s), training of data collectors if appropriate, schedule, data collection forms, and management of data)
   G. Plan for data analysis
      (Analysis of demographic data; analyses for research objectives, questions, or hypotheses; level of significance if appropriate; and other analysis techniques)
   H. Identification of limitations
      (Methodological and theoretical limitations)
   I. Discussion of communication of findings
   J. Presentation of a study budget and timetable

REFERENCES
APPENDICES

theoretical and empirical literature. The theoretical literature provides a background for defining and interrelating relevant study concepts, whereas the empirical literature includes a summary and critique of previous studies. The authors' recommendations, such as changing or expanding a study made by other researchers, are discussed in relation to the proposed study. The depth of the literature review varies and might include only recent studies and theorists' works, or it might be extensive and include a description and critique of a number of past and current studies and an in-depth discussion of theorists' works. The literature review demonstrates that the researcher has command of the current empirical and theoretical knowledge regarding the proposed problem.

This chapter concludes with a summary. The summary includes a synthesis of the theoretical literature and findings from previous research that describe the current knowledge of a problem (Pinch, 1995). Gaps in the knowledge base are also identified, with a description of how the proposed study is expected to contribute to nursing's body of knowledge.

Framework

A framework provides the basis for generating and refining the research problem and purpose and linking them to the relevant theoretical knowledge in nursing or related fields. The framework includes concepts and relationships among concepts, which are sometimes represented in a model or map. The concepts to be studied are conceptually defined and linked to the study variables. If a theorist's or researcher's model from a journal article or book is used in a proposal, letters documenting permission to use this model from the publisher and the theorist or researcher must be included in the proposal appendices.

In some studies, research objectives, questions, or hypotheses are developed to direct the study. The objectives, questions, or hypotheses evolve from the research purpose and study framework and identify the study variables. The variables are conceptually defined to show the link to the framework and operationally defined to indicate the procedures for manipulation or measurement. Other terms relevant

to the study are defined, and assumptions that provide a basis for the study are identified.

Methods and Procedures

The design or general strategy for conducting the study is described, and sometimes a diagram of the design is included. Designs for descriptive and correlational studies are flexible and can be unique to the study being conducted. Because of this uniqueness, designs need to be clearly described, including their strengths and weaknesses. Presenting a design for quasi-experimental and experimental studies involves (1) describing how the research situation will be structured, (2) detailing the treatment to be implemented, (3) describing how the effect of the treatment will be measured, (4) indicating the variables to be controlled and the methods for controlling them, (5) identifying uncontrolled extraneous variables and determining their impact on the findings, (6) describing the methods for assigning subjects to the treatment and control groups, and (7) describing the strengths and weaknesses of a design. The design needs to account for all the objectives, questions, or hypotheses identified in the proposal. If a pilot study is planned, the design should include the procedure for conducting the pilot and for incorporating the results into the proposed study.

The proposal identifies the population to which the study findings will be generalized and the target population from which the sample will be selected. The criteria for selecting a subject and the rationale for these criteria are presented. For example, a subject might be selected according to the following criteria: female aged 20 to 50 years, hospitalized for 2 days, and 1 day after abdominal surgery. The rationale for these criteria might be that the researcher wants to examine the effects of selected pain management interventions on adult females who have recently experienced hospitalization and abdominal surgery. The sampling method and the approximate sample size are discussed in terms of their adequacy and limitations in investigating the research purpose. Usually, a power analysis is conducted to determine an adequate sample size.

A proposal includes a description of the study setting, which frequently includes the name of the agency and the structure of the units or sites where the study is to be conducted. The setting is often identified in the proposal but not in the final research report. The agency selected should have the potential to generate the type and size of sample required for the study. Thus, the proposal usually includes the number of individuals who meet the sample criteria and are cared for by the agency in a given period. In addition, the structure and activities in the agency need to be able to accommodate the proposed design of the study.

Ethical considerations in a proposal include the rights of the subjects and the rights of the agency where the study is to be conducted. Protection of subjects' rights and the risks and potential benefits of the study are described. The steps taken to reduce study risks also need to be addressed. Many agencies require a written consent form, and that form is often included in the appendices of the proposal. The risks and potential benefits of the study for the institution also need to be addressed (Fullwood et al., 1999). If the study places the agency at risk, the steps that will be taken to reduce or eliminate these risks are outlined. The researcher also indicates that the proposal will be reviewed by the thesis or dissertation committee, university human rights review committee, and agency research review committee.

The methods for measuring study variables are described, including each instrument's reliability, validity, methods of scoring, and level of measurement. A plan for examining the reliability and validity of the instruments in the present study needs to be addressed. If an instrument has no reported reliability and validity, a pilot study is usually conducted to examine these qualities. If the intent of the proposed study is to develop an instrument, the process of instrument development is described. A copy of the interview questions, questionnaires, scales, physiological instruments, or other tools to be used in the study is usually included in the proposal appendices. Permission to use copyrighted instruments must be obtained from the authors, and letters documenting that permission has been obtained are included in the proposal appendices.

The data collection plan clarifies what data are to be collected and the process for collecting the data.

In this plan, the data collectors are identified, data collection procedures are described, and a schedule is presented for data collection activities. If more than one person will be involved in data collection, the training of data collectors to ensure consistency is described. The method of recording data is often described, and sample data recording sheets are placed in the proposal appendices. Any special equipment that will be used or developed to collect data for the study is also discussed, and data security is usually addressed, including the methods of data storage.

The plan for data analysis identifies the analysis techniques to be used for summarizing the demographic data and answering the research objectives, questions, or hypotheses. The analysis section is often organized according to these same study objectives, questions, or hypotheses. The analysis techniques identified need to be appropriate for the type of data collected. For example, if an associative hypothesis is developed, correlational analysis must be planned. If a researcher plans to determine differences among groups, the analysis techniques might include a t test or analysis of variance (Munro, 1997). A level of significance ($\alpha = .05$, .01, or .001) is also identified. Often, a researcher projects the type of results that will be generated from data analysis. Dummy tables, graphs, and charts can then be developed for the presentation of these results and included in the proposal appendices. The investigator might also project the possible findings for a study. For example, the researcher might consider what support or nonsupport of a proposed hypothesis would mean in light of the study framework and previous research findings. Projecting a study's findings facilitates logical examination of the findings when the study is complete.

The methods and procedures chapter of a proposal usually concludes with a discussion of the study's limitations and a plan for communication of the findings. Both methodological and theoretical limitations are addressed. Methodological limitations might include areas of weakness in the design, sampling method, sample size, measurement tools, data collection procedures, or data analysis techniques, whereas theoretical limitations set boundaries for the generalization of study findings. For example, the accuracy with which the conceptual definitions and relational statements in a theory reflect reality has a direct impact on the generalization of findings. Theory that has withstood frequent testing provides a stronger framework for the interpretation and generalization of findings. A plan is included for communication of the research through presentations and publications to audiences of nurses, other health professionals, policymakers, and health care consumers.

Frequently, a budget and timetable are included in the proposal appendices. The budget projects the expenses for the study, which might include the cost for data collection tools and procedures, special equipment, consultants for data analysis, computer time, travel related to data collection and analysis, typing, copying, and developing, presenting, and publishing the final report. Funded study budgets frequently include investigators' salaries and secretarial costs. A timetable is needed to direct the steps of the research project and facilitate completion of the project on schedule. A timetable identifies the tasks to be done, who will accomplish these tasks, and when these tasks will be completed.

CONTENT OF A QUALITATIVE RESEARCH PROPOSAL

A qualitative research proposal might include some content similar to that of a quantitative proposal, but the guidelines are usually more flexible and abstract to accommodate the still-emerging design of the study. A qualitative proposal usually includes the following sections or chapters: (1) introduction, (2) research paradigm, (3) research methods, and (4) preliminary findings, limitations, and plans for communication of the study findings (Heath, 1997; Munhall & Boyd, 1999; Sandelowski et al., 1989). Determination of the quality of the proposal is based on the potential scientific contribution of the research to nursing knowledge, the research paradigm guiding the study, the research methods, and the knowledge, skills, and resources available to the investigators (Cohen et al., 1993).

Guidelines for a qualitative research proposal are outlined in Table 28–2.

Introduction

The introduction usually provides a general background for the proposed study by identifying the phenomenon to be investigated and linking this phenomenon to nursing knowledge. The general purpose of the study is identified and indicates the type of qualitative study to be conducted. The purpose is often followed by research questions or aims that direct the investigation (Parse et al.,

---

TABLE 28–2
QUALITATIVE RESEARCH PROPOSAL GUIDELINES FOR STUDENTS

Chapter I. Introduction
  A. Identify the phenomenon to be studied
  B. Identify the study purpose and type of qualitative study
  C. State the study questions or aims
  D. Discuss the study significance
Chapter II. Research Paradigm
  A. Identify the research paradigm for the type of qualitative study to be conducted
  B. Describe the philosophical correlates of the research paradigm
  C. Explain the research assumptions
Chapter III. Research Methods
  A. Demonstrate the researcher's credentials for conducting a particular type of qualitative study
  B. Identify the research method for the study
  C. Select a site and population
  D. Describe the researcher's role
    1. Entry into the site
    2. Selection of informants
    3. Ethical considerations
  E. Detail the data collection process
  F. Describe the data analysis techniques
  G. Plan to document the research process during the study
Chapter IV. Preliminary Findings, Limitations, and Plans for Communication of the Study
  A. Summarize and reference relevant literature as appropriate for the type of qualitative study
  B. Identify biases and previous experiences with research problem
  C. Disclose anticipated findings, hypotheses, and hunches
  D. Discuss procedures to remain open to unexpected information
  E. Discuss limitations of the study
  F. Identify plans for communication of findings
REFERENCES
APPENDICES
  Present the study budget and timetable

1985). These questions or aims focus on real-world problems and dilemmas, such as the following: How do people cope with a new diagnosis of chronic illness? What is it like to live with a chronic illness for 5 or more years? What type of support exists for a person with a chronic illness? What is the impact on the family? An aim might be to describe the burden of the caregiver role in a family with a chronically ill member.

The introduction also includes the significance of the proposed study to practice and policy, as well as the potential contribution that the study will make to nursing knowledge. The discussion of the study's significance often includes how the problem developed, who or what is affected by the problem, and how costly the problem is. Whenever possible, the significance of a study needs to be documented from the literature. Marshall and Rossman (1999) identified the following questions to assess the significance of a study: (1) Who has an interest in this domain of inquiry? (2) What do we already know about the topic? (3) What has not been answered adequately in previous research and practice? and (4) How will this research add to knowledge, practice, and policy in this area? The introduction section concludes with an overview of the remaining sections that are covered in the proposal.

Research Paradigm

This section introduces the reader to the conceptual foundation for qualitative research and addresses the importance of this method of inquiry to the generation of nursing knowledge. Research paradigms vary in qualitative research and may include naturalistic, post-positivism, feminism, and postmodernism types (Miller, 1997). If the reader is familiar with qualitative research, this section can be reduced to the essential elements of philosophy and assumptions of the specific type of qualitative study to be conducted. Because the philosophy varies for the different types of qualitative research (see Chapter 4), the philosophical foundation for the proposed study needs to be described. For example, a phenomenological study might include a discussion of hermeneutics with documentation of appropriate theorists' works. Assumptions about the na-

ture of the knowledge and the reality that underlie the type of qualitative research to be conducted are also identified. The assumptions and philosophy provide a theoretical perspective for the study that influences the focus of the study, data collection and analysis, and articulation of the findings.

Research Methods

Developing and implementing the methodology of qualitative research require a certain expertise that some believe can only be obtained through a mentorship relationship with an experienced qualitative researcher. The role of the researcher and the intricate techniques of data collection and analysis are thought to be best communicated through a one-to-one relationship. Thus, planning the methods of a qualitative study requires knowledge of relevant sources that describe the different qualitative research techniques and procedures (Chenitz & Swanson, 1986; Leininger, 1985; Marshall & Rossman, 1999; Miles & Huberman, 1994; Munhall & Boyd, 1999; Parse et al., 1985), in addition to requiring interaction with a qualitative researcher. The proposal needs to reflect the researcher's credentials for conducting the particular type of qualitative study proposed.

Identifying the methods for conducting a qualitative study is a difficult task because the design of the study is still emerging. Unlike quantitative research, in which the design is a fixed blueprint for a study, the design in qualitative research emerges or evolves as the study is conducted. Thus the researcher must document the logic and appropriateness of the qualitative method and develop a tentative plan for conducting the study. Because this plan is tentative, the researcher reserves the right to modify or change the plan at any point during conduct of the study (Sandelowski et al., 1989). However, the design or plan must be consistent with the study aims, be well conceived, and address prior criticism, as appropriate (Cohen et al., 1993). The tentative plan describes the process for selecting a site and population. The site will allow the researcher entry and will include the subjects necessary to answer the research questions or aims. For the research question "How do individuals cope with a new diagnosis of chronic illness?" the subjects might be identified in hospitals, clinics, practitioners' offices, home care organizations, or rehabilitation facilities, and data collection might be conducted in the subjects' homes.

The methods section includes a detailed description of the proposed researcher's role. The researcher must gain entry into the setting, develop a rapport with the subjects that will facilitate the detailed data collection process, and protect the rights of the subjects (Marshall & Rossman, 1999; Sandelowski et al., 1989). The following questions are addressed in describing the researcher's role: (1) What is the best setting for the study? (2) How will the researcher ease his or her entry into the research site? (3) How will the researcher gain access to the subjects? (4) What actions will the researcher take to facilitate participation and cooperation of the subjects? and (5) What precautions will be taken to protect the rights of the subjects and to prevent the setting and the subjects from being harmed? The process of obtaining informed consent and the actions planned by the researcher to decrease study risks need to be described. The sensitive nature of some qualitative studies increases the risk for subjects, which makes ethical concerns and decisions a major focus of the study.

The primary data collection techniques used in qualitative research are observation and in-depth interviewing. Observations can range from highly detailed, structured notations of behavior to ambiguous descriptions of behavior or events. The interview can also have a range from structured, closed-ended questions to unstructured open-ended questions (Heath, 1997; Marshall & Rossman, 1999). The following questions are addressed when developing a description of the proposed data collection process: (1) Who will collect data and provide any training required for the data collectors? (2) What data will be collected? For example, will the data be field notes from memory, audiotapes of interviews, transcripts of conversations, videotapes of events, or examination of existing documents? (3) What techniques or procedures will be used to collect the data? For example, if interviews are to be conducted, a list of the proposed questions might be attached in the appendix. In historical research,

data are collected through an exhaustive review of published and unpublished literature. (4) What is the anticipated length of time needed to collect data?

The methods section also needs to address how the researcher will document the research process of the study. For example, the researcher might keep progress notes during the course of the study. These notes document the day-to-day activities, methodological events, decision-making procedures, and personal notes about the informants. This information becomes part of the audit trail that is provided to ensure the quality of the study (Heath, 1997).

The methods section of the proposal also includes the analysis techniques and the steps for conducting these techniques. In qualitative research, data collection and analysis often occur simultaneously. The data are in the form of notes, tapes, and other material obtained from observation and interviews. Through qualitative analysis techniques, these data are structured and reduced to determine meaning (Burns, 1989; Miles & Huberman, 1994). Strategies to ensure the credibility, fittingness, and auditability of the findings need to be addressed (Beck, 1993). These qualitative terms are related to the concepts of reliability and validity used in quantitative research and are addressed in Chapter 26. Qualitative analysis techniques are the focus of Chapter 23.

Preliminary Findings, Limitations, and Plans for Communication of the Study

This section of the proposal summarizes and documents all relevant literature that was reviewed for the study. Some qualitative studies involve a literature review before conducting the study. For example, ethnographic research requires a literature review to provide a background for conducting the study, as in quantitative research. Historical research involves a literature review to develop research questions, as does philosophical inquiry to raise philosophical questions. The literature review needs to provide a basis for the aims of the study and clearly indicate how this study will expand nursing knowledge (Cohen et al., 1993).

In phenomenological research, grounded theory research, and critical social theory, the literature review is usually conducted at the end of the research project. The findings from a phenomenological study are compared and combined with findings from the literature to determine current knowledge of the phenomenon. In grounded theory research, the literature is used to explain, support, and extend the theory generated in the study. Study findings obtained through critical social theory are examined in light of the existing literature to determine the current knowledge of a social situation (see Chapter 6).

The researcher needs to describe how the literature reviewed has influenced the proposed research methods. Biases and previous experience with the research problem need to be addressed, as does their potential impact on the proposed study. Often, anticipated findings, hypotheses, and hunches are identified before conduct of the study, followed by a discussion of the procedures that might be used to remain open to new information. Limitations of the study need to be addressed in the context of limitations of similar studies.

The proposal concludes with a description of how the findings will be communicated to a variety of audiences through presentations and publications. Often, a realistic budget and timetable are provided in the appendix. A qualitative study budget is similar to a quantitative study budget and includes costs for data collection tools and procedures, consultants for data analysis, travel related to data collection and analysis, typing, copying, and developing, presenting, and publishing the final report. However, the greatest expenditure in qualitative research is usually the researcher's time. A timetable is developed to project how long the study will take, and often 2 years or more is designated for data collection and analysis (Marshall & Rossman, 1999). The budget and timetable can be used to make decisions regarding funding inasmuch as funding is essential for many qualitative studies.

Content of a Condensed Proposal

The content of proposals developed for review by clinical agencies and funding institutions is usually a condensed version of the student proposal. However, even though these proposals are condensed, the logical links between components of the study need to be clearly demonstrated. A condensed proposal often includes a statement of the problem and purpose; previous research that has been conducted in the area (usually limited to no more than three to five studies); the framework, variables, design, sample, ethical considerations, and plans for data collection and analysis; and plans for dissemination of findings.

A proposal submitted to a clinical agency needs to identify the specific setting clearly, such as the emergency room or intensive care unit, as well as the projected time span for the study. Members of clinical agencies are particularly interested in the data collection process and involvement of institutional personnel in the study. Any expected disruptions in institutional functioning need to be identified, with plans for preventing these disruptions when possible. The researcher must recognize that anything that slows down or disrupts employee functioning costs the agency money and can interfere with the quality of patient care. Indications in the proposal that the researcher is aware of these concerns and has addressed ways to minimize their effect will increase the probability of obtaining approval to conduct the study.

A variety of companies, corporations, and organizations provide funding for research projects. A proposal developed for these types of funding institutions frequently includes a brief description of the study, the significance of the study to the institution, a timetable, and a budget. Most of these proposals are brief and might contain a one-page summary sheet or abstract at the beginning of the proposal that summarizes the steps of the study. The salient points of the study are included on this page in simple, easy-to-read, nontechnical terminology. Some proposal reviewers for funding institutions are laypersons with no background in research or nursing. An inability to understand the terminology might put the reviewer on the defensive or create a negative reaction, which could lead to disapproval of the study. When multiple studies are examined by funding institutions, the summary sheet is often the basis for final decisions about the study. The summary should be concise, informative, and designed to sell the study.

In proposals for both clinical and funding agencies, investigators need to document their research background and supply a curriculum vitae if requested. The research review committee for approval or funding will be interested in previous research, research publications, and clinical expertise, especially if a clinical study is proposed. If the researcher is a graduate student, the committee may request the names of the university committee members and verification that the proposal has been approved by the student's thesis or dissertation committee and the university human subjects review committee.

Content of a Preproposal

Sometimes a researcher will send a preproposal or query letter rather than a proposal to a funding institution. A *preproposal* is a short document of four to five pages plus appendices that is written to explore the funding possibilities for a research project. The parts of the preproposal are logically ordered as follows: "(1) letter of transmittal, (2) proposal for research, (3) personnel, (4) facilities, and (5) budget" (Malasanos, 1976, p. 223). The proposal provides a brief overview of the proposed project, including the research problem, purpose, methodology (brief description), and most important, a statement of the significance of the work to knowledge in general and the funding institution in particular. By developing a preproposal, researchers are able to determine the agencies interested in funding their study and limit submission of their proposals to only institutions that indicate an interest.

SEEKING APPROVAL FOR A STUDY

Initially, proposal reviews were limited to graduate students developing theses or dissertations and researchers seeking grant money. However, as a consequence of stricter rules related to the protection of human subjects, most nursing studies will be reviewed by at least one research committee. *Seeking approval to conduct a study* is an action that should be based on knowledge and guided by purpose. Obtaining approval for a study from a research committee requires understanding the approval process, writing a research proposal for review, and in many cases, verbally defending the

proposal. Little has been written to provide guidance to a researcher who is going through the labyrinth of approval mechanisms. The intent of this section is to provide a background for obtaining approval to conduct a study.

Clinical agencies and health care corporations review studies for the following reasons: (1) to evaluate the quality of the study, (2) to ensure that adequate measures are being taken to protect human subjects, and (3) to evaluate the impact of conducting the study on the reviewing institution (Fullwood et al., 1999). The desired outcomes from a review by an institution are to receive approval to collect data at the reviewing institution and to obtain support for the proposed study.

Approval Process

An initial step in seeking approval is to determine exactly what committees in which agencies must grant approval before the study can be conducted. Researchers need to take the initiative to determine the formal approval process rather than assume that they will be told if a formal review system exists. Information on the formal research review system might be obtained from administrative personnel, special projects or grant officers, chairs of research review committees in clinical agencies, clinicians who have previously conducted research, and university faculty who are involved in research.

Graduate students usually require approval from their thesis or dissertation committee, the university human subjects review committee, and the research committee in the agency where the data are to be collected. University faculty conducting research seek approval through the latter two committees. Nurses conducting research in an agency where they are employed must seek approval only at that agency. If outside funding is sought, additional review committees are involved. Not all studies require full review by the human subjects review committee (see Chapter 9 for the types of studies that qualify for exempt or expedited review). However, the review committee makes the decision about the type of review that the study requires for conduct in that agency.

When multiple committees must review a study,

sometimes an agreement is made, by the respective committees, that review for the protection of human subjects will be done by only one of the committees, with the findings of that committee generally being accepted by the other committees. For example, if the university human subjects review committee reviewed and approved a proposal for the protection of human subjects, funding agencies usually recognize that review as sufficient. Reviews in other committees are then focused on approval to conduct the study within the institution or decisions to provide study funding.

As part of the approval process, the researcher must determine the agency's policy regarding (1) use of the clinical facility's name in reporting findings, (2) presentation and publication of the study, and (3) authorship of publications. The facility's name is used when presenting or publishing a study only with prior written administrative approval. The researcher may feel more free to report findings that could be interpreted negatively in terms of the institution if the agency is not identified. Some institutions have rules about presenting and publishing a study that limit what is presented or published, where it is presented or published, and who is the presenter or author. Before conducting a study, researchers, especially employees of agencies, must clarify the rules and regulations of the agency regarding authorship, presentations, and publications. In some cases, recognition of these rules must be included in the proposal if it is to be approved.

Preparing Proposals for Review Committees

The initial proposals for theses and dissertations are often developed as part of a formal class. The faculty teaching the class provide students with specific proposal guidelines approved by the graduate faculty and assist them in developing their initial proposals. If students elect to conduct a thesis, they ask an appropriate faculty member to serve as chair. With the chair's assistance, the student identifies committee members who will work together to refine the final proposal. This proposal requires approval by the thesis or dissertation committee and the university human rights review committee.

Conducting research in a clinical agency requires approval by the institutional research committee. This committee has the responsibility to (1) provide researchers with copies of institutional policies and requirements, (2) screen proposals for conducting research in the agency, and (3) assist the researcher with the institutional review board process (Vessey & Campos, 1992). The approval process policy and proposal guidelines are usually available from the chair of the research committee. Guidelines established by the committee should be followed carefully, particularly page limitations. Some committees refuse to review proposals that exceed these limitations. Reviewers on these committees are usually evaluating proposals in addition to other full-time responsibilities, and their time is limited.

Investigators also need to be familiar with the research committee's process for screening proposals. Most agency research committees screen proposals for (1) scientific merit, (2) protection of human rights, (3) congruence of the study with the agency's research agenda, and (4) impact of the study on patient care (Vessey & Campos, 1992). Researchers need to develop their proposal with these ideas in mind. They also need to determine whether the committee requires specific forms to be completed and submitted with the research proposal. Other important information can be gathered by addressing the following questions: (1) How often does the committee meet? (2) How long before the next meeting? (3) What materials should be submitted before the meeting? (4) When should these materials be submitted? (5) How many copies of the proposal are required? and (6) What period of time is usually involved in committee review?

Social and Political Factors

Social and political factors play an important role in obtaining approval to conduct a study. The researcher needs to treat the review process with as much care as development of the study. The dynamics of the relationships among committee members is important to assess. This detail is especially important in the selection of a thesis or dissertation committee so that the members selected are willing to work together productively.

Thorough assessment of the social and political situation in which the study will be reviewed and implemented may be crucial to success of the study. Agency research committees may include nurse clinicians who have never conducted research, nurse researchers, and researchers in other disciplines. The reactions of each of these groups to a study could be very different. Sometimes committees are made up primarily of physicians, which is frequently the case in health science centers. Physicians are often not oriented to nursing research methods. The lack of control in nursing studies concerns them, and some believe that the topics of these studies are not important. Sometimes they do not see the nurse researcher as credible because of educational differences, lack of previous experience in research, and few published studies. However, not all physicians view nursing research negatively. Many are strong supporters of nursing research, helpful in suggesting changes in design to strengthen the study, and eager to facilitate access to subjects.

The researcher needs to anticipate potential responses of committee members, prepare the proposal to elicit a favorable response, and consider means of minimizing negative responses. It is wise to meet with the chair of the agency research committee early in the development of a proposal. This meeting could facilitate proposal development, rapport between the researcher and agency personnel, and approval of the research proposal.

In addition to the formal committee approval mechanisms, the researcher will need the tacit approval of the administrative personnel and staff who will be affected in some way by the study. Obtaining informal approval and support often depends on the way in which a person is approached. The researcher needs to demonstrate interest in the institution and the personnel, as well as interest in the research project. The relationships formed with agency personnel should be equal, sharing ones because these people can often provide ideas and strategies for conducting the study that never occurred to the researcher. Support of agency personnel during data collection can also make the difference between a successful or unsuccessful study (Fullwood, et al., 1999).

Conducting nursing research can provide benefits to the institution, as well as to the researcher. Clinicians have an opportunity to see nursing research in action, which can influence their thinking and clinical practice if the relationship with the researcher is positive. These clinicians may be having their first close contact with a researcher, and interpretation of the researcher's role and the study may be necessary. In addition, clinicians tend to be more oriented in the present than researchers are, and they need to see the possible immediate impact that the study findings can have on nursing practice in their institution. Thus, utilization of research findings may be enhanced, and clinicians may even become involved in research activities (Fullwood, et al., 1999). All these activities can add prestige to an institution.

Verbal Defense of a Proposal

Graduate students writing theses or dissertations are frequently required to defend their proposal verbally to their university committee members. Some institutions also require the researcher to meet with the research committee or a subcommittee to defend a proposal. In a verbal defense, reviewers can evaluate the researcher as a person, the researcher's knowledge and understanding of the content of the proposal, and his or her ability to reason and provide logical explanations related to the study. The researcher also has the opportunity to persuade reluctant committee members to approve the study.

Appearance is important in a personal presentation because it can give an impression of competence or incompetence. These presentations are business-like, with logical and rational interactions, so one should dress in a business-like manner. Individuals who are casually dressed might be perceived by the committee as not valuing the review process.

Nonverbal behavior is important during the meeting as well, so appearing calm, in control, and confident projects a positive image. Planning and rehearsing a presentation can reduce anxiety. Obtaining information on the personalities of committee members, their relationships with each other, the vested interests of each member, and their areas of expertise can increase confidence and provide a sense of control. It is important to arrive at the meeting early, assess the environment for the meeting, and carefully select a seat. As the presenter, all members of the committee need to be able to see you. However, selecting a seat on one side of a table with all the committee members on the other side could feel uncomfortable and simulate an atmosphere similar to that of an interrogation rather than a scholarly interaction. Sitting at the side of a table rather than at the head might be a strategic move to elicit support.

The verbal defense usually begins with a brief presentation of the study. The presentation needs to be carefully planned, timed, and rehearsed. Salient points should be highlighted, which can be accomplished by the use of audiovisuals. The presentation is followed by questions from the reviewers, and the researcher needs to be prepared to defend or justify the methods and procedures of the study. Sometimes it is helpful to practice responding to questions related to the study with a friend as a means of determining the best way to defend ideas without appearing defensive. When the meeting has ended, the researcher should thank the members of the committee for their time. If a decision regarding the study has not been made during the meeting, ask when the committee will make a decision.

Revising a Proposal

Reviewers sometimes suggest changes in a proposal; however, some of these changes may be of benefit to the institution but not to the study. In these situations, try to remain receptive to the suggestions, explore with the committee the impact of the changes on the proposed study, and try to resolve the conflict. If the conflict cannot be resolved, the researcher might need to find another setting.

Many times reviewers make valuable suggestions that might improve the quality of a study or facilitate the data collection process. Revision of the proposal is often based on these suggestions before the study is implemented. Sometimes a study requires revision while it is being conducted because of problems with data collection tools or subjects' participation. However, if a proposal has been approved by clinical agency personnel or representatives of funding institutions, the researcher needs to examine the situation seriously before making major changes in the study.

Before revising a proposal, a researcher needs to address three questions: (1) What needs to be changed? (2) Why is the change necessary? and (3) How will the change affect implementation of the study and the study findings? (Diers, 1979). Students need to seek advice from the faculty before revising their studies. Sometimes it is beneficial for seasoned researchers to discuss their proposed study changes with other researchers or agency personnel for suggestions and additional viewpoints.

If a revision is necessary, the researcher should revise the proposal and discuss the change with members of the research committee in the agency where the study is being conducted. The committee members might indicate that the investigators can proceed with the study or that they will have to seek approval for the revised proposal. If a study is funded, the study changes must be discussed with the representatives of the funding agency. The funding agency has the power to approve or disapprove the changes. However, realistic changes that are clearly described and backed with a rationale will probably be approved.

SAMPLE QUANTITATIVE RESEARCH PROPOSAL

A proposal of a quantitative study is provided to direct students in the development of their first research proposal. The proposal was developed by a thesis student to conduct a quasi-experimental study (Ulbrich, 1995). The content of this proposal is very brief and does not include the detail normally presented in a thesis or dissertation.

. . . .

Title: **THE EFFECT OF OPERATOR TECHNIQUE ON TYMPANIC MEMBRANE THERMOMETRY**
Investigator: Sherri L. Ulbrich

CHAPTER 1

Introduction

Temperatures are used to monitor and diagnose infection, inflammation, neoplasia, neurological insults, hypothermia, hyperthermia, and metabolic disorders (Wolff, 1988). Accurate assessment of the body's thermal responses can provide information that results in prompt treatment and may prevent further injury, especially in acute care settings. The tympanic thermometer assesses body temperature by measuring the infrared radiation emitted from the tympanic membrane. Clinical studies have shown the tympanic thermometer to be extremely useful when compared with oral and rectal thermometers (Terndrup, 1992). However, some experts doubt the thermometer's ability to detect fever and others note cases of large differences between tympanic and other core temperature routes (Zinder & Holtel, 1995). Consequently, some health care providers are skeptical about tympanic measurements and adoption in the clinical setting has been delayed.

Some of the skepticism arises from inconsistent measurements and unanswered questions about the technique to be used with tympanic thermometers. Though technique is critical in producing accurate measurements of all vital signs including temperature, little is known about how to best use the tympanic thermometer. Information regarding the operation of this device from the manufacturer and clinical studies is conflicting. In addition, many sources fail to give specific descriptions of operator techniques or only make limited comparisons of these techniques. Currently, few tympanic thermometer technique studies have been conducted on adults (Erickson & Meyer, 1994). If a single, accurate technique for taking tympanic temperatures could be determined, patients and health care providers might benefit from the many advantages of this safe, efficient, and less invasive temperature device. Thus, the purpose of this study is to examine the effects of operator techniques on the measurement of tympanic temperatures in adult critical care patients. This information can be used to develop a research-based protocol, expand the knowledge base about tympanic thermometry, and help meet the demand for better assessment of temperature in critically ill patients.

CHAPTER 2

Review of Relevant Literature

Temperature measurement is an important nursing assessment, especially in critically ill patients. Changes in temperature are physiological cues,

when accurately assessed, that can lead to prompt, effective treatment (Bruce & Grove, 1991; Holtzclaw, 1992). Temperature can be measured by many routes and instruments. The specifications for the development of tympanic thermometers were congruent with the principles and theories in physics, engineering (Fraden, 1991), and physiology.

Research has shown that tympanic thermometers are accurate in healthy and ill patients of all ages in a variety of clinical and hospital settings, except in the cases of inconsistent or poor operator technique (Terndrup, 1992), exposure to low or high ambient temperatures within 20 minutes of measurement (Doyle, Zehner, & Terndrup, 1992; Zehner & Terndrup, 1991), and near complete occlusion of the tympanic membrane by cerumen or severe scarring (Pransky, 1991). Having otitis media, small or moderate amounts of cerumen, and small ear canals in children do not cause significant differences in temperature. Studies have shown tympanic temperatures to be at least as accurate as oral and rectal temperatures and much more accurate than axillary temperatures (Erickson & Yount, 1991; Schmitz, Bair, Falk, & Levine, 1995). However, tympanic temperatures are not as accurate as bladder or pulmonary artery temperatures (Erickson & Meyer, 1994; Milewski, Ferguson, & Terndrup, 1991; Nierman, 1991; Summers, 1991), especially in detecting fever (Zinder & Holtel, 1995). Tympanic thermometers are also less invasive and more time and cost efficient (Alexander & Kelly, 1991a); do not transmit infectious agents among patients (Livornese, Dias, & Samuel, 1992); preserve the patient's modesty; and produce minimal discomfort (Alexander & Kelly, 1991b).

The effect of operator technique on tympanic measurements needs to be investigated carefully. Determining the optimal technique could reduce erroneous and inconsistent measurements in future research and clinical practice (Erickson & Meyer, 1994; Erickson & Woo, 1994; Guthrie & Keunke, 1992; Pransky, 1991). Three elements in tympanic measurement technique have been identified: (1) an eartug to straighten the auditory canal; (2) aiming at the tympanic membrane; and (3) making a snug seal. Additional research is needed that provides control of extraneous variables, use of a core reference temperature, and use of consistent and meaningful analyses for comparison. Multiple techniques have not been previously studied to identify the aspects of technique or combination of techniques that are essential for obtaining the most accurate tympanic temperature measurement. The current study is proposed to expand the knowledge base related to the effects of operator technique on tympanic temperature measurements in critically ill adults. The information obtained from this study can assist nurses in comparing tympanic temperatures with those obtained through bladder or other core temperature routes. (To promote concise coverage of this proposal, only a summary of the theoretical and empirical literature was provided.)

CHAPTER 3

Framework

Thermometry is the science of temperature measurement (Schooley, 1986) and provides the framework for this study. As shown in [Figure 28–1], a linear path of unimpeded heat transfer between the heat source and the thermometer system response results in a temperature measurement under ideal conditions of thermometry. However, in reality, physiological, mechanical, and environmental factors, as well as instrumental error must be controlled or manipulated to facilitate the transfer of

heat and ensure accuracy of the measurement. The extent to which each of these complex factors affects the transfer of heat and temperature measurement has not yet been fully determined. The extent to which operator technique can effectively manipulate or control these factors and influence the transfer of heat to promote optimal accuracy of the thermometer is also unknown.

In this study, the heat sources are the tympanic membrane and urinary bladder. Bladder temperature will be used as the reference core temperature and represents the ideal, accurate temperature measurement. The difference between tympanic temperatures measured using different operator techniques and the accepted standard of measured bladder temperature is the dependent variable in this study. Heat transfer between the heat sources and the thermometer system response occurred by radiation with the tympanic thermometer and conduction with the bladder thermometer. Operator technique is shown in bold face type because it is the concept that represents the independent variables in this study. The three components of operator technique are otoscopic eartug, aim, and seal when using tympanic thermometers. Combinations of these components are the independent variables and will be used to provide additional control over physiological and mechanical factors and thus in-

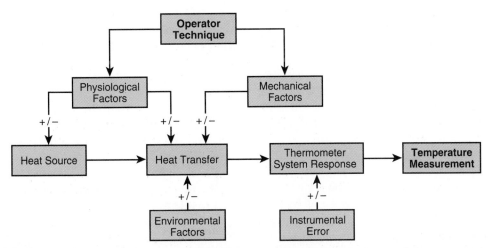

FIGURE 28–1 ■ Thermometry framework. (From Ulbrich, S. L. [1995]. *The effect of operator technique on tympanic membrane thermometry.* Unpublished master's thesis. The University of Texas at Arlington.

fluence the transfer of heat and subsequently, the temperature measurement.

Hypothesis

There is no clinically important difference in tympanic temperature measurements using four operator techniques: (1) an otoscopic eartug with aim and seal, (2) an otoscopic eartug and seal without aim, (3) aim and seal without otoscopic eartug, and (4) seal without otoscopic eartug or aim when compared with bladder temperatures taken in critically ill adults.

Definitions of Independent Variables

Operator Techniques for Tympanic Temperatures

Conceptual definition. Operator techniques are actions used by persons when taking temperatures that affect the physiological and mechanical factors and subsequently influence heat transfer and tympanic temperature measurement.

Operational definition. Each of the combined techniques for taking tympanic temperatures listed in the hypotheses is considered to be a single independent variable. The separate elements of each technique are operationally defined as follows: ▪

Otoscopic eartug is the manipulation of the cartilaginous outer portion of the ear by grasping the auricle firmly but gently, pulling it upward, back, and slightly out in order to straighten the elliptical S-shaped outer canal and improve the view of the lower ear canal and tympanic membrane (Bates, 1983; Erickson & Meyer, 1994).

Aim is aligning the warmest area of the tympanic membrane, the anterior, inferior third, with the tympanic thermometer sensor tip by holding the device level while directing the tip of the probe at the midpoint between the ear and the outer canthus of the eye on the opposite side (Terndrup, 1992).

Seal is leaving no space between the walls of the auditory canal and the covered probe tip by placing the probe tip in the opening of the ear canal and applying gentle but firm pressure to seal the canal from ambient air (Erickson & Yount, 1991).

Definitions of the Dependent Variables

Bladder Temperature

Conceptual definition. Bladder temperature is the approximation of core body heat reflected in the amount of heat in the bladder (Erickson & Meyer, 1994).

Operational definition. Bladder temperature is the numerical measurement of heat in the bladder as detected by Bard thermocath and displayed by Bard and Hewlett Packard monitors using a Fahrenheit scale to the nearest tenth of a degree.

Tympanic Temperature

Conceptual definition. Tympanic temperature is the amount of heat from the tympanic membrane as detected in the auditory canal. This temperature is used as an indicator of core temperature because of its proximity and shared common blood supply with the hypothalamic thermoregulatory center (Fraden, 1991).

Operational definition. Tympanic temperature is the numerical measurement of temperature as determined and displayed by the infrared tympanic thermometer Genius 3000A Model using the Fahrenheit scale to the nearest tenth of a degree. ▪

Attribute Variables

The attribute or demographic variables of this study are age; race; gender; admitting diagnosis to the intensive care unit (ICU); other significant diagnoses or complications; temperature changes in the previous four hours; history of carotid artery disease, stroke, head trauma, or cranial surgery; cranial turban dressing; and type of supplemental oxygenation.

Relevant Terms

Adult is a person over the age of 18 years.
Intensive care is a part of the hospital that deals specifically with life-threatening health problems (American Association of Critical Care Nurses, 1984).

Assumptions

1. Temperature measurement is important in patient care.

2. Accurately measuring temperature is an important nursing responsibility.
3. The optimal thermometer is accurate, precise, safe, efficient, and noninvasive.

CHAPTER 4

Methods and Procedures

This chapter identifies the design, setting, sample, methods of measurement, data collection and analysis plan, and limitations for this proposed study. For conciseness, the key ideas of these sections are presented but not in the detail that usually is included in a thesis.

Design

This study's design is quasi-experimental and includes multiple treatments with nonequivalent dependent variables (see [Figure 28–2]). An attempt will be made to control the carryover effect of the treatments by changing treatment order for each subject (Burns & Grove, 1997). Efforts will be made to control the extraneous variables of environmental temperature, condition of the ear and tympanic membrane, age, activity level, and diurnal effects. A plan was developed for controlling and/or recording essential information regarding each of these extraneous variables.

A protocol was developed to ensure the consistent implementation of the four treatments: tug with aim, tug without aim, aim without tug, and no tug and no aim (see [Appendix 28-A]). The seal is considered essential and will be achieved with all four treatments. The investigator will implement all treatments and obtain and record all measurements according to protocol to ensure consistency. A pilot study will be conducted on five subjects to assess the technique administration, determine the adequacy of the treatment protocol, and discover problems in data collection. Any problems noted in the design and data collection process for the study will be examined and modified as needed.

Setting and Sample

The data will be collected in the ICU of two recently merged, fully accredited, and licensed metropolitan hospitals in north central Texas. The strengths and weaknesses of these units are described. The target population is adult ICU patients who meet the sample criteria and consent to participate in the study. The sample criteria are nonexclusive to gender, ethnic background, diagnosis, or hospital treatment plan. The sample inclusion criteria consist of: (1) being a patient in the ICU, (2) being an adult over 18 years of age, (3) having a Bard Urotrack thermocatheter in place and functioning, (4) having no significant scarring or inflammation of the tympanic membrane, (5) having no bleeding or drainage from the tympanic membrane or ear canal, (6) having no obvious occlusion of the ear canal with cerumen, (7) having not been given antipyretics within the previous three hours, (8) having no exposure to extreme temperatures of 35°C within the past two hours, (9) having not been on a heating or cooling blanket within the past two

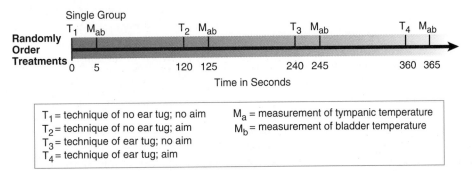

FIGURE 28–2 ■ Multiple treatments with nonequivalent dependent variables design. (From Ulbrich, S. L. [1995]. *The effect of operator technique on tympanic membrane thermometry.* Unpublished master's thesis. The University of Texas at Arlington.

hours, and (10) having a bladder temperature in the range of 96.0–102.0°F or 15.6–43.3°C. The sample size was calculated using a power analysis with a standard power of .8, effect size of .4, and alpha of .05. It was determined that a minimum of 73 subjects will be needed for this study. A nonprobability sample of convenience will be used. However, the design is strengthened by a random selection of right or left ear and a random ordering of treatments. The strengths and weaknesses of this sampling method are described.

Measurement Methods

The tympanic temperatures will be measured using the single First Temp Genius Model 3000A thermometer. This thermometer is equipped with a unique "Peak Select System" that internally records and analyzes 32 separate measurements from the incoming radiation, and displays the average of the highest two readings. The precision, accuracy, sensitivity, and potential error of this thermometer are described.

Bladder temperatures will be measured using Bard Urotrack Foley Catheters, model number 890216/18 sizes 16–18 French, manufactured by Bard Urologic Division of Covington, Georgia. These modified transurethral indwelling Foley catheters, like standard catheters, are made from hydro-gel-coated latex tubes with a five milliliter balloon encircling the catheter just below the tip to anchor the catheter in place within the bladder. . . . The precision, accuracy, sensitivity, and potential error for this catheter are described.

Plan for Data Collection

The treatments will be implemented and data will be collected by the investigator using the protocol outlined in Appendix 28-A. Data will be recorded on the data collection form developed for this study (see [Appendix 28-B]). The investigator will note the consistency of the treatment implementation and the data collection process. When the protocol is not followed consistently, this will be recorded (Egan, Snyder, & Burns, 1992). A complete plan for the data collection process is outlined in [Appendix 28-C]. Raw data and consent forms will be stored

in a locked file drawer in the investigator's house for five years.

Ethical Considerations

Permission to conduct this study will be obtained from the investigator's thesis committee, the Human Rights Review Committee for The University of Texas at Arlington, and the hospital's Institutional Review Board. In addition, verbal approval will be obtained from the ICU managers and the primary physicians of the subjects. Subjects will be provided essential information for informed consent and will sign a consent form (see [Appendix 28-D]). The benefit-risk ratio was assessed for this study, indicating minimal risk and important benefits.

Data Analysis

Data will be input and analyzed by the researcher using Mystat, a software package developed by Munro (1997). All raw data entered in the computer will be checked for errors. Demographic data will be analyzed with frequencies, percents, means, standard deviations, and ranges and presented in a table (see [Appendix 28-E]). The hypothesis will provide direction for the analysis of study data. Means, standard deviations, and ranges will be calculated on the bladder and tympanic temperatures for the four treatments of tug with aim, tug without aim, aim without tug, and no tug and no aim. The Bland-Altman method will be used to compare bladder and tympanic temperatures for each operator technique. Researchers have begun to use this method rather than conventional statistics such as Pearson's product-moment correlations or tests of statistical differences. Bland and Altman (1986) have suggested that conventional statistics are inappropriate when an established method of measurement, such as bladder temperature, is compared to a new method of measurement, such as tympanic temperature. The results will be presented in graphs.

Methodological Limitations

The limitations of this study include that (1) the extraneous variables of environmental and core body temperatures will not be completely con-

TABLE 28-3
STUDY TIMETABLE

TASK TO BE PERFORMED	PERFORMER OF TASK	COMPLETION OF TASK
1. Complete proposal and forms	Researcher	First through sixth months
2. Defend and revise proposal	Researcher	Seventh month
3. Review board approvals	Researcher	Eighth month
4. Equipment gathering and training	Researcher	Eighth month
5. Assemble data collection packets	Researcher	Eighth month
6. Establish potential subject notification with personnel at clinical agency	Researcher	Eighth month
7. Pilot study	Researcher	Ninth month
8. Analyze pilot data and revise	Researcher	Ninth month
9. Data collection	Researcher	Tenth & eleventh months
10. Analyze data	Researcher	Twelfth month
11. Interpret results	Researcher	Twelfth month
12. Final defense	Researcher	Thirteenth month
13. Communicate findings	Researcher	2-3 years

From Ulbrich, S. L. (1995). *The effect of operator technique on tympanic membrane thermometry.* Unpublished master's thesis. The University of Texas at Arlington.

TABLE 28-4
STUDY BUDGET

BUDGET ITEMS	COST PER ITEM	TOTAL COST
1. Printing costs	1500 pages @ .05/page	75.00
2. Consultant costs	Provided by the Center for Nursing Research	.00
3. Statistical software		50.00
4. Genius II tympanic thermometer and probe covers	Provided by Sherwood Medical	.00
5. Bard calibration plug	Provided by Bard Urologic Division	.00
6. Travel costs		150.00
7. Supplies		80.00
8. Communication costs		100.00
	Total	455.00

From Ulbrich, S. L. (1995). *The effect of operator technique on tympanic membrane thermometry.* Unpublished master's thesis. The University of Texas at Arlington.

trolled, (2) nonrandom sample will limit generalizability, and (3) estimation of core body temperature by the bladder thermometer is not quite as accurate as the pulmonary artery catheter, although they correlate at $r = .99$ (Erickson & Meyer, 1994).

Communication of Findings

The study findings will be presented to the thesis committee, hospital research committee, ICU nurses and managers, and the manufacturer of the equipment. In addition, an abstract of the study will be submitted for possible presentation of the research at a national critical care meeting. The study will be submitted for publication in a clinical journal such as *Heart & Lung* or *American Journal of Critical Care.* A study timetable and budget have been developed to direct this project and are presented in Tables [28-3] and [28-4]. (Ulbrich, 1995)

APPENDIX 28-A

DATA COLLECTION PROTOCOL

1. After consent is signed, the data collection form with the corresponding ID No. will be taken to the nursing station.
2. Place the room thermometer in the subject's room.
3. Questions one through ten will be answered by the researcher from information contained within the chart. All demographic questions will be completed prior to experimental data collection.
4. Enter the subject's room, ask any additional questions, and review the procedure if this is appropriate.
5. Record the room temperature from the thermometer left earlier.
6. Place the data collection form, otoscope, tympanic thermometer, and stopwatch on the same side of the patient as the ear selected for intervention.
7. Perform the brief otoscopic examination by gently retracting the subject's ear and inserting the otoscope into the external canal.
8. Note on the data collection form any large amount of cerumen, presence of any trauma, drainage, significant scarring, or severe inflammation. If any of these conditions are present, explain to the subject reasons for exclusion from the study and notify the nursing staff of the findings.
9. Insert the Bard calibration plug into the Urotrack monitor for calibration if applicable.
10. Record the time of day when data collection began.
11. Review the selected treatment order.
12. Remove the tympanic thermometer from its base and place a disposable cover on the probe tip.
13. Manipulate the ear and insert the probe in the *exact* manner outlined below for the first technique.

    T1 (tug: aim)—Gently grasp the superior aspect of the pinna and retract the ear in an upward, outward, and backward motion. Maintain this position and insert the covered tip of the probe, aiming at the point between the bridge of the nose and outer canthus of the eye on the opposite side of the head. Apply gentle pressure with the probe tip to seal the canal.

    T2 (tug: no aim)—Gently grasp the superior aspect of the pinna and retract the ear in an upward, outward, and backward motion. Maintain this position and insert the covered tip of the probe, directing it toward the opposite ear or along the mid-frontal plane of the head. Apply gentle pressure with the probe tip to seal the ear canal.

    T3 (no tug: aim)—Steady the subject's head by placing a hand over the temporal area. Insert the covered probe tip, aiming at the point between the bridge of the nose and outer canthus of the eye on the opposite side of the head. Apply gentle pressure with the probe tip to seal the ear canal.

    T4 (no tug: no aim)—Steady the subject's head by placing a hand over the temporal area. Insert the covered tip of the probe, directing it at the opposite ear or the probe along the mid-frontal plane of the head. Apply gentle pressure with the probe tip to seal the ear canal.

14. Press the SCAN button on the thermometer.
15. Remove the thermometer, release the ear, and dispose of the probe tip cover.
16. Begin the 2-minute interval timer on the stopwatch.
17. Record the temperature in the appropriate blank on the data collection form.
18. Immediately read the bladder temperature from the thermocath monitor.
19. Record the bladder temperature in the appropriate blank on the data collection form.

APPENDIX 28-A

20. Allow the 2 minutes to pass.
21. Repeat steps 12–20 for each of the remaining techniques in the order on the data collection form.
22. Record the time that data collection ended.
23. Thank the subject (if appropriate) for participa-

tion in the study. Answer any questions or address any concerns.
24. Review the data collection sheet for completeness.
25. Gather the equipment and leave the data collection area.

(From Ulbrich, S. L. [1995]. *The effect of operator technique on tympanic membrane thermometry.* Unpublished master's thesis. The University of Texas at Arlington.)

APPENDIX 28-B

DATA COLLECTION FORM

ID No. _____   **Date:** _____

Demographic Data

A. Age _____   B. Gender _____ (1) female   _____ (2) male
C. Race _____ (1) Caucasian   _____ (2) Asian   _____ (3) American Indian
         _____ (4) African American   _____ (5) Hispanic   _____ (6) Other
D. Unit _____ (1) CCU   _____ (2) MICU   _____ (3) SICU   _____ (4) NICU
E. Campus   _____ (1) East   _____ (2) West
F. Admitting/Major diagnosis: _____
G. Other significant diagnoses: _____
H. Supplemental oxygen   _____ (1) NC   _____ (2) vent   _____ (3) FM
                                        _____ (4) FT   _____ (5) other   _____ (6) none
I. Turban cranial dressing   _____ (1) yes   _____ (2) no
J. Hx _____ (1) carotid artery disease   _____ (2) cerebral vascular accident
       _____ (3) major head trauma   _____ (4) cranial surgery
       _____ (5) none
K. Most recent temperature _____ F   Time taken _____
L. Room temperature   _____ F

Experimental Data

M. Ear _____ (1) right   _____ (2) left
N. Noted upon aural exam   _____ (1) large amount of cerumen   _____ (2) trauma
                                        _____ (3) significant scarring   _____ (4) drainage
                                        _____ (5) significant inflammation   _____ (6) hair
                                        _____ (7) other

APPENDIX 28-B

Time data collection began _____

Treatment Order	Tympanic Temp.	Bladder Temp.

Time data collection ended _____

O. Data collection & treatments followed the protocol _____ (1) yes _____ (2) no _____ (3) partial
Explain, if partial _____

Comments:
_____
_____

(From Ulbrich, S. L. [1995]. *The effect of operator technique on tympanic membrane thermometry.* Unpublished master's thesis. The University of Texas at Arlington.)

APPENDIX 28-C

DATA COLLECTION PLAN

1. Locate potential subjects by making a daily phone call or visit to the intensive care units. Potential subjects might also be located by asking staff to notify the researcher by telephone of patients with bladder thermocatheters. The phone number of the researcher is already in the list of numbers in each unit.
2. Assess potential subjects in person using the sample criteria. This information can be gathered from the chart or staff. Timing should be considered in this step to avoid the hours near midnight to 3:00 a.m. and 6:00 a.m. to 8:00 a.m. or when nursing activities can be anticipated (timed dressing changes, scheduled procedures, etc.).
3. If all sample criteria are met, pursue consent to participate from the patient or legal representative.
4. Place the signed consent form in a folder to be kept with the researcher until it can be secured in the safe. Give one copy to the subject and place another in the chart.
5. Gather and record the demographic data from the chart or staff.
6. Follow the specific procedures outlined in the protocol (see [Appendix 28-B]) to implement the procedures and gather the experimental data.
7. Review forms for completeness.
8. Thank the staff and patient (if appropriate) for their participation and assistance.
9. Initiate the entire process with any additional subjects.
10. Gather equipment and return to the office.
11. File and secure all consent and data collection forms.
12. Repeat steps 1–11 until at least 30 subjects are recruited and data are collected.

(From Ulbrich, S. L. [1995]. *The effect of operator technique on tympanic membrane thermometry.* Unpublished master's thesis. The University of Texas at Arlington.)

APPENDIX 28-D

CONSENT FORM

Study Title: The Effect of Operator Technique on Tympanic Membrane Thermometry

Investigator: Sherri L. Ulbrich R.N., B.S.N., CCRN

Subject ID No. _____ **Hospital No.** _____ **Protocol No.** _____

You are invited to be in a research study to determine how different techniques used by nurses in taking tympanic temperatures affect the accuracy of these thermometers in adult patients in the intensive care unit. Over the next four months about 70 participants will be chosen in this nontherapeutic study without regard for race, gender, or socioeconomic status. Since you are already a patient in the intensive care unit and have a special bladder catheter to monitor your temperature, you have been selected as a possible participant. As a benefit, your temperature will be monitored closely and will provide information that might enable nurses to better assess the temperatures of their patients in the future.

The study and its procedures have been approved by the appropriate people and review boards at The University of Texas at Arlington and the hospital. If you were to participate in the study the specially trained researcher would (1) complete a demographic data sheet, (2) perform a brief ear (otoscopic) examination, (3) take a series of tympanic temperatures using different techniques to straighten the ear canal (similar to an ear examination) and aim the instrument, and (4) record the temperature from the special catheter you already have in place. The risk associated with this study is the possibility of injury to the ear canal and/or tympanic membrane. Neither has ever occurred in previous studies. Also, this risk is no greater than with the routine measurement of your temperature with the thermometer that is currently used throughout the hospital. You will be excluded from the study if any abnormalities are found during the ear examination to avoid this risk. Participation in this study will take approximately 10 minutes. You are free to ask any questions about the study or about being a subject and you may call the investigator at (817) 273-2776 if you have further questions.

Your participation in this study is voluntary: You are under no obligation to participate. You have the right to withdraw at any time and the care you receive and your relationship with the health care team will not be affected. Neither you nor the hospital will be charged or incur any expense or compensation for your participation. Although your physician is not an investigator, he or she will be informed of your participation.

The study data will be coded so they will not be linked to your name. Your identity will not be revealed while the study is being conducted, except to the doctors and nurses caring for you, or when the study is reported or published. All study data will be collected by the researcher, stored in a secure place, and will not be shared without your permission. A copy of the consent form will be given to you.

I have read this consent form and voluntarily consent to participate in this study. I understand that I am to rely on the investigator for information regarding the nature and purpose of the research study, the risks involved in the research study, and the possibility of complications, and I have been given an opportunity to discuss these with the investigator.

_____ _____   _____ _____
Subject's Signature   Date   Legally Authorized Representative   Date

I have explained this study to the above subject and have sought his/her understanding for informed consent.

_____ _____
Investigator's Signature   Date

_____

(From Ulbrich, S. L. [1995]. *The effect of operator technique on tympanic membrane thermometry*. Unpublished master's thesis. The University of Texas at Arlington.)

APPENDIX 28-E

DUMMY TABLE TO PRESENT SAMPLE CHARACTERISTICS

DEMOGRAPHIC VARIABLES	SAMPLE STATISTICS* N = 60	
	M *(SD)*	Range
Age		
Most Recent Temperature		
Room Temperature		

	Frequency	Percent
Gender		
male		
female		
Race		
Caucasian		
African American		
Asian		
Hispanic		
American Indian		
Other		
Unit		
CCU		
MICU		
SICU		
NICU		
Primary Diagnosis		
XXXXXXXX		
XXXXXXXX		
XXXXXXXX		
XXXXXXXX		
Other Significant Diagnoses		
XXXXXXXX		
XXXXXXXX		
XXXXXXXX		
XXXXXXXX		
Mechanically Ventilated		
Turban-Type Cranial Dressing		
History of:		
carotid artery disease		
cerebral vascular accident		
major head trauma		
cranial surgery		

*Only selected statistics are used to analyze each variable.

(From Ulbrich, S. L. [1995]. *The effect of operator technique on tympanic membrane thermometry.* Unpublished master's thesis. The University of Texas at Arlington.)

■ SUMMARY

This chapter focuses on writing a research proposal and seeking approval to conduct a study. A research proposal is a written plan that identifies the major elements of a study, such as the research problem, purpose, and framework, and outlines the methods and procedures to conduct a study. A well-written proposal communicates a significant, carefully planned research project, demonstrates the qualifications of the researcher, and generates support for the project. Writing a quality proposal involves (1) developing the ideas logically, (2) determining the depth or detail of the proposal content, (3) identifying the critical points in the proposal, and (4) developing an aesthetically appealing copy.

The content of a proposal needs to be written with the interest and expertise of the reviewers in mind. Proposals are frequently reviewed by faculty, clinical agency members, and representatives of funding institutions. The content of a proposal varies with the reviewers, the guidelines developed for the review, and the type of study (quantitative or qualitative) proposed. A quantitative research proposal usually has four chapters or sections: (1) introduction, (2) review of relevant literature, (3) framework, and (4) methods and procedures. A qualitative research proposal generally includes the following chapters or sections: (1) introduction, (2) research paradigm, (3) research methods, and (4) preliminary findings, limitations, and plans to communicate the study.

The content of a student proposal usually requires greater detail than does a proposal developed for review by clinical agency personnel or funding organizations. Most clinical agencies and funding institutions require a condensed proposal. However, even though these proposals are condensed, the logical links between the components of the study need to be clearly demonstrated. The proposal generally includes a problem, a purpose, previous research conducted in the area, a framework, variables, design, sample, ethical considerations, plan for data collection and analysis, and plan for dissemination of findings.

Sometimes a researcher will send a preproposal or query letter to a funding institution rather than a proposal. A preproposal is a short document of four to five pages plus appendices that is written to explore the funding possibilities for a research project. The parts of the preproposal are logically ordered as follows: (1) letter of transmittal, (2) proposal for research, (3) personnel, (4) facilities, and (5) budget. By using a preproposal, researchers can submit their proposals only to institutions that indicate an interest in their projects.

A research proposal is a formal way to communicate ideas about a proposed study to receive approval for conducting the study or to seek funding. Seeking approval for the conduct or funding of a study is a process that involves submission of a proposal to a selected group for review and, in many situations, verbally defending that proposal. Research proposals are reviewed to (1) evaluate the quality of the study, (2) ensure that adequate measures are being taken to protect human subjects, and (3) evaluate the impact of conduct of the study on the reviewing institution. An initial step in seeking approval to conduct a study is to determine what committees in which agencies must grant approval before the study can be conducted. Receiving approval to conduct a study requires preparing a scholarly proposal, examining the social and political factors in the review committee, and defending the proposal to the committee.

Proposals often require some revision before or during the implementation of a study. Before revising a proposal, a researcher needs to address certain questions: (1) What needs to be changed? (2) Why is the change necessary? and (3) How will the change affect implementation of the study and the study findings? If a change is necessary, the researcher needs to discuss the change with the members of the clinical agency research review committee or the funding agency. The chapter concludes with an example of a brief quantitative research proposal of a quasi-experimental study (Ulbrich, 1995).

REFERENCES

Alexander, D., & Kelly, B. (1991a). Cost effectiveness of tympanic thermometry in the pediatric office setting. *Clinical Pediatrics* (Suppl.), *30*(4), 57–59.

Alexander, D., & Kelly, B. (1991b). Responses of children, parents, and nurses to tympanic thermometry in the pediatric office. *Clinical Pediatrics* (Suppl.), *30*(4), 53–56.

American Association of Critical Care Nurses. (1984). *Definition of critical care nursing.* Newport Beach, CA: AACCN.

American Psychological Association. (1994). *Publication manual of the American Psychological Association* (4th ed.). Washington, DC: Author.

Bates, B. (1983). *A guide to physical examination* (3rd ed.). Philadelphia: Lippincott.

Beck, C. T. (1993). Qualitative research: The evaluation of its credibility, fittingness, and auditability. *Western Journal of Nursing Research, 15*(2), 263–266.

Bland, J. M., & Altman, D. G. (1986). Statistical methods for assessing agreement between two methods of clinical measurement. *Lancet, 1*(8476), 307–310.

Brink, H. (1993). Academic nurse leader's interpretation of concepts and priorities related to the examination of scientific short papers, dissertations and theses: Part 1. *Curationis, 16*(3), 62–67.

Bruce, J. L., & Grove, S. K. (1991). Fever: Pathology and treatment. *Critical Care Nurse, 12*(1), 40–49.

Burns, N. (1989). Standards for qualitative research. *Nursing Science Quarterly, 2*(1), 44–52.

Burns, N., & Grove, S. K. (1997). *The practice of nursing research: Conduct, critique, and utilization* (3rd ed.). Philadelphia: Saunders.

Chenitz, W. C., & Swanson, J. M. (1986). *From practice to grounded theory: Qualitative research in nursing.* Menlo Park, CA: Addison-Wesley.

Cohen, M. Z., Knafl, K., & Dzurec, L. C. (1993). Grant writing for qualitative research. *Image—The Journal of Nursing Scholarship, 25*(2), 151–156.

Dexter, P. (2000). Tips for scholarly writing in nursing. *Journal of Professional Nursing, 16*(1), 6–12.

Diers, D. (1979). *Research in nursing practice.* Philadelphia: Lippincott.

Doyle, F., Zehner, W. J., & Terndrup, T. E. (1992). The effect of ambient temperature on tympanic and oral temperatures. *American Journal of Emergency Medicine, 10*(4), 285–289.

Egan, E. C., Snyder, M., & Burns, K. R. (1992). Intervention studies in nursing: Is the effect due to the independent variable. *Nursing Outlook, 40*(4), 187–190.

Erickson, R. S., & Meyer, L. T. (1994). Accuracy of infrared ear thermometry and other temperature methods in adults. *American Journal of Critical Care, 3*(1), 40–54.

Erickson, R. S., & Woo, T. M. (1994). Accuracy of ear thermometry and traditional temperature methods in young children. *Heart & Lung, 23*(3), 181–195.

Erickson, R. S., & Yount, S. T. (1991). Comparison of tympanic and oral temperatures in surgical patients. *Nursing Research, 40*(2), 90–93.

Fraden, J. (1991). Noncontact temperature measurements in medicine. In D. L. Wise (Ed.), *Bioinstrumentation and biosensors* (pp. 511–549). New York: Marcel Dekker.

Fullwood, J., Granger, B. B., Bride, W., & Taylor, M. C. (1999).

Heart center nursing research: A team effort. *Progress in Cardiovascular Nursing, 14*(1), 25–29.

Guthrie, K. A., & Keunke, N. E. (1992). *Tympanic-based core temperature measurement in relation to thermometer and technique.* Unpublished master's thesis. Portland: Oregon Health Sciences University.

Heath, A. W. (1997, March). The proposal in qualitative research [41 paragraphs]. *The Qualitative Report* [On-line serial], *3*(1). Available at *http://www.nova.edu/ssss/QR/QR3-1/ heath.html* [February 26, 2000].

Holtzclaw, B. J. (1992). The febrile response in critical care: State of the science. *Heart & Lung, 21*(5), 482–501.

Krathwohl, D. R. (1988). *How to prepare a research proposal* (3rd ed.). Syracuse: Syracuse University Press.

Leininger, M. M. (1985). *Qualitative research methods in nursing.* Orlando, FL: Grune & Stratton.

Livornese, L. L., Dias, S., Samuel, C., Romanowski, B., Taylor, S., May, P., Pitsakis, P., Woods, G., Kaye, D., Levison, M. E., et al. (1992). Hospital acquired infection with vancomycin-resistant *Enterococcus faecium* transmitted by electronic thermometers. *Annals of Internal Medicine, 117*(2), 112–116.

Malasanos, L. J. (1976). What is the preproposal? What are its component parts? Is it an effective instrument in assessing funding potential of research ideas? *Nursing Research, 25*(3), 223–224.

Marshall, C., & Rossman, G. B. (1999). *Designing qualitative research* (3rd ed.). New York: Altamira Press.

Miles, M. B., & Huberman, A. M. (1994). *Qualitative data analysis* (2nd ed). Thousand Oaks, CA: Sage.

Milewski, A., Ferguson, K. L., & Terndrup, T. E. (1991). Comparison of pulmonary artery, rectal, and tympanic membrane temperatures in adult intensive care patients. *Clinical Pediatrics* (Suppl.), *30*(4), 13–16.

Miller, S. (1997). Multiple paradigms for nursing. In S. E. Thorne & V. E. Hayes (Eds.). *Nursing praxis: Knowledge and action* (pp. 140–156). Thousands Oaks, CA: Sage.

Munhall, P. L., & Boyd, C. O. (1999). *Nursing research: A qualitative perspective* (2nd ed.). Norwalk, CT: Appleton-Century-Crofts.

Munro, B. H. (1997). *Statistical methods for health care research* (3rd ed.). Philadelphia: Lippincott.

Nierman, D. M. (1991). Core temperature measurement in the intensive care unit. *Critical Care Medicine, 19*(6), 818–823.

Parse, R. R., Coyne, A. B., & Smith, M. J. (1985). *Nursing research: Qualitative methods.* Bowie, MD: Brady.

Pinch, W. J. (1995). Synthesis: Implementing a complex process. *Nurse Educator, 20*(1), 34–40.

Pransky, S. M. (1991). The impact of technique and conditions of the tympanic membrane upon infrared tympanic thermometry. *Clinical Pediatrics* (Suppl.), *30*(4), 50–51.

Rogers, B. (1987). Research proposals: The significance of the study. *AAOHN Journal, 35*(4), 190.

Sandelowski, M., Davis, D. H., & Harris, B. G. (1989). Artful design: Writing the proposal for research in the naturalist paradigm. *Research in Nursing & Health, 12*(2), 77–84.

Schmitz, T., Bair, N., Falk, M., & Levine, C. (1995). A comparison of five methods of temperature measurement in febrile intensive care patients. *American Journal of Critical Care, 4*(4), 286–292.

Schooley, J. F. (1986). *Thermometry.* Boca Raton, FL: CRC Press.

Summers, S. (1991). Axillary, tympanic, and esophageal measurement: Descriptive comparisons in postanesthesia patients. *Journal of Post Anesthesia Nursing, 6*(6), 420–425.

Terndrup, T. E. (1992). An appraisal of temperature assessment by infrared emission detection tympanic thermometry. *Annals of Emergency Medicine, 21*(12), 1483–1492.

Tornquist, E. M. (1986). *From proposal to publication: An informal guide to writing about nursing research.* Menlo Park, CA: Addison-Wesley.

Ulbrich, S. L. (1995). *The effect of operator technique on tympanic membrane thermometry.* Unpublished master's thesis. Arlington, TX: The University of Texas at Arlington.

University of Chicago Press. (1993). *The Chicago manual of style* (14th ed.). Chicago: University of Chicago Press.

Vessey, J. A., & Campos, R. G. (1992). Commentary: The role of nursing research committee. *Nursing Research, 41*(4), 247–249.

Wolff, S. M. (1988). The febrile patient. In J. B. Wyngaarden, & L. H. Smith, (Eds.), *Cecil textbook of medicine* (18th ed., Vol. 2, pp. 1524–1525). Philadelphia: Saunders.

Zehner, W. J., & Terndrup, T. E. (1991). The impact of moderate temperature variance on the relationship between oral, rectal, and tympanic membrane temperatures. *Clinical Pediatrics* (Suppl.), *30*(4), 61–64.

Zinder, D. J., & Holtel, M. (1995). Fever detection in intensive care unit patients using infrared tympanic thermometry. *Critical Care Medicine, 23*(1), A28.

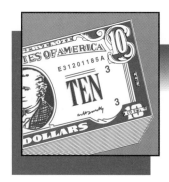

CHAPTER 29

SEEKING FUNDING FOR RESEARCH

Seeking funding for research is important, both for the researcher and for the profession. Well-designed studies can be expensive. As the control of variance and the complexity of the design increase, the cost of the study tends to increase. By obtaining funding, the researcher can conduct a complex, well-designed study. Funding also indicates that the study has been reviewed by others who have recognized its scientific and social merit. In fact, the scientific credibility of the profession is related to the quality of studies conducted by its researchers. Thus, scientific credibility and funding for research are interrelated.

The profession of nursing has invested a great deal of energy in increasing the sources of funding and amount of money available for nursing research. Each award of funding enhances the status of the researcher and increases the possibilities of greater funding for later studies. In addition, funding provides some practical advantages. For example, funding may reimburse part or all of the researcher's salary and therefore release the researcher from other responsibilities to devote time to conducting the study. The availability of research assistants facilitates careful data collection and allows the researcher to use time productively. Thus, skills in seeking funding for research are as important as skills in the conduct of research.

PURPOSES FOR SEEKING RESEARCH FUNDING

Two general types of grants are sought in nursing: developmental (or program) grants and research grants. Developmental grant proposals are written to obtain funding for the development of new programs in nursing, such as a program designed to teach nurses to provide a new type of nursing care or to implement a new approach to patient care. Although these programs may involve evaluation, they seldom involve research. For example, the effectiveness of a new approach to patient care may be evaluated, but the findings can seldom be generalized beyond the unit or institution in which the patient care was provided. The emphasis is on implementing the new approach to care, not on conducting research. Research grants provide funding specifically to conduct a study. Although the two types of grant proposals have similarities, they also have important differences in writing techniques and flow of ideas, as well as content. This chapter focuses on seeking funding for research.

The researcher may have one of two purposes for seeking research funding. First, the funding may allow the researcher to conduct a single study that is of immediate concern or interest. This situation is most common among nursing students who are preparing theses and dissertations. However, nurses in clinical practice may also develop an interest in a single study that has emerged from their clinical situation. Except in unusual circumstances, the person seeking funding for a single study, such as a master's thesis, needs to consider sources of small amounts of money. In most cases, this type of funding will not reimburse for salary and will pay only a portion of the cost of the study. Sources of funding are likely to be those described in the section titled Conducting Research on a Shoestring. These funds may pay for the cost of purchasing or printing instruments, postage, research assistants' salaries, travel to data collection sites, computer analysis, or the services of a statistician, or any combination of these expenses. If the researcher's experience is a positive one, further studies may be conducted later in his or her career. Thus, these small grants can be steppingstones to larger grants.

Another purpose for seeking funding is to initiate or maintain a career of conducting research. This situation is most common among nursing faculty and nurses employed in research positions in health care agencies. An individual planning to continue research activities throughout a career needs to plan a strategy for progressively more extensive funding of research activities. It is unrealistic, even in a university setting, to expect the time and money needed to conduct full-time research without external funding. An aspiring career researcher needs to be willing to invest the time and energy to develop grantsmanship skills. The researcher must also develop a goal to obtain funding for that portion of time that it seems desirable to commit to research activities. This goal is discussed with administrative personnel.

An aspiring career researcher needs to initiate a program of research in a specific area of study, and funding is sought in this area. For example, if the research interest is health promotion in rural areas, a series of studies focusing on rural health promotion needs to be planned. Even more desirable is an interdisciplinary team committed to a research program. Funding agencies are usually more supportive of researchers who focus their efforts in one area of study. Each study conducted within this area will increase the researcher's database and familiarity with the area. Research designs can be built on previous studies. This base of previous research and knowledge greatly increases the probability of receiving further funding. Publication of the studies will also increase the credibility of the researcher.

WAYS TO LEARN GRANTSMANSHIP

Grantsmanship is not an innate skill; it must be learned. Learning the process requires a commit-

ment of both time and energy. However, the rewards can be great. Strategies used to learn grantsmanship are described in the following sections and are listed in order of increasing time commitment, involvement, and level of expertise needed. These strategies are attending grantsmanship courses, developing a reference group, joining research organizations, participating on research committees or review panels, networking, assisting a researcher, and obtaining a mentor.

Attending Grantsmanship Courses

Some universities offer elective courses on grantsmanship. Continuing education programs or professional conferences sometimes offer topics related to grantsmanship. The content of these sessions may include the process of grant writing, techniques for obtaining grant funds, and sources of grant funds. In some cases, representatives of funding agencies will be invited to explain funding procedures. This information is useful for developing skill in writing proposals.

Developing a Reference Group

A reference group consists of individuals who share common values, ways of thinking, or activities, or any combination of these traits. These individuals become a reference group when a person identifies with the group, takes on group values and behavior, and evaluates his or her own values and behavior in relation to those of the group (Cartwright & Zander, 1968). A new researcher moving into grantsmanship may therefore need to switch from a reference group that views research and grant writing to be either over their heads or not worth their time to a group that values this activity. From this group will come the support and feedback necessary to develop grant-writing skills.

Joining Research Organizations

Research organizations are another source of support and new information for grant writing. Regional nursing research associations, located across the United States and internationally, provide many resources useful to the neophyte researcher.

REGIONAL RESEARCH ASSOCIATIONS

Eastern Nursing Research Society
Telephone: (603) 862-2891

Southern Nursing Research Society
http://www.snrs.org/
e-mail: info@snrs.org

Midwest Nursing Research Society
http://www.mnrs.org
e-mail: info@mnrs.org

Western Society of Research in Nursing

INTERNATIONAL NURSING RESEARCH ASSOCIATIONS

Royal Windsor Society for Nursing Research: RNC Research Society
http://www.windsor.igs.net/~nhodgins/
Canadian Association for Nursing Research
http://www.nurseresearcher.com/
This site includes a nurse researcher database that will aid you in finding researchers who can assist you with methodological problems and help establish research networks.
Australia—National Health and Medical Research Council
http://www.health.gov.au/nhmrc/
Canada—Canadian Institutes of Health Research
www.cihr.org/
France—Association of Nursing Research
http://perso.club-internet.fr/giarsi/
Germany—German Nursing Association—Agnes Karll Institute for Nursing Research
http://www.dbfk.de/aki/index.htm
Japan—Japanese Nursing Association
http://www.nurse.or.jp/
The Netherlands—Netherlands Institute for Primary Care
http://www.nivel.nl/
New Zealand—Health Research Council
http://www.hrc.govt.nz/
Norway—Norwegian Nurses Association
www.nosf.no/nsf/nsfweb.nsf
Scotland—Nursing Research Initiative for Scotland
http://www.nris.gcal.ac.uk/

United Kingdom—Research and Development Co-ordination Centre
http://www.man.ac.uk/rcn/rs

OTHER SOURCES OF SUPPORT AND INFORMATION

Sigma Theta Tau Honor Society of Nursing
www.nursingsociety.org/
International Institute for Qualitative Methodology
http://www.ualberta.ca/~iiqm/
Discussion, information, and assistance for qualitative research.

Virginia Henderson Library—Registry of Nursing Knowledge
http://www.stti.iupiu.edu/library/
Human Subjects Protections—National Institutes of Health
http://helix.nih.gov:8001/ohsr/

Specialty nursing organizations have research groups for members interested in conducting studies related to particular nursing specialty.

Serving on Research Committees

Research committees and institutional review boards exist in many work and professional organizations. Through membership on these committees, contacts with researchers can be made. Also, many research committees are involved in reviewing proposals for funding of small grants or granting approval to collect data in an institution. Reviewing proposals and making decisions about funding help researchers become better able to critique their own proposals and revise them before submission for review.

Networking

Networking is a process of developing channels of communication among people with common interests throughout the country. Contacts may be made by computer networks, mail, telephone, or arrangements to meet in groups. Through this process, nurses interested in a particular area of study can maintain contacts made at meetings by exchanging addresses and telephone numbers. These contacts provide opportunities for brainstorming, sharing ideas and problems, and discussing grant-writing opportunities. In some cases, it is possible to write a grant to include members of a network in various parts of the country. When a proposal is being developed, the network, which may become a reference group, can provide feedback at various stages of development of the proposal.

Assisting a Researcher

Volunteering to assist with the activities of another researcher is an excellent way to learn research and grantsmanship. Graduate students can gain this experience by becoming graduate research assistants. Assisting in grant writing and reading proposals that have been funded can be particularly helpful. Examination of proposals that have been rejected can also be useful if the comments of the review committee are available. The criticisms of the review committee point out the weaknesses of the study and therefore clarify the reasons why the proposal was rejected. Examining these comments on the proposal can increase the insight of a new grant writer and also prepare him or her for similar experiences. However, some researchers are sensitive about these criticisms and may be reluctant to share them. If an experienced researcher is willing, it is enlightening to hear his or her perceptions and opinions about the criticisms.

Obtaining a Mentor

Learning effective means of acquiring funding is difficult. Much of the information needed is transmitted verbally, requires actual participation in grant-writing activities, and is best learned in a mentor relationship. A mentor is a person who is more experienced professionally and willing to "teach the ropes" to a less experienced professional. Modeling is an important part of the mentoring process. This type of relationship requires willingness to invest time and energy by both professionals. A mentor relationship has characteristics of both a

teacher-learner relationship and a close friendship. Each must have an affinity for the other, from which a close working relationship can be developed. The relationship usually continues for a long period. However, mentorship is not well developed in nursing, and nurses who have this opportunity should consider themselves fortunate.

Becoming a Funded Researcher

Many of us, as neophyte researchers, have had the fantasy of writing a grant proposal to the federal government or a large foundation for our first study and suddenly achieving "stardom" (100 percent of our salary and everything needed to conduct the ultimate study, including a microcomputer, a secretary, and multiple graduate research assistants). Unfortunately, in reality this scenario seldom occurs for an inexperienced researcher. A new researcher is usually caught in a "Catch-22" situation. One needs to be an experienced researcher to get funded; however, one needs funding to get release time to conduct research. One way of resolving this dilemma is to design initial studies that can realistically be done without release time and with little or no funding. This approach requires a commitment to put in extra hours of work, which is often unrewarded, monetarily or socially. However, these types of studies, when well carried out and published, will provide the credibility one needs to begin the process toward major grant funding.

Some excellent guidance to beginning researchers is provided on BioMedNet's *HMS Beagle* (*http://biomednet.com/hmsbeagle/*) in a section appropriately titled "Adapt or Die." Although the ensuing suggestions were written for someone in an academic career, the same advice holds for researchers in clinical settings. The following guidance is included in "Jump Start: What to Do Before Writing a Grant Proposal" (Reif-Lehrer, 1998a).

. . . .

"Although having a good idea is vital for successfully writing a grant proposal . . . there are other things that will help you get funded: a good reputation in your field, a solid research group, good preliminary data, and good collaborators whose skills and knowledge complement your own. . . . It's good to start building your reputation early. First, make it your business to find out how academia (and your institution) really works. It is true to some extent that what matters is not just what you know, but also who you know. Try to enlist your mentor to help you make your way up the academic career ladder, but don't rely just on her or him. Build relationships with other senior faculty members who are willing to help you attain your goals. The best people in your field often have the most up-to-date information about what is going on. Don't be afraid to approach these people. Talk to them, learn from them, and 'repay' them by mentoring younger people when you reach the appropriate stage of your own career. Build networks with peers in you department, in other departments, and at other universities. Learn how to get the most out of professional meetings. As a graduate student, I found attendance at my first meeting exhausting. I went to ten-minute and one-hour talks all day, every day, for all five days. When I told my research director how I spent the time, he looked me in the eye and said, 'It's not what you learn at the talks, it's what you learn in the hallways that's most important.' Nonetheless, it's important to give good talks at meetings because a large part of your reputation comes from your publications and the talks you give—at professional meetings and when you present seminars at your own and other institutions. Scientists who learn good communications skills early in their education have a substantial professional advantage (p. 1–2).

"You can increase your productivity by getting people around you to help you achieve your goal. Bear in mind that colleagues, administrators, and support staff are more likely to help people who are kind, generous, pleasant, and helpful than those who are selfish, surly, and demanding. Prima donnas may fare well superficially and for a while. But they tend not to do well in the long run—and even when they do, they are often not well liked. Good public relations skills are a great asset, in science as in many other professions. It rarely hurts to become known as a kind patient person who shares, helps others, and is a good mentor." (Reif-Lehrer, 1998a, p. 3) ■

Conducting Research on a Shoestring

Ideas for studies often begin in grandiose ways. You envision the ideal study and follow all the rules in the textbooks and in research courses. However, when you begin to determine what is needed in time and money to conduct this wonderful study, you find your resources sadly lacking. This discovery should not lead you to give up the idea of conducting research. Rather, you need to take stock of your resources to determine exactly what can realistically be done and then modify your study to meet existing constraints. The modified study must remain good research but be scaled down to an achievable level. Such downscaling might involve studying only one aspect of the original study, decreasing the number of variables examined, or limiting the study to a single site. In many cases, a minimal amount of money is needed to conduct small studies. This project can be the pilot study that is essential to attract larger amounts of research funding.

The next step is to determine potential sources of this small amount of money. In some cases, management in the employing institution can supply limited funding for research activities if a good case is presented for the usefulness of the study to the institution. In many universities, funds are available for intramural grants, which are obtained competitively by submitting a brief proposal to a university committee. Some nursing organizations also have money available for research activities. For example, Sigma Theta Tau, the honor society for nurses, provides small grants for nursing research that can be obtained through submission to international, national, regional, or local review committees. Another source is local agencies, such as the American Cancer Society and the American Heart Association. Although grants from the national offices of these organizations require sophistication in research, local or state levels of the organization may have small amounts of funds available for studies in the area of interest of the organization.

Private individuals who are locally active in philanthropy may be willing to provide financial assistance for a small study in an area appealing to them.

One needs to know whom to approach and how and when to make the approach to increase the probability of successful funding. Sometimes this requires knowing someone who knows someone who might be willing to provide financial support. Acquiring funds from private individuals also requires more assertiveness than needed for other approaches to funding (Holmstrom & Burgess, 1982).

Requests for funding need not be limited to a single source. If a larger amount of money is needed than can be supplied by one source, funds can be sought from one source for a specific research need and from another source for another research need. Also, one source may be able to provide funds for a small segment of time, and another source can then be approached to provide funding to continue another phase of the study. A combination of these two strategies can also be used.

Seeking funding from local sources is less demanding in terms of formality and length of the proposal than is the case with other types of grants. Often, the process is informal and may require only a two- or three-page description of the study. The important thing is knowing what funds are available and how to apply for them. Some of these funds go unused each year because nurses are not aware of their existence or think that they are unlikely to be successful in obtaining the money. This unused money leads granting agencies or potential granting agencies to conclude that nurses do not need more money for research.

Small grants are also available nationally. The American Nurses' Foundation and Sigma Theta Tau award a number of grants for less than $5000 on a yearly basis. The grants are competitive and awarded to new investigators with promising ideas, and receiving funding from these organizations is held in high regard. Information regarding these grants is available from the American Nurses' Foundation, Inc. Several federal granting agencies also provide small grants through the Public Health Service. These grants usually limit the amount of money requested to $50,000 to $75,000. Information regarding small grants can be obtained from the *Federal Register*, which is available in local libraries.

Small grants do more than just provide the funds necessary to conduct the research. They are the first step in being recognized as a credible researcher and in being considered for more substantial grants for later studies. Receipt of these grants and your role in the grant need to be listed on curricula vitae or biographical sketches as an indication of first-level recognition as a researcher.

Obtaining Foundation Grants

IDENTIFYING POTENTIALLY INTERESTED FOUNDATIONS

Many foundations in the United States provide funding for research, but the problem is to determine which foundations have interests in a particular field of study. Priorities for funding tend to change annually. When these foundations have been identified, the characteristics of the foundation need to be determined, appropriate foundations selected, query letters sent, a proposal prepared, and if possible, a personal visit made to the foundation. Several publications list foundations and their interests. Bauer and the American Association of Colleges of Nursing (1988) have compiled a list of foundations of particular interest to nursing. A computerized information system, the Sponsored Programs Information Network (SPIN), can also assist researchers in locating the most appropriate funding sources to support their research interests. The database contains approximately 2000 programs that provide information on federal agencies, private foundations, and corporate foundations. Many universities and research institutions have access to SPIN.

DETERMINING FOUNDATION CHARACTERISTICS

When these foundations have been identified, funding information needs to be gathered from each foundation. A foundation might fund only studies by female researchers, or it may be interested only in studies of low-income groups. A foundation may fund only studies being conducted in a specific geographical region. The average amount of money awarded for a single grant and the ranges of awards need to be determined for each foundation. If the average award of a particular foundation is $2500 and if $30,000 is needed, that foundation is not the most desirable source of funds. However, if the researcher has never been funded previously and the project could be conducted with less money, an application to that foundation could be combined with applications to other foundations to obtain the funds needed. The book most useful in determining this information is *The Foundation Directory,* which is available from The Foundation Center, 888 Seventh Avenue, New York, NY 10106.

VERIFYING INSTITUTIONAL SUPPORT

Grant awards are most commonly made to institutions rather than to individuals. Therefore, it is important to determine the willingness of the institution to receive the grant and support the study. This willingness needs to be documented in the proposal. Supporting the study involves appropriateness of the study topic; adequacy of facilities and services; availability of space needed for the study; contributions that the institution is willing to make to the study, such as staff time, equipment, or data processing; and provision for overseeing the rights of human subjects.

SENDING QUERY LETTERS

The next step is to send a query letter to foundations that might be interested in the planned study. The letter is addressed to the person who is the director or head of the appropriate office rather than to an impersonal title such as "Dear Director." Names of directors are available in a number of reference books or can be obtained by calling the organization's switchboard. The letter needs to reflect spontaneity and enthusiasm for the study, with the opening paragraph providing a reason why the letter is being sent to that particular foundation. The query letter should include a succinct description of the proposed study, an explanation of why the study is important, an indication of who will conduct the study, a description of the required facilities, and the estimated duration and cost of the study. The qualifications of the researchers to conduct the study need to be made clear. This is no time to be

modest about credentials or past achievements. The letter should inquire about the foundation's interest in the topic and information regarding how to apply for funds. If a personal visit is possible, the letter should close with a request for an appointment.

PREPARING PROPOSALS

When preparing the proposal, the foundation's guidelines for an application need to be followed carefully. In some cases, funding is sought from several sources. For example, funding requests may be submitted to an agency of the federal government, a nonprofit volunteer agency, and several private foundations. The temptation is to send each source the same proposal rather than retyping it to meet specific guidelines. This tactic can be counterproductive because the proposal will not focus on the interests of each foundation and will not be in the format requested by the foundation, which may lead to rejection of the proposal. Developing a proposal is described in Chapter 28.

MAKING A PERSONAL VISIT

A personal visit to the foundation can be helpful if such contact is feasible and permitted by the foundation. Some foundations wish to see only the written application, whereas others prefer personal contact. A visit should not be made without an appointment. Preparations need to begin for the visit as soon as the appointment has been made, and a fully developed proposal needs to be written before the visit. Such groundwork allows the researcher to have carefully thought through the study and have ideas well developed and organized when he or she goes to the foundation. Friedman suggested the following behavior when visiting foundations: "One, be businesslike; two, be honest; three, know what you mean to do; four, ask questions; and finally, never, never argue with a foundation about the relevance of your proposed project to their program. . . . If they say it doesn't fit, it doesn't" (White, 1975, pp. 219–220).

Although the visit may be informal in a social context, foundation representatives will tend to ask hard, searching questions about the study and planned use of the funding. In a way, this interaction is similar to talking to a banker about a loan. Questions will be geared to help the foundation determine the following: Is the study feasible? Is the institution willing to provide sufficient support to permit the study to be completed? Is the researcher using all available resources? Have other sources of funding been sought? Has the researcher examined anticipated costs in detail and been realistic? What are the benefits of conducting the study? Who will benefit, and how? Is the researcher likely to complete the study? Are the findings likely to be published? If the written proposal has not been submitted, the visit is an appropriate time to submit it. Additional information or notes prepared for the visit can be left with foundation representatives for consideration as the decision is made.

OBTAINING FEDERAL GRANTS

The largest source of grant monies is the federal government—so much so that in effect, the federal government influences what is studied and what is not. Funding can be requested from multiple divisions of the government. Information on funding agencies can be obtained from a document compiled by the federal government, *The Catalog of Federal Domestic Assistance*. This document is available from the U.S. Government Printing Office, Washington, D.C. 20402. Each agency has areas of focus and priorities for funding that change yearly. It is important to know this information and prepare proposals within these areas to obtain funding. Therefore, calling or writing the agency for the most recent list of priorities is essential. An excellent website for identifying sources of funding for nursing research and developing grant proposals was developed by Mary E. Duffy, Ph.D., R.N., FAAN, Director of the Center for Nursing Research at Boston College. The address for this website, Public and Private Grant-Related WWW Resources, is *http://www.nursing.uc.edu/nrm/duffy81598.htm.*

Two approaches can be used to seek federal funding for research. The researcher can identify a significant problem, develop a study to examine it, and submit a proposal for the study to the appropriate federal funding agency. Alternatively, an agency within the federal government can identify a significant problem, develop a plan by which the problem can be studied, and publish a Request for Proposals (RFP) or a Request for Applications (RFA) from researchers.

Reif-Lehrer (1998a) provides some excellent guidance to prepare for seeking federal funding.

. . . .

"To get funding from a major government agency today you need a reasonable amount of good preliminary data. These data must indicate to the reviewers that you can wisely and expediently carry out the project, that the experiments are feasible, and that the data obtained are likely to move the field ahead in some substantive way." (Reif-Lehrer, 1998a, p. 4) ■

Researcher-Initiated Proposals

If the study is researcher initiated, it is useful for the researcher to contact an official within the government agency early in the planning process to inform the agency of the intent to submit a proposal. Each agency has established dates, usually three times a year, when proposals are reviewed. Preparation of the proposal needs to begin months ahead of this deadline, and some agencies are willing to provide assistance and feedback to the researcher during development of the proposal. This assistance may occur through telephone conversation or feedback on a draft of the proposal.

Reviewing proposals that have been funded by that agency can be helpful. Although the agency cannot provide these proposals, they can often be obtained by contacting the principal investigator (PI) of the study personally. In some cases, the researcher may travel to Washington to meet with an agency representative. This type of contact allows modification of the proposal to fit more closely within agency guidelines, thus increasing the probability of funding. In many cases, proposals will fit within the interests of more than one government agency at the time of submission. It is permissible and perhaps desirable to request that the proposal be assigned to two agencies within the Public Health Service.

Requests for Proposals

An RFP is published in the *Federal Register* and usually has a deadline date that is only a few weeks after publication. Therefore, the researcher needs to have a good background in the field of study and be able to write a proposal quickly. Because a number of researchers will be responding to the same RFP and only one or a few proposals will be approved, these proposals are competitive. The agency staff will not be able to provide the same type of feedback as occurs in researcher-initiated proposals. The agency needs to be informed that a proposal is being submitted. Some questions that require clarification about elements of the RFP can be answered; however, other questions cannot be answered because the proposals are competitive and answering might give one researcher an advantage over others. An RFP allows a wide range of creativity in developing a study design to examine the problem of concern.

Requests for Applications

An RFA is similar to an RFP except that with an RFA, the government agency not only identifies the problem of concern but also describes the design of the study. An RFA is a contract for which researchers bid. A carefully written proposal is still required and needs to follow the RFA in detail. After funding, federal agency staff maintain much more control and supervision over the process of the study than is the case with an RFP.

Developing a Proposal

Several excellent sources are available that provide detailed guidelines for the development of grant proposals. For a brief but excellent discussion of this topic, see Tornquist and Funk (1990). A number of books provide more detailed directions for grant proposal development. For example, Bauer (1988, 1989), who has led a number of proposal development workshops in coordination with the American Association of Colleges of Nursing, has developed a grants manual, a series of videotapes, a computer program to guide proposal development,

and a proposal development workbook that can be used to develop skills in proposal writing. The videotapes can be purchased from the American Council on Education, Publications Department, One Dupont Circle, Washington, D.C. 20036. Grant development materials can be ordered from Bauer Associates, 3357 Stadium Court, San Diego, CA 92122, (619) 452-9011.

It is helpful to examine proposals that have been funded as a guide for developing a new proposal. Two proposals have been published to serve as guides in proposal development. Sandelowski and colleagues (1989) provided an example of a qualitative proposal, and Naylor (1990) provided an example of a quantitative proposal.

Set aside sufficient time for careful development of the proposal, including rewriting the text several times. Writing your first proposal on a tight deadline is not wise. We recommend that you plan on 6 to 12 months for proposal development from the point of early development of your research ideas. Contact the agency to obtain written guidelines for development of the proposal and follow them rigidly. Page limitations and type sizes need to be strictly adhered to. Reif-Lehrer (1998b) points out that "the best writing can't turn a bad idea into a good grant proposal, but bad writing can turn a good idea into an unfunded proposal. . . . A good proposal idea must also tweak the reviewers' imagination. . . . Investigators must energetically convey their enthusiasm and sense of excitement about their work and the new research directions they are planning. If the researcher can concretely and clearly describe what is known, and then present a logical leap forward into the unknown, there is great potential for capturing the reviewers' interest" (pp. 1–2). One of the difficult parts of developing a proposal for a grant application is preparing the budget. Beyea and Nicoll (1998) provide excellent guidance on developing the budget section of a grant proposal.

Input from colleagues can be invaluable in refining your ideas. You need individuals whose opinions you trust and who will go beyond telling you globally how magnificent your proposal is. Seek individuals who have experience in grant writing and are willing to critique your proposal thoroughly. After you have used their feedback to revise the proposal, contact a nationally known expert in your research field who will agree to examine your proposal critically. Be prepared to pay a consultant fee for this service.

After revising the proposal again, you are ready to submit it for funding. A number of federal funding agencies are willing to provide feedback on a preliminary draft of a proposal after initial interaction with the researcher by phone. Traveling to make personal contact with agency staff for this feedback is even more helpful. Before making personal contact, the researcher needs to contact a staff member by phone, make an appointment, and send the draft by mail or fax in time for the staff member to review it before the meeting.

Neophytes are least willing to request a critique by colleagues and experts. There is almost a desire to write the proposal in secrecy, submit it quietly, and wait for the letter from the funding agency. That way, if you fail, no one will know about it. If others do know about the proposal development, another strategy is often used. The author furiously writes up to the very last possible deadline and then, in exhaustion, proclaims that there is no time for review before it is submitted. Both these strategies almost guarantee rejection of the proposal. Remember, the critiques of your friends and the expert you have sought are unlikely to be as devastating as that of reviewers at the funding agency. Moreover, you have a chance to make changes after your friends review it. Submission of grant proposals in paper form through the mail is nearing an end. The Public Health Service is currently developing methods for you to apply for grants on-line. In the future, you can expect to submit most of your proposals electronically.

The Federal Grant Review Process

After submission, a grant is assigned to 1 of 90 study sections for scientific evaluation. The study sections have no alignment with the funding agency. Thus, staff in the agencies have no influence on the committee's work of judging the scientific merit of the proposal. The proposal is sent to two or more researchers from the study section who are considered qualified to evaluate the proposal. These scientists prepare a written critique of the study. The proposal is then sent to all the members of the study section. Each member may have 50 to 100 proposals to read in a 1- to 2-month period. A meeting of the full study section is then held. Each application is discussed by those who critiqued the proposal, and other members comment or ask questions. A majority vote determines whether the proposal is approved, disapproved, or deferred.

Approved proposals are assigned a numerical score used to develop a priority rating (White, 1975). A study that is approved is not necessarily funded. The PI will be notified at this point whether the study was approved. At a later time, approved studies are further examined to determine actual funding. Funding begins with the proposal that has the highest rank order and will continue until available funds are depleted. This process can take 6 months or longer. Because of this process, receipt of the money to initiate a grant may not occur for up to a year after submission of the proposal.

Often, researcher-initiated proposals are rejected (or approved but not funded) after the first submission. The critique of the scientific committee is sent to the researcher on a *pink sheet*. Frequently, the agency staff will encourage the researcher to rewrite the proposal with guidance from comments on the pink sheet and resubmit it to the same agency. The probability of funding is often greater the second time if the suggestions are followed.

Review of RFPs or RFAs is slightly different. These applications first go through technical (scientific) evaluation. Proposals that pass the technical review are then evaluated from the standpoint of cost. After the financial review, the contracting officer may negotiate levels of funding with the proposal writers. Funding decisions are based on identification of well-designed proposals that offer the best financial advantage to the government (White, 1975).

PINK SHEETS

The reaction of a researcher to a pink sheet is usually anger and then depression. The proposal is rejected by the researcher, stuffed in a bottom drawer somewhere, and forgotten. There really seems to be no way to avoid the anger and depression after a rejection because of the amount of emotional and time investment required to write a proposal. However, after a few weeks it is advisable to examine the pink sheet again. The comments can be useful in rewriting the proposal for resubmission. The learning experience of rewriting the proposal and evaluating the comments will also provide a background for seeking funding for another study.

A skilled grant writer will have approximately one proposal funded for every five submitted. The average is far less than this. Thus the researcher needs to be committed to repeated efforts of proposal submission to achieve grant funding.

GRANT MANAGEMENT

Receiving notice that a grant proposal has been funded is one of the highlights in a researcher's career and warrants a celebration. However, when the euphoria begins to fade and reality sets in, careful plans need to be made for implementing the study. To avoid problems, consideration needs to be given to managing the budget, hiring and training research personnel, maintaining the promised timetable, and coordinating activities of the study. In addition to the suggestions given in the following sections, Selby-Harrington and associates (1994) provide some excellent guidance in grant management from their experience as PIs of a federally funded grant.

Managing the Budget

Although the supporting institution has ultimate responsibility for dispensing and controlling grant monies, the PI is also responsible for keeping track of budget expenditures and making decisions about how the money is to be spent. If this grant is the first one received, a PI who has no previous administrative experience may need some initial guidance in how to keep records and make reasonable budget decisions. If funding is through a federal agency, interim reports will include reports on the budget, as well as on progress of the study.

Training Research Personnel

When a new grant is initiated, time needs to be set aside for interviewing, hiring, and training grant personnel. The personnel who will be involved in data collection need to learn the process, and then data collection needs to be refined to ensure that each data collector is consistent with the other data collectors. This process helps ensure *interrater reliability*. The PI needs to set aside time to oversee the work of personnel hired for the grant.

Maintaining the Study Schedule

The timetable submitted with the proposal needs to be adhered to whenever possible, which requires some careful planning. Otherwise, other work activities are likely to take precedence and delay the grant work. Unexpected events do happen; however, careful planning can minimize their impact. The PI needs to constantly refer back to the timetable to evaluate progress. If the project falls behind schedule, action needs to be taken to return to the original schedule or to readjust the timetable. Keeping on schedule will be a plus when it is time to apply for the next grant.

Coordinating Activities

During a large study with several investigators and other grant personnel, coordinating activities can be a problem. It is useful to arrange meetings of all grant workers at intervals to facilitate sharing of ideas and problem solving. Records need to be kept of discussions at these meetings. These actions can lead to a more smoothly functioning team.

Submitting Reports

Federal grants require the submission of interim reports according to preset deadlines. The federal agency involved will send written guidelines for the content of the reports, which will consist of a description of grant activities and expenditure of grant monies. Time needs to be set aside to prepare the report, which usually requires compiling figures and tables. In addition to the written reports, it is often useful to maintain phone contact with the appropriate staff at the federal agency.

PLANNING YOUR NEXT GRANT

The researcher should not wait until funding from the first grant has ended to begin seeking funds for a second study because of the length of time required to obtain funding. In fact, it may be wise to have several ongoing studies in various stages of implementation. For example, one could be planning a study, collecting data on a second study, analyzing data on a third study, and writing papers for publication on a fourth study. A full-time researcher could have completed one funded study, be in the last year of funding for a second study, be in the first year of funding for a third study, and be seeking funding for a fourth study. This scenario may sound unrealistic, but with planning, it is not. This strategy not only provides continuous funding for research activities but also facilitates a rhythm of research that prevents time pressures and makes use of lulls in activity in a particular study. To increase the ease of obtaining funding, the studies need to be within the same area of research, each building on previous studies.

■ SUMMARY

Seeking funding for research is important, both for the researcher and for the profession. Researchers may have one of two purposes for seeking research funding. First, the funding may allow the researcher to conduct a single study that is of concern or interest. The second purpose is to initiate or maintain a career of conducting research. To receive funding, grantsmanship skills need to be learned. Strategies used to learn grantsmanship are attending grantsmanship courses, developing a reference group, joining research organizations, participating on research committees or review panels, networking, assisting a researcher, and obtaining a mentor.

Writing a grant proposal for funding requires a commitment to putting in extra hours of work, which are often initially unrewarded, monetarily and socially. The first studies are usually conducted on a shoestring budget. A small amount of money might be obtained from a variety of sources, such as management in employing institutions, universities (intramural grants), or nursing organizations. A study conducted with limited funds that is well carried out and published will often give the credibility one needs to achieve major grant funding.

Larger sums of money can be sought by writing for foundation grants. The researcher initially needs to identify potentially interested foundations and determine the characteristics of these foundations. Foundation grant awards are most commonly made to institutions rather than to individuals. Therefore, it is important to determine the willingness of the institution to receive the grant and support the study. The institution's willingness needs to be documented in the proposal. Query letters are sent to all foundations that might be interested in the planned study. If a foundation is interested, a personal visit, if possible, needs to be made. The grant proposal is developed according to the guidelines of the foundation.

The largest source of grant monies is the federal government. Two approaches can be used to seek federal funding for research. The researcher can identify a significant problem, develop a study to examine it, and submit a proposal for the study to an appropriate federal funding agency. Alternatively, someone within the federal government can identify a significant problem, develop a plan through which the problem can be studied, and publish an RFP or an RFA from researchers.

After submission, grant requests are initially reviewed by staff members of the agency. Researchers who are writing their first federal grant request frequently receive rejection notices or approval-but-not-funded notices. The critique of the scientific committee is sent to the researcher on a pink sheet. Often, the agency staff will encourage the researcher to rewrite and resubmit the proposal after revision guided by comments on the pink sheet.

When a grant proposal is funded, it is a time of celebration for the researcher. However, the researcher then needs to make careful plans for implementing the study. The PI is responsible for keeping up with the budget, training research personnel, keeping up the schedule, and coordinating activities. Federal grants also require the submission of interim reports. A researcher should not wait until funding from the first grant has ended to begin seeking funds for a second study and then a third and then a fourth.

REFERENCES

Bauer, D. G. (1988). *The "how to" grants manual: Successful grantseeking techniques for obtaining public and private grants* (2nd ed.). New York: American Council on Education/Macmillan.

Bauer, D. G. (1989). *Administering grants, contracts, and funds: Evaluating and improving your grants system.* New York: American Council on Education/Macmillan.

Bauer, D. G., & American Association of Colleges of Nursing (1988). In B. K. Redman, & R. Lamothe (Eds.), *The complete grants sourcebook for nursing and health.* New York: American Council on Education/Macmillan.

Beyea, S. C., & Nicoll, L. H. (1998). Debunking research myths—research on a shoestring budget. *AORN Journal, 68*(2), 284.

Cartwright, D., & Zander, A. (1968). *Group dynamics: Research and theory.* New York: Harper & Row.

Holmstrom, L. L., & Burgess, A. W. (1982). Low-cost research: A project on a shoestring. *Nursing Research, 31*(2), 123–125.

Naylor, M. D. (1990). An example of a research grant application: Comprehensive discharge planning for the elderly. *Research in Nursing & Health, 13*(5), 327–348.

Reif-Lehrer, L. (1998b). Going for the gold. *HMS Beagle* (On-line), Issue 29, 5 pages (*http://www.biomednet.com/hmsbeagle/29/labres/adapt.htm*) [Posted May 1, 1998].

Reif-Lehrer, L. (1998a). Jump start: What to do before writing a grant proposal. *HMS Beagle* (On-line), Issue 33, 6 pages (*http://www.biomednet.com/hmsbeagle/33/labres/adapt.htm*) [Posted June 26, 1998].

Sandelowski, M., Davis, D., & Harris, B. (1989). Artful design: Writing the proposal for research in the naturalist paradigm. *Research in Nursing & Health, 12*(2), 77–84.

Selby-Harrington, M. L., Donat, P. L. M., & Hibbard, H. D. (1994). Research grant implementation: Staff development as a tool to accomplish research activities. *Applied Nursing Research, 7*(1), 38–46.

Tornquist, E. M., & Funk, S. G. (1990). How to write a research grant proposal. *Image—The Journal of Nursing Scholarship, 22*(1), 44–51.

White, V. P. (1975). *Grants: How to find out about them and what to do next.* New York: Plenum.

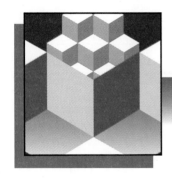

APPENDICES

Appendix A

TABLE OF RANDOM NUMBERS

71510	68311	48214	99929	64650	13229
36921	58733	13459	93488	21949	30920
23288	89515	58503	46185	00368	82604
02668	37444	50640	54968	11409	36148
82091	87298	41397	71112	00076	60029
47837	76717	09653	54466	87988	82363
17934	52793	17641	19502	31735	36901
92296	19293	57583	86043	69502	12601
00535	82698	04174	32342	66533	07875
54446	08795	63563	42296	74647	73120
96981	68729	21154	56182	71840	66135
52397	89724	96436	17871	21823	04027
76403	04655	87277	32593	17097	06913
05136	05115	25922	07123	31485	52166
07645	85123	20945	06370	70255	22806
32530	98883	19105	01769	20276	59402
60427	03316	41439	22012	00159	08461
51811	14651	45119	97921	08063	70820
01832	53295	66575	21384	75357	55888
83430	96917	73978	87884	13249	28870
00995	28829	15048	49573	65278	61493
44032	88720	73058	66010	55115	79227
27929	23392	06432	50201	39055	15529
53484	33973	10614	25190	52647	62580
51184	31339	60009	66595	64358	14985
31359	77470	58126	59192	23371	25190
37842	44387	92421	42965	09736	51873
94596	61368	82091	63835	86859	10678
58210	59820	24710	23225	45788	21426
63354	29875	51058	29958	61221	61200
79958	67599	74103	49824	39306	15069
56328	26905	34454	53965	66617	22137
72806	64421	58711	68436	60301	28620
91920	96081	01413	27281	19397	36231
05010	42003	99866	20924	76152	54090
88239	80732	20778	45726	41481	48277
45705	96458	13918	52375	57457	87884
64274	26236	61096	01309	48632	00431
63731	18917	21614	06412	71008	20255
39891	75337	89452	88092	61012	38072
26466	03735	39891	26362	86817	48193
33492	70485	77323	01016	97315	03944
04509	46144	88909	55261	73434	62538
63187	57352	91208	33555	75943	41669
64651	38741	86190	38197	99113	59694
46792	78975	01999	78892	16177	95747
78076	75002	51309	18791	34162	32258
05345	79268	75608	29916	37005	09213
10991	50452	02376	40372	45077	73706

APPENDIX B

CUMULATIVE NORMAL DISTRIBUTION (Z)

Z	X	Area	Z	X	Area
−3.25	$\mu - 3.25\sigma$	.0006	−1.00	$\mu - 1.00\sigma$	.1587
−3.20	$\mu - 3.20\sigma$	.0007	−.95	$\mu - .95\sigma$	.1711
−3.15	$\mu - 3.15\sigma$	.0008	−.90	$\mu - .90\sigma$	.1841
−3.10	$\mu - 3.10\sigma$	.0010	−.85	$\mu - .85\sigma$	.1977
−3.05	$\mu - 3.05\sigma$	.0011	−.80	$\mu - .80\sigma$	.2119
−3.00	$\mu - 3.00\sigma$	.0013	−.75	$\mu - .75\sigma$	.2266
−2.95	$\mu - 2.95\sigma$	.0016	−.70	$\mu - .70\sigma$	.2420
−2.90	$\mu - 2.90\sigma$	.0019	−.65	$\mu - .65\sigma$	.2578
−2.85	$\mu - 2.85\sigma$	.0022	−.60	$\mu - .60\sigma$	.2743
−2.80	$\mu - 2.80\sigma$	.0026	−.55	$\mu - .55\sigma$	.2912
−2.75	$\mu - 2.75\sigma$	.0030	−.50	$\mu - .50\sigma$	.3085
−2.70	$\mu - 2.70\sigma$	.0035	−.45	$\mu - .45\sigma$	.3264
−2.65	$\mu - 2.65\sigma$	.0040	−.40	$\mu - .40\sigma$	.3446
−2.60	$\mu - 2.60\sigma$	.0047	−.35	$\mu - .35\sigma$	.3632
−2.55	$\mu - 2.55\sigma$	.0054	−.30	$\mu - .30\sigma$	.3821
−2.50	$\mu - 2.50\sigma$	.0062	−.25	$\mu - .25\sigma$	.4013
−2.45	$\mu - 2.45\sigma$	.0071	−.20	$\mu - .20\sigma$	.4207
−2.40	$\mu - 2.40\sigma$	.0082	−.15	$\mu - .15\sigma$	.4404
−2.35	$\mu - 2.35\sigma$	.0094	−.10	$\mu - .10\sigma$	.4602
−2.30	$\mu - 2.30\sigma$	.0107	−.05	$\mu - .05\sigma$	.4801
−2.25	$\mu - 2.25\sigma$	.0122			
−2.20	$\mu - 2.20\sigma$	.0139			
−2.15	$\mu - 2.15\sigma$	.0158	.00	μ	.5000
−2.10	$\mu - 2.10\sigma$	.0179			
−2.05	$\mu - 2.05\sigma$	.0202			
−2.00	$\mu - 2.00\sigma$	.0228	.05	$\mu + .05\sigma$	.5199
−1.95	$\mu - 1.95\sigma$	.0256	.10	$\mu + .10\sigma$	.5398
−1.90	$\mu - 1.90\sigma$	.0287	.15	$\mu + .15\sigma$	.5596
−1.85	$\mu - 1.85\sigma$	.0322	.20	$\mu + .20\sigma$	.5793
−1.80	$\mu - 1.80\sigma$	.0359	.25	$\mu + .25\sigma$	.5987
−1.75	$\mu - 1.75\sigma$	.0401	.30	$\mu + .30\sigma$	.6179
−1.70	$\mu - 1.70\sigma$	.0446	.35	$\mu + .35\sigma$	.6368
−1.65	$\mu - 1.65\sigma$	.0495	.40	$\mu + .40\sigma$	.6554
−1.60	$\mu - 1.60\sigma$	.0548	.45	$\mu + .45\sigma$	.6736
−1.55	$\mu - 1.55\sigma$	.0606	.50	$\mu + .50\sigma$	.6915
−1.50	$\mu - 1.50\sigma$	.0668	.55	$\mu + .55\sigma$	.7088
−1.45	$\mu - 1.45\sigma$	.0735	.60	$\mu + .60\sigma$	.7257
−1.40	$\mu - 1.40\sigma$	.0808	.65	$\mu + .65\sigma$	.7422
−1.35	$\mu - 1.35\sigma$	.0885	.70	$\mu + .70\sigma$	.7580
−1.30	$\mu - 1.30\sigma$	.0968	.75	$\mu + .75\sigma$	.7734
−1.25	$\mu - 1.25\sigma$	.1056	.80	$\mu + .80\sigma$	.7881
−1.20	$\mu - 1.20\sigma$	.1151	.85	$\mu + .85\sigma$	.8023
−1.15	$\mu - 1.15\sigma$	.1251	.90	$\mu + .90\sigma$	.8159
−1.10	$\mu - 1.10\sigma$	.1357	.95	$\mu + .95\sigma$	.8289
−1.05	$\mu - 1.05\sigma$	.1469	1.00	$\mu + 1.00\sigma$	.8413

Table continued on following page

APPENDIX B (*Continued*)

Z	X	Area	Z	X	Area
1.05	$\mu + 1.05\sigma$	.8531	−4.265	$\mu - 4.265\sigma$	.00001
1.10	$\mu + 1.10\sigma$	.8643	−3.719	$\mu - 3.719\sigma$	.0001
1.15	$\mu + 1.15\sigma$	.8749	−3.090	$\mu - 3.090\sigma$	.001
1.20	$\mu + 1.20\sigma$	.8849	−2.576	$\mu - 2.576\sigma$	.005
1.25	$\mu + 1.25\sigma$	.8944	−2.326	$\mu - 2.236\sigma$	.01
1.30	$\mu + 1.30\sigma$	.9032	−2.054	$\mu - 2.054\sigma$	.02
1.35	$\mu + 1.35\sigma$	.9115	−1.960	$\mu - 1.960\sigma$	.025
1.40	$\mu + 1.40\sigma$	.9192	−1.881	$\mu - 1.881\sigma$	.03
1.45	$\mu + 1.45\sigma$	.9265	−1.751	$\mu - 1.751\sigma$	.04
1.50	$\mu + 1.50\sigma$	.9332	−1.645	$\mu - 1.645\sigma$	.05
1.55	$\mu + 1.55\sigma$	.9394	−1.555	$\mu - 1.555\sigma$	.06
1.60	$\mu + 1.60\sigma$	.9452	−1.476	$\mu - 1.476\sigma$	.07
1.65	$\mu + 1.65\sigma$	.9505	−1.405	$\mu - 1.405\sigma$	.08
1.70	$\mu + 1.70\sigma$	.9554	−1.341	$\mu - 1.341\sigma$	.09
1.75	$\mu + 1.75\sigma$	.9599	−1.282	$\mu - 1.282\sigma$	.10
1.80	$\mu + 1.80\sigma$	.9641	−1.036	$\mu - 1.036\sigma$	.15
1.85	$\mu + 1.85\sigma$	.9678	−.842	$\mu - .842\sigma$	.20
1.90	$\mu + 1.90\sigma$	.9713	−.674	$\mu - .674\sigma$	.25
1.95	$\mu + 1.95\sigma$	.9744	−.524	$\mu - .524\sigma$	.30
2.00	$\mu + 2.00\sigma$	.9772	−.385	$\mu - .385\sigma$	.35
2.05	$\mu + 2.05\sigma$	.9798	−.253	$\mu - .253\sigma$	.40
2.10	$\mu + 2.10\sigma$	.9821	−.126	$\mu - .126\sigma$	.45
2.15	$\mu + 2.15\sigma$	.9842	0	μ	.50
2.20	$\mu + 2.20\sigma$	.9861	.126	$\mu + .126\sigma$	.55
2.25	$\mu + 2.25\sigma$	.9878	.253	$\mu + .253\sigma$	.60
2.30	$\mu + 2.30\sigma$	.9893	.385	$\mu + .385\sigma$	.65
2.35	$\mu + 2.35\sigma$	.9906	.524	$\mu + .524\sigma$	.70
2.40	$\mu + 2.40\sigma$	.9918	.674	$\mu + .674\sigma$	.75
2.45	$\mu + 2.45\sigma$	.9929	.842	$\mu + .842\sigma$	.80
2.50	$\mu + 2.50\sigma$	.9938	1.036	$\mu + 1.036\sigma$	.85
2.55	$\mu + 2.55\sigma$	.9946	1.282	$\mu + 1.282\sigma$	.90
2.60	$\mu + 2.60\sigma$	.9953	1.341	$\mu + 1.341\sigma$	.91
2.65	$\mu + 2.65\sigma$	.9960	1.405	$\mu + 1.405\sigma$	.92
2.70	$\mu + 2.70\sigma$	.9965	1.476	$\mu + 1.476\sigma$	.93
2.75	$\mu + 2.75\sigma$	.9970	1.555	$\mu + 1.555\sigma$	.94
2.80	$\mu + 2.80\sigma$	.9974	1.645	$\mu + 1.645\sigma$	.95
2.85	$\mu + 2.85\sigma$	.9978	1.751	$\mu + 1.751\sigma$	.96
2.90	$\mu + 2.90\sigma$	.9981	1.881	$\mu + 1.881\sigma$	.97
2.95	$\mu + 2.95\sigma$	.9984	1.960	$\mu + 1.960\sigma$	.975
3.00	$\mu + 3.00\sigma$	.9987	2.054	$\mu + 2.054\sigma$	.98
3.05	$\mu + 3.05\sigma$	.9989	2.326	$\mu + 2.326\sigma$	.99
3.10	$\mu + 3.10\sigma$	.9990	2.576	$\mu + 2.576\sigma$	.995
3.15	$\mu + 3.15\sigma$	.9992	3.090	$\mu + 3.090\sigma$	.999
3.20	$\mu + 3.20\sigma$	.9993	3.719	$\mu + 3.719\sigma$	.9999
3.25	$\mu + 3.25\sigma$	.9994	4.265	$\mu + 4.265\sigma$	.99999

From Dixon, W. J. & Massey, F. J. Jr. (1969). *Introduction to statistical analysis* (3rd ed). New York: McGraw-Hill.

APPENDIX C

PERCENTAGE POINTS OF STUDENT'S *t* DISTRIBUTION

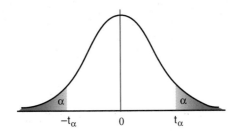

df	α .25 2α .50	.20 .40	.15 .30	.10 .20	.05 .10	.025 .05	.01 .02	.005 .01	.0005 .001
1	1.000	1.376	1.963	3.078	6.314	12.706	31.821	63.657	636.619
2	.816	1.061	1.386	1.886	2.920	4.303	6.965	9.925	31.598
3	.765	.978	1.250	1.638	2.353	3.182	4.541	5.841	12.924
4	.741	.941	1.190	1.533	2.132	2.776	3.747	4.604	8.610
5	.727	.920	1.156	1.476	2.015	2.571	3.365	4.032	6.869
6	.718	.906	1.134	1.440	1.943	2.447	3.143	3.707	5.959
7	.711	.896	1.119	1.415	1.895	2.365	2.998	3.499	5.408
8	.706	.889	1.108	1.397	1.860	2.306	2.896	3.355	5.041
9	.703	.883	1.100	1.383	1.833	2.262	2.821	3.250	4.781
10	.700	.879	1.093	1.372	1.812	2.228	2.764	3.169	4.587
11	.697	.876	1.088	1.363	1.796	2.201	2.718	3.106	4.437
12	.695	.873	1.083	1.356	1.782	2.179	2.681	3.055	4.318
13	.694	.870	1.079	1.350	1.771	2.160	2.650	3.012	4.221
14	.692	.868	1.076	1.345	1.761	2.145	2.624	2.977	4.140
15	.691	.866	1.074	1.341	1.753	2.131	2.602	2.947	4.073
16	.690	.865	1.071	1.337	1.746	2.120	2.583	2.921	4.015
17	.689	.863	1.069	1.333	1.740	2.110	2.567	2.898	3.965
18	.688	.862	1.067	1.330	1.734	2.101	2.552	2.878	3.922
19	.688	.861	1.066	1.328	1.729	2.093	2.539	2.861	3.883
20	.687	.860	1.064	1.325	1.725	2.086	2.528	2.845	3.850
21	.686	.859	1.063	1.323	1.721	2.080	2.518	2.831	3.819
22	.686	.858	1.061	1.321	1.717	2.074	2.508	2.819	3.792
23	.685	.858	1.060	1.319	1.714	2.069	2.500	2.807	3.767
24	.685	.857	1.059	1.318	1.711	2.064	2.492	2.797	3.745
25	.684	.856	1.058	1.316	1.708	2.060	2.458	2.787	3.725
26	.684	.856	1.058	1.315	1.706	2.056	2.479	2.779	3.707
27	.684	.855	1.057	1.314	1.703	2.052	2.473	2.771	3.690
28	.683	.855	1.056	1.313	1.701	2.048	2.467	2.763	3.674
29	.683	.854	1.055	1.311	1.699	2.045	2.462	2.756	3.659
30	.683	.854	1.055	1.310	1.697	2.042	2.457	2.750	3.646
40	.681	.851	1.050	1.303	1.684	2.021	2.423	2.704	3.551
60	.679	.848	1.046	1.296	1.671	2.000	2.390	2.660	3.460
120	.677	.845	1.041	1.289	1.658	1.980	2.358	2.617	3.373
∞	.674	.842	1.036	1.282	1.645	1.960	2.326	2.576	3.291

This table is taken from Table III p. 46 of Fisher, R. A. & Yates, F. (1974). *Statistical tables for biological, agricultural, and medical research* (6th ed.). Published by Longman Group UK Ltd., London. By permission of the authors and publisher).

Appendix D

PERCENTAGE POINTS OF THE *F* DISTRIBUTION

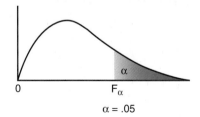

$\alpha = .05$

Degrees of Freedom

V_1

ν_2	1	2	3	4	5	6	7	8	9
1	161.4	199.5	215.7	224.6	230.2	234.0	236.8	238.9	240.5
2	18.51	19.00	19.16	19.25	19.30	19.33	19.35	19.37	19.38
3	10.13	9.55	9.28	9.12	9.01	8.94	8.89	8.85	8.81
4	7.71	6.94	6.59	6.39	6.26	6.16	6.09	6.04	6.00
5	6.61	5.79	5.41	5.19	5.05	4.95	4.88	4.82	4.77
6	5.99	5.14	4.76	4.53	4.39	4.28	4.21	4.15	4.10
7	5.59	4.74	4.35	4.12	3.97	3.87	3.79	3.73	3.68
8	5.32	4.46	4.07	3.84	3.69	3.58	3.50	3.44	3.39
9	5.12	4.26	3.86	3.63	3.48	3.37	3.29	3.23	3.18
10	4.96	4.10	3.71	3.48	3.33	3.22	3.14	3.07	3.02
11	4.84	3.98	3.59	3.36	3.20	3.09	3.01	2.95	2.90
12	4.75	3.89	3.49	3.26	3.11	3.00	2.91	2.85	2.80
13	4.67	3.81	3.41	3.18	3.03	2.92	2.83	2.77	2.71
14	4.60	3.74	3.34	3.11	2.96	2.85	2.76	2.70	2.65
15	4.54	3.68	3.29	3.06	2.90	2.79	2.71	2.64	2.59
16	4.49	3.63	3.24	3.01	2.85	2.74	2.66	2.59	2.54
17	4.45	3.59	3.20	2.96	2.81	2.70	2.61	2.55	2.49
18	4.41	3.55	3.16	2.93	2.77	2.66	2.58	2.51	2.46
19	4.38	3.52	3.13	2.90	2.74	2.63	2.54	2.48	2.42
20	4.35	3.49	3.10	2.87	2.71	2.60	2.51	2.45	2.39
21	4.32	3.47	3.07	2.84	2.68	2.57	2.49	2.42	2.37
22	4.30	3.44	3.05	2.82	2.66	2.55	2.46	2.40	2.34
23	4.28	3.42	3.03	2.80	2.64	2.53	2.44	2.37	2.32
24	4.26	3.40	3.01	2.78	2.62	2.51	2.42	2.36	2.30
25	4.24	3.39	2.99	2.76	2.60	2.49	2.40	2.34	2.28
26	4.23	3.37	2.98	2.74	2.59	2.47	2.39	2.32	2.27
27	4.21	3.35	2.96	2.73	2.57	2.46	2.37	2.31	2.25
28	4.20	3.34	2.95	2.71	2.56	2.45	2.36	2.29	2.24
29	4.18	3.33	2.93	2.70	2.55	2.43	2.35	2.28	2.22
30	4.17	3.32	2.92	2.69	2.53	2.42	2.33	2.27	2.21
40	4.08	3.23	2.84	2.61	2.45	2.34	2.25	2.18	2.12
60	4.00	3.15	2.76	2.53	2.37	2.25	2.17	2.10	2.04
120	3.92	3.07	2.68	2.45	2.29	2.17	2.09	2.02	1.96
∞	3.84	3.00	2.60	2.37	2.21	2.10	2.01	1.94	1.88

APPENDIX **D** *(Continued)*

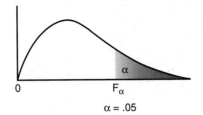

$\alpha = .05$

V_1

10	12	15	20	24	30	40	60	120	∞	v_2
241.9	243.9	245.9	248.0	249.1	250.1	251.1	252.2	253.3	254.3	1
19.40	19.41	19.43	19.45	19.45	19.46	19.47	19.48	19.49	19.50	2
8.79	8.74	8.70	8.66	8.64	8.62	8.59	8.57	8.55	8.53	3
5.96	5.91	5.86	5.80	5.77	5.75	5.72	5.69	5.66	5.63	4
4.74	4.68	4.62	4.56	4.53	4.50	4.46	4.43	4.40	4.36	5
4.06	4.00	3.94	3.87	3.84	3.81	3.77	3.74	3.70	3.67	6
3.64	3.57	3.51	3.44	3.41	3.38	3.34	3.30	3.27	3.23	7
3.35	3.28	3.22	3.15	3.12	3.08	3.04	3.01	2.97	2.93	8
3.14	3.07	3.01	2.94	2.90	2.86	2.83	2.79	2.75	2.71	9
2.98	2.91	2.85	2.77	2.74	2.70	2.66	2.62	2.58	2.54	10
2.85	2.79	2.72	2.65	2.61	2.57	2.53	2.49	2.45	2.40	11
2.75	2.69	2.62	2.54	2.51	2.47	2.43	2.38	2.34	2.30	12
2.67	2.60	2.53	2.46	2.42	2.38	2.34	2.30	2.25	2.21	13
2.60	2.53	2.46	2.39	2.35	2.31	2.27	2.22	2.18	2.13	14
2.54	2.48	2.40	2.33	2.29	2.25	2.20	2.16	2.11	2.07	15
2.49	2.42	2.35	2.28	2.24	2.19	2.15	2.11	2.06	2.01	16
2.45	2.38	2.31	2.23	2.19	2.15	2.10	2.06	2.01	1.96	17
2.41	2.34	2.27	2.19	2.15	2.11	2.06	2.02	1.97	1.92	18
2.38	2.31	2.23	2.16	2.11	2.07	2.03	1.98	1.93	1.88	19
2.35	2.28	2.20	2.12	2.08	2.04	1.99	1.95	1.90	1.84	20
2.32	2.25	2.18	2.10	2.05	2.01	1.96	1.92	1.87	1.81	21
2.30	2.23	2.15	2.07	2.03	1.98	1.94	1.89	1.84	1.78	22
2.27	2.20	2.13	2.05	2.01	1.96	1.91	1.86	1.81	1.76	23
2.25	2.18	2.11	2.03	1.98	1.94	1.89	1.84	1.79	1.73	24
2.24	2.16	2.09	2.01	1.96	1.92	1.87	1.82	1.77	1.71	25
2.22	2.15	2.07	1.99	1.95	1.90	1.85	1.80	1.75	1.69	26
2.20	2.13	2.06	1.97	1.93	1.88	1.84	1.79	1.73	1.67	27
2.19	2.12	2.04	1.96	1.91	1.87	1.82	1.77	1.71	1.65	28
2.18	2.10	2.03	1.94	1.90	1.85	1.81	1.75	1.70	1.64	29
2.16	2.09	2.01	1.93	1.89	1.84	1.79	1.74	1.68	1.62	30
2.08	2.00	1.92	1.84	1.79	1.74	1.69	1.64	1.58	1.51	40
1.99	1.92	1.84	1.75	1.70	1.65	1.59	1.53	1.47	1.39	60
1.91	1.83	1.75	1.66	1.61	1.55	1.50	1.43	1.35	1.25	120
1.83	1.75	1.67	1.57	1.52	1.46	1.39	1.32	1.22	1.00	∞

Table continued on following page

APPENDIX D *(Continued)*

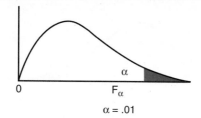

$\alpha = .01$

Degrees of Freedom

ν_1

ν_2	1	2	3	4	5	6	7	8	9
1	4052	4999.5	5403	5625	5764	5859	5928	5982	6022
2	98.50	99.00	99.17	99.25	99.30	99.33	99.36	99.37	99.39
3	34.12	30.82	29.46	28.71	28.24	27.91	27.67	27.49	27.35
4	21.20	18.00	16.69	15.98	15.52	15.21	14.98	14.80	14.66
5	16.26	13.27	12.06	11.39	10.97	10.67	10.46	10.29	10.16
6	13.75	10.92	9.78	9.15	8.75	8.47	8.26	8.10	7.98
7	12.25	9.55	8.45	7.85	7.46	7.19	6.99	6.84	6.72
8	11.26	8.65	7.59	7.01	6.63	6.37	6.18	6.03	5.91
9	10.56	8.02	6.99	6.42	6.06	5.80	5.61	5.47	5.35
10	10.04	7.56	6.55	5.99	5.64	5.39	5.20	5.06	4.94
11	9.65	7.21	6.22	5.67	5.32	5.07	4.89	4.74	4.63
12	9.33	6.93	5.95	5.41	5.06	4.82	4.64	4.50	4.39
13	9.07	6.70	5.74	5.21	4.86	4.62	4.44	4.30	4.19
14	8.86	6.51	5.56	5.04	4.69	4.46	4.28	4.14	4.03
15	8.68	6.36	5.42	4.89	4.56	4.32	4.14	4.00	3.89
16	8.53	6.23	5.29	4.77	4.44	4.20	4.03	3.89	3.78
17	8.40	6.11	5.18	4.67	4.34	4.10	3.93	3.79	3.68
18	8.29	6.01	5.09	4.58	4.25	4.01	3.84	3.71	3.60
19	8.18	5.93	5.01	4.50	4.17	3.94	3.77	3.63	3.52
20	8.10	5.85	4.94	4.43	4.10	3.87	3.70	3.56	3.46
21	8.02	5.78	4.87	4.37	4.04	3.81	3.64	3.51	3.40
22	7.95	5.72	4.82	4.31	3.99	3.76	3.59	3.45	3.35
23	7.88	5.66	4.76	4.26	3.94	3.71	3.54	3.41	3.30
24	7.82	5.61	4.72	4.22	3.90	3.67	3.50	3.36	3.26
25	7.77	5.57	4.68	4.18	3.85	3.63	3.46	3.32	3.22
26	7.72	5.53	4.64	4.14	3.82	3.59	3.42	3.29	3.18
27	7.68	5.49	4.60	4.11	3.78	3.56	3.39	3.26	3.15
28	7.64	5.45	4.57	4.07	3.75	3.53	3.36	3.23	3.12
29	7.60	5.42	4.54	4.04	3.73	3.50	3.33	3.20	3.09
30	7.56	5.39	4.51	4.02	3.70	3.47	3.30	3.17	3.07
40	7.31	5.18	4.31	3.83	3.51	3.29	3.12	2.99	2.89
60	7.08	4.98	4.13	3.65	3.34	3.12	2.95	2.82	2.72
120	6.85	4.79	3.95	3.48	3.17	2.96	2.79	2.66	2.56
∞	6.63	4.61	3.78	3.32	3.02	2.80	2.64	2.51	2.41

APPENDIX D *(Continued)*

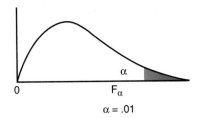

α = .01

				ν_1								ν_2
10	**12**	**15**	**20**	**24**	**30**	**40**	**60**	**120**	**∞**		
6056	6106	6157	6209	6235	6261	6287	6313	6339	6366		1
99.40	99.42	99.43	99.45	99.46	99.47	99.47	99.48	99.49	99.50		2
27.23	27.05	26.87	26.69	26.60	26.50	26.41	26.32	26.22	26.13		3
14.55	14.37	14.20	14.02	13.93	13.84	13.75	13.65	13.56	13.46		4
10.05	9.89	9.72	9.55	9.47	9.38	9.29	9.20	9.11	9.02		5
7.87	7.72	7.56	7.40	7.31	7.23	7.14	7.06	6.97	6.88		6
6.62	6.47	6.31	6.16	6.07	5.99	5.91	5.82	5.74	5.65		7
5.81	5.67	5.52	5.36	5.28	5.20	5.12	5.03	4.95	4.86		8
5.26	5.11	4.96	4.81	4.73	4.65	4.57	4.48	4.40	4.31		9
4.85	4.71	4.56	4.41	4.33	4.25	4.17	4.08	4.00	3.91		10
4.54	4.40	4.25	4.10	4.02	3.94	3.86	3.78	3.69	3.60		11
4.30	4.16	4.01	3.86	3.78	3.70	3.62	3.54	3.45	3.36		12
4.10	3.96	3.82	3.66	3.59	3.51	3.43	3.34	3.25	3.17		13
3.94	3.80	3.66	3.51	3.43	3.35	3.27	3.18	3.09	3.00		14
3.80	3.67	3.52	3.37	3.29	3.21	3.13	3.05	2.96	2.87		15
3.69	3.55	3.41	3.26	3.18	3.10	3.02	2.93	2.84	2.75		16
3.59	3.46	3.31	3.16	3.08	3.00	2.92	2.83	2.75	2.65		17
3.51	3.37	3.23	3.08	3.00	2.92	2.84	2.75	2.66	2.57		18
3.43	3.30	3.15	3.00	2.92	2.84	2.76	2.67	2.58	2.49		19
3.37	3.23	3.09	2.94	2.86	2.78	2.69	2.61	2.52	2.42		20
3.31	3.17	3.03	2.88	2.80	2.72	2.64	2.55	2.46	2.36		21
3.26	3.12	2.98	2.83	2.75	2.67	2.58	2.50	2.40	2.31		22
3.21	3.07	2.93	2.78	2.70	2.62	2.54	2.45	2.35	2.26		23
3.17	3.03	2.89	2.74	2.66	2.58	2.49	2.40	2.31	2.21		24
3.13	2.99	2.85	2.70	2.62	2.54	2.45	2.36	2.27	2.17		25
3.09	2.96	2.81	2.66	2.58	2.50	2.42	2.33	2.23	2.13		26
3.06	2.93	2.78	2.63	2.55	2.47	2.38	2.29	2.20	2.10		27
3.03	2.90	2.75	2.60	2.52	2.44	2.35	2.26	2.17	2.06		28
3.00	2.87	2.73	2.57	2.49	2.41	2.33	2.23	2.14	2.03		29
2.98	2.84	2.70	2.55	2.47	2.39	2.30	2.21	2.11	2.01		30
2.80	2.66	2.52	2.37	2.29	2.20	2.11	2.02	1.92	1.80		40
2.63	2.50	2.35	2.20	2.12	2.03	1.94	1.84	1.73	1.60		60
2.47	2.34	2.19	2.03	1.95	1.86	1.76	1.66	1.53	1.38		120
2.32	2.18	2.04	1.88	1.79	1.70	1.59	1.47	1.32	1.00		∞

From Merrington, M. & Thompson, C. M. (1943). Tables of percentage points of the inverted beta (F) distribution. *Biometrika, 33*(1):73–78.

Appendix E

CRITICAL VALUES OF THE χ^2 DISTRIBUTION

df	$P_{0.5}$	P_{01}	$P_{02.5}$	P_{05}	P_{10}	P_{90}	P_{95}	$P_{97.5}$	P_{99}	$P_{99.5}$
1	.000039	.00016	.00098	.0039	.0158	2.71	3.84	5.02	6.63	7.88
2	.0100	.0201	.0506	.1026	.2107	4.61	5.99	7.38	9.21	10.60
3	.0717	.115	.216	.352	.584	6.25	7.81	9.35	11.34	12.84
4	.207	.297	.484	.711	1.064	7.78	9.49	11.14	13.28	14.86
5	.412	.554	.831	1.15	1.61	9.24	11.07	12.83	15.09	16.75
6	.676	.872	1.24	1.64	2.20	10.64	12.59	14.45	16.81	18.55
7	.989	1.24	1.69	2.17	2.83	12.02	14.07	16.01	18.48	20.28
8	1.34	1.65	2.18	2.73	3.49	13.36	15.51	17.53	20.09	21.96
9	1.73	2.09	2.70	3.33	4.17	14.68	16.92	19.02	21.67	23.59
10	2.16	2.56	3.25	3.94	4.87	15.99	18.31	20.48	23.21	25.19
11	2.60	3.05	3.82	4.57	5.58	17.28	19.68	21.92	24.73	26.76
12	3.07	3.57	4.40	5.23	6.30	18.55	21.03	23.34	26.22	28.30
13	3.57	4.11	5.01	5.89	7.04	19.81	22.36	24.74	27.69	29.82
14	4.07	4.66	5.63	6.57	7.79	21.06	23.68	26.12	29.14	31.32
15	4.60	5.23	6.26	7.26	8.55	22.31	25.00	27.49	30.58	32.80
16	5.14	5.81	6.91	7.96	9.31	23.54	26.30	28.85	32.00	34.27
18	6.26	7.01	8.23	9.39	10.86	25.99	28.87	31.53	34.81	37.16
20	7.43	8.26	9.59	10.85	12.44	28.41	31.41	34.17	37.57	40.00
24	9.89	10.86	12.40	13.85	15.66	33.20	36.42	39.36	42.98	45.56
30	13.79	14.95	16.79	18.49	20.60	40.26	43.77	46.98	50.98	53.67
40	20.71	22.16	24.43	26.51	29.05	51.81	55.76	59.34	63.69	66.77
60	35.53	37.48	40.48	43.19	46.46	74.40	79.08	83.30	88.38	91.95
120	83.85	86.92	91.58	95.70	100.62	140.23	146.57	152.21	158.95	163.64

From Dixon, W. J. & Massey, F. J. Jr. (1969). *Introduction to statistical analysis* (3rd ed.). New York: McGraw-Hill.

APPENDIX F

TABLE OF PROBABILITIES ASSOCIATED WITH VALUES AS SMALL AS OBSERVED VALUES OF *U* IN THE MANN-WHITNEY TEST

$n_2 = 3$			
U \ n_1	1	2	3
0	.250	.100	.050
1	.500	.200	.100
2	.750	.400	.200
3		.600	.350
4			.500
5			.650

$n_2 = 4$				
U \ n_1	1	2	3	4
0	.200	.067	.028	.014
1	.400	.133	.057	.029
2	.600	.267	.114	.057
3		.400	.200	.100
4		.600	.314	.171
5			.429	.243
6			.571	.343
7				.443
8				.557

$n_2 = 5$					
U \ n_1	1	2	3	4	5
0	.167	.047	.018	.008	.005
1	.333	.095	.036	.016	.008
2	.500	.190	.071	.032	.016
3	.667	.286	.125	.056	.028
4		.429	.196	.095	.048
5		.571	.286	.143	.075
6			.393	.206	.111
7			.500	.278	.155
8			.607	.365	.210
9				.452	.274
10				.548	.345
11					.500
12					.579
13					

$n_2 = 6$						
U \ n_1	1	2	3	4	5	6
0	.143	.036	.012	.005	.002	.001
1	.286	.071	.024	.010	.004	.002
2	.428	.143	.048	.019	.009	.004
3	.571	.214	.083	.033	.015	.008
4		.321	.131	.057	.026	.013
5		.429	.190	.086	.041	.021
6		.571	.274	.129	.063	.032
7			.357	.176	.089	.047
8			.452	.238	.123	.066
9			.548	.305	.165	.090
10				.381	.214	.120
11				.457	.268	.155
12				.545	.331	.197
13					.396	.242
14					.465	.294
15					.535	.350
16						.409
17						.469
18						.531

Table continued on following page

APPENDIX F (Continued)

$n_2 = 7$							
n_1 U	1	2	3	4	5	6	7
0	.125	.028	.008	.003	.001	.001	.000
1	.250	.056	.017	.006	.003	.001	.001
2	.375	.111	.033	.012	.005	.002	.001
3	.500	.167	.058	.021	.009	.004	.002
4	.625	.250	.092	.036	.015	.007	.003
5		.333	.133	.055	.024	.011	.006
6		.444	.192	.082	.037	.017	.009
7		.556	.258	.115	.053	.026	.013
8			.333	.158	.074	.037	.019
9			.417	.206	.101	.051	.027
10			.500	.264	.134	.069	.036
11			.583	.324	.172	.090	.049
12				.394	.216	.117	.064
13				.464	.265	.147	.082
14				.538	.319	.183	.104
15					.378	.223	.130
16					.438	.267	.159
17					.500	.314	.191
18					.562	.365	.228
19						.418	.267
20						.473	.310
21						.527	.355
22							.402
23							.451
24							.500
25							.549

APPENDIX F (*Continued*)

					$n_2 = 8$					
n_1										
U	1	2	3	4	5	6	7	8	t	Normal
0	.111	.022	.006	.002	.001	.000	.000	.000	3.308	.001
1	.222	.044	.012	.004	.002	.001	.000	.000	3.203	.001
2	.333	.089	.024	.008	.003	.001	.001	.000	3.098	.001
3	.444	.133	.042	.014	.005	.002	.001	.001	2.993	.001
4	.556	.200	.067	.024	.009	.004	.002	.001	2.888	.002
5		.267	.097	.036	.015	.006	.003	.001	2.783	.003
6		.356	.139	.055	.023	.010	.005	.002	2.678	.004
7		.444	.188	.077	.033	.015	.007	.003	2.573	.005
8		.556	.248	.107	.047	.021	.010	.005	2.468	.007
9			.315	.141	.064	.030	.014	.007	2.363	.009
10			.387	.184	.085	.041	.020	.010	2.258	.012
11			.461	.230	.111	.054	.027	.014	2.153	.016
12			.539	.285	.142	.071	.036	.019	2.048	.020
13				.341	.177	.091	.047	.025	1.943	.026
14				.404	.217	.114	.060	.032	1.838	.033
15				.467	.262	.141	.076	.041	1.733	.041
16				.533	.311	.172	.095	.052	1.628	.052
17					.362	.207	.116	.065	1.523	.064
18					.416	.245	.140	.080	1.418	.078
19					.472	.286	.168	.097	1.313	.094
20					.528	.331	.198	.117	1.208	.113
21						.377	.232	.139	1.102	.135
22						.426	.268	.164	.998	.159
23						.475	.306	.191	.893	.185
24						.525	.347	.221	.788	.215
25							.389	.253	.683	.247
26							.433	.287	.578	.282
27							.478	.323	.473	.318
28							.522	.360	.368	.356
29								.399	.263	.396
30								.439	.158	.437
31								.480	.052	.481
32								.520		

From Mann, H. B. & Whitney, D. R. (1947). On a test of whether one of two random variables is stochastically larger than the other. *Annals of Mathematical Statistics, 18,* 52–54.

APPENDIX G

TABLE OF CRITICAL VALUES OF U IN THE MANN-WHITNEY TEST

TABLE G–1
Critical Values of U for a One-Tailed Test at $\alpha = .001$ or for a
Two-Tailed Test at $\alpha = .002$

n_1 \ n_2	9	10	11	12	13	14	15	16	17	18	19	20
1												
2												
3									0	0	0	0
4		0	0	0	1	1	1	2	2	3	3	3
5	1	1	2	2	3	3	4	5	5	6	7	7
6	2	3	4	4	5	6	7	8	9	10	11	12
7	3	5	6	7	8	9	10	11	13	14	15	16
8	5	6	8	9	11	12	14	15	17	18	20	21
9	7	8	10	12	14	15	17	19	21	23	25	26
10	8	10	12	14	17	19	21	23	25	27	29	32
11	10	12	15	17	20	22	24	27	29	32	34	37
12	12	14	17	20	23	25	28	31	34	37	40	42
13	14	17	20	23	26	29	32	35	38	42	45	48
14	15	19	22	25	29	32	36	39	43	46	50	54
15	17	21	24	28	32	36	40	43	47	51	55	59
16	19	23	27	31	35	39	43	48	52	56	60	65
17	21	25	29	34	38	43	47	52	57	61	66	70
18	23	27	32	37	42	46	51	56	61	66	71	76
19	25	29	34	40	45	50	55	60	66	71	77	82
20	26	32	37	42	48	54	59	65	70	76	82	88

TABLE G–2
Critical Values of U for a One-Tailed Test at $\alpha = .01$ or for a
Two-Tailed Test at $\alpha = .02$

n_1 \ n_2	9	10	11	12	13	14	15	16	17	18	19	20
1												
2					0	0	0	0	0	0	1	1
3	1	1	1	2	2	2	3	3	4	4	4	5
4	3	3	4	5	5	6	7	7	8	9	9	10
5	5	6	7	8	9	10	11	12	13	14	15	16
6	7	8	9	11	12	13	15	16	18	19	20	22
7	9	11	12	14	16	17	19	21	23	24	26	28
8	11	13	15	17	20	22	24	26	28	30	32	34
9	14	16	18	21	23	26	28	31	33	36	38	40
10	16	19	22	24	27	30	33	36	38	41	44	47
11	18	22	25	28	31	34	37	41	44	47	50	53
12	21	24	28	31	35	38	42	46	49	53	56	60
13	23	27	31	35	39	43	47	51	55	59	63	67
14	26	30	34	38	43	47	51	56	60	65	69	73
15	28	33	37	42	47	51	56	61	66	70	75	80
16	31	36	41	46	51	56	61	66	71	76	82	87
17	33	38	44	49	55	60	66	71	77	82	88	93
18	36	41	47	53	59	65	70	76	82	88	94	100
19	38	44	50	56	63	69	75	82	88	94	101	107
20	40	47	53	60	67	73	80	87	93	100	107	114

TABLE G–3
Critical Values of U for a One-Tailed Test at $\alpha = .025$ or for a Two-Tailed Test at $\alpha = .05$

n_1 \ n_2	9	10	11	12	13	14	15	16	17	18	19	20
1												
2	0	0	0	1	1	1	1	1	2	2	2	2
3	2	3	3	4	4	5	5	6	6	7	7	8
4	4	5	6	7	8	9	10	11	11	12	13	13
5	7	8	9	11	12	13	14	15	17	18	19	20
6	10	11	13	14	16	17	19	21	22	24	25	27
7	12	14	16	18	20	22	24	26	28	30	32	34
8	15	17	19	22	24	26	29	31	34	36	38	41
9	17	20	23	26	28	31	34	37	39	42	45	48
10	20	23	26	29	33	36	39	42	45	48	52	55
11	23	26	30	33	37	40	44	47	51	55	58	62
12	26	29	33	37	41	45	49	53	57	61	65	69
13	28	33	37	41	45	50	54	59	63	67	72	76
14	31	36	40	45	50	55	59	64	67	74	78	83
15	34	39	44	49	54	59	64	70	75	80	85	90
16	37	42	47	53	59	64	70	75	81	86	92	98
17	39	45	51	57	63	67	75	81	87	93	99	105
18	42	48	55	61	67	74	80	86	93	99	106	112
19	45	52	58	65	72	78	85	92	99	106	113	119
20	48	55	62	69	76	83	90	98	105	112	119	127

TABLE G–4
Critical Values of U for a One-Tailed Test at $\alpha = .05$ or for a Two-Tailed Test at $\alpha = .10$

n_1 \ n_2	9	10	11	12	13	14	15	16	17	18	19	20
1											0	0
2	1	1	1	2	2	2	3	3	3	4	4	4
3	3	4	5	5	6	7	7	8	9	9	10	11
4	6	7	8	9	10	11	12	14	15	16	17	18
5	9	11	12	13	15	16	18	19	20	22	23	25
6	12	14	16	17	19	21	23	25	26	28	30	32
7	15	17	19	21	24	26	28	30	33	35	37	39
8	18	20	23	26	28	31	33	36	39	41	44	47
9	21	24	27	30	33	36	39	42	45	48	51	54
10	24	27	31	34	37	41	44	48	51	55	58	62
11	27	31	34	38	42	46	50	54	57	61	65	69
12	30	34	38	42	47	51	55	60	64	68	72	77
13	33	37	42	47	51	56	61	65	70	75	80	84
14	36	41	46	51	56	61	66	71	77	82	87	92
15	39	44	50	55	61	66	72	77	83	88	94	100
16	42	48	54	60	65	71	77	83	89	95	101	107
17	45	51	57	64	70	77	83	89	96	102	109	115
18	48	55	61	68	75	82	88	95	102	109	116	123
19	51	58	65	72	80	87	94	101	109	116	123	130
20	54	62	69	77	84	92	100	107	115	123	130	138

From Siegel, S. (1956). *Nonparametric statistics for the behavioral sciences.* New York: McGraw-Hill; as adapted from Auble, D. (1953). Extended tables for the Mann-Whitney Statistic. *Bulletin of Institute of Educational Research at Indiana University* (Vol. 1, No. 2).

APPENDIX H

PERCENTILES OF THE KOLMOGOROV–SMIRNOV TEST STATISTIC

n_1	n_2	One-Sided Test: $\alpha =$ .90 / Two-Sided Test: $\alpha =$ .80	.95 / .90	.975 / .95	.99 / .98	.995 / .99
3	3	.667	.667			
3	4	.750	.750			
3	5	.667	.800	.800		
3	6	.667	.667	.833		
3	7	.667	.714	.857	.857	
3	8	.625	.750	.750	.875	
3	9	.667	.667	.778	.889	.889
3	10	.600	.700	.800	.900	.900
3	12	.583	.667	.750	.833	.917
4	4	.750	.750	.750		
4	5	.600	.750	.800	.800	
4	6	.583	.667	.750	.833	.833
4	7	.607	.714	.750	.857	.857
4	8	.625	.625	.750	.875	.875
4	9	.556	.667	.750	.778	.889
4	10	.550	.650	.700	.800	.800
4	12	.583	.667	.667	.750	.833
4	16	.563	.625	.688	.750	.812
5	5	.600	.600	.800	.800	.800
5	6	.600	.667	.667	.833	.833
5	7	.571	.657	.714	.829	.857
5	8	.550	.625	.675	.800	.800
5	9	.556	.600	.689	.778	.800
5	10	.500	.600	.700	.700	.800
5	15	.533	.600	.667	.733	.733
5	20	.500	.550	.600	.700	.750
6	6	.500	.667	.667	.833	.833
6	7	.548	.571	.690	.714	.833
6	8	.500	.583	.667	.750	.750
6	9	.500	.556	.667	.722	.778
6	10	.500	.567	.633	.700	.733
6	12	.500	.583	.583	.667	.750
6	18	.444	.556	.611	.667	.722
6	24	.458	.500	.583	.625	.667
7	7	.571	.571	.714	.714	.714
7	8	.482	.589	.625	.732	.750
7	9	.492	.556	.635	.714	.746
7	10	.471	.557	.614	.700	.714
7	14	.429	.500	.571	.643	.714
7	28	.429	.464	.536	.607	.643
8	8	.500	.500	.625	.625	.750
8	9	.444	.542	.625	.667	.750
8	10	.475	.525	.575	.675	.700
8	12	.458	.500	.583	.625	.667

APPENDIX H *(Continued)*

n_1	n_2	One-Sided Test: $\alpha =$ .90	.95	.975	.99	.995
		Two-Sided Test: $\alpha =$ .80	.90	.95	.98	.99
8	16	.438	.500	.563	.625	.625
8	32	.406	.438	.500	.563	.594
9	9	.444	.556	.556	.667	.667
9	10	.467	.500	.578	.667	.689
9	12	.444	.500	.556	.611	.667
9	15	.422	.489	.533	.600	.644
9	18	.389	.444	.500	.556	.611
9	36	.361	.417	.472	.528	.556
10	10	.400	.500	.600	.600	.700
10	15	.400	.467	.500	.567	.633
10	20	.400	.450	.500	.550	.600
10	40	.350	.400	.450	.500	.576
11	11	.454	.454	.545	.636	.636
12	12	.417	.417	.500	.583	.583
12	15	.383	.450	.500	.550	.583
12	16	.375	.438	.479	.542	.583
12	18	.361	.417	.472	.528	.556
12	20	.367	.417	.467	.517	.567
13	13	.385	.462	.462	.538	.615
14	14	.357	.429	.500	.500	.571
15	15	.333	.400	.467	.467	.533
16	16	.375	.375	.438	.500	.563
17	17	.353	.412	.412	.471	.529
18	18	.333	.389	.444	.500	.500
19	19	.316	.368	.421	.473	.473
20	20	.300	.350	.400	.450	.500
21	21	.286	.333	.381	.429	.476
22	22	.318	.364	.364	.454	.454
23	23	.304	.348	.391	.435	.435
24	24	.292	.333	.375	.417	.458
25	25	.280	.320	.360	.400	.440

For other sample sizes, let $C = \sqrt{\dfrac{n_1 + n_2}{n_1 n_2}}$, and use as an approximation:

		$1.07C$	$1.22C$	$1.36C$	$1.52C$	$1.63C$

From Marascuilo, L. A. & McSweeney, M. (1978). *Nonparametric and distribution-free methods for the social sciences. Journal of the American Statistical Association, 73*(363), 678–679; as adapted from Massey, F. J. Jr. (1952). *Annals of Mathematical Statistics,* 435–441.

APPENDIX I

TABLE OF CRITICAL VALUES OF *r* IN THE RUNS TEST

Given in the bodies of Table I–1 and Table I–2 are various critical values of *r* for various values of n_1 and n_2. For the one-sample runs test, any value of *r* that is equal to or smaller than that shown in Table I–1 or equal to or larger than that shown in Table I–2 is significant at the .05 level. For the Wald-Wolfowitz two-sample runs test, any value of *r* that is equal to or smaller than that shown in Table I–1 is significant at the .05 level.

TABLE I–1

n_2 \ n_1	2	3	4	5	6	7	8	9	10	11	12	13	14	15	16	17	18	19	20
2											2	2	2	2	2	2	2	2	2
3				2	2	2	2	2	2	2	2	2	3	3	3	3	3	3
4			2	2	2	3	3	3	3	3	3	3	3	4	4	4	4	4
5		2	2	3	3	3	3	3	4	4	4	4	4	4	4	5	5	5
6	2	2	3	3	3	3	4	4	4	4	5	5	5	5	5	5	6	6
7	2	2	3	3	3	4	4	5	5	5	5	5	6	6	6	6	6	6
8	2	3	3	3	4	4	5	5	5	6	6	6	6	6	7	7	7	7
9	2	3	3	4	4	5	5	5	6	6	6	7	7	7	7	8	8	8
10	2	3	3	4	5	5	5	6	6	7	7	7	7	8	8	8	8	9
11	2	3	4	4	5	5	6	6	7	7	7	8	8	8	9	9	9	9
12	2	2	3	4	4	5	6	6	7	7	7	8	8	8	9	9	9	10	10
13	2	2	3	4	5	5	6	6	7	7	8	8	9	9	9	10	10	10	10
14	2	2	3	4	5	5	6	7	7	8	8	9	9	9	10	10	10	11	11
15	2	3	3	4	5	6	6	7	7	8	8	9	9	10	10	11	11	11	12
16	2	3	4	4	5	6	6	7	8	8	9	9	10	10	11	11	11	12	12
17	2	3	4	4	5	6	7	7	8	9	9	10	10	11	11	11	12	12	13
18	2	3	4	5	5	6	7	8	8	9	9	10	10	11	11	12	12	13	13
19	2	3	4	5	6	6	7	8	8	9	10	10	11	11	12	12	13	13	13
20	2	3	4	5	6	6	7	8	9	9	10	10	11	12	12	13	13	13	14

APPENDIX I *(Continued)*

TABLE I–2

n_2 \ n_1	2	3	4	5	6	7	8	9	10	11	12	13	14	15	16	17	18	19	20
2																			
3																			
4				9	9														
5			9	10	10	11	11												
6			9	10	11	12	12	13	13	13	13								
7				11	12	13	13	14	14	14	14	15	15	15					
8				11	12	13	14	14	15	15	16	16	16	16	17	17	17	17	17
9					13	14	14	15	16	16	16	17	17	18	18	18	18	18	18
10					13	14	15	16	16	17	17	18	18	18	19	19	19	20	20
11					13	14	15	16	17	17	18	19	19	19	20	20	20	21	21
12					13	14	16	16	17	18	19	19	20	20	21	21	21	22	22
13						15	16	17	18	19	19	20	20	21	21	22	22	23	23
14						15	16	17	18	19	20	20	21	22	22	23	23	23	24
15						15	16	18	18	19	20	21	22	22	23	23	24	24	25
16							17	18	19	20	21	21	22	23	23	24	25	25	25
17							17	18	19	20	21	22	23	23	24	25	25	26	26
18							17	18	19	20	21	22	23	24	25	25	26	26	27
19							17	18	20	21	22	23	23	24	25	26	26	27	27
20							17	18	20	21	22	23	24	25	25	26	27	27	28

From Siegel, S. (1956). *Nonparametric statistics for the behavioral sciences.* New York: McGraw-Hill; as adapted from Swed, F. S. & Eisenhart, C. (1943). Tables for testing randomness of grouping in a sequence of alternatives. *Annals of Mathematical Statistics, 14,* 83–86.

APPENDIX J

CRITICAL VALUES FOR THE WILCOXON SIGNED-RANKS TEST
($N = 5(1)50$)

One-sided	Two-sided	$N = 5$	$N = 6$	$N = 7$	$N = 8$	$N = 9$	$N = 10$	$N = 11$	$N = 12$	$N = 13$	$N = 14$	$N = 15$	$N = 16$
$p = .05$	$p = .10$	1	2	4	6	8	11	14	17	21	26	30	36
$p = .025$	$p = .05$		1	2	4	6	8	11	14	17	21	25	30
$p = .01$	$p = .02$			0	2	3	5	7	10	13	16	20	24
$p = .005$	$p = .01$				0	2	3	5	7	10	13	16	19

One-sided	Two-sided	$N = 17$	$N = 18$	$N = 19$	$N = 20$	$N = 21$	$N = 22$	$N = 23$	$N = 24$	$N = 25$	$N = 26$	$N = 27$	$N = 28$
$p = .05$	$p = .10$	41	47	54	60	68	75	83	92	101	110	120	130
$p = .025$	$p = .05$	35	40	46	52	59	66	73	81	90	98	107	117
$p = .01$	$p = .02$	28	33	38	43	49	56	62	69	77	85	93	102
$p = .005$	$p = .01$	23	28	32	37	43	49	55	61	68	76	84	92

One-sided	Two-sided	$N = 29$	$N = 30$	$N = 31$	$N = 32$	$N = 33$	$N = 34$	$N = 35$	$N = 36$	$N = 37$	$N = 38$	$N = 39$
$p = .05$	$p = .10$	141	152	163	175	188	201	214	228	242	256	271
$p = .025$	$p = .05$	127	137	148	159	171	183	195	208	222	235	250
$p = .01$	$p = .02$	111	120	130	141	151	162	174	186	198	211	224
$p = .005$	$p = .01$	100	109	118	128	138	149	160	171	183	195	208

One-sided	Two-sided	$N = 40$	$N = 41$	$N = 42$	$N = 43$	$N = 44$	$N = 45$	$N = 46$	$N = 47$	$N = 48$	$N = 49$	$N = 50$
$p = .05$	$p = .10$	287	303	319	336	353	371	389	408	427	446	466
$p = .025$	$p = .05$	264	279	295	311	327	344	361	397	397	415	434
$p = .01$	$p = .02$	238	252	267	281	297	313	329	345	362	380	398
$p = .005$	$p = .01$	221	234	248	262	277	292	307	323	339	356	373

From Wilcoxon, F. & Wilcox, R. A. (1964). *Some rapid approximate statistical procedures* (revised ed.) Pearl River, New York: Lederle Laboratories.

APPENDIX K

TABLE OF PROBABILITIES ASSOCIATED WITH VALUES AS LARGE AS OBSERVED VALUES OF *H* IN THE KRUSKAL–WALLIS ONE-WAY ANALYSIS OF VARIANCE BY RANKS

SAMPLE SIZES					SAMPLE SIZES				
n_1	n_2	n_3	*H*	*p*	n_1	n_2	n_3	*H*	*p*
2	1	1	2.7000	.500	4	3	2	6.4444	.008
								3.6000	.011
2	2	1	3.6000	.200				5.4444	.046
								5.4000	.051
2	2	2	4.5714	.067				4.5111	.098
			3.7143	.200				4.4444	.102
3	1	1	3.2000	.300	4	3	3	6.7455	.010
3	2	1	4.2857	.100				6.7091	.013
			3.8571	.133				5.7909	.046
								5.7273	.050
3	2	2	5.3572	.029				4.7091	.092
			4.7143	.048				4.7000	.101
			4.5000	.067					
			4.4643	.105	4	4	1	6.6667	.010
3	3	1	5.1429	.043				6.1667	.022
			4.5714	.100				4.9667	.048
			4.0000	.129				4.8667	.054
								4.1667	.082
								4.0667	.102
3	3	2	6.2500	.011					
			5.3611	.032	4	4	2	7.0364	.006
			5.1389	.061				6.8727	.011
			4.5556	.100				5.4545	.046
			4.2500	.121				5.2364	.052
								4.5545	.098
3	3	3	7.2000	.004				4.4455	.103
			6.4889	.011					
			5.6889	.029					
			5.6000	.050	4	4	3	7.1439	.010
			5.0667	.086				7.1364	.011
			4.6222	.100				5.5985	.049
								5.5758	.051

Table continued on following page

APPENDIX K *(Continued)*

n_1	n_2	n_3	H	p	n_1	n_2	n_3	H	p
\multicolumn{3}{c}{**SAMPLE SIZES**}			\multicolumn{3}{c}{**SAMPLE SIZES**}			
4	1	1	3.5714	.200				4.5455	.099
								4.4773	.102
4	2	1	4.8214	.057					
			4.5000	.076	4	4	4	7.6538	.008
			4.0179	.114				7.5385	.011
								5.6923	.049
4	2	2	6.0000	.014				5.6538	.054
			5.3333	.033				4.6539	.097
			5.1250	.052				4.5001	.104
			4.4583	.100					
			4.1667	.105	5	1	1	3.8571	.143
4	3	1	5.8333	.021	5	2	1	5.2500	.036
			5.2083	.050				5.0000	.048
			5.0000	.057				4.4500	.071
			4.0556	.093				4.2000	.095
			3.8889	.129				4.0500	.119
								5.6308	.050
5	2	2	6.5333	.008				4.5487	.099
			6.1333	.013				4.5231	.103
			6.1600	.034					
			5.0400	.056	5	4	4	7.7604	.009
			4.3733	.090				7.7440	.011
			4.2933	.122				5.6571	.049
								5.6176	.050
5	3	1	6.4000	.012				4.6187	.100
			4.9600	.048				4.5527	.102
			4.8711	.052					
			4.0178	.095	5	5	1	7.3091	.009
			3.8400	.123				6.8364	.011
								5.1273	.046
5	3	2	6.9091	.009				4.9091	.053
			6.8218	.010				4.1091	.086
			5.2509	.049				4.0364	.105
			5.1055	.052					
			4.6509	.091	5	5	2	7.3385	.010
			4.4945	.101				7.2692	.010
								5.3385	.047

APPENDIX K *(Continued)*

SAMPLE SIZES					SAMPLE SIZES				
n_1	n_2	n_3	H	p	n_1	n_2	n_3	H	p
5	3	3	7.0788	.009				5.2462	.051
			6.9818	.011				4.6231	.097
			5.6485	.049				4.5077	.100
			5.5152	.051					
			4.5333	.097	5	5	3	7.5780	.010
			4.4121	.109				7.5429	.010
								5.7055	.046
5	4	1	6.9545	.008				5.6264	.051
			6.8400	.011				4.5451	.100
			4.9855	.044				4.5363	.102
			4.8600	.056					
			3.9873	.098	5	5	4	7.8229	.010
			3.9600	.102				7.7914	.010
								5.6657	.049
5	4	2	7.2045	.009				5.6429	.050
			7.1182	.010				4.5229	.099
			5.2727	.049				4.5200	.101
			5.2682	.050					
			4.5409	.098	5	5	5	8.0000	.009
			4.5182	.101				7.9800	.010
								5.7800	.049
5	4	3	7.4449	.010				5.6600	.051
			7.3949	.011				4.5600	.100
			5.6564	.049				4.5000	.102

From Siegel, S. (1956). *Nonparametric statistics for the behavioral sciences.* New York: McGraw-Hill; as adapted from Kruskal, W. H. & Wallis, W. A. (1952). Use of ranks in one-criterion variance analysis. *Journal of the American Statistical Association, 47,* 614–617.

APPENDIX L

TABLE OF PROBABILITIES ASSOCIATED WITH VALUES AS LARGE AS OBSERVED VALUES OF χ_r^2 IN THE FRIEDMAN TWO-WAY ANALYSIS OF VARIANCE BY RANKS

TABLE L–1
$k = 3$

χ_r^2	p	χ_r^2	p	χ_r^2	p	χ_r^2	p
N = 2		**N = 3**		**N = 4**		**N = 5**	
0	1.000	.000	1.000	.0	1.000	.0	1.00
1	.833	.667	.944	.5	.931	.4	.954
3	.500	2.000	.528	1.5	.653	1.2	.691
4	167	2.667	.361	2.0	.431	1.6	.522
		4.667	.194	3.5	.273	2.8	.367
		6.000	.028	4.5	.125	3.6	.182
				6.0	.069	4.8	.124
				6.5	.042	5.2	.093
				8.0	.0046	6.4	.039
						7.6	.024
						8.4	.0085
						10.0	.00077

χ_r^2	p	χ_r^2	p	χ_r^2	p	χ_r^2	p
N = 6		**N = 7**		**N = 8**		**N = 9**	
.00	1.000	.000	1.000	.00	1.000	.000	1.000
.33	.956	.286	.964	.25	.967	.222	.971
1.00	.740	.857	.768	.75	.794	.667	.814
1.33	.570	1.143	.620	1.00	.654	.889	.865
2.33	.430	2.000	.486	1.75	.531	1.556	.569
3.00	.252	2.571	.305	2.25	.355	2.000	.398
4.00	.184	3.429	.237	3.00	.285	2.667	.328
4.33	.142	3.714	.192	3.25	.236	2.889	.278
5.33	.072	4.571	.112	4.00	.149	3.556	.187
6.33	.052	5.429	.085	4.75	.120	4.222	.154
7.00	.029	6.000	.052	5.25	.079	4.667	.107
8.33	.012	7.143	.027	6.25	.047	5.556	.069
9.00	.0081	7.714	.021	6.75	.038	6.000	.057
9.33	.0055	8.000	.016	7.00	.030	6.222	.048
10.33	.0017	8.857	.0084	7.75	.018	6.889	.031
12.00	.00013	10.286	.0036	9.00	.0099	8.000	.019
		10.571	.0027	9.25	.0080	8.222	.016
		11.143	.0012	9.75	.0048	8.667	.010
		12.286	.00032	10.75	.0024	9.556	.0060
		14.000	.000021	12.00	.0011	10.667	.0035
				12.25	.00086	10.889	.0029
				13.00	.00026	11.556	.0013
				14.25	.000061	12.667	.00066
				16.00	.0000036	13.556	.00035
						14.000	.00020
						14.222	.000097
						14.889	.000054
						16.222	.000011
						18.000	.0000006

APPENDIX L *(Continued)*

TABLE L–2

$k = 4$

N = 2		N = 3		N = 4			
χ_r^2	p	χ_r^2	p	χ_r^2	p	χ_r^2	p
.0	1.000	.2	1.000	.0	1.000	5.7	.141
.6	.958	.6	.958	.3	.992	6.0	.105
1.2	.834	1.0	.910	.6	.928	6.3	.094
1.8	.792	1.8	.727	.9	.900	6.6	.077
2.4	.625	2.2	.608	1.2	.800	6.9	.068
3.0	.542	2.6	.524	1.5	.754	7.2	.054
3.6	.458	3.4	.446	1.8	.677	7.5	.052
4.2	.375	3.8	.342	2.1	.649	7.8	.036
4.8	.208	4.2	.300	2.4	.524	8.1	.033
5.4	.167	5.0	.207	2.7	.508	8.4	.019
6.0	.042	5.4	.175	3.0	.432	8.7	.014
		5.8	.148	3.3	.389	9.3	.012
		6.6	.075	3.6	.355	9.6	.0069
		7.0	.054	3.9	.324	9.9	.0062
		7.4	.033	4.5	.242	10.2	.0027
		8.2	.017	4.8	.200	10.8	.0016
		9.0	.0017	5.1	.190	11.1	.00094
				5.4	.158	12.0	.000072

From Siegel, S. (1956). *Nonparametric statistics for the behavioral sciences.* New York: McGraw-Hill; as adapted from Friedman, M. (1937). The use of ranks to avoid the assumption of normality implicit in the analysis of variance. *Journal of the American Statistical Association, 32,* 688–689.

APPENDIX M

STATISTICAL POWER TABLES (Δ = EFFECT SIZE)

MASTER TABLE

5% Level, One-Tailed Test

Δ	99	95	90	80	Power 70	60	50	40	30	20	10
0.01	157695	108215	85634	61823	47055	36031	27055	19363	12555	6453	1321
0.02	39417	27050	21405	15454	11763	9007	6764	4841	3139	1614	331
0.03	17514	12019	9511	6867	5227	4003	3006	2152	1396	718	148
0.04	9848	6758	5348	3861	2939	2251	1691	1210	785	404	84
0.05	6299	4323	3421	2470	1881	1440	1082	775	503	259	54
0.06	4372	3000	2375	1715	1305	1000	751	538	349	180	38
0.07	3209	2203	1744	1259	959	734	552	395	257	133	29
0.08	2455	1685	1334	963	734	562	422	303	197	102	23
0.09	1938	1330	1053	761	579	444	334	239	156	81	18
0.10	1568	1076	852	616	469	359	270	194	126	66	15
0.11	1294	889	704	508	387	297	223	160	104	54	13
0.12	1086	746	590	427	325	249	188	135	88	46	11
0.13	924	635	503	363	277	212	160	115	75	39	10
0.14	796	546	433	313	238	183	138	99	65	34	•
0.15	692	475	376	272	207	159	120	86	56	30	•
0.16	607	417	330	239	182	140	105	76	50	27	•
0.17	537	369	292	211	161	124	93	67	44	24	•
0.18	478	328	260	188	144	110	83	60	39	21	•
0.19	428	294	233	169	129	99	75	54	35	19	•
0.20	385	265	210	152	116	89	67	49	32	17	•
0.22	317	218	173	125	96	74	56	40	27	15	•
0.24	265	182	144	105	80	62	47	34	23	12	•
0.26	224	154	122	89	68	52	40	29	19	11	•
0.28	192	132	105	76	58	45	34	25	17	10	•
0.30	166	114	91	66	51	39	30	22	15	•	•
0.32	145	100	79	58	44	34	26	19	13	•	•
0.34	127	88	70	51	39	30	23	17	12	•	•
0.36	113	78	62	45	35	27	20	15	10	•	•
0.38	100	69	55	40	31	24	18	14	•	•	•
0.40	89	62	49	36	28	21	16	12	•	•	•
0.45	69	48	38	28	21	17	13	10	•	•	•
0.50	54	37	30	22	17	13	10	•	•	•	•
0.55	43	30	24	17	14	11	•	•	•	•	•
0.60	34	24	19	14	11	•	•	•	•	•	•
0.65	28	19	16	12	•	•	•	•	•	•	•
0.70	23	16	13	10	•	•	•	•	•	•	•
0.75	18	13	10	•	•	•	•	•	•	•	•
0.80	15	10	•	•	•	•	•	•	•	•	•
0.85	12	•	•	•	•	•	•	•	•	•	•
0.90	•	•	•	•	•	•	•	•	•	•	•

APPENDIX M *(Continued)*

MASTER TABLE

1% Level, One-Tailed Test

Δ	Power 99	95	90	80	70	60	50	40	30	20	10
0.01	216463	157695	130162	100355	81264	66545	54117	42972	32469	22044	10917
0.02	54106	39417	32535	25085	2031	16634	13528	10742	8117	5511	2730
0.03	24040	17514	14456	11146	9026	7391	6011	4773	3607	2449	1214
0.04	13517	9848	8128	6267	5075	4156	3380	2684	2029	1378	683
0.05	8646	6299	5200	4009	3247	2659	2163	1718	1298	882	437
0.06	6000	4372	3609	2783	2254	1846	1501	1192	901	612	304
0.07	4405	3209	2649	2043	1655	1355	1102	876	662	450	224
0.08	3369	2455	2027	1563	1266	1037	843	670	507	344	171
0.09	2660	1938	1600	1234	999	819	666	529	400	272	136
0.10	2152	1568	1295	998	809	663	539	428	324	220	110
0.11	1776	1294	1069	824	668	547	445	354	268	182	91
0.12	1490	1086	897	692	560	459	374	297	225	153	77
0.13	1268	924	763	589	477	391	318	253	191	130	65
0.14	1092	796	657	507	411	337	274	218	165	112	56
0.15	949	692	571	441	357	293	238	190	144	98	49
0.16	833	607	501	387	314	257	209	166	126	86	43
0.17	736	537	443	342	277	277	185	147	112	76	39
0.18	655	478	395	305	247	202	165	131	100	68	34
0.19	587	428	353	273	221	181	148	118	89	61	31
0.20	528	385	318	246	199	163	133	106	81	55	29
0.22	434	317	262	202	164	135	110	87	66	46	24
0.24	363	265	219	169	137	113	92	73	56	38	21
0.26	307	224	185	143	116	95	78	62	47	33	18
0.28	263	192	159	123	100	82	67	53	41	29	16
0.30	227	166	137	106	86	71	58	46	35	25	14
0.32	198	145	120	93	75	62	51	41	31	22	12
0.34	174	127	105	82	66	55	45	36	28	20	11
0.36	154	113	93	72	59	48	40	32	25	18	10
0.38	137	100	83	64	52	43	35	29	22	16	•
0.40	122	89	74	57	47	39	32	26	20	15	•
0.45	94	69	57	44	36	30	25	20	16	12	•
0.50	73	54	45	35	29	24	20	16	13	•	•
0.55	58	43	36	28	23	19	16	13	11	•	•
0.60	47	34	29	23	19	16	13	11	•	•	•
0.65	38	28	23	18	15	13	11	•	•	•	•
0.70	30	23	19	15	12	11	•	•	•	•	•
0.75	25	18	15	12	10	•	•	•	•	•	•
0.80	20	15	12	10	•	•	•	•	•	•	•
0.85	16	12	10	•	•	•	•	•	•	•	•
0.90	12	•	•	•	•	•	•	•	•	•	•

Table continued on following page

APPENDIX M *(Continued)*

MASTER TABLE

5% Level, Two-Tailed Test

Δ	99	95	90	80	Power 70	60	50	40	30	20	10
0.01	183714	129940	105069	78485	61718	48986	38414	29125	20609	12508	4604
0.02	45920	32480	26263	19618	15428	12245	9603	7281	5152	3127	1152
0.03	20403	14431	11669	8717	6855	5441	4267	3236	2290	1390	513
0.04	11472	8115	6562	4902	3855	3060	2400	1820	1288	782	289
0.05	7338	5191	4197	3136	2466	1958	1536	1165	824	501	185
0.06	5093	3602	2913	2177	1712	1359	1066	809	573	348	129
0.07	3739	2645	2139	1598	1257	998	783	594	421	256	95
0.08	2860	2023	1636	1223	962	764	599	455	322	196	73
0.09	2257	1597	1292	965	759	603	473	359	255	155	58
0.10	1826	1292	1045	781	615	488	383	291	206	126	47
0.11	1508	1067	863	645	507	403	316	240	170	104	39
0.12	1265	895	724	541	426	338	266	202	143	88	33
0.13	1076	762	616	461	363	288	226	172	122	75	29
0.14	927	656	531	397	312	248	195	148	105	64	25
0.15	806	570	461	345	272	216	170	129	92	56	22
0.16	707	500	405	303	238	190	149	113	81	50	20
0.17	625	442	358	268	211	168	132	100	71	44	18
0.18	556	394	319	238	188	149	117	89	64	39	16
0.19	498	353	286	214	168	134	105	80	57	35	15
0.20	449	318	257	192	152	121	95	72	52	32	13
0.22	369	261	212	158	125	99	78	60	43	27	11
0.24	308	218	177	133	105	83	66	50	36	23	10
0.26	261	185	150	112	89	71	56	43	31	20	•
0.28	223	159	128	96	76	61	48	37	27	17	•
0.30	193	137	111	83	66	53	42	32	23	15	•
0.32	169	120	97	73	58	46	36	28	21	13	•
0.34	148	105	85	64	51	41	32	25	18	12	•
0.36	131	93	75	57	45	36	29	22	16	11	•
0.38	116	83	67	51	40	32	26	20	15	10	•
0.40	104	74	60	45	36	29	23	18	13	•	•
0.45	80	57	46	35	28	22	18	14	11	•	•
0.50	62	45	36	27	22	18	14	11	•	•	•
0.55	50	35	29	22	18	14	12	•	•	•	•
0.60	40	29	23	18	14	12	10	•	•	•	•
0.65	32	23	19	15	12	10	•	•	•	•	•
0.70	26	19	15	12	10	•	•	•	•	•	•
0.75	21	15	13	10	•	•	•	•	•	•	•
0.80	17	12	10	•	•	•	•	•	•	•	•
0.85	13	10	•	•	•	•	•	•	•	•	•
0.90	10	•	•	•	•	•	•	•	•	•	•

APPENDIX M *(Continued)*

MASTER TABLE

1% Level, Two-Tailed Test

Δ	99	95	90	80	Power 70	60	50	40	30	20	10
0.01	240299	178131	148785	116783	96109	80039	66346	53937	42082	30074	16752
0.02	60064	44525	37190	29191	24024	20007	16584	13483	10520	7518	4188
0.03	26687	19783	16524	12970	10674	8890	7369	5991	4675	3341	1862
0.04	15005	11123	9291	7293	6002	4999	4144	3369	2629	1879	1047
0.05	9598	7115	5943	4665	3840	3198	2651	2155	1682	1202	670
0.06	6661	4938	4125	3238	2665	2220	1840	1496	1168	835	466
0.07	4890	3625	3028	2377	1957	1630	1351	1099	858	613	342
0.08	3740	2773	2316	1819	1497	1247	1034	841	656	469	262
0.09	2952	2189	1829	1436	1182	984	816	664	518	371	207
0.10	2389	1771	1480	1162	956	797	661	537	420	300	168
0.11	1972	1462	1221	959	789	658	545	444	346	248	139
0.12	1654	1227	1025	805	663	552	458	372	291	208	117
0.13	1407	1044	872	685	564	470	390	317	248	177	100
0.14	1212	898	751	590	485	405	336	273	213	153	86
0.15	1054	781	653	513	422	352	292	238	186	133	75
0.16	924	685	573	450	371	309	256	209	163	117	66
0.17	817	606	506	398	328	273	227	185	144	104	58
0.18	727	539	451	354	292	243	202	164	129	92	52
0.19	651	483	404	317	261	218	181	147	115	83	47
0.20	586	435	364	286	235	196	163	133	104	75	42
0.22	482	358	299	235	194	162	134	109	86	62	35
0.24	403	299	250	196	162	135	112	92	72	52	30
0.26	341	253	212	166	137	115	95	78	61	44	26
0.28	292	217	181	143	118	98	82	67	52	38	23
0.30	252	187	157	123	102	85	71	58	45	33	20
0.32	220	163	137	108	89	74	62	51	40	30	18
0.34	193	144	120	95	78	65	54	45	35	26	15
0.36	171	127	106	84	69	58	48	39	31	24	15
0.38	152	113	94	74	62	52	43	35	29	21	13
0.40	135	101	84	67	55	46	38	32	26	19	12
0.45	104	77	65	51	42	36	30	25	20	15	10
0.50	81	61	51	40	33	28	24	20	16	12	•
0.55	64	48	40	32	27	23	19	16	13	10	•
0.60	52	39	32	26	22	19	16	15	11	•	•
0.65	41	31	27	21	18	15	13	11	•	•	•
0.70	33	25	22	17	15	13	11	•	•	•	•
0.75	27	21	17	14	12	10	•	•	•	•	•
0.80	22	17	14	11	•	•	•	•	•	•	•
0.85	17	13	11	•	•	•	•	•	•	•	•
0.90	13	10	•	•	•	•	•	•	•	•	•

From Kraemer, H. C., & Theimann, S. (1987). *How many subjects: Statistical power analysis in research,* Newbury Park, CA: Sage. Reprinted by permission of Sage Publications, Inc.

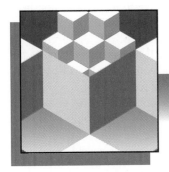

GLOSSARY

abstract. Clear, concise summary of a study, usually limited to 100–250 words.

abstract thinking. Oriented toward the development of an idea without application to or association with a particular instance and independent of time and space. Abstract thinkers tend to look for meaning, patterns, relationships, and philosophical implications.

academic library. Located within institutions of higher learning and containing numerous resources for researchers.

accessible population. Portion of the target population to which the researcher has reasonable access.

accidental or convenience sampling. Subjects are included in the study because they happened to be in the right place at the right time; available subjects are simply entered into the study until the desired sample size is reached.

accuracy in physiological measures. Comparable to validity in that it addresses the extent to which the instrument measured the domain that is defined in the study.

across-method triangulation. Combining research methods or strategies from two or more research traditions in the same study.

action application of research. Using research findings to support the need for change, as an impetus for evaluation of services, and/or as a model for practice.

active rejection. An innovation is examined and a decision is made not to adopt it.

adoption. Full acceptance of the innovation and implementation of the ideas in practice.

Agency for Health Care Policy and Research (AHCPR). Federal government agency created in 1989 to carry out research, demonstration projects, guideline development, training, and dissemination activities with respect to health care services and systems of information regarding the following areas: the effectiveness, efficiency, quality, and outcomes of health services; clinical practice, including primary care; health care technologies, facilities, and equipment; health care costs, productivity, and market forces; health promotion and disease prevention; health statistics and epidemiology; and medical liability.

Agency for Healthcare Research and Quality (AHRQ). New name for the Agency for Health Care Policy and Research that was changed in December 1999.

alpha (α). Level of significance or cutoff point used to determine whether the samples being tested are members of the same population or different populations; alpha is commonly set at .05, .01, or .001.

alternate-forms reliability. Comparing the equivalence of two versions of the same paper-and-pencil instruments.

analysis of covariance (ANCOVA). Statistical procedure designed to reduce the error term (or variance within groups) by partialing out the variance resulting from a confounding variable by performing regression analysis before performing analysis of variance (ANOVA).

analysis of variance (ANOVA). Statistical technique used to examine differences among two or more groups by comparing the variability between the groups with the variability within the groups.

analysis step of critique. Determining the strengths and limitations of the logical links connecting one study element with another.

analysis triangulation. Using two or more analysis techniques to analyze the same set of data for the purpose of validation.

analytical induction. Qualitative research technique that includes enumerative induction, in which a number and variety of instances are collected that verify the model, and eliminative induction, which requires that the hypothesis be tested against alternatives.

analytical preciseness. Performing a series of transformations during which concrete data are transformed across several levels of abstractions to develop a theoretical schema that imparts meaning to the phenomenon under study.

analyzing sources. Involves critiquing studies and comparing across studies to determine the current body of knowledge related to the research problem.

anonymity. Subject's identity cannot be linked, even by the researcher, with his or her individual responses.

applied research. Scientific investigations conducted to generate knowledge that will directly influence or improve practice.

ascendance to an open context. Ability to see depth and complexity within the phenomenon examined and a greater capacity for insight than with the sedimented view. Requires deconstructing sedimented views and reconstructing another view.

assent. A child's affirmative agreement to participate in research.

associative relationship. Identifies variables or concepts that occur or exist together in the real world; thus, when one variable changes, the other variable changes.

assumptions. Statements taken for granted or considered true, even though they have not been scientifically tested.

asymmetrical relationship. If A occurs (or changes), then B will occur (or change), but there may be no indication that if B occurs (or changes), A will occur (or change); A → B.

auditability. Rigorous development of a decision trail that is reported in sufficient detail to allow a second researcher, using the original data and the decision trail, to arrive at conclusions similar to those of the original researcher.

authority. Person with expertise and power who is able to influence opinion and behavior.

autonomous agents. Prospective subjects informed about a proposed study can voluntarily choose to participate or not participate.

autoregressive integrated moving average (ARIMA) model. This model is an equation or series of equations that explain a naturally occurring process and is the most commonly used time-series analysis model in nursing.

backward stepwise regression analysis. Type of stepwise regression analysis in which all the independent variables are initially included in the analysis. Then, one variable at a time is removed from the equation and the effect of that removal on R^2 is evaluated.

basic research. Scientific investigations for the pursuit of knowledge for knowledge's sake or for the pleasure of learning and finding truth.

beneficence, principle of. Encourages the researcher to do good and, above all, to do no harm.

benefit-risk ratio. Researchers and reviewers of research weigh potential benefits and risks in a study to promote the conduct of ethical research.

between-group variance. The variance of the group means around the grand mean (the mean of the total sample) that is examined in analysis of variance (ANOVA).

between-method triangulation. *See* across-method triangulation.

bias. Any influence or action in a study that distorts the findings or slants them away from the true or expected.

bivariate analysis. Statistical procedures that involve comparison of summary values from two groups of the same variable or from two variables within a group.

bivariate correlation. Analysis techniques that measure the extent of the linear relationship between two variables.

Bland-Altman plot. Analysis technique for examining the extent of agreement between two measurement techniques. Generally used to compare a new technique with an established one.

blocking. Design in which the researcher includes subjects with various levels of an extraneous variable in the sample but controls the numbers of subjects at each level of the variable and their random assignment to groups within the study.

body of knowledge. Information, principles, and theories that are organized by the beliefs accepted in a discipline at a given time.

Bonferroni's procedure. Parametric analysis technique that controls for escalation of significance and can be used if various t tests must be performed on different aspects of the same data.

borrowing. Appropriation and use of knowledge from other disciplines to guide nursing practice.

box-and-whisker plots. Exploratory data analysis technique to provide fast visualization of some of the major characteristics of the data, such as the spread, symmetry, and outliers.

bracketing. Qualitative research technique of suspending or laying aside what is known about an experience being studied.

breach of confidentiality. Accidental or direct action that allows an unauthorized person to have access to raw study data.

canonical correlation. Extension of multiple regression with more than one dependent variable.

carryover effect. Application of one treatment can influence the response to following treatments.

case study design. Intensive exploration of a single unit of study, such as a person, family, group, community, or institution.

catalogue. Identifies what is available in the library.

causal hypothesis or relationship. Identifies a cause-and-effect interaction between two or more variables, which are referred to as independent and dependent variables.

causal relationship. Relationship between two variables in which one variable (independent variable) is thought to cause or determine the presence of the other variable (dependent variable).

causality. Includes three conditions: (1) must be a strong correlation between the proposed cause and effect, (2) proposed cause must precede the effect in time, and (3) cause has to be present whenever the effect occurs.

cell. Intersection between the row and column in a table where a specific numerical value is inserted.

central limit theorem. States that even when statistics, such as means, come from a population with a skewed (asymmetrical) distribution, the sampling distribution developed from multiple means obtained from that skewed population will tend to fit the pattern of the normal curve.

change agent. Professional outside a system who enters the system to promote adoption of an innovation.

checklists. Techniques for indicating whether a behavior occurred.

chi-squared test. Used to analyze nominal data to determine significant differences between observed frequencies within the data and frequencies that were expected.

chronolog. A type of unstructured observation that provides a detailed description of an individual's behavior in a natural environment.

cleaning data. Checking raw data to determine errors in data recording, coding, or entry.

clinical decision analysis. A systematic method of describing clinical problems, identifying possible diagnostic and management courses of action, assessing the probability and value of the various outcomes, and then calculating the optimal course of action.

cluster sampling. A sampling frame is developed that includes a list of all the states, cities, institutions, or organizations (clusters) that could be used in a study, and a randomized sample is drawn from this list.

Cochran Q test. Nonparametric test that is an extension of the McNemar test for two related samples.

codebook. Identifies and defines each variable in

a study and includes an abbreviated variable name (limited to 6–8 characters), a descriptive variable label, and the range of possible numerical values of every variable entered into a computer file.

coding. Process of transforming qualitative data into numerical symbols that can be computerized.

coefficient of determination (R^2). Computed from a matrix of correlation coefficients and provides important information on multicolinearity. This value indicates the degree of linear dependencies among the variables.

coercion. An overt threat of harm or excessive reward intentionally presented by one person to another to obtain compliance, such as offering subjects a large sum of money to participate in a dangerous research project.

cognitive application of research. Research-based knowledge is used to affect a person's way of thinking, approaching, and/or observing situations.

cognitive clustering. Comprehensive, scholarly synthesis of scientifically sound research that is evident in integrative reviews of research and meta-analyses.

cohorts. Samples in time-dimensional studies within the field of epidemiology.

coinvestigators. Two or more professionals conducting a study, whose salaries might be paid partially or in full by grant funding.

communicating research findings. Developing a research report and disseminating it through presentations and publications to a variety of audiences.

communication channels. Include one-to-one exchange of information; one individual communicating to several others; or mass media such as books, journals, newspapers, television, and computer networks.

comparative descriptive design. Used to describe differences in variables in two or more groups in a natural setting.

comparison group. The group not receiving a treatment or receiving the usual treatment (standard care) when nonrandom sampling methods are used.

comparison step of critique. The ideal for each step of the research process is compared with the real steps in a study.

compatibility. The degree to which the innovation is perceived to be consistent with current values, past experience, and priority of needs.

complete observer. The researcher is passive and has no direct social interaction in the setting.

complete participation. The researcher becomes a member of the group and conceals the researcher role.

complete review. Extensive review by an institutional review board (IRB) for studies with greater than minimal risk.

complex hypothesis. Predicts the relationship (associative or causal) among three or more variables; thus the hypothesis could include two (or more) independent and/or two (or more) dependent variables.

complexity. The degree to which the innovation is perceived to be difficult to understand or use.

comprehending a source. Involves reading the entire source carefully and focusing on understanding the major concepts and the logical flow of ideas within the source.

comprehension step of critique. Understanding the terms in a research report; identifying study elements; and grasping the nature, significance, and meaning of these elements.

computer searches. Conducted to scan the citations in different databases and identify sources relevant to a research problem.

computerized database. A structured compilation of information that can be scanned, retrieved, and analyzed by computer and can be used for decisions, reports, and research.

concept. A term that abstractly describes and names an object or phenomenon, thus providing it with a separate identity or meaning.

concept analysis. A strategy through which a set of attributes or characteristics essential to the connotative meaning or conceptual definition of a concept are identified.

concept derivation. Process of extracting and defining concepts from theories in other disciplines.

concept synthesis. Process of describing and naming a previously unrecognized concept.

conceptual clustering step of critique. Current knowledge in an area of study is carefully analyzed, summarized, and organized theoretically to maximize the meaning attached to research findings, highlight gaps in the knowledge base, generate research questions, and provide knowledge for use in practice.

conceptual definition. Provides a variable or concept with connotative (abstract, comprehensive, theoretical) meaning and is established through concept analysis, concept derivation, or concept synthesis.

conceptual map. Strategy for expressing a framework of a study that diagrammatically shows the interrelationships of the concepts and statements.

conceptual model. A set of highly abstract, related constructs that broadly explains phenomena of interest, expresses assumptions, and reflects a philosophical stance.

conclusions. Synthesis and clarification of the meaning of study findings.

concrete thinking. Thinking that is oriented toward and limited by tangible things or events observed and experienced in reality.

concurrent relationship. A relationship in which both variables and concepts occur simultaneously.

confidence interval. A range in which the value of the parameter is estimated to be.

confidentiality. Management of private data in research so that subjects' identities are not linked with their responses.

confirmation stage. Stage of the innovation-decision process in which the effectiveness of the innovation is evaluated and a decision is made either to continue or to discontinue the innovation.

confirmatory data analysis. Use of inferential statistics to confirm expectations regarding the data that are expressed as hypotheses, questions, or objectives.

confirmatory factor analysis. Closely related to ordinary least-squares regression analysis or path analysis and based on theory and testing a hypothesis about the existing factor structure.

confirmatory regression analysis. Regression analysis procedures designed to confirm or support a theoretically proposed set of variables.

confounding variables. Variables that are recognized before the study is initiated but that cannot be controlled or variables not recognized until the study is in process.

consensus knowledge building. Outcomes design that requires critique and synthesis of an extensive international search of the literature on the topic of concern, including unpublished studies, studies in progress, dissertations, and theses.

consent form. A written form, tape recording, or videotape used to document a subject's agreement to participate in a study.

consent rate. The percentage of people who indicate a willingness to participate in a study based on the total number of people approached.

construct validity. Examines the fit between conceptual and operational definitions of variables and determines whether the instrument actually measures the theoretical construct that it purports to measure.

constructs. Concepts at very high levels of abstraction that have general meanings.

consultants. People hired for specific tasks during a study.

content analysis. Qualitative analysis technique to classify words in a text into a few categories chosen because of their theoretical importance.

content-related validity. Examines the extent to which the method of measurement includes all the major elements relevant to the construct being measured.

context. The body, the world, and the concerns unique to each person within which that person can be understood. Philosophical element of qualitative research.

context flexibility. Capacity to switch from one context or world view to another in order to shift perception to see things from a different perspective.

contextual variables. Factors that could influence the implementation of an intervention and thus the outcomes of the study or could directly influence the study outcomes.

contingency coefficient. A statistical test that is used with two nominal variables and is the most commonly used of the chi-squared–based measures of association.

contingency tables. Cross-tabulation tables that

allow visual comparison of summary data output related to two variables within a sample.

contingent relationship. Occurs only if a third variable or concept is present.

control. Imposing of rules by the researcher to decrease the possibility of error and increase the probability that the study's findings are an accurate reflection of reality.

control group. The group of elements or subjects not exposed to the experimental treatment. The term is used in studies with random sampling methods.

convenience sampling. *See* accidental or convenience sampling.

correlational analysis. Statistical procedure conducted to determine the direction (positive or negative) and magnitude (or strength) of the relationship between two variables.

correlational coefficient. Indicates the degree of relationship between two variables; coefficients range in value from +1.00 (perfect positive relationship) to 0.00 (no relationship) to −1.00 (perfect negative or inverse relationship).

correlational research. Systematic investigation of relationships between two or more variables to explain the nature of relationships in the world and not to examine cause and effect.

cost-benefit analysis. Analysis technique used in outcomes research that examines the costs and benefits of alternative ways of using resources as assessed in monetary terms and the use that produces the greatest net benefit.

cost-effectiveness analyses. Type of outcomes research in which costs and benefits are compared for different ways of accomplishing a clinical goal, such as diagnosing a condition, treating an illness, or providing a service. The goal of cost-effectiveness analyses is to identify the strategy that provides the most value for the money.

covert data collection. Occurs when subjects are unaware that research data are being collected.

Cramer's V. Analysis technique for nominal data that is a modification of phi for contingency tables larger than 2 × 2.

criterion-referenced testing. Comparison of a subject's score with a criterion of achievement that includes the definition of target behaviors. When the behaviors are mastered, the subject is considered proficient in these behaviors.

critical analysis of studies. Examination of the merits, faults, meaning, and significance of nursing studies by the five steps of comprehension, comparison, analysis, evaluation, and conceptual clustering.

critical social theory. Qualitative research methodology guided by critical social theory; the researcher seeks to understand how people communicate and develop symbolic meanings in a society.

crossover or counterbalanced design. Includes the administration of more than one treatment to each subject, and the treatments are provided sequentially rather than concurrently; comparisons are then made of the effects of the different treatments on the same subject.

cross-sectional designs. Used to examine groups of subjects in various stages of development simultaneously with the intent of inferring trends over time.

cultural immersion. Used in ethnographic research for gaining increased familiarity with such things as language, sociocultural norms, and traditions in a culture.

curvilinear relationship. The relationship between two variables varies depending on the relative values of the variables. The graph of the relationship is a curved line rather than a straight one.

data. Pieces of information that are collected during a study.

data analysis. Conducted to reduce, organize, and give meaning to data.

data coding sheet. A sheet for organizing and recording data for rapid entry into a computer.

data collection. Precise, systematic gathering of information relevant to the research purpose or the specific objectives, questions, or hypotheses of a study.

data collection plan. Details how a study will be implemented.

data reduction. Technique for analyzing qualitative data that focuses on decreasing the volume of data to facilitate examination.

data storage and retrieval. The computer's ability to store vast amounts of data and rapidly retrieve these data for examination and analysis.

data triangulation. Collection of data from multiple sources in the same study.

database. *See* computerized database.

debriefing. Complete disclosure of the study purpose and results at the end of a study.

debugging. Identifying and replacing errors in a computer program with accurate information.

deception. Misinforming subjects for research purposes.

decision stage. Stage in the innovation-decision process when an individual or group chooses to adopt or reject an innovation.

decision theory. Theory that is inductive in nature and based on assumptions associated with the theoretical normal curve. The theory is applied when testing for differences between groups with the expectation that all of the groups are members of the same population.

decision trail. *See* auditability.

Declaration of Helsinki. Ethical code based on the Nuremberg Code that differentiated therapeutic from nontherapeutic research.

deconstructing the sedimented views. Rigorous qualitative research requires that the researcher ascend to an open context and be willing to continue to let go of sedimented views, which involves the process of remaining open to new views. (*See* sedimented view and open context.)

deductive reasoning. Reasoning from the general to the specific or from a general premise to a particular situation.

degrees of freedom (*df*). The freedom of a score's value to vary given the other existing scores' values and the established sum of these scores ($df = N - 1$).

Delphi technique. A method of measuring the judgments of a group of experts for assessing priorities or making forecasts.

demographic variables. Characteristics or attributes of the subjects that are collected to describe the sample.

dependent groups. Groups in which the subjects or observations selected for data collection are in some way related to the selection of other subjects or observations. For example, if subjects serve as their own control by using the pretest as a control, the observations (and therefore the groups) are dependent. Use of twins in a study or matching subjects on a selected variable results in dependent groups.

dependent variable. The response, behavior, or outcome that is predicted or explained in research; changes in the dependent variable are presumed to be caused by the independent variable.

description. Involves identifying and understanding the nature and attributes of nursing phenomena and sometimes the relationships among these phenomena.

descriptive codes. Terms used to organize and classify qualitative data.

descriptive correlational design. Used to describe variables and examine relationships that exist in a situation.

descriptive design. Used to identify a phenomenon of interest, identify variables within the phenomenon, develop conceptual and operational definitions of variables, and describe variables.

descriptive research. Provides an accurate portrayal or account of the characteristics of a particular individual, event, or group in real-life situations for the purpose of discovering new meaning, describing what exists, determining the frequency with which something occurs, and categorizing information.

descriptive statistics. Statistics that allows the researcher to organize the data in ways that give meaning and facilitate insight, such as frequency distributions and measures of central tendency and dispersion.

descriptive vividness. Description of the site, subjects, experience of collecting data, and the researcher's thoughts during the qualitative research process that is presented so clearly that the reader has the sense of personally experiencing the event.

design. Blueprint for conducting a study that maximizes control over factors that could interfere with the validity of the findings.

deterministic relationships. Statements of what always occurs in a particular situation, such as a scientific law.

developmental grant proposals. Proposals written to obtain funding for the development of a new program in a discipline.

dialectic reasoning. Involves the holistic perspective, in which the whole is greater than the sum of the parts, and examining factors that are opposites and making sense of them by merging them into a single unit or idea that is greater than either alone.

diary. Record of events kept by a subject over time that is collected and analyzed by a researcher.

difference scores. Deviation scores obtained by subtracting the mean from each raw score.

diffusion. Process of communicating research findings (innovations) through certain channels over time among the members of a discipline.

diminished autonomy. Subjects with decreased ability to voluntarily give informed consent because of legal or mental incompetence, terminal illness, or confinement to an institution.

direct application. Occurs when an innovation is used exactly as it was developed.

direct measurement. The measurement object and measurement strategies are specific and straightforward, such as those for measuring the concrete variables of height, weight, or temperature.

directional hypothesis. States the specific nature of the interaction or relationship between two or more variables.

discontinuance of an innovation. When using new ideas from research in practice, the individual or organization can decide not to use, or to discontinue the use of, the idea or innovation at any point in time. Discontinuance can be of at least two types: replacement discontinuance and disenchantment discontinuance. Discontinuance is a possibility outlined in the confirmation stage of the innovation-decision process.

discriminant analysis. Designed to allow the researcher to identify characteristics associated with group membership and to predict group membership.

disenchantment discontinuance in utilization

of innovations. Discontinuation of a new idea or innovation because the user is dissatisfied with its outcome.

dissemination of research findings. The diffusion or communication of research findings.

dummy variables. Categorical or dichotomous variables used in regression analysis.

duplicate publication. The practice of publishing the same article or major portions of the article in two or more print or electronic media without notifying the editors or referencing the other publication in the reference list.

dwelling with the data. Immersion in the data as part of the process of data management and reduction in phenomenology.

early adopters of innovations. Opinion leaders in a social system who learn about new ideas rapidly, utilize them, and serve as role models for their use in nursing practice.

early majority in the use of innovations. Individuals who are rarely leaders but are active followers and will readily follow in the use of a new idea in nursing practice.

effect size. The degree to which the phenomenon is present in the population or to which the null hypothesis is false.

eigenvalues. Numerical values generated with factor analysis that are the sum of the squared weights for each factor.

electronic mail. Allows a computer user to rapidly exchange messages, computer files, data, and research reports by satellite networks.

element of a study. A person (subject), event, behavior, or any other single unit of a study.

eliminative induction. Qualitative data analysis technique that is part of a process referred to as analytic induction and requires that the hypothesis generated from the analysis be tested against alternatives.

emic approach. Anthropological research approach of studying behavior from within the culture.

empirical generalization. Statements that have been repeatedly tested through research and have not been disproved. Scientific theories have empirical generalizations.

empirical literature. Includes relevant studies

published in journals and books, as well as unpublished studies, such as master's theses and doctoral dissertations.

empirical world. Experienced through our senses and is the concrete portion of our existence.

enumerative induction. Qualitative data analysis technique that is part of a process referred to as analytic induction in which a number and variety of instances must be collected to verify a model that was developed from the research process.

environmental variable. Type of extraneous variable related to the setting in which a study is conducted.

equivalence. Type of reliability testing that involves comparing two versions of the same paper-and-pencil instrument or two observers measuring the same event.

error score. Amount of random error in the measurement process.

errors in physiological measures. Sources of erroneous measurement with physiological instruments that include environment, user, subject, machine, and interpretation error.

ethical inquiry. Intellectual analysis of ethical problems related to obligation, rights, duty, right and wrong, conscience, choice, intention, and responsibility to obtain desirable, rational ends.

ethical principles. Principles of respect for persons, beneficence, and justice relevant to the conduct of research.

ethical rigor. Requires recognition and discussion by the researcher of the ethical implications related to the conduct of the study.

ethnographic research. A qualitative research methodology for investigating cultures that involves collection, description, and analysis of data to develop a theory of cultural behavior.

ethnonursing research. Emerged from Leininger's theory of transcultural nursing and focuses mainly on observing and documenting interactions with people to determine how daily life conditions and patterns are influencing human care, health, and nursing care practices.

etic approach. Anthropological research approach of studying behavior from outside the culture and examining similarities and differences across cultures.

evaluation step of a critique. Examining the meaning and significance of a study according to set criteria and comparing it with previous studies conducted in the area.

event-partitioning designs. Merger of the longitudinal and trend designs to increase sample size and avoid the effects of history on the validity of findings.

event-time matrix. Qualitative analysis technique that can facilitate comparisons of events occurring in different sites during particular time periods.

evidenced-based practice (EBP). Careful and practical use of current best evidence to guide health care decisions. EBP is based on clinical practice guidelines that evolve from integration of research findings and expert practitioners' opinions.

exclusion criteria. Sampling requirements identified by the researcher that eliminate or exclude an element or subject from being in a sample. Exclusion criteria are exceptions to the inclusion sampling criteria.

execution errors. Errors that occur because of a defect in the data collection procedure.

exempt studies. Studies that have no apparent risks for the research subjects are often designated as exempt from or not requiring institutional review.

existence statement. Declares that a given concept exists or that a given relationship occurs.

expedited review. Review process for studies that have some risk, but the risks are minimal or no greater than those ordinarily encountered in daily life or during the performance of routine physical or psychological examinations.

experimental designs. Designs that provide the greatest amount of control possible to examine causality more closely.

experimental group. The subjects who are exposed to the experimental treatment.

experimental research. Objective, systematic, controlled investigation to examine probability and causality among selected variables for the purpose of predicting and controlling phenomena.

explanation. Achieved when research clarifies the

relationships among phenomena and identifies why certain events occur.

explanatory codes. Developed late in the data collection process after theoretical ideas from the qualitative study have begun to emerge.

explanatory effects matrix. Qualitative analysis technique that can assist in answering questions, such as why an outcome was achieved or what caused the outcome.

exploratory data analysis. Examining the data descriptively to become as familiar as possible with the nature of the data and to search for hidden structures and models.

exploratory factor analysis. Similar to stepwise regression, in which the variance of the first factor is partialed out before analysis is begun on the second factor. It is performed when the researcher has few prior expectations about the factor structure.

exploratory regression analysis. Used when the researcher may not have sufficient information to determine which independent variables are effective predictors of the dependent variable; thus, many variables may be entered into the analysis simultaneously. This type is the most commonly used regression analysis strategy in nursing studies.

external criticism. A method of determining the validity of source materials in historical research that involves knowing where, when, why, and by whom a document was written.

external validity. The extent to which study findings can be generalized beyond the sample used in the study.

extraneous variables. Exist in all studies and can affect the measurement of study variables and the relationships among these variables.

face validity. Verifies that the instrument looked like or gave the appearance of measuring the content.

factor analysis. Analysis that examines interrelationships among large numbers of variables and disentangles those relationships to identify clusters of variables that are most closely linked together. Two types of factor analysis are exploratory and confirmatory factor analysis.

factor rotation. An aspect of factor analysis in which the factors are mathematically adjusted or rotated to reduce the factor structure and clarify the meaning.

factorial analysis of variance. Mathematically, the analysis technique is simply a specialized version of multiple regression; a number of types of factorial ANOVAs have been developed to analyze data from specific experimental designs.

factorial design. Study design that includes two or more different characteristics, treatments, or events that are independently varied within a study.

fair treatment. Ethical principle that promotes fair selection and treatment of subjects during the course of a study.

falsification of research. A type of scientific misconduct that involves manipulating research materials, equipment, or processes or changing or omitting data or results such that the research is not accurately represented in the research record.

fatigue effect. When a subject becomes tired or bored with a study.

feasibility of a study. Determined by examining the time and money commitment; the researcher's expertise; availability of subjects, facility, and equipment; cooperation of others; and the study's ethical considerations.

field research. The activity of collecting the data that requires taking extensive notes in ethnographic research.

findings. The translated and interpreted results from a study.

focus groups. Groups that are designed to obtain participants' perceptions in a specific (or focused) area in a setting that is permissive and nonthreatening.

forced choice. Response set for items in a scale that have an even number of choices, such as four or six, where the respondents cannot choose an uncertain or neutral response and must indicate support for or against the topic measured.

forward stepwise regression analysis. Type of stepwise regression analysis in which the independent variables are entered into the analysis one at a time and an analysis is made of the effect of including that variable on R^2.

foundational inquiry. Research examining the foundations for a science, such as studies that provide analysis of the structure of a science and the process of thinking about and valuing certain phenomena held in common by the science. Debates related to quantitative and qualitative research methods emerge from foundational inquiries.

framework. The abstract, logical structure of meaning that guides development of the study and enables the researcher to link the findings to nursing's body of knowledge.

fraudulent publications. There is documentation or testimony from coauthors that the publication did not reflect what had actually been done.

frequency distribution. A statistical procedure that involves listing all possible measures of a variable and tallying each datum on the listing. The two types of frequency distributions are ungrouped and grouped.

Friedman two-way analysis of variance by ranks. Nonparametric test used with matched samples or in repeated measures.

generalization. Extends the implications of the findings from the sample that was studied to the larger population or from the situation studied to a larger situation.

geographical analyses. Used to examine variations in health status, health services, patterns of care, or patterns of use by geographical area and are sometimes referred to as small area analyses.

gestalt. Organization of knowledge about a particular phenomenon into a cluster of linked ideas. The clustering and interrelatedness enhances the meaning of the ideas.

going native. In ethnographic research, when the researcher becomes part of the culture and loses all objectivity and, with it, the ability to observe clearly.

grant. A proposal developed to seek research funding from private or public institutions.

grounded theory research. An inductive research technique based on symbolic interaction theory that is conducted to discover what problems exist in a social scene and the processes persons use to handle them. The research process involves formulation, testing, and redevelopment of propositions until a theory is developed.

Hawthorne effect. A psychological response in which subjects change their behavior simply because they are subjects in a study, not because of the research treatment.

heterogeneity. The researcher's attempt to obtain subjects with a wide variety of characteristics to reduce the risk of bias in studies not using random sampling.

heuristic relevance. A standard for evaluating a qualitative study in which the study's intuitive recognition, relationship to the existing body of knowledge, and applicability are examined.

hierarchical statement sets. Composed of a specific proposition and a hypothesis or research question. If a conceptual model is included in the framework, the set may also include a general proposition.

highly controlled settings. Artificially constructed environments that are developed for the sole purpose of conducting research, such as laboratories, experimental centers, and test units.

historical research. A narrative description or analysis of events that occurred in the remote or recent past.

history effect. An event that is not related to the planned study but occurs during the time of the study and could influence the responses of subjects to the treatment.

homogeneity. The degree to which objects are similar or a form of equivalence, such as limiting subjects to only one level of an extraneous variable to reduce its impact on the study findings.

homogeneity reliability. Type of reliability testing used with paper-and-pencil tests that addresses the correlation of various items within the instrument.

homoscedastic. Data are evenly dispersed both above and below the regression line, which indicates a linear relationship on a scatter diagram (plot).

human rights. Claims and demands that have been justified in the eyes of an individual or by the consensus of a group of individuals and are protected in research.

hypothesis. Formal statement of the expected relationship between two or more variables in a specified population.

immersed in the culture. Involves gaining increasing familiarity with such things as language, sociocultural norms, traditions, communication patterns, religion, work patterns, and expression of emotion in a selected culture.

implementation stage. Stage in the innovation-decision process when an innovation is used by an individual or group.

implications. The meaning of research conclusions for the body of knowledge, theory, and practice.

inclusion criteria. Sampling requirements identified by the researcher that must be present for the element or subject to be included in the sample.

incomplete disclosure. Subjects are not completely informed about the purpose of a study because that knowledge might alter the subjects' actions. After the study, the subjects must be debriefed.

independent groups. Groups in which the selection of one subject is totally unrelated to the selection of other subjects. An example is when subjects are randomly selected and assigned to the treatment and control groups.

independent variable. The treatment, intervention, or experimental activity that is manipulated or varied by the researcher to create an effect on the dependent variable.

index. Provides assistance in identifying journal articles and other publications relevant to a topic of interest.

indirect measurement. Used with abstract concepts; the concepts are not measured directly, but instead, indicators or attributes of the concepts are used to represent the abstraction.

inductive reasoning. Reasoning from the specific to the general in which particular instances are observed and then combined into a larger whole or general statement.

inferential statistics. Statistics designed to allow inference from a sample statistic to a population parameter; commonly used to test hypotheses of similarities and differences in subsets of the sample under study.

inferred causality. A cause-and-effect relationship is identified from numerous studies conducted over time to determine risk factors or causal factors in selected situations.

informed consent. The prospective subject's agreement to voluntarily participate in a study, which is reached after assimilation of essential information about the study.

inherent variability. Data can be naturally expected to have a few random observations included in the extreme ends of the tails.

innovation. An idea, practice, or object that is perceived as new by an individual or other unit of adoption.

innovation-decision process. Includes the steps of knowledge, persuasion, decision, implementation, and confirmation to promote diffusion or communication of research findings to members of a discipline for use in practice.

innovativeness. The degree to which an individual or other unit of adoption is more willing to adopt new ideas than are the other members of a system.

innovators. Individuals who actively seek out new ideas.

institutional review. A process of examining studies for ethical concerns by a committee of peers.

instrumentation. A component of measurement that involves the application of specific rules to develop a measurement device or instrument.

integrative review of research. Conducted to identify, analyze, and synthesize the results from independent studies to determine the current knowledge (what is known and not known) in a particular area.

intellectual critique of research. Involves a careful examination of all aspects of a study to judge the merits, limitations, meaning, and significance of the study based on previous research experience and knowledge of the topic.

interlibrary loan department. Department that locates books and articles in other libraries and provides the sources within a designated time.

internal criticism. Involves examination of the reliability of historical documents.

internal validity. The extent to which the effects detected in the study are a true reflection of reality rather than being the result of the effects of extraneous variables.

interpretation of research outcomes. Involves

examining the results of data analysis, forming conclusions, considering the implications for nursing, exploring the significance of the findings, generalizing the findings, and suggesting further studies.

interpretive codes. Organizational system developed late in the qualitative data collection and analysis process as the researcher gains some insight into the processes occurring.

interpretive reliability. Assesses the extent to which each judge assigns the same category to a given unit of data.

interrater reliability. The degree of consistency between two raters who are independently assigning ratings to a variable or attribute being investigated.

interrupted time-series designs. These designs are similar to descriptive time designs except that a treatment is applied at some point in the observations.

interval estimate. Researcher identifies a range of values on a number line where the population parameter is thought to be.

interval-scale measurement. Interval scales have equal numerical distances between intervals of the scale in addition to following rules of mutually exclusive categories, exhaustive categories, and rank ordering, such as temperature.

intervention research. New methodology for investigating the effectiveness of a nursing intervention in achieving the desired outcome or outcomes in a natural setting.

intervention theory. This theory includes a careful description of the problem to be addressed by the intervention, the intervening actions that must be implemented to address the problem, moderating variables that might change the impact of the intervention, mediating variables that might alter the effect of the intervention, and expected outcomes of the intervention.

interventions. Treatments, therapies, procedures, or actions implemented by health professionals to and with clients, in a particular situation, to move the clients' conditions toward desired health outcomes that are beneficial to the clients.

interviews. Structured or unstructured verbal communication between the researcher and subject during which information is obtained for a study.

introspection. A process of turning your attention inward toward your own thoughts to provide increased awareness and understanding of the flow and interplay of feelings and ideas.

intuiting. Process of actually looking at the phenomenon in qualitative research; the individual focuses all awareness and energy on the subject of interest.

intuition. An insight or understanding of a situation or event as a whole that usually cannot be logically explained.

intuitive recognition. When individuals are confronted with the theoretical schema derived from the data of a qualitative study, it has meaning within their personal knowledge base.

invasion of privacy. When private information is shared without an individual's knowledge or against his or her will.

inverse linear relationship. Indicates that as one variable or concept changes, the other variable or concept changes in the opposite direction. Also referred to as a negative linear relationship.

investigator triangulation. Exists when two or more research-trained investigators with divergent backgrounds explore the same phenomenon.

justice, principle of. States that human subjects should be treated fairly.

Kendall's tau. Nonparametric test to determine the correlation among variables used when both variables have been measured at the ordinal level.

knowledge stage. The stage in the innovation-decision process when first awareness of the existence of the innovation occurs.

knowledge utilization. The process of disseminating and using research-generated information to make an impact on or change in the existing practices in society.

Kolmogorov-Smirnov two-sample test. Nonparametric test used to determine whether two independent samples have been drawn from the same population.

Kruskal-Wallis test. Most powerful nonparametric analysis technique for examining three independent groups for differences.

kurtosis. The degree of peakedness (platykurtic,

mesokurtic, or leptokurtic) of the curve shape that is related to the spread or variance of scores.

laggards. Individuals who are security oriented, tend to cling to the past, and are often isolates without a strong support system. Term used in the innovation-decision process to describe persons who are reluctant or refuse to adopt innovations.

lambda. Analysis technique that measures the degree of association (or relationship) between two nominal-level variables.

landmark studies. Major projects that generate knowledge that influences a discipline and sometimes society in general. Mark an important stage of development or turning point in a field of research.

late majority. Individuals who are skeptical about new ideas and will adopt them only if group pressure is great. Term used in the innovation-decision process to describe persons who are reluctant to adopt innovations.

latent transition analysis (LTA). Outcomes research strategy used in situations in which stages or categories of recovery have been defined and transitions across stages can be identified. To use this analysis method, each member of the population is placed in a single category or stage for a given point of time.

least-squares principle. The fact that when deviations from the mean are squared, the sum is smaller than the sum of squared deviations from any other value in a sample distribution.

leptokurtic. Term used to describe an extremely peaked-shape distribution of a curve, which means that the scores in the distribution are similar and have limited variance.

level of significance. *See* alpha.

library resources. Includes library personnel, interlibrary loan department, circulation department, reference department, audiovisual department, computer search department, and photocopy services.

life story. A narrative analysis designed to reconstruct and interpret the life of an ordinary person. This methodology emerged from anthropology and more recently from phenomenology.

Likert scale. An instrument designed to determine the opinion or attitude of a subject; it contains a number of declarative statements with a scale after each statement.

limitations. Theoretical and methodological restrictions in a study that may decrease the generalizability of the findings.

linear relationship. The relationship between two variables or concepts will remain consistent regardless of the values of each of the variables or concepts.

linker. An individual who could serve as a connection between the user system and the resource system when research findings are being used in practice.

logic. A science that involves valid ways of relating ideas to promote human understanding and includes abstract and concrete thinking and logistic, inductive, and deductive reasoning.

logistic reasoning. Used to break the whole into parts that can be carefully examined, as can the relationships among the parts.

longitudinal designs. Panel designs used to examine changes in the same subjects over an extended period.

manipulate. Means to move around or to control the movement of, such as the manipulation of a treatment.

Mann-Whitney *U* test. Used to analyze ordinal data with 95% of the power of the *t* test to detect differences between groups of normally distributed populations.

manual search. Involves examining the catalogue, indexes, abstracts, and bibliographies for relevant sources.

map. *See* conceptual map.

matching. This technique is used when an experimental subject is randomly selected and a subject similar in relation to important extraneous variables is randomly selected for inclusion in the control group.

maturation effect. Unplanned and unrecognized changes experienced during a study, such as subjects' growing older, wiser, stronger, hungrier, or more tired, that can influence the findings of a study.

McNemar test. Nonparametric test in which a 2 × 2 table is used to analyze changes that occur in dichotomous variables.

mean. The value obtained by summing all the scores and dividing that total by the number of scores being summed.

mean of means. Statistical value or mean obtained by analyzing the means from many samples obtained from the same population.

measurement. The process of assigning numbers to objects, events, or situations in accord with some rule.

measurement error. The difference between what exists in reality and what is measured by a research instrument.

measures of central tendency. Statistical procedures (mode, median, and mean) for determining the center of a distribution of scores.

measures of dispersion. Statistical procedures (range, difference scores, sum of squares, variance, and standard deviation) for examining how scores vary or are dispersed around the mean.

median. The score at the exact center of the ungrouped frequency distribution.

mediator variables. Variables that bring about the effects of the intervention after it has occurred and thus influence the outcomes of the study.

Medical Treatment Effectiveness Program (MEDTEP). Major research effort initiated by the Agency for Health Care Policy and Research that was implemented to improve the effectiveness and appropriateness of medical practice.

memo. Developed by the researcher to record insights or ideas related to notes, transcripts, or codes during qualitative data analysis.

mentor. Someone who provides information, advice, and emotional support to a novice or protégé.

mentorship. An intense form of role-modeling in which an expert nurse serves as a teacher, sponsor, guide, exemplar, and counselor for a novice nurse.

mesokurtic. Term that describes a normal curve with an intermediate degree of kurtosis and intermediate variance of scores.

meta-analysis design. Merging of findings from several completed studies to determine what is known about a particular phenomenon.

method of least squares. Procedure in regression analysis for developing the line of best fit.

methodological congruence. A standard for evaluating qualitative research in which documentation rigor, procedural rigor, ethical rigor, and auditability of the study are examined.

methodological designs. Used to develop the validity and reliability of instruments to measure research concepts and variables.

methodological limitations. Restrictions in the study design that limit the credibility of the findings and the population to which the findings can be generalized.

methodological triangulation. The use of two or more research methods or procedures in a study, such as different designs, instruments, and data collection procedures.

minimal risk. The risk of harm anticipated in the proposed research is not greater, with regard to probability and magnitude, than that ordinarily encountered in daily life or during the performance of routine physical or psychological examinations.

modal percentage. Appropriate for nominal data and indicates the relationship of the number of data scores represented by the mode to the total number of data scores.

mode. The numerical value or score that occurs with the greatest frequency in a distribution; however, it does not necessarily indicate the center of the data set.

model testing designs. Used to test the accuracy of a hypothesized causal model or map.

moderator variable. Variable that occurs with the intervention (independent variable) and alters the causal relationship between the intervention and outcomes. It includes characteristics of the subjects and the person implementing the intervention.

mono-method bias. More than one measure of a variable is used in a study, but all measures use the same method of recording.

mono-operation bias. Occurs when only one method of measurement is used to measure a construct.

mortality. Subjects drop out of a study before completion, which creates a threat to the study's internal validity.

multicausality. The recognition that a number of interrelating variables can be involved in causing a particular effect.

multicolinearity. Occurs when the independent variables in a regression equation are strongly correlated.

multicomponent treatments, effects of. Occur when a set of treatments are combined to manage a patient problem. Outcomes research designs have been developed to examine the effects of these treatment programs, and some of these designs include treatment package strategy, comparative treatment strategy, dismantling strategy, constructive strategy, factorial ANOVA design, fractional factorial designs, dose-response designs, response surface methodology, and mediational analysis.

multilevel analysis. Used in epidemiology to study how environmental factors and individual attributes and behavior interact to influence individual-level health behavior and disease risk.

multimethod-multitrait technique. When a variety of data collection methods, such as interview and observation, are used and different measurement methods are used for each concept in a study.

multiple regression analysis. Extension of simple linear regression with more than one independent variable entered into the analysis.

multiple triangulation. The use of two or more types of triangulation (theoretical, data, methodological, investigator, and analysis) in a study.

multivariate analysis techniques. Used to analyze data from complex research projects. Techniques included in text are multiple regression, factorial analysis of variance, analysis of covariance, factor analysis, discriminant analysis, canonical correlation, structural equation modeling, time-series analysis, clinical trials, and survival analysis.

natural settings. Field settings or uncontrolled, real-life situations examined in research.

necessary relationship. One variable or concept must occur for the second variable or concept to occur.

negative linear relationship. *See* inverse linear relationship.

nested design. Design that allows the researcher to consider the effect of variables that are found only at some levels of the independent variables being studied.

nested variables. Variables found only at certain levels of the independent variable, such as gender, race, socioeconomic status, and education.

network sampling. Snowballing technique that takes advantage of social networks and the fact that friends tend to hold characteristics in common. Subjects meeting the sample criteria are asked to assist in locating others with similar characteristics.

networking. A process of developing channels of communication between people with common interests throughout the country.

nominal-scale measurement. Lowest level of measurement that is used when data can be organized into categories that are exclusive and exhaustive but the categories cannot be compared, such as gender, race, marital status, and nursing diagnoses.

nondirectional hypothesis. States that a relationship exists but does not predict the exact nature of the relationship.

nonequivalent control group designs. Designs in which the control group is not selected by random means, such as the one-group posttest-only design, posttest-only design with nonequivalent groups, and one-group pretest-posttest design.

nonparametric statistics. Statistical techniques used when the assumptions of parametric statistics are not met and most commonly used to analyze nominal- and ordinal-level data.

nonprobability sampling. Not every element of the population has an opportunity for selection in the sample, such as convenience (accidental) sampling, quota sampling, purposive sampling, and network sampling.

nonrandom sampling. *See* nonprobability sampling.

nonsignificant results. Negative results or results contrary to the researcher's hypotheses that can be an accurate reflection of reality or can be caused by study weaknesses.

nontherapeutic research. Research conducted to generate knowledge for a discipline and in which the results from the study might benefit future patients but will probably not benefit those acting as research subjects.

norm-referenced testing. Test performance standards that have been carefully developed over years with large, representative samples by using standardized tests with extensive reliability and validity.

normal curve. A symmetrical, unimodal bell-shaped curve that is a theoretical distribution of all possible scores, but no real distribution exactly fits the normal curve.

norms. The expected behavior patterns within a social system that affect diffusion of innovations.

null hypothesis. States that there is no relationship between the variables being studied; a statistical hypothesis used for statistical testing and interpreting statistical outcomes.

Nuremberg Code. Ethical code of conduct to guide investigators when conducting research.

nursing process. A subset of the problem-solving process that includes assessment, diagnosis, plan, implementation, evaluation, and modification.

nursing research. A scientific process that validates and refines existing knowledge and generates new knowledge that directly and indirectly influences clinical nursing practice.

oblique rotation. A type of rotation in factor analysis used to accomplish the best fit (best-factor solution) and in which the factors are allowed to be correlated.

observability. The extent to which the results of an innovation are visible to others.

observational measurement. The use of structured and unstructured observation to measure study variables.

observed score. The actual score or value obtained for a subject on a measurement tool.

observer as participant. The researcher's time is spent mainly observing and interviewing subjects and less in the participation role.

one-tailed test of significance. An analysis used with directional hypotheses in which extreme statistical values of interest are thought to occur in a single tail of the curve.

open context. Requires deconstructing a sedimented view to allow one to see the depth and complexity within the phenomenon being examined in qualitative research.

operational definition. Description of how variables or concepts will be measured or manipulated in a study.

operational reasoning. Involves identification and discrimination among many alternatives or viewpoints and focuses on the process of debating on alternatives.

opinion leaders. Those who are in favor of innovations and support change.

ordinal-scale measurement. Yields data that can be ranked but the intervals between the ranked data are not necessarily equal, such as levels of coping.

outcomes research. Important scientific methodology that was developed to examine the end results of patient care. The strategies used in outcomes research are a departure from traditional scientific endeavors and incorporate evaluation research, epidemiology, and economic theory perspectives.

outliers. The extreme scores or values in a set of data that are exceptions to the overall findings.

parallel-forms reliability. *See* alternate-forms reliability.

parameter. A measure or numerical value of a population.

parametric statistical analyses. Statistical techniques used when three assumptions are met: (1) the sample was drawn from a population for which the variance can be calculated, and the distribution is expected to be normal or approximately normal; (2) the level of measurement should be interval or ordinal with an approximately normal distribution; and (3) the data can be treated as random samples.

paraphrasing. Involves expressing clearly and concisely the ideas of an author in your own words.

partially controlled setting. An environment that is manipulated or modified in some way by the researcher.

participant as observer. A special form of observation in which researchers immerse themselves in the setting so they can hear, see, and experience the reality as the participants do. However, the participants are aware of the dual roles of the researcher (participant and observer).

participatory research strategy. A strategy that includes representatives from all groups that will be affected by the change (stakeholders) as collaborators. This strategy facilitates a broad base of support for new interventions for the target population, the professional community, and the general public.

passive rejection. Occurs when an innovation was never seriously considered for use in practice.

path coefficient. The effect of the independent variable on the dependent variable that is determined through path analysis.

patient outcomes research teams (PORTs). Large-scale, multifaceted, and multidisciplinary projects initiated by the Agency for Health Care Policy and Research that are designed to examine the outcomes and cost of current practice patterns, identify the best treatment strategy, and test methods for reducing inappropriate variations.

Pearson's product-moment correlation coefficient. Parametric test used to determine the relationship between variables.

percentage of variance. Value obtained by squaring Pearson's correlation coefficient (r) and the amount of variability explained by the linear relationship.

permission to participate in a study. The agreement of parents or guardians to the participation of their child or ward in research.

personal experience. Gaining knowledge by being personally involved in an event, situation, or circumstance. Benner described five levels of experience in the development of clinical knowledge and expertise: (1) novice, (2) advanced beginner, (3) competent, (4) proficient, and (5) expert.

persuasion stage. Stage in the innovation-decision process when an individual or group forms an attitude toward the innovation.

phenomenological research. Inductive, descriptive qualitative methodology developed from phenomenological philosophy for the purpose of describing experiences as they are lived by the study participants.

phi coefficient. Analysis technique to determine relationships in dichotomous, nominal data.

philosophical analysis. The use of concept or linguistic analysis to examine meaning and develop theories of meaning in philosophical inquiry.

philosophical inquiry. Research using intellectual analysis to clarify meanings, make values manifested, identify ethics, and study the nature of knowledge. Types of philosophical inquiry covered in this text are foundational inquiry, philosophical analysis, and ethical analysis.

philosophy. A broad, global explanation of the world.

physiological measurement. Techniques used to measure physiological variables either directly or indirectly, such as techniques to measure heart rate or mean arterial pressure.

pilot study. A smaller version of a proposed study conducted to develop and/or refine the methodology, such as the treatment, instrument, or data collection process.

pink sheet. A letter indicating rejection of a research grant proposal and a critique by the scientific committee that reviewed the proposal.

plagiarism. A type of scientific misconduct that involves the appropriation of another person's ideas, processes, results, or words without giving appropriate credit, including those obtained through confidential review of others' research proposals and manuscripts.

platykurtic. Term that indicates a relatively flat curve with the scores having large variance among them.

point estimate. A single figure that estimates a related figure in the population of interest.

population. All elements (individuals, objects, events, or substances) that meet the sample criteria for inclusion in a study. Sometimes referred to as a target population.

population-based studies. Important type of outcomes research that involves studying health conditions in the context of the community rather than the context of the medical system.

population studies. Studies that target the entire population.

positive linear relationship. Indicates that as one variable changes (value of the variable increases or decreases), the second variable will also change in the same direction.

post hoc analyses. Statistical tests developed specifically to determine the location of differences after ANOVA. Frequently used post hoc tests are Bonferroni's procedure, the Newman-Keuls test, the Tukey HSD test, the Scheffe test, and Dunnett's test.

poster session. Visual presentation of a study by

using pictures, tables, and illustrations on a display board.

power. The probability that a statistical test will detect a significant difference that exists; power analysis is used to determine the power of a study.

power analysis. Used to determine the risk of a Type II error so that the study can be modified to decrease the risk if necessary.

practical significance of a study. Associated with its importance to nursing's body of knowledge.

practice effect. Occurs when subjects improve as they become more familiar with the experimental protocol.

practice pattern profiling. An epidemiological technique used in outcomes research that focuses on patterns of care rather than individual occurrences of care.

precision. The accuracy with which the population parameters have been estimated within a study. Also used to describe the degree of consistency or reproducibility of measurements with physiological instruments.

prediction. The ability to estimate the probability of a specific outcome in a given situation that can be achieved through research.

prediction equation. Outcome of regression analysis.

predictive design. Developed to predict the value of the dependent variable based on values obtained from the independent variables; one approach to examining causal relationships between variables.

preference clinical trials (PCTs). Studies in which patients choose among all treatments available rather than being randomized into a study group.

preproposal. Short document (four to five pages plus appendices) written to explore the funding possibilities for a research project.

primary source. A source that is written by the person who originated or is responsible for generating the ideas published.

principal component analysis. The second step in exploratory factor analysis that provides preliminary information needed by the researcher so

that decisions can be made before the final factoring.

principal investigator (PI). In a research grant, the individual who will have primary responsibility for administering the grant and interacting with the funding agency.

privacy. The freedom an individual has to determine the time, extent, and general circumstances under which private information will be shared with or withheld from others.

probability sampling. Random sampling techniques in which each member (element) in the population should have a greater than zero opportunity to be selected for the sample; examples include simple random sampling, stratified random sampling, cluster sampling, and systematic sampling.

probability statement. Expresses the likelihood that something will happen in a given situation and addresses relative rather than absolute causality.

probability theory. Theory that addresses relative rather than absolute causality. Thus from a probability perspective, a cause will not produce a specific effect each time that particular cause occurs.

probing. Technique used by the interviewer to obtain more information in a specific area of the interview.

problem-solving process. Systematic identification of a problem, determination of goals related to the problem, identification of possible approaches to achieve these goals, implementation of selected approaches, and evaluation of goal achievement.

problematic reasoning. Involves identifying a problem, selecting solutions to the problem, and resolving the problem.

process-outcome matrix. Qualitative analysis technique that allows the researcher to trace the processes that led to differing outcomes.

projective technique. A method of measuring individuals' responses to unstructured or ambiguous situations as a means of describing attitudes, personality characteristics, and motives of the individuals. An example is the Rorschach inkblot test.

proposal, research. Written plan identifying the major elements of a study, such as the problem, purpose, and framework, and outlining the methods to conduct the study. A formal way to communicate ideas about a proposed study to receive approval to conduct the study and to seek funding.

proposition. An abstract statement that further clarifies the relationship between two concepts.

prospective cohort study. An epidemiological study in which a group of people are identified who are at risk for experiencing a particular event.

prototype. A primitive design that has evolved to the point that it can be tested clinically. Guided by intervention theory, a prototype includes establishing and selecting a mode of delivery of the intervention.

purposive sampling. Judgmental sampling that involves conscious selection by the researcher of certain subjects or elements to include in a study.

Q plot display. Exploratory data analysis technique in which the scores or data are displayed in a distribution by quantile.

Q-sort methodology. A technique of comparative rating in which a subject sorts cards with statements on them into designated piles (usually 7–10 piles in the distribution of a normal curve) that might range from best to worst.

qualitative research. A systematic, interactive, subjective approach used to describe life experiences and give them meaning.

quality practice guidelines. Patient care guidelines that are based on synthesized research findings from meta-analyses, supported by consensus from recognized national experts, and affirmed by outcomes obtained by clinicians.

quantitative research. A formal, objective, systematic process to describe and test relationships, and to examine cause-and-effect interactions among variables.

quasi-experimental designs. Designs with limited control that were developed to provide alternative means for examining causality in situations not conducive to experimental controls.

quasi-experimental research. A type of quantitative research conducted to explain relationships, clarify why certain events happen, and examine causality between selected independent and dependent variables.

query letter. A letter sent to an editor of a journal to determine interest in publishing an article or a letter sent to a funding agency to determine interest in funding a study.

questionable publication. Publication in which no coauthor could produce the original data or no coauthor had personally observed or performed each phase of the research or participated in the research publication.

questionnaire. A printed self-report form designed to elicit information that can be obtained through written responses of the subject.

quota sampling. A convenience sampling technique with an added strategy to ensure the inclusion of subject types likely to be underrepresented in the convenience sample, such as women, minority groups, and the undereducated.

random assignment to groups. A procedure used to assign subjects to treatment or control groups in which the subjects have an equal opportunity to be assigned to either group.

random error. An error that causes individuals' observed scores to vary haphazardly around their true score.

random sampling. *See* probability sampling.

random variation. The expected difference in values that occurs when one examines different subjects from the same sample.

randomized clinical trials. Classic means of examining the effects of various treatments in which the effects of a treatment are examined by comparing the treatment group with the no-treatment group.

range. The simplest measure of dispersion, obtained by subtracting the lowest score from the highest score.

rating scales. Crudest form of measure using scaling techniques; ratings are chosen from an ordered series of categories of a variable assumed to be based on an underlying continuum.

ratio-level measurement. Highest measurement form that meets all the rules of other forms of measure: mutually exclusive categories, exhaustive categories, rank ordering, equal spacing between intervals, and a continuum of values; also has an absolute zero, such as weight.

reasoning. Processing and organizing ideas to

reach conclusions; examples include problematic, operational, dialectic, and logistic.

reconstructing new ideas or views. In qualitative research, researchers examine many dimensions of the area being studied and form new ideas while recognizing that the present reconstructing of ideas is only one of many possible ways of organizing data.

refereed journal. Uses referees or expert reviewers to determine whether a manuscript will be accepted for publication.

referencing. Comparing a subject's score against a standard; used in norm-referenced and criterion-referenced testing.

reflexive thought. Critically thinking through the dynamic interaction between self and the data during the analysis of qualitative data. During this process, the researcher explores personal feelings and experiences that may influence the study and integrates this understanding into the study.

regression line. The line that best represents the values of the raw scores plotted on a scatter diagram, and the procedure for developing the line of best fit is the method of least squares.

reinvention. Adopters modify the innovation to meet their own needs.

rejection. An active or passive decision not to use an innovation.

relational statement. Declares that a relationship of some kind exists between two or more concepts.

relative advantage. The extent to which the innovation is perceived to be better than current practice.

relevant literature. Sources that are pertinent or highly important in providing the in-depth knowledge needed to make changes in practice or to study a selected problem.

reliability. Represents the consistency of the measure obtained.

reliability testing. A measure of the amount of random error in the measurement technique.

replacement discontinuance in the utilization of innovations. Rejection of an innovation identified through research to adopt a better idea.

replication. Reproducing or repeating a study to determine whether similar findings will be obtained.

replication, approximate. An operational replication that involves repeating the original study under similar conditions and following the methods as closely as possible.

replication, concurrent. Involves collection of data for the original study and simultaneous replication of the data to provide a check of the reliability of the original study. Confirmation of the original study findings through replication is part of the original study's design.

replication, exact. Involves precise or exact duplication of the initial researcher's study to confirm the original findings.

replication, systematic. A constructive replication that is done under distinctly new conditions in which the researchers conducting the replication do not follow the design or methods of the original researchers; instead, the second investigative team begins with a similar problem statement but formulates new means to verify the first investigator's findings.

representativeness of the sample. A sample must be like the population in as many ways as possible.

research. Diligent, systematic inquiry or investigation to validate and refine existing knowledge and generate new knowledge.

research grant. Funding specifically for conducting a study.

research hypothesis. The alternative hypothesis to the null hypothesis, stating that there is a relationship between two or more variables.

research objectives. Clear, concise, declarative statements that are expressed to direct a study and are focused on identification and description of variables and/or determination of the relationships among variables.

research misconduct. *See* scientific misconduct.

research problem. An area of concern in which there is a gap in the knowledge base needed for nursing practice. Research is conducted to generate essential knowledge to address the practice concern, with the ultimate goal of providing evidence- or research-based nursing care.

research proposal. *See* proposal, research.

research purpose. A concise, clear statement of the specific goal or aim of the study that is generated from the problem.

research questions. Concise, interrogative statements developed to direct studies that are focused on description of variables, examination of relationships among variables, and determination of differences between two or more groups.

research topics. Concepts or broad problem areas that indicate the foci of essential research knowledge needed to provide evidence-based nursing practice. Research topics include numerous potential research problems.

research tradition. A program of research that is important for building a body of knowledge related to the phenomena explained by a particular conceptual model.

research variables. *See* variables.

respect for persons, principle of. Indicates that persons have the right to self-determination and the freedom to participate or not participate in research.

response set. The parameters within which the question or item is to be answered in a questionnaire.

results. The outcomes from data analysis that are generated for each research objective, question, or hypothesis.

retrospective cohort study. An epidemiological study in which a group of people are identified who have experienced a particular event; for example, studying occupational exposure to chemicals.

review of relevant literature. An analysis and synthesis of research sources to generate a picture of what is known about a particular situation and the knowledge gaps that exist in the situation.

rigor. The striving for excellence in research through the use of discipline, scrupulous adherence to detail, and strict accuracy.

rigor in documentation. Standard for critiquing qualitative research that involves clear, concise presentation of the study elements by the researcher.

robust. Analysis procedure that will yield accurate results even if some of the assumptions are violated by the data being analyzed.

role-modeling. Learning by imitating the behavior of an exemplar or role model.

sample. A subset of the population that is selected for a study.

sample characteristics. Description of the re-

search subjects obtained by analyzing data acquired from the demographic variables.

sampling. Includes selecting groups of people, events, behaviors, or other elements with which to conduct a study.

sampling criteria. A list of the characteristics essential for membership in the target population.

sampling distribution. Determined by using statistical values (such as means) of many samples obtained from the same population.

sampling error. The difference between a sample statistic used to estimate a parameter and the actual but unknown value of the parameter.

sampling frame. Listing of every member of the population with membership defined by the sampling criteria.

sampling method. The process of selecting a group of people, events, behaviors, or other elements that are representative of the population being studied.

sampling plan. Describes the strategies that will be used to obtain a sample for a study and may include either probability or nonprobability sampling methods.

scale. A self-report form of measurement composed of several items that are thought to measure the construct being studied, in which the subject responds to each item on the continuum or scale provided.

science. A coherent body of knowledge composed of research findings, tested theories, scientific principles, and laws for a discipline.

scientific community. A cohesive group of scholars within a discipline who stimulate the creation of new research ideas and the development of innovative methodologies to conduct research.

scientific method. Incorporates all procedures that scientists have used, currently use, or may use in the future to pursue knowledge, such as quantitative research, qualitative research, and outcomes research.

scientific misconduct. Involves such practices as fabrication, falsification, or forging of data; dishonest manipulation of the study design or methods; and plagiarism.

scientific theory. Theory with valid and reliable methods of measuring each concept and relational statements that have been repeatedly tested through research and demonstrated to be valid.

secondary analysis design. Involves studying data previously collected in another study, but different methods of organization of the data and different statistical analyses are used to reexamine the data.

secondary loading. In factor analysis, the lowest loading for a variable when it has high loadings on two factors. When many secondary loadings occur, the factoring is not considered clean.

secondary source. A source that summarizes or quotes content from primary sources.

sedimented view. Seeing things from the perspective of a specific frame of reference, world view, or theory that gives a sense of certainty, security, and control.

seeking approval to conduct a study. A process involving submission of a research proposal to a selected group for review and often verbally defending that proposal.

selectivity in physiological measures. An element of accuracy that involves the ability to identify the signal under study correctly to distinguish it from other signals.

self-determination. Based on the ethical principle of respect for persons, which states that humans are capable of controlling their own destiny. The right to self-determination is violated through the use of coercion, covert data collection, and deception.

semantic differential scale. An instrument that consists of two opposite adjectives with a seven-point scale between them. The subject selects one point on the scale that best describes his or her view of the concept being examined.

seminal study. The first study that prompted the initiation of a field of research.

sensitivity of physiological measures. Related to the amount of change of a parameter that can be measured precisely.

sequential relationship. A relationship in which one concept occurs later than the other.

serendipity. The accidental discovery of something valuable or useful during the conduct of a study.

setting. Location for conducting research, such as

a natural, partially controlled, or highly controlled setting.

sign test. A nonparametric analysis technique developed for data that it is difficult to assign numerical values to but the data can be ranked on some dimension.

significant results. Results that are in keeping with those identified by the researcher.

simple hypothesis. States the relationship (associative or causal) between two variables.

simple linear regression. Parametric analysis technique that provides a means to estimate the value of a dependent variable based on the value of an independent variable.

simple random sampling. Elements are selected at random from the sampling frame for inclusion in a study. Each study element has a probability greater than zero of being selected for inclusion in the study.

skewness. A curve that is asymmetrical (positively or negatively skewed) because of an asymmetrical distribution of scores.

skimming. A quick review of a source to gain a broad overview of the content.

slope. Determines the direction and angle of the regression line within the graph. The value is represented by the letter b.

social system. A set of interrelated units that is engaged in joint problem solving to accomplish a common goal.

Spearman rank-order correlation coefficient. A nonparametric analysis technique for ordinal data that is an adaptation of the Pearson product-moment correlation used to examine relationships among variables in a study.

special library. Contains a collection of materials on a selected topic or for a specialty area, such as nursing or medicine.

split-half reliability. Used to determine the homogeneity of an instrument's items; the items are split in half, and a correlational procedure is performed between the two halves.

stability. Aspect of reliability testing that is concerned with the consistency of repeated measures.

standard deviation. A measure of dispersion that is calculated by taking the square root of the variance.

standard scores. Used to express deviations from

the mean (difference scores) in terms of standard deviation units, such as Z scores, where the mean is zero and the standard deviation is 1.

statement synthesis. The researcher develops statements proposing specific relationships among the concepts being studied. This step is a part of developing a framework for a study.

statistic. A numerical value obtained from a sample that is used to estimate the parameters of a population.

statistical conclusion validity. Concerned with whether the conclusions about relationships and differences drawn from statistical analyses are an accurate reflection of reality.

statistical regression. The movement or regression of extreme scores toward the mean in studies using a pretest-posttest design.

statistical significance. The results are unlikely to be due to chance.

stem-and-leaf displays. Type of exploratory data analysis in which the scores are visually presented to obtain insight.

stepwise regression analysis. Type of exploratory regression analysis in which the independent variables are entered into or removed from the analysis one at a time.

stratified random sampling. Used when the researcher knows some of the variables in the population that are critical to achieving representativeness. These identified variables are used to divide the sample into strata or groups.

stratification. Used in a design so that subjects are distributed throughout the sample by using sampling techniques similar to those used in blocking, but the purpose of the procedure is even distribution throughout the sample.

strength of relationship. The amount of variation explained by the relationship.

structural equation modeling. Analysis technique designed to test theories.

structured interviews. Use of strategies that provide increasing amount of control by the researcher over the content of the interview.

structured observation. Clearly identifying what is to be observed and precisely defining how the observations are to be made, recorded, and coded.

study validity. A measure of the truth or accuracy of a claim that is an important concern throughout the research process.

subjects. Individuals participating in a study.

substantive theory. A theory recognized within the discipline as useful for explaining important phenomena.

substitutable relationship. Relationship in which a similar concept can be substituted for the first concept and the second concept will occur.

sufficient relationship. States that when the first variable or concept occurs, the second will occur regardless of the presence or absence of other factors.

sum of squares. Mathematical manipulation involving summing the squares of the difference scores that is used as part of the analysis process for calculating the standard deviation.

summary statistics. *See* descriptive statistics.

survey. Technique of data collection in which questionnaires or personal interviews are used to gather data about an identified population.

survey design. A design to describe a phenomenon by using questionnaires or personal interviews to collect data.

survival analysis. A set of techniques designed to analyze repeated measures from a given time (e.g., the beginning of the study, onset of a disease, the beginning of a treatment) until a certain event (e.g., death, treatment failure, recurrence of the phenomenon) occurs.

symmetrical relationship. Complex relationship that consists of two statements: If A occurs (or changes), B will occur (or change); if B occurs (or changes), A will occur (or change); A $\leftrightarrow$ B.

symmetry plot. Exploratory data analysis technique designed to determine the presence of skewness in the data.

synthesis of sources. Clustering and interrelating ideas from several sources to form a gestalt or new, complete picture of what is known and not known in an area.

systematic bias or variation. A consequence of selecting subjects whose measurement values are different or vary in some way from the population.

systematic error. Measurement error that is not random but occurs consistently, such as a scale that inaccurately weighs subjects 3 pounds heavier than they are.

systematic sampling. Conducted when an ordered list of all members of the population is available and involves selecting every *k*th individual on the list, starting from a point that is selected randomly.

***t* test.** A parametric analysis technique used to determine significant differences between measures of two samples; *t* test analysis techniques exist for dependent and independent groups.

tails. Extremes of the normal curve where significant statistical values can be found.

target population. A group of individuals who meet the sampling criteria.

tendency statement. Deterministic relationship that describes what always happens in the absence of interfering conditions.

tentative theory. Theory that is newly proposed, has had minimal exposure to critique by the discipline, and has had little testing.

test-retest reliability. Determination of the stability or consistency of a measurement technique by correlating the scores obtained from repeated measures.

testable hypothesis. Contains variables that are measurable or can be manipulated in the real world.

theoretical connectedness. The theoretical schema developed from a qualitative study is clearly expressed, logically consistent, reflective of the data, and compatible with nursing's knowledge base.

theoretical limitations. Weaknesses in the study framework and conceptual and operational definitions that restrict abstract generalization of the findings.

theoretical literature. Includes concept analyses, maps, theories, and conceptual frameworks that support a selected research problem and purpose.

theoretical substruction. A process in which the framework of a published study is separated into component parts to evaluate the logical consistency of the theoretical system and the interaction of the framework with the study methodology.

theoretical triangulation. The use of two or more frameworks or theoretical perspectives in the same study, with development of hypotheses based on the different theoretical perspectives and tested on the same data set.

theory. Consists of an integrated set of defined concepts, existence statements, and relational statements that present a view of a phenomenon and can be used to describe, explain, predict, and/or control that phenomenon.

therapeutic research. Research that provides the patient an opportunity to receive an experimental treatment that might have beneficial results.

time lag. The span of time between the generation of new knowledge through research and the use of this knowledge in practice.

time-dimensional designs. Designs used to examine the sequence and patterns of change, growth, or trends across time.

time-series analysis. A technique designed to analyze changes in a variable across time and thus to uncover a pattern in the data.

traditions. Truths or beliefs that are based on customs and past trends and provide a way of acquiring knowledge.

transformation of ideas. Movement of ideas across levels of abstraction to determine the existing knowledge base in an area of study.

translation. Involves transforming from one language to another to facilitate understanding and is part of the process of interpreting research outcomes where results are translated and interpreted into findings.

treatment. The independent variable that is manipulated in a study to produce an effect on the dependent variable. The treatment or independent variable is usually detailed in a protocol to ensure consistent implementation in the study.

treatment-matching designs. Outcomes research design to compare the relative effectiveness of various treatments.

trend designs. Designs used to examine changes in the general population in relation to a particular phenomenon.

trial and error. An approach with unknown outcomes that is used in a situation of uncertainty when other sources of knowledge are unavailable.

trialability. The extent to which an individual or

agency can try out the idea on a limited basis with the option of returning to previous practices.

triangulation. The use of two or more theories, methods, data sources, investigators, or analysis methods in a study.

true score. Score that would be obtained if there were no error in measurement, but some measurement error always occurs.

two-tailed test of significance. Type of analysis used for a nondirectional hypothesis in which the researcher assumes that an extreme score can occur in either tail.

Type I error. Occurs when the researcher concludes that the samples tested are from different populations (the difference between groups is significant) when in fact the samples are from the same population (the difference between groups is not significant). The null hypothesis is rejected when it is true.

Type II error. Occurs when the researcher concludes that there is no significant difference between the samples examined when, in fact, a difference exists. The null hypothesis is regarded as true when it is false.

unitizing reliability. The extent to which each judge (data collector, coder, researcher) consistently identifies the same units within the data as appropriate for coding.

unstructured interviews. Initiated with a broad question and subjects are usually encouraged to further elaborate on particular dimensions of a topic.

unstructured observations. Involve spontaneously observing and recording what is seen with a minimum of prior planning.

utilization of research findings. The use of knowledge generated through research to guide nursing practice.

validity, design. The strength of a design to produce accurate results, which is determined by examining statistical conclusion validity, internal validity, construct validity, and external validity.

validity, instrument. Determining the extent to which the instrument actually reflects the abstract construct being examined.

validity, study. A measure of the truth or accuracy of a claim; an important concern throughout the research process.

variables. Qualities, properties, or characteristics of persons, things, or situations that change or vary and are manipulated, measured, or controlled in research.

variance. A measure of dispersion that is the mean or average of the sum of squares.

variance analysis. Outcomes research strategy to track individual and group variance from a specific critical pathway. The goal is to decrease preventable variance in process, thus helping patients and their families achieve optimal outcomes.

varimax rotation. A type of rotation in factor analysis used to accomplish the best fit (best-factor solution) when the factors are uncorrelated.

visual analogue scale. A line 100 mm in length with right-angle stops at each end on which subjects are asked to record their response to a study variable.

voluntary consent. The prospective subject has decided to take part in a study of his or her own volition without coercion or any undue influence.

Wald-Wolfowitz runs test. Nonparametric analysis technique used to determine differences between two populations.

Wilcoxon matched-pairs signed-ranks test. Nonparametric analysis technique used to examine changes that occur in pretest/posttest measures or matched-pairs measures.

within-group variance. Variance that results when individual scores in a group vary from the group mean.

within-method triangulation. The use of both quantitative and qualitative research strategies in conducting a study but within one method, such as using only data triangulation in the study or using only theoretical triangulation in the study.

y intercept. The point where the regression line crosses (or intercepts) the y-axis. At this point on the regression line, $x = 0$.

Z scores. Standardized scores developed from the normal curve.

INDEX

Page numbers in *italics* refer to figures; page numbers followed by t refer to tables.